Second Edition

Mosby's
DENTAL
HYGIENE

Concepts, Cases, and Competencies

Susan J. Daniel, RDH, BS D.A.T.E., MS
President, Educational Visions, LLC
Ridgeland, Mississippi
Adjunct Clinical Associate Professor
Department of Dental Ecology
University of North Carolina School of Dentistry
Chapel Hill, North Carolina

Sherry A. Harfst, RDH, BSDH, MS
Consultant
Mobile, Alabama
Adjunct Clinical Associate Professor
Department of Dental Ecology
University of North Carolina School of Dentistry
Chapel Hill, North Carolina

Rebecca S. Wilder, RDH, BSDH, MS
Associate Professor and Director
Graduate Dental Hygiene Education
Department of Dental Ecology
University of North Carolina School of Dentistry
Chapel Hill, North Carolina
Editor in Chief, *Journal of Dental Hygiene*
American Dental Hygienists' Association

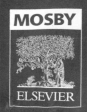

MOSBY
ELSEVIER

11830 Westline Industrial Drive
St. Louis, Missouri 63146

MOSBY'S DENTAL HYGIENE: CONCEPTS, CASES, AND COMPETENCIES

ISBN-13: 978-0-323-04352-6
ISBN-10: 0-323-04352-6

Notice

Knowledge and best practice in this field are constantly changing. As new research and experience broaden our knowledge, changes in practice, treatment and drug therapy may become necessary or appropriate. Readers are advised to check the most current information provided (i) on procedures featured or (ii) by the manufacturer of each product to be administered, to verify the recommended dose or formula, the method and duration of administration, and contraindications. It is the responsibility of the practitioner, relying on their own experience and knowledge of the patient, to make diagnoses, to determine dosages and the best treatment for each individual patient, and to take all appropriate safety precautions. To the fullest extent of the law, neither the Publisher nor the Author assumes any liability for any injury and/or damage to persons or property arising out or related to any use of the material contained in this book.

The Publisher

Library of Congress Cataloging-in-Publication Data
Library of Congress Control Number: 2007921570

Vice President and Publisher: Linda Duncan
Senior Editor: John Dolan
Developmental Editor: Julie Nebel
Publishing Services Manager: Julie Eddy
Project Manager: Laura Loveall
Designer: Margaret Reid

Printed in Canada

Last digit is the print number: 9 8 7 6 5 4 3 2 1

This compilation of teaching and learning materials is dedicated to the faculty who educate the future oral healthcare providers of the world. You carry the responsibility to facilitate more than simple acquisition of knowledge and skills. The profession of teaching the dental hygienists of today and tomorrow is an esteemed honor and, as such, this learning package is dedicated to you.

These printed and electronic materials provide the essential assets to teach the acquisition of knowledge, skills, attitudes, and judgments. They also provide you with the necessary components to assume the role of mentor and guide to all of your students. Serving as a mentor and guide is one of the most important tasks that we can strive for in our careers as dental hygiene educators. Mentoring and serving as a positive role model will facilitate in the development of appropriate attitudes and judgments required of a healthcare professional and nurture the professional and personal development of all the students who journey with us through their dental hygiene education.

The Authors

To my husband, Hugo, who is to be commended for his encouragement and understanding during the development of this edition. Throughout the process, you were always there with wisdom, humor, support, and encouragement.

To my son, Daniel Austin, who provides joy and encouragement with a hug or kind word, you may never know how much that means to me. Thank you.

The display of strength, courage, and caring of my friend and Sherry's husband, David Harfst, during his journey will never be forgotten. Much was learned about life from how he lived his. Thank you.

Susan J. Daniel

Dedication of this work belongs to my husband, David. His vision and passion for people and life was contagious to all who knew him. David Paul Harfst was my friend and mentor. Because of his encouragement, vision, passion and compassion, courage and strength, not to mention irascible stubbornness and incredible wisdom, he will forever be my North Star.

To my daughter, Caroline, from whom I learn daily about the treasures life holds in a moment, and who has always been wise beyond her years. And, finally, to my friends—those very special people who have been the lifejackets in my life who have held me up when I could scarcely swim on my own—I could not ask for a better cheering section.

Sherry A. Harfst

To my husband, Al Wilder, you are truly the *"wind beneath my wings"* in all of my dreams and endeavors. Thanks for being a wonderful husband, father, and best friend.

To my children, Bill, Bradley, Heath, Al, and Scott. You provide such joy in my life and make if all worthwhile.

And, to my mother, Frances Reavis, who was my first and most influential mentor. I will be eternally grateful that she always encouraged me to believe I could do anything I set my mind to do.

Rebecca S. Wilder

Contributors

Martin Addy, BDS, MSc, PhD, FDSRCS (England), FDSRCS (Edinburgh)
Professor of Periodontology and Honorary Consultant in Restorative Dentistry
Department of Oral and Dental Science
University of Bristol
Bristol, United Kingdom

Cathy L. Backinger, PhD, MPH
Acting Chief
Tobacco Control Research Branch
Behavioral Research Program
Division of Cancer Control and Population Sciences
National Cancer Institute
Bethesda, Maryland

Caren M. Barnes, RDH, BS, MS
Professor and Coordinator of Clinical Research
Department of Dental Hygiene
University of Nebraska Medical Center College of Dentistry
Lincoln, Nebraska

Rebecca M. Barry, MEd, RDH
Associate Professor
Chairman of Department of Dental Hygiene
School of Health Related Professions
Assistant Professor
Department of Diagnostic Sciences
School of Dentistry
The University of Mississippi Medical Center
Jackson, Mississippi

Kathy B. Bassett, RDH, BSDH, MEd
Clinic Coordinator, Faculty
Department of Dental Hygiene
Pierce College
Lakewood, Washington

Helene Bednarsh, BS, RDH, MPH
Director, HIV Dental Ombudsperson Program
Boston Public Health Commission
Faculty Member
Forsyth School for Dental Hygiene
Boston University Goldman School of Dental Medicine
Boston Public Health Commission
Boston, Massachusetts

Kristy Menage Bernie, RDH, BS
Owner and Director
Educational Designs, Inc./CareerFlow
San Ramon, California

Kimberly S. Bray, RDH, MS
Professor and Interim Director
Division of Dental Hygiene
University of Missouri-Kansas City School of Dentistry
Kansas City, Missouri

Ann Brunick, RDH, MS
Chair, Department of Dental Hygiene
University of South Dakota
Vermillion, South Dakota

Alan W. Budenz, MS, DDS, MBA
Professor
Department of Anatomical Sciences and Department of Dental Practice
University of the Pacific, Arthur A. Dugoni School of Dentistry
San Francisco, California

Sebastian G. Ciancio, DDS
Distinguished Service Professor and Chair
Department of Periodontics and Endodontics
School of Dental Medicine
University at Buffalo, SUNY
Buffalo, New York

Eve Cuny, MS
President, Eve Cuny Consulting, LLC
Walnut Creek, California

Susan J. Daniel, RDH, BS D.A.T.E., MS
President, Educational Visions, LLC
Ridgeland, Mississippi
Adjunct Clinical Associate Professor
Department of Dental Ecology
University of North Carolina School of Dentistry
Chapel Hill, North Carolina

Christina B. DeBiase, BSDH, MA, EdD
Associate Dean for Academic Affairs
School of Dentistry
West Virginia University
Morgantown, West Virginia

Arthur C. DiMarco, DMD
Assistant Professor
Department of Dental Hygiene
Eastern Washington University
Spokane, Washington

Kathy Eklund, RDH, MHP
Director of Infection Control and Occupational Health
The Forsyth Institute
Boston, Massachusetts
Adjunct Associate Professor
Forsyth School of Dental Hygienists
Massachusetts College of Pharmacy and Health Sciences
Boston, Massachusetts

John D.B. Featherstone, MSc, PhD
Professor and Director
Biomaterials, Biophysical Sciences and Engineering Program
University of California San Francisco
San Francisco, California

Deborah E. Fleming, RDH, MS
Former Clinical Assistant Professor
Dental Hygiene Programs
Department of Dental Ecology
University of North Carolina School of Dentistry
Chapel Hill, North Carolina

Jane L. Forrest, EdD, RDH
Chair
Division of Health Promotion, Disease Prevention &
    Epidemiology
Director
National Center for Dental Hygiene Research
University of Southern California School of Dentistry
Los Angeles, California

Bonnie Francis, RDH, MS
Adjunct Clinical Associate Professor
Department of Dental Ecology
University of North Carolina School of Dentistry
Chapel Hill, North Carolina
Dallas, Texas

Sylvia Frazier-Bowers, DDS, PhD
Assistant Professor
Department of Orthodontics
University of North Carolina School of Dentistry
Chapel Hill, North Carolina

Mary C. George, RDH, BSDH, MEd
Associate Professor, Department of Dental Ecology
University of North Carolina School of Dentistry
Chapel Hill, North Carolina

Joan I. Gluch, PhD, RDH
Director, Community Health
Adjunct Associate Professor
Department of Preventive and Restorative Sciences
University of Pennsylvania
School of Dental Medicine
Philadelphia, Pennsylvania

Maria Perno Goldie, RDH, MS
Editor in Chief, *Modern Hygienist*
San Carlos, California

JoAnn R. Gurenlian, RDH, PhD
President and CEO
Gurenlian & Associates
Haddonfield, New Jersey
Visiting Faculty
Capella University
Minneapolis, Minnesota

Sherry A. Harfst, RDH, BSDH, MS
Consultant
Mobile, Alabama
Adjunct Clinical Associate Professor
Department of Dental Ecology
University of North Carolina School of Dentistry
Chapel Hill, North Carolina

Robert G. Henry, DMD, MPH
Clinical Associate Professor
Director Geriatric Dentistry Section
Public Health Dentistry
University of Kentucky College of Dentistry
Assistant Chief, Dental Service, Department of Veteran Affairs
Lexington, Kentucky

Kristine A. Hodsdon, RDH, BS
Director of RDH eVillage
Speaker, Writer, Consultant
Chester, New Hampshire

Laura Jansen Howerton, RDH, MS
Clinical Associate Professor
Department of Dental Ecology
University of North Carolina School of Dentistry
Chapel Hill, North Carolina

W. Bruce Howerton, Jr., DDS, MS
Oral and Maxillofacial Radiologist
Carolina OMF Radiology
Raleigh, North Carolina

Lynne Carol Hunt, RDH, MS
Adjunct Clinical Faculty
Department of Dental Ecology
University of North Carolina School of Dentistry
Chapel Hill, North Carolina

Carol A. Jahn, RDH, MS
Manager, Professional Education and Communications
Water Pik, Inc.
Fort Collins, Colorado

Katherine Karpinia, DMD, MS
Associate Professor
Department of Periodontology
University of Florida College of Dentistry
Gainesville, Florida

Susan K. Kass, RDH, EdD
Program Director
Department of Dental Hygiene
Miami-Dade College
Miami, Florida

Ralph Howard Leonard, Jr., DDS, MPH
Clinical Professor
Department of Diagnostic Sciences and General Dentistry
University of North Carolina School of Dentistry
Chapel Hill, North Carolina

Annette Ashley Linder, RDH, BS
BS Worldwide Seminars and Consulting
Hobe Sound, Florida

Deborah M. Lyle, RDH, MS
Director of Professional and Clinical Affairs
Marketing
Water Pik, Inc.
Fort Collins, Colorado

Elizabeth Maxbauer, RDH
Office Manager
McNamara, McNamara, Burkhardt, Nolan
Specialists in Orthodontics and Dentofacial Orthopedics
Ann Arbor, Michigan

Robert Ellis Mecklenburg, DDS, MPH
Member, Expert Panel, Tobacco Guideline Update
Center for Tobacco Research and Intervention
University of Wisconsin Medical School
Madison, Wisconsin
Consultant, Expert Panel on Oral Health
Oral Health Program, World Health Organization
Beneva, Switzerland

Syrene A. Miller, BA
Project Manager
National Center for Dental Hygiene Research
University of Southern California School of Dentistry
Los Angeles, California

Samuel Paul Nesbit, DDS, MS
Clinical Associate Professor
Department of Diagnostic Sciences & General Dentistry
University of North Carolina School of Dentistry
Chapel Hill, North Carolina

Patricia J. Nunn, RDH, MS
Professor and Chair
Department of Dental Hygiene
University of Oklahoma College of Dentistry
Oklahoma City, Oklahoma

Pamela B. Overman, BSDH, MS, EdD
Associate Professor and Associate Dean for Academic Affairs
School of Dentistry
University of Missouri–Kansas City
Kansas City, Missouri

Mary R. Pfeifer, RDH, MS, RN, CCRC
Manager, Clinical Research
Department of Medicine, Geriatric
The University of Mississippi Medical Center
Jackson, Mississippi

Dennis N. Ranalli, DDS, MDS
Senior Associate Dean
Professor of Pediatric Dentistry
University of Pittsburgh School of Dental Medicine
Team Dentist, Pittsburgh Panthers
Pittsburgh, Pennsylvania

Jill Rethman, RDH, BA
Adjunct Instructor
Department of Dental Hygiene
University of Pittsburgh
Pittsburgh, Pennsylvania
Editorial Director
Dimensions of Dental Hygiene
Belmont Publications
Kaneohe, Hawaii

David A Reznik, DDS
Director, Oral Health Center, Infectious Disease Program
Chief, Dental Service
Grady Health System
Atlanta, Georgia

Mary Kaye Scaramucci, RDH, MS
Associate Professor
Department of Dental Hygiene
University of Cincinnati, Raymond Walters College
Cincinnati, Ohio

Colleen Schmidt, RDH, MS
Director of Education
American Dental Hygienists' Association
Chicago, Illinois

Francis G. Serio, DMD, MS
Professor and Department Chairman
Department of Periodontics and Preventive Sciences
The University of Mississippi Medical Center
Jackson, Mississippi

Kenneth Shay, DDS, MS
Director, Geriatric Programs
Office of Geriatrics and Extended Care, U.S. Department of
    Veterans Affairs
VA Central Office
Washington, DC
Director, VISN 11 Geriatrics and Extended Care Service Line
Section Chief, Dental Geriatrics
Dental Service
Ann Arbor Veterans Healthcare System
Adjunct Professor of Dentistry
Department of Periodontic, Preventive, and Geriatric
    Dentistry
University of Michigan School of Dentistry
Ann Arbor, Michigan

Barbara J. Smith, PhD, RDH, MPH
Assistant Professor
Department of Periodontics and Oral Medicine
University of Michigan School of Dentistry
Ann Arbor, Michigan

Thomas J. Smith, DDS, MS, JD
Former Associate Dean for Clinical Programs and Professor
Department of Diagnostic Sciences
The University of Mississippi Medical Center
School of Dentistry
Jackson, Mississippi

Ann Eshenaur Spolarich, RDH, PhD
Director of Pharmacy
Arizona School of Dentistry and Oral Health
Mesa, Arizona
Clinical Associate Professor
Course Director of Pharmacology
Department of Dental Hygiene
University of Southern California School of Dentistry
Los Angeles, California

Cynthia A. Stegeman, RDH, M.Ed, RD, CDE
Assistant Professor
Department of Dental Hygiene
University of Cincinnati Raymond Walters College
Cincinnati, Ohio

Deborah Studen-Pavlovich, DMD
Professor and Chair
Department of Pediatric Dentistry
University of Pittsburgh School of Dental Medicine
Pittsburgh, Pennsylvania

William H. Tate, DDS
Associate Professor
Department of Restorative Dentistry & Biomaterials
The University of Texas Health Science Center at Houston,
    Dental Branch
Houston, Texas

George M. Taybos, DDS, MSEd
Professor
Department of Diagnostic Sciences
School of Dentistry
The University of Mississippi Medical Center
Jackson, Mississippi

Karen K. Tiwana, BSc, DDS
Clinical Assistant Professor
Department of Diagnostic Sciences and General Dentistry
University of North Carolina School of Dentistry
Chapel Hill, North Carolina

Peter T. Triolo, Jr., DDS, MS
Clinical Associate Professor
Department of Restorative Dentistry/Comprehensive Care
University of Pittsburgh
School of Dental Medicine
Pittsburgh, Pennsylvania

Victoria C. Vick, RDH, BS
Medical Writer for inVentiv Clinical Solutions
Indianapolis, Indiana

Nicola X. West, BDS, FDSRCS, PhD, RDS (Rest. Dent.)
Senior Lecturer/Honorary Consultant
Department of Restorative Dentistry/Periodontology
Dental School and Hospital
Bristol, United Kingdom

Rebecca S. Wilder, RDH, BSDH, MS
Associate Professor and Director
Graduate Dental Hygiene Education
Department of Dental Ecology
University of North Carolina School of Dentistry
Chapel Hill, North Carolina
Editor in Chief, *Journal of Dental Hygiene*
American Dental Hygienists' Association
Chicago, Illinois

William Woodall, EdD, PT, ATC
Professor
Department of Physical Therapy
School of Health Related Professions
The University of Mississippi Medical Center
Jackson, Mississippi

Douglas A. Young, DDS, MBA, MS
Assistant Professor
Department of Dental Practice
University of the Pacific, Arthur A. Dugoni School of
    Dentistry
San Francisco, California

Reviewers

Preface

This compilation of interactive learning resources was specifically designed to enhance your educational experience in exciting ways. This second edition was developed to engage the learning styles and customs of today's student, providing you with Case Studies, both in the text and on the CD-ROM, and a *Clinical Companion Study Guide* to integrate the learning and shorten the transfer of that learning from lecture and lab to the clinical setting.

These teaching and learning resources were developed with specific assets to accommodate your need to study and learn at times that best fit your schedule outside of the classroom:

- You can peruse CD-ROM exercises and Internet connections as part of an assignment, during class, or for independent study or review.
- The CD-ROM provides real patient learning experiences to assist with the development of evidence-based decision making and problem solving.
- Using the *Clinical Companion Study Guide* will support the development and enhancement of your clinical knowledge and skills.
- The text has specific features that highlight concepts and cases.

It is our sincere desire that this product will provide you with an exciting and productive learning experience that will challenge you to become a competent, knowledgeable, and caring oral healthcare provider.

Who Will Benefit From This Interactive Learning Package?

DENTAL HYGIENE STUDENTS

Whatever your level of study, you will benefit from the depth and range of content and learning features presented in this new edition, which is geared toward the unique requirements of competency-based dental hygiene education. The visual presentation of the book, combined with the interactive CD exercises and review questions, will fully prepare you for the National Board Dental Hygiene Examination and to practice as a professionally-licensed dental hygienist.

FACULTY MEMBERS

The plethora of resources available here will enable you to customize your teaching to match your students' learning style. Plan your lessons using the "Chapter Resources" tables in the *Instructor's Resource Manual*, or create quizzes and examinations efficiently using the Test Bank on the Evolve web site (http://evolve.elsevier.com/Daniel/) and use the CD-ROM exercises to enhance application of knowledge. Be confident that your students will demonstrate competency in every required area!

Why Is This Package Important to the Dental Hygiene Profession?

The textbook, CD-ROM, and other ancillary products that compose this interactive learning resource demonstrate the newest and most comprehensive learning and teaching tools available in the dental hygiene market today. The content covers topics from basic scientific concepts to emerging issues within the profession. By using each element of the interactive resources, students will find themselves fully prepared to emerge from their education with the clinical skills and professional awareness they need to succeed as a dental hygiene professional.

Organization

In this compilation of interactive learning materials, all elements are organized into nine parts, demonstrating the continuum of professional care:

- Part I: Oral Health Care
- Part II: Environmental Ergonomics
- Part III: Patient Assessment
- Part IV: Diagnosis and Planning
- Part V: Prevention Implementation
- Part VI: Therapeutic Implementation
- Part VII: Anxiety and Pain Control
- Part VIII: Care Modifications for Special Needs Patients
- Part IX: Professional Development and Vision

Chapters within each Part address fundamental concepts and contemporary issues and practices in the field of dental hygiene.

New Chapters to This Edition

Several chapters have been moved and reorganized to reflect current educational trends, and seven new chapters are now included:

- **Chapter 4, Evidence-Based Decision Making,** explores clinical practice decision making based on scientific evidence. This chapter walks you through finding and evaluating evidence and then demonstrates how this evidence can be incorporated into patient care.
- **Chapter 6, The Body's Response to Challenge,** reviews the following processes: inflammation, the immune response, hemostasis and wound healing providing an understanding of the impact on patient care.
- **Chapter 36, Esthetics,** presents the evolution of cosmetic dentistry, explaining various rationales behind tooth whitening procedures and other solutions to patients' esthetic problems.

- **Chapter 37, Orthodontics,** provides an overview of common orthodontic profiles and appliances and prepares you for discussing treatment options with patients who may ask about orthodontic treatment.
- **Chapter 38, Oral Malodor Diagnosis and Management,** focuses on the etiology of this common problem and approaches to assist patients in finding solutions.

- **Chapter 47, HIV and AIDS,** reviews the discovery and history of the disease. You will learn about epidemiology, characteristics of HIV and AIDS, oral complications, oral hygiene care and management.
- **Chapter 49, Dental Hygiene Business Practice Management,** reviews basic business skills that you will need to be a productive and contributing member of a healthcare organization.

Special features at the beginning of each chapter help you prepare to learn the content by explaining the WHY, WHAT, and HOW.

WHY: Insight boxes explain the relevance of the chapter content to clinical practice.

HOW: Case Studies help you learn how to relate the content to patient scenarios.

WHAT: Key Terms and Learning Outcomes reinforce new terminology and expectations.

Case Applications appear when chapter content reveals information important in caring for the patient from the Case Study.

Dental Considerations text appears to further connect theoretical content with its clinical relevance.

Special boxes appear next to related text and highlight important thoughts and considerations.

Special icons point out material that is reflected in the CD exercises.

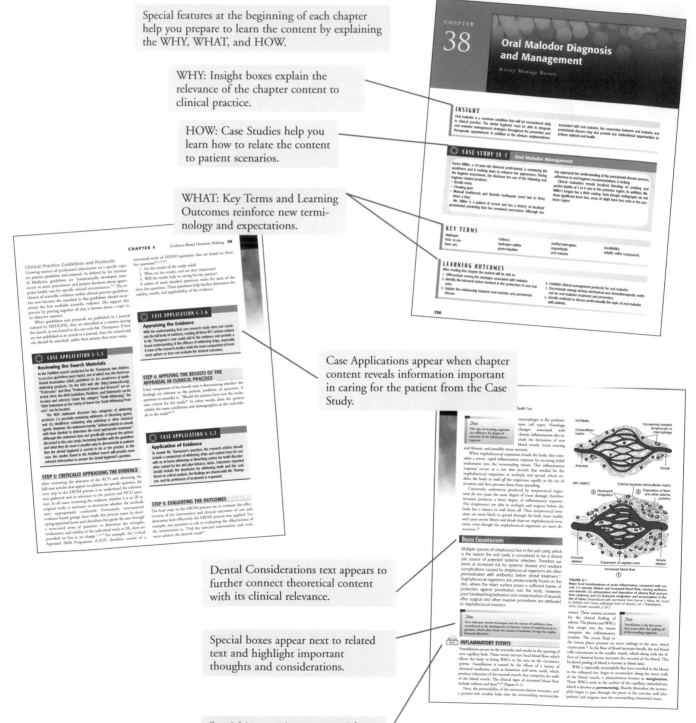

Interactive CD-ROM

The newly-revised CD, packaged with this textbook, includes approximately 300 interactive exercises based on specific chapter content and patient care. Nine distinct and fully-developed patients from all walks of life provide realistic scenarios for you to consider. As you work through each patient exercise, you will learn how their health histories, radiographic and intraoral images, prevention surveys, dental and periodontal charts, and food diaries all factor into making the best decisions for personalized care. Other exercises offer videotaped clips of procedures such as extraoral examination, instrument sharpening, peri-

odontal probing, and powered instrumentation that run following successful completion of the related exercise.

Many of the exercises, once completed, can be saved as reference files for later study.

The Portfolio feature provides a means of storing personal information and recording educational landmarks for later reference and self-assessment in preparation for licensure and writing your resume. Educational achievement and self assessments can be compiled to e-mail to faculty for assessment and review.

Completing CD activities in conjunction with chapter readings will enhance the students' path to competence.

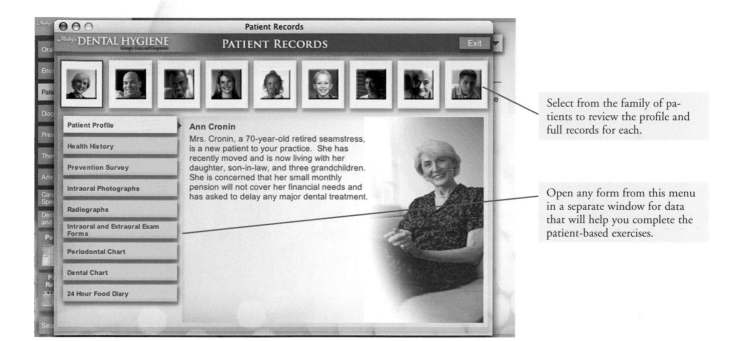

Select from the family of patients to review the profile and full records for each.

Open any form from this menu in a separate window for data that will help you complete the patient-based exercises.

Open specific Portfolio exercises from the main chapter menus, or click on the Portfolio option in the main CD menu to choose from all Portfolio exercises.

Portfolio documents can be edited, printed, or saved to your computer.

My Portfolio lists files that have been completed and saved. Files can be saved under different names as a way to review personal development.

Print Ancillary Products

FOR FACULTY: INSTRUCTOR'S RESOURCE MANUAL

Teaching will be more rewarding than ever with this lesson planning resource—show students how to make the most of the information given to them! This resource manual is organized by chapter and follows a consistent pattern incorporating the following features:

- Chapter Notes
- Of Special Interest
- Chapter Insight Statements (from the text)
- Explanation of the main ideas or concepts behind Case Studies
- Case Applications
- Learning Outcomes list from each chapter
- Chapter Outlines
- Issues to Debate
- Chapter Resources Table—these tables demonstrate the text elements and CD exercises that provide the best teaching opportunities and the learning outcomes associated with each element or exercise.
- Critical Thinking Activities
- Process Performance Forms
- Review Questions with answers and rationales

See the inside front of the Instructor's Resource Manual for a further explanation of how to best use each of these features!

FOR STUDENTS: CLINICAL COMPANION STUDY GUIDE

It is more than a workbook—the conversational format of this new guide shows you how to obtain the most knowledge from each chapter by using the book features and CD-ROM exercises. The *Clinical Companion Study Guide* encourages you to think beyond repetition and memorization!

Take your experiences in the classroom one step further as you prepare for clinical and professional practice.

Working through the exercises and reviewing the outlined resources will provide you with answers to what students *really* want to know:

- WHY do I need to know this chapter information?
- WHAT will I be able to do with this knowledge?
- HOW do I prepare myself to transfer this knowledge to patient care?
- HOW do I perform these skills?
- HOW can I more effectively use this knowledge?
- DO I have all the answers?
- WHERE do I go for more information or support?
- HOW can I keep track of my progress toward competence?

Evolve Resources

The Evolve resources for this compilation of interactive learning resources is available for you to access at http://evolve.elsevier.com/Daniel/.

FOR FACULTY

- **Test Bank**—In addition to a 500-plus question test bank in ExamView that you can use for creating quizzes and examinations to assess your students' progress and prepare them for the National Board Dental Hygiene Examination, you will find the following outstanding assets:
- **Electronic Image Collection**—Includes all the images from the book in various downloadable formats. Use these to prepare presentations and visual class activities quickly and easily!
- **Instructor's Resource Manual available electronically**—Provides easy access to teaching resource tables, outlines, and "Issues to Debate" anywhere, anytime! Resources such as the Outline can be downloaded and modified to meet your specific need.
- **Process Performance Forms**—Can be printed for self, peer and faculty evaluation of clinical progress as each student attains proficiency and reviews clinical skills.
- **Critical Thinking Activity Worksheets** from the *Clinical Companion Study Guide*—Enable you to print out and choose the activities that work best for your students' learning levels.
- **Free access to all the student resources listed in the following section.**

FOR STUDENTS

Both students and faculty will have access to the following additional features on line:

- **Patient Education Handouts** from Mosby's Dental Practice Toolkit, organized by their relevance to text chapters. You can print these and bring them to clinic to practice discussing conditions and treatment approaches with your patients.
- **Patient Record Forms** from the CD-ROM that you can modify and fill out to gain familiarity with creating complete patient files for better treatment planning.
- **Comprehensive Health History Form** from the book that you can use in class and with patients. Combine this with the other record forms to complete a patient profile.
- **Clinical Resource** tables contain helpful information such as lists of state licensing boards, as well as oral healthcare products currently available on the market. Useful items are updated periodically and can be printed for use in clinic.
- **Suggested Agencies and Web Sites** lead you to academic and professional dental hygiene and hygiene-related sites on the Internet. Find contact information for companies, links to educational programs and sites, and web sites of helpful publications.
- **Additional Readings and Resources** point you toward further current and classic sources of information from various books and journals on chapter-specific topics. Use these resource lists for researching papers and projects or for additional learning opportunities on your own time.
- **Competencies for Entry into the Profession of Dental Hygiene** as approved by the 2003 ADEA House of Delegates.

Acknowledgments

There are many things that one does in one's life. Thankfully, all our works are not held to the same value. Few works are conceived, planned, completed, and evaluated without the assistance, insightful input, and continuous encouragement of others.

To my friends and coauthors, Sherry and Becca, your shared insight, energy, expertise, and friendship have left an imprint on this work and my life. Bonnie and Shannon you continue to amaze me with your creative thought and joy for life. I am grateful for your assistance and contributions to this work.

To all who contributed knowledge in the development of chapters; thank you for sharing your expertise with thousands of faculty and students. Without your generosity there would be few works of this nature.

There are many individuals within Mosby who had a role in bringing this publication to market, and I would like to thank all those who had a role in getting this work for dental hygiene education published. Thank you to Penny Rudolph who gave us the opportunity to develop a second edition and to John Dolan for seeing this second edition to completion. Julie Nebel, thank you for your positive attitude, response to inquires, and understanding of the complexities of this work.

Susan J. Daniel

There are many individuals, some within our profession and others with unique areas of expertise, whose insight, dedication, and commitment must be acknowledged as we release the second edition of this text.

Acknowledgment must begin with the extraordinarily talented and gifted team of Susan Daniel Newcomb, Rebecca Wilder, Bonnie Francis, and Shannon Mitchell who worked tirelessly with a vision of excellence that was as inspiring as it was humbling. And to Susan Cieslak, Donna Napiorkowski, Rachel Newingham, Victoria Vick, and Cathy Hopkins, who worked on this and the last edition, I owe a sincere acknowledgement for the patience to get the photography just right, the content on target and cutting-edge, the illustrations clear and concise, and for helping make the CD exercises imaginative without losing the instructional value. What an opportunity and privilege this has been for us all.

Sherry A. Harfst

I have had many mentors in my life and to them I extend a great deal of admiration and humble thanks. First, I wish to thank Susan Daniel and Sherry Harfst for allowing me to work with two intelligent, creative women on a worthwhile project. I want to recognize two others who helped us with this project, Shannon Mitchell and Bonnie Francis. Your abilities and talents are limitless! I wish to thank one of my early mentors, Ms. Margaret Cain, who noticed some potential in me and encouraged me to take the "road less traveled" and expand myself beyond my little world. What a difference that choice has made in my life. Others who have pushed me harder and higher in my life and career are Mary George, Jennifer Reddick, Marilyn Harrington, Maxine Tishk, my colleagues at the University of North Carolina, and the many dental and dental hygiene professionals I have had the privilege of working with through the years. My graduate students have been a huge source of inspiration and continually challenge me to grow and expand. I have many friends in the dental corporate world who strive for excellence in our profession and have been very supportive of us as we have worked on this learning package. My family has been instrumental in helping me accomplish this goal. I am so grateful for the understanding and encouragement they gave to me. I am very grateful to all the contributors who spent countless hours writing, critiquing, and getting it just right! And, finally, I wish to thank the group at Elsevier who pulled it all together!

Rebecca S. Wilder

Contents

The Dental Hygiene Profession

Susan J. Daniel • Mary C. George

CHAPTER

1

INSIGHT

Study of the history of the dental profession provides a window into the past that helps clarify the present. The history of the development of the dental hygiene profession has always emphasized prevention of disease and promotion of health. This rich heritage sets the stage for the profession's contributions as preventive dental care specialists.

CASE STUDY 1-1   Advances in Dental Technology

Pretend for a moment that Irene Newman, the first dental hygiene graduate of Dr. Fones' school in Connecticut, has an opportunity to encounter today's new, modern clinical dental environment. The following section describes the setting that Irene encounters.

Irene arrives at her place of employment and opens the door; her world has been transformed. The area where patients wait is no longer stark with hard, wooden chairs lining the perimeter of the room. Rather, the room is attractive and inviting, with light-colored, soft upholstered chairs. A small sofa, side tables with magazines, and live plants are strategically located in the room. Pleasant artwork adorns the walls, and a dental-related video and monitor for patient viewing occupies a cozy corner.

In awe, Irene proceeds to her work area only to see a totally strange sight. The equipment appears completely foreign. She recognizes what she assumes to be a patient chair, but what is the other chair? She looks at the dental unit and cannot identify the components. She finds neat, small labeled packages containing odd-looking instruments. Next to the unit is a strange boxlike apparatus with a pedal and some type of metal probe protruding from the end of a hose. She notices a large, square box with a glass side attached to something that resembles a typewriter. She is lost in an unfamiliar world.

KEY TERMS

accreditation
American Association for Dental Research
American Association of Public Health Dentistry
American Dental Association
American Dental Education Association
American Dental Hygienists' Association

American Public Health Association
calculus
competence
debridement
disease prevention
evidence-based practice
evidence-based teaching
Health Insurance Portability and Accountability Act

health promotion
Hispanic Dental Association
International Association for Dental Research
International Federation of Dental Hygienists
licensure
National Dental Hygienists' Association
plaque biofilm

regulation
risk assessment
Student American Dental Hygienists' Association
ultrasonic

LEARNING OUTCOMES

After reading this chapter the student will be able to:
1. Appreciate the value of the history of the dental hygiene profession.
2. Understand the process necessary to become a licensed professional.
3. Develop educational goals for the first term of dental hygiene.
4. Create a student portfolio.
5. Develop an appreciation for the profession of dental hygiene and professional associations.

Development of the Profession of Dental Hygiene

Historical accounts detail oral care regimens that have included the cleansing of the teeth and gingiva (gums) with various implements and ingredients. The theory that oral uncleanness or oral diseases result in oral and systemic disease drove modern dentistry to devise methods to rid the mouth of disease-causing agents.

Early records indicate that mechanical and chemical methods of removing tooth deposits have been used throughout time to help prevent oral diseases. Some of the earliest recorded solutions for oral rinsing included alum and vinegar and even myrrh.[24] Hippocrates also advocated the use of whitstone (chalk) as an abrasive. Chalk is still an ingredient in today's dentifrices. Although some of these cleaning protocols seem extreme by current standards, the use of abrasives and instruments to remove deposits forms the basis of many of today's oral care products (Box 1-1).

Modern dentistry has witnessed intermittent exploration but little acceptance of the theory or hypothesis of gum disease causing or compounding systemic disease. Consideration of diseases of the oral cavity has been just that—a disease state considered isolated only to the oral cavity. Systemic sequela has not been a part of the equation. Beginning in the late 1980s, researchers began to explore the relationship between oral and systemic health, reuniting the oral cavity and head with the rest of the body.* The renewed interest in this integrated concept

*References 5-7, 11, 12, 20, 21, 27-31, 33-38, 44.

clearly makes sense; the blood that passes through the oral tissues also circulates to the rest of the body. The humoral response found in host immunity is responsible for circulating antibodies effective against bacterial, parasitic, and viral infections. (See Chapter 6 for more on the humoral response.) Thus an approach to **disease prevention** and **health promotion** based on health risk management is exciting and will certainly affect the practice of dental hygiene. Chapter 2 explores this concept in greater depth.

This chapter explores the following:
- Past and present dental hygiene education and **accreditation**
- Practice behaviors
- Clinical environment
- Technology
- **Licensure** and **regulation**
- Career opportunities
- Pursuit and documentation of maintaining **competence**

History of Dentistry

Figure 1-1 highlights the development of dentistry. History provides a perspective on the richness of the dental hygiene profession, and archeological findings have given dentistry a visual account from ancient cultures.[43] One of the earliest discoveries is a vanity set that includes a toothpick[36] (Figure 1-2). As civilization continued to develop and become more educated, the use of instruments for deposit removal on the teeth was developed. Albucasis was the first to develop a set of instruments and instructions to remove deposits[36] (Box 1-2). Albucasis was an extremely religious Moorish surgeon in Spain and, in

---

BOX 1-1

FIRST DENTIFRICE PRESCRIBED BY HIPPOCRATES

When a woman's mouth smells and her gums are black and unhealthy; one burns, separately, the head of a hare, and three mice, after having taken out the intestines of two of them (not however the liver or kidneys): one pounds in a stone mortar some marble and whitstone, and passes it through a sieve; one then mixes equal parts of these ingredients and with this mixture one rubs the teeth and the interior of the mouth; afterward one rubs them again with greasy wool and one washes the mouth with water. One soaks the dirty wool in honey and with it rubs the gums inside and outside. One pounds dill and anise seeds, 2 aboles (1 abole = 3/4 gram) of myrrh: one immerses these substances in half a cotyle (1 cotyle = 1/4 liter) of pure white wine; one then rinses the mouth with it, holding it in the mouth for some time; this is to be done frequently and the mouth to be rinsed with said preparation fasting and after each meal. The medicament described above cleans the teeth and gives them a sweet smell.

From Hippocrates: *De Morbis Mulierum*, Lib II, 606.

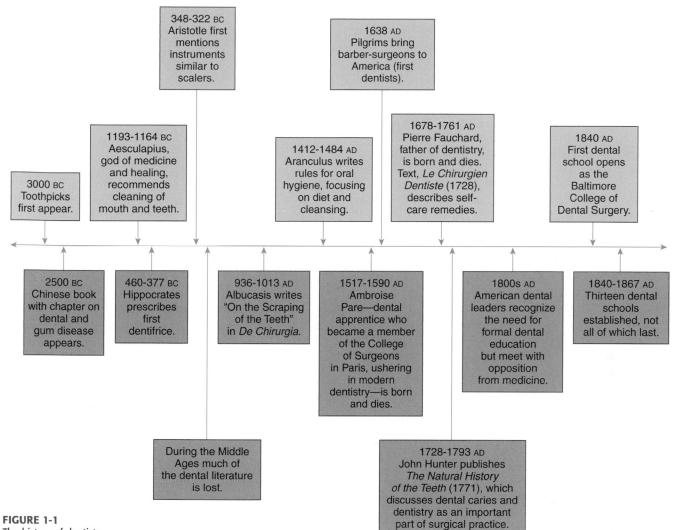

FIGURE 1-1
The history of dentistry.

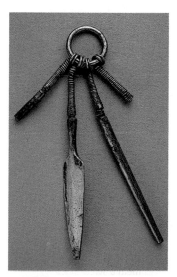

FIGURE 1-2
Vanity set with toothpick. (Courtesy University of Pennsylvania Museum of Archaeology and Anthropology, Philadelphia.)

the Latin treatise *De Chirurgia*, the first individual to recommend a thorough cleaning of the mouth.

Although dentistry has been a surgically oriented profession, its history contains many references to the cleansing of the mouth and the prevention of disease, specifically in the early decades of the 1900s in America.[33] With the focus on disease prevention and mouth cleaning, early leaders in dentistry realized the need for other dental personnel to perform these tasks. By 1906 women were trained to be *dental nurses*. Dr. Alfred

BOX 1-2

ALBUCASIS' WRITTEN INSTRUCTIONS "ON THE SCRAPING OF THE TEETH"

Sometimes on the surface of the teeth, both inside and outside, as well as under the gums, are deposited rough scales, of ugly appearance, and black, green or yellow in color, thus corruption is communicated to the gums, and so the teeth are in process of time denuded. It is necessary for you to lay the patient's head upon your lap and to scrape the teeth and molars, on which are observed either true encrustations, or something similar to sand, and this until nothing more remains of such substances, and also until the dirty color of the teeth disappears, be it black or green or yellowish, or any other color. If a first scraping is sufficient, so much the better, if not, you shall repeat it on the following day or even on the third or fourth day, until the desired purpose is obtained.

Albucasis A: *De Chirurgia* (translated from Latin by Channing S), Oxford, England, 1778.

Fones did not like this name because it carried the connotation of disease. In 1913 he provided a more descriptive name, *dental hygienist;* a dental hygienist is an individual versed in the science of health and the prevention of disease.[19,33]

Education

Formal education of dental hygienists began in the early 1900s with a program for dental nurses at the Ohio College of Dental Surgery. However, because of opposition from the Ohio dentists, the program closed in 1911 and the graduates were never allowed to practice. Figure 1-3 highlights events leading to the prevention movement and the development of dental hygiene. The term *prevention movement* was given to the efforts of a group of prominent dentists who believed in the prevention of oral disease, defined methods for prevention, and wrote and spoke on the subject.

DEVELOPMENT OF FORMAL EDUCATION

After attending a lecture on the benefits of periodic oral prophylaxis, Dr. Alfred C. Fones added this service to his practice. He soon realized the many benefits to his patients' oral health. In 1906, Dr. Fones trained his dental assistant, Irene Newman (the first dental hygiene graduate of his Connecticut school), to scale and polish teeth and to provide general oral self-care instructions to patients. Her education included reading basic and dental science texts and developing scaling and polishing skills.[18,19] The majority of the 27 women in Dr. Fones' first dental hygiene graduating class were employed by the Bridgeport, Connecticut, Board of Education. These first dental

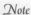

Note

The original role of the dental hygienist was that of disease prevention, specifically dental caries. The disease prevention role forms the basis of current practice.

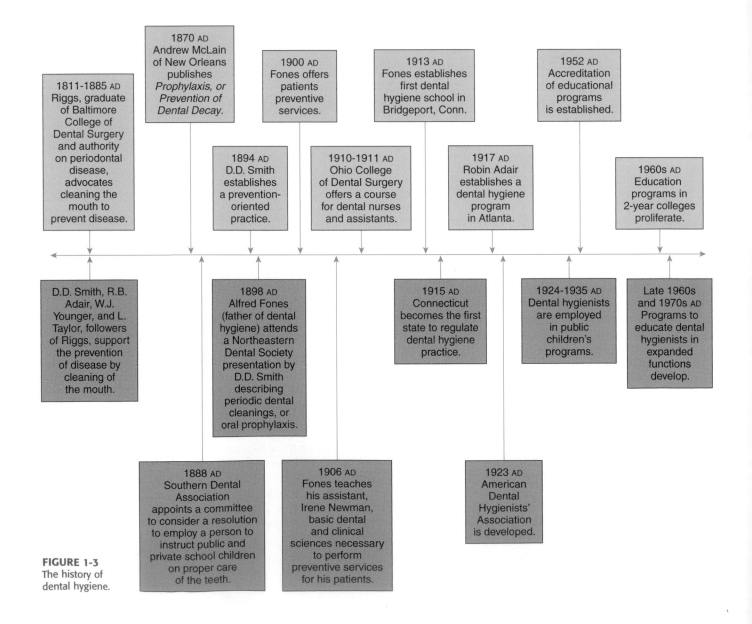

FIGURE 1-3
The history of dental hygiene.

hygienists were credited with helping reduce dental caries by 75% in children participating in their oral care and prevention program. In 1917, Connecticut became the first state to pass licensure laws governing dental hygienists. During this same period, dentists in several other states became disciples of preventive services, including the removal of **plaque biofilm** and hard deposits with specially designed instruments.[18,19]

Many of the early dental hygienists were employed in the public school system and provided educational and preventive services to children.[18] Public health was the primary employment setting for dental hygienists and private practice was secondary, whereas the opposite is true today.

INSTITUTIONAL SETTINGS OF PROGRAMS AND ACCREDITATION

The educational requirements for dental hygienists have changed over the years. Subjective curriculums were replaced with standards and most recently with competencies.[1] Originally, programs were housed in university settings and later in community colleges. In the 1960s the number of programs in 2-year institutions multiplied dramatically. A minimum entry level of education was established as 2 years of college education. The Commission on Dental Education established standards requiring course work in general education; basic, dental, and clinical sciences; and community dental health.

Accredited schools are reviewed every 7 years through a self-study program conducted by the institution, culminating in a site visit by accreditation members. A program accreditation is granted when specified standards are met.

ENTRY LEVEL TO THE PROFESSION AND TYPES OF DEGREES

1-A

Although the minimum educational requirement is 2 years of college with specific standards set forth by the **American Dental Association's** (ADA's) Commission on Dental and Allied Dental Accreditation, not all dental hygiene programs award the same degree. The entry-level dental hygienist can earn a certificate, an associate's degree, or a bachelor's degree. The type of degree awarded depends on the institution and curriculum. Although some 4-year programs might offer expanded functions or concentrations in a subject, no special licensure or functions differentiate a graduate with a certificate or an associate's degree from the individual who has 4 years of education culminating in a bachelor's degree.

Most dental hygiene programs awarding an associate's degree require more than 2 years of college education. Some require a full year of prerequisite courses followed by 2 years of dental hygiene courses. Certificates in dental hygiene are often awarded by an institution (university or college) that recognizes the bachelor's degree as the minimal degree awarded. In the university setting, any less than 4 academic years or equivalent hours usually results in a certificate.

Dental hygiene, as with most professions, is undergoing evaluation, planning, and change. Some would like the entry-level dental hygienist to have a minimum of a bachelor's degree. Additionally, a model curriculum is being planned for the proposed Advanced Dental Hygiene Practitioner (ADHP). This person would have a master's degree and provide direct patient care including diagnostic, preventive, restorative, and therapeutic services in underserved areas.[3]

Changes in Clinical Practice Patterns

PRACTICE ENVIRONMENT

Although dental hygiene remains a prevention-oriented profession, clinical practice behaviors—such as educational requirements—have changed over the years. Approaches to patient education and therapy based on knowledge of origin and treatment modalities have altered the way preventive care is delivered. The practice environment also has changed. Figure 1-4 illustrates an early dental chair. Dentistry has evolved from dental professionals working in a standing position (Figure 1-5) to the ergonomically sound, seated position during patient care (Figure 1-6). Dental equipment has been significantly modified to accommodate this change.

The dental unit was redesigned to allow the seated operator access to the hand piece, suction, and air/water syringe. These components also have undergone modifications. Some equipment changes, known as *engineering controls,* have been developed to protect the operator from infectious diseases, whereas others have been made for operator and patient comfort (ergonomics). More information about engineering controls and ergonomic changes is presented in Chapters 7 and 8.

> *Distinct Care Modifications*
> Equipment modifications to the patient chair allow the patient to be placed in a supine position for the delivery of care by a seated operator.

✷ CASE APPLICATION 1-1.1

Environmental Change

How would you describe the changes in the dental environment to Ms. Newman? What do you think the rationale for these changes has been?

DENTAL CARIES DETECTION AND PREVENTION

Environmental alterations in the clinical practice setting include positioning of the operator, patient, and equipment. Other changes within the setting include the following:
- New terminology
- Discovered etiologies
- Improved detection and management
- Modifications to old and new preventive self-care devices
- Interventions for the treatment of oral diseases

Similarly, protocols used to diagnose oral disease have also changed.

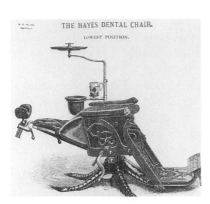

FIGURE 1-4
Early dental chair. (Courtesy James Ulrich, State University of New York, Buffalo, NY.)

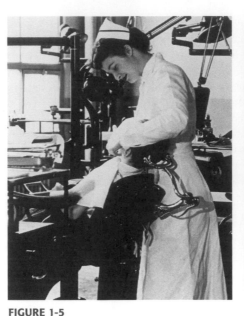

FIGURE 1-5
Dental hygienist during the 1960s working from standing position. (Courtesy Fr. Edward J. Dowling, S.J. Marine Historical Collection, University of Detroit Mercy, Detroit.)

FIGURE 1-6
Contemporary practice setting with the dental hygienist seated.

Distinct Care Modifications

A dental explorer and radiographs were originally the primary tools used to detect dental caries. Because microbes responsible for dental caries have been identified at different stages during lesion development, current literature suggests less use of the explorer and more visual examination with the use of dyes, special illumination, and microbial testing.* Laser technology has been developed for early caries detection and can be operated by the dental hygienist for detection of carious lesions.[27]

*References 10, 13, 15, 23, 26, 39, 40.

Prevention and intervention of dental caries development have improved with the following:

- Knowledge of the remineralization and demineralization processes
- Dental caries **risk assessment** tools (Caries Management by Risk Assessment [CAMBRA] [see Chapter 25])
- Salivary flow rates
- Microbial and enzyme testing of saliva and plaque biofilm
- Topical and systemic fluorides

Treatment has become more conservative with less emphasis placed on the removal of tooth structure and more emphasis on the retention of tooth structure, application of topical fluorides, use of dental sealants, and placement of preventive resins.

CASE APPLICATION 1-1.2

Explaining Changes in Dental Caries Detection

When Ms. Newman was employed as a dental hygienist, there was a limited understanding of the detection and etiology of dental caries. Given the preceding content on change in this area, how would you suggest introducing Ms. Newman to this new way of thinking about dental caries?

ETIOLOGY OF PERIODONTAL DISEASE

Periodontal diseases used to be viewed as a singular disease. Before the late 1960s, only two identified diseases of tooth-supporting structures existed:

- Periodontitis (an inflammatory process requiring gingival tissue or tooth removal)
- Periodontosis (of unknown origin but degenerative with no treatment other than tooth loss)

Knowledge of etiology (quantitative versus qualitative plaque theory), differentiation among several forms of gingival and periodontal diseases, and preventive and conservative therapies have been developed.

Note

Many known forms of periodontal diseases exist and can be differentiated by clinical, microbiological, and patient history risk assessments.

TREATMENT OF PERIODONTAL DISEASE

Treatment modalities for periodontal diseases are more definitive. After the specific form of periodontal disease has been identified, based on existing conditions and oral risk parameters, the appropriate patient-specific prevention, intervention, and therapeutic strategies can be developed (see Chapters 20 through 22). Removing or lowering the bacterial load in the periodontal environment to enable the immune system to trigger wound healing is still the primary therapeutic focus. Although removal of plaque biofilm and calculus are still an objective, dental professionals thought the removal of *all* hard deposits (**calculus**) and the elimination of bacterial plaque biofilm were necessary to prevent gingivitis and periodontitis. This theory did not take into account each individual's immune response to infection. Some individuals with little bacterial plaque or calculus had a higher rate of gingival and periodontal infections than did those with greater amounts of plaque and calculus. Additional research indicated that lowering the amount of deposits is *not* the key to treatment success. The key is to reduce the bacterial load through deposit removal to a level at which the individual's immune system can manage the infection and thereby improve periodontal health.

Current understanding of the disease process and the immune system has changed professional therapeutic strategy. *Powered* instrumentation (sonic and **ultrasonic**) is more frequently used to gain a better healing response than is hand instrumentation. The term **debridement** is used to describe the process of removing deposits. The terms *scaling* and *root planing* are descriptive terms for instrumentation strokes used in the debridement process. Patient self-care habits, use of chemotherapeutic agents, and professional intervention provide greater options in the development of individual strategies to assist the immune response.

CASE APPLICATION 1-1.3

Explaining Change in Periodontics

When Ms. Newman was a dental hygienist, the understanding of an immune system and what it did to keep a person healthy was nonexistent. What can you tell her about the role of the immune system in periodontal health?

RISK ASSESSMENT: DISEASE PREVENTION AND HEALTH PROMOTION

Although the practice of dental hygiene has always focused on prevention, the prevention aspect has expanded to whole-body health.

Careful review of the patient's comprehensive health history, assessment of medications, and interview for signs and symptoms of systemic disease, along with education in the prevention of oral disease, are all part of today's supportive care intervals once referred to as *recall* or *maintenance appointments*.

> **Note**
> The removal of deposits may be the primary concern of the patient, but the practice of dental hygiene is centered on the treatment of the patient as a whole.

Inclusion of all aspects of the patient's health provides insight into the patient's wellbeing:

- Medical and dental history
- Dental caries and periodontal risk
- Fluoride history
- Behaviors and beliefs
- Clinical and radiographic findings
- Current medications
- Oral care routine
- Nutritional habits

Saliva is a bodily fluid teeming with substances that can provide links to health and disease. The processes of identifying the enzymes, proteins, and other substances in saliva are just being discovered. Once obtained and identified, understanding the function and purpose of the identified substances is another part of the puzzle. Chapter 43 begins with an introduction to the role of saliva and some of what we now know about the components in saliva such as the identification of markers associated with breast cancer. Salivary research will continue to evolve and has the potential to position the dental hygienist, who possesses a strong foundation in physiology, biochemistry, and immunology, as a major asset on the healthcare team.

> **Distinct Care Modifications**
> A total risk assessment is essential for disease prevention and health promotion.

Recently, research has linked several systemic conditions with periodontal disease. Lifestyle behaviors such as alcohol use, tobacco use, and improper nutrition affect oral health.

> **Note**
> *Oral Health in America: A Report of the Surgeon General* states the following: "The terms *oral health* and *general health* should not be interpreted as separate entities. Oral health is integral to general health."[41]

CASE APPLICATION 1-1.4

Risk Assessment

Ms. Newman probably never heard of the term, *risk assessment,* or the use of saliva and a person's family history and health behaviors to determine whether there is a risk for certain diseases. How can this knowledge assist you in becoming a better healthcare professional?

The role of the dental hygienist has come full circle from that of an educator primarily in public health settings to clinician in private offices and now returning to educator and specialist in disease prevention and health promotion with roots in public health. The dental hygienist's role is well suited to monitoring the patient's general health with the assessment of vital signs, review of systems in the health history, and oral examination. A dental patient usually sees the dental hygienist periodically for supportive care, possibly more frequently than visiting a physician; therefore the dental hygienist has the opportunity to be the first healthcare provider to discover an undetected illness. Dental hygienists have been educated to note variations from the normal and understand the implications of abnormalities. In addition, dental hygienists develop a rapport with their patients, instilling trust and confidence.

> **Note**
> Oral infections can be the source or first sign of systemic infections.

INFORMED CONSENT AND DOCUMENTATION

Medical legal considerations have received greater emphasis over the years, and informed consent of the patient has become an important issue. Informed consent is the process by which a fully informed patient can participate in choices about his or her health. Treating humans without providing them adequate information about procedures, options, untoward events, and costs is illegal. Simply *informing* a patient of these considerations is not sufficient; the patient or guardian must *understand,*

and the individual's signature must be obtained before procedures are initiated.[25] Documentation in the patient record of all pertinent findings and procedures and the form of documentation are critical. Failure to document patient care meticulously can result in significant legal ramifications. The **Health Insurance Portability and Accountability Act** (HIPAA) (www.hipaa.org) is an enacted federal law that provides comprehensive protection of personal health information. Chapter 3 presents more on ethical and legal considerations.

TECHNOLOGY CHANGES: COMPUTERS

The introduction of computers to dentistry has significantly impacted the provision of dental care. What originally began as a business management tool (e.g., appointment scheduling, patient and insurance billing) has moved into the treatment room. Current use of chairside computers includes the following:

- All patient record keeping
- Charting
- Digital radiography
- Voice-activated periodontal recording
- Dental caries recording

The Internet provides a rapid retrieval system for information that can be used to do the following:

- Enhance patient care
- Better understand treatment modalities and drug interactions
- Locate educational materials for patients
- Provide professional continuing education

RESEARCH

The body of scientific knowledge of dentistry and medicine is growing rapidly. Continued research to identify the disease process and components of the immune response in healing provides evidence for education and practice. Ultimately, the goal is to preserve the oral tissues (hard and soft) and the whole person in health. **Evidence-based teaching** and **evidence-based practice** will assist the dental professional in attaining this goal. Chapter 4 presents more on this subject.

Evidence-based protocols require the use of rapidly changing technology through the evaluation of scientific literature and high-quality continued professional education.

Distinct Care Modifications

Treatment options must be based on the following:
- An assessment of each patient's needs and expectations
- The care providers' clinical experience and scope of expertise
- Sound scientific evidence based on successful treatment outcomes

Licensure and Regulation

1-B

NATIONAL AND STATE OR REGIONAL EXAMINATIONS

Successful progress toward completing an ADA-accredited dental hygiene program permits a candidate to sit for the National Board Dental Hygiene Examination, a written, comprehensive, and objective test required for licensure in all states except Alabama. On successful completion of an accredited program and successful performance on the national board examination, a graduate can then sit for a clinical licensure examination that covers the evaluation of a candidate's application of clinical dental hygiene skills. A regional or state board of examiners or other entity administers the clinical examination. Passing a regional board allows a candidate to apply for licensure in any participating state. All states require each candidate to complete a jurisprudence examination, and some may require other tests of didactic knowledge prior to issuing a dental hygiene license. Passing a state-administered board examination and jurisprudence examination completes the requirements for licensure in each respective state *only*.

LICENSURE BY CREDENTIALS OR RECIPROCITY

Previously, single-state licensing practices required the state-licensing applicant to take another board examination before procuring a license to practice. Realizing the limitations this law created for the dental professionals who are relocating, some state boards have established licensing by credentials and reciprocity avenues as alternatives to the requirement that the candidate must repeat a practical examination. However, the licensing boards in some states do not recognize licensure by credentials or reciprocity and still require the candidate to sit for the practical examination for licensure, regardless of the number of jurisdictions in which the individual is licensed or the number of years of practice experience. Additionally, Florida places limits on the number of years allowed after national board certification to qualify for state licensure.[14] If more than 10 years have elapsed since passing the Dental Hygiene National Board Examination, then the candidate must retake the examination before being allowed to take the Florida clinical examination for licensure.

Groups of educators, practitioners, and examiners believe clinical board examinations are unnecessary if the student graduated from an ADA-accredited program.* In other words, competence as judged by the educational program through the documentation of successful performance should be sufficient to obtain licensure to practice without sitting for a clinical examination.

An alternative course of action for dental licensure under consideration is the use of simulated clinical examinations.[2,13] Currently, each applicant for licensure is required to present one or more patients who meet specific criteria. Selecting appropriate patients and paying transportation, meals, and sometimes lodging and a day's wages are difficult and expensive for the licensure applicant. Using a simulation manikin for the examination sets criteria-based standards, allowing the examination to assess clinical performance more objectively. The Dental Interactive Simulation Corporation (DISC) is working on the development of an interactive simulated national and clinical board examination.[13] The American Board of Dental Examiners is working with other entities to develop a national uniform licensing examination for dentists and

---

*References 9, 16, 17, 22, 27, 32, 42.

dental hygienists. Possibly by the time this text is published, a national examination may exist, which would make it more convenient for professionals to relocate and continue their career without major expense and interruption.

Types of Supervision

Few states allow dental hygienists to practice independently. In most states the practice of dental hygiene is allowed under the supervision of a licensed dentist. Supervision can range from direct to general. States with general supervision language in the practice act may have additional criteria for this form of supervision. Definitions of supervision and business arrangements are identified in Box 1-3.[4]

However, new models for supervision have been developed and are influenced greatly by the number of people who do not receive oral health care. The collaborative practice model in New Mexico has dental hygienists working among other healthcare providers in a *health commons,* which is a site that pools resources from public and private entities to address community health issues among low-income rural areas. In these community healthcare settings the dental hygienist is one of many on the healthcare team who provide direct care in a collaborative environment under the supervision of a physician.[8]

Functions

A dental hygienist's duties vary by state. Universally, dental hygienists assess and record patient histories, perform extraoral and intraoral examinations and chartings, remove deposits on the teeth, expose radiographic film for dental images, place topical fluoride and dental sealants, and teach patients self-care techniques. At the time of this writing, dental hygienists are licensed to administer local anesthesia in 40 jurisdictions within the United States. Other functions delegated to the dental hygienist may include operative procedures such as placing restorations, performing cosmetic whitening, placing or removing sutures or both, making impressions, administering nitrous oxide and oxygen analgesia, and placing subgingival preventive agents. Delegation of procedures varies among the states. Dental hygienists must become familiar with the dental practice act in the states in which they wish to practice.

Will universal licensure, simulated examinations, or licensure based on academic competence occur? Which functions will the dental hygienist perform 50 years from today? Chapters 50 and 51 explore these questions.

Career Mobility and Career Choices

1-2

Dental hygienists are part of an exciting and expanding healthcare environment. Growth in knowledge and technology is being transferred to the educational and career environment. Professional roles assumed by dental hygienists can be found in Figure 1-7. Dental hygienists serve in these roles in many different settings (some of these settings and roles are described in this section).

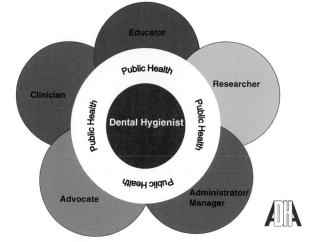

FIGURE 1-7
Professional roles of the dental hygienist. (Courtesy of American Dental Hygienists' Association, Chicago. Reprinted with permission.)

PRIVATE PRACTICE

The private dental practice is the most common site for the employment of dental hygienists. In private practice the hy-

---

BOX 1-3

TYPES AND DEFINITIONS OF DENTAL SUPERVISION

Direct supervision: A dentist must be present in the facility when a dental hygienist performs procedures.

General supervision: A dentist has authorized a dental hygienist to perform procedures and does not need to be present in the treatment facility during the performance of those procedures. As of September 2006, 43 jurisdictions have a form of general supervision.

Independent practice: The dental hygienist owns a dental hygiene practice in this business arrangement—a recognizable incorporated or unincorporated business structure that can be bought and sold. An independent practitioner may have a supervisory relationship with a dentist. An unsupervised dental hygienist may be employed to work in a dental office or other entity.

Collaborative practice: This is similar in scope to the independent practice. The state of New Mexico defines this practice as "the science and prevention of oral disease through the provision of educational, assessment, preventive, clinical, and other specified therapeutic services in a cooperative working relationship with a consulting dentist without general supervision."*

Independent contracting: With this tax status, the dental hygienist does not maintain an employee relationship with a dentist for whose patients the hygienist provides dental hygiene services. As nonemployees, dental hygienists pay their own withholding taxes and Social Security taxes, and the dentist does not pay worker's compensation or unemployment insurance on their behalf.

*Extracted from the New Mexico Administrative Code 16.5.17.

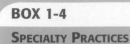

BOX 1-4

SPECIALTY PRACTICES IN DENTISTRY

Dental public health
Endodontics
Oral and maxillofacial radiology
Oral and maxillofacial surgery
Oral pathology
Orthodontics
Pediatric dentistry
Periodontics
Prosthodontics

---

gienist typically functions as a clinician and patient educator, providing preventive services to patients. Dental hygienists are most often employed in a general dental practice, but some choose to work in a dental specialty practice (Box 1-4). In some practices the dental hygienist may assume any of the following administrative or managerial roles:

- Office or practice manager
- Infection-control manager
- Tobacco cessation intervention coordinator

Sometimes the dental hygienist will assume any one of these roles in addition to the responsibilities of providing patient care. Each of these roles requires specific skills and knowledge.

EDUCATION

Dental hygienists holding advanced degrees may become dental hygiene educators. The type of institution and dental hygiene degree being awarded by the program dictate the level of degree required of full-time faculty members. Academic responsibilities of a dental hygiene faculty member vary according to the type of institution (e.g., community college, university) and its mission. In some institutions, faculty members are required to teach, provide community service, and conduct research and publish. Some institutions also require clinical patient care. Continued activity in these areas assists the dental hygiene educator in maintaining competence. Students are only as competent as the educators who facilitate learning.

PUBLIC HEALTH

Dental hygienists may be employed by the public health division of state governments to perform oral screenings of school children for dental diseases and provide preventive services in local clinics.

The U.S. Public Health Service and the Indian Health Service (IHS) of the federal government employ dental hygienists to work in dental clinics nationwide. Dental hygienists with bachelor's degrees can become commissioned officers in the U.S. Public Health Service. The IHS is also responsible for the Dental Health Aide Therapist, a member of the Alaska model who provides oral healthcare services to the rural native Alaskan population. Individuals from various tribes are selected and educated for 2 years in New Zealand. On return, they function under general supervision providing preventive services, simple restorative procedures, and extractions.[42]

Other employment opportunities are available within the Veteran's Administration Hospitals' dental clinics and the federal and state prison systems. Many larger institutions have dental clinic facilities on their premises.

DENTAL PRODUCT SALES AND MARKETING

Corporations employ dental hygienists to market products to private offices, retail stores, and institutions. The dental hygienist's knowledge and use of preventive products are most beneficial for the companies that employ them, not only in teaching consumers about the product but also in developing educational materials for use in pharmaceutical and medical sales, which are also options for the dental hygienist. The basic science foundation within the hygienist's educational curriculum provides the understanding needed to market these types of products effectively. Dental hygienists within the dental product industry can be found in administrative and managerial roles.

INSURANCE INDUSTRY

The insurance industry employs dental hygienists as dental claim reviewers. Knowledge of the following provides the dental hygienist with the foundation to be an asset in the insurance industry:

- Radiographic imaging
- Treatment codes
- Pathology
- Ethical behavior
- Treatment needs

DENTAL RESEARCH

The quest for new knowledge provides another opportunity for employment and career extension. Investigation of ideas and questions is the genesis of tomorrow's education and practice—evidence supporting which treatment to provide and when, why, and how. Dental hygienists employed as researchers work independently, whereas others are part of a group of investigators. Most dental hygiene researchers have obtained advanced degrees or specific training to understand the research process and to prepare them for research presentation and publication skills. Research activity without publication of the findings is of little value to anyone other than perhaps those directly involved in the investigative activity. Publishing research findings adds to the body of literature and provides supportive evidence for educational and clinical practice knowledge and techniques. Using research findings in education and practice assists in the quest for continued competence.

Maintaining Competence

CONTINUING EDUCATION

Although maintaining competence is necessary in all fields, it is especially important in health care. Healthcare providers should desire continued learning. Due to the rapid changes in knowledge and technology in medicine and dentistry, continuing education is critical to maintaining competence. One measure of competence is to assess continually or annually the amount (in hours) and content of education a healthcare provider receives. Almost all state dental licensing boards specifically mandate continuing education hours for a given time to allow for the licensee to retain active licensure and practice. Continuing education hours may be obtained in many forms, and each state identifies the type of format it will accept, which includes class sessions or workshops; courses on video, CD, or on line; and offerings within professional journals.

1-D PROFESSIONAL ORGANIZATIONS

Maintaining competence can be time-consuming. Isolation allows complacency and dissatisfaction with the care being rendered and its outcomes. Dental hygienists often report feeling isolated when working in a single dental practice. Becoming a member and participating in a professional organization facilitates discussion among peers who frequently experience or have experienced similar situations. Professional organizations allow for the sharing of ideas, offer support and encouragement, and provide a forum for formal learning experiences through seminars and other continuing educational activities. Membership in professional associations or groups in the healthcare profession is important to maintain a sense of belonging and to increase knowledge about the profession.

Dental hygienists have various professional associations from which to choose, and many dental hygienists have membership in more than one professional association. The **American Dental Hygienists' Association** (ADHA) was organized in 1923 and is the professional association representing only dental hygienists. The association office is located in Chicago, Illinois. Members, officers, and staff provide representation for dental hygiene in national governmental affairs and in other associations, especially in the ADA's Commission on Dental and Allied Dental Accreditation and the **American Dental Education Association** (ADEA). The ADHA develops recommendations for dental hygiene practice and supports dental hygiene activities nationwide. The official publications of the ADHA are the *Journal of Dental Hygiene* and *Access*.

A student member status also exists in ADHA, and each dental hygiene program can establish a chapter. The student group is referred to as the **Student American Dental Hygienists' Association** (SADHA).

Many countries have national professional organizations for dental hygienists. An international association exists for national organizations and individual members. The **International Federation of Dental Hygienists** (www.ifdh.org) comprises 21 national organizations (Box 1-5).

The Canadian Dental Hygienists' Association (CDHA) was formed in 1964 and represents approximately 14,000 dental hygienists in Canada. The official publication of CDHA is the *Canadian Journal of Dental Hygiene.*

The ADEA is the professional association representing dental and allied dental educators. The association provides continuing educational opportunities for dental, dental hygiene, dental assisting, and dental laboratory technology faculty and supports dental and allied dental education in other healthcare and governmental affairs. Educators have an opportunity to share and learn what other educators are doing in their respective programs. Additionally, members of the association, through committees, develop subject guidelines for program curricula. Research in dental, allied dental, and health services research is often presented at the annual ADEA meeting. The official publications are the *Journal of Dental Education* and the *Bulletin of Dental Education.*

The **American Association for Dental Research** (AADR) is the research association for scientists conducting research in dental- and allied dental–related topics in the United States. Other countries also have their own dental research associations. Membership in the AADR has reciprocal membership with the **International Association for Dental Research** (IADR). Similar to other professional organizations, the AADR/IADR provide a forum to showcase dental research. This exchange of ideas, theories, and original research findings assists with the development of improved treatment and prevention regimens and forms the basis of future educational curricular change.

The **American Association of Public Health Dentistry** (AAPHD) and the **American Public Health Association** (APHA) are organizations providing support and innovations in dental public health and public health, respectively. These associations address general and oral health issues, their effect on the population, and measures to alleviate and prevent disease.

Other professional associations and organizations in which dental hygienists can become members include the **National Dental Hygienists' Association** (NDHA) and the **Hispanic Dental Association** (HDA). These organizations support and encourage oral health promotion for their respective minorities. The important aspect is to remain a part of a professional organization that promotes oral and systemic health and supports the role of dental hygienists in the pursuit of improved oral health care for all.

BOX 1-5

ASSOCIATION MEMBERS OF THE INTERNATIONAL FEDERATION OF DENTAL HYGIENISTS

Australia	Japan	Slovakia
Austria	Korea	South Africa
Canada	Latvia	Spain
Denmark	Lithuania	Sweden
Finland	Netherlands	Switzerland
Germany	New Zealand	United Kingdom
Ireland	Nigeria	United States of
Israel	Norway	America
Italy	Portugal	

✦ CASE APPLICATION 1-1.5

Professionalism

With dental hygiene education as the beginning of a professional career, what measures will you take and what behaviors will you exhibit that define professionalism?

PROFESSIONAL PORTFOLIO

Of the many responsibilities of being a healthcare provider, maintaining competence is possibly the most important. Many avenues exist for documentation, but the most comprehensive is the portfolio.

Documentation of continuing education and other professional activities of the dental hygienist is important for use in assessing the dental hygienist's career progress and attainment of goals. Additionally, this documentation can be used to provide support of competence and expertise in dental hygiene. The dental hygienist's portfolio may include the following information:

- Continuing education courses attended, hours attained, and pertinent information about the courses
- Information on community service activities performed individually or with other professionals
- Professional meetings attended
- Documentation of patient care for those with systemic and oral diseases, oral risks identified, strategies used, and treatment successes

This information will assist with future patient care and self-evaluation of effectiveness and perhaps provide the information required for a salary increase or to procure future employment.

STUDENT PORTFOLIO

1-E
1-F

The portfolio of the dental hygiene student is similar to other professional portfolios and forms the basis for continuation of the professional portfolio. Each dental hygiene program may devise its own mechanism for evaluating the progress through the academic program. The portfolio is one mechanism for obtaining the information that can be used to determine a student's progress. Students within an academic program must obtain the competencies of that specific dental hygiene program. These competencies can usually be placed into categories such as the following:

- Patient care
- Professional growth and development
- Health promotion and disease prevention
- Community involvement

These categories can be used to develop the framework for the student portfolio. Once competencies have been identified, faculty can determine the level of achievement required of a student at given points in the program (i.e., academic terms or more frequently). The student can set goals for each term and begin to record and document the performance toward meeting those goals. Working with a faculty advisor for goal setting can be beneficial in guiding the student toward realistic goals. At the end of the evaluation period the student should perform a self-evaluation of performance using documentation in each category. The documentation is reviewed at the end of the designated term, and the information is compared with established goals. The student determines whether the documentation is sufficient to establish whether the goals have been met. If the goals have been met, then new ones can be established. If goals have not been met, then it is important to determine the deficiency and prioritize the steps toward meeting the goals within the next evaluation period. The faculty mentor can provide an evaluation of the student achievement based on the same process the student uses, but the faculty member will also take into consideration the validity of the student's self-evaluation.

Another level of evaluation—peer evaluation—can also be placed into the evaluation profile or equation. This third component should be developed at the beginning of the semester with the assignment of a pair of students to work with each other. Each student provides an evaluation of the other based on the goals established at the beginning of the semester, documented achievement, and self-evaluation as described in the previous paragraph.

A format for converting the evaluation to a measurement can be developed by the faculty and shared with students at the beginning of the academic term. The ownership of the student's progress is clear with the establishment of goals in each of the categories. Some academic terms may be weighted more heavily in clinical development and less so in service, or service may be weighted a specified amount for all academic terms. Preclinical development may have vastly different goals from clinical development. Professional growth and development begins when entering the program and continues throughout a provider's career. Observing and documenting personal and professional growth and development can be insightful and rewarding. Whether or not the academic program is using a portfolio, setting goals and recording actions that indicate the goals are being pursued or met (or both) is a worthwhile self-assessment. This process is advocated throughout an oral healthcare provider's career. Beginning that process now will serve the dental hygienist well.

The remainder of this text details information necessary to become a dental hygienist. Providing preventive oral health care is becoming increasingly important as more links are discovered between oral and systemic health. This is an exciting time to embark on a career in dental hygiene. Dental hygienists should always search for ways to improve themselves and those they serve; this text, its accompanying CD-ROM, Clinical Companion Study Guide, and Evolve web site provide a rich foundation for those goals.

References

1. American Dental Association: *Accreditation standards for dental hygiene education,* Chicago, 1998, Commission on Dental Accreditation, The Association.
2. American Dental Association House of Delegates: Resolution 64RC, 2000.
3. American Dental Hygienists' Association: *Dental hygiene: focus on advancing the professions,* Chicago, 2005, ADHA.
4. American Dental Hygienists' Association: *House of delegates manual: definition of commonly used terms,* Chicago, 1999, ADHA.
5. Beck JD et al: Evaluation of oral bacteria as risk indictors for periodontitis in older adults, *J Periodontol* 63:93-99, 1992.
6. Beck JD et al: Periodontal disease and cardiovascular disease, *J Periodontol* 67:1123-1137, 1996.

7. Beck JD et al: Periodontitis: a risk factor for coronary heart disease, *Ann Periodontol* 3(1):127-141, 1998.

8. Beestra S et al: A "health commons" approach to oral health for low-income populations in a rural state, *Am J Public Health* 92(1):12-13, 2002.

9. Buchannan RN: Problems related to the use of human subjects in clinical evaluation/responsibility for follow-up care, *J Dent Educ* 55:797-798, 1991.

10. Colston BW et al: Imaging of hard- and soft-tissue structure in the oral cavity by optical coherence tomography, *Applied Optics* 37:3582-3585, 1998.

11. Dasanayake AP: Poor periodontal health of the pregnant woman as a risk factor for low birth weight, *Ann Periodontol* 3(1):206-211, 1998.

12. Davenport ES et al: The East London study of maternal chronic periodontal disease and preterm low birth weight infants: study design and prevalence data, *Ann Periodontol* 3(1):213-221, 1998.

13. Dental Interactive Simulation Corporation: *DISC dental simulations,* Aurora, Colo, 2001, The Corporation. Available at: http://www.uiowa.edu/dentistry-disc/index.html.

14. Department of Health, Board of Dentistry, Division of Medical Quality Assurance: *Florida Statutes and Rule 64B5, Florida Administrative Code,* Tallahassee, 2000, The Department.

15. Everett MJ et al: Non-invasive diagnosis of early caries with polarization sensitive optical tomography (PS-OCT). In Featherstone JD, editor: *Lasers in dentistry v. proceedings of SPIE,* Bellingham, Wash, 1999, SPIE.

16. Feil P, Meeske J, Fortman J: Knowledge of ethical lapses and other experiences on clinical licensure examinations, *J Dent Educ* 63:453-458, 1999.

17. Field MJ, editor: *Dental education at the crossroads: challenges and change,* Washington, DC, 1995, National Academy Press.

18. Fones AC: *Mouth hygiene,* ed 2, Philadelphia, 1921, Lea & Febiger.

19. Fones AC: The origin and history of the dental hygienist movement, *J Am Dent Assoc* 13:1809-1821, 1926.

20. Grau AJ et al: Association between acute cerebrovascular ischemia and chronic and recurrent infection, *Stroke* 28:1724-1729, 1997.

21. Grossi SG, Genco RJ: Periodontal disease and diabetes mellitus: a two-way relationship, *Ann Peridontol* 3(1):51-61, 1998.

22. Guarino KS: Licensure and certification of dentists and accreditation of dental schools, *J Dent Educ* 59:205-236, 1995.

23. Hall FA et al: Dye-enhanced laser fluorescence method. In Stookey, GK, editor: *Early detection of dental caries: proceedings of the 1st Annual Indiana Conference,* Indianapolis, 1996, Indiana University School of Dentistry.

24. Hippocrates: *De Morbis Mulierum,* Lib II, 606.

25. Justice Cardozo BN: Doctrine of informed consent. *Schloendorff v. Society of New York Hospital,* 211 N.Y. 125, 105 N.E. 92, 1914.

26. KaVo Corporation, Lake Zurich, Ill: DIAGNOdent (equipment for detecting dental caries). Available at: http://www.kavo.com. Accessed 2001.

27. Linz AM: Dental licensure, *J Am Dent Assoc* 123:9-10, 1992.

28. Loesche W, Pohl A, Karapetow F: Plasma lipids and blood glucose in patients with marginal periodontitis, *J Dent Res* 76:408, 1997.

29. Mattila KJ et al: Association between dental health and acute myocardial infarction, *Br Med J* 298:779-781, 1989.

30. Mattila KJ et al: Dental infections and coronary atherosclerosis, *Atherosclerosis* 103:205-211, 1993.

31. Mattila KJ et al: Dental infection and the risk of new coronary events: prospective study of patients with documented coronary artery disease, *Clin Infect Dis* 20:588-592, 1995.

32. Meskin LH: Dental licensure revisited, *J Am Dent Assoc* 127:292-294, 1996.

33. Motley WE: *History of the American Dental Hygienists' Association 1923-1982,* Chicago, 1983, American Dental Hygienists' Association.

34. Offenbacher S et al: Periodontal infection as a possible risk factor for preterm low birth weight, *J Periodontol* 67:1103-1113, 1996.

35. Offenbacher S et al: Potential pathogenic mechanisms of periodontitis-associated pregnancy complications, *Ann Periodontol* 3(1):233-250, 1998.

36. Ring ME: *Dentistry: an illustrated history,* St Louis, 1985, Mosby.

37. Schlossman M et al: Type 2 diabetes mellitus and periodontal disease, *J Am Dent Assoc* 121:532-536, 1990.

38. Syrjanen J et al: Dental infections in association with cerebral infarction in young and middle-aged men, *J Intern Med* 25:179-184, 1989.

39. ten Bosch JJ: General aspects of optical methods in dentistry, *Adv Dent Res* 1:5-7, 1987.

40. ten Bosch JJ, Angmar-Mansson B: A review of quantitative methods for studies of mineral content of intra-oral incipient caries lesions, *J Dent Res* 70:2-14, 1991.

41. US Department of Health and Human Services: *Oral health in America: a report of the surgeon general,* Rockville, Md, 2000, The Department, National Institute of Dental and Craniofacial Research, National Institutes of Health.

42. US Public Health Service: *Alaska dental health aide program background,* prepared for the American Dental Association. A Brief for the ADA 10/16/03. Available at: http://dhfs.wisconsin.gov/health/Oral_Health/taskforce/pdf/alaskaprogram.pdf

43. Weinberger BW: *An introduction to the history of dentistry in America,* vol I, St Louis, 1948, Mosby.

44. Zambon JJ et al: Identification of periodontal pathogens in atheromatous plaques, *J Dent Res* 76:408, 1997.

Health Promotion:
A Basis of Practice

Kimberly S. Bray • Joan I. Gluch

INSIGHT

The dental hygienist's role in health care is exemplified as one who can promote health through prevention and intervention. Possessing knowledge of health theory, health behavior, and the mechanism for change is key to health promotion in the dental hygiene practice. This chapter provides dental hygienists with the foundation for their roles as the promoters of appropriate healthcare habits and behaviors for patients.

✦ CASE STUDY 2-1   Expanding the Definition of Health

Elizabeth Marino, age 57, visits her dental office for a routine supportive care appointment, during which she expects to have a dental prophylaxis, radiographic studies completed, and intraoral and extraoral examinations. Ms. Marino's health history indicates a recent diagnosis of type 2 diabetes and mild hypertension. She reports her diabetes is managed with diet and exercise.

Her vital signs, taken at the appointment, indicate a blood pressure of 140/85 mm Hg with a faint pulse of 86 beats per minute. She reports no additional illness or medication. Her personal history indicates that she is overweight (5 feet tall and 155 pounds) and lacks daily physical exercise. After reviewing her chart before the appointment, the dental hygienist notices that the patient has not been in for

an appointment in almost 2 years.

Clinically, Ms. Marino exhibits several areas of attachment loss and generalized bleeding on probing. Because Ms. Marino does not monitor her own blood glucose levels, the hygienist recommends and the patient consents to a chair-side finger-stick blood glucose check. The glucometer reports 236 mcg/dl blood glucose. The relationship between periodontal infection and diabetes is explained, and Ms. Marino is informed that today's blood glucose findings will be shared with her physician. The dental hygienist also recommends an appointment with the physician within the next 2 days. In what ways has the hygienist promoted concepts of health to Ms. Marino?

KEY TERMS

behavior intent	epidemiologic surveys	health promotion	intention
burden of disease	health	health theory	

LEARNING OUTCOMES

After reading this chapter the student will be able to:
1. Determine working definitions for *health* and *health promotion*.
2. Discuss the paradigm shift with regard to health promotion in dental hygiene.
3. Apply theoretical models of health behavior to plan interventions aimed at changing health behaviors.

4. State general demographic parameters of an epidemiologic survey.
5. Describe the burden of oral disease in the U.S. population.
6. Discuss the two national health planning reports and their implications for dental hygienists for improving both individual and population health.

Link between Dentistry and Human Health

One of the many benefits of becoming a member of a health-care profession is the personal and professional satisfaction gained in patient interaction. As a member of the dental health-care team, the role of the dental hygienist is critical in the promotion of general health, as well as oral health.

As healthcare providers, dental hygienists are in a key position to discuss and promote oral health, systemic health, and general well-being. Dental hygienists examine some populations of patients on a more consistent basis and more frequently than do most other healthcare professionals. Dental hygienists have the opportunity to touch a patient's life and, through a thorough assessment and patient-specific interventions, significantly affect the behaviors and beliefs of those seeking care. For example, when dental hygienists routinely complete blood pressure measurements with patients, they may be in a position to detect elevated readings for referral and evaluation by a physician. In addition, when dental hygienists routinely complete oral examination procedures, they may also be in a position to detect potentially fatal oral cancerous lesions and refer their patients for evaluation by the oral maxillofacial specialist. Especially when dental hygienists recommend tobacco cessation activities for their patients, they can make a significant difference in improving their patients' health status. These three actions of dental hygienists illustrate the essential and critical role this healthcare professional can play with his or her patients in promoting general health and in preventing disease beyond the oral cavity.

In 2002 the Institute of Medicine released an influential report, "The Future of the Public's Health in the 21st Century." This report emphasized the critical role that collaboration and partnerships play to ensure the health of the population.[30] Rather than simply relying on government and public health agencies, this report emphasized the cooperation and interaction of many groups to promote and protect the safety and well-being of the nation. Figure 2-1 graphically illustrates the six groups and their interactions that can ensure optimal health of the population. When dental hygienists provide clinical services, they are working as part of the healthcare delivery system from a clinical perspective to promote population health. Dental hygienists can also promote health from a community perspective when they participate as consumer advocates, educators, and health promoters in the following five groups: (1) academia, (2) governmental public health infrastructure, (3) media, (4) community, and (5) business.

Health Promotion Definitions

In the current era in which the focus is on wellness and in which oral health professionals assume an expanded role, the definition of **health promotion** takes on a new meaning. In addition, **health** can no longer be defined as the mere absence of disease. The World Health Organization (WHO) defines health promotion as follows:

. . . the process of enabling people to increase control over, and to improve, their health. To reach a state of complete physical, mental and social well-being, an individual or group must be able to identify and to realize aspirations, to satisfy needs, and to change or cope with the environment. Health is, therefore, seen as a resource for everyday life, not the objective of living. Health is a positive concept emphasizing social and personal resources, as well as physical capacities. Therefore, health promotion goes beyond healthy life-styles to well-being.[66]

The Institute of Medicine also incorporates a broader perspective into the definition of health, emphasizing that the key focus is the health of the population:

. . . the health of the population as measured by health status indicators and as influenced by social, economic and physical environments, personal health practices, individual capacity and coping skills, human biology, early childhood development and health services.[30]

Dental hygienists need to understand this multidimensional view of health to provide more appropriate and realistic health promotion strategies and activities for their patients. For example, disparities in oral health status exist for a variety of reasons. These reasons include biological, social, and economic factors, and dental hygienists can work in an advocacy role with their patients and in the community to ensure increased access to oral health services for the underserved population.

National Health Promotion Guidelines

As the focus of general and oral health moves from the elimination of disease to the restoration and promotion of health and well-being, the role of the dental hygienist is clarified. Dental hygienists continue to participate in providing the necessary oral health services to identify, treat, and restore health. Their primary focus, however, is on the promotion of general and oral health. Although this focus might be considered a challenging and diffuse goal, two national reports provide guidance and direction for a national effort in promoting population health.

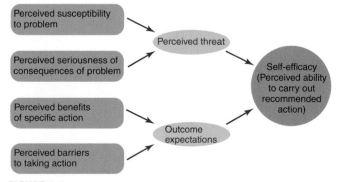

FIGURE 2-1
Health Belief Model. (Adapted from Nutbeam D, Harris E: *Theory in a nutshell: a practitioner's guide to commonly used theories and models in health promotion,* Sydney, 1998, University of Sydney, Department of Public Health and Community Medicine, National Centre for Health Promotion.)

The first report, *Healthy People 2010,* is the national planning document that sets goals, specific objectives, and priorities for the national health services. The second report, *Report of the Surgeon General on Oral Health,* provides the specific linkage for oral health as essential in general health, and it sets priorities and direction for action.

HEALTHY PEOPLE 2010

"Healthy people in healthy communities"[8] is the vision for the *Healthy People 2010* initiative, which is a national health promotion and disease prevention program that brings together federal, state, and local government agencies; nonprofit, voluntary, and professional organizations; and businesses, communities, and individuals. With the overall mandate to improve the health of all Americans, two major goals have been identified: (1) eliminate disparities in health, and (2) improve the quality of the years of a healthy life. The nation's progress in achieving these goals is monitored through 467 objectives in 28 focus areas (Box 2-1). Many objectives focus on interventions designed to reduce or eliminate illness, disability, and premature death among individuals and communities. Others focus on broader issues, such as improving access to quality health care, strengthening of public health services, and improving the availability and dissemination of health-related information. Each objective has a target for specific improvements to be achieved by the year 2010. Together, these objectives reflect the depth of scientific knowledge and the breadth of diversity in the nation's communities. More importantly, these objectives are designed to help the nation achieve its two platform goals and realize the vision of healthy people living in healthy communities.

Oral Health Goals for 2010

The overall oral health goal of the *Healthy People 2010* initiative is to prevent and control oral and craniofacial diseases, conditions, and injuries

> ### BOX 2-1
>
> #### HEALTHY PEOPLE 2010 FOCUS AREAS
>
> Access to quality health services
> Arthritis, osteoporosis, and chronic back conditions
> Cancer
> Chronic kidney disease
> Diabetes
> Disability and secondary conditions
> Educational and community-based programs
> Environmental health
> Family planning
> Food safety
> Health communication
> Heart disease and stroke
> HIV
> Immunization and infectious diseases
> Injury and violence prevention
> Maternal, infant, and child health
> Medical product safety
> Mental health and mental disorders
> Nutrition and obesity
> Occupational safety and health
> Oral health
> Physical activity and fitness
> Public health infrastructure
> Respiratory diseases
> Sexually transmitted diseases
> Substance abuse
> Tobacco use
> Vision and hearing

and to improve access to related services. Specific to this goal, the *Healthy People 2010* conference established the following 17 distinct objectives:

1. Reduce the proportion of children and adolescents who have dental caries experience in their primary or permanent teeth.

	Baseline	Target Goal
Young children—primary teeth	18%	11%
Young children—primary and permanent teeth	52%	42%
Adolescents—permanent teeth	61%	51%

2. Reduce the proportion of children, adolescents, and adults with untreated dental decay.

	Baseline	Target Goal
Young children—primary teeth	16%	9%
Young children—primary or permanent teeth	29%	21%
Adolescents—permanent teeth	20%	15%
Adults—permanent teeth	27%	15%

3. Increase the proportion of adults who have never had a permanent tooth extracted because of dental caries or periodontal disease.

	Baseline	Target Goal
Adults	31%	42%

4. Reduce the proportion of older adults who have had all their natural teeth extracted.

	Baseline	Target Goal
Older adults	26%	20%

5. Reduce periodontal disease.

	Baseline	Target Goal
Gingivitis	48%	41%
Destructive periodontal disease	22%	14%

6. Increase the proportion of oral and pharyngeal cancers detected at the earliest stages.

	Baseline	Target Goal
All	35%	50%

7. Increase the proportion of adults who, in the past 12 months, report having had an examination to detect oral and pharyngeal cancer.

	Baseline	Target Goal
Adults	14%	35%

8. Increase the proportion of children who have received dental sealants on their molar teeth.

	Baseline	Target Goal
Children, age 8 years	23%	50%
Adolescents, age 14 years	15%	50%

9. Increase the proportion of the U.S. population served by community water systems with optimally fluoridated water.

	Baseline	Target Goal
All	62%	75%

10. Increase the proportion of children and adults who use the oral health care system each year.

	Baseline	Target Goal
Children and adults	65%	83%

11. Increase the proportion of long-term care residents who use the oral health care system each year.

	Baseline	Target Goal
Long-term care residents	19%	25%

12. Increase the proportion of children and adolescents under age 19 years at or below 20% of the federal poverty level who received any preventive dental service during the past year.

	Baseline	Target Goal
Children and adolescents under age 19	20%	57%

13. Attain a developmental increase in the proportion of school-based health centers with an oral health component.

	Baseline	Target Goal
None available	N/A	N/A

14. Increase the proportion of local health departments and community-based health centers, including community, migrant, and homeless health centers, that have an oral health component.

	Baseline	Target Goal
Community-based health centers	34%	75%

15. Increase the number of states, including the District of Columbia, that have a system for the recording and referral of infants and children with cleft lips, cleft palates, and other craniofacial anomalies to craniofacial anomaly rehabilitative teams.

	Baseline	Target Goal
All states	23 States	All states

16. Increase the number of states, including the District of Columbia, that have an oral and craniofacial health surveillance system.

	Baseline	Target Goal
All states	0	All states

17. Increase the number of Tribal, State (including the District of Columbia), and local health agencies that serve jurisdictions of 250,000 or more individuals that have in place an effective dental health program directed by a dental professional with public health training.

Baseline		Target Goal
In development	In development	In development

REPORT OF THE SURGEON GENERAL ON ORAL HEALTH

The first surgeon general's report on oral health in May 2000 was designed to alert Americans to the full meaning of oral health and its importance to general health and well-being. The often-repeated quote by former Surgeon General C. Everett Koop, "You're not healthy without good oral health,"[63] set the tone for this landmark report that continues to be influential with policymakers, clinicians, and consumers alike. The in-depth report covers questions such as "What is oral health?" and "What are the needs and opportunities to enhance oral health?" It includes a summary document of findings at the conclusion of most chapters[45] (Box 2-2).

The report offers a framework for action, outlining needs and opportunities to enhance oral health as follows:

- *Change the perceptions regarding oral health and disease so that oral health becomes an accepted component of general health.* Perceptions need to change on three levels: (1) public, (2) policymakers, and (3) health providers.
- *Accelerate the building of the science and evidence base, and apply science effectively to improve oral health.* The acceleration of research and the effective transfer of research findings to the public and health professions are keys to this part of the plan.
- *Build an effective health infrastructure that meets the oral health needs of all Americans and effectively integrates oral health for all.* Because of cutbacks, limited personnel, equipment, and facilities, disease prevention programs are not being implemented in many communities. Coupled with the lack of racial and ethnic diversity in the oral health workforce, those populations most in need of health promotion receive the least. Shortages also exist in oral health education, research, and practice.
- *Remove known barriers between people and oral health services.* Use public-private partnerships to improve the oral health of those who still disproportionately suffer from oral disease.

Specifically, the dental professional was charged with the following responsibilities:

- Stay abreast of technologic advances in dental and medical science.
- Continue to be responsive to the expectations of patients.
- Explore partnerships with medicine as the knowledge base regarding the relationship between oral health and systemic health increases.
- Expand the community disease–based prevention programs to meet emerging needs.
- Continue to seek solutions to questions of access and barriers to care.
- Understand the profound relationship between oral health and the quality of life.

In 2003 the surgeon general issued a "Call to Action," which reemphasized the critical role of oral health in general health and asked for a renewed commitment to the framework for action.[65] The dental hygiene community has embraced this report and has implemented multiple strategies to capitalize on the opportunities provided by this "Call to Action." Increased collaboration with physicians, nurses, and healthcare professionals; innovative strategies to increase access to care; and increased funding for oral health programs are some concrete examples of activities that have been initiated and facilitated by this report. A renewed emphasis on the essential nature of oral health provides many challenges for dental hygienists to embrace a broadened view of health and health promotion and to understand the vast opportunity to promote optimal health for all.

BOX 2-2

ORAL HEALTH IN AMERICA: A REPORT OF THE SURGEON GENERAL

Major Findings, Executive Summary

- *Oral disease and disorders in and of themselves affect health and well-being throughout life.* Dental disease affects patient life. The patient may be among a particularly vulnerable population. The **burden of disease** is extensive and may include the following:
  - Oral lesions
  - Candidiasis
  - Birth defects
  - Chronic facial pain
  - Oral cancers

  Many of these conditions and their treatments may undermine self-image and self-esteem, discourage normal social interaction, cause other health problems, lead to chronic stress and depression, and incur great financial cost. They also may interfere with vital functions such as breathing, food selection, eating, swallowing, and speaking, as well as with activities of daily living such as work, school, and family interactions.

- *Safe and effective measures exist to prevent the most common dental diseases—dental caries and periodontal diseases.* Community water fluoridation is safe and effective in the prevention of dental caries in both children and adults. Water fluoridation benefits all residents served by community water supplies, regardless of their social or economic status. Professional and individual measures, including the use of fluoride mouth rinses, gels, dentifrices, and dietary supplements and the application of dental sealants, are additional means to prevent dental caries. Gingivitis can be prevented with good personal oral hygiene including brushing and flossing.

- *Lifestyle behaviors that affect general health, such as tobacco use, excessive alcohol use, and poor dietary choices, affect oral and craniofacial health as well.* These individual behaviors are associated with increased risk for craniofacial birth defects, oral and pharyngeal cancers, periodontal disease, dental caries, and candidiasis, among other oral health problems. Opportunities exist to expand the public's knowledge and practices of oral disease prevention and health promotion through community programs and in healthcare settings. All healthcare providers can help promote healthy lifestyles by incorporating tobacco-cessation programs, nutritional counseling, and other health promotion efforts into their practices.

- *Profound and consequential oral health disparities exist within the U.S. population.* Disparities for various oral conditions may relate to income, age, sex, race or ethnicity, or medical status. Although common dental diseases are preventable, not all members of society are informed about or able to use appropriate oral health–promoting measures. Similarly, not all healthcare providers may be aware of the services needed to improve health. In addition, oral health care is not fully integrated into many care programs. Social, economic, and cultural factors and changing population demographics affect the ways in which health services are delivered and used, as well as the ways in which people care for themselves. Reducing disparities requires wide-ranging approaches that target populations at highest risk for specific oral diseases and improve access to existing care. One approach includes more available dental insurance for Americans. Public coverage for dental care is minimal for adults, and programs for children have not reached the many eligible beneficiaries.

- *More information is needed to improve America's oral health and to* eliminate health disparities. Adequate data do not exist for health, disease, and health practices and care for the U.S. population as a whole and its diverse segments, which include racial and ethnic minorities, rural populations, individuals with disabilities, the homeless, immigrants, migrant workers, the very young, and frail older adults. In addition, sufficient data do not exist that explore health issues in relation to sex or sexual orientation. Data on state and local populations, essential for program planning and evaluation, are rare or unavailable and reflect the limited capacity of the U.S. health infrastructure for oral health. Health services research, which could provide much-needed information on the cost, cost-effectiveness, and outcomes of treatment, is also sorely lacking. Finally, measurement of disease and health outcomes is needed. Although progress has been made in the measurement of oral health–related quality of life, more needs to be done, and measures of oral health *per se* do not exist.

- *The mouth reflects general health and well-being.* The mouth is a readily accessible and visible part of the body and provides healthcare providers and individuals with a window to their patients' general health status. As the gateway of the body, the mouth senses and responds to the external world and at the same time reflects what is happening deep inside the body. The mouth may show signs of nutritional deficiencies and serve as an early warning system for diseases such as HIV infection and other immune system problems. The mouth can also show signs of general infection and stress. As the number of substances that can be reliably measured in saliva increases, it may well become the diagnostic fluid of choice, enabling the diagnosis of specific disease and the measurement of the concentration of a variety of drugs, hormones, and other molecules of interest. Cells and fluids in the mouth may also be used for genetic analysis to help uncover risks for disease and predict outcomes of medical treatments.

- *Oral diseases and conditions are associated with other health problems.* Oral infections can be the source of systemic infections in people with weakened immune systems, and oral signs and symptoms are often part of a general health condition. Associations between chronic oral infections and other oral health problems, including diabetes, heart disease, and adverse pregnancy outcomes, also have been reported.* Ongoing research may uncover mechanisms that strengthen the current findings and explain these relationships.

- *Scientific research is key to further reduction in the burden of diseases and disorders that affect the face, mouth, and teeth.* The science base for dental diseases is broad and provides a strong foundation for further improvements in prevention. For other craniofacial and oral health conditions, the base has not yet reached the same level of maturity. Scientific research has led to a variety of approaches to improve oral health through prevention, early diagnosis, and treatment. Through investigation, the public and the healthcare professions can take these prevention measures further into ways that develop more targeted and effective interventions and devise ways to enhance their appropriate adoption. The application of powerful new tools and techniques is important. Their use in research into genetics and genomics, neuroscience, and cancer has permitted rapid progress in these fields. An intensified effort to understand the relationships between oral infections and their management and other illnesses and conditions is warranted, along with

---

*References 3, 5-7, 9-12, 15-17, 24, 28-36, 38, 54, 55.

BOX 2-2

ORAL HEALTH IN AMERICA: A REPORT OF THE SURGEON GENERAL—CONT'D

the development of oral-based diagnostics. These developments hold great promise.

Craniofacial Complex

Natural selection has served *Homo sapiens* well in the evolution of a craniofacial complex with remarkable functions and abilities to adapt, enabling the organism to meet the challenges of an ever-changing environment. An examination of the various tissues reveals elaborate designs that have evolved to serve the basic needs and functions of a complex mammal, as well as those that are uniquely human, such as speech. The rich distribution of nerves, muscles, and blood vessels in the region and the extensive endocrine and immune system connections indicates the vital role of the craniofacial complex in adaptation and survival over a long life span. The following features are of particular interest:

- Genes controlling the basic patterning and segmental organizations of human development, and specifically the craniofacial complex, are highly conserved in nature. Mutated genes affecting human development have counterparts in many simpler organisms.
- Considerable reserve capacity or redundancy exists in the cells and tissues of the craniofacial complex. Consequently, if they are properly cared for, then the structures should function more than a lifetime.
- The salivary glands and saliva subserve tasting and digestive functions and also participate in the mucosal immune system, a mainline defense against pathogens, irritants, and toxins.
- Salivary components protect and maintain oral tissues through antimicrobial components, buffering agents, and a process by which dental enamel can be remineralized.

Magnitude of the Problem

- Over the last 5 decades, major improvements in oral health have been noted nationally for most Americans.
- Despite improvements in oral health status, profound disparities remain in some population groups as classified by sex, income, age, and race or ethnicity. For some disease and conditions, the magnitude of the differences in oral health status among population groups is striking.
- Oral diseases and conditions affect individuals throughout their life. Nearly every American has experienced the most common oral disease, dental caries.
- Conditions that severely affect the face and facial expression, such as birth defects, craniofacial injuries, and neoplastic diseases, are more common in the young and older adult populations.
- Orofacial pain can greatly reduce quality of life and restrict major functions. Pain is a common symptom for many of the conditions affecting orofacial structures.
- National and state data for many oral and craniofacial diseases and conditions and for population groups are limited or nonexistent. Available state data reveal variations within and among states in patterns of oral health and disease among population groups.
- Research is needed to develop improved measures of disease and health, to explain differences among population groups, and to develop interventions targeted at eliminating disparities.

Diseases and Disorders

- Microbial infections, including those caused by bacteria, viruses, and fungi, are the primary cause of the most prevalent oral diseases.

These include dental caries, periodontal diseases, herpes labialis, and candidiasis.

- The cause and pathogenesis of diseases and disorders affecting the craniofacial structures are multifactorial and complex, involving interplay among genetic, environmental, and behavioral factors.
- Many inherited and congenital conditions affect the craniofacial complex, often resulting in disfigurement and impairments that may involve many body organs and systems and affect millions of children worldwide.
- Tobacco use, excessive alcohol use, and inappropriate dietary practices contribute to many diseases and disorders. In particular, tobacco use is a risk factor for oral cavity and pharyngeal cancers, periodontal diseases, candidiasis, and dental caries, among other diseases.
- Some chronic diseases, such as Sjögren's syndrome, exhibit primary oral symptoms.
- Orofacial pain conditions are common and often have complex causes.

Linkages with General Health

- Many systemic diseases and conditions have oral manifestations that may be the initial sign of clinical disease and, as such, serve to inform healthcare professionals and individuals of the need for further assessment.
- The oral cavity is a portal of entry and the site of disease for microbial infections that affect general health status.
- The oral cavity and its functions can be adversely affected by many pharmaceutical medications and other therapies commonly used to treat systemic conditions. The oral complications of these therapies can compromise patient compliance with treatment.
- Immunocompromised and hospitalized individuals are at great risk for general morbidity because of oral infections.
- Individuals with diabetes are at greater risk for periodontal diseases.[*]
- Animal- and population-based studies have demonstrated associations between periodontal diseases and diabetes, cardiovascular disease, stroke, and adverse pregnancy outcomes.[†]
- Further research is needed to determine the extent to which these associations are causal or coincidental.

Effects on Well-Being and Quality of Life

Examination of efforts to characterize the functional and social implications of oral and craniofacial disease reveals the following findings:

- Oral health is related to the well-being and quality of life as measured along functional, psychosocial, and economic dimensions. Diet, nutrition, sleep, psychologic status, social interactions, school, and work are affected by impaired oral and craniofacial health.
- Cultural values influence oral and craniofacial health and well-being and can play an important role in care-use practices and in the perpetuation of acceptable oral health and facial norms.
- Oral and craniofacial diseases and their treatment place a burden on society in the form of lost days and years of productive work. Acute dental conditions contribute to a range of problems for employed adults, including restricted activity, bed days, and work loss, with children losing days of school. In addition, conditions such as oral and pharyngeal cancers contribute to premature death and can be measured by years of life lost.

---

*References 5, 7, 13, 22, 25, 42, 47, 51, 56, 57, 60.
†References 6, 7, 9, 10, 14-16, 22, 24, 25, 28, 30-34, 38, 39, 54, 55.

Continued

BOX 2-2

ORAL HEALTH IN AMERICA: A REPORT OF THE SURGEON GENERAL—CONT'D

- Oral and craniofacial diseases and conditions contribute to compromised abilities to bite, chew, and swallow foods; limitations in food selection; and poor nutrition. These conditions include tooth loss, diminished salivary functions, orofacial pain conditions such as temporomandibular disorders, alterations in taste, and functional limitations of prosthetic replacements.
- Orofacial pain, as a symptom of untreated dental and oral problems and as a condition in and of itself, is a major source of diminished quality of life. Orofacial pain is associated with sleep deprivation, depression, and multiple adverse psychosocial outcomes.
- Self-reported effects of oral conditions on social function include limitations in verbal and nonverbal communication, social interaction, and intimacy. Individuals with facial disfigurements resulting from craniofacial diseases and conditions and their treatments may experience loss of self-image and self-esteem, anxiety, depression, and social stigma; these, in turn, may limit educational, career, and marital opportunities and affect other social relations.
- Reduced oral health–related quality of life is associated with poor clinical status and reduced access to care.

Community and Other Approaches to Promote Oral Health and Prevent Oral Disease
- Community water fluoridation, an effective, safe, and ideal public health measure, benefits individuals of all ages and socioeconomic strata. Unfortunately, more than one third of the U.S. population (100 million individuals) are without this critical public health measure.
- Effective disease prevention measures exist for use by individuals, practitioners, and communities. Most of these measures focus on dental caries prevention, such as fluorides and dental sealants, in which a combination of services is required to achieve optimal disease prevention. Daily oral hygiene practices, such as brushing and flossing, can prevent gingivitis.
- Community-based approaches for the prevention of other oral diseases and conditions, such as oral and pharyngeal cancers and orofacial trauma, require intensified developmental efforts.
- A gap exists between research findings and the oral disease prevention and health promotion practices and knowledge of the public and healthcare professions.
- Disease prevention and health promotion approaches, such as tobacco control, appropriate use of fluoride for dental caries prevention, and folate supplementation for neural tube defect prevention, highlight opportunities for partnerships between community-based programs and practitioners and collaborations among healthcare professionals.
- Many community-based programs require a combined effort among social service, health care, and educational services at the local or state level.

Personal and Provider Approaches to Oral Health
- Achieving and maintaining oral health require individual action, complemented by professional care and community-based activities.
- Individuals can take actions for themselves and for persons under their care to prevent disease and maintain health. Primary prevention of many oral diseases is possible with appropriate diet, nutrition, oral hygiene, and health-promoting behaviors, including the appropriate use of professional services. Individuals should use a fluoride dentifrice daily to help prevent dental caries and should brush and floss daily to prevent gingivitis.
- All primary care providers can contribute to improved oral and craniofacial health.
- Interdisciplinary care is needed to manage the oral health–general health interface. Dentists, as primary care providers, are uniquely positioned to play an expanded role in the detection, early recognition, and management of a wide range of complex oral and general diseases and conditions.
- Nonsurgical interventions are available to reverse disease progression and to manage oral diseases as infections.
- New knowledge and the development of molecular and genetically based tests will facilitate risk assessment and management and improve the ability of healthcare providers to customize treatment.
- Healthcare providers can successfully deliver tobacco-cessation and other health-promotion programs in their offices, contributing to both overall health and oral health.
- Biocompatible rehabilitative materials and biologically engineered tissues are being developed to enhance greatly the treatment options available to providers and their patients.

Provision of Oral Health Care
- Dental, medical, and public health delivery systems each provide services that affect oral and craniofacial health in the U.S. population. A private practice workforce predominantly provides clinical oral health care.
- Dental services alone made up 4.7% of the nation's health expenditures in 1998, $53.8 billion of $1.1 trillion.[2] These expenditures underestimate the true costs to the nation, however, because data are unavailable to determine the extent of the expenditures and services provided for craniofacial health care by other providers and institutions.
- The public health infrastructure for oral health is insufficient to address the needs of disadvantaged groups, and the integration of oral and general health programs is lacking.
- Expansion of community-based disease prevention initiatives and the lowering of barriers to personal oral health care are needed to meet the needs of the population.
- Insurance coverage for dental care is increasing but still lags behind medical insurance. For every child age 18 years or younger without medical insurance, at least two children are without dental insurance. For every adult 19 years or older without medical insurance, three are without dental insurance.
- A narrow definition of the phrase *medically necessary dental care* currently limits oral health services for many insured persons, particularly older adults.
- The dentist-to-population ratio is declining, creating concern as to the capability of the dental workforce to meet the emerging demands of society and to provide required services efficiently.
- An estimated 25 million individuals reside in areas lacking adequate dental care services, as defined by Health Professional Shortage Areas (HPSA) criteria.
- Educational debt has increased, affecting both career choices and practice location.

BOX 2-2

ORAL HEALTH IN AMERICA: A REPORT OF THE SURGEON GENERAL—CONT'D

- Disparities exist in the oral health profession workforce and career paths. The number of underrepresented minorities in the oral health professions is disproportionate to their distribution in the general population.
- Current and projected demand for dental school faculty positions and research scientists is not being met. A crisis in the number of faculty members and researchers threatens the quality of dental education; oral, dental, and craniofacial research; and, ultimately, the health of the public.
- Reliable and valid measures of outcomes for oral health care need to be developed, validated, and incorporated into practice and programs.

Factors Affecting Oral Health Over the Life Span

- The major determinants of oral and general health and well-being are individual biologic and genetic factors and the environment, which includes its physical and socioeconomic aspects; personal behaviors and lifestyle; access to care; and organization of health care. These factors interact over the life span and determine the health of individuals, population groups, and communities—from neighborhoods to nations.

- The burden of oral disease and conditions is disproportionately borne by individuals with low socioeconomic status at each life stage and by those who are vulnerable because of poor general health.
- Access to care makes a difference. A complex set of factors underlies access to care and includes the need to have informed public and policymakers, integrated and culturally competent programs, and resources to pay and reimburse for the care. Among other factors, the availability of insurance increases access to care.
- Preventive interventions, such as protective head and mouth gear and dental sealants, exist but are not uniformly used or reinforced.
- Nursing homes and long-term care and other institutions have a limited capacity to deliver necessary oral health services to their residents, most of whom are at increased risk for oral diseases.
- Anticipatory guidance and risk assessment and management facilitate care for children and for the older adult population.
- Federal and state assistance programs for selected oral health services exist; however, the scope of these services is severely limited, and their reimbursement level for oral health services is low compared with the usual fee for care.

Modified from U.S. Department of Health and Human Services: *Oral health in America: a report of the surgeon general,* Rockville, Md, 2000, The Department, National Institute of Dental and Craniofacial Research, National Institutes of Health.

Focus on Oral Health: Burden of Oral Disease

Both the *Healthy People 2010* initiative and the *Report of the Surgeon General on Oral Health* include detailed descriptions of the current status of oral health, which exerts a tremendous burden on the health of both individuals and communities. Those considering the cost of dental care in our nation may tend to calculate the cost of the placement and replacement of fillings, tooth extractions, and treatment of gum disease. However, closer evaluation allows for the appreciation of oral disease as progressive, cumulative, and complex. Strictly based on dental needs, our nation's dental bill was approximately $80 billion in 2004.[2] Added to this initial figure are billions of dollars in medical care associated with chronic craniofacial pain from conditions such as temporomandibular disorders, trigeminal neuralgia, shingles, burning mouth syndrome, cleft lip and palate, oral and pharyngeal cancers, autoimmune diseases, and injury.[17] To the cost of dental and medical expenses is added the cost of social, psychologic, and economic consequences.

Although major oral health improvements have been made in the last 50 years, disparities remain in some subgroups as classified by sex, income, age, and race and ethnicity.[40] An understanding of the state of the nation's oral health is captured through the evaluation of epidemiologic data for specific oral conditions.

EPIDEMIOLOGY OF ORAL DISEASES

Evaluating the health of a nation and then determining which health promotion actions should be taken is a huge task involving thousands of research participants, volunteers, and hours. Several of the major studies from which status data are drawn are listed in the following sections. Population samples from which these types of data are drawn are usually large, nationally representative surveys of the U.S. civilian, noninstitutionalized population and are referred to as **epidemiologic surveys.**

National Health and Nutrition Examination Survey

The most recent survey, the National Health and Nutrition Examination Survey (NHANES) III, was conducted between 1999 and 2002 by the National Center for Chronic Disease Prevention and Health Promotion and the Division of Oral Health at the Centers for Disease Control and Prevention (CDC). Trained interviewers gathered demographic and related health data. Selected individuals then were invited to a mobile examination center for health assessments, including an oral examination by a trained dentist.

National Oral Health Surveillance System

Conducted in 1999, the most recent National Oral Health Surveillance System (NOHSS) is a collaborative effort between the CDC and the American State and Territorial Dental Directors. This survey includes data on the following oral health indicators:

- Most recent dental visits
- Teeth cleaning
- Complete tooth loss
- Fluoridation status and pharynx
- Dental caries experience
- Untreated tooth decay
- Dental sealants
- Cancer of the oral cavity

FINDINGS

Dental Caries in Children

Dental caries is one of the most common childhood diseases and is five times more common than asthma and seven times more common than hay fever. Among children ages 2 through 11 years, 41% have experienced dental caries in their primary teeth, with 21% identified with untreated tooth decay in their primary teeth. Approximately 42% of children and adolescents ages 6 through 19 years have experienced dental caries in their permanent teeth, with 14% identified with untreated tooth decay in their permanent teeth. Dental decay rates are increasing for children living in families with incomes less than 200% of the federal poverty level and also for children of black and Hispanic-American descent.[63] Figures 2-2 through 2-4 and Box 2-3 offer detailed information regarding economic and racial disparities in oral health status in children.

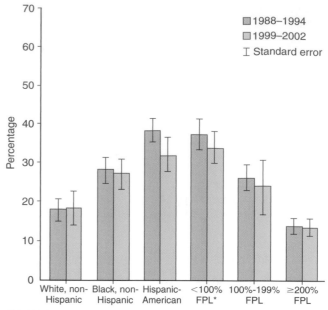

FIGURE 2-3
Untreated dental caries in primary teeth. Prevalence of untreated tooth decay in primary teeth among children aged 2 through 11 years by selected characteristics—United States, National Health and Nutrition Examination Survey, 1988-1994 and 1999-2002. (Modified from Beltrán-Aguilar ED et al: Surveillance for dental caries, dental sealants, tooth retention, edentulism, and enamel fluorosis—United States, 1988-1994 and 1999-2002, Centers for Disease Control and Prevention, *MMWR* 54[3]:1-44, 2005.) *Federal poverty level.

Dental Caries in Adults

Approximately 91% of adults have experienced dental caries in their lifetime, with 23% of adults identified with untreated dental decay. From 1999 to 2002, adults of every age group showed declines in the prevalence and severity of dental caries from previous epidemiologic surveys. Despite these overall gains, disparities still exist with increased caries rates witnessed in non-Hispanic black and Hispanic participants, as well as those with family incomes less than 200% of the federal poverty level (Figures 2-5 and 2-6; Box 2-4).

Periodontal Diseases

One method used to measure periodontal disease clinically is through the calculation of attachment loss, which accounts for the way in which much of the supporting structure has been lost. The greater the attachment loss, the more severe the disease. Attachment loss varies by age, sex, and racial and ethnic group. Most adults 25 years and older have at least one site of 2 mm or more loss of attachment. The percentage of adults with 6 mm or more of attachment loss increases with age (Figure 2-7); 19% of 55- to 64-year-old adults and 23.4% of 65- to 74-year-old adults showed an attachment loss of 6 mm or more at one or more sites.[63]

More men than women are likely to have at least one tooth exhibiting a 6-mm loss of attachment (Figure 2-8). More non-Hispanic black adults have had at least one tooth site exhibiting

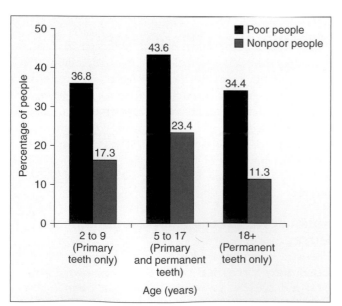

FIGURE 2-2
Untreated dental caries. A higher percentage of people living at the poverty level have at least one untreated decayed tooth. (Modified from U.S. Department of Health and Human Services, National Center for Health Statistics: *Third national health and nutrition examination survey, 1988-94*. Public use data file no. 7-0627, Hyattsville, Md, 1997, Centers for Disease Control and Prevention.)

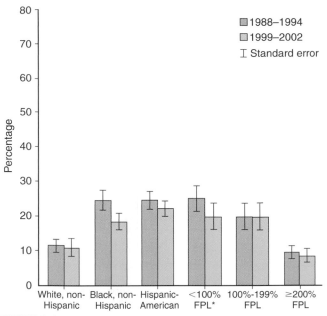

FIGURE 2-4
Untreated dental caries in permanent teeth. Prevalence of untreated tooth decay in permanent teeth among children and adolescents aged 6 through 19 years by selected characteristics—United States, National Health and Nutrition Examination Survey, 1988-1994 and 1999-2002. (Modified from Beltrán-Aguilar ED et al: Surveillance for dental caries, dental sealants, tooth retention, edentulism, and enamel fluorosis—United States, 1988-1994 and 1999-2002. Centers for Disease Control and Prevention, *MMWR* 54[3]:1-44, 2005.) *Federal poverty level.

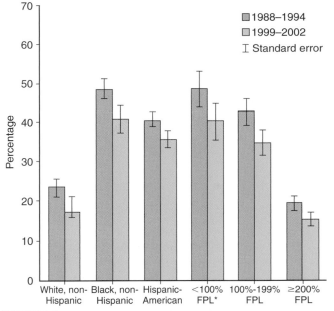

FIGURE 2-5
Untreated dental caries in adults. Prevalence of untreated tooth decay among dentate adults aged 20 years or older by selected characteristics. Adults living in poverty have a higher percentage of untreated decayed teeth than other adults—United States, National Health and Nutrition Examination Survey, 1988-1994 and 1999-2002. (Modified from Beltrán-Aguilar ED et al: Surveillance for dental caries, dental sealants, tooth retention, edentulism, and enamel fluorosis—United States, 1988-1994 and 1999-2002. Centers for Disease Control and Prevention, *MMWR* 54[3]:1-44, 2005.) *Federal poverty level.

6 mm or more of attachment loss as compared with Hispanic-Americans and non-Hispanic white adults (Figure 2-9). Those of the lowest socioeconomic status demonstrated at least one site with attachment loss of 6 mm or more, compared with those at a higher socioeconomic standing[62] (Figure 2-10).

Tooth Loss and Edentulism

Edentulism affects approximately 8% of adults over the age of 20 years. Families living below the poverty level are more likely to be edentulous than those living above it. By age 17 years, more than 7.3% of children in the United States have lost at

---

BOX 2-3

BURDEN OF ORAL DISEASE IN CHILDREN

- Cleft lip and cleft palate affects an estimated 1 of 600 live births for whites; 1 out of 1850 live births for blacks.
- Other devastating birth defects, such as ectodermal dysplasia, cause ongoing, lifetime problems.
- Dental caries is the single most common chronic childhood disease—5 times more common than asthma and 7 times more common than hay fever.
- More than 50% of 5- to 9-year-olds have at least one area of dental caries or filling. This figure increases to 78% among 17-year-old adolescents.
- Income levels create disparities in dental disease. Poor children suffer twice as much from dental caries, and their diseases are more likely to remain untreated. One of four children is born into poverty; children living below the poverty line (annual income of $17,000 for a family of four) have more severe or untreated dental caries or both.

- Head, neck, and mouth are common sites of unintentional injuries in children.
- Tobacco-related oral lesions are prevalent in adolescents who use smokeless (spit) tobacco.
- Professional care is necessary to maintain oral health. Approximately 25% of poor children have not been examined by a dentist before entering kindergarten.
- Uninsured children are 2.5 times less likely to receive dental care and have 3 times the dental needs of children with public or private insurance. For every child with medical insurance, 2.6 children exist without it.
- More than 41 million school hours are lost each year to dental-related illness. Poor children suffer 12 times more restricted-activity days than do children from higher income families.

From U.S. Department of Health and Human Services: *Oral health in America: a report of the surgeon general,* Rockville, Md, 2000, The Department, National Institute of Dental and Craniofacial Research, National Institutes of Health.

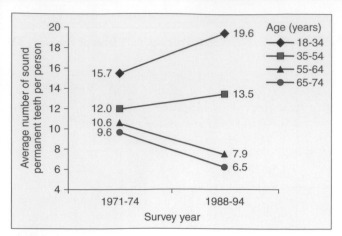

FIGURE 2-6
Since 1971 through 1974, the average number of permanent teeth without decay or fillings has increased among 18- to 54-year-old **adults.** (Modified from U.S. Department of Health and Human Services, National Center for Health Statistics: *Third national health and nutrition examination survey, 1988-94.* Public use data file no. 7-0627, Hyattsville, Md, 1997, Centers for Disease Control and Prevention.)

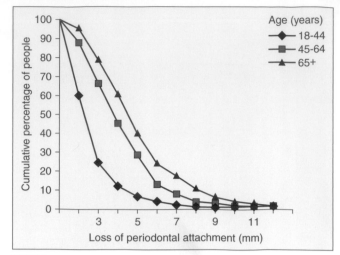

FIGURE 2-7
Periodontal attachment loss by age. Although older adults have more periodontal attachment loss than do younger adults, severe loss is observed among a small percentage of individuals at every age. (Modified from U.S. Department of Health and Human Services, National Center for Health Statistics: *Third national health and nutrition examination survey, 1988-94.* Public use data file no. 7-0627, Hyattsville, Md, 1997, Centers for Disease Control and Prevention; Burt BA, Eklund SA: *Dentistry, dental practice, and the community,* ed 6, St Louis, 2005, WB Saunders.)

BOX 2-4

ADULTS: SUMMARY FINDINGS

- Most adults show signs of periodontal or gingival disease.
- Clinical symptoms of viral infections (herpes labialis, oral ulcers) are common in adulthood, affecting approximately 19% of adults 25 to 44 years of age.
- Chronic disabling diseases, such as the following, affect millions of Americans, compromising oral health and function:
  - Temporomandibular disorders
  - Sjögren's syndrome
  - Diabetes
  - Osteoporosis
- Approximately 22% of adults reported some form of chronic craniofacial pain in the previous 6-month period.

- Of the patients undergoing treatment for oral and pharyngeal cancers, more than 400,000 will develop complications annually.
- Immunocompromised patients are at greater risk for oral problems.
- Employed adults lose more than 164 million hours of work each year as a result of dental-related problems (e.g., treatments, diseases).
- For every adult age 19 years or older without medical insurance, three are without dental insurance.
- Less than two thirds of adults visited a dentist in the previous 12-month period.
- Approximately 23% of 65- to 74-year-olds have severe periodontal disease.

From U.S. Department of Health and Human Services: *Oral health in America: a report of the surgeon general,* Rockville, MD, 2000, The Department, National Institute of Dental and Craniofacial Research, National Institutes of Health.

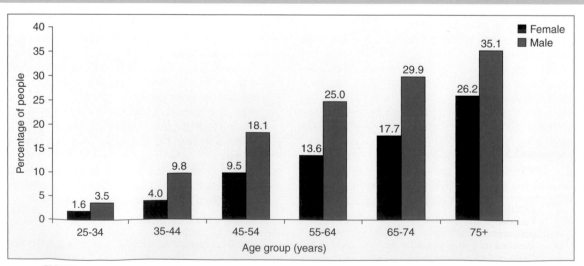

FIGURE 2-8
Periodontal attachment loss by gender. Men are more likely than women to have at least one tooth site with 6 mm or more of periodontal loss of attachment. (Modified from U.S. Department of Health and Human Services, National Center for Health Statistics: *Third national health and nutrition examination survey, 1988-94.* Public use data file no. 7-0627, Hyattsville, Md, 1997, Centers for Disease Control and Prevention; Burt BA, Eklund SA: *Dentistry, dental practice, and the community,* ed 6, St Louis, 2005, WB Saunders.)

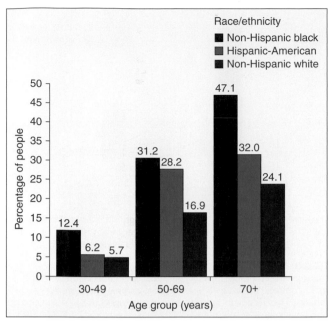

FIGURE 2-9
Periodontal attachment loss by race. Non-Hispanic black adults are more likely than other groups to have at least one tooth site with 6 mm or more of periodontal loss of attachment. (Modified from U.S. Department of Health and Human Services, National Center for Health Statistics: *Third national health and nutrition examination survey, 1988-94.* Public use data file no. 7-0627, Hyattsville, Md, 1997, Centers for Disease Control and Prevention.)

least one permanent tooth because of dental caries. By age 50 years, Americans have lost an average of 12.1 teeth, including their third molars. Complete tooth loss varies by race and ethnicity, smoking status, and poverty status[62] (Figure 2-11).

Oral and Pharyngeal Cancers

In 2004, 28,300 new cases of oral and pharyngeal cancers were documented, which accounted for 2.1% of all cancers.[1] Approximately 7200 individuals die from oral cancers annually. Oral cancer is twice as prevalent in men than it is in women; the median age of diagnosis is 64 years of age, and the occurrence increases with age (Figure 2-12). The overall 5-year survival rate for individuals with oral and pharyngeal cancers is 52%. Although the 5-year survival rate is 81.3% for individuals with oral cancers detected at an early stage, only 35% of oral and pharyngeal cancers are diagnosed at this stage. Unfortunately, racial and ethnic disparities exist in relation to oral and pharyngeal cancer because the incidence is 39.6% higher for black individuals than it is for white adults. Overall, the incidence rate of oral and pharyngeal cancer is decreasing. The largest annual decline in incidence rates is documented for lip cancers. The incidence of tongue cancer, however, may be increasing among young men.[62] The most related risk factor for cancers of the oral cavity and pharynx is the use of tobacco (Figure 2-13). Both smoking and smokeless (spit) tobacco account for more than 90% of cancers of the oral cavity and pharynx (see Chapter 29).

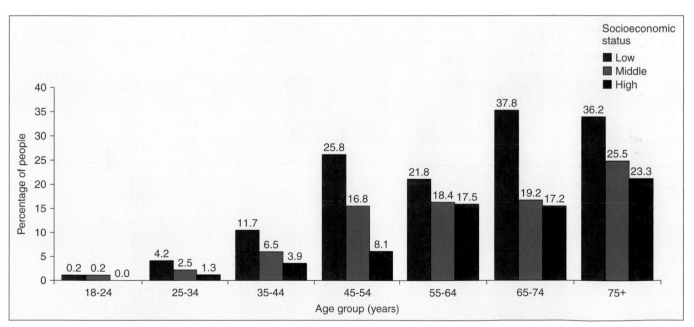

FIGURE 2-10
Periodontal attachment loss by socioeconomic status. Proportion of adults with at least one site with loss of periodontal attachment of 6 mm or more. By age and socioeconomic status, United States, 1988-1994.
(Modified from U.S. Department of Health and Human Services, National Center for Health Statistics: *Third national health and nutrition examination survey, 1988-94.* Public use data file no. 7-0627, Hyattsville, Md, 1997, Centers for Disease Control and Prevention; Burt BA, Eklund SA: *Dentistry, dental practice, and the community,* ed 6, St Louis, 2005, WB Saunders.)

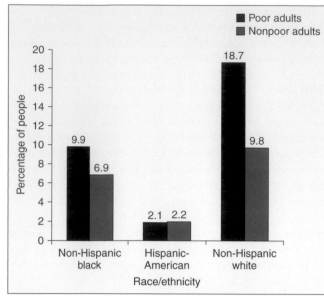

FIGURE 2-11
Tooth loss by race. Complete tooth loss varies by race and ethnicity and by poverty status. A higher percentage of poor and nonpoor, non-Hispanic white adults (18 years and older) have no teeth, compared with non-Hispanic blacks and Hispanic-American adults. (Modified from U.S. Department of Health and Human Services, National Center for Health Statistics: *Third national health and nutrition examination survey, 1988-94.* Public use data file no. 7-0627, Hyattsville, Md, 1997, Centers for Disease Control and Prevention.)

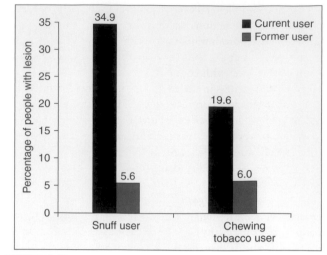

FIGURE 2-13
Tobacco-related oral lesions by age. Tobacco-related oral lesions are more common in 12- to 17-year-old adolescents who currently use spit tobacco. (Modified from Tomar SL et al: Oral mucosal smokeless tobacco lesions among adolescents in the United States, *J Dent Res* 76:1277-1286, 1997.)

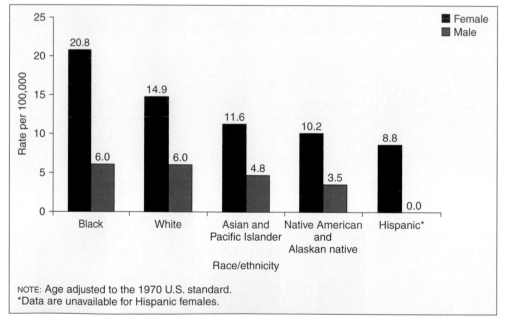

FIGURE 2-12
Oral and pharyngeal cancer by gender. Men have higher incidence rates of oral and pharyngeal cancers than do women. (Modified from Wingo PA et al: Annual report to the nation on the status of cancer, 1973-1996, with a special section on lung cancer and tobacco smoking, *J Natl Cancer Inst* 91:675-690, 1999.)

Health Promotion: Broadening the Paradigm for Dental Hygiene

The renewed emphasis on general and oral health promotion demands changes in the conceptual role of the dental hygienist. Although the promotion of oral health through patient educa-

tion has provided an underlying philosophy of the practice of dentistry and dental hygiene over the past century, the reality of clinical dental hygiene practice has been in the delivery of preventive and therapeutic services—essentially, hands-on treatment rendered by the dental professional. However, in light of the goals of the *Healthy People 2010* report[62] and the mandate from the Surgeon General's report on oral health in America,[63] the dental hygiene actions need to be redefined in terms of education, health promotion, and health advocacy when working with patients at the individual level, as well as working at the population level with community groups.

Significant progress in the reduction of the incidence, prevalence, and severity of common oral diseases have clearly heralded the age of *prevention* in dentistry. This growing body of knowledge, however, does not guarantee a higher quality of life for the population at large or for individual patients. Scientific advances must be shared and implemented. The oral health objectives of *Healthy People 2010* and the framework for action in the *Report of the Surgeon General on Oral Health* provide structure for identifying, prioritizing, and implementing actions at the community level to promote health. However, simply imparting information at the community level and with individual patients is not enough to overcome barriers to a change in health behavior. Disparity exists between *knowledge* about prevention of disease and preventive *actions taken.*[34,62] Based on the WHO definition, the determinants of health are not solely based on knowledge but on complex interactions between the individual and his or her environment. Effective and sustainable health promotion must concomitantly address the cause of the disease and the psychologic, sociologic, anthropologic, educational, and epidemiologic context of health.[1] A number of multidisciplinary health theories and conceptual models describe this complex interaction. Dental hygienists are in key positions to effect changes in health behavior. Improving a client's health behavior may in fact be one of the most challenging tasks.

> *Barriers to Health Promotion*
> * Lack of access to care that still plagues the United States
> * Limited income
> * Limited or no insurance benefits
> * Lack of transportation
> * Inability to schedule free time for health issues
> * Complex issues surrounding medical conditions
> * Physical, emotional, and mental disabilities
> * Low priority with policymakers

Applying Theory in Health Promotion

An understanding of **health theory** can be applied to guide the various stages of assessing, planning, implementing, and evaluating health behavior in the context of the dental hygiene process of care. Theory serves as a pattern for approximating the interrelated nature of health behavior. It helps explain the dynamics of the behavior, the process for changing the behavior, and the effects of the multiple levels of influence on the behavior. Health promotion succeeds when the appropriate theory is matched to the practice strategy. Theories are designed to reach people at the individual, community, or system level.

An understanding of different health theories and the ability to apply them skillfully in practice is what distinguishes a professional from someone simply carrying out a set of activities. Similar to an expert chef, theoretically grounded health education professionals do not blindly follow a cookbook recipe; rather, they constantly create new theories, depending on

the circumstances. For example, a patient who routinely exhibits moderate marginal plaque biofilm may not benefit from yet another demonstration of the modified Bass brushing technique. The clinician must reveal the determinants of behavior that are influencing this patient's ambivalence toward oral hygiene practice. Similar to the determinants of health, health education and health behavior theories that describe patient interactions are broad and varied. No single theory applies to all situations. Selecting the most useful theory will depend on the target audience (e.g., individual, group, community) and the type of behavior influenced; that is, repetitive maintenance behaviors, habitual behaviors, or those concerning brand choice.

Individual Cognitive Behavioral Models

HEALTH BELIEF MODEL

The clinical practice of the dental hygienist focuses largely on influencing health maintenance behaviors of patients. The Health Belief Model (HBM) is widely used to describe the determinants for change or for the maintenance of behaviors in an individual. The basic premise of the model is that individuals will take action to engage in health behaviors if:
* They regard themselves as susceptible.
* They believe the consequences are serious.
* They believe proposed health practices will reduce or eliminate their susceptibility to the disease or condition (see Figure 2-1).

An investigation of the role of a patient's health belief in relation to compliance with daily brushing recommendations revealed compliance was significantly related to his or her perceived benefits of the action.[3,4] Race, sex, and age differences all influence oral health beliefs. Self-care and utilization patterns of white American women can best be predicted by their perception of the importance of the health behavior.[9] The female sex, higher educational level, and better self-rated health are significant indicators of positive oral health beliefs.[39] In general, older individuals have less favorable beliefs and attitudes regarding oral health.[18,33] Older individuals in one investigation were less knowledgeable about periodontal disease than their younger counterparts.[34]

Self-efficacy is a key construct in this model. In other words, individuals must have confidence in their ability to take action. The dental hygienist can build this confidence by providing training and guidance in performing the action, setting progressive goals associated with the benefits of the action, providing reinforcement, and reducing anxiety associated with performing the action. Application of the HBM has predicted glycemic control among persons with type 2 diabetes. Perceived severity and perceived barriers were related to glycemic status and predicted reductions in glycated hemoglobin. Based on these observations, interventions aimed at supporting beliefs in the severity of diabetic complications and efforts that demonstrated the barriers to therapeutic behavior helped assist patients with type 2 diabetes in managing their disease.[11,60]

THEORY OF REASONED ACTION AND THEORY OF PLANNED BEHAVIOR

The Theory of Reasoned Action (TRA) model attempts to capture the relationship between attitudes and behavior (Figure 2-14). According to the theory, **behavior intent** is the most important determinant of a patient's behavior.[61] The person's **intention** to perform a behavior is a series of linked concepts. The TRA proposes that an individual's attitude toward performing the behavior and the subjective norm determine intention. Under this construct, *attitude* consists of a person's belief that a behavior leads to certain results and also to his or her evaluations of the results. Concomitantly, *subjective norm* is determined by an individual's belief that specific individuals or groups think they should perform the behavior and his or her motivation to comply with these groups.

The Theory of Planned Behavior (TPB) model adds a third dimension to HBM, suggesting behavioral intent is also determined by perceived behavioral control. Perceived behavioral control is influenced by an individual's belief that he or she has the opportunity, knowledge, skill, and resources to perform the behavior.

Adherence to oral self-care activities when analyzed in relation to the TPB model indicates that attitude and subjective norm concerning toothbrushing were important for the intention to brush teeth. Consistent with the model, the intention to brush teeth was indeed related to reported frequency of brushing.[54,56] Diabetes adherence was strongly influenced by subjective norm for oral health behaviors and attitude. These findings give credibility to the role of physicians, dental hygienists, family, coworkers, and other significant others and how they might help strengthen the subjective norms and attitudes concerning oral health behavior among individuals with diabetes.

Applying the TRA model to understand an adolescent's decision for sugar consumption revealed that the immediate pleasurable taste of sugar outweighed and deferred the recognition of dangers associated with its consumption. However, the role of parental figures, dental experience, and knowledge all acted as important influences and can be used when setting food choice goals with teenagers.[21] The TRA has also been used to determine the effects of knowledge and attitudes on oral preventive measures. Results indicate that knowledge was great among younger individuals and that women were more likely to have a more positive attitude toward prevention.[49]

TRANSTHEORETICAL MODEL AND STAGES OF CHANGE

The Transtheoretical Model (TTM) describes how individuals make intentional changes or acquire positive health behaviors. The central construct of the transtheoretical model is the "Stages of Change." The different stages represent the decision-making process required to change behavior. The stages are divided into the following six levels:

- Precontemplation
- Contemplation
- Preparation
- Action
- Maintenance
- Relapse

Precontemplation is the entry stage of the model during which no foreseeable intent to change is evident (Figure 2-15). *Contemplation* represents the next stage of the model in which an intent to change is first considered. By continuing in a forward direction of change, an individual makes *preparations* to take *action* to change. Once the change in behavior has been adopted for 6 months, individuals are then considered in the *maintenance* stage. *Termination* of the model occurs with sus-

---

★ CASE APPLICATION 2-1.1

Stages of Change

Consider Ms. Marino's case once again. In what stage of change is Ms. Marino regarding the control of her blood glucose levels? How might the TTM be used to teach Ms. Marino the relationship between diabetes and periodontal disease? What other strategies to improve Ms. Marino's diabetes adherence are suggested by the other models presented?

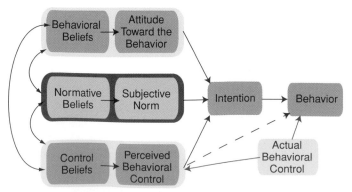

FIGURE 2-14
Theory of Reasoned Action and Theory of Planned Behavior. (Redrawn from Theory of Planned Behavior, copyright ©2006 Icek Ajzen. Accessible on-line at http://www.people.umass.edu/aizen/tpb.html)

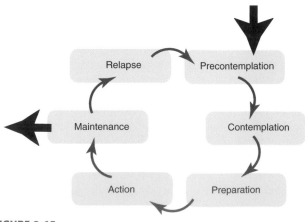

FIGURE 2-15
Stages of change.

tained change. The TTM is dynamic, and relapse can occur at any time, allowing an individual to re-enter the model at various stages. Table 2-1 characterizes each stage of change and offers techniques to facilitate progress toward the desired behavior. The TTM has also been studied and used extensively to develop effective interventions to promote behavioral change associated with reduced harm or abstinence from substance misuse such as tobacco cessation.

SOCIAL COGNITIVE THEORY

The Social Cognitive Theory (SCT) explains how individuals acquire and maintain certain behavioral patterns while also providing the basis for intervention strategies.[3] According to SCT, people, their environment, and their behavior are constantly interacting and influencing each other. The model proposes a number of determinants that influence health behavior.[24] (Box 2-5

BOX 2-5

SOCIAL COGNITIVE THEORY

- *Environment.* Factors physically external to the person; provide opportunities and social support
- *Situation.* Perception of the environment; correct misperceptions and promote healthful forms
- *Behavioral capability.* Knowledge and skill to perform a given behavior; promote mastery learning through skills training
- *Expectations.* Anticipatory outcomes of a behavior; model positive outcomes of healthful behavior
- *Expectancies.* Values that the person places on a given outcome, incentives; present outcomes of change that have functional meaning
- *Self-control.* Personal regulation of goal-directed behavior or performance; provide opportunities for self-monitoring, goal setting, problem solving, and rewarding self

- *Observational learning.* Behavioral acquisition that occurs by watching the actions and outcomes of others' behavior; includes credible role models of the targeted behavior
- *Reinforcements.* Responses to a person's behavior that increase or decrease the likelihood of reoccurrence; promote self-initiated rewards and incentives
- *Self-efficacy.* Person's confidence in performing a particular behavior; approach behavioral change in small steps to ensure success
- *Emotional coping responses.* Strategies or tactics that are used by an individual to deal with emotional stimuli; provide training in problem solving and stress management
- *Reciprocal determinism.* The dynamic interaction of the person, the behavior, and the environment in which the behavior is performed; consider multiple avenues to behavioral change, including environmental, skill, and personal change

From Glanz K, Rimer BK, Lewis FM: *Health behavior and health education theory, research, and practice,* ed 3, New Jersey, 2002, Jossey-Bass.

Table 2-1 Stages of Change

STAGE OF CHANGE	CHARACTERISTICS	TECHNIQUES
Precontemplation	• Is not currently considering change; "Ignorance is bliss."	• Validate lack of readiness. • Clarify that decision is theirs. • Encourage re-evaluation of current behavior. • Encourage self-exploration, not action. • Explain and personalize risk.
Contemplation	• Is ambivalent about change; " . . . is sitting on the fence." • Is not considering change within the next month.	• Validate lack of readiness. • Clarify that decision is theirs. • Encourage evaluation of pros and cons of behavioral change. • Identify and promote new, positive outcome expectations.
Preparation	• Some have experience with change and are trying to change; "I am testing the waters." • Is planning to act within 1 month.	• Identify and assist in problem solving regarding obstacles. • Help patient identify social support. • Verify that patient has underlying skills for behavioral change. • Encourage small initial steps.
Action	• Is practicing new behavior for 3 to 6 months.	• Focus is on restructuring cues and social support. • Bolster self-efficacy for dealing with obstacles. • Combat feelings of loss, and reiterate long-term benefits.
Maintenance	• Have continued commitment to sustaining new behavior after 6 months to 5 years.	• Plan for follow-up support. • Reinforce internal rewards. • Discuss coping with relapse.
Relapse	• Have resumed old behaviors; "I have fallen from grace."	• Evaluate trigger for relapse. • Reassess motivation and barriers. • Plan stronger coping strategies.

summarizes the constructs and intervention strategies associated with each construct.) Application of the model for health education consists of setting desirable outcomes, identifying the variables likely to influence each behavior, and designing interventions to modify SCT variables.

The SCT was applied to promote the performance of health-protective behaviors. The interventions derived from the model included health education, skills training, and self-monitoring activities. Each of three experiments added social support, intensive contact, or flexible goal setting. Regardless of the additional intervention, excellent adherence was observed in the study; unfortunately, little change was sustained at follow-up.[37]

⁂ CASE APPLICATION 2-1.2

Social Cognitive Theory

Ms. Marino's physician politely replies that he is aware of her type 2 diabetes and is managing her condition with diet and exercise. After completing nonsurgical periodontal therapy, Ms. Marino achieves little reduction in pocket depths or bleeding on probing. Her plaque biofilm index, however, is reduced by 55%. She is encouraged to hear that her efforts to follow the oral hygiene regimen are effective, but she is disappointed in her clinical response. Once again, a finger-stick blood test reveals her blood glucose is only slightly improved at 185 mcg/dl. The dental hygienist indicates that these results will once again be shared with her physician. This time, the letter to her physician indicates that Ms. Marino's consistently higher-than-normal blood glucose levels are interfering with the outcomes of her periodontal therapy. The individual health behavior models are reviewed, and the methods used to apply each model to Ms. Marino's case are discussed with her physician.

Historical Perspective on Health Promotion

MILESTONES

Beginning with the successful adoption of preventive methods to control dental caries led by dental professionals, the United States has witnessed significant improvement in oral health. Community water fluoridation can clearly be cited as one of the greatest achievements of public health in the twentieth century—an inexpensive means to improve oral health that benefits all community residents, regardless of age or socioeconomic status. Other community strategies for primary prevention of dental caries have included school-based programs of fluoride use (e.g., mouthrinses, dietary fluoride tablets), sealant programs, and screening and referral programs. These types of science application to a generalized, severe oral health problem have given the profession an opportunity to evaluate methods to affect human health positively in other areas (Box 2-6).

COMMUNITY LEVEL STRATEGIES TO REACH HEALTH OBJECTIVES

Community level health promotion attempts to screen for and prevent disease in susceptible populations by fostering healthful lifestyles or by reducing or eliminating hazards. Similar to

effecting change in an individual, community level models for change rely on creating an environment for change. These strategies are often initiated in institutions or organizations (e.g., schools, worksites, government agencies, community health advocacy groups, healthcare settings) with an interest in protecting and improving health. Prolonged community health promotion relies not only on change at the individual level but also on public advocacy and policy development. (Examples of community level health promotion are presented in Box 2-6.)

⁂ CASE APPLICATION 2-1.3

Identifying Additional Risk

Considering the *burden of oral disease* in the U.S. population, should the dental hygienist discuss any additional health promotion topics with Ms. Marino? Is she possibly at risk for oral manifestations of reported diseases and medications? Is she at risk for systemic manifestations as a result of oral disease?

COMMUNITY ORGANIZATION

Unlike the models for individual health promotion, *community organization* does not refer to one unified model; rather, community organization represents several models that describe how community groups are assisted in identifying common problems or goals, mobilizing resources, and developing and implementing strategies for reaching the health goals they have collectively set.[64] Despite varying designs, community organizing approaches can be dichotomized on the basis of needs or strengths. They may be heavily process-oriented models such as those that emphasize consensus building and collaboration. By contrast, heavily task-oriented models (conflict) emphasize the problem-solving abilities of a community or assign an outside expert. These models rely on advocacy and ally-building strategies. Several models use a combination of process- and task-oriented approaches. Despite diverse modeling, community organization relies on similar key constructs (Table 2-2).

DIFFUSION OF INNOVATION

The Diffusion of Innovation Theory (DIT) addresses how new ideas, products, and social practices spread in a society or from one society to another. DIT describes the communication process required to bring a new idea to the implementation level of a peer group. The diffusion process consists of a passive spread of planned efforts to make the innovation become routine. The steps of diffusion are as follows[46]:

- Gaining the knowledge
- Making the decision from persuasion to adopt or reject the innovation
- Implementing the innovation to bring about confirmation of the need for the innovation

This theory is applicable at the community level when the decision to adopt a new health promotion tool or strategy, such as recommended use of xylitol gum to reduce dental caries, is made on behalf of an organization or community.

Addressing characteristics of innovation can enhance the likely adoption of the innovation. The greater the perceived relative

BOX 2-6

COMMUNITY STRATEGIES FOR PRIMARY PREVENTION OF KEY ORAL DISEASES AND CONDITIONS

Dental Caries
- Community-wide health promotion interventions*
- Fluoride use
  - Community water fluoridation
  - Dental caries prevention and control is one area for which effective interventions have been developed and evaluated. Community water fluoridation is perhaps the most successful community level strategy resulting in median dental caries reduction of 50.7%.
  - School-based dietary fluoride tablets
  - School-based fluoride mouthrinse
- School-based and school-linked sealant programs
- Sealants are applied in school-based or school-linked programs to children of various socioeconomic status and levels of risk. The median decrease in occlusal dental caries in posterior teeth among children ages 6 to 17 years is 60%.
- School-linked screenings and referrals

Periodontal Disease
- Community-wide health promotion interventions*
  - School-based personal hygiene

- Reinforcement of personal and oral hygiene habits in Head Start or primary school classrooms
- School-linked screenings and referrals

Head and Neck Cancers
- Community-wide health promotion interventions*
  - Cancer screening programs (e.g., health fairs)
  - Crete Declaration on Oral Cancer Prevention represents the unified commitment from 57 countries to support the work of national and international health authorities, research institutions, nongovernmental organizations, and civil society for the effective control of oral cancer.[45]

Inherited Disorders
- Early detection programs

Trauma
- Community-wide health promotion interventions*

---

*Community-wide health promotion interventions (e.g., educational, political, regulatory, organizational) are directed toward the public, practitioners, and policymakers to create a healthful environment, reduce risk factors, inform target groups, and improve knowledge and behaviors.

---

advantage of the innovation, the more likely it will be implemented. *Compatibility* accounts for how consistent the innovation is with the norms of potential adopters. The concept of *complexity* promotes the idea that the easier the innovation is to use, the greater the chance that it will be adopted. *Trialability* describes the opportunity for testing before implementation. *Observability* promotes the idea that the more visible the innovation is to the peer group, the more likely it will be adopted. (Each characteristic and relative applications are presented in Table 2-3.)

Other community level models describe the nature of health promotion at the organizational level. Many of these models are based in organizational development theory. Obviously, change will be most successful if it is planned with consideration for the sometimes-complex layering in the organization. Discussion of organizational development theory is beyond the scope of this text. Practitioners facilitating health promotion at the organizational level are encouraged to secure additional resources for further study of this approach.

Table 2-2	Community Organization	
CONCEPT	**DEFINITION**	**APPLICATION**
Empowerment	Process of gaining mastery and power over self and the community to produce change	Give individuals and communities tools and responsibility for making decisions that affect them.
Community Competence	Community's ability to engage in effective problem-solving activities	Work with community to identify problems. Create consensus and reach goals.
Participation and Relevance	Learners' ability to be active participants; work should "start where the people are"	Help community set goals within the context of preexisting goals, and encourage active participation.
Issue Selection	Identifying winnable, simple, and specific concerns as the focus of action	Assist community in examining how it can communicate concerns and whether success is likely.
Critical Consciousness	Developing understanding of root causes of problems	Guide consideration of health concerns in broad perspective of social problems.

From Glanz K, Rimer BK, Lewis FM: *Health behavior and health education theory, research, and practice,* ed 3, New Jersey, 2002, Jossey-Bass.

Table 2-3	Diffusion of Innovations Theory	
CONCEPT	**DEFINITION**	**APPLICATION**
Relative Advantage	Degree to which an innovation is seen as better than the idea, practice, program, or product it replaces	Point out unique benefits: monetary value, convenience, time saving, and prestige.
Compatibility	Degree to which the innovation is consistent with values, habits, experience, and needs of potential adopters	Tailor innovation for the intended audience's values, norms, or situations.
Complexity	Degree to which the innovation is difficult to understand or use or both	Create program, idea, or product to be uncomplicated, easy to use, and easy to understand.
Trialability	Extent to which the innovation can endure experimentation before a commitment to adopt is required	Provide opportunities to try on a limited basis (e.g., free samples, introductory sessions, money-back guarantee).
Observability	Extent to which the innovation provides tangible or visible results	Ensure visibility of results in the areas of feedback or publicity.

Summary: Oral Cavity Is a Mirror of the Health of the Body

FIRST PORTAL OF ENTRY FOR POTENTIAL PATHOGENS

As a portal of entry, the mouth serves as a gateway through which any number of potential pathogens can pass, primarily bacteria, viruses, parasites, and fungi. Once the pathogen enters the oral cavity, protective mechanisms are immediately released. When the oral tissues are not compromised, the invader is swiftly defeated. Most dental infections are opportunistic in that microorganisms commonly found in the mouth are the cause. If, however, oral tissues are compromised, then an opportunity for infection is present. In this way, the mouth can actually serve as a source for diseases and pathologic processes that can affect other organ systems and become a source for contagion to others.

In the last 10 years, intriguing research studies have been accumulating evidence regarding the connection between oral health and diabetes, cardiovascular diseases, respiratory diseases, preterm delivery and low birth weight, and human immunodeficiency virus (HIV) and acquired immunodeficiency syndrome (AIDS).*

PERIODONTAL DISEASE AND DIABETES

In 1993, Dr. Harald Löe defined periodontitis as the sixth complication of diabetes.[35] Both insulin-dependent and non–insulin-dependent diabetes increase both the incidence and severity of periodontal disease by approximately two to five-fold.[11, 60] The severity of periodontal disease observed in patients with diabetes is a result of the increased production of inflammatory mediators, dysfunction of neutrophils, and alterations of connective tissue, all based on the presence of bacterial pathogens. Patients who receive periodontal care can reduce their risks for more severe periodontal disease. New

evidence indicates that the stabilization of periodontal health can help maintain optimal blood glucose levels, pointing to a potential bidirectional relationship between periodontal health and diabetes control.[32,59,61]

ORAL INFECTION, HEART DISEASE, AND STROKE

Studies suggest a link between oral infections and the risk for cardiovascular disease.[16,31,55] Studies initiated in the 1980s and recently confirmed suggest a correlation between periodontal disease and cardiovascular disease. Specific organisms of *Streptococcus sanguis* and *Porphyromonas gingivalis,* identified as two pathogens in the complex cause of periodontal disease, have the potential to produce platelet aggregation, promoting thrombus formation.[28]

Mechanisms of action that have been examined include a direct infection of the blood vessel walls with bacteria or viruses originating in tissues such as the oral mucosa, causing local inflammation and injury contributing to atherosclerosis. White blood cells or platelets become integrated into the atherosclerotic plaque, triggering inflammatory pathways (i.e., the release of prostaglandins, interleukins, thromboxane, and tumor necrosis factor-alpha). Under these conditions, the liver may be stimulated to produce additional inflammatory responses. Tissue factor, another proinflammatory element released by the presence of bacteria in the blood, is responsible for coagulation. During coagulation, more platelets become entrapped by the developing thrombus. As the lumen of the coronary vessels narrows, blood supply to the cardiac muscle diminishes. When the artery fully occludes, a myocardial infarction (i.e., heart attack) occurs. If blood supply is not returned, then the cardiac muscle dies, resulting in profoundly diminished cardiac function or death.[10]

RESPIRATORY DISEASES

Several epidemiologic and microbiologic studies have suggested associations between poor oral health and bacterial plaque biofilm and respiratory diseases such as chronic obstructive pulmonary disease (COPD) and nosocomial pneumonia.[41] One such study suggested some resident bacteria in the mouth are likely

---

*References 7, 13-15, 20, 25, 31, 32, 38, 40, 55.

aspirated along with respiratory pathogens and may affect the adhesion of pathogenic organisms and cause infection in the respiratory epithelium. These studies provide early evidence of an association that must be explored through further research.

PERIODONTAL DISEASES AND ADVERSE BIRTH OUTCOMES

Prematurity and low–birth-weight infants threaten to increase infant mortality rates and to contribute to a wide variety of functional disorders for surviving infants.[36,48,51,52] Examinations of the inflammatory pathways involved in the preterm delivery of low–birth-weight infants have found them to be consistent with the inflammatory pathways caused by the gram-negative infections of periodontal disease.[12,14-15,43-44] These early associations between oral disease and systemic health show promising results and require comprehensive, in-depth studies to determine whether a causal relationship exists and will thus become the next dental frontier.

HUMAN IMMUNODEFICIENCY VIRUS AND ACQUIRED IMMUNODEFICIENCY SYNDROME

> *Note*
> Oral health is an essential part of general health, especially for patients with existing medical conditions.

Over 95% of patients with HIV or AIDS will have oral manifestations of symptomatic infection. The most common HIV-related oral diseases include candidiasis, oral warts, hairy leukoplakia, periodontitis, herpes simplex, varicella zoster, recurrent aphthous stomatitis, bacterial infections, and Kaposi's sarcoma. (See Chapter 47 for more information.)

✦ CASE APPLICATION 2-1.4

Applying the Theory of Planned Behavior Model

At her 3-month maintenance interval, Ms. Marino exhibits a generalized 1-mm pocket-depth reduction and a 57% reduction in bleeding on probing. She indicates that her physician prescribed an oral medication to help regulate her blood glucose levels and has her monitoring her levels daily. She reports her usual blood glucose to be 135 mcg/dl. Clearly, Ms. Marino's intent to perform regular oral hygiene was influenced by her belief that she could perform the daily regimen and by the subjective norms associated with her physician's casual management of her diabetes. Accordingly, the TPB model provided a framework plan and a health promotion strategy targeted to her specific needs, enabling the factors that were influencing Ms. Marino's intent to perform oral hygiene behaviors to be observed and addressed.

References

1. American Cancer Society: *Cancer facts and figures,* Atlanta, 1999, The Society.
2. Baker SL: *US national health spending* [Internet], 2004, University of South Carolina, Arnold School of Public Health, Dept. of Health Services Policy and Management, HSPM J712. Available at: http://cdc.gov/nchs/data.
3. Bandura A: *Self-efficacy: the exercise of control,* New York, 1997, WH Freeman.
4. Barker T: Role of health beliefs in patient compliance with preventive dental advice, *Community Dent Oral Epidemiol* 22(5 Pt 1):327-330, 1994.
5. Belting CM, Hiniker JJ, Dummett CO: Influence of diabetes mellitus on the severity of periodontal disease in diabetics, *J Periodontol* 35:476-480, 1964.
6. Boggess KA et al: Maternal periodontal disease in early pregnancy and risk for a small-for-gestational-age infant, *Am J Obstet Gynecol* 194(5):1316-1322, 2006.
7. Bridges RB et al: Periodontal status of diabetic and non-diabetic men: effects of smoking, glycemic control, and socioeconomic factors, *J Periodontol* 67(11):1185-1192, 1996.
8. Centers for Disease Control and Prevention: *The guide to community preventive services (community guide),* Atlanta, 2002, CDC.
9. Chen M, Tatsuoka M: The relationship between American women's preventive dental behavior and dental health beliefs, *Soc Sci Med* 19(9):971-978, 1984.
10. Chun YH et al: Biological foundation for periodontitis as a potential risk factor for atherosclerosis, *J Periodontal Res* 40(1):87-95, 2005.
11. Cohen DW et al: Diabetes mellitus and periodontal disease: two-year longitudinal observations—I, *J Periodontol* 41(12):709-712, 1970.
12. Collins JG et al: Effects of *Escherichia coli* and *Porphyromonas gingivalis* lipopolysaccharide on pregnancy outcome in the golden hamster, *Infect Immun* 62(10):4652-4655, 1994.
13. Daniel M, Messer LC: Perceptions of disease severity and barriers to self-care predict glycemic control in aboriginal persons with type II diabetes, *Chronic Dis Can* 23(4):130-138, 2002.
14. Dasanayake AP: Poor periodontal health of the pregnant woman as a risk factor for low birth weight, *Ann Periodontol* 3:206-212, 1998.
15. Davenport ES et al: The east London study of maternal chronic periodontal disease and preterm low birth weight infants: study design and prevalence data, *Ann Periodontol* 3:213-221, 1998.
16. DeStefano F et al: Dental disease and risk of coronary heart disease and mortality, *Br Med J* 306(6879):688-691, 1993.
17. de Wet FA: The prevention of orofacial sports injuries in the adolescent, *Int Dent J* 31:313-319, 1981.
18. Diehnelt D, Kiyak HA, Beach BH: Predictors of oral health behavior among elderly Japanese Americans, *Spec Care Dent* 10:114-120, 1990.
19. Emrich LJ, Shlossman M, Genco RJ: Periodontal diseases in non–insulin-dependent diabetes mellitus, *J Periodontol* 62(2):123-131, 1991.
20. Firatli E: The relationship between clinical periodontal status and insulin-dependent diabetes mellitus. Results after 5 years, *J Periodontol* 68(2):136-140, 1997.
21. Freeman R, Sheiham A: Understanding decision-making processes for sugar consumption in adolescence, *Community Dent Oral Epidemiol* 25(3):228-232, 1997.
22. Galea H, Aganovic I, Aganovic M: The dental caries and periodontal disease experience of patients with early onset insulin-dependent diabetes, *Int Dent J* 36(4):219-224, 1986.
23. Genco RJ: Current view of risk factors for periodontal diseases, *J Periodontol* 67(10 Suppl):1041-1049, 1996.

24. Glanz K, Rimer BK, Lewis FM: *Health behavior and health education theory, research and practice,* ed 3, New Jersey, 2002, Jossey-Bass.

25. Grossi SG, Genco RJ: Periodontal disease and diabetes mellitus: a two-way relationship, *Ann Periodontol* 3(1):51-61, 1998.

26. Grossi SG et al: Response to periodontal therapy in diabetics and smokers, *J Periodontol* 67(10 Suppl):1094-1102, 1996.

27. Haber J: Cigarette smoking: a major risk factor for periodontitis, *Compend Cont Educ Dent* 15:1002-1014, 1994.

28. Herzberg MC, Brintzenhofe KL, Clawson CC: Aggregation of human platelets and adhesion of *Streptococcus sanguis, Infect Immun* 39(3):1457-1469, 1983.

29. Hildebolt CF et al: Attachment loss with postmenopausal age and smoking, *J Periodontal Res* 32(7):619-625, 1997.

30. Institute of Medicine: *Dental education at the crossroads: challenges and change,* Washington, DC, 1995, National Academy Press.

31. Khader YS, Albashaireh ZS, Alomari MA: Periodontal diseases and the risk of coronary heart and cerebrovascular diseases: a meta-analysis, *J Periodontol* 75(8):1046-1053, 2004.

32. Kiran M et al: The effect of improved periodontal health on metabolic control in type 2 diabetes mellitus, *J Clin Periodontol* 32(3):266-272, 2005.

33. Kiyak HA, Miller RR: Age differences in oral health attitudes and dental service utilization, *J Public Health Dent* 42:29-41, 1982.

34. Lee J, Kiyak HA: Oral disease beliefs, behaviors, and oral health status of Korean-Americans, *J Public Health Dent* 52:131-136, 1992.

35. Löe H: Periodontal disease: the sixth complication of diabetes mellitus, *Diabetes Care* 16(1):329-334, 1993.

36. Lowry RB, Thunem NY, Uh SH: Birth prevalence of cleft lip and palate in British Columbia between 1952 and 1986: stability of rates, *Can Med Assoc J* 140(10):1167-1170, 1989.

37. McCaul KD, Glasgow RE, O'Neill HK: The problem of creating habits: establishing health-protective dental behaviors, *Health Psychol* 11(2):101-110, 1992.

38. Moliterno LF et al: Association between periodontitis and low birth weight: a case-control study, *J Clin Periodontol* 32(8):886-890, 2005.

39. Nakazono TT, Davidson PL, Andersen RM: Oral health beliefs in diverse populations, *Adv Dent Res* 11(2):235-244, 1997.

40. National Center for Health Statistics: Preliminary data from the Centers for Disease Control and Prevention, *Mon Vital Stat Rep* 46(Suppl 2), 1997.

41. National Center for Health Statistics: *Prevalence of selected chronic conditions: United States 1990-92.* DHHS Pub No PH-S97-1522, Hyattsville, Md, January 1997, US Department of Health and Human Services, CDC.

42. Nishimura FK et al: Periodontal disease as a complication of diabetes mellitus, *Ann Periodontol* 3:20-29, 1998.

43. Offenbacher S et al: Periodontal infection as a possible risk factor for preterm low birthweight, *J Periodontol* 67(10 Suppl):1103-1106, 1996.

44. Offenbacher S et al: Potential pathogenic mechanisms of periodontitis-associated pregnancy complications, *Ann Periodontol* 3(1):233-250, 1998.

45. Petersen PE: Strengthening the prevention of oral cancer: the WHO perspective, *Community Dent Oral Epidemiol* 33:397-399, 2005.

46. Rogers EM: *Diffusion of innovations,* ed 4, New York, 1995, Free Press.

47. Safkan-Sappala B, Ainamo J: Periodontal conditions in insulin dependent diabetes mellitus, *J Clin Periodontol* 19:24-29, 1992.

48. Schulman J et al: Surveillance for and comparison of birth defect prevalences in two geographic areas—United States, 1983-1988, *MMWR Morb Mortal Wkly Rep* 42(1):1-7, 1993.

49. Schwarz E, Lo EC: Dental health knowledge and attitudes among the middle aged and elderly in Hong Kong, *Community Dent Oral Epidemiol* 22:358-363, 1994.

50. Seppala B, Ainamo J: A site-by-site follow-up study on insulin-dependent diabetes mellitus, *J Clin Periodontol* 21(3):161-165, 1994.

51. Seppala B, Seppala M, Ainamo J: A longitudinal study on insulin-dependent diabetes mellitus, *J Clin Periodontol* 21(3):161-165, 1994.

52. Shapiro S et al: Relevance of correlates of infant deaths for significant morbidity at 1 year of age, *Am J Obstet Gynecol* 136(3):363-373, 1980.

53. Shlossman M et al: Type 2 diabetes mellitus and periodontal disease, *J Am Dent Assoc* 121(4):532-536, 1994.

54. Skully C: Herpes simplex virus (HSV). In Millard HD, Mason DK, editors: *World workshop on oral medicine,* Chicago, 1989, Year Book.

55. Southerland JH et al: Commonality in chronic inflammatory diseases: periodontitis, diabetes, and coronary artery disease, *Periodontol 2000* 40:130-143, 2006.

56. Syrjalal AM, Niskanen MC, Knuuttila ML: The theory of reasoned action in describing tooth brushing, dental caries and diabetes adherence among diabetic patients, *J Clin Periodontol* 29:427-432, 2002.

57. Szpunar SM, Ismail AI, Eklund SA: Diabetes and periodontal disease: analyses of NHANES I and HHANES, *J Dent Res* 68 (special no):164-438, 1989.

58. Talal N: Sjögren's syndrome: historical overview and clinical spectrum of disease, *Rheum Dis Clin North Am* 18(3):507-515, 1992.

59. Talbert J et al: The effect of periodontal therapy on TNF-alpha, IL-6 and metabolic control in type 2 diabetics, *J Dent Hyg* 80(2):7, 2006.

60. Taylor GW et al: Severe periodontitis and risk for poor glycemic control in patients with non-insulin dependent diabetes mellitus, *J Periodontol* 67:1085-1093, 1996.

61. Tedesco LA, Keffer MA, Fleck-Kandath C: Self-efficacy, reasoned action, and oral health behavior reports: a social cognitive approach to compliance, *J Behav Med* 14:341-355, 1991.

62. US Department of Health and Human Services: *Healthy people 2010: understanding and improving health,* Washington DC, 2000, The Department.

63. US Department of Health and Human Services: *Oral health in America: a report of the surgeon general,* Rockville, Md, 2000, US Department of Health and Human Services, National Institute of Dental and Craniofacial Research, National Institutes of Health.

64. US Department of Health and Human Services: Community, provider, and individual strategies for primary prevention of key oral diseases and conditions. In *Oral health in America: a report of the surgeon general,* Rockville, Md, 2000, The Department, National Institute of Dental and Craniofacial Research, National Institutes of Health.

65. US Department of Health and Human Services: *National call to action to promote oral health,* Rockville, Md, US Department of Health and Human Services, Public Health Service, National Institutes of Health, National Institute of Dental and Craniofacial Research. NIH Publication No. 03-5303, Spring 2003.

66. World Health Organization: *International classification of disease and stomatology: ICD-DA,* ed 3, Geneva, 1994, The Organization.

Legal and Ethical Considerations

Pamela B. Overman • Thomas J. Smith

INSIGHT

Society places trust in health professionals, and with that trust comes a set of expectations that the professional will work for the good of the public he or she serves. Some of these expectations are codified into laws and regulations, and some are spelled out in professional standards of conduct. As with other health professionals, the conduct of a dental hygienist is bound by legal statutes, regulations, and ethical guidelines.

✦ CASE STUDY 3-1   Ethics and the Law

Gloria Allen has been a dental hygienist for 15 years. She is presently working in a general practice for Dr. Randolph Peters in a state in which the dental **practice act** includes the following dental hygiene services:

- Complete prophylaxis, including removal of all hard and soft deposits from all surfaces of human teeth to the junctional epithelium, polishing of natural and restored teeth, and root planing
- Preventive measures such as oral prophylaxis and application of fluorides and other recognized topical agents for the prevention of oral disease or discomfort
- Examination of soft and hard tissue of the head, neck, and oral cavity; notation of deformities, defects, and abnormalities
- Application of pit and fissure sealants
- Fabrication of athletic mouthguard appliances
- Polishing of amalgam restorations
- Removal of excess cement from crown and orthodontic bands
- Exposure and processing of radiographic films

Before accepting her current position, Gloria worked for Dr. Samuel Ray in a state in which the dental practice act permits the following services to be performed by a dental hygienist:

- Oral prophylaxis, including scaling and polishing of the dentition
- Application of pit and fissure sealants
- Information gathering for patients' medical histories
- Application of topical fluoride
- Instruction of patients in the performance of oral hygiene techniques
- Placement and condensing of amalgam and tooth-colored restorations
- Impressions for diagnostic models

- Preparation of teeth for bonding
- Exposure and processing of radiographic films
- Application of topical anesthetic agents
- Recording of patients' vital signs
- Placement and removal of rubber dam
- Administration of local anesthetics and nitrous oxide
- Placement of periodontal sutures

Situation One

Gloria is an excellent clinician who enjoys chatting with all her patients. On Monday, her third patient was Mr. Alex Fenten, a 54-year-old architect for whom she has provided dental hygiene services during the past 5 years. She complimented Mr. Fenten on his excellent oral hygiene. She cited her first patient of the day, Mrs. Amelia Gray, a nurse. Gloria described Mrs. Gray's terrible periodontal disease resulting from improper care of her oral tissues. She also told Mr. Fenten that Mrs. Gray was going through an awful divorce after her husband had run off with his secretary and that Mrs. Gray was recently diagnosed with cancer.

After listening to Gloria describe Mrs. Gray's plight, Mr. Fenten explained that Mrs. Gray is his sister. Gloria expressed surprise, changed the subject, and completed her work.

Situation Two

The next Friday afternoon, Gloria was completing a prophylaxis for her last patient of the day, Mrs. Betty Walters. Dr. Peters was out of town attending a continuing dental education program. As Gloria was scaling Mrs. Walters' anterior teeth, she accidentally removed the restoration on tooth #8, leaving a rather unsightly gap between teeth #8 and #9. Gloria explained to Mrs. Walters what happened and that

CASE STUDY 3-1   Ethics and the Law—cont'd

she would have to return on Monday to have Dr. Peters replace the restoration. Mrs. Walters saw her smile in the mirror and was horrified. She explained that she and her husband were attending a dinner party that evening at the home of her husband's employer and that she absolutely could not attend with her tooth in such a condition. She then pleaded with Gloria to fix the tooth. Feeling responsible for Mrs. Walters' dilemma and knowing that she had completed such restorations while working with Dr. Ray, Gloria used Dr. Peters' treatment room to replace a restoration on tooth #8. She then explained to Mrs. Walters that this was only a temporary measure and that she would have to return to the office to have Dr. Peters replace the filling.

Situation Three
The following week Gloria had lunch with her friend Elisa Jensen. Elisa is also a dental hygienist who works for another dentist in the same office complex. Elisa told Gloria that her mother has been seriously ill for the past 6 months. She explained that she has been so busy caring for her mother that she did not have the time to attend continuing dental hygiene education courses and feared the loss of her license. In an attempt to console her friend, Gloria explained that she had attended far more dental hygiene education programs than she needed for relicensure and would be happy to give Elisa the documentation of attendance for them.

Situation Four
After lunch, Gloria's first patient was Mr. Jonas Black, whom she had not seen for 3 years. An oral assessment indicated that Mr. Black has advanced periodontal disease. Heavy generalized calculus deposits were on both maxillary and mandibular arches. His oral tissue was edema-

tous, with profuse bleeding on probing, which revealed 5- to 8-mm pocketing on teeth #2, #3, #14, #15, #16, #18, #19, #30, and #32 and 4- to 6-mm pocketing on teeth #6, #9, #23, #27, and #28. Gloria, fearing that she did not have adequate time to treat Mr. Black, immediately began scaling with the ultrasonic scaler on the maxillary right quadrant but did not scale any teeth to completion. When she finished, Gloria explained to Mr. Black that because he had not received a dental prophylaxis in more than 3 years, the procedure had taken her longer than normal to complete; therefore the charges for his appointment would be higher than the usual cost. Gloria also explained that she was able to complete only one quadrant of his mouth and that he must return for at least four visits to complete the treatment. Mr. Black left, announcing he was on his way to his attorney's office.

Before reading this chapter, the reader is encouraged to answer the following questions regarding this case. After reading the chapter, an assessment of the answers should be made to determine whether any of the responses would change. The case applications for these questions are found near the end of the chapter.

1. Is Gloria's conversation with Mr. Fenten a breach of duty? If so, describe the breach. Was this a breach of *ethics* or a *legal duty*?
2. In view of Mrs. Walters' dilemma and Dr. Peters' absence, was Gloria justified in placing the restoration? If so, by what authority? If not, what was the violation?
3. Was the friendly exchange between Gloria and Elisa illegal, unethical, or neither?
4. Considering Mr. Black's periodontal disease, was Gloria justified in proceeding with treatment? Why would Mr. Black consult his attorney? What advice will Mr. Black's attorney give him?

CASE STUDY 3-2   Ethical Decision-Making Model

A month ago, Mary Cardwell, a registered dental hygienist (RDH), started a new full-time dental hygiene position. In her interview with the prospective employer, Mary believed she and the dentist, Dr. Frawley, held similar values about providing quality care for patients. At the interview, Mary and Dr. Frawley discussed patient scheduling, and Mary was pleased that patients with periodontal disease were to be scheduled and treated according to their needs, rather than based on time limits. Now, 4 weeks into her employment with Dr. Frawley, Mary is concerned. She identified a patient with chronic periodontitis last week and developed a treatment plan to reflect the dental

hygiene diagnosis. Dr. Frawley came in during Mary's first visit with the patient, did a quick examination, and then assured the patient her gums were fine but she needed a few fillings. He went on to tell the patient that Mary would be finishing her tooth cleaning today, and the next appointment would be scheduled to begin work on her restorations. Mary excused herself from the patient and explained her recommended treatment to Dr. Frawley. Dr. Frawley disagreed, and suggested Mary use ultrasonic instrumentation to complete treatment during the first session and allow him to begin the dental phase of treatment.

KEY TERMS

adjudication	compensatory damages	liability	punitive damages
arbitration	contracts	libel	*res judicata*
assault	deceit	malpractice	slander
autonomy	defamation	mediation	*stare decisis*
battery	doctrine of informed consent	negligent malpractice	statutes
beneficence	ethics	nonmaleficence	tort
breach of confidentiality	justice	practice act	veracity

When seeking health care, members of society expect that their healthcare providers will practice in an ethical and legal manner. The laws that apply to healthcare providers are enforced perhaps with more vigor today than they were historically. Consumers are more aware of reasonable expectations from their healthcare providers. When treatment does not go as planned, consumers who believe they have been wronged may take legal action by filing suit against the practitioner or by filing a complaint with the appropriate regulatory agency. Consequently, dental healthcare providers must be aware of and consistently apply the laws that govern their practice, ensuring they are always in compliance.

Note

Dental hygienists are fully responsible healthcare providers who must assess and minimize their exposure to risk in practice.

Although dental hygienists have often perceived their own exposure to liability as nonexistent or at least significantly less than that of the dentist, this perception is not true. The scope of dental hygiene practice has changed and expanded; therefore dental hygiene practitioners must accept their legal responsibility in providing care and hold themselves legally accountable.

Laws affect and control the direct delivery of dental and dental hygiene services. Examples are the manner in which communication among healthcare professionals is conducted and between dental hygienists and patients transpires and the way in which information acquired during those communications is used.

Discussions of the dental hygienist's legal responsibility in providing dental hygiene care usually include the hygienist's ethical responsibilities. The law denotes the legal practice of the profession; the ethical code of a profession tends to lend guidance for acceptable behavior when a direct legal component does not exist. Failure to abide by professional standards of conduct might disappoint a patient but may not carry the force of law. For example, refusing to accept patients on Medicaid as part of a practice is considered by many to be unethical, but it is not against the law.

Dental hygienists must assess and minimize their exposure to risk in practice. They must manage risks through improved patient-practitioner communication, informed consent, and treatment that always meets or exceeds standards. Thorough and accurate documentation is also a critical component of any risk management program.

This chapter presents the ethical responsibilities of dental hygienists and reviews the legal responsibilities of both the patient as the recipient of care and the dental hygienist as the provider of dental hygiene care.

Brief Overview of the Legal System

A brief review of the fundamentals of how the legal system in the United States operates is important before learning about how the dental hygienist must successfully function within the system. Law defines the minimal acceptable level of conduct for a society; morality requires more. Society expects more than this minimum from healthcare providers such as dental hygienists. The Code of Ethics for Dental Hygienists[1] was created to address this expectation. Laws must be obeyed and followed; otherwise, the result is legal consequences (Box 3-1).

Note

Law is a system of principles and rules devised by organized society for the purpose of controlling human conduct and avoiding conflict between individuals (i.e., civil law) and between government and individuals (i.e., criminal or quasi-criminal law).

The foundation of the U.S. legal system is the common law or the law that was common in England. It originated in England after the Norman invasion in 1066 and was used in the early United States. The doctrine of *stare decisis* was developed by this common law system. **Stare decisis** enables courts to examine past disputes involving similar facts to determine the outcome of the current case on the basis of earlier decisions. Courts are given some flexibility in modifying the legal rule when the facts vary from the precedent or previous case, or they may completely overturn their own earlier decisions. *Stare decisis* generally applies vertically to higher courts but not to equal or lower courts in the same system or to other courts in other systems. This application means that courts make decisions based on previous decisions by their own court or by courts above them in the same jurisdiction.

BOX 3-1

GENERAL CATEGORIES OF LAW

- *Public law.* Public law concerns itself with the government and its relationships with individuals and business organizations. It defines, regulates, and enforces rights where any part or agency of government is involved. The three primary sources of public law are:
  - *Constitutions.* Two types of constitutions, the U.S. Constitution and state constitutions, exist. The U.S. Constitution limits the powers of the legislative, executive, and judicial branches of the federal government; it contains 27 amendments, the first 10 of which are the Bill of Rights. Individual state constitutions, which are subordinate to the U.S. Constitution, are more comprehensive and detailed.
  - *Statutory enactments.* Statutory enactments are laws created by legislative bodies (e.g., Congress, state legislatures, local govern-

ments). These enactments create and empower governmental agencies.
  - *Administrative rules and regulations.* Administrative rules and regulations are created and enforced by governmental agencies. These rules and regulations play a significant role in governing the practice of dentistry.
- *Private law.* Private law contains rules and principles, which define and regulate rights and duties between or among persons or private businesses. Judicial decisions, which are subordinate to constitutions and statutes, are the primary source of private law.

A court may look to courts in other jurisdictions for guidance, but it does not have to abide by their decisions even if it has never made a similar decision in its own court. **Res judicata** is another important common law concept. *Res judicata* means that once a legal dispute has been decided by a court and all appeals exhausted within higher courts in that jurisdiction, the same parties may not later bring suit regarding matters that have already been decided by the court. Without *res judicata,* few cases would ever be brought to conclusion.

Risk Management

The English common law system usually redressed acts after an event occurred using very harsh and specific rules; consequently, England developed a separate court, the Court of Chancery, and the concept of equity. Courts of equity created new remedies and were able to enforce moral obligations of fairness and justice when the common law courts could not. Today, equity is administered by most U.S. courts and is able to provide preventive relief before a wrong occurs. An injunction, which restrains a party from doing certain acts until a final legal solution is provided, is an example of a preventive equitable remedy. The process of risk management used in health care is similar in that it also is proactive or preventive, rather than reactive after an event. Risk management continuously measures levels of legal risk and is designed to protect the financial resources of a business from losses resulting from legal actions. Three activities commonly associated with risk management are (1) identifying areas of legal vulnerability, (2) instituting corrective or preventive measures, and (3) purchasing liability insurance. Liability insurance of this sort does not provide protection against criminal or quasi-criminal allegations. Quasi-criminal allegations are those made by governmental agencies.

Functions that can place the dental hygienist at risk include the following:

- Assessing a patient's oral condition
- Delivering care
- Communicating with patients
- Maintaining confidentiality

Dispute Resolution

Legal disputes may be resolved by employing the following methods:

- Legal actions filed in court systems
- Adjudication
- Arbitration
- Mediation

COURT SYSTEMS

Chiefly, 52 court systems exist: 1 federal, 50 states, and 1 for the District of Columbia. Most court systems have three levels of jurisdiction. The first, courts of original jurisdiction, includes U.S. district courts and state trial courts where actions are initiated and usually heard first. The intermediate appellate courts, U.S. courts of appeal and state courts of appeal, represent the second level, where decisions by the courts of original jurisdiction or administrative agencies are reviewed. The third level is represented by the U.S. Supreme Court or state supreme courts, which decide final appeals.

ADJUDICATION

Adjudication, a second method of resolving legal disputes, is performed by administrative agencies, such as state boards of dental licensure, when settling disputes controlled by administrative law. Adjudication is used more frequently than legal actions filed in court systems to settle disputes.

ARBITRATION

Arbitration, a third method, is the submission of a dispute for settlement to a third person or to a panel of experts outside the judicial trial process. This method is quicker and less complicated and is therefore less expensive than submitting a case to the courts. Various types of arbitration are available.

MEDIATION

Mediation, the last method of resolving legal disputes, has no power to require a settlement, but it uses a third-party mediator to attempt to persuade adverse parties to agree to settle their differences. The dental peer-review process, which usually uses dental providers as mediators when attempting to resolve disputes between dentists and their patients, is an example of mediation.

STAGES OF CIVIL LITIGATION

When it has been determined that a legal dispute is to be decided in a court of law, six primary stages in the civil litigation process take place.

Stage 1: A plaintiff commences the lawsuit by filing a complaint, and the court issues a summons notifying the defendant to appear in court to defend the complaint. In general, most jurisdictions require that a tort complaint against a healthcare provider arising out of professional services be filed within 2 years from the date of discovering the alleged injury.

Stage 2: The defendant responds by filing an answer to the complaint, admitting, denying, or pleading ignorance of the allegations. The defendant may also ask the court to dismiss the complaint.

Stage 3: Methods used for pretrial discovery include:
- Depositions
- Interrogatories
- Inspecting and copying the opponent's documents
- Performing physical or mental examinations
- Requesting the admission of certain facts by the other party

Depositions are written records of oral testimony given before a public officer and commonly used in a lawsuit. A deposed person should always tell the truth and answer only the questions that are asked during a deposition. Interrogatories are written questions that may be directed to anyone having information about a case; these questions are answered under oath and in writing. Each party in a case is entitled to inspect and copy an opponent's documents, may request physical or mental examinations of those involved, or may request an admission of certain agreed-on facts during the discovery stage.

Stage 4: Once the discovery stage is completed, the trial commences. Issues of law and facts are presented to a judge, judges, or jury during the trial. Either side may make objections to any improper or illegal matter or proceeding. The outcomes of these objections may later be used when appealing a case.

Stage 5: Appeals are generally based on questions of law, not facts.

Stage 6: Once all appeals are exhausted, a writ of execution, which entitles the seizure of the defendant's property if necessary, is issued to enforce the final judgment of the court.

Causes of Action

A discussion of the most common civil causes of action affecting dentistry must first begin by explaining the differences between criminal or quasi-criminal and civil law. These differ particularly with the parties involved, resulting penalties, and standards of proof.

A violation of criminal law (i.e., **statutes** written by a legislative branch of government) might result in imprisonment or death. A felony is an offense usually punishable

> *Note*
> Criminal law, for example, involves the state against a citizen, whereas civil law involves a citizen against a citizen.

by death or imprisonment for a term exceeding 1 year. A misdemeanor, which is any criminal offense other than a felony, may be punishable by imprisonment up to 1 year. Quasi-criminal cases involve the state against a citizen and represent violations of administrative law (i.e., rules and regulations written by administrative agencies) and may include any criminal penalty but will exclude imprisonment or death.

Penalties in civil law usually result only in monetary damages or compensation. Criminal convictions require the highest standard of proof, beyond a reasonable doubt (i.e., any doubt based on reason). Quasi-criminal cases (i.e., cases involving administrative law violations) require only substantial evidence (i.e., adequate evidence) to issue penalties. Civil cases require a preponderance of evidence (i.e., a degree of proof that is more probable than not).

> *Note*
> A violation of a state board of dental licensure rule or regulation could result in loss or suspension of a license to practice, mandatory psychological counseling, drug rehabilitation, mandatory continuing education, or fines.

Contracts and Torts

The most common civil causes of action brought against dentists and dental hygienists are divided into two groups: contracts and torts. The penalties differ between these two causes of action. A contract cause of action can result only in compensatory damages, whereas a tort cause of action can result in both compensatory and **punitive damages. Compensatory damages** compensate a plaintiff for an injury; punitive damages are intended to punish the defendant and act as a deterrent to future similar cases.

Contracts are promises or sets of promises between two parties, for breach of which the law gives remedy. A breach occurs when one party who has a duty to perform does not perform according to the terms of the contract. Contracts can be either expressed or implied between patients and healthcare providers. A **tort,** or twisted conduct, occurs when a legal duty other than a contract that is owed to a plaintiff is violated. Two types of torts exist: intentional and unintentional.

The four common intentional torts that can occur in dental practice are assault and battery, deceit, defamation, and breach of confidentiality. These behaviors are intentional and unlawful.

1. **Assault** and **battery.** An assault occurs when a believable threat to harm with no bodily contact is expressed. A battery is an unpermitted or unauthorized touching or contact. When a dentist exceeds a patient's consent and extracts the wrong tooth, a battery occurs. Assault and battery usually exist together and are both a tort and a crime.

2. **Deceit.** Deceit is a knowingly untrue statement used to trick another into acting. For example, informing a patient that periodontal surgery is required to save a patient's teeth when it is not is deceit.
3. **Defamation.** Defamation, a third intentional tort, includes both libel and slander. **Libel** is any false publication that is injurious to the reputation or good name of another. **Slander** is the speaking of a false and defamatory statement concerning another to a third person.
4. **Breach of confidentiality.** Breach of confidentiality occurs when information obtained from or about a patient in confidence is shared with another outside the scope of the patient's care. Exceptions to these privileged communications, such as requirements to report communicable diseases, are often included in various state statutes.

MEDICAL MALPRACTICE

Malpractice is a term of common usage referring to certain types of misconduct or improper performances of professional duties by a dentist or other healthcare provider, for which he or she becomes legally liable to compensate a patient who is the victim of these wrongful acts.

Negligent malpractice, which is the failure to perform a duty that the law imposes on one person for the benefit of another, is the predominant cause of action in medical malpractice cases. A plaintiff must prove each of the following four elements to recover from a negligence cause of action:

> *Note*
>
> Medical malpractice, an unintentional tort, is the most common example of a cause of action in dentistry and therefore should be of the greatest interest to dental hygienists.

1. Existence of a legal duty
2. Breach of that duty
3. Causation or a connection between the breach and injury
4. Injury (i.e., emotional or physical harm to the plaintiff)

These four elements can serve as a checklist during risk management evaluations and when being threatened by a negligence lawsuit.

Informed Consent

> *Note*
>
> In 1914 a New York court decision written by Justice Cardozo stated, "Every human being of adult years and sound mind has a right to determine what shall be done with his own body."[15]

The legal **doctrine of informed consent** says that before a physician or dentist, or his or her agent, may administer any treatment, the patient must be adequately informed about the proposed therapy and its effects and must freely consent to being treated. *Respondeat superior,* or vicarious **liability,** is the legal doctrine that makes it important for the dental hygienist to understand and apply the doctrine of informed consent. *Respondeat superior* holds that an employer is liable for the tortious acts committed by his or her agent or employee when acting within the scope of employment. The

legal duty of informed consent or negligent nondisclosure was first applied in 1972 in *Cobbs v Grant,*[4] which said that to be effective, a patient's consent to treatment must be an informed consent. This case referenced a minority opinion in a 1914 case, *Schloendorff v N.Y. Hospital,*[15] which says that "every human being of adult years and sound mind has a right to determine what shall be done with his [or her] own body; and a surgeon who performs an operation without the patient's consent commits an assault for which he [or she] is liable in damages."

Successful application of the legal duty of informed consent in practice can be ensured by following Meisel's Model of Informed Consent,[13] which states that, "When information is disclosed by a physician to a competent person, that person will understand the information and voluntarily make a decision to accept or refuse the recommended medical procedure." This model, which can be applied in dentistry as well, contains five elements.

1. *Disclosure.* The nature of the procedure to be performed, its risks and hazards, the benefits of treatment, any alternatives to the procedure, and the consequences of no treatment must be disclosed.
2. *Competence.* To be competent, a patient must be free of mental illness and must not be a minor as defined by the jurisdiction when consenting to treatment.
3. *Understanding.* Understanding cannot be satisfied when a patient is chemically influenced by drugs or alcohol or is intellectually compromised.
4. *Voluntariness.* To ensure that consent is voluntary, a patient must not be coerced with severe threats or the information must not be manipulated by altering the actual choices of treatment. An example of manipulation would be withholding possible choices of treatment. Persuasion, which is the intent to influence a patient through appeals to reason, is permissible.
5. *Decision making.* Once all of the previous elements are satisfied, the patient must make a decision before starting any treatment. Decisions are usually implied by patient actions or are expressed either in writing (Figure 3-1) or verbally.

Satisfying all these elements is required in most jurisdictions. Informed consents, especially when they are complicated, are often videotaped or audiotaped.

When a patient alleges in a negligent nondisclosure lawsuit that the legal requirement of informed consent was not properly used, the material risk standard of proof usually must be satisfied. This standard of proof asks whether, by a preponderance of the evidence, a reasonable person in the patient's position would have refused treatment had he or she been informed of a disclosed risk.

The following are exceptions to informed consent:

- *Emergency.* Informed consent may not be possible when an emergency occurs such as when a patient is unconscious and his or her life is in danger.
- *Therapeutic privilege.* This is often used when, in the physician's judgment, a patient's health would be compromised if certain negative information were disclosed; that

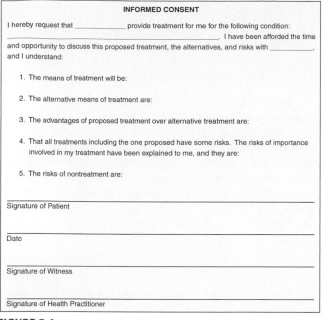

INFORMED CONSENT

I hereby request that _____ provide treatment for me for the following condition: _____. I have been afforded the time and opportunity to discuss this proposed treatment, the alternatives, and risks with _____, and I understand:

1. The means of treatment will be:

2. The alternative means of treatment are:

3. The advantages of proposed treatment over alternative treatment are:

4. That all treatments including the one proposed have some risks. The risks of importance involved in my treatment have been explained to me, and they are:

5. The risks of nontreatment are:

Signature of Patient

Date

Signature of Witness

Signature of Health Practitioner

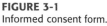
FIGURE 3-1
Informed consent form.

is, the information is withheld for the protection of the patient.
- *Incompetence.* Although it is not necessary to obtain consent from a patient when a patient is incompetent, it is necessary to use a proxy or surrogate in these instances.
- *Waiver.* A patient may waive the privilege of giving an informed consent. Courts caution against using waiver as a reason or defense for not complying with the doctrine.

The healthcare provider may use these exceptions when defending against a negligent nondisclosure cause of action.

The legally created doctrine of informed consent is a dynamic process that should take place before treatment and during every patient visit. Informed consent is not simply a form to be signed by a patient authorizing treatment. If any of the other four elements of the doctrine have not been satisfied, then a patient's decision to authorize treatment is not enough and will subject the healthcare professional to a possible lawsuit. Continuous communication with patients using excellent speaking and listening skills will often prevent lawsuits such as those involving lack of proper informed consent.

Health Insurance Portability and Accountability Act

The Health Insurance Portability and Accountability Act (HIPAA) was signed into law in 1996 and took effect on October 16, 2002; it covers three primary areas:
1. Patient privacy
2. Patient rights
3. Administrative requirements of personnel and institutions in the healthcare industry

All individuals who are provided any form of health care must sign a protected health information (PHI) form before treatment. This form informs the patient of how his or her health information will be protected and to whom the healthcare provider or administrative personnel can provide personal health information. (Box 3-2 provides information on the application of HIPAA in the dental environment.)

> *Note*
> The dental hygienist must become familiar with the application of HIPAA.

Ethical Principles in Health Professions

The public generally holds health professionals in high regard. Similar to members of any profession, health professionals undergo extensive training, study a unique body of knowledge, master the competencies of the profession, and pass licensure examinations established by external agencies.[3] Healthcare professionals are unique in that health professionals are expected to use their knowledge and skill to benefit their patients, whether the patients are individuals or communities. This commitment to serving the needs of the patient is one of the hallmarks of a health profession. More than simply obeying the law, health professionals are expected to do what is right when making decisions for the health of their patients. Ethical guidelines offer health professionals a set of principles of conduct to help determine what is good or right when ethical dilemmas exist.

In today's complex society, healthcare professionals are faced with challenging issues with no clear-cut answers. Cloning, death and dying, abortion, stem cell research, and distribution of scarce healthcare resources are only a few of the issues that face healthcare providers and bioethicists. To help resolve these issues and provide guidance for clinicians, health professional organizations typically articulate a set of ethical principles or code of **ethics.** Certain ethical principles are almost universally mentioned when describing the ethical standards that guide the behavior of health professionals. They include *autonomy, beneficence, nonmaleficence,* and *justice.*[2,14]

These principles appear to be straightforward and easy to apply, but everyday circumstances faced by healthcare practitioners often place the principles of autonomy, beneficence, autonomy, and justice in conflict with each other. For example, a new patient visits the office and desires teeth whitening and other types of cosmetic dentistry. Examination of the patient reveals advanced periodontal disease. The need for therapy (e.g., nonsurgical periodontal procedures requiring multiple visits) before cosmetic whitening is explained to the patient, but the patient is firm in her desire to have teeth whitening immediately. The clinician offers what she believes to be the treatment plan that is in the best interest of the patient (**beneficence**). Patient **autonomy** suggests the patient has a role in deciding what is to be done after having heard the risks and benefits of the various options. Failing to get the periodontal disease under control has the potential of causing harm to the patient; consequently, the principle of **nonmaleficence** may

BOX 3-2

HOW THE HEALTH INSURANCE PORTABILITY AND ACCOUNTABILITY ACT WILL AFFECT YOUR NEXT DENTAL VISIT

The U.S. Department of Health and Human Services has issued national health information privacy standards. The Health Insurance Portability and Accountability Act, a federally mandated law known as HIPAA, is designed to:
- Provide protection for the privacy of certain identifiable health data (called *protected health information [PHI]*)
- Ensure health insurance coverage when changing employers
- Provide standards for facilitating electronic transfers of healthcare-related information

While the privacy of a personal PHI will remain confidential, certain aspects of this law will permit disclosures of a PHI to facilitate public health activities. The following charts review the types of health data disclosure allowed under HIPAA:

PHI Disclosure with Authorization
Patients may request a limitation or restriction on the disclosure of this information. Patients have the right to:
- Request a restriction or limit of any of the above disclosures used for treatment, payment, or office operations
- Inspect and copy information that may be used to make decisions about patient care
- Request an amendment of this information if the patient believes it is incorrect or incomplete

- Request an accounting of disclosures made that were not related to treatment, payment, or operations of the dental office

These requests must be submitted in writing to the office manager; the patient will be informed of the specifics that are required for this request.
- *Treatment.* PHI will be used to provide appropriate treatment either by the dental office or other healthcare providers or by diagnostic or fabrication laboratories.
- *Payment.* PHI will be used to facilitate payment for treatment rendered. The patient health plan requires this information to bill, collect payments, or obtain approval before treatment.
- *Healthcare Operations.* To ensure all patients receive timely and quality care, PHI is used to facilitate the daily operations of the dental practice. These operations include but are not limited to:
  - Clinical and research studies to improve the dental practice
  - Appointment reminders via telephone calls or mailings
  - Sign-in sheets used to notify the dental office of patient arrival
  - Posted appointment schedules
  - Information regarding patient treatment options or related benefits and services
  - Communications with family or friends that are involved in patient care or payment for patient care

PHI Disclosure without Authorization

As required by law	Judicial and administrative proceedings	Oversight PHI can be disclosed to a health oversight agency as authorized by law for audits, investigations, inspections, and licensure.
Public health	Lawsuits and disputes	Workers' compensation PHI may be released to workers' compensation or similar programs that provide benefits for work-related injuries or illness.
Public health risks	Law enforcement	Military and veterans
Health research PHI disclosures are permitted when required by federal, state, tribal, or local laws.	Coroners and medical examiners Release of PHI to officials will occur: • In response to a court order, subpoena, discovery request, or summons • To identify a suggested fugitive, witness, or missing person • If a victim of crime is unable to be found to obtain permission • To identify a deceased person to determine cause of death or to confirm whether the death is the result of criminal conduct • If criminal conduct has occurred at the practice • In emergency situations	National security and intelligence activities
Abuse, neglect, or domestic violence PHI can be disclosed to prevent a threat to patient health and safety or to ensure the health and safety of others.	Cadaver organ, eye, or tissue donations PHI disclosure can be made to organ banks as necessary to facilitate organ or tissue donation and transplantation.	Protective services for the president and others PHI may be released as authorized by law when requested by military command authorities, federal officials for national security, and protection of the president and other heads of state.

From Harfst DP, Candio SJ: *Dental practice tool kit*, St Louis, 2004, Elsevier.

also be involved. In fact, distinguishing the two principles is not always easy. Failing to act in the best interest of the patient may also cause the patient harm. Some authors link the two principles. For clarity, this text will refer to them separately.[14] The principle of **justice** in this case would indicate that the patient should have access to the best quality oral health care. However, is performing the cosmetic whitening prior to treating the periodontal disease the best quality oral health care?

Practitioners face these types of dilemmas on a regular basis. An understanding of the appropriate professional code of ethics helps practitioners clarify the issues in these situations. In addition to providing guidance to health professionals when ethical dilemmas arise, codes of ethics also announce to those who are served by the profession that its members are concerned with the well-being of their patients. A third reason for the importance of ethical codes is that they serve as a valuable tool in educating those entering the profession about what its members believe constitutes the standards of the profession. Ethical codes do not dictate how specific situations should be handled; rather, they provide a framework for decision making.

Ethical Principles in Dental Hygiene

Dental hygienists are professionals dedicated to disease prevention and health promotion for individual patients and for communities of patients. The professional organization of dental hygienists, the American Dental Hygienists' Association (ADHA),

has established a code of ethics that incorporates the core values of beneficence, nonmaleficence, justice, and autonomy (Box 3-3). In addition, the ADHA code of ethics includes additional values: confidentiality, societal trust, and **veracity**; dental hygienists are obligated to tell the truth and expect that others will do the same. The code of ethics further lists a set of "Standards of Professional Responsibility" that clarifies how the ethical dental hygienist practices and the duties that exist when a dental hygienist relates to patients, employers, other professionals, and the community.[1] Although the professional expectations for dental hygienists are clearly spelled out in the ADHA's code, the challenge is implementing the ethical guidelines on a day-by-day basis in their professional activities.

Codes of ethics and their principles are most valuable when considered in the context of actual clinical situations in which competing interests arise. In a survey of members of ADHA, Gaston and colleagues reported on the ethical dilemmas that were most frequently encountered by dental hygienists in clinical practice.[8] These included the following:

- Witnessing behaviors that do not conform to standard infection control guidelines
- Failing to refer patients to a specialist
- Failing to diagnose dental disease

Beemsterboer identified eight categories of ethical dilemmas that can occur in dental hygiene practice settings:[3]

- Substandard care
- Overtreatment (provision of excessive services)

BOX 3-3

DENTAL HYGIENE CODE OF ETHICS

1. Preamble
As dental hygienists, we are a community of professionals devoted to the prevention of disease and the promotion and improvement of the public's health. We are preventive oral health professionals who provide educational, clinical, and therapeutic services to the public. We strive to live meaningful, productive, satisfying lives that simultaneously serve us, our profession, our society, and the world. Our actions, behaviors, and attitudes are consistent with our commitment to public service. We endorse and incorporate the Code into our daily lives.

2. Purpose
The purpose of a professional code of ethics is to achieve high levels of ethical consciousness, decision making, and practice by the members of the profession. Specific objectives of the Dental Hygiene Code of Ethics are as follows:
- To increase our professional and ethical consciousness and sense of ethical responsibility
- To lead us to recognize ethical issues and choices and to guide us in making more informed ethical decisions
- To establish a standard for professional judgment and conduct
- To provide a statement of the ethical behavior the public can expect from us

The Dental Hygiene Code of Ethics is meant to influence us throughout our careers. It stimulates our continuing study of ethical issues and challenges us to explore our ethical responsibilities. The Code establishes concise standards of behavior to guide the public's expectations of our profession and supports dental hygiene practice, laws, and regulations. By holding ourselves accountable to meeting the standards stated in the Code, we enhance the public's trust, on which our professional privilege and status are founded.

3. Key Concepts
Our beliefs, principles, values, and ethics are concepts reflected in the Code. They are the essential elements of our comprehensive and definitive code of ethics and are interrelated and mutually dependent.

4. Basic Beliefs
We recognize the importance of the following beliefs that guide our practice and provide context for our ethics:
- The services we provide contribute to the health and well-being of society.
- Our education and licensure qualify us to serve the public by preventing and treating oral disease and helping individuals achieve and maintain optimal health.

Approved and ratified by the ADHA House of Delegates, 1995.
Reprinted with permission from the American Dental Hygienists' Association, homepage (www.adha.com).

Continued

BOX 3-3

DENTAL HYGIENE CODE OF ETHICS—CONT'D

- Individuals have intrinsic worth, are responsible for their own health, and are entitled to make choices regarding their health.
- Dental hygiene care is an essential component of overall health care, and we function interdependently with other healthcare providers.
- All people should have access to health care, including oral health care.
- We are individually responsible for our actions and the quality of care we provide.

5. Fundamental Principles

These fundamental principles, universal concepts, and general laws of conduct provide the foundation for our ethics.

Universality

The principle of universality expects that if one individual judges an action to be right or wrong in a given situation, other people considering the same action in the same situation would make the same judgment.

Complementarity

The principle of complementarity recognizes the existence of an obligation to justice and basic human rights. In all relationships, it requires considering the values and perspectives of others before making decisions or taking actions affecting them.

Ethics

Ethics are the general standards of right and wrong that guide behavior within society. As generally accepted actions, they can be judged by determining the extent to which they promote good and minimize harm. Ethics compel us to engage in health promotion and disease prevention activities.

Community

This principle expresses our concern for the bond among individuals, the community, and society in general. It leads us to preserve natural resources and inspires us to show concern for the global environment.

Responsibility

Responsibility is central to our ethics. We recognize that there are guidelines for making ethical choices and accept responsibility for knowing and applying them. We accept the consequences of our actions or the failure to act and are willing to make ethical choices and publicly affirm them.

6. Core Values

We acknowledge these values as general for our choices and actions.

Individual autonomy and respect for human beings

People have the right to be treated with respect. They have the right to informed consent prior to treatment, and they have the right to full disclosure of all relevant information so that they can make informed choices about their care.

Confidentiality

We respect the confidentiality of client information and relationships as a demonstration of the value we place on individual autonomy. We acknowledge our obligation to justify any violation of a confidence.

Societal trust

We value client trust and understand that public trust in our profession is based on our actions and behavior.

Nonmaleficence

We accept our fundamental obligation to provide services in a manner that protects all clients and minimizes harm to them and others involved in their treatment.

Beneficence

We have a primary role in promoting the well being of individuals and the public by engaging in health promotion and disease prevention activities.

Justice and fairness

We value justice and support the fair and equitable distribution of healthcare resources. We believe all people should have access to high-quality, affordable oral health care.

Veracity

We accept our obligation to tell the truth and expect that others will do the same. We value self-knowledge and seek truth and honesty in all relationships.

7. Standards Of Professional Responsibility

We are obligated to practice our profession in a manner that supports our purpose, beliefs, and values in accordance with the fundamental principles that support our ethics. We acknowledge the following responsibilities.

To ourselves as individuals . . .

- Avoid self-deception and continually strive for knowledge and personal growth.
- Establish and maintain a lifestyle that supports optimal health.
- Create a safe work environment.
- Assert our own interests in ways that are fair and equitable.
- Seek the advice and counsel of others when challenged with ethical dilemmas.
- Have realistic expectations for ourselves and recognize our limitations.

To ourselves as professionals . . .

- Enhance professional competencies through continuous learning in order to practice according to high standards of care.
- Support dental hygiene peer-review systems and quality-assurance measures.
- Develop collaborative professional relationships and exchange knowledge to enhance our own lifelong professional development.

To family and friends . . .

- Support the efforts of others to establish and maintain healthy lifestyles and respect the rights of friends and family.

To clients . . .

- Provide oral health care, using high levels of professional knowledge, judgment, and skill.
- Maintain a work environment that minimizes the risk of harm.

BOX 3-3

DENTAL HYGIENE CODE OF ETHICS—CONT'D

- Serve all clients without discrimination and avoid action toward any individual or group that may be interpreted as discriminatory.
- Hold professional client relationships confidential.
- Communicate with clients in a respectful manner.
- Promote ethical behavior and high standards of care by all dental hygienists.
- Serve as an advocate for the welfare of clients.
- Provide clients with the information necessary to make informed decisions about their oral health and encourage their full participation in treatment decisions and goals.
- Refer clients to other healthcare providers when their needs are beyond our ability or scope of practice.
- Educate clients about high-quality oral health care.

To colleagues . . .
- Conduct professional activities and programs and develop relationships in ways that are honest, responsible, and appropriately open and candid.
- Encourage a work environment that promotes individual professional growth and development.
- Collaborate with others to create a work environment that minimizes risk to the personal health and safety of our colleagues.
- Manage conflicts constructively.
- Support the efforts of other dental hygienists to communicate the dental hygiene philosophy and preventive oral care.
- Inform other healthcare professionals about the relationship between general and oral health.
- Promote human relationships that are mutually beneficial, including those with other healthcare professionals.

To employees and employers . . .
- Conduct professional activities and programs, and develop relationships in ways that are honest, responsible, open, and candid.
- Manage conflicts constructively.
- Support the right of our employees and employers to work in an environment that promotes wellness.
- Respect the employment rights of our employers and employees.

To the dental hygiene profession . . .
- Participate in the development and advancement of our profession.
- Avoid conflicts of interest and declare them when they occur.
- Seek opportunities to increase public awareness and understanding of oral health practices.
- Act in ways that bring credit to our profession while demonstrating appropriate respect for colleagues in other professions.
- Contribute time, talent, and financial resources to support and promote our profession.
- Promote a positive image for our profession.
- Promote a framework for professional education that develops dental hygiene competencies to meet the oral and overall health needs of the public.

To the community and society . . .
- Recognize and uphold the laws and regulations governing our profession.

- Document and report inappropriate, inadequate, or substandard care and/or illegal activities by a healthcare provider to the responsible authorities.
- Use peer review as a mechanism to identify inappropriate, inadequate, or substandard care provided by dental hygienists.
- Comply with local, state, and federal statutes that promote public health and safety.
- Develop support systems and quality-assurance programs in the workplace to assist dental hygienists in providing the appropriate standard of care.
- Promote access to dental hygiene services for all, supporting justice and fairness in the distribution of healthcare resources.
- Act consistently with the ethics of the global scientific community, of which our profession is a part.
- Create a healthful workplace ecosystem to support a healthy environment.
- Recognize and uphold our obligation to provide pro bono service.

To scientific investigation . . .
We accept responsibility for conducting research according to the fundamental principles underlying our ethical beliefs in compliance with universal codes, governmental standards, and professional guidelines for the care and management of experimental subjects. We acknowledge our ethical obligations to the scientific community:
- Conduct research that contributes knowledge that is valid and useful to our clients and society.
- Use research methods that meet accepted scientific standards.
- Use research resources appropriately.
- Systematically review and justify research in progress to ensure the most favorable benefit-to-risk ratio to research subjects.
- Submit all proposals involving human subjects to an appropriate human subject review committee.
- Secure appropriate institutional committee approval for the conduct of research involving animals.
- Obtain informed consent from human subjects participating in research that is based on specification published in Title 21 Code of Federal Regulations Part 46.
- Respect the confidentiality and privacy of data.
- Seek opportunities to advance dental hygiene knowledge through research by providing financial, human, and technical resources whenever possible.
- Report research results in a timely manner.
- Report research findings completely and honestly, drawing only those conclusions that are supported by the data presented.
- Report the names of investigators fairly and accurately.
- Interpret the research and the research of others accurately and objectively, drawing conclusions that are supported by the data presented and seeking clarity when uncertain.
- Critically evaluate research methods and results before applying new theory and technology in practice.
- Be knowledgeable concerning currently accepted preventive and therapeutic methods, products, and technology and their application to our practice.

Approved and ratified by the ADHA House of Delegates, 1995.
Reprinted with permission from the American Dental Hygienists' Association, homepage (www.adha.com).

- Scope of practice (practitioner exceeds his or her legally established role)
- Fraud (false claims for reimbursement)
- Confidentiality
- Impaired professional
- Sexual harassment
- Abuse

These situations may present illegal or unethical practices and no clear-cut options. What is the dental hygienist's responsibility to the patients, to the dentist, and to the profession in situations such as these? The various alternatives should be carefully weighed. Options that might be considered include the following:

- Discussing the situation with the dentist
- Reporting the situation to an appropriate peer-review group or other agency
- Expressing concerns to the patient
- Leaving the practice

Having an ethical decision-making model and discussing choices can help the dental hygienist decide on a plan of action when situations such as these arise.

Ethical Decision Making in Dental Hygiene Practice

An ethical dilemma occurs when a situation presents one or more opposing ethical principles. For example, informing a patient about a diagnosis of advanced cancer may cause pain (a harm), yet withholding the information would violate the patient's right to autonomy and the clinician's obligation to tell the truth. Potential ethical dilemmas may be further complicated by the patient's cultural background, because the nation's population is increasingly from cultures other than white, non-Hispanic residents. Dental hygiene educators and researchers have proposed a six-step ethical decision-making model[3,11]:

1. Identify the problem.
2. Collect information about the problem.
3. State the options or alternatives.
4. Apply ethical principles to the various options.
5. Make the decision.
6. Implement the decision.

Because dental hygienists have reportedly been confronted with a variety of ethical dilemmas, developing the necessary skills to apply the decision-making model is helpful before the dental hygienist is actually confronted with the problematic situation.

Patients' Rights and Responsibilities in Dental Care

Duties or responsibilities are integral to any discussion of patients' rights because each patient's right creates a duty on the part of a healthcare provider. Dental healthcare providers have

---

✦ CASE APPLICATION 3-2.1

Ethical Decision-Making Model

The first step in ethical decision making is to identify the issues. Mary is concerned that the patient has periodontal disease requiring extensive scaling and root planing. Rushing through to complete the dental hygiene treatment will not allow time for patient education and meticulous debridement. She is also disappointed with Dr. Frawley's recommendation that she "finish the tooth cleaning today," because she and Dr. Frawley discussed this issue during her preemployment interview. Dr. Frawley believes Mary has made an incorrect diagnosis and that he is living up to his commitment to provide the best care possible for patients. He is concerned that the restorative phase of care be completed to get the dental caries under control. No clear-cut answers are found in ethical dilemmas. Mary might identify the ethical issues as a matter of failing to diagnose periodontal disease or providing substandard care. On the other hand, Dr. Frawley might believe that quadrant scaling and root planing are overtreatments for this patient.

The next steps in the ethical decision-making model are to collect information and state the options. Mary identifies the following options: (1) She can attempt to complete the patient's treatment as thoroughly as possible in the allotted time and place the patient on a shortened recall. (2) She can take the record to Dr. Frawley and explain the rationale for her recommended treatment and ask him to reconsider. (3) Mary could recommend that the patient seek a second opinion about her possible periodontal disease.

After the options are identified, applying the ethical principles to each of the options is important. The first option, completing the dental hygiene phase of care quickly but as thoroughly as possible in the limited time, addresses beneficence and nonmaleficence, the obligation to provide care in a manner that protects the patient. The first requirement of a health professional is to "do no harm," and rushing through treatment could hinder Mary's ability to provide care in a manner that protects the patient and acts in her best interest.[3] The second option, taking the record to Dr. Frawley and asking him to reconsider, involves the ethical principles of veracity and trust. By honestly conveying her conclusions and recommendations to Dr. Frawley, Mary is telling him what she believes to be the truth. This open communication can build mutual trust between Dr. Frawley and Mary; however, a risk that it will not foster collegiality is also a possibility. The final option, recommending the patient seek a second opinion, involves beneficence because Mary believes having a second opinion will promote the well-being and oral health of the patient. This option also will involve the ethical principle to trust. By acting in what she considers the best interest of the patient, Mary may act in direct opposition to the recommended treatment plan of Dr. Frawley. This option may help protect the patient from the harm of undiagnosed periodontal disease (nonmaleficence), but it could seriously impair the future working relationship between Dr. Frawley and Mary.

The final steps in the ethical decision-making model are to make and implement the decision. Although not formally part of the decision-making model, it is important that the practitioner also evaluate the decision to foster life-long learning and application of the ethical decision-making process.

the ethical and legal duty to ensure that their patients' rights are protected.

FIRST AMENDMENT RIGHTS

Because the First Amendment protects religious beliefs, courts have found that the decision to refuse medical treatment need not be rational but the reasoning process should be. What seems to be irrational reasoning is protected if it is based on a religious belief. The belief must be held by a sufficient number of people, for an extended time, or be similar to beliefs held by other religious groups considered to be orthodox. In a 1965 case, *Aste v Brooks,* a woman informed her physician that she would not permit a blood transfusion because of her faith, despite the consequences of her refusal. The court held[2]:

> Even though we may consider the appellant's beliefs unwise, foolish, or ridiculous, in the absence of an overriding danger to society we may not permit interference . . . in the waning hours of her life for the sole purpose of compelling her to accept medical treatment forbidden by her religious principles and previously refused by her with full knowledge of the probable consequence.

The First Amendment to the US Constitution provides that "Congress shall make no law respecting an establishment of religion, or prohibiting the free exercise thereof" (referred to as the *establishment clause* or the *free exercise clause*). Historically in Europe and in the early days of the United States, individuals were punished in cruel and inhumane ways if they did not conform their religious beliefs to those held by the most powerful in society. Constitutional separation of church and state protected religious freedom from government control and was a critical component of the concept of individual freedom, which the drafters of the US Constitution sought to preserve.

Countless court decisions have addressed the issues surrounding First Amendment protection. One of these decisions was *Cantwell v Connecticut*. The court addressed the free-exercise clause by stating[5]:

> The Amendment embraces two concepts, freedom to believe and freedom to act. The first is absolute but, in the nature of things, the second cannot be. Conduct remains subject to regulation for the protection of society.

For example, the courts upheld decisions to require vaccinations[9] and prohibit polygamous marriages[10] despite claims of interference with the free-exercise clause because society has an overriding interest in protecting the lives of its citizens, and conduct may be regulated to ensure this protection.

Another example of the way in which conduct may be regulated relates to the protection of children. Members of religious groups that restrict medical care are not always permitted to do so on behalf of their children. Courts have held that parents may not exercise the power of life and death over their children. The court will often appoint a guardian *ad litem* for the purpose of making medical decisions on behalf of the child and for

the best interest of the child. The child is sometimes removed from the home but usually is not. With the exception of decision making regarding medical treatment, parents maintain control of the child. Parents' authority to control their children is also restricted under state child abuse and neglect statutes. Parents may not deprive their children of the basic necessities of life, including housing, clothing, food, education, and medical care. Neglect regarding medical care may be extended to dental care. The state may exercise its authority and take custody of a child to ensure basic needs are met, or, in the case of abuse, the child may be removed from a harmful environment. Therefore children have a right to the protection of society for basic needs, and dental healthcare providers have a duty to report suspected cases of child abuse to the appropriate state authorities.

PATIENT SELF-DETERMINATION

When professionals provide material information regarding treatment choices, communication is enhanced. Increased communication and participation of patients in making informed decisions relating to dental treatment is beneficial. The first and foremost benefit is patient satisfaction with the care they receive. This satisfaction produces a harmonious patient-provider relationship. Healthcare providers do not have a duty to continue to treat a patient who repeatedly refuses to follow their recommendations.

> *Note*
>
> Patients have the right to direct the medical or dental care they receive, and this direction includes the participation in treatment choices.

In the past, patients with terminal diseases were not always informed that the recommended treatment might not greatly expand their life expectancy, nor were they informed of their fatal condition. The courts and members of society now generally agree that withholding this type of information is not ethical or legal. A physician may not exercise control over decisions relating to the life and death of a patient. For personal or religious reasons, patients must have the opportunity to control their last hours, days, weeks, months, or years.

The U.S. Congress determined that a patient's right of self-determination regarding health care is an essential individual right to be upheld throughout his or her life, if desired. In 1990, Congress passed the Patient Self-Determination Act. This law was enacted to require healthcare institutions to inform patients regarding their rights under state law in making decisions related to medical care (i.e., the right to accept or refuse medical treatment and to execute advanced directives). An advanced directive is a living will or durable power of attorney for health care (called *healthcare surrogates* in some states). Each institution must have a written policy regarding the implementation of these rights and must provide the patient a copy of such policy. Each patient's record must include information as to whether the patient has executed an advanced directive of any kind. Under a durable power of attorney, an agent (usually a trusted friend, family member, or spouse) is designated to make decisions relating to medical treatment when the person is unable to make such decisions (Figure 3-2). A living will defines an individual's wishes regarding the termination of life-sustaining treatment (Figure 3-3). These two documents are included in this text to demonstrate the difference between the two but are not meant to be legal documents; the legal requirements regarding content vary from state to state.

PATIENT DUTIES AND RESPONSIBILITIES

The bulk of what has been discussed in this text refers to the rights of the patient. Patients also have duties or responsibilities in the patient-provider relationship. Because the professional is responsible for informed consent, the patient bears the duty to ask questions and address any concerns relating to treatment to ensure that the consent may be truly informed. In addition, the

patient owes a duty to disclose personal medical information. Treatment risks may be determined only by a full disclosure of the patient's health. Patients have the duty to comply with professional recommendations relating to their health. A patient has the duty to pay the healthcare provider a fee for services rendered. A patient's refusal to comply with any of these duties may be the basis for the termination of the patient-provider relationship by the healthcare provider.

ABANDONMENT

A healthcare provider generally has no legal or ethical duty to provide care and may refuse to provide care for any reason except on the basis of discriminatory reasons. However, once the patient-provider relationship is created, the healthcare provider has a duty not to abandon the patient.

In *Domurad v Hill*,[7] the court ruled that a dentist is held to the same standard as a physician. More specifically, when a dentist terminates a dentist-patient relationship, the dentist must provide due notice to the patient and give the patient an opportunity to secure other dental services. Such notice should be in writing and include the reason for the termination. A copy should be retained in the patient's file. All patient treatment that has started should be completed. Therefore between the time that notice is given and the termination date, the dentist should try to complete any dental treatment in progress. The dentist should also be available to provide emergency care during this time to ensure that the transition to a new dentist does not compromise the patient's oral health. In addition, dental professionals are strongly urged to contact their lawyers to ensure that all their state's legal requirements are met.

DURABLE POWER OF ATTORNEY FOR HEALTH CARE

If I should have an incurable and irreversible condition that will, without the administration of life-sustaining treatment, in the opinion of my attending physician, cause my death within a relatively short time, and I am no longer able to make or communicate decisions regarding my medical treatment, I appoint _____, whose address is _____, or, if he or she is not reasonably available or is unwilling to serve, _____, whose address is _____, to act as my attorney in fact to make decisions on my behalf regarding any and all healthcare decisions, including the type of treatment, location of treatment, and in addition, the right to refuse or decline life-prolonging treatment and to decide whatever care I receive solely to alleviate pain.

Signed this _____ day of _____,_____.
Signature:_____
Address:_____
Witness to Signature:_____   Address:_____
Witness to Signature:_____   Address:_____
STATE OF _____
COUNTY OF _____
_____ personally appeared before me and acknowledged the execution of this power of attorney for the purposes set forth herein.
Dated:_____

_____
Notary Public

FIGURE 3-2
Durable power of attorney for health care form.

LIVING WILL DECLARATION

If I should have an incurable and irreversible condition that will, without the administration of life-sustaining treatment, in the opinion of my attending physician, cause my death within a relatively short time, and I am no longer able to make or communicate decisions regarding my medical treatment, I direct my attending physician to withhold or withdraw treatment which only prolongs the process of dying and is not necessary for my comfort or to relieve pain.

If it is permissible under the laws of the jurisdiction in which I may be hospitalized, I direct that the physicians supervising my care upon a terminal diagnosis to discontinue artificially administered nutrition and/or hydration should the continuation of either or both be judged to result in prolonging a natural death.

I release any and all hospitals, physicians, and others both for myself and for my estate from any and all liability for complying with this declaration to the fullest extent provided by law.

I authorize my spouse,_____, or any individual who may become responsible for my health to effectuate my transfer from any hospital or other healthcare facility in which I may be receiving care should that facility decline or refuse to effectuate the instructions given herein.

Signed this _____ day of _____,_____.
Signature:_____
Address:_____
Social Security Number:_____
Witness to Signature:_____   Witness to Signature:_____
Address:_____   Address:_____

FIGURE 3-3
Living will declaration form.

Dental Hygienists' Responsibilities in Providing Care

PRACTICING WITHIN THE LIMITS OF THE LAW

Individuals who meet all the criteria for licensure in a particular state and are granted a valid license must recognize that licensure is a privilege, not a legal right. To maintain that privilege, the dental hygienist must practice within the law. The dental hygiene practitioner cannot exceed the legally delegable scope of practice for dental hygiene in a particular state.

Additionally, dental hygienists must practice with the legally required level of supervision. Dental hygienists, as licensed dental professionals, must accept their legally delegated responsibility to provide competent dental hygiene care. This responsibility requires that contemporary dental hygiene care always meets or exceeds the standard of care. The standard of care is generally recognized as that degree of skill, care, and knowledge possessed and exercised by dental hygienists in similar situations. This standard may be affected by and derived from a multitude of professional sources, including criteria developed in educational programs for health professionals and professional organizations. For example, "Patient Bill of Rights" developed for a school of dentistry (Box 3-4) establishes a basis for the standards of care relating to patient services.

BOX 3-4

PATIENT BILL OF RIGHTS

- You have the right to the most appropriate care we can provide for your problem, without regard to race, sex, color, religion, marital status, age, national origin, or disability.
- You have the right to receive treatment that meets or exceeds the standards of care that exist in the dental community.
- You have the right to be addressed by your proper name and without undue familiarity and to be assured that your individuality will be respected and that your treatment will be confidential.
- You have the right to know the names of the providers who are directly responsible for your care.
- You have the right to ask questions and to receive answers at any time concerning any aspect of your dental condition or care.
- You have the right to voluntarily consent to or refuse any treatment and to expect that the nature of each dental treatment procedure, its alternatives, its risks and benefits, and the risks and benefits of no treatment be disclosed prior to your decision.
- You have the right to request and receive an estimate of the cost of all planned dental treatment and to be informed of any changes in the cost before any treatment begins.
- You have the right to withdraw consent and to discontinue treatment at any time.
- You have the right to receive all planned dental treatment in a timely manner.
- You have the right to receive immediate care in the case of a dental emergency.

In return for these considerations we have a just claim, or right, to expect that you, the patient, will fulfill the following responsibilities in order to help us accomplish our mutual goal of providing you with the best dental treatment possible.

- We have the right to expect that you will provide complete and accurate information regarding your past and current health status and any medications that you are currently receiving.
- We have the right to expect that you will be available for and keep scheduled appointments and arrive for appointments on time.
- We have the right to expect that you will understand that fees will be charged for each dental treatment procedure and that you will pay for treatment as treatment is provided.
- We have the right to expect that you will cooperate with and follow the instructions of the providers directly responsible for your care and that you will ask questions if you do not understand those instructions.
- We have the right to expect that you will express concerns, complaints, or problems as soon as they arise to providers directly responsible for your care.
- We have the right to expect that you will be respectful and considerate of providers, staff, and other patients.
- We have the right to expect that you will understand that there are limits to the success or permanence of dental treatment.

A court may find healthcare professionals liable for harm to patients when the services they provide fall below the standards of care. Historically, tracking lawsuits against dental hygienists has been difficult because many complaints filed ended in settlement and were not concluded in trial. Case law demonstrates that dental hygienists have been held accountable for their actions in addition to their dentist employers by patients who believed they sustained injury as a result of the dental hygiene care received.[16] Patients are also more likely than in the past to file complaints against dental hygiene licensees, complaining about the care they received. A national unpublished survey completed by the ADHA Governmental Affairs Division during 1987 and 1988 indicated that the complaints most often filed against dental hygienists were based on the following:

- Practice without a license
- Performance of procedures beyond the role of practice
- Substance abuse or dependency
- Practice while under the influence
- Performance of duties outside required supervision

Adverse action (e.g., revocation, suspension) against a healthcare professional's license to practice and legal action against the healthcare professional must be reported to the National Data Bank. The National Data Bank is a result of the Health Care Quality Improvement Act of 1986. The purpose of the Bank is to monitor professional practice to ensure that healthcare professionals who have been disciplined in one state will not find it easy to obtain a license in another state. The National Data Bank may be accessed for information by state licensing agencies and professional societies. Individual practitioners may access the Bank only as it relates to actions taken against them.

Prevention

The dental hygienist should review the dental practice act and dental hygiene rules and regulations whenever he or she begins to practice in a new licensing jurisdiction. This review will ensure that the dental hygienist is practicing within the law in that state.

CONTINUING DENTAL HYGIENE EDUCATION

As professionals, dental hygienists must assume the responsibility for keeping themselves apprised of changes in professional practice. As state laws change, the dental hygienist is responsible for gaining the knowledge of these changes. Participation in professional meetings and organizations is one of the best ways for a practitioner to maintain an up-to-date knowledge base of the practice. Often, members of a dental hygiene organization will specifically receive notification of changes in the laws affecting practice through association newsletters or as a part of a continuing education (CE) course in dental hygiene. The number of hours for renewal varies from state to state. Some states additionally require that a portion of the hours be directed toward certain topics such as infection control or that all courses be related to clinical care. As the scope of practice for dental hygiene changes or increases in various states, the CE requirements often increase as well.

RISK MANAGEMENT FOR THE DENTAL HYGIENIST

Dental hygienists can exercise appropriate risk management with effective communication, accurate assessments, appropriate treatment, and ethical behaviors. Effective communication in practice is essential to maintain good patient relations, minimize misunderstanding between the provider and the patient, and prevent unrealistic expectations. Patients who are adequately informed in an honest and caring manner are far less likely to harbor unrealistic expectations regarding the progression or outcome of their treatment. In the event of an undesired outcome, which can happen in the face of excellent technique and adequate patient compliance, a patient who has had the opportunity to make an informed decision about care through an informed consent process will more likely continue to work with the practitioner. As a result, this patient will be less likely to pursue administrative or legal recourse against a practitioner or the practice in which the dental hygienist is employed. The practitioner should keep patients apprised of the progress of their treatment, including unforeseen consequences, rather than misinform or fail to inform them.

Although good communication begins with the interaction between the patient and the dental hygienist, the result of those communications and the decisions made should be thoroughly documented in the patient record. The entire process from assessment of the patient's presenting condition, including the treatment provided and the evaluation after treatment, should be documented in the patient treatment record. This record should reflect what was done, how it was done, and why it was done in as complete and understandable manner as possible, making the occurrences clear to any third party. A standard system of documentation should be developed for the dental office, and all providers should adhere to that system. Failure to implement such a system usually results in an unorganized and incomplete document. The patient treatment record is significant because it documents treatment provided and is a legal document that may be used in the event of a future dispute between practitioner and patient. Poorly documented or inaccurate patient records are one of the major problems in litigation against dental hygienists or dentists.

Dental hygienists must accurately record in the dental treatment record and prevent any attempt to alter an entry. If an error is made during the entering of information into the record, then it should be acknowledged as an entry and the correct information entered. For example, a practitioner forgets to enter pertinent information regarding patient assessment or treatment and remembers it at a later date. In this case, the dental hygienist should date and enter the information when remembered. The dental hygienist should clearly sign all entries with the full name.

Because the treatment record is a legal document, it must accurately reflect all aspects of patient assessment, treatment, and compliance and must be written in a professional, factual manner. For example, including subjective comments about a patient's psychologic state or derogatory statements about the patient is inappropriate. Entries should be factual and describe the circumstances surrounding the care received as objectively as possible.

OWNERSHIP AND ACCESS TO DENTAL TREATMENT RECORDS

As in all healthcare records, ownership of the dental treatment record lies with the owner dentist of the practice. Patients have a legal right to access a copy of their record at their request. Because of state confidentiality laws, the release of a dental treatment record should be with the patient's written consent or as otherwise required by law. Patients may be charged a reasonable fee for copying their records but cannot legally be denied access to records because they have outstanding balances for treatment received.

RESPECT FOR THE PATIENT-PRACTITIONER RELATIONSHIP

A professional relationship exists between the patient and dental hygienist that requires the dental hygienist to keep the information acquired in confidence as a part of the relationship. Improper disclosure of information learned as part of this relationship may lead to liability for breach of confidentiality on the part of the dental healthcare provider.

✦ CASE APPLICATION 3-1.1

Ethics and the Law

Case Study 3.1 incorporates many of the legal and ethical issues regarding dental hygiene practice addressed in this chapter. The following summarizing comments address each of the questions presented at the end of the case study and discuss the legal and ethical implications associated with each:

1. Gloria, the dental hygienist, breached her duty to keep all learned information confidential as a part of the patient–dental hygienist relationship when she disclosed information regarding one patient to another without the legal authority to do so. She had not received written consent to disclose this information, nor was she required to disclose it under the law. The breach represents both a violation of law and a breach of ethics.

2. Dental hygienists must practice within the law in the state in which they practice, regardless of their educational preparation or experience. Although Gloria may have the expertise to provide dental therapies not legally allowed, she practiced in violation of the law when she provided these services when such responsibilities were not legally delegable in her state. Arguably, Gloria was attempting to assist the patient in the dilemma that had occurred—the loss of a restoration. Ethically, she may have considered what she was doing a service to the patient, specifically because she felt adequately trained to perform the procedure.

CASE APPLICATION 3-1.1-cont'd

3. The friendly exchange between the two dental hygienists involving the renewal of their licenses and the continuing dental education requirement for nonrenewal was both illegal and unethical. Although Gloria may have thought she was helping a colleague, she was in fact assisting her in committing misrepresentation to the state board. State dental boards often perform audits or reviews of this documentation, and if the board discovered that Elisa had falsified her information regarding renewal, her actions would be considered fraud. Misrepresentation and fraud are illegal and unethical. The requirement for CE is in place to promote additional education for the dental hygienist to assist these practitioners in practice. Gloria was promoting a behavior inconsistent with certain principles of the ADHA Code of Ethics (see Box 3-3).

4. The situation that occurred with Mr. Black presents several issues. Gloria's oral assessment indicated significant disease in Mr. Black's mouth. The disease may have been so severe that its treatment warranted an immediate referral to a periodontist for a complete diagnosis before the initiation of treatment. Without proper diagnosis, an appropriate treatment plan cannot be developed. Dental hygiene care provided without an accurate diagnosis may fall below the standard of care.

Another issue is whether Mr. Black's periodontal problem has gone undiagnosed and untreated because of the negligence of the office, including Gloria, over the course of the past 3 years. If this has occurred, then the patient may have a legal cause of action based on negligence, in this case a concept known as *supervised neglect*. These may be reasons that Mr. Black would seek the advice of an attorney.

Finally, the increase in cost assessed Mr. Black because the treatment took longer is not illegal. However, the manner in which this information was presented to the patient did not promote patient acceptance and understanding. Gloria should have developed a treatment plan based on an accurate diagnosis and presented it to the patient for acceptance before the implementation of any treatment. She should have made a full disclosure to Mr. Black and obtained informed consent before proceeding with dental hygiene care. Mr. Black's attorney may review this issue in considering whether Mr. Black actually owes the office the fee charged.

In addition, this scenario involves ethical considerations. By starting treatment immediately, Gloria may actually have done harm to Mr. Black. This action is in direct violation of the ADHA Code of Ethics because dental hygienists are to practice nonmaleficence and promote beneficence to the patients for whom they provide dental hygiene care.

The ADHA Code of Ethics also incorporates the core values of individual autonomy and respect for human beings: nonmaleficence, beneficence, justice, and fairness.[1] These core values are acknowledged as general for the dental hygienist's choices and actions in providing care. Nonmaleficence dictates that the dental professional has a fundamental obligation to provide services in a manner that protects the patient and results in minimal harm; beneficence is the promotion of well-being of both individuals and the public by engaging in health promotion and disease prevention activities. Furthermore, justice and fairness emphasize the fair and equitable distribution of healthcare resources and incorporate a belief that all people should have access to high-quality, affordable oral health care.

References

1. American Dental Hygienists' Association: *Code of ethics,* Chicago, 1995, The Association.
2. *Aste v Brooks,* 32 Ill 2d 361, 205 NE 2d 435 (Ill 1965).
3. Beemsterboer PL: *Ethics and law in dental hygiene,* Philadelphia, 2001, WB Saunders.
4. *Canterbury v Spence,* 464 F2d 722 (DC Cir 1972).
5. *Cantwell v Connecticut,* 310 US 296, 60 SCt 900 (Conn 1940).
6. Chiodo GT, Tolle SW: Ethical dilemmas in dental hygiene practice, *Gen Dent* 43(4):322-324, 1995.
7. *Domurad v Hill,* 605 NE 2d 858 (Mass 1993).
8. Gaston MA, Brown D, Waring MB: Survey of ethical issues in dental hygiene, *J Dent Hyg* 64(5):217-224, 1990.
9. *Hales v Pittman,* 576 P2d 493 (Ariz 1978).
10. *Jacobson v Massachusetts,* 25 SCt 358 (Mass 1905).
11. Kimbrough VJ, Lautar CJ: *Ethics, jurisprudence, and practice management in dental hygiene,* Upper Saddle River, NJ, 2002, Prentice Hall.
12. McCormick TR: *Bioethics in medicine.* Available at http://eduserv.hscer.washington.edu. Accessed 8/23/05.
13. Meisel A, Roth L: What we do and do not know about informed consent, *JAMA* 246(21):2473-2477, 1981.
14. Rule JT, Veatch RM: *Ethical questions in dentistry,* ed 2, Chicago, 2004, Quintessence Publishing.
15. *Schloendorff v Society of New York Hospital,* 211 NY 125, 105 NE 92 (NY 1914).
16. *Truman v Truman,* 165 Cal Rptr, 611 P2d 902 (Cal 1980).

Evidence-Based Decision Making

Jane L. Forrest • Syrene A. Miller

INSIGHT

The decisions made about clinical care must incorporate the best available scientific evidence to maximize the potential for successful patient care outcomes. Because practitioners rely on the publication of findings from well-designed research studies, the scientific literature is an essential tool for making evidence-based decisions to solve problems.

This chapter defines the basic concepts and skills that enable dental hygiene practitioners to find, evaluate, and incorporate effectively the evidence and to access resources that are available to help advance evidence-based decision-making (EBDM) skills.

CASE STUDY 4-1 — Comparison of In-Office and At-Home Bleaching Techniques

A new patient, Mr. Kevin Thompson, is a 33-year-old architect. His chief complaint is the discoloration of his teeth. He would like them whitened within 2 weeks before he attends his best friend's wedding.

A review of his health history and oral health habits reveals that Mr. Thompson is a tea drinker and pipe smoker. From his examination, his only treatment needs are determined to be preventive care and the suggestion that the discoloration be re-evaluated after this appointment because the stain could be the result of both intrinsic and extrinsic factors. If additional treatment is needed, then vital bleaching can be provided in the office or custom trays can be made for use with an at-home whitening system.

After the re-evaluation at the end of the appointment, Mr. Thompson still believes his teeth need to be whitened. The bleaching procedure options, their safety and efficacy, and related fees are presented to the patient. He then questions the dental hygienist about the new whitening strips that do not require a tray. From what he has heard advertised on television, these strips are as effective as and less costly than the bleaching options presented.

The dental hygienist's lack of familiarity with the most recent scientific literature on whitening strips makes it impossible to answer Mr. Thompson's questions. Therefore the hygienist offers to investigate whitening strips to provide both Mr. Thompson and the dental hygienist with the most current information on which to base a decision. In addition, this information would be valuable to know when questioned by other patients.

The situation described in this case is commonly encountered by dental hygienists and underscores the importance of keeping current with the scientific information related to new products, techniques, and other areas of practice. The proliferation of whitening products on the market is one example of new self-care options consumers have available to them and, in turn, will seek professional advice regarding effectiveness. This case is used to illustrate the five steps in the evidence-based decision-making process to answer this clinical question and to assist patients in making better-informed decisions. This same structured process and related skills serve as a model for developing the skills to integrate evidence-based decision making.

KEY TERMS

biomedical databases
case series
Cochrane Database of Systematic Reviews
cohort studies

evidence-based decision making
evidence-based journals
evidence-based medicine
levels of evidence

meta-analysis
PICO
primary sources
PubMed

randomized controlled trials
secondary sources
systematic review
traditional literature reviews

What Is Evidence-Based Decision Making?

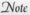

PURPOSE AND DEFINITION OF EVIDENCE-BASED DECISION MAKING

Using evidence from the medical literature to answer questions and guide practice was pioneered at McMaster University in Ontario, Canada, in the 1980s. As clinical research and the publication of findings increased, so did the need to use the medical literature to direct clinical action. The old clinical problem-solving model based on individual experience or the use of information gained by consulting authorities (e.g., colleagues, textbooks) gave way to a new methodology for practice and restructured the way in which more effective clinical problem solving should be conducted. This new methodology was termed **evidence-based medicine** (EBM).[16]

> *Note*
>
> EBM is defined as "the integration of the best research evidence with clinical expertise and patient values."[35]

Inherent in this definition is the recognition that evidence derived from valid research is a valued component of the clinical decision-making process. In other words, the use of current best evidence does *not* replace clinical skills, judgment, or experience; rather, it provides another dimension to the decision-making process[11,15,23] (Box 4-1). It is this decision-making process that is termed **evidence-based decision making** (EBDM).

BOX 4-1

FIVE SKILLS AND ABILITIES NEEDED TO APPLY THE EBDM PROCESS[33]

1. Convert information needs and problems into clinical questions to enable them to be answered.
2. Conduct a computerized search with maximum efficiency for finding the best external evidence with which to answer the question.
3. Critically appraise the evidence for its validity and usefulness (clinical applicability).
4. Apply the results of the appraisal, or evidence, in clinical practice.
5. Evaluate the process and performance of the dental hygienist.

PRINCIPLES OF EVIDENCE-BASED DECISION MAKING

EBDM recognizes that clinicians can never be completely current with all conditions, medications, materials, or available products; therefore EBDM provides a mechanism for assimilating current research findings into everyday practice to answer questions and to stay current with innovations in dentistry and dental hygiene. Initially, the focus of EBM emphasized the use of randomized clinical trials (RCT) and other quantifiable methods. Yet, as EBM has evolved, so has the realization that the evidence from clinical research is only one key component of the decision-making process; EBDM does not tell a practitioner what to do.[19]

EBDM is about solving clinical problems and involves two fundamental principles:

1. Evidence alone is never sufficient to make a clinical decision.
2. Hierarchies of quality and applicability of evidence exist to guide clinical decision making.[17]

In contrast to EBDM, traditional decision making relies more on intuition and unsystematic ways of evaluating clinical experience or making observations, which

> *Note*
>
> EBDM is a structured process that incorporates a formal set of rules for interpreting the results of clinical research.

may lead to inaccurate conclusions. In addition, not all physiologic observations result in desirable patient outcomes when tested using a rigorous research design such as an RCT.[17,30] For example, the use of sodium fluoride increases trabecular vertebral body density, which would appear to be helpful for patients with osteoporosis and to prevent vertebral fractures. However, when actually tested using an RCT, the results demonstrated that the fluoride-treated group had 3.2 times the number of fractures than the placebo group.[17]

Need for Evidence-Based Decision Making

Forces driving the need for EBDM to improve the quality of care are the following:

- Variations in practice patterns[6,14,21]
- Clinicians' difficulty in assimilating scientific evidence into practice[11,15,37]

VARIATIONS IN PRACTICE PATTERNS

Substantial advances have been made in the knowledge of effective disease prevention measures and of new therapies, diagnostic tests, materials, techniques, and delivery systems; yet, the translation of this knowledge into practice has not been fully applied. Variations far too often occur as a result of a gap between the time that current research knowledge becomes available and its application to care. Consequently, adopting useful procedures and discontinuing ineffective or harmful ones are delayed.[2,13,18,22] The reason this integration of new evidence has been slow is partially explained in terms of the traditional approach to learning and practice with its reliance on *authority*, rather than seeking the most current empirical evidence. Coupled with the reliance on authority, clinicians tend to practice the same as they were taught in school. Consequently, trends indicate that the longer clinicians are out of school, the bigger the gap in their knowledge of modern care.[32,34]

> **Note**
> The longer clinicians are out of school, the bigger the gap in their knowledge of modern care.

Another explanation for the delay in integrating new evidence is the need for translating it into information that is useful for each decision maker and his or her patient. Using a standard, unbiased method to evaluate information is considered better and necessary because the number of new scientific insights that emerge each year is overwhelming. In addition, contributing to variations in practice is the lack of or weak scientific evidence for answering specific clinical questions,[15] including those related to the most frequent treatments in dentistry and dental hygiene.[4,24] In these cases, an evidence-based approach serves another purpose by helping inform the profession and investigators of needed research.

ASSIMILATING EVIDENCE INTO PRACTICE

> **Note**
> Using the evidence-based process has been recognized as one solution to better assimilate scientific evidence into practice. It requires using the Internet and electronic databases, such as MEDLINE (PubMed) and the Cochrane Database of Systematic Reviews, to search for published scientific articles.

Traditionally, practitioners have tried to keep current with dental innovations through extensive reading and attending courses. However, with the proliferation of clinical studies and journal publications, keeping up to date with relevant research is challenging. Consequently, substantial advances made in the knowledge of prevention, health promotion, and clinical dental hygiene have not been translated into practice or fully applied to ensure that patients receive the total benefit.

As a result, practitioners need more efficient and effective question formulation and on-line searching skills to find relevant evidence, as well as the critical appraisal skills to evaluate and sort rapidly what is useful and what is not.[31]

Translating the EBDM process into action is based on five abilities and skills (see Box 4-1). The following text describes each of these abilities and skills and their application to Mr. Thompson's case.

STEP 1: ASKING GOOD QUESTIONS— PICO PROCESS

The first step in the evidence-based approach is forming a well-built clinical question based on the patient's chief concern, problem, or informational needs. Converting the concern, problem, or needs into a clinical question is a difficult skill to learn; yet, asking good questions is fundamental to evidence-based practice. The process almost always begins with the patient's question or problem. A *well-built* question should identify the following four parts:

- P—patient problem or population
- I—intervention
- C—comparison
- O—outcome(s)

These parts are referred to as **PICO**.[33] Once these four components are clearly and succinctly identified, the following format can be used to structure the question:

"For a patient with _____ (P), will _____ (I) as compared with _____ (C) increase/decrease/provide better/in doing _____ (O)?"

The formality of using PICO to frame the question serves three key purposes:

1. The clinician is forced to focus on what he or she and the patient believe to be the most important single issue and outcome.
2. The clinician must identify key terms related to the case that facilitates the next step in the process—the computerized search.[33]
3. The clinician is directed to identify clearly the problem, results, and outcomes related to the specific care provided to that patient. This, in turn, allows the type of evidence and information required to solve the problem to be identified, as well as includes considerations for measuring the effectiveness of the intervention and the application of the EBDM process.

Thus EBDM supports continuous quality improvements through measuring outcomes of care and self-reflection.

⋆ CASE APPLICATION 4-1.1

Applying the PICO Process

The first step in developing a well-built question is to identify the patient problem (P) by describing the patient's chief complaint, problem, or information needs. In Mr. Thompson's case, the chief

★ CASE APPLICATION 4-1.1—cont'd

complaint is *discoloration of his teeth.* We know that *tea and pipe tobacco* are contributing factors. In addition to the chief complaint, the patient's age, current habits, and previous behaviors may influence the decision as to which treatment might be most appropriate. In this case, research that used participants with tea or pipe-tobacco stains in the study of tooth whitening effectiveness is desired. Therefore the P is the following: *For a patient with tooth discoloration caused by tea and pipe-tobacco stains, . . .*

Identifying the intervention *(I)* is the second step in the PICO process. The intervention is the main consideration for that patient and is typically the focus of concern for the patient, which keeps the focus of the question *patient centered.*[33] In Mr. Thompson's case, the intervention being considered is *over-the-counter whitening strips.* The intervention is then phrased as the following: *. . . will over-the-counter whitening strips, . . .*

The next step in formulating the question is the comparison *(C)*, which is the main alternative intervention or treatment being considered.[33] The comparison should be specific and limited to one alternative choice or the gold standard of care to facilitate an effective computerized search. The comparison is the only optional component in the PICO question because an alternative may not be available. In this case, a *custom tray for at-home bleaching* is the main alternative. The comparison is then phrased as follows: *. . . as compared with custom trays for use with an at-home whitening or bleaching system, . . .*

The final part of the PICO question is the outcome *(O)*. This component specifies the result or results of what should be accomplished, improved, or affected, and it should be measurable. Outcomes may consist of relieving or eliminating specific symptoms, improving or maintaining function, or enhancing esthetics. In Mr. Thompson's case, evidence is needed to demonstrate the effectiveness of each whitening or bleaching treatment under a given set of conditions. Therefore the outcome component is then phrased as the following: *. . . be more effective in whitening teeth within 2 weeks and, secondarily, be less expensive?* Outcomes yield better search results when defined in specific terms. *More effective* is not acceptable unless it describes how the intervention is more effective. For this example, more effective in whitening teeth within *2 weeks* and *less expensive* are the desired outcomes.

Based on the case information, the four PICO components are summarized as follows:
- P—tooth discoloration caused by tea and pipe-tobacco stains
- I—over-the-counter whitening strips
- C—custom trays for use with an at-home whitening or bleaching system
- O—more effective in whitening teeth within 2 weeks and less expensive

Using these four components, the PICO question can be structured to read as follows:

For a patient with tooth discoloration caused by tea and pipe-tobacco stains (P), will over-the-counter whitening strips (I), as compared with custom trays for use with an at-home whitening or bleaching system (C), be more effective in whitening teeth within 2 weeks and, secondarily, be less expensive (O)?

STEP 2: SEARCHING FOR AND ACQUIRING THE EVIDENCE

The first step, formulating the PICO question, provides the foundation for the search terms used in the database. By identifying the treatments under consideration (the *intervention* and *comparison*) for this problem, as well as knowing the specific outcome(s), a set of citations that will potentially provide an answer to the question being posed can be quickly pinpointed.

> *Note*
> Finding relevant evidence requires conducting a focused search of the peer-reviewed professional literature.

★ CASE APPLICATION 4-1.2

Selection of Search Terms

Key words from Mr. Thompson's case that can be used for the search include *tooth whitening, tooth bleaching, whitening strips, Whitestrips, custom tray bleaching,* and *night guard bleaching.* From this example, it is clear that an evidence-based search requires a shift in thinking from looking for everything on a topic (i.e., tooth whitening and bleaching, which would include brush-on gels, use of lasers, whitening dentifrices, or other aspects of tooth bleaching such as pulpal bleaching or bleaching of tetracycline-stained teeth) to something very specific (i.e., whitening strips and custom tray bleaching for tooth discoloration caused by tea and pipe-tobacco stains).

What Constitutes the Evidence?

Clinical evidence typically comes from studies related to questions about treatment and prevention, diagnosis, origin, harm, and prognosis of disease. Once synthesized, evidence can help inform the clinician to make decisions about whether a specific method of diagnosis or a treatment is effective as compared with other methods of diagnosis or with other treatments and under what circumstances.

> *Note*
> Evidence is considered the synthesis of all valid research that answers a specific question, which distinguishes it from a single research study.[20]

★ CASE APPLICATION 4-1.3

Treatment Options

In Mr. Thompson's case study, two treatments are under consideration—whitening strips and custom trays—for use with an at-home whitening and bleaching system, with the requirement that the treatment works within 2 weeks and is less expensive. Staying current with the scientific literature becomes increasingly important because the body of evidence evolves over time as more research is conducted and synthesized with previous research.

4-3

Levels of Evidence

A hierarchy is used to identify the highest level of evidence related to the clinical question being asked and is based on the notion of cause and effect and on the need to control bias [25,26] (Box 4-2). Level 1, the highest level of evidence, is the **systematic review** (SR) and **meta-analysis** (i.e., more than one human RCT). These types of review are considered the *gold standard* for evidence because they provide a summary of multiple research studies that have investigated the same specific question. Meta-analysis is a statistical process commonly used with SRs when the statistical analyses of several individual studies can be combined into one analysis. Combining several studies increases the sample size and power. As a result, the combined effect can increase the precision of estimated treatment effects and exposure risks.[28]

SRs and meta-analyses and individual RCTs are followed by **cohort studies** (Level 2); case-control studies (Level 3); **case series** (Level 4); **traditional literature reviews** without critical appraisal, ideas, editorials, and opinions (Level 5); to studies not involving human subjects (Level 6).[7] In the absence of scientific evidence, a consensus of experts in appropriate fields of research and clinical practice is used (see Box 4-2).

Although each level may contribute to the total body of knowledge, "…not all levels are equally useful for making patient care decisions."[26] In progressing up the pyramid, the number of studies and, correspondingly, the amount of available literature both decrease, while at the same time their relevance to answering clinical questions increases. The *Guide to Research Methods* and the Evidence Pyramid at SUNY's Downstate Medical Research Library's web site[36] (http://library.downstate.edu) offer further information and a graphic review of research designs and **levels of evidence.**

4-4
to
4-6
4-A

Where to Look

Primary and secondary types of evidence-based sources are available:

- **Primary sources** are original research publications that have not been filtered or synthesized and include **randomized controlled trials,** cohort studies, and case studies.

- **Secondary sources** are synthesized publications of the primary literature. These include SRs and meta-analyses, evidence-based article reviews, and clinical practice guidelines and protocols.

Both primary and secondary sources can be found by conducting a search using **biomedical databases** such as MEDLINE (PubMed), HealthSTAR, and CINAHL (Cumulative Index to Nursing and Allied Health Literature). In addition, the Cochrane Collaboration provides access to SRs (http://www.cochrane.org).

Primary sources of evidence

To assist professionals in quickly finding both primary and secondary research sources, free on-line access to MEDLINE and the National Library of Medicine's premier bibliographic database, which covers the fields of medicine, nursing, dentistry, veterinary medicine, and the healthcare system, are available through PubMed (http://pubmed.gov).

PubMed provides access to bibliographic citations and author abstracts from more than 4800 biomedical journals published in the United States and in 70 other countries, with more than 12 million citations dating back to 1966. This total number of citations grows each year with more than 520,000 new documents added annually.[29]

Using PICO to search PubMed

Although on-line databases provide quick access to the literature, knowing how databases filter information and having an understanding of how to use PICO to best use database features allows a more efficient search to be conducted. These concepts are applied to the case study as illustrated on the "History" page of the PubMed search (Figure 4-1). A more detailed understanding of searching PubMed can be gained by completing the on-line PubMed tutorial (http://www.nlm.nih.gov/bsd/pubmed_tutorial/m1001.html).

Using the key terms identified in the PICO question and combining them using the Boolean operators, *OR* and *AND,** the number of relevant articles relating to whitening strips *OR* Whitestrips (65 articles) *AND* custom tray bleaching *OR* night guard bleaching (36 articles) have been narrowed from 101 articles to a manageable 8. Reviewing 101 abstracts or articles would have been unmanageable, and reviewing the 1325 articles that would have been listed if the search stopped after tooth bleaching *OR* tooth whitening would have been even more unwieldy.

Knowing what constitutes the highest levels of evidence and how to apply evidence-based limits and filters are necessary skills when searching the literature with maximum efficiency.[26] The search can be further refined using the "Limits" feature, which allows the user to search for publication types such as meta-analyses, RCTs, clinical trials, and practice guidelines.

BOX 4-2

HIERARCHICAL LEVEL OF EVIDENCE

Highest	Level 1	Systematic reviews
		Meta-analysis
		Randomized controlled trials
	Level 2	Cohort studies
	Level 3	Case-control studies
	Level 4	Case series
	Level 5	Traditional literature reviews
Lowest	Level 6	Studies without human participants

---

*These words are used by MEDLINE to combine, eliminate, or cross-reference more than one term.

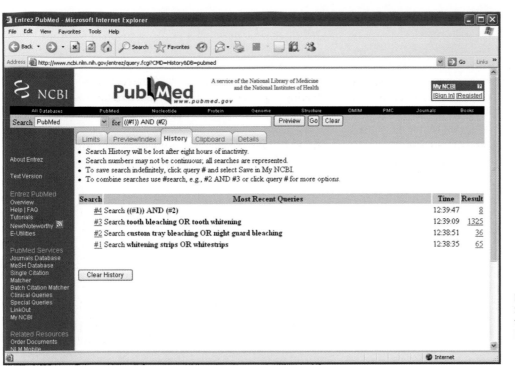

FIGURE 4-1
Sample search history showing terms and results found on PubMed.

CASE APPLICATION 4-1.4

Narrowing the Search

In this case, the search results indicate there are no meta-analyses, three RCTs that compare whitening strips and Whitestrips with custom tray and night guard bleaching, and one additional study that was identified when limiting the search to a clinical trial. This number of articles is certainly manageable to review. If none of these abstracts were applicable, then the user would have reviewed the other three citations not identified before applying the "Limits" feature. In addition, two results were found when limiting "tooth bleaching" OR "tooth whitening" to *Practice Guidelines*. Fortunately, seven to nine abstracts are still a manageable number to review.

Secondary Sources of Evidence

Evidence-based groups are developing many resources for busy practitioners to access easily because finding relevant studies is recognized as being difficult. These resources include SRs and summaries of SRs or individual research articles and clinical practice guidelines and protocols.

Systematic reviews and summaries of research articles

Evidence-based journals are an emerging resource designed specifically to assist clinicians. Two journals are published related to dental practice: the *Journal of Evidence-Based Dental Practice* (http://www.sciencedirect.com/science/journal/15323382) and *Evidence-Based Dentistry* (http://www.nature.com/ebd/index. html). Both journals provide concise and easy-to-read summa-

ries from both original research articles and SRs selected from the biomedical literature. A one- to two-page structured abstract along with an expert commentary highlighting the most relevant and practical information is generally provided. In addition to summaries with commentaries of SRs, selected abstracts of new SRs from the Cochrane Collaboration are provided.

The Cochrane Collaboration is an international, volunteer, non-profit organization made up of more than 50 specialist review groups from 15 countries.[10] To date, the Cochrane Collaboration Oral Health Group has produced over 100 SRs and protocols (i.e., studies being conducted) covering specific questions related to disease prevention interventions and different general dentistry and dental specialty topics. A complete listing of topics and their abstracts can be accessed free of charge from the **Cochrane Database of Systematic Reviews** (http://www. cochrane.org/reviews/en/topics/84.html).

SRs facilitate decision-making by providing a clear summary of the current state of the existing evidence on a specific topic and provide a way of *managing large quantities of information*,[28] making it easier to keep current with new research. SRs also support the development of guidelines by putting together all that is known about a topic in an objective manner. SRs, however, should not be confused with traditional literature reviews. They differ significantly in that SRs concentrate on answering a specific clinically focused question, narrowing them in scope to a greater extent than a literature review. Generally, a multidisciplinary team of experts who are trained in searching, appraising, and summarizing all research, whether published or unpublished, conducts the review.[3,5,26] This team uses formal and explicit methods and specifies criteria for including or excluding studies in the review, which is designed to reduce bias. The methods used to conduct an SR surpass what can be reasonably expected from any one individual.

In contrast to SRs, traditional literature or narrative reviews are directed by an individual using personal experience to define a hypothesis or research question, who then selects and summarizes the literature. The traditional approach deals with a broad range of issues on a given topic rather than answering a specific question in depth. In addition, the traditional literature approach is less systematic and more subjective in that the preestablished criteria for selecting literature are not specified and the search usually does not include unpublished literature or use critical analysis procedures.[9] Typically, a literature review does not include combining data or statistically analyzing it. A comparison of SRs and literature reviews is given in Table 4-1.

Unfortunately, the already appraised evidence does not cover many topics. In these cases, using the EBDM process is necessary to conduct a search for primary studies with the scientific databases, such as PubMed.

Table 4-1	Comparison of Systematic Reviews and Literature Reviews	
CHARACTERISTIC	**SYSTEMATIC REVIEW**	**LITERATURE REVIEW**
Focus of the Review	• *Specific problem or patient question:* Narrow focus • *Example:* Is fluoride varnish, as compared with fluoride gels, more effective in the prevention of dental caries in children and adolescents?	• *Range of issues on a topic:* Broad focus • *Example:* Dental caries prevention • *Sealants:* Xylitol gum, topical fluorides (gels, mouthrinses, toothpastes, varnishes); may or may not make comparisons between methods
Who Conducts?	• Trained multidisciplinary team	• Individual
Selection of Studies to Include	• Search strategy is rigorous, thorough, and reproducible. • Search includes database searching, reference searching, hand searching through journals, "gray" (unpublished) research, and contacting researchers to clarify studies. • Preestablished inclusion and exclusion criteria are based on validity of study design, interventions, and outcome measures. • More than one reviewer determines whether studies meet inclusion or exclusion criteria. • Bias is minimized based on selection criteria.	• Criteria are not preestablished or reported in methods. Range of issues is used in the search. • One reviewer determines whether studies or other literature are included. May include literature other than scientific studies. • May include or exclude studies based on personal bias or support for the hypothesis, if one is stated. • Inherent bias with lack of criteria.
Reported Findings	• Description of search strategy and databases searched • Number of studies identified • Number of studies that met criteria; number of studies excluded and why • Description of study design, subjects, length of trial, state of health and disease, procedures, outcome measures, and indices	• Literature review format crafted by the individual author • Search strategy, databases, total number of studies pro and con not usually identified • Descriptive in nature reporting the outcomes of studies rather than their study designs
Synthesis of Selected Studies	• Description of the critical analysis of included studies • Determination of whether results could be statistically combined; if so, how was meta-analysis conducted?	• Reporting of studies that support a procedure or position and those that do not rather than combining data or conducting a statistical analysis
Main Results	• Summary of trials, total number of subjects • Definitive statements about the findings in relation to the specified objectives and outcome measures • Numbers needed to treat and confidence interval • Results updated at regular intervals	• Summary of the findings by the author in relation to the purpose of the literature review and specific objectives • Results not updated
Conclusions or Comments	• Discussion of the key findings with an interpretation of the results, including potential biases and recommendations for future trials	• Discussion of the key findings with interpretation of the results, including limitations and recommendations for future trials

©2003 Forrest & Miller, NCDHR.

Clinical Practice Guidelines and Protocols

Growing sources of synthesized information on a specific topic are *practice guidelines and protocols*. As defined by the Institute of Medicine, guidelines are "systematically developed statements to assist practitioner and patient decisions about appropriate health care for specific clinical circumstances."[11] The inclusion of scientific evidence within clinical practice guidelines has now become the standard in that guidelines should incorporate the best available scientific evidence. SRs support this process by putting together all that is known about a topic in an objective manner.

When guidelines and protocols are published in a journal indexed by MEDLINE, they are identified as a citation during the search, as was found in the case with Mr. Thompson. If they are not published as an article in a journal, then the related web site should be searched, rather than assume that none exists.

CASE APPLICATION 4-1.5

Reviewing the Search Materials

In the PubMed search conducted for Mr. Thompson, two citations to practice guidelines were found, one of which was the American Dental Association (ADA) guidelines for the acceptance of tooth-whitening products. On the ADA web site (http://www.ada.org), "Profession" and then "Professional Issues and Research" are selected. Here, the *ADA Guidelines, Positions, and Statements* can be located and selected. Under the category "Tooth Whitening," the "ADA Statement on the Safety of Home-Use Tooth Whitening Products" can be located.

The ADA statement discusses two categories of whitening products: (1) peroxide-containing whiteners or bleaching agents, and (2) dentifrices containing only polishing or other chemical agents. However, the statement merely "advises patients to consult with their dentists to determine the most appropriate treatment." *Although this statement does not specifically compare the options discussed in the case study, becoming familiar with the guidelines and what they do cover is another way to demonstrate to patients that the dental hygienist is current in his or her practice. In this case, the studies found in the PubMed search will provide more relevant information to answer the dental hygienist's question.*

STEP 3: CRITICALLY APPRAISING THE EVIDENCE

After reviewing the abstracts of the RCTs and obtaining the full-text articles that appear to address the specific question, the next step in the EBDM process is to understand the information gathered and its relevance to the patient and PICO question. In all cases, reviewing the evidence, whether it is an SR or original study, is necessary to determine whether the methods were appropriately conducted. Fortunately, international evidence-based groups have made this process easier by developing appraisal forms and checklists that guide the user through a structured series of questions to determine the strengths, weaknesses, and validity of the individual study or SR; these are provided on line at no charge.[1,12,27] For example, the Critical Appraisal Skills Programme (CASP) checklists consist of a

structured series of *YES/NO* questions that are based on three key questions[8,12,17,35]:

1. Are the results of the study valid?
2. What are the results, and are they important?
3. Will the results help in caring for the patient?

A subset of more detailed questions exists for each of the three key questions. These questions help further determine the validity, results, and applicability of the evidence.

CASE APPLICATION 4-1.6

Appraising the Evidence

With the understanding that one research study does not constitute the full body of evidence, reading all three RCT articles related to Mr. Thompson's case could add to the evidence and provide a broad understanding of the efficacy of whitening strips, especially if none of the research studies make the exact comparison of treatment options or does not evaluate the desired outcomes.

STEP 4: APPLYING THE RESULTS OF THE APPRAISAL IN CLINICAL PRACTICE

A key component of the fourth step is determining whether the findings are relevant to the patient, problem, or question. A question to consider is, "Would the patient have met the inclusion criteria for the study?" In other words, does the patient exhibit the same conditions and demographics as the individuals in the study?[8,12]

CASE APPLICATION 4-1.7

Application of Evidence

To answer Mr. Thompson's question, the research articles should include a comparison of whitening strips and custom trays for use with an at-home whitening or bleaching system for tooth discoloration caused by tea and pipe-tobacco stains. Outcomes reported should include the timeframe for whitening teeth and the cost. Based on critical analysis, the findings are shared with Mr. Thompson, and his preference of treatment is requested.

STEP 5: EVALUATING THE OUTCOMES

The final steps in the EBDM process are to evaluate the effectiveness of the intervention and clinical outcomes of care and determine how effectively the EBDM process was applied. For example, one question to ask in evaluating the effectiveness of the intervention is, "Did the selected intervention and treatment achieve the desired result?"

CASE APPLICATION 4-1.8

Evaluation of a Case Using the PICO Process

In Mr. Thompson's case, the question to ask is, "Did the treatment selected (either the whitening strips or the custom tray whitening or bleaching system) whiten his teeth within 2 weeks and at a lower cost?"

Using an EBDM approach requires the understanding of new concepts and developing new skills. Questions that parallel each step in the EBDM process can be asked in evaluating self-performance. For example, "How well was the PICO question formulated to ensure that key terms were easily identified for conducting the search?" As with most learning, time and practice are essential to mastering new techniques.

Benefits and Conclusions

An EBDM approach closes the gap between clinical research and the realities of practice by providing dental practitioners with the skills to find, efficiently filter, interpret, and apply research findings to ensure that what is known is reflected in the care provided. This approach assists dental hygienists in keeping current with conditions a patient may have by providing a mechanism for addressing gaps in knowledge to provide the best care possible.

> **Note**
>
> By integrating good science with clinical judgment and patient preferences, clinicians enhance their decision-making ability and enhance the potential for successful patient care outcomes.

As EBDM becomes standard practice, individuals must be knowledgeable about what constitutes the evidence and how it is reported. Understanding evidence-based methods and the distinctions among different types of articles, such as SRs and literature reviews, allows the clinician to judge more accurately the validity and relevance of reported findings. To assist practitioners with this endeavor, SRs are being conducted to answer specific clinical questions, and new journals devoted to evidence-based practice are being published, which will alert readers to important advances in a concise and user-friendly manner.

References

1. Altman D et al: The revised CONSORT statement for reporting randomized trials: explanation and elaboration, *Ann Intern Med* 134:663-694, 2001. CONSORT statement available at: http://www.consort-statement.org. Accessed August 23, 2005.
2. Anderson G, Allison D: Intrapartum electronic fetal heart rate monitoring: a review of current status for the task force on the periodic health examination. In Goldbloom RG, Lawrence RS, eds; *Preventing disease: beyond the basics,* New York, 1990, Springer-Verlag.
3. Bader J, Ismail A: A primer on outcomes in dentistry, *J Publ Health Dent* 59(3):131-135, 1999.
4. Bader J, Ismail A: Survey of systematic reviews in dentistry, *J Am Dent Assoc* 135:464, 2004.
5. Bader J, Ismail A, Clarkson J: Evidence-based dentistry and the dental research community, *J Dent Res* 78(9):1480-1483, 1999.
6. Bader JD, Shugars DA: Variation in dentists' clinical decisions, *J Public Health Dent* 55(3):181-188, 1995.
7. Centre for Evidence-Based Medicine: *Levels of evidence and grades of recommendations.* Updated May 2001. Available at: http://www.cebm.net/levels_of_evidence.asp. Accessed August 23, 2005.
8. Centre for Evidence-Based Medicine: *Critical appraisal.* Available at: http://www.cebm.net/critical_appraisal.asp. Accessed August 23, 2005.
9. Chalmers I, Altman D: *Systematic reviews,* London, 1995, BMJ Publishing Group.
10. Cochrane Collaboration: *What is the Cochrane Collaboration?* Available at: http://www.cochrane.org. Accessed August 23, 2005.
11. Committee on Quality of Health Care in America IOM: *Crossing the quality chasm: a new health system for the 21st century,* Washington DC, 2000, The National Academy of Sciences. Available at: http://www.nap.edu/catalog/10027.html. Accessed August 23, 2005.
12. Critical Appraisal Skills Programme: *10 Questions to help make sense of the literature,* CASP Institute of Health Sciences, Updated March 9, 2005. Available at: http://www.phru.nhs.uk/casp/appraisa.htm. Accessed August 23, 2005.
13. Crowley P, Chalmers I, Keirse M: The effects of corticosteroid administration before preterm delivery: an overview of the evidence from controlled trials, *Br J Obstet Gynaecol* 97:11-25, 1990.
14. Ecenbarger W: How honest are dentists? *Reader's Digest,* 50-56, February 1997.
15. Eisenberg J: *Statement of health care quality before the house subcommittee on health and the environment, 105th Congress, presented on 10/28/97.* Agency for Health Care Policy and Research Archive. Available at: http://www.ahcpr.gov/news/test1028.htm. Accessed August 23, 2005.
16. Evidence-based Medicine Working Group: Evidence-based medicine: a new approach to teaching the practice of medicine, *JAMA* 268:2420-2425, 1992.
17. Evidence-based Medicine Working Group: *Users' guides to the medical literature, a manual for EB clinical practice,* Chicago, 2002, AMA Press.
18. Frazier P, Horowitz A: *Prevention: a public health perspective. Oral health promotion and disease prevention,* Copenhagen, 1995, Munksgaard.
19. Greco P, Eisenberg J: Changing physicians' practices, *N Engl J Med* 329:1271-1273, 1993.
20. Greenhalgh T: "Is my practice evidence-based?" Should be answered in qualitative, as well as quantitative terms, *Br Med J* 313(7063):957-958, 1996.
21. Grembowski D, Milgrom P, Fiset L: Dental decision making and variation in dentist service rates, *Soc Sci Med* 32(3):287-294, 1991.
22. Grimes DA: Introducing evidence-based medicine into a department of obstetrics and gynecology, *Obstet Gynecol* 86(3):451-457, 1995.
23. Haynes R: Some problems in applying evidence in clinical practice, *Ann N Y Acad Sci* 703:210-224, 1999.
24. Institute of Medicine: *Dental education at the crossroads: challenges, and change,* Washington, DC, 1995, National Academy Press.
25. Long A, Harrison S: The balance of evidence. Evidence-based decision making, *Health Serv J* (Glaxo Wellcome Supplement) 6:1-2, 1995.

26. McKibbon A, Eady A, Marks S: *PDQ, evidence-based principles and practice,* Hamilton, Ontario, 1999, BC Decker.

27. Moher D et al: Improving the quality of reports of meta-analyses of randomised controlled trials: the QUOROM statement, *Lancet* 354:1896-1900, 1999. QUOROM statement available at: http://www.consort-statement.org/QUOROM.pdf. Accessed August 23, 2005.

28. Mulrow C: Rationale for systematic reviews, *Br Med J* 309(6954):597-599, 1994.

29. National Library of Medicine, NCBI: *PubMed overview,* Electronic citation, 2001, National Library of Medicine, NIH.

30. NHS Centre for Reviews and Dissemination, University of York: *Undertaking systematic reviews of research on effectiveness.* Available at University of York web site: http://www.york.ac.uk. Updated March 2001. Accessed August 23, 2005.

31. Palmer J, Lusher A, Snowball R: Searching for the evidence, *Genitourin Med* 73(1):70-72. 1997.

32. Ramsey P, Carline J, Inui T: Changes over time in the knowledge base of practicing internists, *JAMA* 266:1103-1107, 1991.

33. Sackett D et al: *Evidence-based medicine: how to practice and teach EBM,* New York, 1997, Churchill Livingstone.

34. Sackett D et al: Evidence-based medicine: what it is and what it isn't, *Br Med J* 312:71-72, 1996.

35. Sackett D, Straus S, Richardson W: *Evidence-based medicine: how to practice and teach EBM,* ed 2, London, 2000, Churchill Livingstone.

36. SUNY Health Sciences: *A guide to research methods, the evidence pyramid.* Evidence Based Medicine Course, State University of New York, Downstate Medical Center, Medical Research Library of Brooklyn. Available at: http://library.downstate.edu/ebm/2100.htm. Accessed August 23, 2005.

37. Verdonschot E et al: Developments in caries diagnosis and their relationship to treatment decisions and quality of care. ORCA Saturday Afternoon Symposium 1997, *Caries Res* 33(1):32-40, 1999.

CHAPTER

5

Communication

Rebecca S. Wilder • Susan H. Kass

INSIGHT

Effective communication skills are vital to excellent patient care. Although a dental hygienist may have good clinical skills, when the professional is unable to communicate effectively with the patient through verbal and nonverbal mechanisms, the overall experience for the patient will be limited.

CASE STUDY 5-1   Team Approach to Communication

Andrea Miller is a dental hygienist and has worked in Dr. Justin Joy's dental practice for 10 years. During this time she has developed exceptional professional and interpersonal skills. As a result of Andrea and Dr. Joy's attention to both patients and other dental team members, the practice has grown.

Together with the dental team, Andrea has helped Dr. Joy create a philosophy of practice and patient care that demonstrates high professional standards. Patients are at the heart of the mission of the practice, and the values displayed daily attest to this mission.

Today, Andrea is running 30 minutes behind schedule with her morning patients. A family of four was scheduled for the day's first set of appointments, but they arrived late. Andrea has been trying to catch up, but she is still behind schedule. Andrea's next patient, Todd McPherson, has arrived, and Andrea is not ready to seat him. Mr. McPherson is getting a little irritated. How might his needs, as well as the needs of the family members that Andrea is treating, be satisfied without creating additional stress while still maintaining the integrity of the office?

A different scenario may control a potentially volatile situation. When Mr. McPherson arrives, the receptionist, Julie Rodriguez, has the appointment schedule in front of her and has anticipated his arrival. Julie leaves her desk and greets Mr. McPherson in the reception room:

Julie: Hi, Mr. McPherson. Thank you for being prompt. I know how difficult it can be to get away from work and make it downtown at this time of day. I need to let you know that I tried calling you earlier, but your assistant told me that you had already left your office. She gave me your cell phone number, but I was unable to get through to you.

The reason for the call was to let you know that Andrea is running about 30 minutes behind schedule this morning.

Mr. McPherson: Oh, swell . . . just when I have a critical lunch meeting on the other side of town. I do appreciate the attempts to call, but what are we going to do now?

Julie: I am terribly sorry for this inconvenience. I'm sure that this is very frustrating for you. I know it would be the same for me *[with empathy in her voice]*. What I would suggest, Mr. McPherson, is that we get you settled into the treatment room right away and have Ann Jenkins get all the necessary paperwork completed. Ann, our assistant, as you know, has worked with you before. Andrea can check on you. As soon as she is finished with her current patient, she can pick up where Ann left off. I think we would save quite a bit of time, and, depending on the time you have available at that point, we can make a decision as to how far to take your treatment today. Is this agreeable with you?

Mr. McPherson: What are my other options?

Julie: The alternative that I see is that we reschedule your appointment for another time, perhaps the same time next week. I would feel badly if all this effort were wasted, however.

Julie is quietly looking at Mr. McPherson while he considers what she has said. He seems perplexed and still a little upset.

Julie: Why don't you have a glass of water and think about it for a minute or two? I'll see how Ann and Andrea are progressing and then come back to see what you want to do. The decision is your choice, whatever suits you best.

Julie brings Mr. McPherson a glass of water and makes certain that he is comfortable in a chair in the reception area. She looks at him again to see how he is doing as she walks to the door and back to the treatment room. She quickly confers with Andrea. Julie tells Andrea about her conversation with Mr. McPherson and the options that she has offered him. Andrea agrees with the plan (it is consistent with their philosophy) and asks Julie to check with Ann regarding her readiness to help. Ann has been in this situation before and knows what needs to be done.

Julie returns to the reception area. Mr. McPherson is sitting deep in thought.

Julie: Well, Mr. McPherson, what would you like to do?

Mr. McPherson: [standing up and squaring his shoulders, looking Julie in the eyes and smiling] Why don't we go with plan A? I know how efficient Ann is, and I am certain that Andrea will get to me just as soon as she can.

Julie smiles back at Mr. McPherson and asks him to accompany her to the treatment room. She allows him to lead the way while she accompanies him with an attending manner.

As they arrive at the treatment room, Ann is already waiting. Ann greets Mr. McPherson and expresses her appreciation for being flexible with his schedule. She makes certain that he gets comfortably into the chair and asks him whether he would like a magazine. He states that everything is fine. As Mr. McPherson reclines in the chair, he notices the absence of a lot of equipment and instruments and recognizes the enlarged pictures of the staff's family members.

Mr. McPherson: Nice photos [gazing around the room]. Which family is yours?

Ann: This is my family [taking a color picture down from the wall]— my two sons, my daughter, and my husband, Tom. The boys are 11 and 12 years old, and Emily is 14. Tom works at the local bank.

Mr. McPherson: Nice-looking family. I also deal with the bank where your husband works.

Placing the picture back on the wall, Ann gets Mr. McPherson settled into the chair. Andrea walks in, greets her patient, and states how happy she is that he decided to keep the appointment. She adjusts her stool to ensure that she is at a comfortable eye level with him.

Andrea: I realize how busy you are and what an inconvenience even 15 minutes can be in your schedule.

As she is speaking with him, she observes his face to see that he is attending to her and recognizing that she is being sincere.

Andrea: I am so sorry about the delay, Mr. McPherson. We will do everything feasible to get back on schedule. I need to spend another 5 minutes with my previous patient, and then we can begin. Ann will have everything ready so that we can finish in ample time for your lunch appointment.

She tells him this while she is scanning his face, again making sure that she is exuding sincerity.

Mr. McPherson: Andrea, thanks for taking a minute to be with me. I'm sure Ann will take good care of me. I will be ready when you come back. I wonder, though, can I call my office and let them know the situation?

Andrea: Certainly. Let me get our portable telephone, so you don't have to get up [moving the overheard light and getting the phone].

Just as Andrea begins her assessment, Dr. Joy comes into the room.

Dr. Joy: Hi, Mr. McPherson, it's good of you to be so patient with us. I'm certain Andrea will do everything she can to get your treatment completed thoroughly in comfort and in a reasonable timeframe. If there is anything we can do for you, let me know. I'll stop in before you leave.

The treatment continues. Julie and Ann did what they needed to do to minimize Mr. McPherson's stress. Andrea reassured him that they can get quite a bit accomplished, and Dr. Joy appreciated his patience and understanding. Mr. McPherson felt he was treated well. His needs were recognized, options were provided, comfort was ensured, and he was made to feel like he was the integral person to several successful outcomes.

Which elements of this case demonstrate effective communication?

Jorges Selinta, a dental hygienist employed in a periodontal practice, is attentive to his patients. After a patient is greeted by the receptionist and made comfortable, Jorges appears to prepare her for treatment. Jorges greets her warmly, politely using her surname, and asks about her preparedness for the appointment. Jorges observes the patient as she walks toward the room. He notes any particular postural or gait issues that might foretell problems getting into the chair. While walking back to the room, Jorges may assist the patient if he notes gait issues by allowing his patient to hold his arm for stability while he guides her to the treatment room. Once there, he helps the patient into the chair and makes sure that she is comfortably settled in before proceeding. Then, after ensuring that he is at the patient's eye level, Jorges asks her questions about her health and any concerns she has.

What does Jorges do that sets him apart from other professionals? He is actively involved with his patients, which is, perhaps, the key dimension in effective communication. Active involvement means being *in* communication *with* another. It does not mean communicating *to* another. The "*in*" communication denotes empathy for another person. Rapport is established.

KEY TERMS

attending	director	listening	relator
behavioral styles	distance	observing	social distance
communication	empathy	personal distance	socializer
cultural competence	intimate distance	public distance	thinker
cultural sensitivity	jargon	rapport	

LEARNING OUTCOMES

After reading this chapter the student will be able to:

1. Recognize that effective communication skills can be learned.
2. Identify the stages in the acquisition of new skills: knowledge, interest, belief, commitment, practice, and habituation.
3. Distinguish among the three key attributes of effective communication: listening, observing, and attending.
4. Explain the function of space, time, culture, context, and language in the establishment of rapport.
5. Identify and explain the importance of core nonverbal behaviors such as facial expression, body language, and eye contact.
6. Explain and demonstrate key elements of deepening rapport: empathy, respect, warmth, concreteness, genuineness, and self-disclosure.
7. Become a better communicator by providing positive feedback, using "I" messages, and practicing active listening.
8. Evaluate with discernment the principles of communication.
9. Explain how a patient's behavioral style influences the communication process.

Communication poses many frustrating challenges. Unclear communication can be unproductive and sometimes offensive. Clear communication is difficult to achieve at times but is ultimately satisfying to all parties involved.

The purpose of this chapter is to foster better understanding of the art of communication in both professional and personal relationships. Effective, healthy, forthright, and clear communication is the catalyst used to establish, maintain, and enhance relationships, wherever they may be found.

Self-Evaluation

Figure 5-1 lists 10 questions to consider about communication. This survey has no right or wrong answers. Individuals should read each question in the context of their natural communication style and circle the number corresponding to the degree that best describes them. The score is derived as follows: points are totaled and divided by 10. A score lower than 2.5 is associated with a successful communication style. However, a score of 4.5 and greater suggests a need to pay particular attention to the concepts in this chapter and to practice the lessons that follow with a peer. A score between 2.5 and 4.5 is typical. However, as the score approaches 4.5, more attention is required to an individual's communication style.

After completing this brief questionnaire, readers should review their responses and ask, "How do I know this is true?" Capturing examples and feelings can bring personal insight to behavior that can pave the way for change.

Working Definition

Adler and Towne state the following[1]:

> . . . all that ever has been accomplished by humans and all that ever will be accomplished involves communication with others. Many social and organizational problems derive from unsatisfactory relationships brought about by inadequate communication between people.

Communication is a process between at least two people beginning with one person's desire to convey some information to another. It originates as a mental image, such as a picture, idea, thought, or emotion. However, what is communicated is not always what was intended.

Effective communication is dynamic; that is, messages and images flow almost instantaneously between the sender and the receiver. Communication involves a vast range of sounds, words, pictures, and gestures; some are clearly articulated and some are perceived only subtly. A message stated in one context may be perceived differently in another context. The context of the dental office generates a message of its own. The office context can include the colors chosen for a treatment room, the textures of fabric for the chair in the reception room, the paintings hanging on the wall, or the dental instruments on the tray.

Both nonverbal and verbal actions relay important messages. Sometimes these messages are misunderstood.

Steps toward Changing Communication Behaviors

INFLUENTIAL COMMUNICATORS: MODELS FOR LEARNED COMMUNICATION

Can a person really learn how to communicate more effectively, or is it a skill that is predominantly inborn? Actually, the skills pertaining to effective communication can be learned. Helen Keller—a girl unable to hear, see, or speak—became an influential figure in the twentieth century. She was able to communicate using tactile and kinetic symbols and acquired speech. Her writings were published. Helen Keller still influences the lives of many people who are living with physical challenges today.

1. Is it difficult for you to talk comfortably with other people?

1	2	3	4	5	6
It is very easy for me.					It is very difficult for me.

2. Are you aware of how your tone of voice may affect others?

1	2	3	4	5	6
I am conscious of my tonality.					I am not aware at all.

3. Is it difficult for you to accept constructive criticism from others?

1	2	3	4	5	6
It is not a problem.					I do not do well with it at all.

4. When you are working with a patient, are you able to put yourself in his or her shoes?

1	2	3	4	5	6
I do so all the time.					What shoes?

5. Do you become uncomfortable when a patient asks you a difficult question?

1	2	3	4	5	6
Not at all					Usually

6. Do you find yourself becoming impatient with people who don't seem to understand what you are trying to explain?

1	2	3	4	5	6
I am very patient.					I get really frustrated.

7. Do your patients and other team members listen to you when you are talking?

1	2	3	4	5	6
I believe that others listen to me.					Many times I feel as if I am not heard.

8. In conversation with a patient, can you tell the difference between what a person is saying and what that person may be feeling?

1	2	3	4	5	6
Yes, readily.					I usually misperceive.

9. In conversation, do you let the other person finish talking before responding to what he or she says?

1	2	3	4	5	6
Always					Never happens

10. Generally, are you able to trust others?

1	2	3	4	5	6
Almost always					Almost never

FIGURE 5-1
Self-evaluation of communication skills.

Mother Teresa of Calcutta is another example—a small woman of immense stature who communicated her message of love for the poor through the use of her physical size, actions, and deeds without a lot of words. She was and still is the symbol of the powerful message she delivered to the world.

Think, too, of Stephen Hawking, the renowned physicist who has been confined to a wheelchair because of a motor neuron disease (amyotrophic lateral sclerosis [ALS]) and yet has been hailed as the most brilliant theoretical physicist since Einstein. In 1985 after finishing the first draft of his best-selling book, *A Brief History of Time,*[9] Hawking developed pneumonia, resulting in a tracheotomy that removed his ability to speak. Although Hawking is neither able to move his body nor speak except through a synthesized program, he continues to communicate effectively to audiences on the issues of time and space.

Thousands of inspirational stories attest to the courage of the human spirit and show how, given the determination, time, and practice, anyone can become more effective in communication.

COMMUNICATION ASSETS

Considering the examples previously mentioned, are seeing, hearing, vocalizing, and moving essential to communication? Obviously, the answer is no, but they make communication a lot easier. Some basic physical structures are helpful to the communication process: ears, complete with intact inner ear structures; a larynx with a functional set of vocal chords; eyes, with the attending rods, cones, and nerve endings; and an intact set of neural pathways with an alert and conscious brain. The ability to move arms, hands, fingers, head, shoulders, or the whole body helps create gestures to support (or not support) verbal communication.

Assuming that the physical structures used to communicate are intact and fully functioning, what can improve communication skills? The following model is helpful; it has been used to explain how behaviors are learned. This model suggests an upward, stepwise approach toward communication. The first step is acknowledgment of the need for change. The next step is a willingness to act on this knowledge. The desire to act and improve one's communication skills must be a conscious decision.

> *Note*
> Improving a skill may mean "unlearning" an old skill. In other words, an existing behavior may need to be replaced with a new behavior.

UNLEARNING POOR COMMUNICATION HABITS

Improving a skill may mean "unlearning" an old skill. In other words, an existing behavior may need to be replaced with a new behavior. For example, to improve communication skills, a shy person might try to make direct eye contact, a difficult task for such a person. In a different example, when someone makes sounds while speaking that others find distracting to the conversation, this individual first must become aware of the distracting habit so that effective communication can be maintained. Figure 5-2 is a model for communication, listing the steps to better communication.

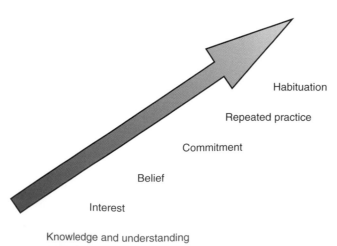

Habituation

Repeated practice

Commitment

Belief

Interest

Knowledge and understanding

FIGURE 5-2
Model for communication enhancement.

RECOGNIZING THE NEED FOR BETTER COMMUNICATION

Recognizing when communication skills need improvement is an important first step. Patients' facial expressions may communicate, "What in the world are you talking about?" A child's blank stare may say, "You're not making sense again." Rolling of the eyes may indicate a lack of communication.

Communication breakdown may occur when either the right message is not sent or the right message is sent in an unclear manner, whether by spoken words, written words, or gestures. Communication requires constant monitoring to ensure that the receiver of the message is indeed receiving the correct message.

INTEREST

Mere recognition of a communication breakdown is not enough to inspire a change in communication tactics. Interest is also required. Individuals must intensify their interest in how others perceive their communication message.

A realistic assessment of communication skills is necessary in different settings, under different conditions, and with different people. What are the strengths and weaknesses of an individual's communication skills?

BELIEF

Believing in positive results is necessary for anyone desiring to change a behavior. Belief reflects personal values. Where communication is concerned, values of family, satisfaction in work, good friendships, and professional growth are critical.

COMMITMENT

Commitment describes a pledge of devotion to something. Verbalizing the intent to improve communication states a person's commitment. The next step is preparation for action.

ACTION

Action is the quantum leap in the acquisition of new skills or the enhancement of old skills. All the knowledge, interest, belief, and commitment mean little without action. Being proactive may include the purchase of a book on more effective communication, a request for input from colleagues, a request for feedback from a spouse, a request for the supervisor to restate the intended message, or the checking up on children to see whether they followed instructions.

REPEATED ACTION AND HABITUATION

Effective change demands practice. Performing a new skill once does not ensure mastery. Every interaction is an opportunity to practice new skills. Conscious attention to the need for change and method of change will help.

Key Elements of Communication

5-1
5-4
to
5-7

Using four key elements of communication ensures effective communication and supports the development of working relationships. These important ingredients are **listening,** observing, **attending,** and understanding **behavioral styles.** The first three interrelated behaviors occur almost simultaneously in an effective interpersonal exchange. The fourth element, understanding behavioral styles to enhance communication, comes from experience with the person with whom an individual is communicating, with consideration given to the needs and desires of the other person.

LISTENING

A patient may say to a dental staff member who has poor communication skills, "You are not listening to me," or "You didn't hear a thing I said." Sometimes patients speak softly, and some sounds are not heard as clearly as others. Low-pitch sounds tend to fade. Soft voices compete with background "noise." On the other hand, excitement results in a loud speaking voice. The noise is so profound that the other person is unable to hear what is being said. Listening and speaking are inextricably linked, and both are important elements in effective communication.

OBSERVING AND ATTENDING

Listening well is an art. For example, Sally, a dental hygienist and an effective listener, attends to the speaker. She acknowledges the person's comments with a nod of her head or by verbally rephrasing what she believes the other person has said. In doing so, Sally engenders warmth and empathy. She watches her communication partners, looks at their eyes, and stands far enough back to observe their posture. Sally knows when she has been heard. If she believes that she has not been heard, then she asks for comments. She chooses easily understood words and ensures that the background noise is not overwhelming. Her

gestures support her words, but she makes certain not to be overbearing with them. Her colleagues leave a meeting believing with certainty that they were heard. Sally builds relationships.

Understanding Behavioral Styles

Patients respond to dental situations depending on their own behavioral style. Behavioral style or type is defined as a pattern, a group of recurring habits, centering on how an individual deals with people and situations. Alessandra and O'Connor have identified four behavioral types: **director, socializer, relater,** and **thinker.**[2] When the dental hygienist begins to form a relationship with a patient, the behavioral type can be easily identified. Because each behavioral type prefers to be communicated with according to his or her type, the dental hygienist can enhance the relationship by adapting to the preferences of the individual patient (Box 5-1).

The four behavioral types are as follows:

- *Director.* This behavioral type is very determined and assertive in meeting his or her needs through directing or dominating others. They can be decisive at one end and defiant at the other. They can be perceived as results-oriented, forceful, and practical or as overbearing, insensitive, and distrusting. To communicate effectively with a *director,* the dental hygienist needs to be prepared, organized, fast-paced, and to the point. The dental hygienist needs to greet the patient in a professional and businesslike manner. The dental hygienist needs to find out what the patient wants to accomplish and what he or she wants to change. If possible, options need to be provided and the patient is allowed to make the decisions. The *director*

BOX 5-1

STRATEGIES FOR WORKING WITH THE FOUR BEHAVIORAL TYPES

Director
- Plan to be prepared, organized, fast-paced, and to the point.
- Meet these patients in a professional and businesslike manner.
- Find out what these patients hope to accomplish. What are the goals for their oral health?
- Get to the point.
- Provide options and let the patient make the decisions.
- Verify that the intention is not to waste their time.

Socializer
- Show interest in these patients. Let them talk—within limits. Show enthusiasm.
- Make introductions in a friendly and informal manner.
- Illustrate suggestions with stories, pictures, and visual stimulation.
- Summarize any details regarding treatment. Direct these patients toward mutually agreeable steps to improve oral health.
- Provide testimonials.
- Give these patients written instructions to take home.

Relater
- Personally get to know these patients.
- Approach them in a friendly, nonthreatening manner.
- Develop trust and friendship at a slow pace.
- Explain the plan to these patients so that they know what to expect.
- Do not force them into a quick decision about their care.
- Practice consistent and predictable follow-up.

Thinker
- Greet these patients cordially but with no personal or social talk.
- Ask logical, fact-oriented questions.
- If the answer to a question is not known, then attempt to find the answer and follow up.
- Emphasize logic, consistency, accuracy, and quality when describing treatment options.
- Describe the process of care in detail and how it will produce the results they seek.
- Avoid rushing these patients into making decisions.

Adapted from Alessandra T, O'Connor MJ: *People smarts,* San Diego, 1994, Pfeiffer & Co, pp 175-193.

likes to be in control, and he or she fears being taken advantage of by others.

- *Socializer.* This behavioral type is entertaining and motivated to interact with others. These patients are people oriented and like to share personal feelings and opinions. They can be perceived as invigorating or as overly subjective and superficial. To communicate effectively with the *socializer,* the dental hygienist needs to be upbeat, friendly, and complimentary. Because the *socializer* likes to talk and socialize, the dental hygienist will need to direct him or her toward the objective of the appointment. The patient responds to *feeling* words and testimonials. This type typically has so many interests that it is hard for him or her to focus. The *socializer* has a keen desire to be liked and seeks approval. Because the *socializer* finds it difficult to focus, sending written material or instructions home with this patient is prudent.

- *Relater.* This behavioral type tends to approach situations in a slow, methodical manner, ensuring known action and results. These patients tend to be very dependable and cooperative. They desire personal stability and do not like change unless it is absolutely necessary. They prefer specific, structured appointment schedules. This style can be indecisive and overly systematic, needing an increased amount of explanation before making decisions. When possible, the *relater* should be given the time to make decisions. This type of style is also extremely motivated by appreciation and positive feedback.

- *Thinker.* This behavioral type tends to be precise, reserved, and concerned about performing tasks the correct way. These patients can be creative and inquisitive, or they can be viewed as overly perfectionistic, overly demanding of themselves and others, and aloof. Patients of this type do not need a lot of social interaction. The dental hygienist should speak to them in a logical, fact-oriented manner, asking only relevant questions. The *thinker* expects the professional to be prepared, proceed quickly to the task, and explain thoroughly how and why something applies to them. They also need time to think and make decisions. Working with this style may demand patience on the part of the professional because the *thinker* likes to know all the pros and cons of a situation or treatment before he or she can make a final decision.

ESTABLISHING RAPPORT

Miller and Steinberg describe **rapport** as a state of being with mutual openness, trust, and spontaneity. Rapport is characterized by an "absence of defensiveness and freedom from censored speech."[12] Developing rapport is critical to the maintenance of effective patient management, performance of treatment, and obtaining patient compliance.

> ### Note
> Developing rapport is critical to the maintenance of effective patient management, performance of treatment, and obtaining patient compliance. Patients have a better sense of how they are being treated than they do of the quality of the actual procedures.

Patients have a better sense of how they are being treated than they do of the quality of the actual procedures.

Communication is easier in an accepting, noncritical environment. With friendships, rapport develops over time through many varied experiences. In the dental setting, the time is brief and the setting is consistently within the practice. Achieving rapport in the dental setting is demanding. How can it be achieved in a short period and in a potentially stressful environment? (See Box 5-2.)

Personal Space

The dental hygienist should find a **distance** from the other person that is neither threatening nor too distant to be heard. In his book, *The Hidden Dimension,*[8] Hall discusses four distances and their appropriateness for certain relationships. He asserts that the violation of the distance or inappropriate encroachment on another person's space results in tension.

The four zones are as follows:

1. **Intimate distance** (0 to 18 inches) is usually reserved for individuals who know one another well. An individual's physical presence tends to be powerful within this space. Trying to communicate within this proximity is extremely difficult, unless the communication conforms to or mirrors the space. Listening is hard in close proximity.

2. **Personal distance** (18 inches to 4 feet) is typically reserved for close friends. Physical presence is not a problem between them. They are able to listen attentively with seemingly little effort. (Various cultures may have different categories or definitions for personal space.)

3. **Social distance** (4 to 7 feet) is apparent when in public places. An example is the distance between groups of people in shopping malls or cafeterias. Social distance is a comfortable space between strangers. Interestingly, most restaurants, movie theaters, and many other public places do not provide this amount of space.

4. **Public distance** (more than 12 feet) suggests formality and status. However, public distance is rarely found in professional offices or public settings.

Each person has a unique need for personal space. Individuals do not like to have others "invade their space." They know when they feel encroached upon and when others are getting too close for comfort. People request tables in the backs of

> ### BOX 5-2
> #### ACHIEVING RAPPORT IN THE DENTAL SETTING
> - Understand personal space concerns:
>   - Intimate distance
>   - Personal distance
>   - Social distance
>   - Public distance
> - Be culturally sensitive.
> - Use the context appropriately.
> - Use time effectively.
> - Use language appropriately.
> - Read nonverbal cues correctly.

> ### Distinct Care Modifications
> The dental hygienist should find a distance from the other person that is neither threatening nor too distant to be heard.

restaurants to ensure added privacy. They walk around groups of people to give themselves and others more room; they push away from overwhelming hugs or pull closer when they are feeling comfortable.

In the dental setting, the professional is continually invading the patient's space. The nature of dental work does not allow for public distance. On entering the practice, the patient begins to lose personal space. When seated in the dental chair, the patient has personal space of only a few inches. To minimize tension, personal space should be reduced slowly.

★ CASE APPLICATION 5-2.1

Rapport

Jorges greets his seated patient and kneels down to achieve eye contact. Distance is close as they move to the treatment room. Jorges realizes that he will be invading the intimate space as demanded by dental treatment and wants to take some time to ensure the patient's comfort.

Patients realize that dental treatment demands close physical proximity. They are willing to tolerate this briefly until the need for more space becomes too great. Providing time between treatment phases can relieve tension during this intense encounter.

Cultural Competence and Sensitivity

The United States Census Bureau estimates that racial and ethnic minorities in the United States will make up approximately 48% of the total population by the year 2050; 14.4% will be black, 22.5% Hispanic, 9.7% Asian, 0.9% Native American, and 52.5% white.[14] The complexities associated with providing informed and sensitive health care in such a diverse society requires cultural competence on the part of the practitioner. **Cultural competence** includes developing a set of skills, attitudes, and knowledge that allows the dental hygiene practitioner to work effectively with diverse racial, ethnic, and social groups with sensitivity and responsiveness to cultural differences and according to the cultural demands of a given situation. The development of cultural competence is a life-long process requiring introspection and an appreciation for the similarities and differences among humans. It requires that dental care providers carefully examine their own cultural assumptions and identities to increase awareness of personal values and biases.[3]

Personal attributes of cultural competency articulated through the National Association for Social Work Standards for Cultural Competence in Social Work Practice apply equally to the dental hygiene practitioner and include "qualities that reflect genuineness, empathy, and warmth; the capacity to respond flexibly to a range of possible solutions; an acceptance of and openness to differences among people; a willingness to learn to work with clients from different backgrounds; an articulation and clarification of stereotypes and biases and how these may accommodate or conflict with the needs of diverse client groups; and personal commitment to alleviate racism, sexism, homophobia, ageism, and poverty."[13]

Culture plays an important role in the way people attend to one another. Some cultures are more reserved than others. **Cultural sensitivity,** as part of communication, implies an awareness of and accounting for cultural differences during human interaction. Cultures differ in dynamic ways (i.e., differences in expression, gender roles, dress, dietary intake), which can affect interpersonal communication.

> **𝒩ote**
> In developing cultural competence and sensitivity, self-assessment is an important first step in gaining perspective and encouraging the exploration of issues of prejudice and bias without judgment by others.

Linguistic differences are also a consideration. The number of individuals who speak English as a second language is increasing. Language may be only one barrier to overcome. Other considerations may include issues of gender, attitudes toward preventive medicine and dentistry, wellness and health promotion, territoriality, eye contact, nutrition, and temporal issues.

In developing cultural competence and sensitivity, self-assessment is an important first step in gaining perspective and encouraging the exploration of issues of prejudice and bias without judgment by others. The dental professional must consider family origins, culture, and beliefs and then consider how personal values may be similar or different from other groups. Spending time learning about different cultures including health beliefs, customs, rituals, and practices increases understanding. Seeking out and participating in cultural competency training sessions will provide invaluable experience.[3]

Dental office culture

A culture also exists in the dental practice. The dental environment has a language with a set of norms and customs that govern behavior and its unique physical context. The members of the staff take this culture for granted. They know their roles, their responsibilities, and their colleagues' dispositions and expectations. Practices that have maintained the same staff members for a long period become like families in which behaviors are taken for granted. Communication flows with the ease of a family gathering, and few words are necessary to make requests or explain actions.

Members of the dental culture typically share similar values. Beliefs about professionalism, family, community, well-being, and patient care are readily shared. These values are visible in the décor of the office, the information given to patients as they arrive (e.g., *Patient's Bill of Rights* [see Chapter 3]) or leave, the information posted on walls, pictures, and patient information. The culture becomes a powerful ally to the technical care of the patient when the behaviors that reflect those values are evident to patients.

Cultures do not spring into existence overnight; they must be built with care over time. Discussing the evolving culture helps focus its energies on those areas where values are in conflict or where personal action is not consistent with the values expressed. Developing a consistent practice philosophy should be an ongoing activity.

The language of the dental office culture includes unique terminology or **jargon.** This vocabulary is necessary to convey critical information among members of the professional staff. Although the dental team understands dental terminology, it can be confusing to a patient. Disease processes (such as gingivitis or periodontitis) or treatment modalities (such as pulpectomy) hold specific meaning to the professional. They may, however, convey a different meaning to the patient and may carry emotional overtones. Therefore practitioners should select words that patients will understand. Using more common terms and ensuring that the terms are understood enhance positive patient comprehension and subsequent behavioral compliance.

Context

Social conversation differs from professional conversation. Maintaining communication consistent with the context in which it takes place helps ensure active listening and enhance understanding. For example, a dental professional should not discuss items of intimate personal interest or share inappropriate jokes.

The dental team members can create the context they believe necessary to reflect their culture. How an office and its treatment rooms are decorated speaks volumes to the values that the staff members share. Cool colors create a sense of warmth and well-being. Comfortable chairs in the reception room help minimize anxiety. Appropriate reading material can help the patient focus on personal health-related interests. An orderly, clean treatment room reflects the cleanliness values of the staff members.

Time

The duration of the appointment is less important than the quality of the interaction during the visit. However, respecting the time set for an appointment helps ease patients' anxiety. Effective use of time can ease the patient into the treatment setting. A receptionist who is quick to attend to the patient can set the tone for what follows. Visiting with the patient briefly before moving to the treatment room helps stage the visit. Taking time to become acquainted with what has occurred during the interval between visits eases the transition to treatment. Effectively and judiciously suggesting the time needed to devote to a particular treatment will help frame the patient's expectations.

Zunin,[15] who writes about the importance of time, particularly short time periods, proposes that relationships grow or fail depending on what occurs in the first 4 minutes of the encounter. Zunin asserts that each new encounter has the potential to create a new relationship or enhance an existing one, regardless of age, gender, status, profession, or occupation.

Communication encounters are influenced by outside events. For example, a staff member has a fight with his spouse and is still fuming when he arrives at work. An employer misplaces a dental record she took home with her over the weekend and realizes that the file belongs to the first patient of the day. The second patient of the day is 15 minutes late, and the dental hygienist realizes she is already running behind schedule. A patient needs to make an emergency appointment although the schedule includes no available time. How these common and human experiences are expressed in the first few seconds will set the tone for the day.

The following are ways dental hygienists can make use of this time concept:

- Attend to patients quickly.
- Smile at colleagues even when it is difficult.
- Withhold criticism or derogatory comments about a colleague rather than engage in gossip.
- Open the conversation with a patient in a friendly, warm manner.

The response may be surprising. The expressed behavior in the first few seconds and minutes within an encounter can make or break the chance to establish rapport.

Language

The previous section highlighted the importance of the use of words patients understand and the avoidance of the profession's jargon. Consideration should also be given to words that may convey strong emotion to patients. Words such as *needle, drill, explore, bleed, scalpel, probe, cut,* and *oops* may result in strong emotional reactions. Although avoidance of these words is not always possible, observance and attendance to patients' responses to them can help manage the emotion. Momentary pausing in a procedure or discussion to validate the response also reduces the emotional potential.

Words that are relative or equivocal can also be confusing. Consider the phrase, "It's only a small amount of decay." The word *only* minimizes the importance of the problem, and the patient has no reference point for the word *small.* Relative words need further explanation. Being specific is a better tactic. Practitioners should break down complex thoughts and messages into smaller and understandable segments. Being clear, specific, and forthright helps build trust and compliance.

> *Distinct Care Modifications*
>
> Consideration should be given to words that may convey strong emotion to patients. Words such as *needle, drill, explore, bleed, scalpel, probe, cut,* and *oops* may result in strong emotional reactions.

Other words and expressions make people immediately defensive. When a person is contradicted, criticized, ridiculed or shamed, threatened, or lectured, the person tends to "turn off and tune out" what is being said. For example, patients are not likely to improve their toothbrushing technique based on a dental hygienist's condescending statement, "Gee, you haven't gotten it right yet."

Nonverbal Cues

Effective listening is not a passive process. It involves attendance to both verbal and nonverbal cues throughout the encounter. The sender of the message must be acknowledged. Restating words spoken in a questioning tone can enhance the meaning of what has been said. Asking open-end questions rather than closed-end questions will allow the speaker to provide more information than "yes" or "no." Nonverbal cues such as a nod of the head or the turn of one's face toward the person speaking can encourage elaboration. Responses such as "I don't understand what you mean," "Oh, I see," and "Hmmm" can also encourage a person to provide additional information.

> **Note**
>
> In normal conversation between two people, nonverbal behaviors provide almost two thirds of the total social meaning expressed by them.[10]

Although much information is transmitted through vocalization, only a limited amount of meaning about the information comes from the spoken word. Nonverbal cues fill in the blank spaces. Greeting the patient with a firm handshake, good eye contact, and a genuine smile evokes confidence within the patient for the dental hygienist (Figure 5-3). Tilting the head toward the communication partner elicits attention, whereas tilting it away lessens the demand for attention. Arm and hand gestures provide considerable information about the importance of the message. Too many gestures are bewildering, and gestures that appear to be incongruous with what is being said can be confusing. The dental hygienist providing feedback while looking out the window shows a lack of interest in the patient.

Facial expressions tend to provide the most information about people's attitudes, beliefs, and emotions. Knapp suggests that in normal conversation between two people, nonverbal behaviors provide almost two thirds of the total social meaning expressed by them.[10] And Ekman states that "the primary emotions of anger, sadness, happiness, surprise, fear, and disgust are communicated by means of facial expression that are quite uniform across cultures."[4,5]

Becoming reasonably adept at the understanding of body language and facial cueing is an important skill in the professional setting, particularly when the ability to obtain patients' verbal responses is often difficult. The concept of verbal-nonverbal congruity is essential to understanding. Congruity implies that a patient's nonverbal response supports or is in alignment with what is vocalized. For example, a dental hygienist asks, "Is this hurtful to you?" The patient replies, "No!" but the patient's fingers may be wrapped tightly on the arm of the chair and the patient is wincing. These nonverbal cues suggest incongruity (Figure 5-4).

Of all the nonverbal cues, eye contact is perhaps the most important and the most difficult to sustain over long periods. Ekman and Friesen suggest that the average length of eye contact in an interpersonal setting lasts about 3 seconds.[5] The speaker usually maintains eye contact twice as long as the listener. As the distance between people increases, so will eye contact.

Eye contact is also cultural. People from more introverted cultures tend to display less eye contact.[5] Eye contact is also gender based; women tend to gaze into space more than men and more quickly avoid mutual eye contact. Eye contact, according to Ekman and Friesen, regulates verbal communication, reflects interest in what is being discussed, mediates and helps build rapport, expresses emotions, reflects status, and reflects personal characteristics.[5] Maintaining eye contact is particularly important in the dental environment because of the use of personal protective barriers. Facemasks worn during treatment prevent the patient from observing the dental hygienist's smile. Therefore the expression in a dental hygienist's eyes is a critical asset to the development of rapport.

Regulating Verbal Communication

The clues are obvious when a person becomes disinterested in a conversation and stops listening. The person's eyes glaze over and begin drifting away. As this happens, the dental hygienist may wonder whether the person is confused or simply not paying attention. Was the patient upset by something that was said? Was the dental hygienist using words that were not understood? Was the dental hygienist's rate of speaking too fast? Is the patient tired? Answers to these questions will affect the outcome of the interaction.

Reflecting Interest in the Discussion

Dental hygienists have the challenge of conveying instructions with interest for mundane tasks. For example, when providing toothbrushing instructions to a teenager, a dental hygienist may observe the teenager's lack of eye contact or fidgeting. As the patient's eyes glaze over, the importance of the message is lost. The dental hygienist relays this information frequently; however,

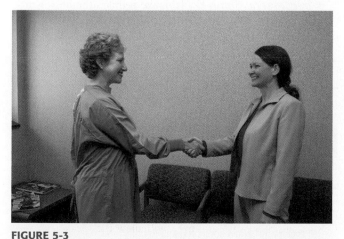

FIGURE 5-3
The dental hygienist greets a patient with a firm handshake, good eye contact, and a genuine smile.

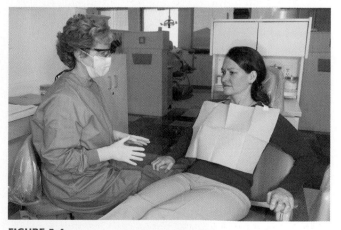

FIGURE 5-4
Patient is displaying discomfort through nonverbal cues.

expressing it with interest is more effective. The patient's continued focused gaze and nodding head suggest interest and attention. Only time will tell whether that interest leads to commitment and subsequent action. The dental hygienist should try to enhance the patient's interest by sitting at eye level to the patient and focusing on the conversation while the patient is talking. The dental hygienist should avoid turning away from the patient during an explanation by the patient. This nonverbal communication reflects a lack of interest on the part of the dental hygienist (Figure 5-5).

Expressing Emotion

A common saying is, "The eyes are the windows to the soul." This adage is true in the dental office. Expression in the eyes tells the dental staff how the patient is feeling. Pupils constricting and eye muscles tightening are evidences of pain. The dental hygienist should observe the patient's eyes while explaining the treatment planned for the day, particularly when using words such as *drill, needle, prophylaxis, decay,* or *gingivitis* or the phrase, "This may hurt a little." The dental hygienist should immediately pause, identify, and attempt to assuage negative emotions.

Reflecting Status and Describing Personal Characteristics

Extroverted, more self-confident people tend to be more direct in their eye contact than those who are introverted and more self-conscious. Authority figures tend to maintain eye contact. People who are in trouble or frightened look away.

The previous statements are generalizations. However, recognition of these characteristics within the dental practice may be helpful. Some patients like to be in control. Their eyes are penetrating, which may make others, including dental staff members, uncomfortable. Dental professionals can deal with this lack of comfort by taking a deep breath while maintaining eye contact.

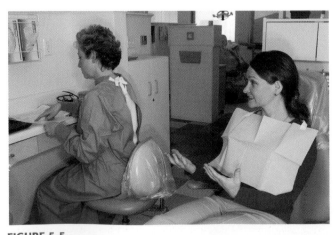

FIGURE 5-5
Physically turning away from the patient during the conversation reflects a lack of interest in the patient.

DEEPENING RAPPORT AND ESTABLISHING ONGOING RELATIONSHIPS

In 1975, George Gazda and his colleagues presented information on the importance of six interpersonal skills needed to create and enhance positive relationships: they are empathy, respect, warmth, concreteness, genuineness, and self-disclosure.[6] More than 30 years later, these skills are more important than ever. Practicing them deepens the hygienist-patient relationship. The following text provides a description of and practice scenarios for these techniques.

RESPONDING WITH EMPATHY

Empathy means a deep understanding of another person's feelings, thoughts, or attitudes. In the dental setting, empathy is often shared among team members. For example, one team member displays emotions, which others recognize, label, and respond to appropriately. Empathy also should be present in the treatment room. For example, a dental hygienist demonstrates empathy by pausing to reassure a patient who is gripping the arms of the dental chair.

In addition to attending to patients, dental hygienists must also be conscious of themselves and their environment.

Example of Effective Communication: Empathy

A comment to a seemingly anxious co-worker demonstrates empathy: "Mary, you seem so upset about misplacing Mr. Randolph's chart. Let me help you look for it. Where should we begin to look?" This comment shows concern for Mary's feelings and a willingness to help her resolve the problem. The following statements demonstrate empathy among dental office team members and patients:

- *Hygienist to receptionist:* Boy, am I tired today. My son was up all night with a fever. I finally got the fever down, and he fell asleep. My sitter was able to come over early, but I don't know how things are going to work out this afternoon. What words could be used to describe the hygienist's feelings?
- *Hygienist to dentist:* Dr. Jankowski, this is the fourth time someone has misplaced Mr. Randolph's charts. How in the world does something like this happen in this office? I thought we had a good system for chart management. We should have a meeting on this. What do you think? What words could be used to describe the hygienist's feelings?

DEMONSTRATING RESPECT

Respect is not automatic; it is earned. Respect for the skills of others on the dental team involves verbal acknowledgment of tasks well performed and other non–work-related activities that help create the desired office culture. Respect is earned when patients are greeted in a timely manner, treated with utmost sensitivity, and listened to empathetically. Gossip and lack of interest diminish respect.

Example of Effective Communication: Respect

The following statements demonstrate ways in which the dental team members can demonstrate respect among themselves and toward their patients:

- *Hygienist to patient:* Mr. Brownstein, I am delighted to see that your oral hygiene has improved since your last visit. You have been able to maintain a plaque-free condition, and your gums look super. You have really spent time with your brush and floss these past 3 months, haven't you?

   What has the hygienist said to demonstrate respect?

- *Hygienist to patient:* Hi, Tommy! I'm so happy to see you again. How is that throwing arm doing? Your mom told me that you were getting ready to play first base on your T-ball team. Sounds exciting, good for you! Let me sit down to get a good look at you so I can see that handsome smile of yours.

   What has the hygienist said to demonstrate respect?

- *Dentist to hygienist:* Maria, I am delighted with the progress of the Martin family's oral hygiene. The whole family seems to have taken your instructions very well. Now that they are responding, I am sure even more can be done for them if other members of the team can get involved. Why don't you get the group together to discuss this and report back at our next regularly scheduled office meeting?

   What has the dentist said to demonstrate respect?

EXPRESSING EMOTIONAL WARMTH

Warmth is actively demonstrated through facial expression, gestures, and touch. As the dental team members become more comfortable with one another, they more readily disclose their beliefs and thoughts.

Touch is one of the most sensitive means of communication, conveying feelings impossible to express verbally. A light touch on someone's arm during a heated exchange demonstrates understanding and eases tension. A firm hand on the back of a frail patient engenders reassurance.

Example of Effective Communication: Emotional Warmth

How could the dental hygienist demonstrate warmth in the following situations?

1. While the hygienist is cleaning his teeth, an adult patient suddenly digs his hands into the sides of the chair and his eyes become closed tight.

2. A patient is arguing with the receptionist. Both people are standing by the counter. Neither seems to be listening to the other.

3. One of the dental assistants in the office was visibly upset by a particularly difficult procedure. Now she is about to set up the hygienist's treatment room. The hygienist's patient is waiting.

4. A 10-year-old boy is squirming in the chair. He is restless but not belligerent.

BEING DIRECT

The possibility of misperceiving, mistaking, misrepresenting, misstating, and misunderstanding is always present. These errors usually occur as a result of incomplete, insufficient, or unclear information. It is important to use language consistent with the level of understanding of the patient. Providing new information in small amounts helps patients listen. Giving examples and showing pictures or models reinforce the verbal messages and make difficult concepts more understandable. For example, a straightforward, stepwise approach helps ensure patient compliance with oral hygiene techniques. Dental hygienists should start at the beginning and "walk" the patient through the experience. Asking the patient to demonstrate the behavior in the dental office allows for correction of any mistaken ideas.

BEING CONCRETE

In a similar manner, being clear and precise with each dental team member helps enhance the team member's job performance. Clarity of expression also promotes a healthy work culture. For example, when asked where Mr. Randolph's chart is located, a dental hygienist could respond with a precise location rather than stating, "It's somewhere in the treatment room."

Example of Effective Communication: Being Direct and Concrete

The following statements help demonstrate how the patient and dental team member can be direct and concrete:

- *Patient to hygienist:* I have been coming to see you on a regular basis for the past 2 years, but my gums are still bleeding. Do you think I should be using a different toothbrush or brushing a new way?

   What should the hygienist say? What should he or she do?

- *Hygienist to dental assistant:* Mary is really a pill today. I've never seen her so worked up! If we don't get her under control, we'll have our hands full for the rest of the day. She is going to drive us all crazy.

   What could the hygienist do to find out what is bothering Mary? What words might the hygienist choose to ensure that Mary hears and understands?

BEING GENUINE

Each person is unique. Dental hygienists each carry his or her own special set of values, beliefs, attitudes, likes, dislikes, wishes, and dreams. Sharing them appropriately with patients and colleagues helps build an interpersonal rapport.

Humans are fallible, and dental hygienists are, of course, no exception. Making mistakes and learning from them is an important part of life. Dental staff members should not feel obligated to hide errors but rather to be genuine, admitting errors and finding remedies as soon as possible.

Being genuine also demands caring about the whole person; the patient's general health and health of the patient's family is critical. Dental hygienists should be interested in the work patients do, where they live, what schools they attend, what they like to do for recreational activities, and what they do not like. They should respect patients' intelligence and their ability to make choices. Dental hygienists should recognize they are not superior to patients but simply have an expertise different from that of their patients.

Example of Effective Communication: Being Genuine

The following statements help demonstrate ways in which the patient and dental team member can be genuine in their interactions:

- *Patient to hygienist:* Did you know that every time I make an appointment here, I am kept waiting? It's not your fault, but I get so frustrated and you know how stressed I get about being here anyway.

  What could the hygienist say to the patient to let her know that the hygienist is empathetic and genuine?

- *Hygienist to patient:* The dental hygienist observes that the patient has not followed any of the oral hygiene instructions. His oral condition has significantly deteriorated since his last visit. The patient has been provided with ample instruction and feedback in the past.

  How should the hygienist introduce this observation? What words could the hygienist use to demonstrate the extent of the problem? What other communication aids might be useful?

PRACTICING SELF-DISCLOSURE

In his book, *Of Human Interaction,* Luft suggests that openness engenders openness in others.[11] Openness is a reciprocal and dynamic experience. Sharing a tale of joy or sorrow inspires others to share similar stories.

Establishing relationships in the practice community introduces the opportunity and risk of exposing the true self. For example, sharing too much personal information too quickly may be somewhat disconcerting to others. Therefore the level of existing and growing trust in the practice setting governs the rate at which patients and dental professionals share personal information.

Example of Effective Communication: Self-Disclosure

The following statements help demonstrate ways in which the dental team member and patient can disclose personal information to facilitate communication:

- *Patient to hygienist:* Mary, I am so glad you are my dental hygienist. You always seem to care about me. You know,

when I was younger I was really very scared of going to the dentist. Now I'm not fearful at all.

  How could the hygienist share personal experiences with this patient?

- *Patient to hygienist:* Time is so crucial for me. I'm pleased that this office respects that. Some offices keep you waiting forever. Life is so hectic nowadays, and I always feel so rushed.

  How could the hygienist share personal experiences with this patient?

- *Pediatric patient to hygienist:* This is a neat place. You have some great stuff for me to play with while I'm waiting. I really like the Legos.

  How could the hygienist share personal experiences with this patient?

Developing these skills helps deepen the rapport between the dental team members and their patients. Carefully providing feedback, actively listening, and using appropriately framed "I" messages that are complemented by congruent nonverbal cues of facial expression, gestures, and touch enhance relationships.

PROVIDING FEEDBACK USING THE "I" MESSAGE

Critical to a healthcare professional's success is the ability to provide personal and professional feedback effectively. Feedback should both enhance relationships and correct problems. The term *feedback* is borrowed from the early days of rocket engineering when an intricate feedback loop was designed to control rocket operations.

Feedback occurs constantly in a variety of situations. In the professional environment, feedback occurs either among members of the dental team or between the dental professional and patient. For example, the dental hygienist is discussing a new concept in oral hygiene practice, and the dental assistant wants a more detailed description. The dental hygienist stops and provides the description. Another example is a patient interrupting the practitioner's presentation on toothbrushing techniques to ask a question about a new mechanical brush she has heard about. The dental hygienist stops talking about toothbrushing techniques and discusses the benefits of these devices.

This exchange of information has all the risks involved in any other communication. The following guidelines are useful in adequately providing feedback in the professional setting (Box 5-3):

- *Consider the needs of others.* Although this maxim sounds relatively easy, it is among the most difficult guidelines to follow. Often the dental hygienist is so intent on the procedure that the patient's needs are inadvertently ignored. Instructions on oral health should consider the patient's frame of reference. How knowledgeable is the patient about dental disease and the ability to control it? Does he seem to care? What values drive the patient to better oral health? Is she concerned more with function than cosmetics? How do his cultural values affect his behavior? What emotions are expressed during the discussion on oral self-care? How can the dental hygienist assuage negative emotion? Is the dental hygienist choosing words that are ap-

---

BOX 5-3

PROVIDING FEEDBACK

- Consider the needs of others.
- Avoid using jargon.
- Use straightforward language to describe only the patient's behaviors—not attitudes, beliefs, or faults—when attempting to interpret them.
- Focus on behaviors that can be changed.
- Be specific.
- Wait for feedback to be solicited.
- Be nonjudgmental.

- Provide feedback immediately after the behavior has been exhibited.
- Allow freedom to change or not to change.
- Define expectations.
- Specify the value of the acquisition of the new behavior in real terms.
- Structure the skill in manageable steps.
- Coach for success.
- Provide rewards for successful outcomes.
- Express feelings directly.

---

propriate to the patient's level of knowledge? The dental professional should begin with the patient's frame of reference. If the professional has truly taken the time to understand the patient's background, emotion, and level of understanding, then the interaction should be successful. Emotion can make or break the success of an interaction. When patients are feeling anxious or fearful, they will not fully attend to instructions.

- *Avoid using jargon.* Dental staff members should use words the patient understands. Although patients may be impressed with the dental vocabulary of the dental professional, it often interferes with successful feedback. Less complicated words facilitate understanding.

- *Use straightforward language to describe only the patient's behaviors—not attitudes, beliefs, or faults—when attempting to interpret them.* Dental hygienists should be descriptive rather than interpretive. Visual aids may help descriptions. Examples help clarify answers to questions.

- *Focus on behaviors that can be changed.* Attempting to help patients overcome unsurpassable obstacles is frustrating. Breaking large-scale changes into smaller, achievable steps will enhance the patient's ability to acquire the new skill. The change will probably not be immediate. Acquiring fine motor skills related to effective flossing, for example, takes time and practice similar to changing one's diet. The professional has to consider whether the patient can adopt the new behavior, identify the patient's interest level in changing behavior, and determine whether the patient will practice the new behavior.

- *Be specific.* Using vague descriptions and explanations will not be helpful. Patients' questions should be thoroughly answered within the practitioner's knowledge base. This approach is particularly important with young patients. The more specific and direct the dental hygienist is with children, the better they will follow direction.

- *Wait for feedback to be solicited.* When possible, the practitioner should wait for the patient to make the first move. A first move may be as simple as the question, "What should I do?" However, the feedback may be solicited without words, such as a quizzical look or confused frown. These nonverbal cues can be used to advance discussion and instruction.

- *Be nonjudgmental.* Patients flee from criticism. They are willing to hear the bad news but do not want to be judged as being bad. Focusing on behavior, skills, and conditions in understandable language with gentle tones allows patients to remain open to the communication. Harsh criticism is an obstacle to communication and rapport. Defensive patients will not respond well to instruction or advice.

- *Provide feedback immediately after the behavior has been exhibited.* Flossing skills can be taught and evaluated in the dental office. Immediately providing feedback corrects any errant flossing behaviors before they become habitual. Allowing too much time to intervene between the behavior and the feedback diminishes learning potential.

- *Allow freedom to change or not to change.* Most dental professionals probably have strong beliefs about oral hygiene and oral health. Understandably, they desire positive outcomes from patient education. However, patients will typically behave in ways that are comfortable to them. They may not want to change their behaviors in the direction prescribed. The patient always has choices, and these choices should be honored. However, to maximize the chance of changing patients' oral health and hygiene behaviors, the following guidelines are recommended:

1. *Define expectations.* Dental personnel should be explicit and help the patient set goals relative to the expectations. Patients should participate in setting these goals.

2. *Specify the value of the acquisition of the new behavior in real terms.* Dental hygienists may want to discuss what will happen to the patient's dentition without a behavioral change. Contrasting the consequence of no change in the behavior with the adoption of the new or different technique may be a helpful persuasive tool. Pictures, diagrams, or models may enhance the discussion.

3. *Structure the skill in manageable steps.* Breaking down instruction into manageable steps makes it easier for the patient to follow.

4. *Coach for success.* Positive feedback, "I" statements that reflect success and approval, specific feedback during

the learning process, and continuing support are effective coaching techniques.

5. *Provide rewards for successful outcomes.* Meeting a challenge provides its own internal reward. A small token may help reinforce the new behavior. It can be something as simple as a certificate showing successful completion of an oral self-care program, including the name of the patient and signature of dentist or dental hygienist.

6. *Express feelings directly.* Using "I" messages allows ownership of feelings without excessive emotionality. The listener's feedback will determine what is said next. Expressing feelings to patients may be more difficult, but appropriate phrasing and avoidance of harsh criticism should help.

The concept of active listening and the use of "I" messages is best described in a book written by Thomas Gordon and published in 1970. In the book, *Parent Effectiveness Training,* and its several sequels, Gordon presents a very powerful model for communicating with children and adults.[7] This model is particularly useful when the message that needs to be conveyed is negative or unpleasant. Gordon challenges the senders of messages to focus on themselves as the *owners* of the attending feelings, rather than on the explicit behavior of the other person. The "I" message contains the following four components:

1. Description of the unpleasant or uncomfortable behavior
2. Statement of the feelings concerning the effects of the unpleasant behavior
3. Description of the consequences of the behavior
4. Statement of the request or preference

In the professional setting, unpleasant behavior may relate to a patient's continual refusal to floss after meals, or it may relate to the receptionist's unwillingness to avoid scheduling a supportive care appointment during the hygienist's lunch break.

In brief, the "I" message reads as follows:

• *When I . . .* —Dental professionals should state the unpleasant feeling, behavior, or situation and condition. For example, "When I look into your mouth and see all the plaque accumulated around your teeth and your gums bleeding as I probe around them, I . . .

• *I feel* (or sense, experience, believe, understand, think) *. . .* —Dental professionals should state what is felt, experienced, believed, understood, or thought. For example, "I feel worried."

• *Because . . .* —Dental professionals should state the consequences of the feeling, behavior, situation, or condition. For example, "I am at a loss as to what else we can do. Perhaps we can use a different technique and use some mechanical devices."

• *I prefer that . . .* or *It would be helpful to me if . . .* —Dental professionals should state the alternative action. For example, "I prefer that you use dental floss after every meal."

Examples of Effective Communication: "I" Messages

Dr. Felix Hertz has a habit of always picking the same person to lead the discussion on office morale, thus arousing feelings of discomfort in that individual. In such a situation, the "I" message may take the following form:

1. "Dr. Hertz, when you ask me to get the discussion started on staff morale…"
2. "I really feel uncomfortable and anxious…"
3. "It puts me in a very difficult position with everyone else. I believe that they think I have the answer to everything. This makes me very uncomfortable."

"I" statements are helpful in dealings with sensitive issues. Giving positive "I" messages also builds relationships.

When a patient has been particularly successful with her oral hygiene, the dental hygienist might say, "Jane, I am very excited about the progress you have been making with your plaque control. There is quite a difference in your oral health from a month ago. You are making real progress."

> ### *Note*
> "I" messages facilitate team cohesiveness, enhance compliance behaviors, and reinforce the behavior. An example is showing appreciation for assistance given by one of the staff members: "Mary, I really appreciate that you were able to fill in for me last week. It made life a lot easier for my family."

✦ CASE APPLICATION 5-1.2

The Use of "I" Messages

The dental team in the scenario at the beginning of the chapter used "I" messages. The patient, Mr. McPherson, is on time for his scheduled appointment, but the hygienist is 30 minutes behind schedule. The entire dental team takes the time to express their thoughts and feelings to Mr. McPherson to help ensure a positive outcome in a potentially stressful situation.

Active listening expands the "I" message concept. Active listening involves the taking of positive steps to ensure correct interpretation of the speaker's words. In other words, active listening conveys to the speaker the knowledge that the listener understands what the speaker is saying. (Nonverbal cues for effective listening are discussed earlier in this chapter.)

Although these aids encourage communication, dental hygienists may find the following two specific behaviors especially helpful:

1. *Paraphrase to reflect understanding.* After patients ask their questions or make statements about their health, practitioners can restate these statements using their own words and asking whether they correctly understood the patients.

2. *Prepare to listen.* A little preparation for active listening helps ensure continuing high-quality communication. Two considerations are suggested: (1) Preparation includes reflection on the agenda for the meeting, review of the

cases for the day, or thoughts about what to say to a patient. (2) Distractions such as superfluous noise, clutter, and competing thoughts interfere with the attention owed to the communicating partner. The listener must also be able to see the speaker's nonverbal cues. Examples of reducing distractions include placing oneself at the eye level of a pediatric patient or moving the chair back to observe sufficiently the body language of a senior patient.

Example of Effective Communication: Paraphrasing

A patient is concerned about his new dentures becoming loose. He says, "I'm going to a fancy dinner party tonight. I know they are going to have some real special foods there, and I really like the way the hostess prepares her meals. I guess I better just stay with the soft foods, huh?" A sincere and knowing response might be, "Mr. Lentz, it sounds like you are worried that you might eat something that will loosen your new dentures. Is this the concern you have?"

As another example, a mother might ask about a procedure her child is about to undergo, "Danielle, is it common for the doctor to take out healthy teeth before placing braces?" Danielle might respond, "You seem concerned about the need to remove permanent teeth. Let's see whether Dr. Smith has a moment to talk with you about this concern."

Paraphrasing comments made by dental team members also helps keep communication on track. A receptionist said, "Every time I get a new system in place, our doctor reverts to the old one. I don't know what I have to do to train him to use the new system." Paraphrasing this statement to express understanding may reduce the tension. For example, the dental hygienist might say, "I hear that you are frustrated in getting us to adopt and manage the new filing system. It's hard for us and particularly for Dr. Fernandez to adapt to these new behaviors. Maybe I can help in the transition."

References

1. Adler R, Towne N: *Looking out/looking in,* ed 2, New York, 1978, Holt, Rinehart & Winston.
2. Alessandra T, O'Connor MJ: *People smarts,* San Diego, 1994, Pfeiffer & Co.
3. Cross T et al: *Towards a culturally competent system of care,* vol 1, monograph on effective services for minority children who are severely emotionally disturbed. Washington, DC, 1989, CASSP Technical Assistance Center, Georgetown University Child Development Center.
4. Ekman P: Facial expression. In Seigman AW, Feldstein S, eds: *Nonverbal behavior and communication,* Hillsdale, NJ, 1978, Erlbaum.
5. Ekman P, Friesen WV: Nonverbal leakage and clues to deception, *Psychiatry* 32:88-106, 1969.
6. Gazda GM et al: *Human relations development: a manual for health sciences,* Boston, 1975, Allyn and Bacon.
7. Gordon T: *Parent effectiveness training,* New York, 1970, Plume.
8. Hall ET: *The hidden dimension,* Garden City, NJ, 1969, Doubleday.
9. Hawking S: *A brief history of time,* New York, 1988, Bantam.
10. Knapp ML: *Essentials of nonverbal communication,* New York, 1980, Holt, Rinehart & Winston.
11. Luft J: *Of human interaction,* Palo Alto, Calif, 1969, Natural Press Books.
12. Miller GR, Steinberg M: *Between people: a new analysis of interpersonal communication,* Chicago, 1975, SRA.
13. NASW Standards for Cultural Competence in Social Work Practice. Prepared by the NASW National Committee on Racial and Ethnic Diversity. Available at: http://www.socialworkers.org. Accessed December 4, 2005.
14. US Bureau of the Census: *Statistical Abstract of the United States,* Washington, DC, 1995, The Bureau.
15. Zunin L: *Contact: the first four minutes,* New York, 1972, Ballantine Books.

The Body's Response to Challenge

Ann Eshenaur Spolarich

INSIGHT

The body is continually exposed to a variety of microbes, many of which are normally found in the body and others that pose a significant threat for causing infection and disease. The human body is capable of responding to these threats with a variety of complex, highly regulated processes that allow the body to rid itself of invaders and resultant infections and by facilitating repair. This chapter reviews the processes of inflammation, immune response, hemostasis, and wound healing. Normal events, as well as alterations in response and associated pathophysiology, are also discussed. Understanding these concepts is essential for the dental hygienist because these topics make up the framework of host response mechanisms critical for function and survival.

CASE STUDY 6-1   New Patient Indicates Allergy to Novocaine

A new patient schedules dental hygiene treatment and indicates that she is allergic to Novocaine on her medical history form. On questioning, the patient states that she developed hives, dizziness, and difficulty breathing after receiving an injection of dental anesthetic while undergoing restorative dental care in another office 15 years earlier. Approximately 2 years ago, she visited another dentist for emergency treatment after breaking a tooth while on vacation. She reports that she did not have any difficulty with the local dental anesthetic that she received from the second dentist. Further questioning reveals that her adverse reaction to the first local dental anesthetic was treated with "a shot of something that made my heart race. Afterward, I had to see my physician to make sure that I was all right. I never went back to that office again. I do not want any shots while I am here." Interviewing the patient also reveals an allergy to shellfish and iodine dyes.

6-1

KEY TERMS

activated partial thromboplastin
   time test
acute-phase proteins
adaptive immunity
angiogenesis
antibody
antigens
B lymphocytes
chemokines
chemotaxis
cortisol
cytokines

cytotoxic T cells
diapedesis
embolus
growth factors
helper T cells
hemostasis
hormones
immunity
immunoglobulin
immunologic tolerance
inflammation
innate immunity

International Normalized Ratio
leukocytes
leukocytosis
leukemia
leukopenia
lysosomes
margination
mediators
opsonins
opsonization
pavementing

phagocytosis
phagosome
platelets
platelet count
primary intention
prostaglandins
prothrombin time test
secondary intention
suppressor T cells
thrombus
T lymphocytes

White Blood Cells

TYPES OF WHITE BLOOD CELLS

White blood cells (WBCs), also known as **leukocytes,** are the primary elements of the body's protective response and are formed in either bone marrow or lymphoid tissues. Following are types of WBCs found in the blood:

- Polymorphonuclear neutrophils (PMNs)
- Polymorphonuclear eosinophils
- Polymorphonuclear basophils
- Monocytes
- Lymphocytes
- Plasma cells

Polymorphonuclear WBCs are also known as granulocytes because of their granular appearance and *polys* because they have multiple nuclei. WBCs are transported in the blood to areas of infection and inflammation and produce a rapid response against invasion.[16]

Granulocytes and monocytes are formed only in the bone marrow and are primarily responsible for **phagocytosis,** or the ingestion of invading organisms. These WBCs are stored within the bone marrow with three times the number of cells stored as compared with the number that circulate in the bloodstream. Granulocytes and monocytes remain stored until they are needed, with marrow stores of these cells accumulating to an equivalent of a 6-day supply. Once released from the bone marrow, granulocytes survive for 4 to 8 hours in the blood and from 4 to 5 days in the tissues, unless they are destroyed sooner during the inflammatory process.[16]

Monocytes survive for up to 10 hours in the blood before entering the tissues. At this point, monocytes are immature cells with little ability to fight invading organisms. However, on entering the tissues, monocytes swell in size and become macrophages. **Lysosomes,** which are intracellular sacs that contain toxins used during phagocytosis, fill up the cytoplasm of macrophages, enabling the macrophage to kill a variety of invaders within the tissues. Macrophages survive for months in tissues and provide the basis for ongoing tissue defense against infections. Macrophages normally die as a result of their phagocytic activity.[16]

Lymphocytes and plasma cells are produced by lymph tissues found in the lymph glands, spleen, thymus, and tonsils. Patches of lymphoid tissue can also be found throughout the body, notably underneath the epithelium in the gastrointestinal (GI) tract, known as Peyer's patches. Lymphocytes are stored in all of these tissues, with small numbers circulating in the bloodstream. Lymphocytes enter and leave the circulatory system via the lymphatic system; as a result, continuous circulation of these cells occurs. The life span of a lymphocyte ranges from weeks to months, depending on the need. Lymphocytes and plasma cells play significant roles in the immune response.

Eosinophils make up a small percentage of the total number of WBCs and play only a minor role in the body's defense against infection (Table 6-1). However, these cells proliferate in patients infected with parasites. Eosinophils destroy invading parasites by attaching to them with special surface molecules and then releasing a variety of lethal substances that kill them. These substances include hydrolytic enzymes, highly reactive forms of oxygen, and a polypeptide molecule known as the *major basic protein.*[16]

Eosinophils are more commonly known for their role in the body's allergic reaction response; mast cells and basophils release an eosinophil chemotactic factor that causes eosinophils to migrate toward inflamed tissues. Thus eosinophils are found in large numbers in the tissues where allergic reactions have occurred.[16] Typically, these sites include the tissues surrounding the lungs and in the skin. Eosinophils detoxify inflammatory substances released by mast cells and basophils and destroy allergen-antibody complexes, preventing the spread of local inflammation.[16]

Basophils are found in the circulating blood and share many similarities to mast cells, which are found outside of the capillaries. Both basophils and mast cells are associated with allergic reactions, especially those involving immunoglobulin E (IgE), which attaches itself to these cells, triggering the release of a variety of chemical mediators that produce the vascular and tissue reactions associated with allergy (see Allergy and Hypersensitivity Reactions later in this chapter). In addition, basophils and mast cells secrete heparin into the blood to prevent coagulation[16] (see Hemostasis and Blood Clotting later in this

Table 6-1	Differential White Blood Cell Count
TEST	**RANGE OF NORMAL VALUES (in percentages)**
Segmented Neutrophils	56.0
Lymphocytes	34.0
Monocytes	4.0
Bands	3.0
Eosinophils	2.7
Basophils	0.3

Modified from Wynn RL, Meiller TF, Crossley HL: *Drug information handbook for dentistry,* ed 10, Hudson, Ohio, 2005, Lexi-Comp.

chapter). Basophils comprise the smallest quantity of WBCs present in the blood (see Table 6-1).

> *Note*
> An elevated WBC count is a characteristic sign of infection and is known as **leukocytosis.**[31]

The normal quantity of WBCs in the blood is 7000 per microliter of blood, with a range from 4500 to 11,000.[45] PMNs comprise approximately 60% of the total number of WBCs, followed by lymphocytes at 30%[16] (see Table 6-1). When infection is present, the bone marrow and lymph tissues increase the production and release of leukocytes, which may elevate the WBC count to 30,000 or higher per microliter of blood.

> *Note*
> Uncontrolled production of WBCs results in **leukemia.** Cancerous mutation of either myelogenous or lymphogenous cells causes leukemia.

When the bone marrow produces few WBCs, the patient develops **leukopenia.** When the WBC count drops, bacteria that normally inhabit the body begin to invade the tissues. In as few as 2 days after the suppression of WBC production, the patient may develop mouth ulcers, ulceration of the colon, and life-threatening respiratory infections. Without medical intervention, death may occur within 1 week after total leukopenia has developed. Leukopenia is also caused by irradiation and is a rare side effect of certain medications.[45] Patients may respond favorably with transfusion and drug therapies.[16]

Lymphocytic leukemias begin in lymph tissues and spread to other parts of the body. Myelogenous leukemias begin in the bone marrow and spread throughout the body, resulting in WBC production in many organs including lymph nodes, spleen, and liver. Myelogenous leukemias exhibit two distinct presentations. First, the cancer produces cells that are partially differentiated; as a result, the cells resemble normal WBCs. These types of differentiated leukemias are labeled according to the cell types to which they most closely resemble, for example, basophilic leukemia. Second and more frequently, the leukemia cells are undifferentiated and do not in any way resemble normal WBCs. Acute leukemias are associated with undifferentiated cells and progress rapidly without treatment. Chronic leukemias are associated with more differentiated cells and develop slowly, with a disease course that often spans several decades. WBCs formed during leukemia do not provide the body with a defense against infection.[16]

DEFENSE PROPERTIES OF WHITE BLOOD CELLS

Neutrophils and macrophages exit the blood vessel by squeezing through pores, a process known as **diapedesis.** The cells become temporarily constricted as they enter the pores because the diameter of the pores is smaller than the cells. These cells normally travel through the blood and then migrate into the tissues where they are needed to fight invaders.

> *Note*
> Neutrophils and macrophages are primarily responsible for destroying invading organisms.

Macrophages that travel throughout the body in this manner are known as *mobile macrophages.*

Upon entering the tissues, neutrophils and macrophages move in a unidirectional path toward the inflamed area. Chemical substances in the tissue attract the cells to migrate in this direction, a process known as **chemotaxis.** These chemical substances include bacterial and viral toxins, inflammatory tissue by-products, reactive products from the complement cascade (e.g., C5a), products of the lipoxygenase pathway (e.g., leukotriene B_4), and reaction products associated with clotting. The concentration of these chemical substances is greatest at the source; thus chemotaxis is most effective in areas with a high concentration gradient. However, chemotaxis is still effective at up to 100 micrometers away from the site of inflamed tissue. No tissue in the body is more than 50 micrometers away from a capillary; for this reason, the body is able to mobilize large numbers of WBCs quickly and efficiently into the area.[16]

Neutrophils and macrophages destroy invading organisms through ingestion, a process known as *phagocytosis.* These cells must be able to differentiate between normal cells and structures versus invading organisms. The following three criteria assist phagocytes with selection:

1. Surface texture
2. Outer coatings
3. Recognition

First, naturally occurring structures have a smooth surface texture, which resists phagocytosis; thus the more rough or irregular the surface, the greater the susceptibility to phagocytes. Second, naturally occurring structures have protective coatings that repel phagocytes; invading organisms and dead tissues do not have these coatings. Third, antibodies against invading organisms adhere to their membranes, thus increasing their susceptibility to phagocytes. **Antibody** molecules combine with C3 molecules formed by the complement cascade and then attach themselves to receptors on the phagocyte membrane, which initiates phagocytosis. This process is called **opsonization. Opsonins** are specific proteins, such as **immunoglobulin** antibodies and plasma lectins, which are recognized by specific receptors on leukocytes.[16]

Once in the tissues, neutrophils can immediately initiate phagocytosis because they are already mature cells. They can phagocytize up to 20 bacteria before dying themselves. Neutrophils are limited by the fact that they cannot phagocytize organisms larger than bacteria. Conversely, macrophages are more powerful phagocytes and can destroy up to 100 bacteria. They can also ingest larger particles; after digestion, they often survive and function for several months.

Important to note, some bacteria possess coatings that surround and protect the organism from death by digestion via lysosomal enzymes because these enzymes cannot penetrate or destroy these coatings. Thus both neutrophils and macrophages also contain oxidizing agents that perform bactericidal actions to these coated organisms. These oxidizing agents are lethal to most bacteria.[16]

Unlike their more mobile counterparts, other macrophages become attached to tissues, where they may remain for long periods until they are stimulated by the immune system and are known as *attached* or *adherent* macrophages. They perform the same functions as other macrophages, and once stimulated, they can break away from their attachments and become mobile, respond to chemotaxis, and perform phagocytosis of large particles. Adherent tissue macrophages are found throughout the body, most notably in the skin and lungs, along the GI tract, and in the liver and spleen.[16]

Macrophages found in the skin respond to invading organisms that enter the tissue through a break in the integrity of the skin, which normally prevents such invasion. Invading organisms in the tissue that survive the local response enter into the lymph system, where they are destroyed by macrophages in the lymph nodes.

Particles that enter the lungs are engulfed by macrophages in the alveoli. If the particles are ingestible, then they are destroyed and their digestive products are released into the lymph. If the particle is not ingestible, then the macrophage forms a *giant cell* capsule that surrounds the particle until it can be dissolved. These capsules are formed around inhaled dust, asbestos, carbon particles, and tuberculosis bacilli.[16]

Macrophages are also found in the liver and destroy particles that enter the liver via the portal circulation. This system effectively prevents bacteria that enter the blood via the GI tract from entering the general circulation. If bacteria manage to enter the general circulation, then tissue macrophages in the spleen and bone marrow are able to perform phagocytosis.[16]

Inflammation

Common causes of inflammation include the following[31]:

- Trauma
- Pathogenic organisms
- Allergens
- Foreign substances
- Extreme thermal changes such as burns
- Chemical exposure

In response to injury, the body produces both vascular and cellular reactions that are mediated by a number of chemical factors. These chemicals are derived from plasma proteins or cells that are produced in response to or are activated by the inflammatory stimulus.[16,24]

Inflammation is characterized by vasodilation, increased capillary permeability, edema, clotting of fluid in the interstitial space, and migration of large numbers of granulocytes and monocytes into the tissue.[16,24] These vascular and cellular changes are associated with the following five cardinal signs of inflammation:

1. Redness (rubor) as a result of increased vascularity
2. Swelling (tumor) caused by the accumulation of fluid exudates
3. Heat (calor) as a result of increased blood flow to the area and the release of inflammatory mediators
4. Pain (dolor) as a result of the stimulation of pain receptors and nerves by inflammatory exudates and the release of chemical mediators
5. Loss of function (function laesa) from the combination of all these effects[24]

DENTAL CONSIDERATIONS

Dental hygienists assess the oral cavity for signs of inflammation associated with disease. Redness and swelling of the gingiva reflect periodontal infection caused by bacteria. These visual markers are also used to determine the extent and severity of the disease. Pain is more likely to occur with acute forms of gingivitis versus chronic forms of the disease. The absence of pain and the patient's ability to function with damaged periodontal tissues do not alert the patient to the presence of periodontal disease. Some patients will seek an oral evaluation only when chronic tissue destruction results in pain, tooth mobility, and tooth loss.

Blood clots, which are made up of fibrinogen, seal off the tissue spaces and lymphatic vessels in the inflamed area to prevent fluid from entering or exiting the tissue spaces. This mechanism helps limit the area of inflammation

and reduces the spread of infection to other parts of the body.[16]

Inflammation can be acute or chronic in nature, and the degree of severity of the response is typically proportional to the degree of tissue injury.[16] Rapid onset with a short duration of action characterizes acute inflammation. PMNs are the most common WBC associated with this type of response. Chronic inflammation exhibits longer duration, with lymphocytes and macrophages as the predominant cell types. Histologic changes associated with chronic inflammation also include the formation of new blood vessels, tissue scarring and fibrosis, and possible tissue necrosis.

When staphylococcal organisms invade the body, they stimulate a severe, rapid inflammatory response by excreting lethal endotoxins into the surrounding tissues. This inflammatory response occurs at a rate that exceeds that needed for the staphylococcal organisms to multiply and spread, which enables the body to *wall off* the organisms rapidly at the site of invasion and thus prevent them from spreading.

Conversely, endotoxins produced by streptococcal organisms do not cause the same degree of tissue damage; therefore invasion produces a lesser degree of inflammatory response. The streptococci are able to multiply and migrate before the body has a chance to wall them off. Thus streptococcal invasions are more likely to spread through the body more readily and cause severe illness and death than are staphylococcal invasions, even though the staphylococcal organisms are more destructive.[16]

DENTAL CONSIDERATIONS

Multiple species of streptococci live in the oral cavity, which is the reason the oral cavity is considered to be a distant site source of potential systemic infection. Therefore patients at increased risk for systemic disease and resultant complications caused by streptococcal organisms are often premedicated with antibiotics before dental treatment.[11] Staphylococcal organisms are predominantly found on the skin, where the intact surface poses a sufficient barrier of protection against penetration into the body. However, poor handwashing behaviors and contamination of wounds after surgical and other invasive procedures are attributed to staphylococcal invasion.

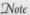 **6-2** **INFLAMMATORY EVENTS**

Vasodilation occurs in the arterioles and results in the opening of new capillary beds. These events increase local blood flow, which allows the body to bring WBCs to the area via the circulatory system. Vasodilation is caused by the effects of a variety of chemical mediators, such as histamine and nitric oxide, which produce relaxation of the smooth muscle that comprises the walls of the blood vessels. The clinical signs of increased blood flow include redness and heat[16,24] (Figure 6-1).

Next, the permeability of the microvasculature increases, and a protein-rich exudate leaks into the surrounding extravascular

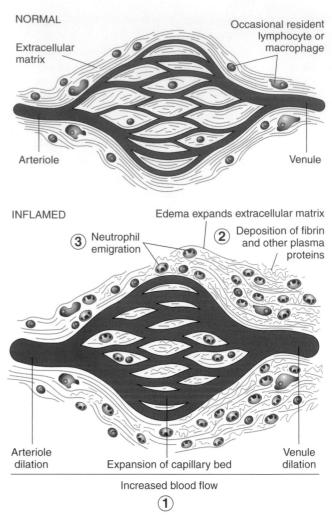

FIGURE 6-1
Major local manifestations of acute inflammation, compared with normal: (1) vascular dilation and increased blood flow, causing erythema and warmth; (2) extravasation and deposition of plasma fluid and proteins (edema); and (3) leukocyte emigration and accumulation in the site of injury. (Reproduced with permission from Kumar V, Abbas AK, Fausto N: *Robbins and Cotran pathologic basis of disease*, ed 7, Philadelphia, 2005, Elsevier Saunders, p 50.)

tissues. These actions account for the clinical finding of edema. The plasma and WBCs that escape into the tissues comprise the inflammatory exudate. The excess fluid in

the tissues places pressure on nerve endings in the area, which causes pain.[31] As the flow of blood increases locally, the red blood cells concentrate in the smaller vessels, which along with the effects of chemical factors increases the viscosity of the blood. This localized *pooling* of blood is known as *blood stasis*.

WBCs, especially neutrophils that have traveled in the blood to the inflamed site, begin to accumulate along the inner walls of the blood vessels, a phenomenon known as **margination.** These WBCs stick to the surface of the capillary endothelium, which is known as **pavementing.** Shortly thereafter, the neutrophils begin to pass through the pores in the vascular wall (diapedesis) and migrate into the surrounding interstitial tissue.

As previously mentioned, these neutrophils are already mature cells and can immediately begin the processes of killing bacteria and performing phagocytosis. During the first 6 to 24 hours of the inflammatory response, neutrophils predominate in the inflammatory infiltrate.

Importantly, within minutes of the onset of inflammation, local tissue macrophages, already present in the area, begin phagocytosis as well. Products of infection and inflammation activate these macrophages, which then enlarge in size; many break away from their attachments and become mobile. Although they provide some degree of defense during the first hour of inflammation, the actual number of macrophages in the area is too few to mount a significant defense.[16]

Along with the neutrophils, monocytes also migrate from the blood into the surrounding inflamed tissue. Once in the tissue, these monocytes enlarge and become macrophages. However, the number of monocytes in the circulating blood is low, and the number of monocytes stored in the bone marrow is also considerably less than the number of stored neutrophils. In addition, it may take up to 8 hours for monocytes to swell and enlarge to the degree where they develop adequate quantities of lysosomes, at which point they can act as macrophages.[16]

Inflammatory chemicals activate these macrophages, which produces significant growth and accumulation of these cells in the area. After several days, the neutrophils in the inflamed tissue are replaced by macrophages. The increased number of monocytes produced by the bone marrow also influences the increased number of macrophages present. In response to activated macrophages and T cells, the following three factors are produced in inflamed tissues, which stimulate the bone marrow to produce more granulocytes and monocytes:

1. Granulocyte-monocyte colony-stimulating factor (GM-CSF)
2. Granulocyte colony-stimulating factor (G-CSF)
3. Monocyte colony-stimulating factor (M-CSF)

These factors enable the body to produce more WBCs to aid in the defense.[16]

Once in the tissues, neutrophils and macrophages migrate toward the area of tissue damage via chemotaxis. These cells then destroy the invading organism via phagocytosis. Extensions of the phagocyte's cytoplasm flow around the organism to be ingested, resulting in complete enclosure of the organism within a **phagosome** created by the plasma membrane of the cell in a process known as *engulfment.* Lysosomal enzymes then kill the organism.

Phagocytosis is an essential mechanism of ridding the body of invading organisms.

As previously described, neutrophils phagocytize up to 20 bacteria; macrophages destroy up to 100 bacteria, as well as toxins and necrotic tissue before they eventually die (apoptosis).[16] Substances released from the dead cells liquefy the tissue. This liquid, including inflammatory exudate and dead neutrophils and macrophages, is known as *pus.* Bacteria that cause pus formation are called *pyogenic bacteria,* and inflammation with pus formation is known as *suppuration.*[31] The pus is gradually autolyzed over a few days, the end-products of which are absorbed into the surrounding tissues.[16] The inflammatory exudate contains *fibrin,* a plasma protein essential for the formation of a blood clot, the first stage in wound healing.

> **Note**
> Tissue repair cannot begin until all bacteria have been destroyed.[31]

CHEMICAL MEDIATORS OF THE INFLAMMATORY PROCESS

Multiple chemicals play important roles in facilitating the processes of inflammation and immunity. These chemicals are derived from either plasma or cells, and the presence of microbial products or host proteins trigger their production.[24] Chemical mediators bind to specific receptors on target cells and initiate responses via direct enzymatic activity or by mediating oxidative reactions. Once activated, the presence of these chemicals is short lived; however, their presence often produces detrimental effects. Plasma-derived mediators, such as complement proteins and kinins, are in precursor form and require activation before exerting their effects. Cell-derived mediators include the following:

- Histamines
- Prostaglandins (PGs)
- **Cytokines,** which come from a variety of cell types including the following:
  - Mast cells
  - Monocytes and macrophages
  - Neutrophils
  - Platelets[24]

Chemicals involved with inflammation, immunity, and wound healing can be classified into four categories.[29] A cytokine is a low–molecular-weight, biologically active protein that alters the cellular function of either the cell that released it or adjacent cells. Different cytokines have either similar or diverse activities, and their effects may be synergistic or inhibitory. **Hormones** are biologically active substances that are released into the circulation and produce an effect in cells that are distant from the site of secretion. **Mediators** are proteins from the plasma protein systems (discussed in the text that follows) or are released from mast cells. **Growth factors** are molecules that initiate cellular signaling mechanisms and regulate growth, proliferation, and maturation of cells.[29]

Histamine is stored in the granules of mast cells and causes vasodilation, increased vascular permeability, and contraction of bronchial and intestinal smooth muscles.[1]

> **Note**
> After phagocytosis, lysosomal enzymes and other leukocyte products are released into the surrounding area, causing local tissue damage and damage to the endothelium. This action is the reason the process of inflammation is both helpful and yet detrimental to the body. Long-term exposure to this leukocyte infiltrate is harmful to the body and is associated with many chronic diseases.[24]

> **Note**
> Histamine and serotonin are known as vasoactive amines, based on their actions on blood vessels.

> **Note**
> Histamine is best known for its role in allergic reactions.

Serotonin is found in platelets and enterochromaffin cells and causes increased vascular permeability during immunologic reactions.[24]

A variety of plasma proteins are produced through three distinct systems (Figure 6-2):

- Complement
- Kinin
- Clotting

The complement system is made up of 20 proteins, which collectively cause increased vascular permeability, chemotaxis, and opsonization. Of the 20 proteins, C3 and C5 play the most important roles in mediating inflammation. C3a, C4a, and C5a stimulate histamine release from mast cells. They are also referred to as *anaphylatoxins* because they also produce similar effects in anaphylaxis. C5a activates leukocytes, promotes leukocyte adhesion, and initiates chemotaxis. C5a is a chemoattractant for neutrophils, monocytes, eosinophils, and basophils. C3b is an opsonin that facilitates phagocytosis.[24]

The kinin system produces vasoactive peptides from a group of plasma proteins known as *kininogens*. Kininogens make kinins via the action of proteases called *kallikreins,* which are released during tissue destruction. The most predominant member of this class of chemicals is *bradykinin,* which causes the following actions:

- Vasodilation
- Increased vascular permeability
- Leukocyte chemotaxis
- Contraction of smooth muscle

The activation of kinins is triggered by the activation of the Hageman factor, also known as *factor XII of the intrinsic clotting pathway* (see Hemostasis and Blood Clotting later in this chapter). The actions of bradykinin are short lived and are inactivated by kininase.[24]

The clotting system forms a variety of chemicals that play important roles in both inflammation and wound healing, including thrombin, fibrinopeptides, and factor X (see Hemostasis and Blood Clotting later in this chapter). Substances that are released during tissue destruction activate this system. These substances include the following:

- Collagenase
- Proteinases
- Kallikreins
- Bacterial endotoxins

> **Note**
> Bradykinin is also a potent stimulant of sensory nerve endings and thus induces pain associated with inflammation.

> **Note**
> The complement, clotting, and kinin systems interact together because a protein from one system can activate one or both of the other systems.

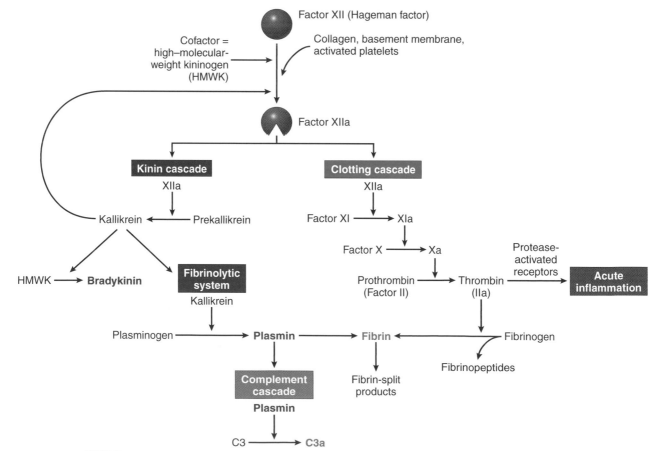

FIGURE 6-2
Interrelations among the four plasma mediator systems triggered by activation of factor XII (Hageman factor). Thrombin induces inflammation by binding to protease-activated receptors on platelets, endothelium, smooth muscle cells, and other cells. (Reproduced with permission from Kumar V, Abbas AK, Fausto N: *Robbins and Cotran pathologic basis of disease,* ed 7, Philadelphia, 2005, Elsevier Saunders, p 214.)

As previously discussed, the clotting system assists with walling off the invading organism at the onset of inflammation to prevent the spread of infection, which also facilitates phagocytosis. Clotting factors are also essential for hemostasis and wound healing. Other actions include neutrophil chemotaxis and increased vascular permeability.[24]

The two arms of the arachidonic acid cascade are responsible for the formation of a variety of chemical mediators necessary for inflammation, immunity, and blood clotting (Figure 6-3). Arachidonic acid is a locally acting hormone that is rapidly synthesized from cell membrane phospholipids via the action of phospholipases. Arachidonic acid is converted into other chemical substances by two different enzymes, lipoxygenase and cyclooxygenase (COX).

> *Note*
>
> The leukotrienes cause intense vasoconstriction, bronchospasm, and increased vascular permeability, all of which contribute to the pathophysiology of asthma.

The 5-lipoxygenase pathway forms the leukotrienes, which are associated with respiratory diseases such as asthma and chronic allergies. Leukotriene A4 forms leukotriene B4, which is involved in chemotaxis. Leukotrienes D4 and E4 are components of the slow-reacting substance of anaphylaxis, the receptors for which are the targets for the site of action of the respiratory drug zafirlukast (Accolate) (see Allergy and Hypersensitivity Reactions later in this chapter). Montelukast (Singulair) is another selective leukotriene-receptor antagonist medication used to block the action of cysteinyl leukotrienes for the relief of symptoms of asthma and allergy[45] (see Figure 6-3).

The 12-lipoxygenase pathway forms lipoxins that produce vasodilation, which is the opposing effect of the leukotrienes. Lipoxins also inhibit leukocyte recruitment and neutrophil chemotaxis. Lipoxins stimulate monocyte adhesion to endothelium[24] (see Figure 6-3).

Two basic types of prostaglandins are present: (1) those that are cytoprotective and help maintain homeostasis and (2) those that mediate inflammation. Prostaglandins that mediate inflammation (PGD_2, PGE_2, $PGF_{2\alpha}$) cause the following actions:

- Vasodilation
- Increased vascular permeability
- Chemotaxis

> *Prevention*
>
> The cyclooxygenase (COX) pathway is responsible for the conversion of arachidonic acid to prostaglandins. **Prostaglandins** are potent mediators of numerous different physiologic processes. Blocking COX prevents the formation of prostaglandins.[24,45]

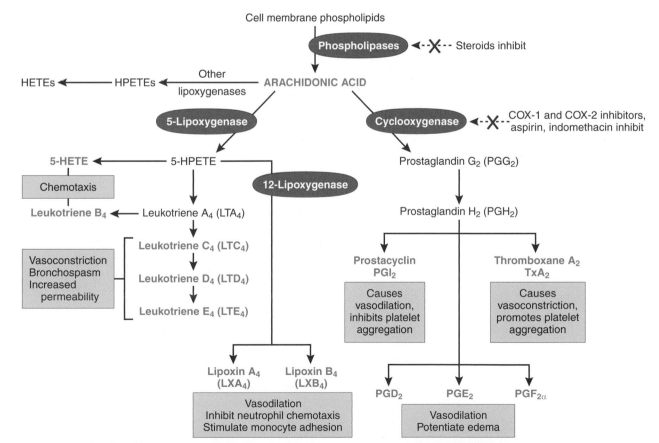

FIGURE 6-3
Generation of arachidonic acid metabolites and their roles in inflammation. The molecular targets of action of some antiinflammatory drugs are indicated *(red X)*. *COX,* Cyclooxygenase; *HETE,* hydroxyeicosatetraenoic acid; *HPETE,* hydroperoxyeicosatetraenoic acid. (Reproduced with permission from Kumar V, Abbas AK, Fausto N: *Robbins and Cotran pathologic basis of disease,* ed 7, Philadelphia, 2005, Elsevier Saunders, p 69.)

These prostaglandins are also responsible for the clinical signs of pain, fever, and swelling associated with inflammation.

Drugs such as aspirin; nonselective, nonsteroidal antiinflammatory drugs (NSAIDs), such as COX-1 inhibitors (ibuprofen); and selective NSAIDs, such as COX-2 inhibitors (celecoxib, rofecoxib, valdecoxib), act to reduce the signs and symptoms of inflammation by blocking the action of COX.

Prostaglandins further give rise to prostacyclin (PGI_2) and thromboxane A_2 (TxA_2), which produce opposing actions to each other in vasoactive activity and platelet aggregation. Prostacyclin causes vasodilation and inhibits platelet aggregation, whereas TxA_2 causes vasoconstriction and promotes platelet aggregation. These substances are integral to clot formation and wound healing[24] (see Figure 6-3) (see Hemostasis and Blood Clotting later in this chapter).

> **Note**
>
> Tumor necrosis factor-α (TNF-α) and interleukin-1 (IL-1) are two major cytokines that mediate inflammation.

These cytokines are produced mainly by monocytes and macrophages and also by T cells (see Chemical Mediators of Innate Immunity later in this chapter). These chemicals are responsible for endothelial activation and the synthesis of endothelial adhesion molecules and chemical mediators. In addition, these chemicals activate monocytes and macrophages and participate in leukocyte chemotaxis.

These cytokines also produce enzymes associated with matrix remodeling known as *matrix metalloproteinases* (MMPs), stimulate osteoclasts that destroy connective tissue and bone, and activate T cells.[24,32]

These cytokines also contribute to the induction of systemic acute-phase responses of infection and injury that include the following:

- Fever
- Loss of appetite
- Release of neutrophils
- Increased production and secretion of corticotropin and corticosteroids (see the next section, Chronic Inflammation)

Interleukin-6 (IL-6) is found in T cells, monocytes, macrophages, fibroblasts, and epithelial cells, and it increases the production of IL-1, PGE_2, and MMPs. It also assists with the process of B-cell differentiation (see Adaptive [Acquired] Immunity later in this chapter). Interleukin-8 is found in epithelial cells and promotes chemotaxis and transepithelial migration of PMNs. PGE_2 is found in monocytes, macrophages, and fibroblasts; it stimulates osteoclasts and increases the production of MMPs. Both MMP-1 (found in fibroblasts, monocytes, macrophages, and epithelial cells) and MMP-8 (found in PMNs) stimulate collagenase, which destroys connective tissue and bone.[32]

Chemokines are small proteins that act as chemoattractants for leukocytes and help control the normal migration of cells through the tissues. Nitric oxide (NO) is released from endothelial cells, is microbicidal, and causes vasodilation. Neuropeptides, such as substance P and neurokinin A, participate in the initiation and propagation of inflammation and promote pain. Platelet-activating factor (PAF) is a lipoprotein derived from plasma membrane phospholipids that increases vascular permeability and activation of platelets. It also increases leukocyte adhesion to endothelium, chemotaxis, and degranulation, as well as the synthesis of other chemical mediators.[24]

Finally, monocytes and neutrophils contain lysosomal granules that contain a variety of enzymes necessary for phagocytosis. These enzymes include lysozyme, collagenase, alkaline phosphatase, and elastase, among others, and are responsible for tissue destruction that occurs after phagocytosis.

> **Note**
>
> Oxygen-derived free radicals are also released from leukocytes after phagocytosis and are potent inflammatory mediators. Free radicals damage multiple cell types, including endothelial cells and red blood cells, and they cause increased vascular permeability.[24]

CHRONIC INFLAMMATION

Persistent infections, prolonged exposure to toxic agents, and autoimmunity cause chronic inflammation.[24] The classic outcome of chronic inflammation is tissue damage, which may be extensive or limit the afflicted person's ability to function or both. The body's attempt to heal itself results in connective tissue damage and fibrosis (Figure 6-4). Classic inflammatory diseases include arthritis, chronic obstructive pulmonary disease (COPD), cardiovascular disease, and periodontitis. (For a full discussion of chronic inflammatory diseases associated with autoimmunity, see Chapter 46.)

Histologically, macrophages, lymphocytes, and plasma cells predominate in the inflammatory infiltrate associated with chronic disease. In addition, a predominance of fibroblasts and other vascular elements increases the production of connective tissue. These cells produce a granulomatous inflammation characterized by focal accumulation of activated macrophages.[24] Activated lymphocytes and macrophages secrete inflammatory

> **Note**
>
> The chemical products of the inflammatory mediators destroy the injurious organisms or particles and help initiate repair; however, they are also responsible for much of the tissue damage associated with chronic inflammation (see Figure 6-4).

> **Distinct Care Modifications**
>
> Tetracycline drugs, such as doxycycline, are used to kill the pathogens associated with periodontal disease. Tetracyclines have a high affinity for bone, and they are excreted into the gingival crevicular fluid, where bacteria live in the gingival crevice. Antibiotics support the body's natural defense systems by killing invading bacterial organisms. Antibiotics are useful adjunctive therapies for the management of aggressive forms of periodontal disease and in patients with a genetic susceptibility to disease. Sublethal doses of doxycycline are given to patients with periodontal disease to suppress collagenase activity, thereby stopping the destruction of the gingival connective tissue and surrounding bone. Triclosan, an antimicrobial agent included in Colgate Total dentifrice, has also been shown to inhibit IL-1 and TNF-α, thereby exhibiting antiinflammatory properties as well.

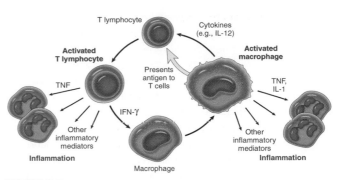

FIGURE 6-5
Macrophage-lymphocyte interactions in chronic inflammation. Activated lymphocytes and macrophages influence each other and also release inflammatory mediators that affect other cells. (Reproduced with permission from Kumar V, Abbas AK, Fausto N: *Robbins and Cotran pathologic basis of disease,* ed 7, Philadelphia, 2005, Elsevier Saunders, p 82.)

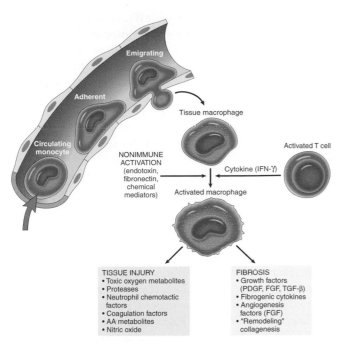

FIGURE 6-4
Roles of activated macrophages in chronic inflammation. Macrophages are activated by cytokines from immune-activated T cells, particularly IFN-γ, or by nonimmunologic stimuli such as endotoxin. The products made by activated macrophages that cause tissue injury and fibrosis are indicated. *INF-γ,* Interferon-γ; *AA,* arachidonic acid; *PDGF,* platelet-derived growth factor; *FGF,* fibroblast growth factor; *TGF-β,* transforming growth factor–β. (Reproduced with permission from Kumar V, Abbas AK, Fausto N: *Robbins and Cotran pathologic basis of disease,* ed 7, Philadelphia, 2005, Elsevier Saunders, p 80.)

mediators that influence each other, as well as other adjacent cells (Figure 6-5).

The end result of these processes is an ongoing battle between tissue destruction and tissue repair, with a final result of insufficient, incomplete wound healing that alters function.

DENTAL CONSIDERATIONS

The continual production of and exposure to inflammatory chemicals not only destroys local tissues but also, in time, affects tissues at distant sites away from the source of chemical production.[29] For example, the chronic inflammation of periodontal disease has been associated with cardiovascular disease; diabetes; respiratory diseases; and preterm, low–birth-weight babies.*

---

*References 2, 3, 10, 14, 15, 33-37, 39, 40, 42-44.

The lymphatic system assumes a greater role by providing a secondary line of defense by draining the excessive fluid that accumulates in the extravascular space.[24]

Several notable acute-phase responses correspond to the systemic effects of inflammation, also known as the *systemic inflammatory response syndrome.* The first acute reaction is fever, which is produced in response to pyrogens that stimulate prostaglandin synthesis. **Acute-phase proteins** are produced by the body in response to inflammation and include C-reactive protein (CRP),

fibrinogen, and serum amyloid A (SAA) protein. These substances bind to microbial cell walls and act as opsonins. Prolonged activation results in a secondary amyloidosis in chronic inflammation. Elevated levels of CRP and fibrinogen have been shown to increase the risk for adverse cardiovascular events.[6,12,38]

Other acute-phase responses include leukocytosis, which is commonly found in bacterial infections (see the section, White Blood Cells, earlier in this chapter). Cell counts in leukocytosis may rise from 15,000 to 20,000/mm³ (normal range is 4500 to 11,000/mm³) or to extremes of 40,000/mm³ and higher.[24] In severe bacterial infections, large quantities of cytokines, especially TNF-α and IL-1, produce thrombosis and coagulation. Multiple organs can be affected by chronic exposure to inflammatory chemicals and intravascular thrombosis. Other symptoms include high temperature, hypoglycemia, and cardiovascular failure. This condition is known as *septic shock* or *sepsis* and can result in death without immediate medical attention.[24]

ROLE OF STEROIDS IN REDUCING INFLAMMATION

Steroid medications are often used to combat the adverse effects of inflammation and mimic the effects of cortisol, the endogenous steroid secreted by the adrenal cortex. **Cortisol** demonstrates multiple antiinflammatory properties and is extensively used for the treatment of chronic inflammatory diseases (see Chapter 46). Administering cortisol can block the formation of inflammation or reverse many of its effects once inflammation has started. Cortisol also increases the rate of healing[16] (Box 6-1).

One of the most important antiinflammatory effects of

> **BOX 6-1**
>
> **FUNCTIONS OF CORTISOL**
>
> - Increases rate of healing
> - Stabilizes lysosomal membranes
> - Decreases capillary permeability, which prevents edema and swelling
> - Decreases production of leukotrienes and prostaglandins
> - Suppresses immune system
> - Reduces fever
> - Decreases degree of severity of inflammation and quantity of inflammatory by-products released

cortisol is that it stabilizes lysosomal membranes, making it more difficult for these membranes to rupture. Thus most of the lysosomal enzymes that are released from damaged cells and initiate inflammation are kept contained within the lysosome, or the quantity that is released into the tissues is greatly reduced.[16]

Cortisol decreases capillary permeability, which prevents edema and swelling. Cortisol decreases WBC migration into inflamed tissues and decreases phagocytosis. These effects are attributed to the fact that cortisol decreases the production of leukotrienes and prostaglandins.[16]

Cortisol suppresses the immune system, especially T lymphocytes, which reduces the number of T cells and antibodies in the inflamed area. This effect reduces the severity of the tissue reactions that promote inflammation. Finally, cortisol lowers fever by reducing the release of IL-1 from the WBCs. Decreased temperature reduces the degree of vasodilation.[16]

Cortisol does not affect the basic antigen-antibody response associated with an allergic reaction. However, because the inflammatory response associated with allergic reactions can be severe and life-threatening, the administration of cortisol will reduce the degree of severity of inflammation, as well as reduce the quantity of inflammatory products released. In this manner, cortisol can be used as a component of the treatment protocol to prevent shock or death from anaphylaxis.[16]

Cortisol also decreases the number of eosinophils and lymphocytes in the circulation, which is observed shortly after injection and becomes more pronounced several hours later. One of the primary adverse effects associated with steroids is that large quantities produce significant atrophy of the lymphoid tissues throughout the body. This effect decreases the production of T cells and antibodies from the lymph tissues, which decreases immunity and increases susceptibility to infection (see the following section, Immunity). However, the ability to suppress immunity makes steroids useful medications for preventing the rejection of organ transplants[16] (see Immune Reactions for Transplanted Tissues later in this chapter).

CASE APPLICATION 6-1.1

Assessing a Patient's Use of Steroids

Dental hygienists should assess use of steroids when reviewing a patient's medical history. Steroids are often used to manage diseases associated with chronic inflammation, including asthma, arthritis, and autoimmune diseases. Long-term use of steroid medications can increase the patient's risk for infection and lowers the patient's ability to fight stress. Taking steroid medications suppresses the body's own production of cortisol, which increases the risk for adrenal crisis during physiologic stress (e.g., infection or surgery) or psychologic stress (e.g., fear or anxiety). These patients may require a stress-reduction protocol prior to receiving invasive dental procedures, which includes the administration of supplemental steroids, such as hydrocortisone. A physician consultation prior to initiating invasive dental hygiene procedures may be warranted to prevent this medical emergency in patients undergoing ‑term steroid therapy.

Immunity

Immunity is defined as resistance to infectious disease. The cells, tissues, and molecules that make up the immune system act together to mediate resistance to disease in a process known as the *immune response*. The function of the immune system is to prevent and eliminate infections.[1]

Innate Immunity

Two aspects of human immunity exist: **innate immunity** and **adaptive immunity.** Innate immunity, also known as *natural immunity,* provides the initial protection against infection by preventing the entry of microorganisms into the body and by destroying any microorganisms that do manage to enter the body tissues. The mechanisms of innate immunity share one similar characteristic: they all respond to microorganisms but do not react to nonmicrobial substances. Innate immunity also responds to host cells that are infected with or are damaged by invading microorganisms. These characteristics distinguish innate immunity from adaptive immunity, which is an immune response that must be stimulated by and adapted to the presence of microorganisms before it can effectively destroy them. Adaptive immunity also differs in that it responds to both microorganisms and nonmicrobial **antigens.**[1]

The components of the innate immune system recognize structures that are found in a variety of microorganisms but are not produced by host cells. For example, phagocytes have receptors that recognize bacterial lipopolysaccharide (LPS), better known as an *endotoxin,* which is a waste product produced by bacteria but not by host cells.[1]

DENTAL CONSIDERATIONS

An LPS produced by periodontal pathogens is a known trigger for the immune response and resultant inflammatory reaction observed in the mouth after bacterial infection of the periodontium.

The innate immune system can recognize structures that are essential for bacteria to both survive and cause infection. The innate immune response recognizes and destroys bacteria by their structural and functional components; thus bacteria cannot avoid the innate immune response. Bacteria cannot mutate or stop the expression of these functional structures because they lose their viability and ability to infect the host. However, microorganisms can sometimes evade the adaptive immune response by mutating the antigens expressed on the surface of the organism that are recognized by lymphocytes. These antigens are not usually required for the

Note

Every time the innate immune system encounters a microorganism, the system responds in the same way. Conversely, the adaptive immune system responds more efficiently and effectively with repeated exposure to an organism. The adaptive immune system *remembers* past encounters with an organism, which allows the human body to react defensively against repeated or persistent infections.[1]

survival of the organism and thus are not targeted by the innate immune response either.[1]

Neither the innate nor the adaptive immune system reacts against the host. The innate immune system recognizes microbial structures versus host cells, and regulatory molecules expressed by host cells prevent innate immune reactions from destroying them. Lymphocytes that possess the ability to recognize self-antigens produced by host cells are an important aspect of the adaptive immune system; these lymphocytes are destroyed or inactivated when they encounter self-antigens[1] (see Self-Tolerance later in this chapter).

COMPONENTS OF INNATE IMMUNITY

Many components make up innate immunity (Figure 6-6). First, neutrophils and macrophages are recruited to the sites of infection, where they recognize the invading microorganisms by several receptors. These WBCs destroy bacteria via phagocytosis, secrete cytokines, and assist in tissue repair.

Second, hydrochloric acid in the stomach and other digestive enzymes destroy bacteria that enter the body via the GI tract.[1,16]

Third, the most common portals of entry into the body, notably the skin, the GI tract, and the respiratory tract, are lined with a continuous layer of epithelium that acts as a physical barrier to microbial invasion. The epithelial cells that compose this barrier secrete endogenous peptide antibiotics that also kill bacteria; thus the epithelium acts as a chemical barrier as well. Intraepithelial lymphocytes also provide additional protection that assists in preventing infections.[1,16]

Fourth, specialized lymphocytes known as natural killer (NK) cells produce interferon-γ (IFN-γ), a powerful cytokine that activates the microbicidal function of macrophages. This action enables macrophages to kill phagocytosed microorganisms. NK

cells also kill host cells that have become infected by intracellular microorganisms, including viruses. By killing infected host cells, NK cells eliminate potential sources of infection from the body.[1]

Fifth, chemicals found in the blood attach to and destroy microorganisms or toxins. These chemicals include lysozymes, basic polypeptides, and complement proteins.[1,16] Twenty complement proteins are normally present among the plasma proteins in the blood, as well as among the proteins that leak out of capillaries into the surrounding tissue spaces. Complement proteins opsonize microorganisms for phagocytosis, trigger inflammation, and destroy the organisms via lysis. Many of these proteins are enzyme precursors; in other words, they form other enzymes on activation. Of the 20 complement proteins, approximately 11, named C1 through C9, a, b, and d, are the primary components of the complement system. The enzyme precursors are normally inactive until they are activated by one of three pathways[1,16] (Figure 6-7).

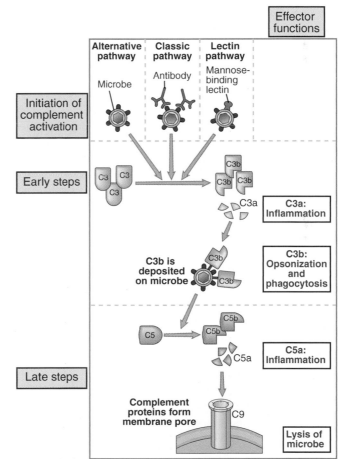

FIGURE 6-7
Pathways of complement activation. Three distinct pathways, all of which lead to the production of C3b (the early steps), may initiate the activation of the complement system. C3b initiates the late steps of complement activation, culminating in the production of numerous peptides and polymerized C9, which forms the *membrane attack complex,* so named because it creates holes in plasma membranes. The principal functions of proteins produced at different steps are shown. (Reproduced with permission from Abbas AK, Lichtman AH: *Basic immunology: functions and disorders of the immune system,* ed 2, Philadelphia, 2004, Elsevier, p 33.)

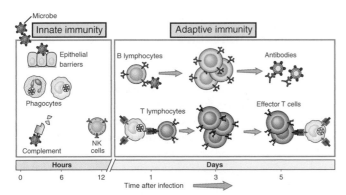

FIGURE 6-6
The principal mechanisms of innate and adaptive immunity. The mechanisms of innate immunity provide the initial defense against infections. Some of the mechanisms prevent infections (e.g., epithelial barriers) and others eliminate microbes (e.g., phagocytes, NK [natural killer] cells, complement system). Adaptive immune responses develop later and are mediated by lymphocytes and their by-products. Antibodies block infections and eliminate microbes, and T lymphocytes eradicate intracellular microbes. The kinetics of the innate and adaptive immune responses are approximations and may vary in different infections. (Reproduced with permission from Abbas AK, Lichtman AH: *Basic immunology: functions and disorders of the immune system,* ed 2, Philadelphia, 2004, Elsevier, p 3.)

PATHWAYS OF COMPLEMENT ACTIVATION

Two of the three pathways of complement activation are associated with innate immunity (see Figure 6-7). The *alternative pathway* is triggered when complement proteins are activated on microbial surfaces. This activation cannot be controlled because complement regulatory proteins are found only on host cells, not on invading microorganisms. The *lectin pathway* is activated when a mannose-binding lectin, a plasma protein, binds to surface receptors of microorganisms. This pathway is initiated in the absence of antibodies, which makes it a component of innate immunity.[1]

The *classic pathway* of complement activation is a component of adaptive immunity and is activated in an antigen-antibody reaction (see Figure 6-7) (see the discussion under Adaptive [Acquired] Immunity later in this chapter). When an antibody binds to an antigen, a series of enzymatic reactions is initiated, beginning with the activation of the proenzyme C1. C1 enzymes that are formed cause a sequential activation of other enzymes in increasingly large quantities, resulting in the formation of multiple end-products and the death of the invader.[16]

The complement system serves many functions in host defense. C3b coats microorganisms (opsonization), promotes binding of these coated organisms to phagocytes, and activates phagocytosis by neutrophils and macrophages. By-products of complement proteins, including fragment C5a, serve as chemoattractants, promoting chemotaxis of phagocytes and inflammation. These by-products also alter the surface texture of microorganisms, allowing them to adhere to one another in a process known as *agglutination*. Fragments C3a, C4a, and C5a activate mast cells and basophils, causing the release of histamine, heparin, and other substances locally. This action increases blood flow and edema and triggers local tissue reactions that inactivate the invading organisms.

Complement enzymes and by-products also attack the structures of some viruses, which decreases virulence and their ability to cause viral infections.

Prevention

The inflammatory effects triggered by complement by-products help prevent the movement of the invading organism through the tissues.[16]

Prevention

The most important by-product of the complement cascade is the formation of the lytic complex, C5b6789, a protein complex that inserts into the cell membrane of the invading organism, which ruptures the cell membrane. The rupture creates an opening that allows for the influx of water and ions into the organism, causing death.[1,16]

CHEMICAL MEDIATORS OF INNATE IMMUNITY

When macrophages recognize microorganisms, they become activated and secrete cytokines (Figure 6-8). Activated macrophages are the major source of cytokines in innate immune responses. These cytokines are produced in small amounts and generally act on either the cells that produce them or the adjacent cells.[1]

Cytokines mediate inflammation (e.g., TNF, IL-1, chemokines), activate NK cells (IL-12), activate other macrophages (IFN-γ), and prevent viral infections via type 1 interferon (IFN-1). IFN-1 inhibits viral replication and prevents the spread of viral infection to other uninfected cells. Dental hygienists recognize the synthetic form of IFN-1, known as *interferon-α (IFN-α)*, a medication used to treat patients with chronic viral hepatitis.[1]

In addition to the circulating complement proteins, other plasma proteins contribute to host defense as well. The number of these plasma proteins increases quickly after infection. These proteins are also known as *acute-phase proteins* and include surfactant proteins that protect the lungs and CRP that is produced by the liver (see Chronic Inflammation earlier in this chapter). Acute-phase proteins and complement proteins mediate phagocytosis of extracellular bacteria and fungi.

Note

Cytokines communicate with phagocytes and NK cells to destroy intracellular bacteria and viruses.[1]

Adaptive (Acquired) Immunity

The adaptive immune response, also known as *acquired immunity*, often uses the basic mechanisms of innate immunity (e.g., phagocytosis, cell lysis) to eliminate infections. Thus these two forms of immunity work together to provide optimal defense for the body against invaders.[1]

Note

Innate immunity provides the early defense against infection and instructs the adaptive immune response how to respond to different organisms most effectively.

The adaptive immune system destroys the microorganisms that have evolved to resist the innate immune system. The adaptive immune system recognizes both microorganisms and noninfectious molecules. Lymphocytes are the primary cells involved in the adaptive immune system, which express specific receptors that recognize different substances produced by organisms and molecules, known as *antigens*. Antigens are typically large proteins or polysaccharides that are unique from other compounds. Adaptive immune responses are triggered only when antigens break through the epithelial barrier and travel through the bloodstream to the lymph organs of the body. Once in the lymph tissues, the lymphocytes recognize these antigens, which triggers a response that is appropriate to combat the invading organism and potential infection.[1,16]

Lymphocytes are predominately located in the lymph nodes but are also found in the spleen, GI tract, and bone marrow. Lymph tissues are found in regions of the body where they can intercept invading organisms. Invading organisms or substances typically enter the tissue fluids of the body, where they are transported via the lymphatic system to the lymph nodes or lymph organs. Antigens that enter the peripheral tissues of the body are transported to the lymph tissue in the lymph nodes.

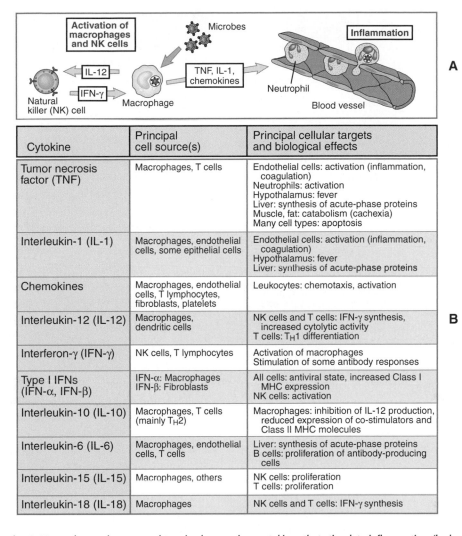

FIGURE 6-8
Cytokines of innate immunity. **A,** Macrophages that respond to microbes produce cytokines that stimulate inflammation (leukocyte recruitment) and activate NK cells to produce the macrophage-activating cytokine, IFN-γ. **B,** Some important characteristics of the major cytokines of innate immunity are listed. IFN-γ is a cytokine of both innate and adaptive immunity. The name, *tumor necrosis factor* (TNF), arose from an experiment showing that a cytokine induced by lipopolysaccharide killed tumors in mice. This effect is the result of TNF-induced thrombosis of tumor blood vessels, which is an exaggerated form of reaction observed in inflammation. The name, *interferon*, arose from the ability of these cytokines to interfere with viral infection. IFN-γ is a weak antiviral cytokine compared with Type I IFNs. *T$_H$,* Helper T lymphocyte; *MHC,* major histocompatbility complex. (Reproduced with permission from Abbas AK, Lichtman AH: *Basic immunology: functions and disorders of the immune system,* ed 2, Philadelphia, 2004, Elsevier, p 35.)

Antigens that enter the body via the GI tract are destroyed by the lymphocytes that are housed in the lymph tissues in the GI submucosa. The tonsils and adenoids trap antigens that enter the body through the upper respiratory tract. The spleen and bone marrow trap any antigens that manage to bypass these other defensive routes and enter the bloodstream.[16]

CELL-MEDIATED IMMUNITY

> **Note**
> There are two forms of adaptive immunity: (1) cell-mediated immunity and (2) humoral immunity (Figure 6-9).

Defense against invaders that live inside of infected host cells is called *cell-mediated immunity* and is mediated by **T lymphocytes.** T lymphocytes recognize antigens produced by intracellular micro-

organisms. Lymphocytes that form activated T lymphocytes are preprocessed in the thymus gland, thus the *T* designation. T lymphocytes are originally formed in the bone marrow and then migrate to the thymus gland where they develop reactivity for specific antigens. While in the thymus gland, the T lymphocytes are also exposed to the body's self-antigens, which act as a protective mechanism that prevents the T lymphocytes from attacking the host's body. If a T lymphocyte reacts to a self-antigen while still in the thymus, then it is phagocytized instead of being released into the body. This preexposure to self-antigens ensures that the T lymphocytes recognize and destroy only antigens that come from a foreign source outside of the body. On leaving the thymus gland, these lymphocytes travel through the bloodstream and lodge in the lymph tissues of the body.[16]

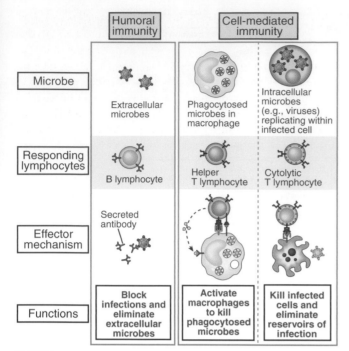

FIGURE 6-9
Types of adaptive immunity. In humoral immunity, B lymphocytes secrete antibodies that eliminate extracellular microbes. In cell-mediated immunity, T lymphocytes either activate macrophages to destroy phagocytosed microbes or kill infected cells. (Reproduced with permission from Abbas AK, Lichtman AH: *Basic immunology: functions and disorders of the immune system,* ed 2, Philadelphia, 2004, Elsevier, p 5.)

HUMORAL IMMUNITY

> *Note*
>
> Proteins known as *antibodies,* which are produced by B lymphocytes, mediate humoral immunity (see Figure 6-9).

B lymphocytes are preprocessed in the liver during fetal life and in the bone marrow after birth. B lymphocytes differ from T lymphocytes in that instead of the entire cell having specificity for a particular antigen, B lymphocytes secrete antibodies that are the reactive agents. B lymphocytes can form millions of types of antibodies with different reactivity against specific antigens; consequently, they are more diverse than T lymphocytes. After preprocessing, B lymphocytes travel in the bloodstream and lodge in lymph tissues. B and T lymphocytes are housed in different compartments of the lymph tissues but within reasonable proximity to one another, which allows for communication between the cell types.[1,16]

Antibodies are immunoglobulins that make up approximately 20% of all of the plasma proteins. Five classes of antibodies are found, and each antibody is specific for a particular antigen (Table 6-2). Antibodies are secreted into the blood and mucosal fluids, where they directly attack and kill invaders or neutralize toxins or both. These circulating and mucosal antibodies prevent invaders found on the surface of mucosa from infecting the host cells and entering the underlying connective tissue.[1] For example, salivary immunoglobulins help protect the oral mucosa from microbial invasion. Antibodies also prevent infection by activating the complement system. (The reader is

Table 6-2	Functions of Immunoglobulins
TEST	**CHARACTERISTICS**
IgG	Most abundant immunoglobulin Opsonization
IgA	Two forms: secretory (body fluids), serum Last immunoglobulin to appear in childhood
IgM	Restricted to the intravascular space First immunoglobulin produced Activates complement
IgE	Increases in parasitic and atopic diseases Mediates type I hypersensitivity reactions
IgD	Found in serum Little immunologic importance

Modified from Little JW et al: *Dental management of the medically compromised patient,* ed 6, St Louis, 2002, Mosby, p 318.

referred back to the discussion of the classic pathway of complement activation [see Pathways of Complement Activation] earlier in this chapter). Antibodies from B lymphocytes mediate defense against extracellular microorganisms and toxins; antibodies do not have access to intracellular invaders.[1,16]

SPECIFICITY

The immune system has the ability to distinguish millions of different antigens or portions of antigens. Preformed lymphocytes stored in the lymph tissues have the ability to form either one type of antibody or one type of T cell with a single type of specificity. When a specific antigen comes in contact with either a T lymphocyte or a B lymphocyte, the lymphocyte becomes *activated.* Activated T lymphocytes and the antibodies formed from activated B lymphocytes react to the specific antigen that triggered their development. Only the specific type of antigen with which it can react can activate the lymphocyte. Once activated, these lymphocytes begin to replicate in large numbers. These duplicate lymphocytes are known as *lymphocyte clones.* B lymphocyte clones will secrete the same type of antibody into the circulation. T lymphocyte clones are highly specific T cells that circulate throughout the blood, tissue fluids, and lymph system for many months to years.[16]

Each lymphocyte clone responds to a single type of antigen. When the antigen presents itself to the lymphocyte, it immediately attaches to the cell membrane, triggering activation. B lymphocytes contain more than 100,000 surface antibodies on their cell membranes for antigen binding. T lymphocytes contain surface-receptor proteins for antigen binding, with as many as 100,000 surface-receptor sites on a single T cell.[16]

Most antigens activate both B lymphocytes and T lymphocytes simultaneously. A specialized form of T lymphocytes known as **helper T cells** secrete lymphokines, which are substances that help activate the B lymphocytes. Without the assistance of helper T cells, the number of antibodies produced by activated B lymphocytes is low (see Specialized T Cells later in this chapter).

Macrophages also play a role in lymphocyte activation. When an invading organism enters the lymph tissue, the millions of macrophages that are also housed there recognize, phagocytize, and partially digest the organism. Antigen by-product is then contained in the macrophage cytosol, which is then passed on to the neighboring lymphocyte via cell-to-cell communication. This contact with the antigen activates the lymphocyte. Furthermore, macrophages secrete IL-1, a substance that activates and promotes the growth of lymphocytes.[16]

Activated B lymphocytes and their clones enlarge to form lymphoblasts, which further differentiate into plasmablasts and eventually form plasma cells. Plasmablasts rapidly divide and proliferate, forming 500 cells for every 1 original plasmablast. Plasma cells rapidly produce gamma globulin antibodies, which are secreted into the lymph fluid and circulation. This process of proliferation and secretion of antibodies persists for several weeks until the plasma cells eventually die.[16]

Activated T lymphocytes and their clones also proliferate as whole activated T cells are released into the lymph fluid and circulation. These cells are then distributed throughout the body via the bloodstream and pass through the capillary walls and into the tissue spaces where they once again enter the lymph fluid. These cells continually circulate through the body in this manner for many months to years.[16]

MEMORY

Repeated exposure to the same antigen creates a larger and more effective immune response. The initial exposure to an antigen is called the *primary response*. The primary response is mediated by lymphocytes that are encountering the antigen for the first time. Repeated exposures to the same antigen initiate the *secondary response,* which is a more rapid and larger reaction that is able to eliminate the antigen more efficiently.[1]

Several of the activated B lymphocyte clones do not differentiate into plasma cells; rather, they form new B lymphocytes that circulate throughout the body and reside in the lymph tissues. These cells remain dormant until they encounter the same antigen that triggered their original activation. Once again, these new B lymphocytes become activated, but this time they produce a greater, more powerful antibody reaction. These cells are called *memory cells* and are able to produce a more potent response because more memory cells are present in the lymph tissues than are original B lymphocyte clones.[16]

T lymphocyte memory cells are formed in a similar manner. When an antigen activates a T lymphocyte clone, many of the newly formed T cells remain stored in the lymph tissue and later become new T cells of the original clone. Repeated exposure to the same antigen triggers a more rapid and powerful release of activated T cells as compared with the primary response.[16]

Immunologic memory enables the body to combat persistent or recurrent infections because with each subsequent exposure to the antigen, new memory cells are formed and existing memory cells become activated. Immunologic memory is the justification for immunization for disease prevention.[1]

Immunization

Several methods can induce immunity in the body. An individual who is exposed to an antigen that triggers an immune response to eliminate the infection will later develop resistance to that antigen. This resistance is a form of active immunity. Active immunity can also be acquired through vaccination.[1] Dead organisms that still possess their chemical antigens but are no longer capable of producing disease are injected into the body. An example of this method of active immunity is vaccination against diphtheria and other forms of bacterial infections. Toxins that have been treated with chemicals, but still possess their antigens, are also used for vaccinations (i.e., immunizations against tetanus or botulism). An injection with live organisms, grown in special cultures or passed through a series of animals that mutate to the point where they cannot cause disease but still possess their antigens, are the form of immunization used to fight poliomyelitis, smallpox, and other viral organisms.[16]

The process of immunizing an individual is based on the understanding of the primary and secondary response to exposure to an antigen. After the initial exposure to an antigen, the primary response for forming antibodies is slow, with antibody production lasting for only a few weeks. However, with subsequent exposure to the antigen, the secondary response is faster and has a greater magnitude, with antibody formation lasting for several months. For this reason, some immunizations require the injection of antigen in multiple doses over a period of several weeks or months between injections.[16] Dental hygienists will recognize this strategic approach to immunization against the hepatitis B virus.

Finally, passive immunity can be acquired for short periods by transferring lymphocytes or antibodies from one individual who is immune to an infection to another individual. This type of immunity occurs when an infant acquires immunity from its mother; the infant receives maternal antibodies through the placenta and breast milk. This type of immunity is useful for newborns who are not able to mount an active immune response because their immune systems are not yet fully developed. It is important to note, however, that passive immunity does not lead to life-long immunity or long-term resistance to infection.[1]

Stages of the Immune Response   6-3

Immunity occurs in five sequential stages (Figure 6-10). The first stage is the *recognition phase,* when specific lymphocytes recognize microbial antigens.

The second stage is the *lymphocyte activation phase,* which requires two types of signals. The first signal is the initiation of the immune response, which is triggered by antigens binding to antigen receptors on lymphocytes. The second signal is the recognition of microbes mediated by the innate immune system. This signal ensures that a foreign microbial invader rather than a noninfectious antigen triggers the immune response. During the activation phase, lymphocyte clones are formed and multiply. Some of these lymphocyte clones differentiate into effector lymphocytes that function to eliminate the antigen.[1]

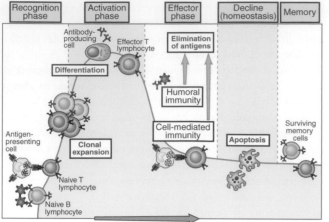

FIGURE 6-10
Phases of adaptive immune responses. Adaptive immune responses consist of sequential phases, recognition of antigen by specific lymphocytes, activation of lymphocytes (consisting of their proliferation and differentiation into effector cells), and the effector phase (elimination of antigen). The response declines as antigen is eliminated, and most of the antigen-stimulated lymphocytes die by apoptosis. The antigen-specific cells that survive are responsible for memory. The duration of each phase may vary in different immune responses. The y axis represents an arbitrary measure of the magnitude of the response. These principles apply to humoral immunity (mediated by B lymphocytes) and cell-mediated immunity (mediated by T lymphocytes). (Reproduced with permission from Abbas AK, Lichtman AH: *Basic immunology: functions and disorders of the immune system,* ed 2, Philadelphia, 2004, Elsevier, p 8.)

The third stage is the elimination of the antigen. During this stage the B lymphocytes differentiate into plasma cells that secrete antibodies and T lymphocytes differentiate into specialized killer cells that eliminate infected host cells. This stage is also known as the *effector phase.*[1]

The fourth stage is designated as the *decline phase,* during which the infection has been cleared and thus the stimulation for the activation of lymphocytes has been eliminated. Cells that were activated by antigens die via apoptosis and are then cleared from the body via phagocytosis.

The fifth and last stage is the formation of memory as the only cells that remain are the memory lymphocytes. These memory cells remain in the body in a dormant state until activated by a repeat exposure to the microorganism.[1]

Specialized T Cells

The three specialized forms of T lymphocytes are (1) helper T cells, (2) **cytotoxic T cells,** and (3) **suppressor T cells.** Each of these specialized cells performs a unique set of functions.

Helper T cells make up the majority of specialized T cells and regulate the functions of the immune system. These cells form and secrete lymphokines, which are protein mediators that act on other cells of the immune system and on the bone marrow. The most important of these lymphokines are IL-2, IL-3, IL-4, IL-5, IL-6, GM-CSF, and IFN-γ.[16] This list supports the fact that the major source of cytokines for adaptive immunity comes from helper T cells.

IL-2 stimulates the growth and proliferation of cytotoxic and suppressor T cells. Most of the interleukins stimulate the B lymphocyte response. IL-4, IL-5, and IL-6 produce the most potent stimulatory effects on B lymphocytes and are collectively known as *B-cell–stimulating factors.* Interleukins also activate macrophages to increase the efficiency of phagocytosis. IL-2 has a feedback mechanism that stimulates the activation of additional helper T cells, which amplifies the entire immune response against invading antigens.[16]

Cytotoxic T cells are also known as *killer cells.* As the name implies, these cells kill invading microorganisms and occasionally host cells. After binding to an antigen on an invading organism, these cells secrete *perforins,* which are proteins that create holes in the cell membrane of the microorganism, allowing for fluid influx that eventually destroys the organism. Cytotoxic T cells are also able to secrete toxic substances directly into the microorganism, causing the cell to dissolve. Cytotoxic T cells are especially effective at killing cells that are infected with viruses, as well as cancerous cells and foreign cells from transplanted tissues. After these actions, cytotoxic T cells detach themselves from the invading organism and continue to survive in the tissues for extended lengths of time.[16]

Suppressor T cells suppress the actions of helper T cells and cytotoxic cells and are thus believed to play a role in regulating immune reactions. It is believed that these cells prevent extreme immune reactions that could potentially damage the host's tissues. Suppressor cells also prevent the body from attacking itself and thus contribute to the protective function of self-tolerance.[16]

Self-Tolerance

The immune system normally recognizes the difference between the host's own tissues and foreign invaders. Few T lymphocytes and antibodies are formed against self-antigens. This ability to recognize self-antigens is called **immunologic tolerance.** When individuals lose their immune tolerance, the body begins to attack itself, resulting in tissue damage and altered physiologic function. This condition is known as *autoimmunity* and occurs more often in the elderly and in genetically susceptible individuals. After tissue destruction, the release of an increased quantity of self-antigens occurs, which may trigger the adaptive immune response via activated T lymphocytes or antibodies.[1,16] (For a complete discussion of autoimmune diseases, the reader is referred to Chapter 46.)

Immune Reactions for Transplanted Tissues

Transplanted tissues from a donor are recognized by the recipient as foreign and trigger immune reactions. Portions of or whole organs (i.e., autografts) donated and transplanted in the same body (e.g., skin grafting) and transplanted tissues between members of the same species (i.e., allografts) all contain antigens that are able to survive for long periods in the donor recipient when given an adequate blood supply. Tissues that are transplanted from one species to another species (e.g., from an animal to a human) almost always trigger an immune response, and, without intervention, will cause rejection of the graft within weeks of transplantation.[16]

To prevent organ rejection, several strategies are used to prevent severe antigen-antibody reactions. Tissue typing assesses human leukocyte antigens (HLAs) that are present on the surface of cell membranes. However, considering that more than 150 different types of these antigens exist that yield more than a trillion possible combinations, finding an identical match between two people is statistically impossible. Immunity against any one of these antigens can cause organ rejection.[16]

HLAs are also found on the surfaces of WBCs, which allow for tissue typing to be performed on lymphocytes separate from a blood sample from both the potential donor and recipient. Not all HLAs are severely antigenic, which allows for finding the "best" or "closest" tissue match, increasing the likelihood of a successful transplant.

Only identical twins have the same six HLAs; therefore tissues donated from one twin to the other (i.e., isografts) have the greatest chance for successful transplantation. Tissue rejection rarely occurs between twins. Organ donations between siblings and between parent and child are also more likely to be successful.[16]

Drugs that suppress T cells are used to prevent rejection. These drugs include corticosteroids, which suppress the growth of lymph tissues and thus decrease T cells and antibodies from B lymphocytes. Azathioprine (Imuran) prevents the formation of antibodies and T cells by targeting the lymph tissues. Cyclosporine (Sandimmune) inhibits the formation of helper T cells and is the most valuable drug for the prevention of rejection. The use of these and other related medications increases the individual's susceptibility to infections because of extreme immunosuppression.

Allergy and Hypersensitivity Reactions

One adverse effect of immunity is the development of allergies or immune hypersensitivity. Some individuals demonstrate an *allergic tendency* because of their unusual immune system response. This tendency is inherited and is characterized by the presence of large quantities of IgE antibodies in the blood. Although immunoglobulin G (IgG) is the most abundant immunoglobulin in the body, IgE mediates the more commonly occurring reactions to environmental triggers, foods, and medications[16,27] (see immunoglobulins listed in Table 6-2).

IgE antibodies are also known as *reagins* or sensitizing antibodies and have a strong tendency to attach to basophils and mast cells. When an allergen (i.e., an antigen that binds to an IgE antibody) enters the body, an allergen-reagin reaction occurs, which triggers an allergic reaction. Binding of an allergen to IgE antibodies that are already bound to a basophil or mast

cell triggers the rupture of the basophil or mast cell, resulting in the release of their granular contents into the tissue. Sometimes the cell does not rupture but secretes other substances that are not already formed in its granules.[16]

Substances that are immediately released or are secreted afterward from basophils and mast cells include the following[16] (Figure 6-11):

- Histamine
- Protease
- Slow-reacting substance of anaphylaxis
- Eosinophil chemotactic substance
- Neutrophil chemotactic substance
- Heparin
- Platelet-activating factors

These chemicals produce a variety of effects including vasodilation, edema from increased capillary permeability, attraction of WBCs to the site of the reaction, local tissue damage by protease, and smooth muscle contraction. The type of tissue effects varies with the type of tissue in which the allergen-reagin reaction occurs.[16]

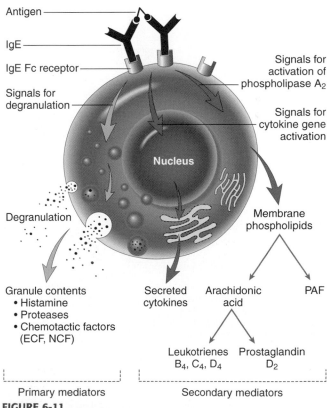

FIGURE 6-11
Activation of mast cells in immediate hypersensitivity and release of their mediators. *ECF,* Eosinophil chemotactic factor; *NCF,* neutrophil chemotactic factor; *PAF,* platelet-activating factor. (Reproduced with permission from Kumar V, Abbas AK, Fausto N: *Robbins and Cotran pathologic basis of disease,* ed 7, Philadelphia, 2005, Elsevier Saunders, p 208.)

Type I hypersensitivity reactions are associated with the humoral immune system and typically occur after the second exposure to the antigen. This type of reaction is associated with exposure to common allergens such as dust mites, pollen, molds, animal dander, and food. This type of reaction is also associated with drug allergies, which may occur after repeated contact with a drug such as penicillin.[23,27]

When a specific antigen is injected into the circulation, it causes widespread reactions throughout the body by interacting with basophils in the blood and with mast cells in the tissues surrounding the microvasculature that have already been sensitized by attachment of IgE reagins (Figure 6-12).

Without intervention, the individual may die from anaphylactic shock, which results from circulatory collapse from the plasma loss. Slow-reacting substance of anaphylaxis, a mixture of leukotrienes, is also released from the mast cells, causing smooth muscle spasms resulting in bronchoconstriction and eventually respiratory failure. Anaphylaxis occurs within minutes of exposure to the allergen, and respiratory and circulatory depression occurs early in the course of the reaction.

> **Note**
> The immediate injection of epinephrine is the treatment for anaphylaxis, which causes vasoconstriction and dilation of the bronchial airways.[16,23,27]

> **Note**
> *Urticaria,* also known as *hives,* is a superficial skin lesion caused by an antigen entering the skin, triggering a localized anaphylactoid reaction.

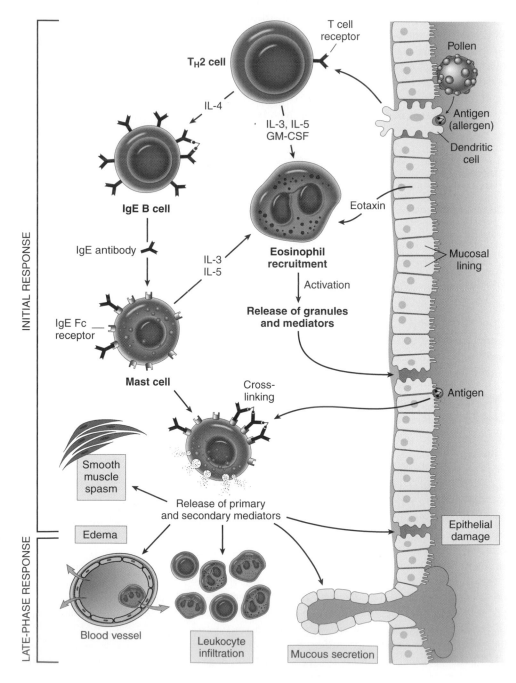

FIGURE 6-12
Pathogenesis of immediate (type I) hypersensitivity reaction. The late-phase reaction is dominated by leukocyte infiltration and tissue injury. T_H2, T helper type 2 CD4 cells; *GM-CSF,* granulocyte-moncyte colony-stimulating factor; *IgE,* immunogloblin E; *IgE Fc,* receptor for IgE antibody; *IL-3,* interleukin 3; *IL-4,* interleukin 4; *IL-5,* interleukin 5. (Reproduced with permission from Kumar V, Abbas AK, Fausto N: *Robbins and Cotran pathologic basis of disease,* ed 7, Philadelphia, 2005, Elsevier Saunders, p 207.)

Antigen-antibody binding triggers the release of histamine from mast cells, resulting in vasodilation and increased vascular permeability. These effects of histamine cause the redness and localized swellings of hives. The treatment of hives includes the administration of an antihistamine such as diphenhydramine (Benadryl).[23,27,45]

Angioneurotic edema is a lesion that occurs in the deeper layers of the skin and in other tissues that include the tongue and larynx.

Dental Considerations

Dental professionals may observe angioneurotic edema in the lips, tongue, or oropharynx from exposure to a topical medication or anesthetic agent in the oral cavity.

The onset of angioneurotic edema is fairly rapid but painless and may last for several days. Exudates from the surrounding blood vessels cause the swelling. Treatment with the antihistamine diphenhydramine (Benadryl) is administered for up to 3 days.[23,27]

Hay fever is the result of allergen-reagin reactions that occur in the nose. Inhaled pollen or other known triggers cause the release of histamine locally in the nose. The effects include intranasal vasodilation and increased capillary permeability and pressure, leading to swelling of the nasal passages, increased secretions, and sneezing. Hay fever and seasonal allergies are treated with a variety of antihistamines.[16,23,27]

People with asthma often exhibit an allergic tendency, and the allergen-reagin reaction occurs in the bronchial passages. The slow-reacting substance of anaphylaxis from mast cells produces the unwanted bronchoconstrictor effects and difficulty breathing. These symptoms persist until the products from the allergic reaction have been removed. Antihistamines are not effective interventions for an asthma attack because the reaction is not mediated by histamine. β-2 agonists, such as albuterol, are powerful bronchodilators that serve as rescue medications to reverse the unwanted bronchoconstriction during an asthma attack. Albuterol is a required rescue medication for all dental emergency kits. Leukotriene-receptor antagonist medications may also be helpful in preventing these symptoms in people with asthma.[23,27,45]

Type II hypersensitivity reactions are IgG- or IgM-mediated cytotoxic reactions. This type of reaction occurs when a person receives the incorrect blood type during a transfusion. Type III hypersensitivity reactions occur in blood vessels and are also known as *immune complex–mediated hypersensitivity*. These reactions manifest as vasculitis, such as the reaction caused by systemic lupus erythematosus. Type IV hypersensitivity reactions involve the cellular immune system and include contact dermatitis, organ transplant rejection, and graft-versus-host disease. Type IV reactions have a delayed onset, and signs and symptoms may appear in 48 to 72 hours after exposure to the antigen.[23,27]

Hemostasis and Blood Clotting

Hemostasis is the prevention of blood loss from the body.[16] Trauma to a blood vessel, such as a cut or rupture, immediately causes the vessel to contract, which reduces the loss of blood. In large vessels, direct damage to the vascular wall induces most of the contraction, which is influenced by neural input, spasm, and locally released humoral factors. In smaller vessels, platelets are responsible for inducing vasoconstriction with the release of TxA_2.

Platelets are fragments of megakaryocytes that are synthesized in the bone marrow and play an essential role in blood clotting. The number of platelets normally found in the blood is approximately 300,000 per microliter of blood. Platelets are

---

Distinct Care Modifications

Dental professionals must quickly respond when a patient exhibits the signs of anaphylaxis.
- Emergency medical service (EMS) should be immediately contacted for assistance.
- The patient is then placed in a supine position with careful positioning to ensure that the airway remains open.
- Supplemental oxygen should be administered to facilitate breathing.
- The patient's pulse, respiration, and blood pressure should be continually monitored for changes. If respiration is absent or no pulse is present (or both), then rescue breathing and CPR will be required.
- Between 0.3 and 0.5 mL of 1:1000 epinephrine is immediately injected intramuscularly (IM) into the patient's tongue.
- If the patient does not respond, then a second injection at the same dose of 1:1000 epinephrine is administered.

Prevention

Epinephrine is a required rescue medication for all dental emergency kits.[27]

CASE APPLICATION 6-1.2

Questioning Patients about Adverse Reactions to Medication

Dental hygienists must question their patients about any adverse reactions that they have experienced related to medication use or other substances known to trigger these reactions. It is important to note that many patients who experience food allergies are also more likely to experience drug allergies. Many patients are allergic to preservatives, including the sulfites that are used in dental local anesthetics; sulfites are added to prevent oxidation of the vasoconstrictor. Patients who report adverse reactions should be questioned about the nature of the reaction. The clinical signs and symptoms described by the patient should be noted and may include the following:

- Itching
- Hives
- Localized swelling
- Difficulty breathing
- Anaphylaxis

Patients should be asked whether medical intervention was necessary at the time of the reaction, as well as the time between exposure and onset of symptoms, and any medications that were used to reverse the reaction. Patients with known allergies, such as allergies to drugs or bee stings, should carry an EpiPen with them in case of exposure to manage the onset of an anaphylactic reaction.

active cells that synthesize prostaglandins, which are hormones that produce vascular and other local tissue reactions; proteins that assist with blood coagulation; growth factors that aid in vascular repair; and enzymes that form adenosine triphosphate (ATP) and adenosine diphosphate (ADP). Glycoproteins that coat the cell surface of platelets prevent them from adhering to normal vascular endothelium but allow for adherence to injured endothelium or exposed collagen in the vessel wall. Platelet-membrane phospholipids help activate the process of blood clotting. Platelets have a limited life span and are eliminated from the body via removal by macrophages in the spleen. Platelets are replaced in the body approximately every 10 days; thus 30,000 platelets are formed each day for each microliter of blood.[16]

When platelets come into contact with injured vascular endothelium, the platelets immediately begin to swell. They form an irregular shape and become sticky to facilitate adherence to collagen and to a protein called the *von Willebrand factor,* which spreads throughout the plasma. The platelets excrete ADP and TxA_2, which activate other platelets in the vicinity. In turn, these activated platelets adhere to the original platelets, forming a platelet plug.

If the opening in the vessel wall is small, then the platelet plug itself may be sufficient to stop the bleeding. However, if the wound is large, then a blood clot is also needed to stop the bleeding. Activator substances from the damaged vessel wall, from platelets and from blood proteins, initiate the clotting process. More than 50 substances in the blood affect blood coagulation by acting as either procoagulants or anticoagulants. If the trauma is severe, then the clot begins to form within 15 to 20 seconds; if the trauma is minor, then clotting occurs more slowly, typically within 1 to 2 minutes.[16]

Trauma to the vessel wall and surrounding tissues or blood contacting damaged endothelium triggers the formation of prothrombin activator. Prothrombin activator is formed via the extrinsic pathway, from trauma to the vascular wall and surrounding tissues, or via the intrinsic pathway that begins in the blood itself.[16]

In both pathways, blood-clotting factors, when converted to their active forms, cause a series of enzymatic reactions that result in clotting (Figure 6-13).

Once formed, prothrombin activator in the presence of sufficient quantities of calcium causes the conversion of prothrombin to thrombin. In turn, thrombin causes polymerization of fibrinogen molecules into fibrin fibers. Fibrin fibers attach tightly to platelets, forming a meshwork that allows the platelets, blood cells, and plasma to form a clot. Platelets themselves also influence the conversion of prothrombin to thrombin. Much of the prothrombin that is formed attaches to prothrombin receptors found on the platelets that have already adhered to the damaged tissue. As the platelet-binding action accelerates, the formation of thrombin from prothrombin increases locally in the area where the clot is needed.

Importantly, vitamin K is necessary for the liver formation of five important clotting factors: factor II (prothrombin), factor VII, factor IX, factor X, and protein C.

Reduced vitamin K is a necessary cofactor in the gamma

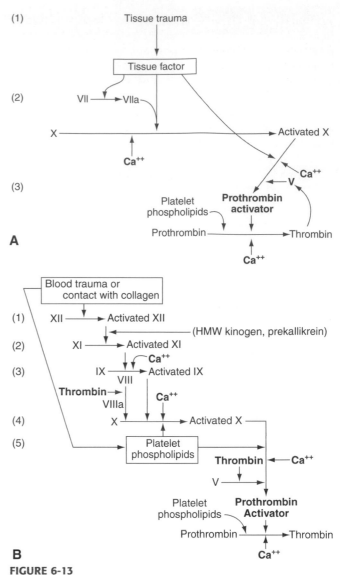

FIGURE 6-13
A, Extrinsic pathway for initiating blood clotting. **B,** Intrinsic pathway for initiating blood clotting. *HMW,* High–molecular weight. (Reproduced with permission from Guyton AC, Hall JE: *Textbook of medical physiology,* ed 10, Philadelphia, 2000, WB Saunders, p 424.)

carboxylation of these vitamin K–dependent clotting factors. Precursors to these clotting factors undergo vitamin K–dependent modification to produce their active forms.

Warfarin (Coumadin) binds to the liver microsomal enzyme vitamin K 2,3-epoxide reductase and inhibits the production of the reduced form of vitamin K. By inhibiting the formation of reduced vitamin K, *coumarins* prevent the activation of these clotting factors. Thus the clotting factors remain as inactive molecules that cannot participate in the clotting process, thereby stopping the formation of thrombin and fibrin. Warfarin also depresses proteins C and S, which are endogenous anticoagulants. Levels of these two proteins may be depressed by warfarin before the other clotting factors, resulting in a dangerous state of hypercoagulation for a short period. For this reason, heparin therapy usually overlaps warfarin therapy for at least the first 2 days of oral anticoagulant therapy to allow for the warfarin to take effect and to achieve an optimal therapeutic range of anticoagulation.[4,9]

Normal Anticoagulant Mechanisms

The three most important endogenous anticoagulant mechanisms for preventing clotting in the vasculature are the following:

1. Smoothness of the endothelium surface, which prevents activation of the intrinsic pathway by preventing contact of the platelets with vascular wall collagen
2. Mucopolysaccharide glycocalyx layer on top of the endothelium, which repels platelets and clotting factors
3. Thrombomodulin, which is a protein bound to the endothelial membrane that binds thrombin to slow the clotting process

Binding thrombomodulin to thrombin also activates protein C, a powerful anticoagulant in the blood that inactivates activated factors V and VIII.[16]

Several chemicals that remove thrombin from the blood act as powerful anticoagulants in the body. Fibrin fibers in the clot absorb as much as 85% of the thrombin formed from prothrombin, which reduces the amount of thrombin in the blood, thereby preventing excessive spreading of the clot. The remaining thrombin that is not absorbed combines with antithrombin III, which blocks the effects of thrombin on fibrinogen and inactivates any remaining thrombin in approximately 20 minutes.

Many cells in the body produce heparin, but it is primarily produced by mast cells found in the connective tissue surrounding capillaries in the body. These mast cells continually produce small quantities of heparin that diffuses into the circulation. Basophils in the blood also release heparin into the plasma. The concentration of heparin in the blood is normally low and produces significant anticoagulant effects under only specific circumstances. Heparin is medically used in high concentrations to prevent intravascular clotting.[16]

When heparin combines with antithrombin III, it increases the effectiveness of antithrombin III at removing thrombin by up to a thousandfold. Large quantities of heparin assist antithrombin III in removing circulating-free thrombin from the blood almost instantaneously. In addition to removing thrombin, the heparin–antithrombin III complex removes activated blood coagulation factors IX, X, XI, and XII, promoting additional anticoagulation.[16]

Laboratory Testing to Evaluate Bleeding Time

Multiple laboratory tests are available to assess bleeding status and help determine potential risk for bleeding complications caused by medications, diseases, or invasive procedures. The most common laboratory tests include the following[28]:

- Platelet count
- Bleeding time
- Prothrombin time
- International Normalized Ratio (INR)
- Activated partial thromboplastin time

The **platelet count** is a measure of the number of platelets in the systemic circulation and is used to evaluate and monitor bleeding disorders.[22,28] Liver disease, pathologic conditions such as leukemia, and drugs are implicated in altering the number of platelets, either by destruction or by increasing or de-creasing platelet production. This test is not useful in measuring platelet function; however, reduced numbers of platelets can suggest the degree of risk for bleeding. The normal platelet count range is 150,000 to 450,000 per microliter of blood.

The oldest test is the bleeding time (BT) test, which is a technique-sensitive test primarily used to assess the capillary function, platelet number and function, and ability of platelets to adhere to a vessel wall and form a plug.[22] The technique involves placing a blood pressure cuff on the arm; it is then inflated and adjusted to 40 mm Hg. The skin of the arm is held taut and two approximately 3-mm deep puncture wounds are made in the inner surface of the forearm; immediately afterward, a stopwatch is started. At 30-second intervals, the drops of blood are blotted away. When bleeding stops, the stopwatch is stopped. The time to clotting depends largely on the depth of the wound and the technique used. The normal BT range is 1 to 6 minutes. Lack of clotting factors, lack of platelets, platelet dysfunction, aspirin use, and poor technique can all alter normal BT.[5,7,13,30] Because obvious sensitivity and reproducibility limitations exist, this test is seldom used in the clinical setting.[16,22]

The **prothrombin time** (PT) **test** is a simple test that evaluates the extrinsic pathway of coagulation as it assesses reduced levels or activity of factors II, V, VII, X and fibrinogen. Blood that is taken from the patient is immediately oxalated to ensure that none of the prothrombin can convert to thrombin. Calcium and thromboplastin are then added to the blood; the time it takes for clot formation to occur is measured in seconds. The thromboplastin that is added is extracted from animal tissues and contains tissue factor and phospholipids necessary for factor VII to activate factor X. The normal PT range is 10 to 13 seconds.[22]

Before the 1980s, thromboplastins used in medical laboratories varied considerably, as to source of species, tissues used, and the method of preparation, which resulted in a lack of sensitivity of the thromboplastins to detect clotting-factor deficiencies.[17,22] Through the 1970s, initial target therapeutic ranges for anticoagulation therapy were based on a PT ratio (PTR) (patient's PT:laboratory control), with values between 2.0 and 2.5.[17] However, although the sensitivity of the thromboplastins in use varied, the values of the target range remained the same. This greatly affected between-laboratory comparability of test results and often resulted in PT test results that were artificially low or beneath the targeted therapeutic range.[41] Consequently, physicians prescribing anticoagulant therapies inadvertently used doses that resulted in anticoagulation at levels that were in actuality much higher than originally intended, increasing the risk for hemorrhage.[8,17,22]

Warfarin (Coumadin) is used for long-term anticoagulation therapy; the goal is to reduce morbidity and prevent mortality without causing hemorrhage. In the past, the PT test was used to control the dose of warfarin; typically, warfarin was administered at a dose that prolonged the PT to twice that of normal control plasma. This regimen produced excessive anticoagulation, a practice that is no longer used.[22]

To address overanticoagulation and the variation in the sensitivity of thromboplastins used in laboratory testing, the International Council for Standardization in Haematology

(ICSH) and the International Committee on Thrombosis and Haemostasis (ICTH) adopted in 1983 the **International Normalized Ratio (INR)** system as the test of choice for monitoring warfarin therapy.[22] This testing system uses the World Health Organization (WHO) international reference preparation of thromboplastin as the laboratory standard. The system also requires the calibration of all commercial thromboplastins against the WHO reference preparation. The International Sensitivity Index (ISI) is a rating given to each thromboplastin reagent based on the responsiveness of that agent to the reduction in vitamin K–dependent clotting factors. To improve the precision of the INR, thromboplastins with an ISI of less than 1.5 (ideally less than 1.2) are recommended as reagents for PT tests.[22]

The INR is the patient's PT divided by the mean normal PT for the laboratory (PTR), with additional adjustment made for the reactivity of the reagents (ISI), based on the following formula:

$$INR = PTR^{ISI}$$

The INR makes it possible to target the same therapeutic ranges while using different laboratory reagents.[17-20] The INR is an adjusted PTR and always has a higher value than the PTR.[17] An INR of 2.0 to 3.0 is recommended for all conditions with the exception of patients with prosthetic heart valves, whose INR will range from 2.5 to 3.5.[18-20,22]

Although more physicians, dentists, and laboratories have universally adopted the INR, problems persist with its use and interpretation. Some laboratories continue to use thromboplastins with higher ISI values than recommended or use different methods than those recommended by the manufacturers.[21,25,26] Patients taking warfarin usually have an INR obtained every 4 to 6 weeks.

Finally, the **activated partial thromboplastin time (aPTT) test** evaluates the intrinsic coagulation cascade. It is primarily used to monitor anticoagulation with heparin therapy and to aid in the diagnosis of hemophilia; congenital deficiencies in intrinsic

factors II, V, VIII, IX, X, XI, and XII; vitamin K deficiency; and various congenital clotting abnormalities. The test uses a contact activator that is added to the patient's blood to measure the ability of the blood to clot. A control sample is always performed for comparison. Under normal circumstances the blood should clot within 25 to 35 seconds. The effects of heparin are to prolong the aPTT. Different reagents and instruments used can affect the aPTT response to heparin. Test sensitivity is most influenced by the reagent used, whereas test precision is most affected by the type of instrument used.[22,28]

Thromboembolic Conditions

A **thrombus** is an abnormal clot that forms in a blood vessel. When the velocity of the blood flowing past the clot breaks the clot free from its attachment to the vessel wall, the free-floating clot is referred to as an **embolus.** Clots that originate on the left side of the heart on the arterial side of the circulation clog arteries and arterioles that feed organs, resulting in ischemia and permanent damage to the organ tissue. Clots that originate on the venous side of the circulation or on the right side of the heart flow through the pulmonary arteries to the lungs, resulting in pulmonary embolism.

Risk for pulmonary embolism is high for patients who are immobile or bedridden because intravenous clotting forms in the legs as a result of blood pooling in the lower extremities. This condition is known as *deep vein thrombosis* (DVT), a problem that can also occur in those traveling for long periods who are seated in a motor vehicle or airplane. The risk is that a portion of or the entire clot itself will break free and flow back to the right side of the heart and into the pulmonary arteries. If both branches of the pulmonary artery are blocked by emboli, then the patient dies immediately from massive pulmonary embolism. If only one of the branches is blocked, then risk for death remains high because of further growth of the clot in the vessel. However, life-saving thrombolytic drugs, such as tissue plasminogen activator (t-PA), can be used to increase survival[16] (see Clot Lysis and Thrombolytic Agents later in this chapter).

Arteriosclerosis, infections, or trauma to the blood vessels roughens the surface of the endothelium, triggering the process of clotting as previously described. Atherosclerotic plaques, the most frequent cause of ischemic coronary heart disease, can also trigger clotting.[16] A thrombus is formed where the atherosclerotic plaque has broken through the endothelium and is in direct contact with the blood. The surface of the plaque itself is rough, which allows platelets, as well as fibrin and red blood cells, to adhere, thus forming the clot. The clot itself can occlude the coronary artery or can break free from its attachment to the atherosclerotic plaque and block another peripheral branch of the coronary artery. Atherosclerotic plaques may also cause local spasm of the vascular smooth muscle wall, leading to a secondary thrombosis of the artery.[16]

Clotting also occurs in vessels where blood travels more slowly, as in veins and venules, which is another reason why venous thrombosis is problematic. Small amounts of thrombin and other procoagulants are continually formed in the blood; when blood flows slowly, the local concentration of these coagulants rises to a level that is high enough to initiate clotting. Not surprisingly, mast cells that secrete heparin are found in large numbers in areas that receive many embolic clots from slow-flowing venous blood, especially around the lungs and liver. The presence of heparin in these vascular beds prevents the further growth of and potential damage caused by these clots. Conversely, in vessels where blood flows rapidly, the procoagulants are mixed with a large volume of blood, which limits their clotting action until they are eventually removed from the blood by the liver.[16]

Excessive amounts of traumatized or dead tissues in the body secrete large quantities of tissue factor into the bloodstream, initiating the clotting cascade via the extrinsic clotting pathway. In addition, circulating bacteria and bacterial endotoxins can activate clotting mechanisms as well, such as that seen in septic shock. These conditions produce small but numerous clots that plug blood vessels in the peripheral limbs, depriving many tissues of oxygen and other essential nutrients.[16]

Clot Lysis and Thrombolytic Agents

Within several minutes of clot formation, the clot begins to contract. Platelets trapped in the clot release procoagulant factors that cause increased cross-linking of fibrin fibers and activate contractile proteins that compress the clot into a smaller mesh. As the clot retracts, most of the fluid is expressed from the clot, and the edges of the damaged vessel are pulled together, resulting in hemostasis.

After hemostasis has been reestablished, the clot needs to be removed. Clot dissolution, also known as *lysis,* occurs as a result of the action of plasmin. The plasma contains a substance called *plasminogen,* which, when activated, forms the enzyme *plasmin.* Injured tissues and damaged endothelium release t-PA, which catalyzes the conversion of plasminogen to plasmin. Plasmin destroys fibrin fibers, as well as many coagulant substances including fibrinogen; factors V, VIII, and XII; and prothrombin. Thus when plasmin is formed, it causes lysis of the clot by destroying many of the clotting factors in the blood.[16]

Plasmin also reopens small vessels that become occluded with clots, especially those smaller vessels found in the peripheral limbs. This important protective function ensures good blood flow. Genetically engineered t-PA (i.e., alteplase) is used to manage acute myocardial infarction for lysis of thrombi in the coronary arteries and for the management of acute massive pulmonary embolism. This type of synthetic t-PA can be directly delivered into a thrombosed area of the heart via a catheter; by triggering the conversion of plasminogen to plasmin, multiple intravascular clots can be quickly dissolved. If administered within the first hour of blockage of the coronary artery, major damage to the heart muscle can often be prevented.[16]

Streptokinase (Streptase) is a thrombolytic agent used in the treatment of recent severe or massive DVT, pulmonary embolism, myocardial infarction, and occluded arteriovenous cannulas.[45] Specific types of β-hemolytic streptococci produce streptokinase. It activates the conversion of plasminogen to plasmin and is effective both outside and inside of the thrombus or embolus.[16,45] Bleeding is the major adverse effect associated with both t-PA and streptokinase. Hemorrhage can occur at any site, and the risk for hemorrhage is dependent on many factors, including dose, concurrent use of multiple agents that may alter hemostasis, and patient predisposition. Concurrent use of oral anticoagulants, heparin, low–molecular-weight heparins, and drugs that alter platelet function all increase the risk of bleeding complications.[45]

Wound Healing

After injury, tissues must be repaired or replaced via a complex process that involves the growth of new cells and tissues to replace damaged or lost structures (Figure 6-14). Wound healing occurs in response to trauma, inflammation, or cellular necrosis, and by either tissue regeneration or scar formation. Tissue repair and regeneration are influenced by local factors, such as residual infection or the presence of foreign material in the wound, and by systemic factors, such as drugs and disease.[24]

Wound healing begins early in the process of inflammation with the formation of granulation tissue. Granulation tissue is pink in color with a grainy surface texture; it forms the initial covering of the wound. Granulation tissue formation is associated with the formation of new microvasculature and the proliferation of fibroblasts.[24]

Successful wound healing is dependent on an adequate blood supply to the newly formed tissues. **Angiogenesis** is the process of forming new blood vessels derived from existing blood vessels found in close proximity to the wound. Growth and maturation of these new blood vessels is influenced by growth factors such as vascular endothelial growth factor (VEGF) and endothelial progenitor cells (EPCs) from the bone marrow.[24]

Vasodilation and increased vascular permeability in blood vessels adjacent to the wound allows for the local delivery of tissue factors that facilitate angiogenesis. Extracellular matrix (ECM) proteins secreted by fibroblasts, including integrins and matricellular proteins, direct the migration and maturation of endothelial cells, which eventually remodel into new capillary tubes. These ECM proteins also recruit periendothelial cells into the newly formed capillary tubes and assist with the maturation of the new blood vessel.[24]

Several processes are involved in scar formation. Growth factors released from platelets, inflammatory cells, and activated

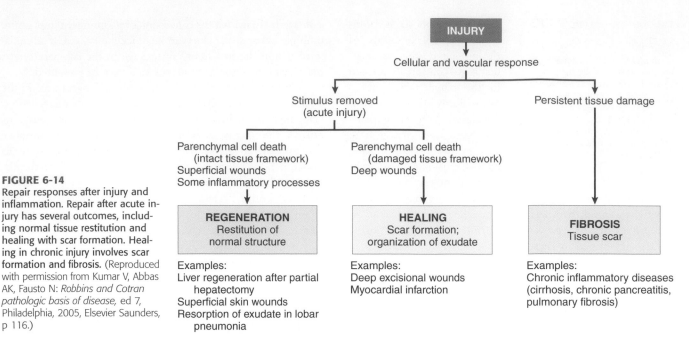

FIGURE 6-14
Repair responses after injury and inflammation. Repair after acute injury has several outcomes, including normal tissue restitution and healing with scar formation. Healing in chronic injury involves scar formation and fibrosis. (Reproduced with permission from Kumar V, Abbas AK, Fausto N: *Robbins and Cotran pathologic basis of disease,* ed 7, Philadelphia, 2005, Elsevier Saunders, p 116.)

endothelium trigger the migration of fibroblasts to the site of injury. These growth factors also contribute to the proliferation in the number of fibroblasts at the site. Fibroblasts begin forming 3 to 5 days after injury and continue to proliferate for several weeks. These same growth factors also stimulate fibroblasts to synthesize ECM proteins, which are used to form fibrillar collagens that make up the structural components of the healing wound and add strength to the newly formed tissue. Granulation tissue is converted into a scar, which is made up of fibroblasts, dense collagen, fragments of elastic tissue, and other ECM protein components. The once vascular granulation tissue transforms into a pale, avascular scar.[24]

MMPs produced by fibroblasts, neutrophils, macrophages, synovial cells, and epithelial cells degrade the ECM protein components, which triggers the process of tissue remodeling. Secretion of MMPs is influenced by growth factors, physical stress, and phagocytosis. Steroids and other growth factors in the body inhibit the activity of MMPs.[24]

Wound healing can occur by either primary or secondary intention (Figure 6-15). Healing by **primary intention,** also known as *primary union,* occurs when a narrow incisional space fills with clotted blood, resulting in clot formation and a scab that covers the wound. In this instance, the edges of the wound are brought together in close approximation, for example, with the use of sutures or tissue adhesives. Within 24 hours, neutrophils appear along the margins of the incision and move toward the clot. Within 48 hours, epithelial cells move from the edges of the wound to fuse in the midline beneath the scab. This activity causes closure of the wound and the formation of a basement membrane.[24]

Within 72 hours, the neutrophils are replaced with macrophages and granulation tissue begins to form. Collagen fibers form along the margins of the incision, and epithelial cells proliferate and thicken the newly formed epidermal layer. Within

5 days, the incisional space is filled with granulation tissue, with collagen fibers forming a bridge across the incision. Surface keratinization appears on the maturing epidermal layer. By 2 weeks, fibroblasts continue to proliferate and collagen continues to form. The inflammatory process is essentially complete. By 4 weeks, the scar is made up of connective tissue and an intact epidermal layer, with increased strength of the repaired wound.[24]

Healing by **secondary intention,** also known as *secondary union,* is associated with wounds that have separated edges, such as tissue craters from tooth extractions or traumatic injuries that remove large pieces of tissue. In this type of healing, extensive granulation tissue is formed from the base of the wound and grows in from the margins to complete the repair process. The associated inflammatory response is of greater magnitude as a result of the presence of a larger clot and the fact that more necrotic tissue debris and exudates exist, which require removal from the wound. Myofibroblasts that resemble smooth muscle cells assist with the contraction of large surface wounds. Healing by secondary intention occurs more slowly than healing by primary intention and is usually associated with substantial scar formation and a thinning of the surrounding epidermis.[24]

After the initial healing process, the strength of the newly formed tissues continues to improve over a period of 2 months. Tissue strength

Prevention

Suturing is used to approximate the edges of the incision made during periodontal surgery to encourage healing by primary intention. Periodontal dressings are often placed on top of the sutured wound to keep bacteria and debris out of the surgical site and to prevent infection (see Chapter 34). Patients are instructed not to sip liquids through a straw to prevent dislodging the clot from the tooth socket. A *dry socket* that does not contain a clot cannot heal properly and is often associated with infection.

HEALING BY FIRST INTENTION

HEALING BY SECOND INTENTION

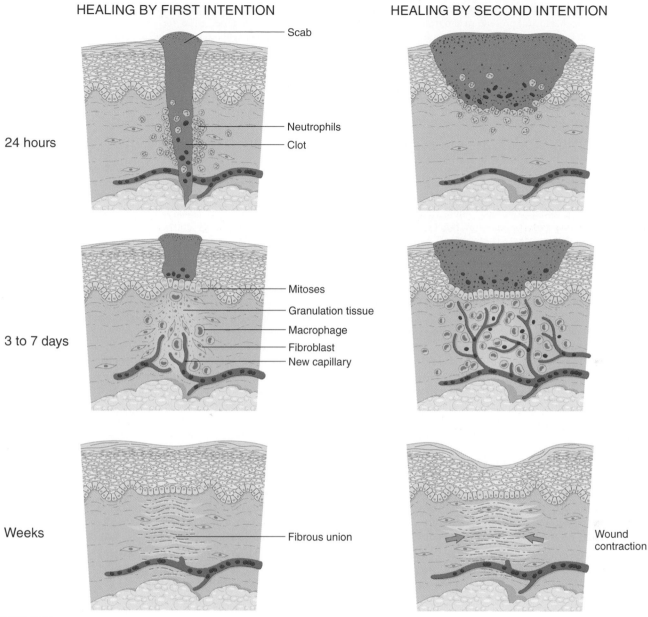

24 hours — Scab — Neutrophils — Clot

3 to 7 days — Mitoses — Granulation tissue — Macrophage — Fibroblast — New capillary

Weeks — Fibrous union — Wound contraction

FIGURE 6-15
Steps in wound healing by first intention *(left)* and second intention *(right)*. Large amounts of granulation tissue and wound contraction in healing by second intention are noted. (Reproduced with permission from Kumar V, Abbas AK, Fausto N: *Robbins and Cotran pathologic basis of disease,* ed 7, Philadelphia, 2005, Elsevier Saunders, p 112.)

is increased as a result of collagen synthesis and structural changes in the collagen fibers that make up the new connective tissue. Occasionally, complications arise during the wound healing process that alter scar formation. When a scar extends beyond its intended boundaries and does not regress with time, the scar is known as a *keloid.* Scars that remain raised above the epidermal layer are known as *hypertrophic scars.* Deformity of the wound and surrounding tissues caused by an exaggeration of the normal contraction process is typically found in patients with extensive burn injuries. Inadequate blood supply to the wound during healing may result in inadequate closure or ulceration of the wound. Excessive formation of scar tissue is known as *fibrosis* and is associated with chronic inflammatory diseases and autoimmune disease.[24]

References

1. Abbas AK, Lichtman AH: *Basic immunology: functions and disorders of the immune system,* ed 2, Philadelphia, 2004, Elsevier.
2. Aldridge JP et al: Single-blind studies of the effects of improved periodontal health on metabolic control in type I diabetes mellitus, *J Clin Periodontol* 22:271-275, 1995.
3. American Academy of Periodontology: Periodontal diseases and human health: new directions in periodontal medicine, *Ann Periodontol* 3:1-387, 1998.

4. American College of Chest Physicians: Sixth ACCP guidelines for antithrombotic therapy for prevention and treatment of thrombosis, *Chest* 119(1 suppl):1S-2S, 2001.

5. Barber A et al: The bleeding time as a preoperative screening test, *Am J Med* 78:761-764, 1985.

6. Blake GJ, Ridker PM: Inflammatory bio-markers and cardiovascular risk prediction, *J Intern Med* 252:283-294, 2002.

7. Bowie EJW, Fass DN, Owen CA: Hemostatic effect of transfused Willebrand factor in porcine von Willebrand's disease: similarities to the human disease, *Haemostasis* 9:352-365, 1980.

8. Bussey HI et al: Reliance on prothrombin time ratios causes significant errors in anticoagulation therapy, *Arch Intern Med* 152:278-281, 1992.

9. Choonara IA et al: The relationship between inhibition of vitamin K_1 2,3-epoxide reductase and reduction of clotting factor activity with warfarin, *Br J Clin Pharmacol* 25:1-7, 1988.

10. Cianciola LJ et al: Prevalence of periodontal disease in insulin-dependent diabetes mellitus (juvenile diabetes), *J Am Dent Assoc* 104:653-660, 1982.

11. Dajani AS et al: Prevention of bacterial endocarditis: recommendations by the American Heart Association, *JAMA* 277:1794-1801, 1997.

12. Danesh J et al: Association of fibrinogen, C-reactive protein, albumin, or leukocyte count with coronary heart disease: meta-analysis of prospective studies, *JAMA* 279:1477-1482, 1998.

13. Deykin D, Janson P, McMahon L: Ethanol potentiation of aspirin-induced prolongation of the bleeding time, *N Engl J Med* 306:852-854, 1982.

14. Emrich LJ, Shlossman M, Genco RJ: Periodontal disease in non-insulin dependent diabetes mellitus, *J Periodontol* 62:123-131, 1991.

15. Grossi SG et al: Treatment of periodontal disease in diabetics reduces glycated hemoglobin, *J Periodontol* 68:713-719, 1997.

16. Guyton AC, Hall JE: *Textbook of medical physiology,* ed 10, Philadelphia, 2000, WB Saunders.

17. Herman WW, Konzelman JL, Sutley SH: Current perspectives on dental patients receiving coumarin anticoagulant therapy, *J Am Dent Assoc* 128:327-335, 1997.

18. Hirsh J: Optimal intensity and monitoring warfarin, *Am J Cardiol* 75(6):39B-42B, 1995.

19. Hirsh J et al: Oral anticoagulants: mechanism of action, clinical effectiveness, and optimal therapeutic range, *Chest* 102(Suppl):312S-326S, 1992.

20. Hirsh J, Fuster V: Guide to anticoagulant therapy: part 2—oral anticoagulants, *Circulation* 89:1469-1480, 1994.

21. Hobbs FD et al: Is the international normalized ratio reliable? A trial of comparative measurements in hospital laboratory and primary care settings, *J Clin Pathol* 52:494-497, 1999.

22. Jacobs SD et al: *Laboratory test handbook,* Hudson, Ohio, 1996, Lexi-Comp.

23. Kay AB: Allergies and allergic diseases, *N Engl J Med* 344:30-37, 2001.

24. Kumar V, Abbas AK, Fausto N: *Robbins and Cotran pathologic basis of disease,* ed 7, Philadelphia, 2005, Elsevier Saunders.

25. Lassen JF, Brandslund I, Antonsen S: International normalized ratio for prothrombin times in patients taking oral anticoagulants: critical difference and probability of significant change in consecutive measurements, *Clin Chem* 41:444-447, 1995.

26. Lassen JF et al: Interpretation of serial measurements of international normalized ratio for prothrombin times in monitoring oral anticoagulant therapy, *Clin Chem* 41(8 Pt 1):1171-1176, 1995.

27. Little JW et al: *Dental management of the medically compromised patient,* ed 6, St Louis, 2002, Mosby.

28. Lockhart PB et al: Dental management considerations for the patient with an acquired coagulopathy: part 1—coagulopathies from systemic disease, *Br Dent J* 195:439-445, 2003.

29. Mariotti A: A primer on inflammation, *Compendium* 25(Suppl 1):7-15, 2004.

30. Mielke CH: Aspirin prolongation of the template bleeding time: influence of venostasis and direction of incision, *Blood* 60:1139-1142, 1982.

31. Mulvihill ML et al: *Human diseases: a systemic approach,* ed 5, Upper Saddle River, NJ, 2001, Prentice Hall.

32. Rowland RW: Immunoinflammatory response in periodontal diseases. In Rose LF et al, eds: *Periodontics: medicine, surgery, and implants,* St Louis, 2004, Elsevier Mosby.

33. Saremi A et al: Periodontal disease and mortality in type 2 diabetes, *Diabetes Care* 28:27-32, 2005.

34. Scannapieco FA, Bush RM, Paju S: Associations between periodontal disease and risk for atherosclerosis, cardiovascular disease and stroke: a systematic review, *Ann Periodontol* 8:38-53, 2003.

35. Scannapieco FA, Bush RM, Paju S: Associations between periodontal disease and risk for nosocomial bacterial pneumonia and chronic obstructive pulmonary disease: a systematic review, *Ann Periodontol* 8:54-69, 2003.

36. Scannapieco FA, Bush RM, Paju S: Periodontal disease as a risk factor for adverse pregnancy outcomes: a systematic review, *Ann Periodontol* 8:70-78, 2003.

37. Seppälä B, Seppälä M, Ainamo J: A longitudinal study on insulin-dependent diabetes mellitus and periodontal disease, *J Clin Periodontol* 20:161-165, 1993.

38. Shah SH, Newby LK: C-reactive protein: a novel marker of cardiovascular risk, *Cardiol Rev* 11:169-179, 2003.

39. Shlossman M et al: Type 2 diabetes mellitus and periodontal disease, *J Am Dent Assoc* 121:532-536, 1990.

40. Smith GT et al: Short-term responses to periodontal therapy in insulin-dependent diabetic patients, *J Periodontol* 67:794-802, 1996.

41. Steinberg MJ, Moores JF: Use of INR to assess degree of anticoagulation in patients who have dental procedures, *Oral Surg Oral Med Oral Pathol* 80:175-177, 1995.

42. Stewart JE et al: The effect of periodontal treatment on glycemic control in patients with type 2 diabetes mellitus, *J Clin Periodontol* 28:306-310, 2001.

43. Taylor GW et al: Severe periodontitis and risk for poor glycemic control in patients with non-insulin dependent diabetes mellitus, *J Periodontol* 67(10 suppl):1085-1093, 1996.

44. Thorstensson H, Hugoson A: Periodontal disease experience in adult long-duration insulin-dependent diabetes, *J Clin Periodontol* 20:352-358, 1993.

45. Wynn RL, Meiller TF, Crossley HL: *Drug information handbook for dentistry,* ed 10, Hudson, Ohio, 2005, Lexi-Comp.

Exposure Control and Prevention of Disease Transmission

Kathy B. Bassett • Kathy Eklund

INSIGHT

The dental hygiene professional has the ethical responsibility to integrate many principles into practice: basic science, principles of safety, and professional standards of care and policy, as well as to comply with numerous federal, state, and local regulations applied to infection control in the healthcare setting. Once this responsibility is understood, dental hygienists then must provide their patients oral healthcare services in a way that protects the health of both the patients and dental healthcare personnel.

✷ CASE STUDY 7-1 | Infection Control and Nonclinical Personnel

Ruth Levine is in her early 50s and works as an office manager in a small dental practice. She is a hard-working and supportive member of the staff. Her primary duties are at the front desk.

Ruth has been suffering from significant fatigue, chronic fever, and swollen glands for several weeks. She has been examined by her physician and has had multiple tests performed with no significant findings. At her last appointment the physician expressed concern about Ruth's liver function tests. After additional studies were performed with no conclusive findings, Ruth was referred to a liver specialist for evaluation. The specialist decided to perform a liver biopsy. However, on the day of the procedure, the physician postponed the biopsy to run one more test; Ruth's blood sample was taken.

✷ CASE STUDY 7-2 | Sterilization Cycle Failure

While cleaning her treatment area after a patient appointment, a second-year dental hygiene student noticed that the cycle indicator on the sterilization bag for the instruments she had just used had not changed color, which meant that the physical parameters for sterilization had not been met.

On further investigation, she discovered that two loads of instruments had been distributed without indication that appropriate sterilization had taken place. The instruments appeared to have been used during a student laboratory (in which students practiced on one another), and some had been used on general clinic patients. At least one patient was confirmed to have been exposed to unsterilized instruments, and no other students were able to confirm whether the instruments they used during that session were from the unsterilized load. A few remaining unused instrument packs were located, repackaged, and returned for proper sterilization. The patients on whom the instruments were used (the source of contamination) all appeared to be first-year dental hygiene students and had been patients in the second-year clinic the previous day.

✷ CASE STUDY 7-3 | Safe Handling of Sharps

As the dental hygienist withdrew a curet from a patient's mouth, a significant mass of blood and debris adhered to the blade of the instrument. Without giving it a second thought, the hygienist picked up a 2×2 gauze square and wiped the instrument clean with a pinching motion before returning to work.

CASE STUDY 7-4   Patient Protection

Jim Birdwell woke one morning with a sore eye. He complained of a "grainy sort of feeling," as if he had a piece of sand in his eye. He rubbed his eyes, thinking that it was just a "sleeper," which increased his discomfort. Mr. Birdwell assumed that it would eventually wash its way out and ignored the feeling. After a couple of hours the pain increased. His attempts to flush out his eye with water were unsuccessful.

After evaluation by a physician, Mr. Birdwell was referred to an ophthalmologist. Mr. Birdwell's diagnosis was an infection on the outer surface of his eye, just out of his line of sight. The grainy feeling he experienced was the formation of scar tissue. The ophthalmologist speculated that some type of bacterial matter had entered his eye, causing the infection.

KEY TERMS

acquired immunodeficiency
    syndrome
aerosols
autogenous
bioburden
biofilm
biohazardous materials
blood-borne pathogen
Centers for Disease Control and
    Prevention
contaminated
decontamination
dental health care personnel

direct transmission
droplets
engineering controls
Environmental Protection
    Agency
exposure control plan
exposure incident
guidelines
hazard abatement
healthcare-associated infections
host reservoirs
host susceptibility
human immunodeficiency virus

indirect transmission
occupational exposure
Occupational Safety and Health
    Administration
parenteral
pathogenic
personal protective equipment
recommendations
regulations
resident flora
Resource Conservation and
    Recovery Act

routes of transmission
source individual
standard operating procedures
standard precautions
standards
universal precautions
U.S. Food and Drug
    Administration
virulence
waterborne
work-practice controls

LEARNING OUTCOMES

After reading this chapter the student will be able to:

1. State the basic principles and science of disease transmission and common infectious diseases of humans, infection control in the dental workplace, and safety as it applies to biohazards in the dental workplace.
2. Identify the names of state and federal regulatory and advisory agencies that concern infection control practices and the management of biohazardous materials.
3. Integrate basic science, clinical practice, professional standards of care, and regulatory standards for infection control and work-

practice safety to prevent disease transmission and protect the health of both employees and patients in the dental workplace.
4. Apply effective principles of infection control and safe handling of biohazardous materials to provide a safe environment for dental hygienists, co-workers, patients in the dental workplace, and household members.
5. Comply with federal, state, and local standards and regulations for the dental workplace.

Infection Control and Disease Prevention

To help understand and apply the principles and implications of infection control procedures and professional responsibility, the four case histories at the beginning of this chapter represent four actual events.

Infectious disease transmission can pose serious problems in the dental workplace. All **dental health care personnel*** (DHCP) must understand the basic principles of disease transmission, infection control, and safety to minimize the risks associated with exposure to biohazardous agents. DHCP must pay close attention to basic sciences and integrate safety practices to comply with the numerous guidelines, standards of

---

*The Centers for Disease Control and Prevention (CDC) states that the term *dental health care personnel* refers to all paid and unpaid personnel in the dental health care setting who might be occupationally exposed to infectious materials, including body substances and contaminated supplies, equipment, environmental surfaces, water, or air. This group of dental professionals includes dentists, dental hygienists, dental assistants, dental laboratory technicians (e.g., in-office, commercial), students and trainees, contractual personnel, and other individuals not directly involved in patient care but potentially exposed to infectious agents (e.g., administrative, clerical, housekeeping, maintenance, volunteers).[19] The Occupational Safety and Health Administration uses the term *dental health care worker*. For the purposes of this text, the term *dental health care personnel* will be used.

care, and regulations initiated to protect the health of patients and healthcare workers.

To ensure an understanding of the risks presented and to implement safe work practices, federal regulations require that all health-care personnel (HCP) participate in specific training in infection control practices for the exposure to and handling of **biohazardous materials.** Training programs must include the following elements:

- Basics of disease transmission
- Epidemiologic characteristics of infectious diseases
- Modes of transmission for infectious agents
- Exposure prevention
- Precautionary measures

Factors in Disease Transmission

Disease transmission is influenced by a number of factors (Table 7-1). To fully understand the process, DHCP must consider the nature and source of infectious microorganisms, the ways in which these agents are transmitted to a new host, and the factors that affect infection once they reach the new host. In addition, understanding the ways in which microorganisms vary in their resistance to destruction by the host immune system or by other means is important. To control disease transmission in the dental environment, DHCP must appropriately apply the principles of infection control and associated factors to work situations.[66,95]

NATURE OF MICROORGANISMS AND INFECTIOUS AGENTS

Not all microorganisms found on or in tissues are considered capable of producing disease, or **pathogenic,** by nature. Many microorganisms, referred to as **resident flora,** are normally found in humans and are necessary to routine body functions. Included in this category are microorganisms normally found in the oral cavity.[66] The human body has adapted to and can even

Table 7-1	Basic Elements of Disease Transmission	
HOST SOURCE	**ESCAPE FROM HOST**	**ENTRY INTO NEW HOST**
Surface Skin	Natural oral activity (speech, cough, sneeze)	Inhalation
Oral Tissues	Natural oral activity (speech, cough, sneeze)	Ingestion
Saliva	Artificial (hands, instruments, aerosols, spatter)	Contact with mucous membranes
Blood	Artificial (hands, instruments, aerosols, spatter)	Penetration of intact skin

benefit from their presence. Although both nonpathogenic and pathogenic organisms are present in the oral environment, even resident flora can be pathogenic if they increase in numbers greater than normal or are transferred to sites in the body where these specific microorganisms are not normally present.

Three basic categories of microorganisms can be found in the oral environment and are easily spread through oral contact and dental procedures. To aid in this discussion, the definitions in Box 7-1 are taken from *Mosby's Dictionary of Medicine, Nursing, and Allied Health* (sixth edition).

RESERVOIRS OR SOURCES OF PATHOGENIC MICROORGANISMS

A reservoir or source allows a pathogen to survive and multiply. **Host reservoirs** in the dental environment include both patients and DHCP. Pathogenic microorganisms may be found on the surfaces of the skin and in body tissues and fluids (e.g., blood, saliva).

BOX 7-1

CATEGORIES OF MICROORGANISMS FOUND IN THE ORAL ENVIRONMENT

Virus. Minute parasitic microorganism much smaller than a bacterium that, having no independent metabolic activity, may replicate only within the cell of a living plant or host animal. Consists of a core of nucleic acid (deoxyribonucleic acid [DNA] or ribonucleic acid [RNA]) surrounded by a coat of antigenic protein sometimes and then surrounded by an envelope of lipoprotein. Examples include common cold viruses, herpes, hepatitis, HIV, measles, and rubella.

Bacteria. Any of the small unicellular microorganisms of the class Schizomycetes. They vary morphologically, are sphere shaped (cocci), rod shaped (bacilli), spiral shaped (spirochetes), or comma shaped (vibrios). The nature, severity, and outcome of any infection caused by a bacterium are characteristic of that species. Examples of infectious bacteria include TB, *Staphylococcus* strains, *Streptococcus* strains,

Neisseria gonorrhoeae, and *Legionella* strains.

Fungi (mushrooms, yeasts, molds). General term for a group of eukaryotic, thallous-forming organisms that require an external carbon source. They lack both chlorophyll and chemolithotrophic systems, can be saprophytes (i.e., organisms living on dead organic material) or parasites, reproduce by budding (e.g., simple fungus) or spore formation (e.g., multicellular fungus), and may invade living organisms including humans and nonliving organic substances. Approximately 100,000 species have been identified, 100 common in humans and 10 pathogenic. Examples of fungal infections include *Pneumocystis carinii* pneumonia, *Cryptococcus neoformans, Candida albicans,* and histoplasmosis.

HIV, Human immunodeficiency virus; *TB,* tuberculosis.

MODES OF TRANSMISSION

Microorganisms can escape the host reservoir and spread through natural occurrences, such as during speaking, coughing, sneezing, or another oral activity; through artificial means, such as carried on hands, instruments, and equipment; or through aerosols and spatter.

Once the microorganisms have escaped one host, they can spread to a new host through established *primary modes of transmission.*[10,95]

The **Centers for Disease Control and Prevention** (CDC) has defined these primary modes of transmission in the *Guidelines for Infection Control in Dental Health-Care Settings—2003.* This document states the following:

> These organisms can be transmitted in dental settings through (1) direct contact with blood, oral fluids, or other patient materials; (2) indirect contact with contaminated objects (e.g., instruments, equipment, or environmental surfaces); (3) contact of conjunctival, nasal, or oral mucosa with droplets (e.g., spatter) containing microorganisms generated from an infected person and propelled a short distance (e.g., by coughing, sneezing, or talking); and (4) inhalation of airborne microorganisms that can remain suspended in the air for long periods.[19]

Visit www.cdc.gov/OralHealth/infectioncontrol/guidelines/index.htm to view the 2003 guidelines.

Direct transmission describes the transfer of microorganisms from a specific person or host reservoir (source) directly to another person (host). Blood-borne microorganisms are transmitted by direct contact with blood, through blood products, and in blood-contaminated saliva.

Indirect transmission describes transfer of microorganisms from a specific person or host reservoir (source) to an inanimate object, such as a surface or item, and the subsequent transfer to another person (host).

Droplets (e.g., spatter) describe the transfer of microorganisms from a person or host reservoir (source), subsequently incorporated into materials that become airborne, and ultimately transferred to a person (host). Spatter or droplets are considered visible particles greater than 50 microns. This method can lead to both cross-infection or autogenous infection (i.e., back to the source).[11,28]

Aerosols describe the suspension of microorganisms within invisible particles less than 50 microns in size (usually less than 5 microns) than can be inhaled.[11,28]

Two other mechanisms of transmission, although not considered primary routes, are worthy of consideration:

- **Autogenous** (self-infection) transfer can result from any of the routes of transmission previously discussed. It involves introduction of a microorganism from one area of the body to another. Although the microorganism may be nonpathogenic in one part of the body, it may be pathogenic when introduced to another susceptible site. Examples include a transient bacteremia induced during subgingival scaling. A bacteremia peaks in approximately 15 minutes and from the initial point of contact is normally cleared from the body in 20 to 30 minutes with no harm to the host. Infective endocarditis, however, can develop in susceptible individuals with severe outcomes to the host.
- **Waterborne** transfer describes a subject of more recent concern—transmission of microorganisms through contaminated dental unit waterlines.[2,5] A film of microorganisms can attach tenaciously to the inner surface of waterline tubing, a formation known as a **biofilm.** A number of causes and contributing factors are cited for how this phenomenon occurs. When portions of this biofilm dislodge, they are carried through the waterline and can be expelled into the patient's mouth during dental procedures. If the organisms are pathogenic and the patient is a susceptible host, then an infection can develop. As many as 40 different microorganisms have been identified in contaminated waterlines.[98] Although several of these can be pathogenic, two are of significant concern for dentistry: *Legionella pneumophila* and *Pseudomonas aeruginosa.*[6,98]

PATHOGEN PORTAL OF ENTRY TO A NEW HOST

Entry into a new host is considered a completed transmission, usually occurring in the dental environment through contact with mucous membranes through one of the following:

- **Parenteral** inoculation
- Inhalation
- Breaks in the skin
- Ingestion of microorganisms carried in blood, saliva, or oral tissues

For a **blood-borne pathogen** such as hepatitis B or **human immunodeficiency virus** (HIV) to infect the host, it must gain access to the bloodstream via blood or serum body fluids. In the case of tuberculosis (TB), the portal of entry is the respiratory system via inhalation of airborne droplet nuclei.

After exposure and transmission of pathogenic microorganisms, a number of additional factors affect whether the infection will occur (Figure 7-1), including the **virulence** of the pathogen,

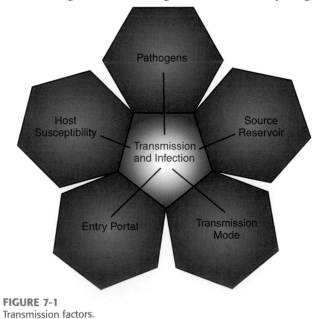

FIGURE 7-1
Transmission factors.

dose of microorganisms transmitted, and the new host's ability to resist infection.[66] The virulence or nature of a microorganism determines its pathogenicity, its degree of infectiousness, and the conditions necessary for infection to occur. Regarding dose, some highly pathogenic organisms require a small dose to initiate an infection, whereas others require a large-dose exposure before infection is likely. For example, hepatitis B is significantly more virulent than HIV. (The probability that an infection will occur is demonstrated in Figure 7-2.)

$$Infection = \frac{Virulence \times Dose\ of\ Pathogens}{Host\ Susceptibility}$$

FIGURE 7-2
Infection equation.

HOST SUSCEPTIBILITY

Also of importance in the disease transmission equation are factors not directly related to the microorganism itself. The body has a number of protective barriers and systems to help prevent infection. Intact skin is the primary physical barrier of the body. Physiologic characteristics of the respiratory system also function as primary barriers or filters to infectious agents. If these physical barriers fail, then the body's next line of defense is the immune system.

The status of the host's immune system, defined as the body's ability to resist infection, is important in the prevention of infection. **Host susceptibility** is affected by (1) the individual's general state of health (i.e., a healthy host with an intact immune system that can protect itself from many infections) and (2) the ability to resist infection (i.e., a host with a compromised immune system that is susceptible to infectious agents). When an immune system becomes compromised (immunosuppression) as a result of the presence of other conditions, diseases, or infections (co-infection), the body is less able to resist infection and is at an increased risk for developing disease. In addition to co-infection by a systemic disease, host immunosuppression can be induced by physical defects (e.g., heart valve damage, prosthetic joints), immunosuppressive drugs (e.g., chemotherapeutic agents), organ transplants with associated antirejection drugs, and the natural physiologic processes associated with stress, fatigue, and aging.[66]

Host immunity can be increased through natural or acquired immunity (i.e., having had the disease) or artificial immunity (i.e., immunization). Natural and acquired immunity varies among individuals and is a direct reflection of the person's general health.[86] (See Chapter 6 for more information on the immune system.)

Chain of Infection
The CDC explains:

Infection through any of these routes [of transmission] requires that all of the following conditions be present:
- Pathogenic organism of sufficient virulence and in adequate numbers to cause disease;

- Reservoir or source that allows the pathogen to survive and multiply (e.g., blood);
- Mode of transmission from the source to the host;
- Portal of entry through which the pathogen can enter the host; and
- Susceptible host (i.e., one who is not immune).

Occurrence of these events provides the chain of infection. Effective infection-control strategies prevent disease transmission by interrupting one or more links in the chain.[19]

Risk of Exposure in the Dental Environment

Oral healthcare procedures by nature challenge the body's natural barrier and defense systems, creating an *at-risk* environment. Theoretically, infectious agents may be passed from patient to DHCP, from DHCP to patient, to other staff members, and then carried home to associates, friends, spouses, children, and other family members. DHCP are frequently exposed to blood and blood-contaminated saliva during dental procedures. These procedures involve repeated contact with blood, saliva, oral mucous membranes, and tissues; the use of sharp instruments and needles with a danger of injury; and a wide variety of routinely performed procedures. These procedures create a greater risk of infection with a blood-borne pathogen for DHCP than for their patients.

The occurrence of infection after exposure to pathogenic organisms depends on a number of factors with respect to host resistance. Pathogenic microorganisms carried by one individual without any clinically evident or significant disease could infect and lead to disease in another individual.

Microbial Resistance

To reduce the risk of infection and spread of pathogenic microorganisms in the dental environment, understanding the nature of the organism in relationship to environmental survival time, methods of decontamination, and sterilization is necessary. For example, HIV remains viable (capable of transmitting infection) on environmental surfaces (Table 7-2) for merely minutes, whereas without appropriate decontamination, hepatitis B virus remains viable for days to weeks.[66] In addition, some microorganisms are more resistant to decontamination than others; for example, bacterial endospores (e.g., TB) are the most resistant to destruction by disinfection and sterilization procedures, whereas vegetative bacteria are the least resistant[66,81] (Figure 7-3).

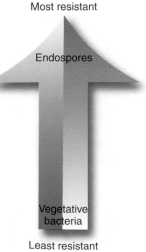

Most resistant

Endospores

Vegetative bacteria

Least resistant

FIGURE 7-3
Microbial resistance.

Table 7-2 — Modes of Transmission of Microorganisms

AGENT (DISEASE)	ROUTE(S)
Bacterial	
Mycobacterium tuberculosis (tuberculosis)	Saliva, sputum
Staphylococcus aureus (staphylococcal infections)	Saliva, skin, exudates
Streptococcus pyogenes (streptococcal endocarditis)	Open wound, blood
Treponema pallidum (syphilis)	Direct contact with lesions
Viral	
Respiratory viruses (influenza, colds, pneumonia)	Salivary secretions
Hepatitis A virus	Blood, feces, saliva
Hepatitis B virus	Blood, saliva, other body fluids
HIV (HIV-related diseases, AIDS)	Blood, other body fluids
HSV 1 and 2 (recurrent herpes, herpetic whitlow, herpetic conjunctivitis)	Saliva, secretions

Modified from Nisengard RJ, Newman MG: *Applied microbiology and immunology,* ed 2, Philadelphia, 1988, WB Saunders.
AIDS, Acquired immunodeficiency syndrome; *HIV,* human immunodeficiency virus; *HSV,* herpes simplex virus.

This knowledge enables the healthcare provider to apply appropriate measures for disinfection and sterilization to items contaminated by these organisms.

Infectious Diseases of Concern for Dental Health Care Providers

Understanding the nature of the organisms, specific transmission factors, symptoms of infection, and effects of infection can reinforce the importance for control of exposure to and transmission of infectious agents (Table 7-3). (See the suggested agencies and web sites on the Evolve site.)

> *Note*
>
> Of significant concern in the dental environment are several diseases that can be transmitted by bacteria, viruses, and fungi.*
>
> *References 10, 21, 45, 66, 83, 88, 95.

DISEASES CAUSED BY VIRAL AGENTS

The diseases listed in the following sections are caused by infection with viral agents.[10,66,95] (See suggested agencies and web sites on the Evolve site.)

Hepatitis Infection

The transmission of hepatitis in healthcare settings is a significant concern. The **Occupational Safety and Health Administration** (OSHA) has determined that healthcare workers are at great risk of contracting hepatitis B virus because any exposure may result in infection.[78]

> *Note*
>
> Hepatitis infection is a viral liver infection caused by a group of viruses.

To manage exposure to hepatitis, understanding the various types of the disease, associated routes of transmission, and prevention strategies is necessary (Table 7-4). To date, seven different hepatitis viruses have been identified: hepatitis A virus (HAV), hepatitis B virus (HBV), hepatitis C virus (HCV), hepatitis D virus (HDV), hepatitis E virus (HEV), and hepatitis G virus (HGV).* Hepatitis F virus (HFV) has been reported but not confirmed, and little is known about it. The most common symptoms of hepatitis infection are influenza-like symptoms that include fatigue; diarrhea; fever; muscle and joint pain; nausea; abdominal discomfort; and jaundice, a classic symptom of hepatitis infection. Persistent and chronic infection can lead to severe liver damage and death. (See the suggested agencies and web sites on the Evolve site.)

Hepatitis A virus

HAV is the most prevalent hepatitis infection.[10,50,51,88] It is transmitted through oral-fecal cross-contamination, ingestion of foods or water contaminated by an infected person, or close person-to-person contact. Incubation is typically 30 days after exposure but can occur between 15 and 50 days. Proper handwashing techniques are the most effective means to prevent transmission.

Screening for the antibody is the test for HAV. Vaccination to prevent HAV infection is available and can provide long-term protection against the disease. An immune globulin injection can help prevent HAV infection if it is administered within 14 days of exposure for individuals who have not been vaccinated or previously infected. Infected persons do not necessarily experience all the symptoms; in many cases, children may not experience symptoms at all. Adult infection usually causes severe illness that can last several months.

Hepatitis E virus

HEV infection shares some of the characteristics of HAV, such as a lack of a chronic phase.[51,88] Incubation is typically 2 to 9 weeks after the initial exposure and mild symptoms. Laboratory screening is the test for HEV. Immune globulin injection has not been shown to be useful in the prevention of infection after exposure, and no vaccination is currently available. HEV is primarily found in underdeveloped countries with contaminated water supplies. Outbreaks have not been observed in the United States.

Hepatitis B virus

HBV infection is transmitted through blood, blood products, or body fluids (including saliva) or a combination of all three.[10,33,48,88]

The viral life span of HBV on inanimate objects can be from 7 to 14 days, with virulence remaining high. Incubation can be from 1 to 6 months after initial exposure. A number of laboratory tests are performed to detect anti-

> *Note*
>
> HBV is the most significant hepatitis of concern in healthcare settings. A large number of these cases develop into a carrier state, with the host being contagious but not showing any clinical symptoms of disease.

*References 10, 12, 46, 51, 66, 89, 95.

Table 7-3	Summary of Significant Infectious Diseases

DISEASE	PATHOGEN	TRANSMISSION	RELATED MANIFESTATIONS	SERIOUS COMPLICATIONS
Caused by Viral Agents				
HUMAN IMMUNODEFICIENCY VIRUS	HIV	B, OBF, SC	Secondary oral infections (viral, bacterial, fungal, neoplasms)	AIDS, opportunistic infections, death
CHICKENPOX	VZV	S, B, AD	Oral lesions, latent shingles	Conjunctivitis, shingles, encephalitis
COMMON COLD	Rhinoviruses (others)	S, B, AD	Sore throat, respiratory infection	Temporary disability
CYTOMEGALOVIRUS	CMV	S, B	Adults—mononucleosis-like syndrome	Birth defects with immunosuppression, death
HEPATITIS A, E	HAV, HEV	Oral-fecal	*	*
HEPATITIS B	HBV	S, B, AD	Jaundice	Chronic disability, carrier state, hepatocellular carcinoma, co-infection, death
HEPATITIS C	HCV	S, B, AD	Liver inflammation	
HEPATITIS D	HDV	B	*	*
HERPES, OCULAR	HSV 1	S, B, AD	Herpes conjunctivitis	Potential blindness
HERPES SIMPLEX (1 OR 2)	HSV 1 or HSV 2	S, B, SC	Primary gingivostomatitis, oral herpes, herpetic whitlow	Painful lesions, disability
INFECTIOUS MONONUCLEOSIS	EBV	S, B, AD	Sore throat, oral ulcers	Temporary disability, latent disease
INFLUENZA	Influenza viruses	S, AD	Sore throat, respiratory infection	Pneumonia, death
MEASLES, RUBELLA	Rubella virus	S, NR, AD	Vascular rash	Congenital defects, infant death
MEASLES, RUBEOLA	Rubeola virus	S, NR, AD	Vascular rash	Temporary disability, encephalitis
MUMPS	Mumps virus	NR	Parotitis	Temporary disability, male sterility
PNEUMONIA, VIRAL	Cold and influenza viruses	B	Respiratory infection	Respiratory arrest
SARS	SARS-CoV	S, AD, NR, direct	Cough, difficulty breathing, hypoxia and radiographic evidence of pneumonia	Respiratory arrest
WEST NILE VIRUS	WNV	Mosquito	Fever, headache, skin rash, swollen lymph nodes, neck stiffness, stupor, disorientation, coma, tremors, muscle weakness and paralysis	Encephalitis, meningitis, death

*Content between symbols applies to all forms of hepatitis.
AD, Aerosol or droplets; *AIDS*, acquired immunodeficiency syndrome; *B*, blood, *CMV*, cytomegalovirus; *EBV*, Epstein-Barr virus; *HAV*, hepatitis A virus; *HBV*, hepatitis B virus; *HCV*, hepatitis C virus; *HDV*, hepatitis D virus; *HEV*, hepatitis E virus; *HIV*, human immunodeficiency virus; *HSV*, herpes simplex virus; *NR*, nasal or respiratory; *OBF*, other body fluids; *S*, saliva; *SARS*, severe acute respiratory syndrome; *SARS-CoV*, SARS-associated coronavirus; *SC*, sexual contact; *VZV*, varicella-zoster virus.

Continued

Table 7-3	Summary of Significant Infectious Diseases—cont'd			
DISEASE	**PATHOGEN**	**TRANSMISSION**	**RELATED MANIFESTATIONS**	**SERIOUS COMPLICATIONS**
Caused by Bacterial Agents				
GONORRHEA	*Neisseria gonorrhoeae*	SC	Gonococcal pharyngitis	Arthritis, female sterility, infant blindness
LEGIONNAIRES' DISEASE	*Legionella pneumophila*	NR	Respiratory infection	Respiratory arrest
PNEUMONIA, BACTERIAL	*Staphylococcus aureus, Streptococcus pyogenes*	NR, B	Respiratory infection	Respiratory arrest
STAPHYLOCOCCAL INFECTIONS	*S. aureus*	S, AD, nosocomial, direct	Skin lesions	Skin lesions, bacteremia, endocarditis, death
STREPTOCOCCAL INFECTIONS	*S. pyogenes*	S, B, AD	Streptococcal pharyngitis, "strep throat," skin lesions	Rheumatic heart disease, pneumonia, endocarditis, kidney problems, death
SYPHILIS	*Treponema pallidum*	SC, congenital	Primary chancre, oral ulcers	Central nervous system damage, death
TUBERCULOSIS	*Mycobacterium tuberculosis*	S, AD	Productive cough more than 3 weeks	Disability, death
Caused by Fungal Agents				
CANDIDIASIS	*Candida albicans*	S, AD, direct	Oral thrush, cutaneous infection	Opportunistic infection

bodies against the HBV-surface antigen (HBsAg); antibodies often appear before symptoms develop and may be detectable 6 months after recovery. As many as 90% of HBV infections are subclinical cases, and a large number of these cases develop into a carrier state, with the host being contagious but not showing any clinical symptoms of disease. HBV infection and its sequela continue to be a major cause of death in the world population.

The greatest concentration of HBV intraorally is in the gingival sulcus, a common site of bleeding during many dental procedures. Past studies have shown nearly twice the prevalence of HBV among dental healthcare providers when compared with the general public.[33]

The CDC recommends that all HCP who are at risk for exposure to blood-borne pathogens receive the HBV immunization.[19,27] This vaccine has proven to provide effective immunity to HBV infection. OSHA requires that employers offer immunization to employees before assigning them to work-related tasks that place them at risk of exposure. Studies performed in the 1980s identified a 8% to 15% decrease over an 8-year period in the number of dental personnel naturally infected with HBV, demonstrating effective protection with HBV immunization.[33]

Hepatitis C virus

HCV infection is transmitted through blood, blood products, or body fluids or a combination of all three.* Incubation can be from 2 to 6 months after initial exposure, and many people show no symptoms at all. HCV has become a significant concern in healthcare settings. No vaccine currently exists.

HCV has been successfully treated with the drug interferon. Recently, additional combination therapy injections are showing promise for the treatment of chronic HCV infection.

> **Note**
> Subclinical cases of HCV can establish a carrier state in which the host is contagious but shows no clinical symptoms of disease. Approximately 95% of individuals infected with HCV show no symptoms at all.

Hepatitis D virus

HDV infection is transmitted through blood, blood products, or body fluids or a combination of all three.[10,50,52,88] The host must first be infected with acute or chronic HBV for HDV infection to occur. HDV infection is the most severe form of viral hepatitis and is acquired only as a co-infection with HBV.

Hepatitis G virus

HGV infection (also known as *HGBV-C*)[50,53] is transmitted through blood, blood products, or body fluids or a combination of all three. HGV is considered a distant relative of HCV. Currently, only sophisticated laboratory testing can identify HGV. The nature, risk factors, means of prevention, and frequency of HGV infection are unclear.

Table 7-4		**Summary Comparison of Human Hepatitis Viruses**					
Hepatitis viruses—basic factors							
VIRAL AGENT	**INCU-BATION PERIOD**	**HOST RESERVOIR**	**PRIMARY TRANS-MISSION**	**CHRONIC CARRIER STATE**	**SERUM MARKERS**	**TERMINOLOGY**	**SIGNIFICANCE IN DIAGNOSIS**
HAV	2 to 7 wk	Feces, saliva, blood	Oral-fecal	No	Anti-HAV	Antibody to HAV	Detectable at onset of symptoms; persists for lifetime
					IgM anti-HAV	IgM class antibody to HAV	Indicates recent infection; detectable for 4-6 mo after infection
HBV	6 wk-6 mo	Blood, other body fluids (serum-derived, [e.g., saliva])	Parenteral, sexual, peri-natal	Yes	HBsAg	HB surface antigen	Surface antigen HBV; detectable in large quantity in serum
					HBeAg	HBe antigen	Soluble antigen of HBV; correlates with viral replication and infectivity
					Anti-HBs	Antibodies to HBsAg	Indicates past infection, immunity, passive immunity, or immunization
					Anti-HBe	Antibodies to HBeAg	Presence in serum of carrier; indicates low titer
					Anti-HBc	Antibodies to HBcAg	Indicates past infection; undetermined time period
					IgM anti-HBc	IgM antibodies to HBsAg	Indicates recent infection; detectable for 4-6 mo after infection
HCV	2 wk-6 mo	Blood	Parenteral	Yes	Anti-HCV	Antibodies to HCV	Delayed detection; no distinction between acute and chronic infection; persists for lifetime; does not indicate immunity
HDV	3-7 wk	Blood	Parenteral	Yes	HDAg	HD antigen	Detectable in early acute delta infection
			Sexual		Anti-HDV	Antibodies to HDV	Indicates past or present infection
HEV	2-9 wk	Feces	Oral-fecal	No	Anti-HEV	Antibodies to HEV	Clinical tests for HEV unavailable; diagnosis by exclusion
HGV	2-7 wk	Blood	Parenteral Perinatal	Unknown	Anti-HGV HGV RNA	Antibodies to HGV Hepatitis G RNA	Detectable in infection Present in early infection; persists at least 1 yr
						AST	Indicates liver damage; may increase with HGV infection; possible correlation to early infection

Modified from Centers for Disease Control (ACIP), Protection against viral hepatitis, *MMWR* 39(RR-2):6-7, 1990.
AST, Alanine aminotransferase; *HAV,* hepatitis A virus; *HBcAg,* hepatitis B core antigen; *HBeAg,* hepatitis B e antigen, *HBsAg,* hepatitis B virus surface antigen; *HBV,* hepatitis B virus; *HCV,* hepatitis C virus; *HDAg,* hepatitis D antigen; *HDV,* hepatitis D virus; *HEV,* hepatitis E virus; *HGV,* hepatitis G virus; *IgM,* immunoglobulin M, *RNA,* ribonucleic acid.

Transmission through blood transfusion has been documented, as has perinatal infection. Other modes of transmission are possible but have not been well documented. An increased prevalence of HGV exists among individuals with frequent exposure to blood or blood products, and co-infection with HBV or HCV (or both) is common (representing similar modes of transmission). The disease state caused by HGV infection remains unclear, and no significant evidence exists that proves HGV infection has any important sequela; however, it seems to worsen with co-infection. No proven treatment or commercial screening tests are currently available.

In addition, many other viral agents can be responsible for acute inflammatory diseases of the liver that mimic a hepatitis infection, such as herpes simplex virus (HSV), cytomegalovirus (CMV), and Epstein-Barr virus (EBV).

Patient Education Opportunity

Body piercing and tattooing have become popular fashion trends in Western industrialized nations in recent years. Risks involved with such trends include chronic infection, prolonged bleeding, scarring, chipped teeth, abscesses or boils, and speech impediments. More serious risks include the transmission of HBV and HCV, tetanus, and even HIV.* Currently, 26% of the states have regulatory authority over body-piercing establishments, whereas only four states exercise such authority.† With little or no regulation and little incentive for employees in such facilities to take precautions against infections or health hazards, dental hygiene services must include prevention and education of such risks. Body-piercing and tattoo education can be incorporated into any disease prevention discussion and protocol.

Certain practices can make body piercing and tattooing safer, including the cleanliness of the shop and the equipment used for the procedure. Are the same **standard precautions** followed in dental hygiene care? Practices such as wearing disposable masks and gloves, using single-use needles and subsequently disposing of them properly, and sterilizing every item that comes near the patient are important disease-prevention and transmission standards that should be followed in body-piercing and tattoo establishments. Follow-up instructions and care also should be emphasized. The treated area should be kept clean with soap, not alcohol, and the individual should not pick or tug at the area. If oral piercing has been done, then an antibacterial mouthwash should be used after eating to reduce infection. Care should be taken to ensure healing, with close observation of any signs of infection or complication. A physician should be contacted immediately if the area becomes sore, irritated, or infected.

*Folz BJ et al: Hazards of piercing and facial body art: a report of three patients and literature review, *Ann Plast Surg* 45(4):374-381, 2000.

†Braithwaite RL et al: Risks associated with tattooing and body piercing, *J Public Health Policy* 20(4):459-470, 1999.

Herpes Viruses

The eight types of human herpes viruses (HHV) are identified as the following†:

- HHV-1
- HHV-2 (HSV-1 and HSV-2)
- HHV-3 (varicella-zoster virus [VZV])
- HHV-4 (EBV)
- HHV-5 (CMV)
- HHV-6 (has been associated with roseola)

*References 10, 32, 49, 54, 55, 57, 89.
†References 10, 45, 61, 66, 89, 95.

- HHV-7 (sequela for which is unknown)
- HHV-8 (has been associated with Kaposi's sarcoma)[63,89]

HHV-1 through HHV-5 are discussed later in this chapter.

Viral agents are responsible for herpetic diseases, which are transmitted in saliva, blood, and droplets and through sexual contact; some diseases can be acquired through respiratory exposure. The incubation periods vary for each type of infection.

A characteristic of viruses of this family is the ability to establish a latent state (i.e., dormant with a potential for recurrent infection) in the host cells they infect. Each such virus has been implicated in central nervous system infection, specifically meningitis and meningoencephalitis.

> **Human Herpes Viruses**
> Herpetic infections cause recurrent diseases that exhibit vesicular skin lesions found on the skin surface, in the oral cavity, and on the genitalia.

> **Note**
> Primary infection may be clinically evident; 80% to 90% of primary infections are asymptomatic.

Herpes lesions are observed frequently in HIV-infected individuals and manifest as significant infections with painful, persistent oral lesions or asymptomatic shaggy white plaques on the tongue known as *hairy leukoplakia*. CMV and EBV have been associated with oral malignancies related to **acquired immunodeficiency syndrome** (AIDS), CMV with Kaposi's sarcoma, and EBV with AIDS-associated lymphoma.[45]

Herpes simplex virus

HSV has an affinity for epithelial cells and commonly attacks mucous membranes, skin, eyes, and the nervous system.[10,66,95] Transmission is through contact with contaminated saliva, and the incubation period is 2 to 12 days. Transient shedding of the virus, even with a lack of symptoms, is common.

After primary infection takes place, the virus persists in the neural ganglia that innervate the site as a latent infection, with symptoms recurring at a later time. Between episodes of infection, HSV remains dormant in the ganglia. In response to stimuli, recurrent lesions appear in the initially infected area, causing a wide variety of chronically occurring diseases. (See the suggested agencies and web sites on the Evolve site.)

HSV-1 and HSV-2 infections are most easily differentiated by the site of infection. HSV-1 infections are most commonly noted in the oral cavity, whereas HSV-2 infections are generally transmitted sexually and noted on the genitalia. Both types can exhibit skin infections, such as recurrent perioral infections and herpes labialis, the most frequent manifestation.

Other manifestations of herpes infection include herpetic whitlow, which most frequently develops around fingernail beds; ocular herpes or herpetic keratitis, which can be primary or recurrent, causing corneal ulcerations or lesions of the conjunctiva (or both); genital infections; and neonatal infections.

Herpes Simplex Virus Type 1

Only an estimated 10% of patients infected with HSV-1 show symptoms. Primary infection of HSV-1 most commonly occurs in the mouth, usually in children between ages 6 months and 6 years. Specific caution should be exercised around children with broken skin or lesions because they are highly susceptible to infection. Although the majority of primary infections are subclinical, some develop into gingivostomatitis. Pain, fever, and lymphadenopathy usually accompany this infection. The lesions generally spontaneously heal in 1 to 2 weeks.

> ## $\mathcal{HSV}$-1
> HSV-1 is the most significant viral disease affecting the oral mucosa.

Herpes labialis is characterized by recurrent lesions on the lips and, occasionally, within the oral cavity. In younger patients, lesions can be observed on the buccal mucosa, tongue, soft palate, lips, and gingiva. Lymphadenopathy in cervical and submandibular nodes is frequent with primary infection.

Herpetic gingivostomatitis is characterized by the presence of vesicles and ulcerations on oral mucosa that is attached to the periosteum, such as the gingiva.

Herpetic conjunctivitis (keratitis) and ocular herpes infection are the leading causes of blindness in the United States as a result of corneal infections. Ocular herpes infection can occur alone or simultaneously with oral infection; it almost always exhibits unilaterally and begins as conjunctivitis, with vesicles on the eyelids.

Herpetic whitlow is characterized by swelling, redness, and tenderness, with subsequent vesicle formation on the fingers. This infection is often observed around the cuticles and nail beds, occurring where small breaks in the skin are present. Herpetic whitlow was more commonly documented in dental personnel (and subsequently transmitted to patients) before the universal use of gloves.

Herpes encephalitis appears most commonly during periods of nonepidemic viral encephalitis and is caused by HSV.

Herpes Simplex Virus Type 2

> ## $\mathcal{HSV}$-2
> HSV-2 exhibits as herpes genitalia and is the most common genital disease in women.

Oral lesions can also occur from HSV-2 infection. (See the suggested agencies and web sites on the Evolve site.)

Cytomegalovirus

CMV is transmitted congenitally and through blood, saliva, crevicular fluids, sexual transmission, and possibly respiratory exposure. Incubation ranges from 3 to 12 weeks. CMV has a propensity for salivary glands. The majority of the adult population has been infected with CMV, resulting in life-long latent association in the host. Reactivation can result in severe infection in immunosuppressed hosts.

Infection may involve multiple organ systems, and acute infection may mimic infectious mononucleosis or hepatitis. The most common clinical presentation of CMV infection in the compromised individual is that of a mononucleosis-like syndrome, with the next most common syndrome being pneumonia. No effective therapy exists for the treatment of CMV pneumonitis. CMV infection can be severe in cases of neonatal transmissions. (See the suggested agencies and web sites on the Evolve site.)

Epstein-Barr Virus

EBV may be excreted into saliva during the infectious stage of mononucleosis and for weeks after infection. It is acquired primarily by oral contact, through contact with saliva, and less commonly through blood transfusion.

> ## $\mathcal{EBV}$
> During the incubation period, EBV can replicate in the oropharynx for 4 to 7 weeks while the individual continues to be infectious.

EBV may persist in blood lymphocytes for years after infection and exhibit symptoms in latent disease. Clinical symptoms include fever, pharyngitis, and cervical lymphadenopathy. EBV also has been found in the white hairy plaque on the tongue of HIV-infected persons, known as *hairy leukoplakia*.

Infectious mononucleosis is the primary EBV infection in young adults. More than 90% of adults have been exposed to EBV, and differentiation from other causes of mononucleosis is made through antibody testing. (See the suggested agencies and web sites on the Evolve site.)

Varicella-Zoster Virus

VZV enters the body via the respiratory tract and is transmitted by airborne water particles through sneezing and coughing and by direct contact with skin lesions. After a 2-week incubation period, cutaneous vesicles develop—a primary infection known as *chickenpox*. During primary infection, VZV migrates to the dorsal root ganglia and along sensory nerves, establishing a latent infection known as *shingles*.

Chickenpox is a viral exanthematous disease (exhibiting cutaneous lesions). The incubation period is 10 to 21 days. Chickenpox is usually benign in healthy children, but in immunocompromised children the disease can become life-threatening. The varicella vaccine is available to prevent chickenpox. Most people who get the vaccine will not get chickenpox or will have a milder form of the disease.[1] The most obvious clinical symptom is small vesicles on the skin that go through three distinctive phases—from fluid-filled vesicles, to pustules, to dry-crusted lesions—and can be found anywhere on the body including the oral cavity. (See the suggested agencies and web sites on the Evolve site.)

Shingles is the result of latent or persistent VZV infection, established in spinal cord ganglia similar to other herpes viral infections. This recurrent infection, herpes zoster (shingles), is painful and can be severe or life-threatening. (See the suggested agencies and web sites on the Evolve site.)

Human Immunodeficiency Virus Infection and Acquired Immunodeficiency Syndrome

A viral agent present in the blood and body fluids of the infected host transmits the HIV infection. The incubation period for HIV varies; the clinical onset of symptoms has been noted from a few weeks to several months. The severity of HIV-related diseases and the development of AIDS are directly related to the

sions are the following:

- Fungal (candidiasis, histoplasmosis)
- Viral (hairy leukoplakia, HSV)
- Bacterial (gingival, periodontal)
- Neoplastic (Kaposi's sarcoma, lymphoma)
- Other lesions (parotitis)

Co-infections may pose a greater hazard than HIV itself. With the use of protease inhibitors in the treatment of HIV infection, a decline has been noted in the most common oral lesions associated with HIV, such as hairy leukoplakia and oral candidiasis. However, at the same time, a significant increase has been noted in oral warts linked directly to the use of protease inhibitors.[68]

HIV-related diseases and AIDS include a vast number of associated opportunistic infections, and the course of disease identifies its classification. The CDC has established a classification system for HIV infection. (See the Clinical Resources asset on the Evolve site.) This system lists the vast, clinically identified secondary infections and laboratory test factors involved in the diagnosis and management of HIV disease.

Although HIV is not considered a high-risk hazard in dentistry with the appropriate use of standard precautions, an **exposure incident** is a concern if it does occur. Appropriate follow-up is critical (see Postexposure Management on page 145 of this chapter). (Because of the extensive information on HIV and AIDS, the suggested agencies and web sites on the Evolve site should be consulted for study on HIV, AIDS, and related infections. See Chapter 47 for more specific content on this disease.)

Measles

Rubeola (hard measles) is a viral infection that was once widespread and highly communicable in children before the introduction of a vaccination.[10,32,66] A second form of measles, known as *rubella* (German measles), exhibits milder symptoms than rubeola.[10,66,95] Transmission is airborne, through water droplets, or via direct contact with nasal and throat secretions of an infected host. The incubation period for rubeola is 7 to 18 days; for rubella, incubation is 14 to 23 days. Symptoms include fever, conjunctivitis, cough, and Koplik's spots on the buccal mucosa, followed by a red, blotchy rash on the face that spreads to the body.

Vaccination is required in the United States for all infants, with booster shots administered to school-aged children. (See the suggested agencies and web sites on the Evolve site.)

degree of immune system dysfunction. Numerous opportunistic infections and cancers can develop in the HIV-infected host; the five primary types of HIV-associated lesions are the following:

Respiratory Diseases

A number of respiratory diseases are acquired primarily through respiratory transmission.[10,66,95]

Common cold

The common cold is the most frequently occurring infection worldwide.

The incubation period for the common cold is 48 to 72 hours. The three primary **routes of transmission** are via virions suspended in droplets that are sneezed or coughed directly onto a new host; by aerosols that can remain airborne for long periods, being inhaled and then inoculated onto the nasal mucosa; and by direct contact and transfer through contaminated hands, with inoculation into the nose or mucosa of the eye. Colds are cited as the most common reason for absenteeism in the workplace, and transmission is promoted in crowded conditions such as school classrooms. In the United States, adults typically experience two to four colds per year, whereas children experience six per year. If acute oropharyngitis is present, then a secondary infection by *Streptococcus pyogenes* can lead to rheumatic heart disease. Pneumonia is another secondary infection with serious complications. (See the suggested agencies and web sites on the Evolve site).

Influenza

Influenza infection (commonly known as the *flu*) is generally attributed to exposure to two primary types of viruses: influenza types A and B.[24,25]

The predominant mode of transmission is direct contact through airborne water droplet exposure.

Incubation is short, generally 1 to 5 days. A vaccine is valuable for high-risk groups, such as the elderly, individuals with immunosuppressive diseases, and healthcare workers. (See the suggested agencies and web sites on the Evolve site.)

Haemophilus influenzae type B (HIB) is a highly contagious bacterial infection known to cause life-threatening infections in children younger than 5 years of age. Importantly, this bacterium is not a cause of influenza.

Antibiotics such as ampicillin are no longer effective against HIB as a result of bacterial resistance; however, HIB can be prevented by vaccination.[24,25]

Mumps

Mumps infection occurs when its virus enters the upper respiratory tract via saliva or other secretions. The incubation period is 16 to 18 days, and the virus may be present in saliva for 6 to 7 days before clinical symptoms appear. The main clinical manifestation of mumps is inflammation of the salivary glands and clinical swelling of the parotid glands, although the virus spreads throughout the body. Mumps viral infection can be prevented by immunization. (See the suggested agencies and web sites on the Evolve site.)

Viral pneumonia

Viral pneumonia can develop as a secondary complication to any viral infection, such as colds, influenza, and lower respiratory tract infections, as well as a sequela to measles and chickenpox. Transmission factors primarily include person-to-person contact via droplet aerosols and with contaminated hands. A pneumonia vaccine is available.

Emerging and Reemerging Infectious Diseases

The top three infectious diseases emerging worldwide are AIDS, malaria, and TB. Although not considered a *significant risk* for DHCP, notable emerging diseases include severe acute respiratory syndrome (SARS) and West Nile virus (WNV).

Severe acute respiratory syndrome

SARS was first identified in late 2002 in Asia. The virus responsible for SARS is a coronavirus.

The illness manifests as respiratory distress ranging from mild to extreme (e.g., cough, difficulty breathing, hypoxia) with fever and radiographic evidence of pneumonia. The virus is spread by close contact with someone who is infected with SARS through droplets from coughing, sneezing, kissing, embracing, sharing eating and drinking utensils, and close conversation.[16]

> *SARS*
> To date, no tests can definitively diagnose the SARS coronavirus; therefore the diagnosis is made from clinical data.

West Nile virus

An infected mosquito transmits WNV. WNV may be asymptomatic (mild infection) in some individuals, to severe (1 in 150 infections) in others, resulting in encephalitis, meningitis, or meningoencephalitis.

The incubation period in humans is from 3 to 14 days after exposure. Symptoms are fever; headache; body aches; sometimes a skin rash; swollen lymph nodes; and in more severe cases headache, high fever, neck stiffness, muscle weakness, tremors, paralysis, disorientation, stupor, and coma. No specific treatment for WNV exists unless the illness is severe, at which time hospitalization is often necessary as a result of the symptoms. Treatment can include intravenous fluids, pain control, respiratory support, and the prevention of secondary infections.[18]

DISEASES CAUSED BY BACTERIAL AGENTS

The diseases discussed in the following sections are caused by infection with bacterial agents.[10,66,95] (See the suggested agencies and web sites on the Evolve site.)

Gonorrhea

Gonorrhea is an infection caused by the species *Neisseria gonorrhoeae*. Transmission is through contact with exudates from mucous membranes of infected persons and almost always results from sexual activity with an infected individual.

> *Gonorrhea*
> Gonorrhea can be infectious for months in untreated asymptomatic individuals.

The incubation period ranges from 2 to 7 days. (See the suggested agencies and web sites on the Evolve site.)

Legionella

Legionella species appears as two distinct acute bacterial infections: legionnaires' disease and Pontiac fever.[6,10,29] Several strains of the causative agent, *Legionella* species, have been identified. Transmission is usually airborne from aerosol-producing devices and air-conditioning units.

> *Legionella*
> Person-to-person transmission of *Legionella* has not been documented.

The incubation period is 2 to 10 days for legionnaires' disease and 24 to 48 hours for Pontiac fever. (See the suggested agencies and web sites on the Evolve site.)

Bacterial Pneumonia

Bacterial pneumonia can follow acute lower respiratory tract infection with *Streptococcus pneumoniae*. Several other bacterial agents (including oral bacteria) have also been implicated in pneumonia infections. The most common types of infection vary between adults and children. Transmission is spread through airborne water droplets or direct oral contact or indirectly from articles freshly soiled with respiratory discharges. Incubation for bacterial pneumonia may be as short as 1 to 3 days. Infection is characterized by a sudden onset of chills and fever.

> *Bacterial Pneumonia*
> Pneumonia is a serious secondary illness and a noted cause of death in infants, the elderly, and immunocompromised individuals.

Staphylococcus Infections

Staphylococcus microorganisms,[81] such as *S. aureus* and *S. epidermidis,* are part of the normal resident flora of the body for many individuals.

S. aureus is a major cause of nosocomial and community-acquired infections and is exhibited in a number of ways, including skin infec-

> *Staphylococcus*
> As high as 50% of the population harbors *Staphylococcus* organisms, with higher percentages noted for hospital personnel.

tions such as impetigo and gastrointestinal tract infections that cause vomiting and diarrhea. *S. aureus* is also responsible for the acute febrile disease infection known as *toxic shock syndrome*.

Autoinfection is responsible for at least one third of infections, with draining lesions and purulent discharge being the most common sources of epidemic spread. Transmission is by contact with a person who either has lesions or is asymptomatic (i.e., harboring pathogenic strains in the anterior nasal passages). The hands are the most common vehicle of transmission. The incubation period is most commonly 4 to 10 days but varies and can be indefinite. *Staphylococcus* is communicable as long as lesions continue to drain or a carrier state persists, and autoinfection may continue during the period of nasal colonization or throughout the duration of active lesions.

Currently, many *S. aureus* infections do not respond to common antibiotic treatment because of the emergence of resistant strains. As high as 80% of *S. aureus* strains are resistant to penicillin. Such strains have developed resistance to most aggressive types of antibiotics available, such as methicillin and vancomycin. These strains pose serious challenges for healthcare providers. (See the suggested agencies and web sites on the Evolve site.)

Streptococcus Infections

Bacterial agents that cause *Streptococcus* infections are group A

> **Streptococcus**
>
> *Streptococcus* infections are rarely transmitted by indirect contact with objects or hands, and casual contact rarely leads to infection.

(S. pyogenes) and group B *(S. agalactiae)* streptococci. Group A is the causative agent for a variety of diseases (e.g., sore throat, scarlet fever, impetigo), whereas group B is responsible for two distinct and serious forms of infections in newborn infants. The primary mode of transmission is through direct or intimate contact with carriers. Microorganisms harbored in the nasal passage are particularly likely to transmit infection.

The incubation period is short, usually 1 to 3 days, whereas the infectious period lasts for 10 to 21 days in mild cases. More aggressive cases that include purulent discharge can remain infectious for weeks. Bacteria may be present on the skin 1 to 2 weeks before the development of impetigo lesions. (See the suggested agencies and web sites on the Evolve site.)

Syphilis

> **Cause of Syphilis**
>
> The bacterial agent, *Treponema pallidum*, causes syphilis.

Syphilis transmission is through direct contact with infectious exudates from obvious or concealed moist lesions of skin and mucous membranes, body fluids, and secretions (e.g., saliva, semen, blood, vaginal discharge) of infected individuals during sexual contact. Transmission can occur through blood transfusion when the donor is in the early stages of infection. The incubation period is 10 days to 3 months, with the individual being

infectious indefinitely; latent infection is expected. (See the suggested agencies and web sites on the Evolve site.)

Tetanus

Tetanus is an infection, induced by the tetanus bacillus *Clostridium tetani* at the site of an open wound injury.

The presence of necrotic tissue or foreign bodies sup-

> **Tetanus Transmission**
>
> Tetanus is usually transmitted through puncture wounds contaminated by soil, dust, or feces.

ports the growth of this anaerobic pathogen. The incubation period for tetanus is 3 to 21 days. Highly contaminated wounds may develop infection more rapidly with more severe symptoms and a poorer prognosis. Tetanus infection can be prevented with a tetanus immunization, the effects of which last approximately 10 years. Booster shots are recommended at 10-year intervals or after a contaminated injury.

Tuberculosis

TB is an infection acquired by respiratory exposure to *Mycobacterium tuberculosis*.[*]

The incubation period for TB is 4 to 12 weeks from infection to primary lesions or a significant tuberculin test reaction. Clinical illness most

> **Tuberculosis**
>
> TB is spread through airborne droplet nuclei, escaping the source during oropharyngeal activities such as coughing, sneezing, and singing and can remain airborne for some time.

commonly develops within 6 to 12 months of infection. Symptoms of pulmonary TB include a persistent cough, fever, night sweats, fatigue, and loss of appetite. Pulmonary TB is more common than extrapulmonary disease, affecting structures such as the lymph nodes, skin, kidneys, bones, and joints.

Healthcare employees exposed to acute cases of infection or having repeated, long-term exposure through day-to-day, close contact with an active carrier are at particular risk for developing TB. Over time, TB is walled off in the body and considered inactive. During latent disease, if the host immune system is compromised, then TB can reactivate and shed the infectious agent again. A positive skin test does not indicate that the host is infectious but rather that the individual has been infected at some time. A positive TB skin test can result even with an inactive, latent infection.

CDC has guidelines and recommendations for TB exposure prevention and management in healthcare settings.[16a] These guidelines and requirements are applied as indicated, based on the frequency of exposure and the number of cases geographically present. Guidelines are more commonly applied in medical healthcare facilities but may be applied in dental facilities if the risk of significant exposure is present. Most dental facilities fall into the *low risk* category. Screening (PPD screening) of personnel in low risk settings is indicated to establish a baseline and further testing is not required unless exposure occurs or the

---

*References 7, 9, 20, 23, 24, 34-39, 94.

dental healthcare setting TB risk changes to a medium or potential transmission risk category.[16a]

DISEASES CAUSED BY FUNGAL AGENTS

Although several diseases are caused by infection with fungal agents, candidiasis is a significant infection.[10,66,95] (See the suggested agencies and web sites on the Evolve site.)

Candidiasis

The fungal agent *Candida albicans,* which is often part of the normal oral flora, causes candidiasis. Transmission is through contact with secretions of the mouth, skin, or feces of an infected host and from mother to infant during childbirth. Candidiasis, also known as *thrush,* is a common oral condition in newborns. The incubation period is 2 to 5 days in infants, but otherwise it varies.

> *Note*
>
> Candidiasis is communicable when lesions are present. Clinical infection usually occurs when host immune defenses are low, such as in immunocompromised states.

Infection usually is confined to superficial layers of the skin and mucous membranes, exhibiting clinically as oral thrush. Candidiasis may also exhibit ulcerations or pseudomembranes in the esophagus and gastrointestinal tract.

Government Agencies: Regulations, Standards, and Guidelines

Because of the diverse nature of the practice of dentistry, several federal, state, and local agencies contribute to the regulations, standards, guidelines, and practices that affect the dental workplace. To integrate the recommendations and requirements of each with the concepts of basic science and microbiology, an understanding of the focus of each agency is important.

REGULATORY TERMINOLOGY

> *Note*
>
> The terms *regulations* and *standards* are often interchanged, as are *guidelines* and *recommendations,* in discussions of the provisions of governing agencies.

Defining the nature of the authority and the influence of each agency or organization is important to compliance. The following terminology explains the intent of the documents and authority of each agency:

- **Regulations** are governmental orders carrying the force of law.
- **Standards** indicate an expectation of compliance with a level of requirement.
- **Guidelines** are policies or rules intended to give practical guidance.
- **Recommendations** are intended to give advice or counsel.

CENTERS FOR DISEASE CONTROL AND PREVENTION

The CDC is a federal agency that studies and monitors the etiology and epidemiologic characteristics of diseases world-wide. It is the primary source of updated and current information on infectious diseases for DHCP. The CDC issues guidelines recommending procedures for the control of disease transmission for public health,[27] including immunization recommendations, infection control and injury prevention, and postinjury or postexposure protocols. (See the suggested agencies and web sites on the Evolve site.) The CDC only issues guidelines; it is not considered an enforcement agency. It is the primary source of scientific evidence on which specific standards for healthcare issues are based. (See the suggested agencies and web sites on the Evolve site.)

The CDC's *Guidelines for Infection Control in Dental Health-Care Settings—2003*[19] is the current key document that sets the minimum standards for infection control practices in dentistry. The following text is taken from the introduction to the guidelines:

This report consolidates recommendations for preventing and controlling infectious diseases and managing personnel health and safety concerns related to infection control in dental settings. This report 1) updates and revises previous CDC recommendations regarding infection control in dental settings; 2) incorporates relevant infection-control measures from other CDC guidelines; and 3) discusses concerns not addressed in previous recommendations for dentistry. These updates and additional topics include the following:

- application of standard precautions rather than universal precautions;
- work restrictions for health-care personnel (HCP) infected with or occupationally exposed to infectious diseases;
- management of occupational exposures to bloodborne pathogens, including postexposure prophylaxis (PEP) for work exposures to hepatitis B virus (HBV), hepatitis C virus (HCV), and human immunodeficiency virus (HIV);
- selection and use of devices with features designed to prevent sharps injury;
- contact dermatitis and latex hypersensitivity;
- sterilization of unwrapped instruments;
- dental water-quality concerns (e.g., dental unit waterline biofilms; delivery of water of acceptable biological quality for patient care; usefulness of flushing waterlines; use of sterile irrigating solutions for oral surgical procedures; handling of community boil-water advisories);
- dental radiology;
- aseptic technique for parenteral medications;
- preprocedural mouth rinsing for patients;
- oral surgical procedures;
- laser/electrosurgery plumes;
- tuberculosis (TB);
- Creutzfeldt-Jakob disease (CJD) and other prion-related diseases;
- infection-control program evaluation; and
- research considerations.

OCCUPATIONAL SAFETY AND HEALTH ADMINISTRATION

OSHA, a division of the U.S. Department of Labor, exists to ensure the protection of employee safety through the enforcement of standards or regulations. It exercises federal regulatory authority for compliance by employers. The development and enforcement of standards for healthcare employees is based on the CDC's recommendations and guidelines.

OSHA standards[78] protect each employee's right to a safe workplace, including the following:

- Practices that help reduce risk of exposure to blood-borne pathogens
- Provision and maintenance of proper personal protection
- Rules for handling any item **contaminated** with body fluids or potentially infectious agents
- Instruction in the proper use and storage of chemical products
- Requirement that an employee be informed of the hazardous nature and all risks inherent to a work assignment

Each employer must ensure that infection control and workplace safety is implemented and monitored. (See the suggested agencies and web sites on the Evolve site.)

DHCP must remain current with proposed OSHA regulations and revisions that may affect dentistry. Of significant concern are upcoming revisions and final standards in the areas of indoor air quality; use of new **engineering controls,** which stress the use of devices for the management of contaminated needles and other sharp instruments; as well as ergonomics. Directives in each of these areas will have a direct effect on dentistry. (See the suggested agencies and web sites on the Evolve site.)

ENVIRONMENTAL PROTECTION AGENCY

The **Environmental Protection Agency** (EPA) is the federal organization responsible for regulating the use and disposal of products and waste that may adversely affect the environment. The EPA can provide information on the classification of chemical agents used in dentistry to help DHCP select appropriate products for each specific task, such as when to use high- or intermediate-level disinfectants. It can also help interpret manufacturers' labeling and label claims for the proper use and handling of a product. All chemical products used for disinfection, sterilization, and decontamination must be registered with the EPA. Some products require EPA or U.S. Food and Drug Administration registrations or both, considerations that should be noted in product selection.

For many states the EPA is the primary authority o n acceptable disposal of medical, infectious, hazardous, and toxic wastes. Each state and local government may have primary jurisdiction over waste disposal. Knowing all the agencies with regulatory authority in the area in which a workplace is located is necessary. The most stringent regulations must be applied. Even in states with their own regulations on hazardous waste, the EPA can take precedence if its regulations are more stringent or if the waste causes environmental contamination.

The **Resource Conservation and Recovery Act** (RCRA) designates the generator of the waste as ultimately responsible, no matter where the waste ends up (with or without knowl-

edge). This party must pay for the clean-up costs for any improper disposal of hazardous waste, a concept known as *cradle-to-grave liability* that is meant to ensure the appropriate disposal of the waste generated. (See the suggested agencies and web sites on the Evolve site.)

U.S. FOOD AND DRUG ADMINISTRATION

The **U.S. Food and Drug Administration** (FDA) regulates products and equipment that affect living tissue—by ingestion, contact, inhalation, or exposure—including chemical products, drugs, food, medical devices, and accessories to medical devices (e.g., sterilizers, radiology equipment, gloves used for medical care). A specific branch in the FDA deals with the numerous infection control items used in the healthcare industry. The FDA reviews all safety and efficacy data submitted by the manufacturer before granting permission to market a product. The FDA provides consumer, radiation safety and hygiene, and quality assurance information on request.

The Safe Medical Devices Act of 1990 (SMDA) is a law that requires device-user facilities and distributors, as well as manufacturers of medical devices, to report certain device-related problems to the FDA. (See the suggested agencies and web sites available on the Evolve site.)

STATE AGENCIES

Individual state agencies may mandate aspects of infection control policy and practices in dentistry, such as state-based OSHA plans, licensing boards, dental quality assurance commissions, or state public health departments. An even greater number of states regulate the disposal of infectious and hazardous medical waste through state EPA offices, local boards of health, and public health departments. Some state guidelines are more stringent than the federal regulations and current professional standards or guidelines.

Local authorities also may place limits on the disposal of medical waste and wastewater, particularly if the community is served by septic systems or if the current municipal facilities are affected. All agencies concerned with medical waste should be contacted and their regulations reviewed before making any decision on waste hauling and disposal.

PROFESSIONAL ASSOCIATIONS

A number of professional associations representing medicine, dentistry, science, health care, and education set standards of care, regulations, education, and training in infection control. They serve as resources for healthcare professionals and include but are not limited to the following:

- *Organization for Safety and Asepsis Procedures* (OSAP) is dedicated to the establishment, implementation, and maintenance of scientifically valid and reliable standards for infection control. OSAP is a unique organization of practitioners, educators, and industry members who collaborate to share ideas and information promoting sound policies, practices, and technology for infection control. (See the suggested agencies and web sites available on the Evolve site.)

- *Association for Professionals in Infection Control and Epidemiology* (APIC) is a multidisciplinary voluntary international organization designed to influence, support, and improve the quality of health care through the practice and management of infection control and the application of epidemiologic findings in all healthcare settings. (See the suggested agencies and web sites on the Evolve site.)
- *American Dental Association* (ADA) takes an active role in setting standards of care and interpreting external regulations for dentistry. Although the ADA affects professional guidelines regarding the prudent and safe practice of dentistry, it does not have any direct regulatory authority. However, DHCP are expected to follow these basic standards for patient care based on CDC-published guidelines and OSHA standards. (See the suggested agencies and web sites on the Evolve site.)
- *American Dental Education Association* (ADEA) is the leading national organization for dental education. Members include all U.S. and Canadian dental schools, advanced general dentistry education programs, hospital programs, and allied dental education programs, as well as corporations, faculty, and students. ADEA's mission is to lead the dental education community by addressing contemporary issues influencing education, research, and public health. Included in this commitment is the development of curricular guidelines for dental education regarding infection control.[80,90] (See the suggested agencies and web sites on the Evolve site.)

STATE AND LOCAL PROFESSIONAL ASSOCIATIONS AND SOCIETIES

Local professional associations for dental hygiene, dental, dental assisting, dental laboratory technology, and denturist professionals can be excellent resources for specific state and local regulations. These organizations have affiliations with many of the national associations previously discussed.

Advisory and Regulatory Terminology and Explanations

Over the past decade, new terminology has been applied in the field of infection control. This terminology is defined in federal standards set by OSHA for **occupational exposure** to blood-borne pathogens. The primary concept, *exposure control,* incorporates the basic science and concepts of infection control with a focus on prevention of initial exposure to blood-borne pathogens and the transmission of infectious disease.

To help integrate the CDC's *Guidelines for Infection Control in Dental Health-Care Settings—2003,*[19] the CDC developed operational definitions. These definitions can be found in Appendix C and should become part of your professional vocabulary.

Note

Although the term *exposure control* is commonly interchanged with *infection control,* readers should understand that exposure control is a primary goal of infection control.

GLOSSARY OF SELECTED OSHA TERMS

To help integrate OSHA's standard for exposure control with the basic principles of dental infection control, the following OSHA definitions from the *OSHA Bloodborne Pathogens Standard, Section 29 CFR 1910.1030*[78] are applied:

Blood: Human blood, human blood components, and products made from human blood.

Blood-borne pathogens: Pathogenic microorganisms, which include but are not limited to HBV and HIV, present in human blood and capable of causing disease in humans.

Contaminated: Presence or the reasonably anticipated presence of blood or other potentially infectious materials (OPIM) on an item or surface.

Contaminated sharps: Any contaminated object that can penetrate the skin, including but not limited to needles, scalpels, broken glass, broken capillary tubes, and exposed ends of dental wires.

Exposure incident: Specific eye, mouth, other mucous membrane, nonintact skin, or parenteral contact with blood or OPIM that occurs during the performance of an employee's duties.

Handwashing facilities: Places providing an adequate supply of running potable water, soap, and single-use towels or hot-air–drying machines.

Hazard abatement: Policies, procedures, and pieces of equipment that reduce the risk of occupational exposures to blood-borne pathogens, including OSHA's eight primary categories of control:

1. **Universal precautions:** This approach to infection control treats all human blood and certain human body fluids as if they were known to be infected with HIV, HBV, and other blood-borne pathogens and all material as if it were potentially infected with blood-borne pathogens.
2. **Personal protective equipment** (PPE): Specialized clothing or equipment that is worn by an employee for protection against a hazard. General work clothes, not intended to function as protection against a hazard, are not considered PPE. In oral health care, PPE refers to those barriers that protect the employee from exposure to infectious and potentially infectious or hazardous materials.
3. **Work-practice controls** (WPCs): These controls reduce the likelihood of exposure by altering the manner in which a task is performed, including methods of performing a task (e.g., actions, behaviors) that reduce the chance of an exposure incident. WPCs ensure that a task is performed in the safest way possible.
4. *Engineering controls* (ECs): These controls isolate or remove the blood-borne pathogen hazard from the workplace and may involve an actual device or a method of use provided by available technology. The purpose of ECs is to reduce the risk by confining or isolating infectious materials. ECs must be regularly examined and maintained or replaced to ensure effectiveness.

5. *Housekeeping:* These methods, procedures, and tasks ensure that the workplace is maintained in a clean and sanitary condition. The employer shall determine and implement a written schedule for cleaning, including the methods, procedures, and tasks to be performed and the materials and products to be used.

6. *Signs and labels:* These items are used to identify an immediate or recognized hazard. Examples include the universal biohazard label and symbol, chemical hazard information, fire hazard and evacuation signs, and others.

7. *Record keeping:* Documents must be kept to verify employment practices and training, such as employee medical records maintained for the duration of employment plus 30 years, including immunization records and injury and incident records. Training records are maintained for 3 years. Informed refusal and declination records of HBV immunization and vaccination and other specified or indicated immunizations are also required. Postexposure evaluation and follow-up records, including the informed refusal and declination of postexposure follow-up are maintained. Material safety data sheets (MSDS), which are part of the OSHA hazards communication standard and not the blood-borne pathogen standard, are kept.

8. *Information and training:* All employees with occupational exposure are required to participate in a training program that is provided at no cost to the employee during working hours.

Source individual: Any individual, living or dead, whose blood or OPIMs may be sources of occupational exposure.

OTHER RELATED TERMINOLOGY

To further understand the application of basic infection control language, the following terminology is provided:

Exposure control plan (ECP): Written statement of specific procedures and tasks to be performed for the prevention of initial exposure to biohazardous materials and substances. The ultimate goal of an exposure control plan is to prevent any exposure, therefore eliminating the *initial* transmission of infectious agents that can lead to subsequent infection.

Infection control policy (ICP): Written directive for infection control efforts and implementation of individual exposure control procedures that reduce or eliminate hazards to which students, employees, and patients may be exposed via direct or indirect contact with infectious body fluids.

Performance-based (or procedural-based) choices: Considers the actions and consequences involved in the performance of a task or a procedure, in contrast to choices based on beliefs or presumptions about patient risk factors related to disease transmission.

Standard operating procedures (SOPs): Documented practices that are followed during the performance of any risk-related task or procedure.

Techniques, Procedures, and Supportive Evidence

Infection control is a system of policies, procedures, and practices that when successfully implemented will minimize the risk of transmission of pathogenic microorganisms.

The primary goal of infection control is to prevent **healthcare-associated infections** for HCP and patients using a variety of strategies. These strategies are designed to break the chain of infection at one or more points by reducing or preventing the risk of transmitting infectious agents in dental healthcare settings.

Evidence-based strategies for disease prevention and risk reduction make up the foundation for an effective program and should be used to develop and implement policies, procedures, and practices designed to prevent healthcare-associated infections for HCP and patients. Site-specific SOPs facilitate DHCP in the day-to-day implementation of the program. The CDC's 2003 guidelines[19] are based on recommendations categorized on the basis of existing scientific data, theoretical rationale, and applicability.

The categories in Box 7-2 are based on the system used by CDC's Healthcare Infection Control and Prevention Advisory Committee (HICPAC) to categorize recommendations.

GOAL OF AN INFECTION CONTROL PROGRAM

The ultimate goal of procedures defined by the ECP is to eliminate cross-contamination and potential exposure to pathogenic microorganisms for patients and DHCP during the provision of dental care. Infection control is an outcome of exposure control; through the reduction of exposure to infectious agents few infections should occur. To achieve this goal, both the DHCP and the patient must be aware of the potential risks associated with the delivery and receipt of oral healthcare services and accompanying procedures used to reduce these risks significantly.

The primary focus of all exposure control procedures is to prevent or reduce the risk of exposure to infectious agents and to minimize the risk of infection from any exposure that occurs during routine tasks.

Prevention

The steps to reduce risk of exposure and minimize risk of infection are as follows:

- Reduce the number of pathogenic microorganisms present, eliminate cross-contamination, and stop the spread of infection. When primary exposure levels are reduced, the body's normal resistance mechanisms should prevent infection.
- Increase host resistance. Following published immunization protocols for healthcare employees is important.
- Treat each potential exposure situation as though disease transmission can occur, and take appropriate measures to alter the situation to reduce the risk of exposure. Treat all patients as if they were carriers of an infectious disease, applying standard precautions.
- Implement and follow practices that are intended to protect patients, DHCP, and their families from infection and the subsequent effect of income loss and possible liability.

BOX 7-2

CDC AND HICPAC CATEGORIES OF RECOMMENDATION FOR INFECTION CONTROL

Category IA. Strongly recommended for implementation and strongly supported by well-designed experimental, clinical, or epidemiologic studies.

Category IB. Strongly recommended for implementation and supported by experimental, clinical, or epidemiologic studies and a strong theoretical rationale.

Category IC. Required for implementation as mandated by federal or state regulations or standards. When Category IC is used, a second rating can be included to provide the basis of existing scientific data, theoretical rationale, and applicability. Because of state differences, the reader should not assume that the absence of a category IC implies the absence of state regulations.

Category II. Suggested for implementation and supported by suggestive clinical or epidemiologic studies or a theoretical rationale.

Unresolved issue. No recommendation. Insufficient evidence or no consensus exists regarding efficacy.

CDC, Centers for Disease Control and Prevention; *HICPAC,* Healthcare Infection Control and Prevention Advisory Committee.

PUTTING HAZARD ABATEMENT AND STANDARD OPERATING PROCEDURES TO WORK

The integration of science with regulatory demands and **hazard abatement** is necessary for effective implementation of safe work practices and SOPs, requiring careful consideration of basic science, disease transmission and infection, and the actual risks for infection.[27,67,78] Many infection control measures protect the health of both patients and DHCP, including the use of PPE (e.g., protective eyewear, gloves, facemasks for DHCP; protective eyewear for patients), WPCs, and ECs (e.g., environmental surface decontamination or barriers to prevent cross-contamination) and the use of disposable or sterilizable, reusable items for all procedures in the oral cavity. All these SOPs address the various OSHA hazard abatement strategies. (See the suggested agencies and web sites on the Evolve site.)

Assessing the potential for disease transmission throughout the workplace is essential and should be followed by the development of SOPs to meet workplace needs. Examples of SOPs for dentistry can be acquired from sources such as the CDC (*Guidelines for Infection Control in Dental Health-Care Settings—2003*[19] and *Practical Infection Control in the Dental Office: A Workbook for the Dental Team*[26]) and OSAP (*OSAP Infection Control in Dentistry Guidelines*[67]). (See the suggested agencies and web sites on the Evolve site.)

Principles of Infection Control

As DHCP prepare to implement guidelines and recommendations, keeping the following basic principles in mind is important:

- Take action to stay healthy.
- Avoid contact with blood.
- Make objects safe for use.
- Limit the spread of contamination.

Each policy or action placed into practice should apply these principles.

Appropriate SOPs integrate a number of safety concepts recommended by the CDC[19] and OSHA.[78] These concepts include the previously defined eight OSHA primary hazard abatement strategies to reduce the risk of occupational exposures to blood-borne disease (Box 7-3).

Standard Precautions

Given the limitations of routine health history information, DHCP cannot be certain of the health status of each patient. DHCP cannot assume that a lack of disease history and clinical findings indicates that the patient is presently free of infectious disease or will remain so on subsequent clinical visits. Many individuals are unaware that they are infected with a disease, which their blood or saliva may be capable of transmitting. Although the current infection may be subclinical or the patient may be asymptomatic (without symptoms), the individual is contagious, as with chronic carriers of HBV or HCV. Individuals may be unaware of their exposure and may transmit disease or withhold information about the existence of a transmissible disease or condition because of embarrassment, privacy, or discrimination concerns.

Ultimately, DHCP are responsible for the delivery of services in a manner that ensures appropriate care is rendered in the safest way possible, regardless of the health status of the patient. Standard precautions apply not only to direct patient care procedures, but also to those procedures performed as support and routine maintenance for patient care.

As previously stated, the goal is to approach each situation as if a risk is known and to apply each hazard abatement strategy routinely and

Note

In applying standard precautions, DHCP must assume that every direct contact with body fluids or items that may be potentially infectious is capable of transmitting infection and requires protection and procedures as though such body fluids were infected with HBV or HIV.

7-1

BOX 7-3

OSHA PRIMARY HAZARD ABATEMENT STRATEGIES

1. UPs
2. PPE
3. WPCs
4. ECs
5. Housekeeping
6. Signs and labels
7. Record keeping
8. Information and training

ECs, Engineering controls; *OSHA,* Occupational Safety and Health Administration; *PPE,* personal protective equipment; *UPs,* universal precautions; *WPCs,* work-practice controls.

comprehensively. This philosophy or approach should be applied to all aspects of dental care and should serve as an example of WPCs to meet OSHA requirements (Figure 7-4).

Host Immunity and Immunizations

One approach to standard precautions is not only to protect the individual from exposure but also to increase host resistance to infectious diseases should an exposure occur,[10] as in the following examples:

- *Natural immunity:* When an individual is exposed to a disease-producing pathogen, natural immunity stimulates the immune system to produce specific antibodies to that pathogen. If this process is successful, then the pathogen

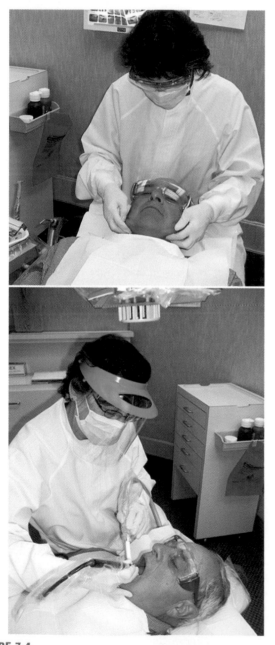

FIGURE 7-4
Proper PPE and WPCs for HCP, patient, and environment, including use of shield with aerosol-prone procedures.

is destroyed by the host immune system or suppressed to a minor or subclinical state. Once the infection resolves, antibodies remain present in the body and continue to suppress or destroy dormant organisms in the host system. If the individual is once again exposed to or infected by the same pathogen, then these antibodies are again stimulated. Numerous childhood diseases, such as rubella (German measles), mumps, rubeola, and chickenpox, stimulate natural immunity to the invading pathogen. Another pathogen that stimulates natural immunity is HAV. In addition, HBV infection may produce natural immunity or the immune system response may be unsuccessful in destroying the virus, in which case a chronic carrier state may develop. In this state the host continues to be infectious. Natural immunity may last a lifetime, provided the immune system is not damaged or suppressed.

- *Artificial or active immunity:* Vaccines and immunizations that exogenously stimulate the immune system to produce specific antibodies without the individual actually having the disease creates an artificial or active immunity. Artificially stimulated immunity may last a lifetime, or a booster dose of the vaccine may be necessary to maintain ongoing protection, such as with childhood immunizations for measles, mumps, and rubella.

- *Passive immunity:* Infants who received antibodies passed from the mother have developed passive immunity. The protection is temporary, and when the antibodies are shed from the infant's system, immunization is required to stimulate artificial immunity.

Recommendations for Immunizations

All DHCP who have contact with patients or materials that are potentially infectious should receive HBV immunization or show evidence of immunity from a previous vaccination or an actual infection. OSHA requires that this immunization be offered at no cost to each "at-risk" employee. Additionally, DHCP should remain current on immunizations and health screenings as recommended by the CDC (Table 7-5), including vaccination for HBV; tetanus and diphtheria (DPT); measles (rubeola), mumps, and rubella (MMR); poliomyelitis; pneumonia; and annual influenza, as well as testing for exposure to TB with a purified protein derivative (PPD) tuberculin skin test.[14,19] (See the suggested agencies and web sites on the Evolve site.)

Restricting Duties of Healthcare Employees during Illness

Taking care of one's own health while reducing the risk of exposure to the patient is also an important aspect of the DHCP's ECP. Healthcare professionals at times should withdraw from direct patient contact and indirect contact activities when exhibiting symptoms of some infectious disease. (See Table 7-6 and the Clinical Resources asset on the Evolve web site.) This concept involves but is not limited to the following conditions:

- Chickenpox
- CMV
- Conjunctivitis
- Diarrheal diseases (acute stage)

Table 7-5	Immunizations Strongly Recommended for Healthcare Personnel			
VACCINE	**DOSE SCHEDULE**	**INDICATIONS**	**MAJOR PRECAUTIONS AND CONTRAIN-DICATIONS**	**SPECIAL CONSIDERATIONS**
Hepatitis B Recombinant Vaccine*	Three-dose schedule administered IM in the deltoid; 0, 1, 6; second dose administered 1 month after first dose; third dose administered 4 months after second dose. Booster doses are not necessary for persons who have developed adequate antibodies to anti-HBs.	HCP at risk for exposure to blood and body fluids.	History of anaphylactic reaction to common baker's yeast. Pregnancy is not a contraindication.	No therapeutic or adverse effects on HBV-infected persons; cost-effectiveness of prevaccination screening for susceptibility to HBV depends on costs of prevalence of immunity in the group of potential vaccines; healthcare personnel who have ongoing contact with patients or blood should be tested 1-2 months after completing the vaccination series to determine serologic response. If vaccination does not induce adequate anti-HBs (>10 mIU/mL), a second vaccine series should be administered.
Influenza Vaccine (Inactivated)[†]	Annual single-dose vaccination IM with current vaccine.	HCP who have contact with patients at high risk or who work in chronic-care facilities; HCP aged ≥ 50 years or who have high-risk medical conditions.	History of anaphylactic hypersensitivity to eggs or to other components of the vaccine.	Recommended for women who will be in the second or third trimesters of pregnancy during the influenza season and women in any stage of pregnancy who have chronic medical conditions that are associated with an increased risk of influenza.[‡]
Measles Live-Virus Vaccine	One dose administered SQ; second dose ≥ 4 weeks later.	HCP who were born during or after 1957 without documentation of: 1) receipt of two doses of live vaccine on or after their first birthday; 2) physician-diagnosed measles; or 3) laboratory evidence of immunity, including those born before 1957.	Pregnancy; immunocompromised[§] state (including HIV-infected persons with severe immunosuppression); history of anaphylactic reactions after gelatin ingestion or receipt of neomycin; or recent receipt of antibody-containing blood products.	MMR is the recommended vaccine if recipients are also likely to be susceptible to rubella or mumps; persons vaccinated during 1963-1967 with: 1) measles killed-virus vaccine alone, 2) killed-virus vaccine followed by live-virus vaccine, or 3) a vaccine of unknown type, should be revaccinated with two doses of live-virus measles vaccine.

*A federal standard issued in December 191 under the Occupational Safety and Health Act mandates that hepatitis B vaccine be made available at the employer's expense to all HCP occupationally exposed to blood or other potentially infectious materials. The Occupational Safety and Health Administration requires that employers make available hepatitis B vaccinations, evaluations, and follow-up procedures in accordance with current CDC recommendations.

[†]A live attenuated influenza vaccine (LAIV) is FDA-approved for healthy persons aged 5-49 years. Because of the possibility of transmission of vaccine viruses from recipients of LAIV to other persons and in the absence of data on the risk of illness and among immunocompromised persons infected with LAIV viruses, the inactivated influenza vaccine is preferred for HCP who have close contact with immunocompromised persons.

[‡]Vaccination of pregnant women after the first trimester might be preferred to avoid coincidental association with spontaneous abortions, which are most common during the first trimester. However, no adverse fetal effects have been associated with influenza vaccination.

[§]Persons immunocompromised because of immune deficiencies, HIV infection, leukemia, lymphoma, generalized malignancy; or persons receiving immunosuppressive therapy with corticosteroids, alkylating drugs, antimetabolites; or persons receiving radiation.

anti-HBs, hepatitis B surface antigen; *HBV,* hepatitis B virus; *HCP,* healthcare personnel; *HIV,* human immunodeficiency virus; *IM,* intramuscularly; *MMR,* measles, mumps, rubella; *SQ,* subcutaneously.

Modified from Centers for Disease Control and Prevention: Appendix B: immunizations strongly recommended for health-care personnel (HCP), *MMWR Recomm Rep* 52(RR17):65, 2003.

Continued

Table 7-5	**Immunizations Strongly Recommended for Healthcare Personnel—cont'd**			
VACCINE	**DOSE SCHEDULE**	**INDICATIONS**	**MAJOR PRECAUTIONS AND CONTRAIN-DICATIONS**	**SPECIAL CONSIDERATIONS**
Mumps Live-Virus Vaccine	One dose SQ; no booster.	HCP believed susceptible can be vaccinated; adults born before 1957 can be considered immune.	Pregnancy; immunocompromised[§] state; history of anaphylactic reaction after gelatin ingestion or receipt of neomycin.	MMR is the recommended vaccine.
Rubella Live-Virus Vaccine	One dose SQ; no booster.	HCP, both male and female, who lack documentation of receipt of live vaccine on or after their first birthday, or lack of laboratory evidence of immunity can be vaccinated. Adults born before 1957 can be considered immune, except women of childbearing age.	Pregnancy; immunocompromised[§] state; history of anaphylactic reaction after receipt of neomycin.	Women pregnant when vaccinated or who become pregnant within 4 weeks of vaccination should be counseled regarding theoretic risks to the fetus; however, the risk of rubella vaccine-associated malformations among these women is negligible. MMR is the recommended vaccine.
Varicella-Zoster Live-Virus Vaccine	Two 0.5 mL doses SQ 4-8 weeks apart if aged ≥13 years.	HCP without reliable history of varicella or laboratory evidence of varicella immunity.	Pregnancy; immunocompromised[§] state; history of anaphylactic reaction after receipt of neomycin or gelatin; recent receipt of antibody-containing blood products; salicylate use should be avoided for 6 weeks after vaccination.	Because 71-93% of U.S.-born persons without a history of varicella are immune, serologic testing before vaccination might be cost-effective.

- HAV
- HBV
- HCV
- HSV (orofacial, whitlow)
- Measles
- Meningococcal infections
- Rubella
- Shingles
- *Staphylococcus aureus* infections
- Active streptococcal group A infections
- TB (active)
- Viral respiratory infections

Each condition should be assessed to determine the nature of contact for activities such as direct-patient procedures, tasks in treatment areas, instrument and cleaning procedures, and avoidance or modification of work assignments to meet the best interests of all parties. Additional conditions and updates are included as a Clinical Resource table on the Evolve web site.

Patient Health History

The first step in any infection control plan is to review the patient's health history thoroughly, an important tool used to determine any conditions that may require modifications in infection control products or procedures.

Screening patients as carriers of possible infectious disease is acceptable, but only as it relates to the prescription of appropri-

ate treatment, during postexposure management when necessary (e.g., if an exposure incident occurs that involves the patient).

The patient's health history, combined with a thorough oral assessment, may indicate the need for referral to another appropriate healthcare provider for differential diagnosis of an infectious disease. Such a referral does not mean that the individual is *infected*, but that the person's present state of health must be determined to ensure that appropriate treatment can be administered.

Of critical note: The patient's health history is a

Distinct Care Modifications

Patients with health problems such as iodine allergies, alcohol sensitivity, and latex allergies require modifications to standard infection control procedures that use products containing iodine, alcohol, or latex materials. Examples of such products include iodophor disinfectants; preprocedural mouthrinses containing alcohol; and the use of any items made from latex, including but not limited to rubber dams, rubber polishing cups, nitrous nose hoods, and gloves.

Patient Health History

The patient health history is *not* a tool for use to screen patients as *infectious disease risks* or to justify increases in infection control measures. Such practices are both unethical and illegal.

confidential document requiring informed consent of the patient before the disclosure of any information to other parties. Federal laws such as the Health Insurance Portability and Accountability Act (HIPAA) and specific state laws on patient-medical confidentiality should be consulted.

Extraoral and Intraoral Examinations

A comprehensive patient examination may identify lesions possibly associated with systemic disease. It is important that the patient be referred for definitive diagnosis of the lesion and any related systemic conditions.

Personal Hygiene and Appearance

All individuals with patient contact should adhere to high standards of personal hygiene, dressing in a clean, professional manner appropriate for the tasks performed. These expectations may vary among different workplaces, but some basic principles should be universally followed. Although these issues may seem obvious, attention to the basics of healthcare delivery is necessary as a foundation for the appropriate use of required PPE and sound infection control practices.

Hair

Hair should be kept off the face and should not touch the patient, instruments, or work surfaces. Decorative hair accessories can become contaminated by aerosols from procedures and are considered inappropriate. Facial hair also is easily contaminated by aerosols from procedures and should be covered by a facemask or shield.

Personal jewelry

Personal jewelry should not be worn during work. Direct contact and aerosols can easily contaminate personal jewelry (e.g., rings, watches, earrings, decorative pins). Jewelry harbors higher levels of bacteria than does the skin and is difficult to clean.[60] Total bacterial counts are higher when rings are worn, and such jewelry can cause damage to gloves, leaving small breaks in the barrier protection. In addition, microorganisms can be carried home on these items.

Hand care

> *Hands*
>
> DHCP *must* take care of their hands and skin to maintain the natural protective function for the health of both themselves and their patients.

Hand care is important for the healthcare worker.[60,67,72] The skin of the hands, wrists, and forearms should be healthy and free of inflammation. Although the skin is the primary physical barrier against entry of microorganisms into the body, it can also be a primary vehicle for transmitting infections acquired from microorganisms on the hands.

Nails

Keeping nails short is important because the majority of flora on the hands are found under and around the fingernails. The CDC recommends that DHCP keep fingernails short with smooth, filed edges to allow DHCP to thoroughly clean underneath them and prevent glove tears. Sharp nail edges or broken nails are also likely to increase glove failure.[19]

> *Nails*
>
> Nails should be kept clean and short, making cleaning the hands easier.

DHCP should not wear hand or nail jewelry if it makes donning gloves more difficult or compromises the fit and integrity of the glove. Long nails can make donning gloves more difficult and can cause gloves to tear more readily. Use of artificial nails is usually not recommended. The presence of gram-negative organisms has been determined to be greater among wearers of artificial nails, both before and after handwashing. Artificial fingernails or extenders have been epidemiologically implicated in multiple outbreaks involving fungal and bacterial infections in hospital intensive-care units and operating rooms in hospitals. Studies indicate that freshly-applied nail polish on natural nails does not increase the microbial load from periungual skin if fingernails are short; however, chipped nail polish can harbor added bacteria.[19]

Broken Skin

Caution should be particularly exercised in patient treatment to reduce the risk that either party may acquire or transmit a secondary infection through broken skin. This issue should be considered along with other conditions that may limit patient contact (Table 7-6) and other duties.

> *Skin*
>
> Broken skin resulting from dry, chapped, and cracked skin; injury; skin erosions; eczema; or dermatitis should be a concern for DHCP.

Hand Hygiene

Proper hand hygiene is essential to prevent contamination that can occur when the hands touch any object not designated as clean, thus causing cross-contamination. Such objects include DHCP's hair, work clothing, glasses, and masks contaminated during routine patient procedures.

> *Prevention*
>
> Hand hygiene is the most important and effective procedure for preventing the transmission of many infectious organisms on the hands.

Hand hygiene is mandatory before and after patient contact, after any contact with potential sources of microorganisms (e.g., body fluids and substances, mucous membranes, nonintact skin, inanimate objects that are likely to be contaminated), after removing gloves, and before and after treatment room setup and cleanup after treatment. When in doubt about any kind of contamination, DHCP should wash their hands. The three basic levels of handwashing protocol for health care are shown in Table 7-7.

Handwashing procedures in health care vary relative to the tasks to be performed. The recommended basic handwashing procedure for routine dental procedures begins with the wetting of hands under cool-to-warm running water, followed by the application of an appropriate handwashing agent distrib-

Table 7-6	Suggested Work Restrictions for Healthcare Personnel*	
DISEASE OR INFECTION	**SUGGESTED RESTRICTION**	**DURATION OF RESTRICTION**
Conjunctivitis	From patient contact and patient environment	Until lesions dry and crust
Cytomegalovirus	None	–
Diarrhea Diseases, Acute Stage	From patient contact, patient environment, and food handling	Until symptoms resolve
Hepatitis A	From patient contact, patient environment, and food handling	Until 7 days after onset of jaundice
Hepatitis B (Surface Antigenemia)	None; refer to state regulations	
Hepatitis C	None[†]	Unresolved
Herpes Simplex, Orofacial	Evaluate need to restrict from care of patients at high risk.	
Herpes Simplex, Whitlow	From patient contact and patient environment	Until lesions heal
Measles (Active)	Exclusion from duty	Until 7 days after rash appears
Meningococcal Infection	Exclusion from duty	Until 24 hr after start of effective therapy
Rubella (Active)	Exclusion from duty	Until 5 days after rash appears
Staphylococcus aureus, Active	From patient contact, patient environment, and food handling	Until lesions have resolved
Streptococci Group A	From patient contact, patient environment, and food handling	Until 24 hr after adequate treatment started
Tuberculosis (Active)	Exclusion from duty	Until proved noninfectious
Varicella (Active)	Exclusion from duty	Until lesions dry and crust
Viral Respiratory Infection, Acute Febrile	Consider excluding from care of patients with high risk and patient environment[‡]	Until acute symptoms resolve
Zoster (Shingles)—Localized	Restrict from patients at high risk[§]; cover lesions	Until all lesions dry and crust
Zoster (Shingles)—Generalized	Restrict from patient contact	Until all lesions dry and crust

Adapted from Kohn WG et al: Guidelines for infection control in dental health care settings, *MMWR Recomm Rep* 52(RR-17):1-61, 2003; and Bolyard EA: Hospital infection control practices advisory committee. Guidelines for infection control in health care personnel, *Am J Infect Control* 26:289-354, 1998.
*Modified from recommendations of the Advisory Committee on Immunization Practices (ACIP).
[†]Unless epidemiologically linked to transmission of infection.
[‡]Patients at high risk as defined by ACIP.
[§]Those susceptible to and at increased risk of varicella.

uted thoroughly over the hands. For most procedures, a vigorous rubbing together of all the surfaces of premoistened lathered hands and fingers for at least 15 seconds, followed by rinsing under a stream of cool or tepid water, is recommended.[19] Hands should always be thoroughly dried before donning gloves. The combined mechanical action and thorough rinsing are critical for the removal of **bioburden** (the microbiologic load of microorganisms present), with special attention given to the fingertip area, not just the palms.

Hand antisepsis is required for oral surgical procedures. Oral surgical procedures involve the incision, excision, or reflection of tissue that exposes the normally sterile areas of the oral cavity. Examples include biopsy, periodontal surgery, apical surgery, implant surgery, and surgical extractions of teeth. DHCP should perform surgical hand antisepsis by using an antimicrobial product (e.g., antimicrobial soap and water, or soap and water followed by alcohol-based hand scrub with persistent activity) before donning sterile surgeon's gloves.[19]

Table 7-7	**Hand-Hygiene Methods and Indications**			
METHOD	**AGENT**	**PURPOSE**	**DURATION (MINIMUM)**	**INDICATION***
Routine Hand Wash	Water and nonantimicrobial soap (e.g., plain soap)[†]	Remove soil and transient microorganisms.	15 seconds[‡]	Before and after treating each patient (e.g., before glove placement and after glove removal); after barehanded touching of inanimate objects likely to be contaminated by blood or saliva; before leaving the dental operatory or the dental laboratory; when visibly soiled; before regloving after removing gloves that are torn, cut, or punctured.
Antiseptic Hand Wash	Water and antimicrobial soap (e.g., chlorhexidine, iodine and iodophors, chloroxylenol [PCMX], triclosan)	Remove or destroy transient microorganisms and reduce resident flora.	15 seconds[‡]	
Antiseptic Hand Rub	Alcohol-based hand rub	Remove or destroy transient microorganisms and reduce resident flora.	Rub hands until the agent is dry.[§]	
Surgical Antisepsis	Water and antimicrobial soap (e.g., chlorhexidine, iodine and iodophors, PCMX, triclosan)	Remove or destroy transient microorganisms, and reduce resident flora (persistent effect).	2-6 min Follow manufacturer's instructions for surgical hand-scrub product with persistent activity[‖]	Before donning sterile surgeon's gloves for surgical procedures[¶]

Reference numbering corresponds to the complete document: Guidelines for Infection Control in Dental Health-Care Settings—2003, *MMWR Recomm Rep* 52(RR-17):1-61, 2003.
*References 7, 9, 11, 13, 113, 120-123, 125, 126, 136-138.
[†]Pathogenic organisms have been found on or around bar soap during and after use.[139] Use of liquid soap with hands-free dispensing controls is preferable.
[‡]Time reported as effective in removing most transient flora from the skin.
[§]Alcohol-based hand rubs should contain 60% to 95% ethanol or isopropanol and should not be used in the presence of visible soil or organic material.
[‖]After application of alcohol-based surgical hand scrub product with persistent activity as recommended, allow hands and forearms to dry thoroughly and immediately don sterile surgeon's gloves.[144,145] Follow manufacturer instructions.[122,123,137,146]
[¶]Before beginning surgical hand-scrub, remove all arm jewelry and any hand jewelry that may make donning gloves more difficult, cause gloves to tear more readily, or interfere with glove usage (e.g., ability to wear the correct-sized glove or altered glove integrity).[142,143]

Products used for handwashing, surgical scrubs, and hand care should be carefully selected with consideration given to the purpose for use, advantages and disadvantages of the agent, overall cost, and acceptance (biocompatibility) of the product by users. Reusable cloth towels are not recommended for hand drying in healthcare facilities. Single-use paper towels or air dryers are preferred.

If an alcohol-based hand rub is used, then an adequate amount is applied to the palm of one hand and the hands are rubbed together, covering all surfaces of the hand and fingers until hands are dry. Manufacturers' recommendations should be followed regarding the volume of product to use. Alcohol-based hand rubs are excellent antiseptics, but not good cleaning agents. These products should only be used on hands that are clean (e.g., free of visible debris and bioburden).

Hand Lotions

Although the use of hand lotions is often suggested as a way to reduce the effects on the skin from repeated handwashing, lotion can become contaminated and act as a reservoir for microorganisms.[60] Concern also has risen regarding the use of petroleum-based lotions because of their potential to weaken the protective ability of latex gloves by increasing surface permeability and allowing microorganisms to enter. In addition, some questions remain as to the compatibility of lotion and antiseptic products; some lotions have been shown to reduce the antiseptic's ability to disperse bacteria from the skin.[60]

Soaps

Soaps used for handwashing are the basic component of infection control, and a number of antiseptic agents are available for use in healthcare facilities. The benefits and limitations of each product should be considered in the selection process. Some products can cause skin irritation over time and therefore are not suitable for repeated use. Certain DHCP may be sensitive to specific products. Irritation to the skin will reduce its integrity. If an irritation continues or becomes serious, then a dermatologist should be consulted for recommendations. (See Table 7-7 for a list of the active ingredients of the most commonly used agents.) Several products have been shown to provide continued or *residual* antiseptic protection on the skin to extend throughout the day, known as *substantivity,* a significant benefit.

Storage and Dispensing of Hand-Care Products

> **Note**
>
> Reusable containers can become contaminated and serve as reservoirs for microorganisms and should be thoroughly washed and dried before refilling.

Appropriate storage and dispensing guidelines must be followed to prevent contamination. Liquid products should be stored in closed containers. Disposable containers are best, but if they cannot be used, then routine maintenance schedules should be followed.

7-2 Personal Protective Equipment

PPE provides protection from hazards including contact with blood or OPIMs (including saliva) that can be reasonably anticipated during the performance of normal work tasks. The selection of PPE is based on the procedures and tasks expected to be performed.

> **Note**
>
> The intent of PPE is to provide protection to the skin, eyes, nose, mucous membranes, and clothing from exposure to biologic, physical or parenteral, and chemical hazards in the workplace.[67,78,79]

Other DHCP such as the receptionist may be exposed indirectly to these risks or occasionally have direct contact and must also be trained to use appropriate PPE. For routine procedures in dentistry, this equipment includes but is not limited to the use of the following:

- Gloves
- Masks
- Face shields
- Protective eyewear
- Protective attire
- Clinic gowns or uniforms as indicated by the tasks the employee is required to perform (Figures 7-5 and 7-6).

The use and care of procedurally indicated PPE also integrates the concepts of WPCs and ECs recommended by OSHA. For example, the use of antimicrobial soap to wash contaminated eyewear is an action (i.e., WPC) meant to decontaminate PPE, while at the same time the use of a special antimicrobial agent in the soap enhances such effects (i.e., EC). Together, this process meets three OSHA strategies for safety.

Throughout the following paragraphs the reader should search for ways that practice and science can work together to create the safest work situation possible, reflecting the link between WPCs and ECs. Individual actions are combined with scientific developments, working together to achieve safe working practices.

Gloves

Gloves should be worn in addition to but not as a substitute for handwashing. They are required for contact with oral mucous membranes, saliva, blood, or OPIMs. Most oral health services involve direct contact with the oral cavity, which poses biologi-

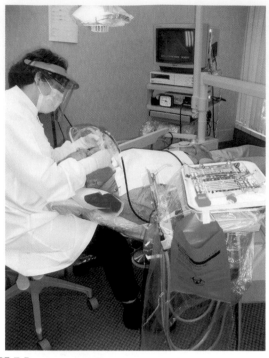

FIGURE 7-5
Proper use of WPCs and PPE.

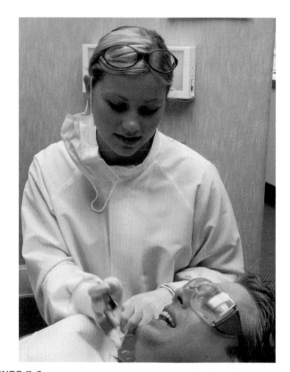

FIGURE 7-6
Unacceptable use of PPE.

cal hazards, whereas infection control practices require the routine use of disinfectant agents, which pose chemical hazards, and the handling of sharp instruments, which poses physical hazards.

> **Note**
>
> Although not all procedures are performed in a blood-contaminated field, it must be stressed that saliva in dentistry is also defined as a fluid for which standard precautions apply.

The types of gloves used should be selected based on the tasks to be performed and the individual needs of the person wearing them. Employers must provide appropriate gloves for each employee. A number of different types of gloves are indicated and available for protection against biological, chemical, and physical hazards anticipated in the workplace.

The procedures and inherent hazards should be considered. For biological hazards, nonsterile examination gloves or sterile surgeons' gloves are indicated; for chemical hazards, nitrile rubber utility gloves are needed. In handling of hot trays, equipment, or instruments after sterilization, heat-resistant mitts provide the needed physical protection, and puncture-resistant gloves are indicated during cleanup of contaminated instruments after patient procedures.

> **Prevention**
> Gloves are the single most effective element of PPE for the reduction of disease transmission in dentistry.

Examination or Procedure Gloves

Examination gloves are available in several types, including sterile neoprene and nonsterile latex or vinyl, latex-free synthetic, powdered and nonpowdered, nitrile rubber examination and utility gloves, and right-left paired or ambidextrous versions.

Nonsterile gloves are dispensed in bulk and should be obtained with clean hands and placed on cleaned hands. Examination gloves should *not* be washed and reused, even for the same patient.

Sterile surgeon's gloves should be selected when sterile conditions are required. These are packaged by size in pairs (right and left) and sealed in sterile packs. A sterile technique is required to don the gloves so as not to contaminate them before use. After the wrapper is opened, only the outside of the wrapper should be touched before the gloves are removed; only the inner surface of the gloves should be touched as the fingers slide between the cuff and palm or back of the gloved hand. Care must be taken to prevent contact with the outer surface of the gloves with the hands or the inner surface of the gloves with the outer surface of the gloves to avoid contamination before use.

Over Gloves

CDC has recommendations regarding the use of over gloves; they are not to be worn for treatment procedures. Over gloves are thin vinyl or co-polymer gloves (e.g., food handlers' gloves) placed over the examination glove to prevent cross-contamination. The use of over gloves, worn over treatment gloves, can reduce cross-contamination when DHCP touch any surface out of the direct treatment area—for example, to retrieve additional supplies from a drawer, use a pen to make a treatment notation, or press an activation button when exposing a radiographic film.

Utility Gloves

Utility gloves are heavy unlined gloves worn during the handling of any chemicals or infectious waste; cleaning of contaminated surfaces, instruments, or materials; and environmental surface cleaning and disinfection. Gloves made of nitrile rubber have an increased resistance to instrument punctures and can be autoclaved. They should be discarded when visibly worn or damaged. Alternatives include reusable utility gloves that can be disinfected after each use, similar to dishwashing gloves. Procedures used to store utility gloves must include washing and disinfecting after each use.

Factors for Appropriate Use

Disposable gloves must be worn whenever contact with blood, saliva, or mucous membranes is present and when materials, substances, or surfaces are potentially contaminated. A new pair of examination gloves must be used for each patient. Gloves should be removed and hands washed when tasks are completed, before the employee leaves the treatment room, and between patients. If damage to gloves is possible, then DHCP should remove their gloves and wash their hands. Contaminated gloves should not be washed between patients or removed and reused later on the same patient. Removing the gloves and washing them can damage the integrity of the material, leaving microtears or pinholes that may permit the passage of infectious agents. To prevent contamination of gloves during the donning of PPE, the facemask and protective eyewear should be placed and adjusted before handwashing and gloving.

> ### ✷ CASE APPLICATION 7-1.1
>
> #### Use of Gloves
> Ruth's primary duties involve the front desk. She is a valued team member and known to be helpful when the staff members are behind schedule. Although staff members appreciate that Ruth will help clean up treatment rooms, she has not had training in SOPs. Ruth admits that she does not always wear gloves when she helps clean up treatment rooms.

Gloves made of alternative materials (e.g., vinyl) should be available for personnel with sensitivity to glove materials such as latex. Individuals with dermatitis related to glove use should seek medical attention to determine appropriate modifications to hand care.

Experience dictates the size glove that fits best. A glove should fit tightly all around the hand, with no excess, folds, or wrinkling at the fingertips or webs of the hand. However, the glove should allow an easy spread of the fingers and should not pull the hand and fingers into the center of the palm. Gloves should cover the cuffs of long-sleeved gowns to cover exposed skin.[79]

> **Distinct Care Modifications**
> Double gloving (two pairs worn at once) may be indicated under certain circumstances, such as when DHCP have a cut or lesion on their hands. Double gloving provides inner and outer barriers for potentially infectious agents.[67,78,79]

> **Note**
> Medical gloves sold in the United States are regulated by the FDA.

Recent studies have shown that the use of right- or left-hand ambidextrous gloves may be linked to the development of neuromuscular injuries to the hands of dental professionals.[82] Paying careful attention to the proper fit of a glove and sampling several manufacturers and sizes is the best way to meet individual needs.

Latex Allergies

> *Latex Allergy*
>
> As standard precautions have been implemented, the use of gloves and the incidences of latex allergy appear to have increased. Surveys have reported that approximately 40% of DHCP demonstrate sensitivity to latex.[44]

Examination and surgical gloves are predominately made from latex products.*

A number of conditions can predispose an individual to latex allergy, such as multiple allergic conditions; multiple surgeries; and food allergies to banana, kiwi, and avocado—to name a few. A thorough medical history is critical to help identify patients and employees at risk.

Type I latex allergy symptoms (e.g., immediate hypersensitivity) typically first exhibit as localized skin reactions; more serious reactions can develop as severe respiratory and systemic symptoms. Latex allergies can progress from a simple localized dermatitis into a life-threatening allergy or anaphylaxis.

An allergy specialist should assess any possible latex reaction to define the specific nature of the reaction and appropriate treatment. Although differentiating among reactions to other irritants (e.g., powders inside the gloves) from actual latex-specific allergies can be quite difficult, an accurate diagnosis of the problem is critical to the selection of appropriate alternatives and, if necessary, the creation of a latex-free environment for the protection of the affected employee.

Several alternatives to latex gloves, as well as powder free latex gloves, are available. Any problem with latex products should be closely monitored because of the potential severe health problems that may result. No cure exists for latex allergy, and the reactions can increase in severity and may even be delayed (e.g., type IV hypersensitivity) to long after the initial contact. Reducing or eliminating latex products in the environment is critical in the presence of latex-allergic patients or DHCP. (See the suggested agencies and web sites on the Evolve site.)

Protective eyewear

> *Note*
>
> Protective eyewear is required for all procedures that have the potential to create aerosols or spatter.

Protective eyewear should provide protection from contamination and traumatic injuries resulting from flying debris, aerosols or spatter of OPIMs, and chemicals.

Several styles of protective eyewear are available; the user should select the most comfortable version for extended wear. Many styles can be worn over prescription glasses, or personal prescription lenses can be made to fit safety frames for adequate eye protection.

---

*References 13, 14, 41, 44, 73, 76, 92.

Safety Glasses

Safety glasses or goggles with top and side coverage provide the highest degree of protection. Standard eyewear models lack side and top protection and may not meet the impact requirements for safety glasses (see Figures 7-5 and 7-6).

Face Shields

Face shields may be used in place of safety glasses, particularly for procedures in which significant spatter is anticipated, such as ultrasonic use and air-powder polishing procedures. Reusable face shields should be decontaminated between patients.

Patient Eye Protection

Protection for the patient should also be provided because the same eye hazards exist for the patient during procedures as those for the DHCP (Figure 7-7).

Eye Protection

Mr. Birdwell's ophthalmologist speculated that bacterial matter had gotten into his eye and caused an infection. Careful questioning traced the most probable cause to Mr. Birdwell's recent dental treatment. At that visit, Mr. Birdwell did not recall being offered safety glasses to wear to protect his eyes from potential mouth spatter.

Laser and High-Intensity Lights

Laser and high-intensity lights used to cure dental materials can cause injury to the eye with repeated exposure. Special light-filter glasses and shields should be used during operation of

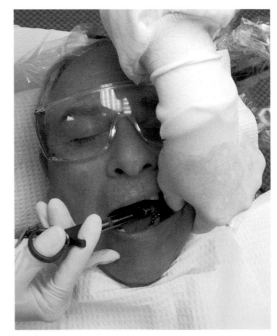

FIGURE 7-7
Safety glasses for patient protection.

these light sources. The manufacturer's instructions should be consulted for safety specifications.

Factors for Appropriate Use and Care

Protective eyewear and face shields should be put on and adjusted before gloves are donned. Protective eyewear must meet the guidelines of the American National Standards Institute (ANSI) as shatter resistant. (See the suggested agencies and web sites on the Evolve site.) Approved eyewear features the ANSI symbol printed on the frame. Other required elements for OSHA approval require that the eyewear have solid side shields with recommended top and bottom rims.

Proper size and fit for each individual is important to minimize the need to adjust eyewear during use, taking care not to push eyewear up with a contaminated glove. Pushing up glasses, adjusting a facemask, or touching the face and hair can promote cross-contamination to or from the gloves and should be avoided.

Routine infection control procedures should include decontamination of safety lenses with soap and water at a minimum. Caution should be taken when chemical disinfectants are used because many of these chemicals may cause irritation to the skin or eyes. Use of an antimicrobial soap to wash eyewear between patients reduces both surface contamination and the risk of chemical irritation.

Facemasks

The CDC recommends that DHCP wear a surgical mask and eye protection with solid side shields or a face shield to protect mucous membranes of the eyes, nose, and mouth during procedures likely to generate splashing or spattering of blood or other body fluids.[19]

A surgical facemask is worn as part of standard precautions and provides a barrier to the mucous membranes of the nose and mouth. This type of facemask protects against microorganisms generated by the wearer, with >95% bacterial filtration efficiency, and it also protects DHCP from large-particle droplet spatter that might contain bloodborne pathogens or other infectious microorganisms. The mask's outer surface can become contaminated with infectious droplets from spray of oral fluids or from touching the mask with contaminated fingers. When a mask becomes wet from the moist breath exhaled by the DHCP, the resistance to airflow through the mask increases, causing more airflow to pass around the edges of the mask. The CDC recommends that DHCP change masks between patients and during patient treatment if it becomes wet.[19]

Types and Fit

Masks come in several sizes and styles, including molded dome, flat, pleated paper, and variations on both with elastic straps, ear loops, or ties. Masks are available in several types of materials and surface textures, all designed to prevent or reduce passage of moisture and microorganisms.

To maximize protection, a facemask must cover the nose, mouth, and facial hair, fitting snugly with no gaps at the bridge of the nose or sides of the face. Properly fitted facemasks create

a seal for the nose and mouth, reducing the risk of exposure of the respiratory system. For example, when a facemask is worn over only the mouth but not the nose, no protection is provided. Gaps along the side of the mask or the bridge of the nose will allow airborne contamination to be inhaled.

Factors for Appropriate Selection and Use

DHCP must use science and logic to determine the most appropriate mask for the tasks to be performed. The mask must be able to provide protection against spatter that may contain microorganisms and particles and still function in a moist environment created from the interior by the operator when exhaling and speaking and from the exterior by dental procedures.

Some masks are made of materials or contain dyes that may irritate the skin or eyes. Others may be comfortable to wear but are insufficiently thick and do not provide appropriate particle filtration protection in a wet environment.

To maintain the integrity of the mask surface, DHCP should avoid touching the mask with contaminated hands or gloves and must remove the mask before leaving the treatment area.

Protective garments

Protective garments are to be changed daily or when visibly soiled. As with other PPE, a number of protective garments are available. Selection should be based on the tasks to be performed and the level of protection needed. Moisture-resistant garments are designed to provide additional protection to skin and clothing from potentially saturating contamination.

> *Note*
>
> Appropriate clinical attire should always be used for dental procedures to protect the skin and underlying clothing from contamination.[56]

Garments that are long enough to cover the lap area during sitting, with long sleeves, high necks, tight cuffs, and simple styling, are usually best. When surgical scrubs are worn, the jacket and pants are considered part of the PPE and must be handled accordingly. Protective garments are intended for use during exposure-prone tasks and should not be worn outside of the general treatment area, a practice that allows for cross-contamination of areas not normally decontaminated between patients.

OSHA requires that employers provide and maintain protective garments. This includes laundering of reusable protective garments and proper disposal of disposable garments.

Implementation of Work-Practice and Engineering Controls

Numerous WPCs and ECs are aimed at reducing exposure to hazards during dental procedures and are tailored to the individual workplace.

Combining these practices with the use of appropriately designed products and equipment is the goal of WPCs and ECs—where science and practice meet.*

---

*References 3, 8, 16, 66, 92.

Controls that can be routinely applied by DHCP to reduce cross-contamination and support the concept of standard precautions[19] include but are not limited to the practices discussed in the following sections.

Barrier protection

The use of barriers has become a universal practice in dentistry to prevent contact with infectious agents and contamination of environmental surfaces.

PPE is essentially the use of individual or personal barrier protection to prevent exposure to the skin, mucous membranes, and clothing of DHCP and to reduce the risk of inhalation of infectious agents. Both surface and personal barriers, such as gloves and masks (e.g., PPE), are designed to be disposed of after each patient and replaced with fresh ones. A rubber dam is another effective barrier recommended for use during exposure-prone procedures.[11,26,28,31] Although environmental barriers protect surfaces from contamination, a rubber dam is a *reverse* barrier to reduce spattering and aerosolization of oral fluids and blood and should be used whenever possible (Figure 7-8).

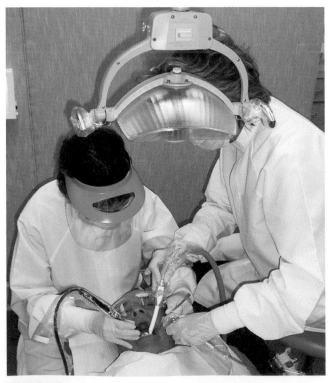

FIGURE 7-8
Good implementation of PPE includes gloves over cuffs of laboratory coat, well-fitted masks, use of shield, and environmental barriers.

High-velocity evacuation

High-velocity evacuation (HVE) should be used whenever procedures generating aerosols or spatter are performed, such as the use of high-speed hand pieces, ultrasonic or sonic scalers (Figure 7-9), or water spray from the air/water syringe.

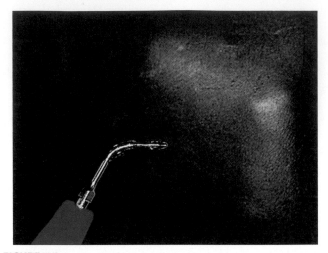

FIGURE 7-9
Halo of spray from ultrasonic scaler.

Reduction of microbial load

Reducing the number of microorganisms in the oral environment is one means to reduce the potential for microbial contamination. Asking the patient to brush the teeth before the appointment may reduce the available microorganisms in the oral cavity.

A second approach is to ask the patient to rinse with an antimicrobial mouthrinse before treatment; again, the goal is to reduce the volume of available microorganisms.

Several mouthrinses are available for selection as a pretreatment rinse, all of which chemically reduce the number of oral microbes in the oral environment. Rinsing with a chemical agent that has substantivity (e.g., chlorhexidine) extends the duration of residual antimicrobial activity.

X-ray equipment

Many times, x-ray films are taken in the same room in which the treatment is provided. Therefore the basic treatment room setup includes the use of protective coverings and disinfection procedures for the x-ray equipment, including the x-ray tube head and activation button (Figure

7-10). Care should be taken to touch only the covered surfaces of the x-ray tube head during alignment. After exposure,

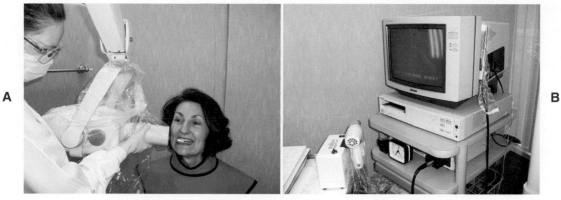

FIGURE 7-10
A, Appropriate use of surface barriers (WPC) for environmental protection in radiology area. **B,** Protected technology.

film packets must be appropriately handled to prevent cross-contamination.

Each office's SOPs must address WPCs designed to manage contaminated film packets during transportation, processing procedures, and disposal of waste. Once the x-ray films have been exposed, they are taken to a darkroom or other area for developing; caution is needed to prevent cross-contaminating this area. Gloves must be worn at all times while handling contaminated packets, and film packets must be disposed of as potentially infectious waste resulting from contamination by saliva.

Disposable items

> *Note*
>
> Items dispensed for single use must **NEVER** be reused. Reuse of such items is a violation of FDA regulations for approved devices.

The use of disposable items can significantly increase the efficiency of surface disinfection, sterilization, and treatment room management. Disposable items should be discarded immediately after use to prevent contaminating other items.

Chairside safety

Examples of chairside WPCs include the presence of over gloves for reaching into drawers for supplies or writing on charts and the inclusion of an extra pair of cotton pliers with each setup to retrieve extra supplies from clean areas.

> *Prevention*
>
> When DHCP are present at chairside for patient treatment, the risk of exposure or injury is ever present. Careful consideration of available ECs and WPCs can minimize these risks.

Supply-dispensing techniques should prevent contamination of bulk supplies. DHCP need to plan ahead for supplies rather than contaminating supply containers. The goal is to minimize the number of surfaces and items that may be touched with contaminated hands during an appointment.

Use of transfer forceps

Instruments or supplies not individually wrapped or protected by a bulk wrapping may be stored in sterile jars and removed from storage with transfer forceps. Similarly, items that have

been immersed in liquid disinfectants are also handled with transfer forceps.

Dental Unit Waterline Management

Over the past decade, the presence of biofilm accumulation in dental unit waterlines (DUWL) has been investigated and procedures developed for biofilm control.*

Biofilm

Biofilm describes colonies of cell growth that attach to the wet inner surfaces of small tubing[96,98] (Figure 7-11). This matrix of organisms may form a mass up to 400 mm thick. In simple terms, biofilm forms *slime,* which becomes a microenvironment that can sustain microbial growth of both aerobic and anaerobic organisms and may serve as a reservoir for the transmission of pathogens. This formation of biofilm appears rapidly and adheres to the wet surface by an extracellular polysaccharide fiber matrix and is tightly bound to the surface of the DUWL tubing.

Biofilm may become resistant to chemical disinfection and poses a significant challenge to the management of DUWL.

Risk

Exposure to the majority of microorganisms recovered from contaminated DUWL, such as various strains of *Pseudomonas* species, can be managed by a healthy immune system. Of greater concern has been the isolation of *Legionella* species.[29] If conditions are altered in the transmission equation, then documentation exists that suggests an infection can follow exposure to the organisms expelled from the waterline during dental procedures.

Management

The CDC recommends that dental facilities use water that meets EPA regulatory standards for drinking water (i.e., ≤500 CFU/mL of heterotrophic water bacteria) for routine dental treatment output water. Several technologies are now available to meet this standard. DHCP should consult with the dental unit manufacturer for appropriate methods and equipment to maintain the recommended quality of dental water. It is important to follow recommendations for monitoring water quality

*References 2, 4, 5, 7, 20, 26, 41, 57, 60, 64, 74, 96-98.

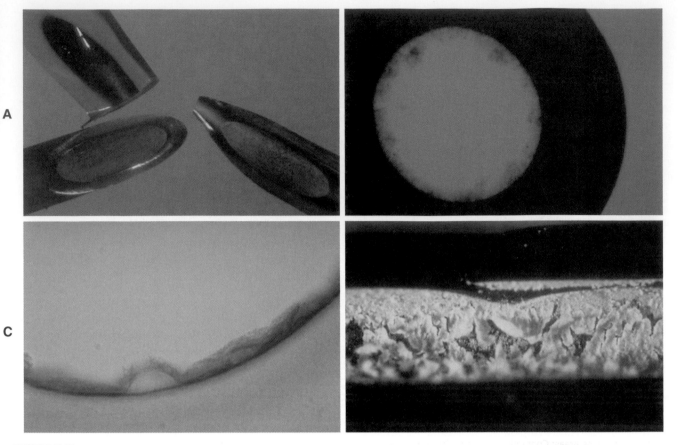

FIGURE 7-11
Dental waterline biofilm. **A,** Diagonal cut of lumen. **B,** Cross-section of tubing with biofilm. **C,** Close-up view of biofilm on inner surface of tubing. **D,** Dried biofilm removed from tubing.

provided by the manufacturer of the unit or waterline treatment product.[19]

The CDC still recommends that DHCP discharge water and air for a minimum of 20-30 seconds after each patient, from any device connected to the dental water system that enters the patient's mouth. This is necessary because patient material (e.g., oral microorganisms, blood, and saliva) can enter the dental water system during patient treatment. Recently manufactured dental units are engineered to prevent retraction of oral fluids, but some older dental units are equipped with antiretraction valves that require periodic maintenance. Users should consult the owner's manual or contact the manufacturer to determine whether testing or maintenance of antiretraction valves or other devices is required. Even with antiretraction valves, the CDC still recommends flushing devices for a minimum of 20-30 seconds after each patient.[19]

General Environmental and Equipment Procedures

Comprehensive infection control practices include preprocedure and postprocedure, as well as direct patient procedure management. Any surface, nonsterilizable equipment, or material that may potentially become contaminated during the course of dental care must be considered.

Work zones

The CDC recommends dividing environmental surfaces into clinical contact surfaces and housekeeping surfaces (Figures 7-12 and 7-13). Because housekeeping surfaces (e.g., floors, walls, and sinks) have limited risk of disease transmission, they can be decontaminated with less rigorous methods than those used on dental patient-care items and clinical contact surfaces. Strategies for cleaning and disinfecting surfaces in patient-care areas should consider the following: 1) potential for direct patient contact; 2) degree and frequency of hand contact; and 3) potential contamination of the surface with body substances or environmental sources of microorganisms (e.g., soil, dust, or water).[19]

Daily preparation

Cleaning is a form of decontamination that renders the environmental surface safe by removing organic matter, salts, and visible soils, all of which interfere with microbial inactivation. The physical action of scrubbing with detergents and surfactants and rinsing with water removes substantial numbers of microorganisms. If a surface is not cleaned first, the

Note
To ensure that the treatment area is ready at the start of the day, SOPs should be followed to prepare the treatment room.

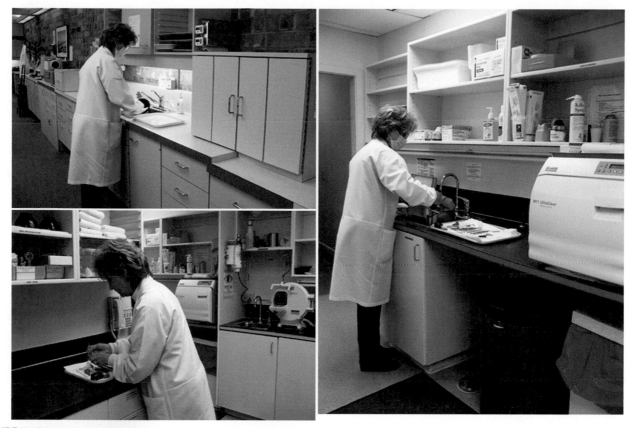

FIGURE 7-12
Instrument reprocessing areas: Contaminated zones *(labeled with red at the front of the counters)* and areas of caution *(labeled with yellow at the front of the counters)* are shown.

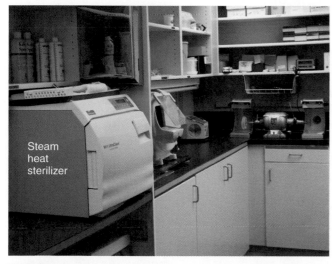

FIGURE 7-13
Steam heat sterilizer, laboratory work area, and work zones: Contamination zones *(labeled with red)* and areas of caution *(labeled with yellow)* are shown.

success of the disinfection process can be compromised. Removal of all visible blood and inorganic and organic matter can be as critical as the germicidal activity of the disinfecting agent.

The CDC recommends using surface barriers to protect clinical contact surfaces, particularly those that are difficult to clean (e.g., switches on dental chairs).[19] These barriers should be removed after each patient, and new barriers should be placed. There is not need to clean and disinfect the underlying surface between patients unless it has become contaminated.

The CDC recommends cleaning and disinfecting clinical contact surfaces (e.g., smooth hard surfaces) that are not barrier-protected and that can be adequately cleaned between patients. Disinfectants appropriate for dental health-care settings are EPA-registered hospital germicides with a low-level (i.e., HIV and HBV label claims) to intermediate-level (i.e., tuberculocidal claim) activity. Use of an intermediate-level disinfectant is recommended if the surface is visibly contaminated with blood. It is important to follow the specific manufacturers' directions for correct use of cleaning and EPA-registered hospital disinfecting products.[19]

Environmental surface protection

The following surfaces are considered potential areas of contamination and should be cleaned and sanitized at the start of each day:

- All smooth surfaces in the treatment area (i.e., countertops, tops of cubicle unit partitions)
- Operator, assistant, and patient chairs (including the base of the patient chair and the height adjustment handles)

7-3
7-4

> *Note*
>
> In this section SOP for cleaning environmental surfaces helps eliminate all but the most virulent microorganisms and serves as an example of the general housekeeping component of the office procedures.

- Light pole
- Arm
- Handles
- Switch
- Light cover (cleaning the cover *only* according to the manufacturer's instructions)
- Mobile carts (all switches, hoses, attachments, and nozzles on the power cart)
- X-ray view box, sink unit
- X-ray tube head
- Any other items or surfaces that may be touched during patient care[3,19,67]

Once these surfaces have been prepared for the day, disposable barriers are placed on difficult-to-clean items and those best managed with barriers. These include the following:

- Headrest and upper back of the dental chair
- Light adjustment handles
- Power cart with necessary switches, hand pieces, and tubing
- Evacuation tips
- Air/water syringe
- Patient tray (Figure 7-14)

Preparing the treatment room for patient treatment

The following items are generally considered part of the basic initial preparation:

- Tray and cover
- Patient bib
- Disposables, including gauze squares and cotton swabs
- Treatment supplies (i.e., prophy paste, cups, floss)
- Patient home-care supplies

- Chairside biohazard segregation bag or chairside waste bag (see Figure 7-14)

In addition, gloves, masks, safety glasses (both operator and patient), over gloves, and patient chart should be easily available.

If possible, charts should be left outside the treatment area. A *no-glove policy* for handling charts can reduce the risk of contamination. Some microorganisms can remain virulent on environmental surfaces for a significant time (see Table 7-2), potentially transmitting infectious agents to any individual who handles a contaminated chart. This caution also applies to the use of pens or pencils that may have been handled with contaminated hands.

Note

To prepare for patient treatment, the DHCP should gather the necessary supplies and organize them in the treatment room according to the work zones defined for that workspace.

Prevention

Clinical DHCP must ensure that patient charts are managed safely and not contaminated by handling with contaminated hands and subsequently circulated to front-office employees.

✴ CASE APPLICATION 7-1.2

Handling of Charts

Ruth regularly handles patient charts, filing, billing, and insurance matters. She is often the first person to receive the patient's chart immediately after the appointment is completed. Ruth has missed several weeks of work, showing lingering signs of a systemic illness. She is extremely fatigued, running a chronic fever, and appears to have some liver dysfunction.

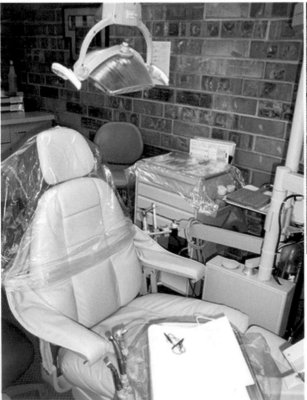

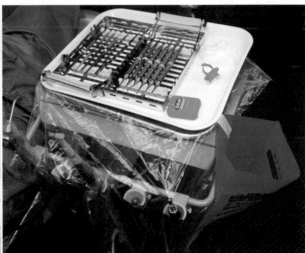

FIGURE 7-14
Appropriate use of surface barriers (WPC) for environmental protection in patient treatment area.

Once all necessary items are set up chairside and barrier covers are placed, the patient chair and other equipment should be positioned to enable the patient to sit down easily. The operator's stool should be adjusted to prevent contact with the height and back support adjustment handles during the appointment. Mobile and power carts must be carefully prepared, with all surfaces that may be touched during treatment covered, including hand pieces, the air/water syringe, suction tubes, and switches (see Figure 7-14). Inserting suction tips, burs, prophy cups, saliva ejector, and other similar items after barriers are placed on tubes and hand pieces is a good practice. Although the instrument tray is a flat, smooth surface and easy to clean, disposable covers also may be used on trays to reduce cleanup time between patients (see Figure 7-14). When work zones are defined (see Figure 7-13), a section of the counter area should be designated *clean* and should contain items that are not to be touched with contaminated hands. The treatment area should be double-checked to ensure that the x-ray view box is set up with the patient's x-ray films ready to go.

Treatment room cleanup

> **Prevention**
> Wearing nitrile rubber utility gloves can reduce exposure to contaminated items and injury from sharp objects and provide protection from contact with chemical agents.

Treatment room cleanup routinely involves the handling of sharp instruments and contaminated waste and the use of chemicals. DHCP should pay close attention when handling these contaminated items.

A systematic approach ensures that all contaminated surfaces are cleaned, that instruments and equipment are safely transported for processing, and that waste is properly disposed.

All surfaces in the treatment room must be cleaned, be disinfected, and have their disposable covers changed between patients (see Figure 7-14).

End of day

The manufacturer's instructions should dictate cleanup for all chemicals being used.

Daily equipment routines include flushing the evacuation system to reduce debris accumulation in the lines and performing the end-of-day procedures for clean water delivery systems. An appropriate cleaning solution always should be used, and manufacturer's instructions should be followed *exactly* for both systems.

> **Note**
> DHCP should remove all surface barriers at the end of the day and clean and disinfect the treatment room.

Decontamination, Disinfection, and Sterilization Procedures

Decontamination of surfaces and instruments after patient treatment requires a variety of procedures.* These procedures vary based on the surface area and size of the item, the type of equipment or instruments, the materials from which those instruments

*References 40, 68, 70, 81, 91, 95.

Table 7-8	**Spaulding Classifications and Chemical Agent Use**			
SPAULDING RISK CATEGORY	**EXPECTED CONTACT**	**EXPOSURE RISK**	**LEVEL OF DECONTAMINATION**	**METHOD OF DECONTAMINATION**
Critical	Direct contact Invasive procedures, penetration of mucous membranes, contact with bone *Example:* Periodontal scalers	Mucous membranes, oral fluids, blood, saliva	Sterilization	Heat sterilization preferred Chemical sterilant (glutaraldehyde)
Semicritical	Direct or indirect contact Contact with mucous membranes, penetration of mucous membranes not anticipated. *Examples:* Dental mouth mirror, dental hand pieces*	Mucous membranes, oral fluids, blood, saliva	Sterilization High-level disinfection	Heat sterilization Chemical sterilant High-level disinfectant (alcohols, chlorines, iodophors, synthetic phenolics, synergized quaternaries,† sodium bromide, and chlorine)
Noncritical	Direct or indirect contact Contact with intact skin, mucous membranes or penetration not anticipated *Example:* Radiograph head or cone	Indirect exposure to oral fluids, blood, saliva	Sanitization Low- to intermediate-level disinfection Barriers	Surface cleaner Intermediate-level disinfectant High-level disinfectant (alcohols, chlorines, iodophors, synthetic phenolics, synergized quaternaries,† sodium bromide, and chlorine)

*Although considered a semicritical item, a dental hand piece should always be sterilized between uses and not high-level disinfected.
†Indicates newer-generation products; previous formulations were not acceptable surface disinfectants.
The CDC adopted the Spaulding system in 2002.

are manufactured, and the intended uses. The determination as to which procedures are required to ensure that the surface or item is safe to touch and reuse becomes one of risk versus benefit.

The risk of cross-contamination (Table 7-8) during reuse of an item or contact with the surface must be determined to be noncritical (e.g., seat of the dental chair), semicritical (e.g., working surfaces, suction devices), or critical (e.g., instruments used in the oral cavity, known to be contaminated by blood or saliva). Appropriate measures then must be taken to treat the item in a way that renders it safe for use.[81,86,91]

Understanding that both chemical and physical decontamination activities take time and that the microorganisms are not all killed at the same rate is an important issue.[81] Complete destruction of the target microorganisms requires a series of events over time. Precleaning treatment surfaces to reduce the bioburden becomes an important element in an efficient system. Organic matter is capable of neutralizing disinfecting agents and can physically shelter microbes from the agent. Physical cleaning may be appropriate for some situations, whereas heat sterilization is required for others. The three most common processes for decontamination in the dental setting are sanitization, disinfection, and sterilization.

Sanitization

Sanitization provides the lowest level of safety and does not target any particular microorganism. Sanitization is intended for general housekeeping of noncritical surfaces or for devices made of materials that may deteriorate with the use of stronger agents.

> ### Note
> Sanitization is the process by which the number of microorganisms is reduced to a relatively safe level, with the focus being on reduction of the *microbial load*.

Chemical agents designed for sanitization are considered low-level disinfectants capable of inactivating vegetative bacteria but *not* spores, TB, or nonlipid viruses. Low-level cleaners and disinfectants are not used to decontaminate potentially infectious agents because they are not EPA-registered as effective against TB and therefore not suitable for use in postprocedure cleanup of semicritical or critical surfaces.

Disinfection

Disinfection is the destruction of pathogenic and other kinds of microorganisms by physical or chemical means. However, some thermal disinfection processes also are available.

Chemicals designed for intermediate- and high-level disinfection destroy microorganisms by causing protein denaturation, damaging cell membranes, inhibiting enzymes, or altering nucleic material, most with a combination of these actions.

> ### Note
> Disinfection is less lethal than sterilization because it destroys the majority of recognized pathogenic microorganisms, but not necessarily all microbial forms (e.g., bacterial spores). Disinfection does not assure the degree of safety associated with sterilization processes.

Intermediate-level disinfectants inactivate all organisms except spores and kill most vegetative bacteria (e.g., TB) and viruses (poliomyelitis II, South African [SA] rotavirus). These chemicals are used for surface decontamination, where a breach in a surface barrier may have occurred, and to treat surfaces not covered with barriers. Disinfectants used in healthcare settings must be registered with the EPA as hospital disinfectants. Low-level disinfectants are labeled hospital disinfectants and intermediate-level disinfectants are labeled as hospital disinfectants and have a tuberculocidal claim. (See Clinical Resources on Evolve for additional CDC Guidelines on sterilization and disinfection.)

> ### Prevention
> Manufacturers' directions are different for disinfection and sterilization, a vital concept, and immersion for longer times is required for sterilization. In addition, the dilution ratios are different for some products. DHCP should always follow specific manufacturers' instructions.

High-level disinfectants designed for use in dentistry are capable of inactivating spores when specific contact time recommendations are followed.

These chemicals are used to treat heat-sensitive items (e.g., plastics) and the process often is referred to as *immersion sterilization,* terminology that is important to understand. Many of these products, when used for different lengths of time, may be either disinfectants or chemical immersion sterilants. These chemicals should not be used for applications other than those indicated in their label instructions. Misapplications include use as an environmental surface disinfectant or instrument-holding solution.[19] High-level disinfectants and immersion chemical sterilants are regulated by the FDA.

Chemical Germicide Selection Criteria

A suggested ideal disinfectant agent would[40,62,64]:
- Be effective against a broad spectrum of organisms with a short contact time
- Not be inhibited by physical factors such as bioburden
- Not damage materials on repeated contact
- Have a residual effect on treated surfaces
- Be easy to use
- Be odorless
- Be economical

When choosing a disinfection and immersion chemical sterilant product, DHCP must always read the entire label, the most important step in the use of any chemical in the workplace. To be effective, agents must be used consistently with the manufacturers' specifications. Identifying and understanding the following information is necessary for the appropriate use of any chemical agent:
- Storage and shelf life
- Mixing and concentration necessary for proper use
- Special activation
- Effects of temperature and time on effective use
- Shelf life after mixing or dispensing
- Requirements for precleaning (e.g., Is the agent also a cleaner? Is a separate precleaning agent needed?)
- Whether the product is intended for surface or immersion use
- Contact time for tuberculocidal action
- Label's warnings

DHCP always should take the time to determine whether any potential toxic effects or precautions or special handling instructions are necessary for the disposal of used solutions. Chemical disinfectants for noncritical environmental surfaces in dentistry include alcohols, chlorine compounds, iodine compounds, phenolics, and hydrogen peroxide.

7-5 Sterilization

Heat sterilization has long been considered the most effective method of sterilization and is particularly effective when combined with steam or chemical vapor pressure (see Figure 7-13). Because sterilization equipment and chemical sterilants are considered medical devices, the FDA regulates them. All equipment and chemicals used for sterilization should be registered and approved as medical devices by that organization.

> **Note**
> Sterilization is the process by which microorganisms, including spore-forming organisms, are destroyed.[81,95]

Each practice setting must examine the type of equipment used, the available space and ventilation needs of the equipment, and the time-management issues of instrument reprocessing. No one method can meet all the needs of every practice setting.

Consequently, the following criteria should be considered in the selection of appropriate methods and equipment:

- Materials and items to be sterilized must be compatible with each method of sterilization.
- Volume of items to be processed at any one time is limited by the chamber capacity of the equipment.
- Time for reprocessing and cycle time needed for each method must be considered.
- Packaging materials must be compatible with the method and equipment used.
- Process indicators and biological monitors must be available for each method.

The most common methods of sterilization[81,86] in dentistry are: 1) steam, 2) chemical vapor, 3) dry heat, and 4) other low-temperature methods.

Steam Sterilization

Steam sterilization is also known as *autoclaving*. Steam sterilization, which is dependable and economical, is the most widely used for critical and semicritical items that are not sensitive to heat and moisture. This sterilization method requires exposure of each item to direct steam contact at a required temperature and pressure for a specified time needed to kill microorganisms. Specific manufacturers' instructions should be followed for all time and temperature parameters.

The gravity displacement and the high-speed prevacuum sterilizer are the two basic types of steam sterilizers sold in the United States. The majority of tabletop sterilizers used in a dental practice are gravity displacement sterilizers, although prevacuum sterilizers are becoming more widely available. In gravity displacement steam sterilizers, steam is admitted through steam lines, a steam generator, or self-generation of steam within the chamber. Unsaturated air is forced out of the chamber through a vent in the chamber wall. Trapping of air is a concern when using saturated steam under gravity displacement; errors in packaging items or overloading the sterilizer chamber can result in cool air pockets and items not being sterilized.

Prevacuum steam sterilizers require less time than gravity displacement types to sterilize instruments. They are fitted with a pump to create a vacuum in the chamber and ensure air removal from the sterilizing chamber before the chamber is pressurized with steam. Relative to gravity displacement, this procedure allows faster and more positive steam penetration throughout the entire load. Prevacuum sterilizers should be tested periodically for adequate air removal, as recommended by the manufacturer. Air not removed from the chamber will interfere with steam contact. If a sterilizer fails the air removal test, it should not be used until inspected by sterilizer maintenance personnel, and it passes the test. Manufacturer's instructions, with specific details regarding operation and user maintenance information, should be followed.

Chemical Vapor Sterilization

Unsaturated chemical-vapor sterilization requires heating a chemical solution of primarily alcohol with 0.23% formaldehyde in a closed pressurized chamber. Unsaturated chemical vapor sterilization of carbon steel instruments (e.g., dental burs) causes less corrosion than steam sterilization because of the low level of water present during the cycle. Instruments should be dry before sterilizing. State and local authorities should be consulted for hazardous waste disposal requirements for the sterilizing solution.

Dry Heat Sterilization

Dry heat is used to sterilize materials that might be damaged by moist heat (e.g., high carbon steel and certain hinged orthodontic instruments). Although dry heat has the advantages of low operating cost and being noncorrosive, it is a prolonged process and the high temperatures required are not suitable for certain patient-care items and devices.

> **Prevention**
> Chemical sterilization is accepted for non-heat tolerant semicritical items but should not be used for critical items (see Table 7-8).

There are two basic types of dry-heat sterilizers used in dentistry static-air and forced-air types:

- The static-air type is commonly called an *oven-type sterilizer*. Heating coils in the bottom or sides of the unit cause hot air to rise inside the chamber through natural convection.
- The forced-air type is also known as a *rapid heat-transfer sterilizer*. Heated air is circulated throughout the chamber at a high velocity, permitting more rapid transfer of energy from the air to the instruments, thereby reducing the time needed for sterilization. The forced-air sterilization cycle is much faster than the static-air type.

Other Sterilization Methods

Heat-sensitive critical and semicritical instruments and devices can be sterilized by immersing them in liquid chemical germicides registered by FDA as sterilants. The CDC cautions that when using a liquid chemical germicide for sterilization, certain poststerilization procedures are essential. Items need to be: 1) rinsed with sterile water after removal to remove toxic or irritating residues; 2) handled using sterile gloves and dried with sterile towels; and 3) delivered to the point of use in an aseptic manner. If stored before use, the instrument should not be considered sterile, and it should be sterilized again just before use. In addition, the sterilization process with liquid chemical sterilants cannot be verified with biological indicators.[19] The CDC discourages the use of liquid chemical germicides. Due to the many limitations of these chemicals, the CDC recommends replacing heat-sensitive semicritical items with heat tolerant or disposable items.[19]

Low-temperature sterilization with ethylene oxide gas (ETO) has been used extensively in larger health-care facilities. Its primary advantage is the ability to sterilize heat-sensitive and moisture-sensitive patient-care items with reduced damaging effects. Due to extended sterilization times of 10 to 48 hours, potential hazards to patients, and DHCP requiring stringent health and safety requirements, this method is impractical for most private-practice settings. It should be noted that, currently, dental handpieces cannot be effectively sterilized with this method because of decreased penetration of ETO gas flow through a small lumen in the devices.

Bead sterilizers have been used in dentistry to sterilize small metallic instruments (e.g., endodontic files). FDA has determined that a risk of infection exists with these devices because of their potential failure to sterilize dental instruments and has required their commercial distribution cease unless the manufacturer files a premarket approval application. If a bead sterilizer is employed, DHCP assume the risk of employing a dental device FDA has deemed neither safe nor effective.

Sterilization monitors

An essential part of instrument sterilization is monitoring, which is performed at a variety of levels to ensure proper operation of sterilization equipment and instruments.

Physical Cycle Monitor

The first level of monitoring includes physical checks of equipment during processing, such as confirmation that cycle indicators come on at appropriate times to signal that the equipment is operating properly. Sterilizers have a number of *readout* methods, depending on the age of the equipment, that range from dials and gauges, to lights, to liquid crystal display (LCD) panels and printers.

Goal

This level of monitoring allows the operator to determine whether the equipment is running at appropriate temperature, pressure, and time parameters.

For each load, monitors for fluid levels, temperature, pressure, and time should be checked. Physical controls, such as pressure gauges and thermometers, are used widely but should be considered secondary methods used to monitor the efficacy of sterilization.

Chemical Indicators

Chemical indicators, internal and external, use sensitive chemicals to assess physical conditions (e.g., time and temperature) during the sterilization process. Chemical indicators do not prove sterilization has been achieved, but they can alert the DHCP that the parameters for sterilization have not been met. Chemical indicator test results are received when the sterilization cycle is complete. These results can provide an early indication of a problem and where in the process the problem might exist. There are two basic types of chemical indicators internal and external.

External indicators are applied to the outside of a package (e.g., chemical indicator tape or special markings on the packaging material itself), change color rapidly when a specific parameter is reached, and they verify that the package has been exposed to the sterilization process. Internal chemical indicators should be used inside each package to ensure the sterilizing agent has penetrated the packaging material and actually reached the instruments and items inside. A single-parameter internal chemical indicator provides information regarding only one sterilization parameter (e.g., time or temperature). Multiparameter internal chemical indicators are designed to react to ≥ 2 parameters (e.g., time and temperature; or time, temperature, and the presence of steam) and can provide a more reliable indication that sterilization conditions have been met. At the date of this publication, multiparameter internal indicators are available only for steam sterilizers (i.e., autoclaves).

The CDC recommends that DHCP place a chemical indicator on the inside of each package of instruments prior to sterilization. If the internal indicator is not visible from the outside, also place an exterior chemical indicator on the package. If either mechanical indicators or internal or external chemical indicators detect inadequate processing, items in the load should not be used until they are re-packaged with a new chemical indicator(s) and re-sterilized.[19]

✳ CASE APPLICATION 7-2.1

Sterilization Monitoring

The first indication of a problem was when the student noticed that the cycle integrator on the sterilization bag for the instruments she had just used had not changed color, indicating that the physical parameters for sterilization had not been met. Without this monitor, she would not be able to determine whether the pack had been exposed to a sterilization cycle.

Further checking of processing records identified the individuals who had operated the sterilizer for the two batches in question, and an interview revealed that they had not been present to monitor each initial physical check when the sterilizing unit had been started. They were unable to confirm that the equipment appeared to be operating properly. At this point, two levels of monitoring indicated a potential problem.

Biologic Indicators

A biologic indicator (BI) is a strip or vial impregnated with non-pathogenic bacterial spores. The BI is used to verify sterilization and is a quality control tool for heat sterilizers. *Geobacillus stearothermophilus* is the BI organism appropriate for steam heat and chemical vapor sterilization methods. *Bacillis pumilus* is used for dry heat. The CDC recommends that DHCP monitor sterilizers at least weekly by using a biological indicator with a matching control (i.e., biological indicator and control from same lot number). The CDC also recommends using a biological indicator for every sterilizer load that contains an implantable device and to verify results before using the implantable device, whenever possible.[19]

> ### Biological Indicators
> The biological indicators most reliable level of monitoring sterilization procedures is the use of biological indicators that are placed throughout the load before it is placed in the sterilization chamber.

To assess sterilization, test strips are placed with a load of instruments before initiating a normal cycle. If the load contains wrapped items, then a test pack should be prepared containing a spore strip and should be positioned in the center of the sterilizer load. Then the sterilizer should be operated in accordance with manufacturer's instructions. After the sterilization cycle is complete, the BIs are incubated with a control and monitored for microbial growth. This monitor testing is usually sent to an off-site monitoring service; in-office test kits are also available.

If complete sterilization has occurred, then the processed test will show no growth; the unsterilized control indicates microbial growth. Failure of a sterilizer to sterilize the BI successfully should initiate a recall of all materials processed in that machine. Follow-up through verification (a repeat of the BI testing) should be performed. Before an assumption is made that the error is mechanical, the WPC should be reviewed to determine whether the error was operator based, such as through overloading of the sterilizer, a common cause of sterilization failure.

BI testing is required as a part of routine equipment maintenance and office infection control practices and is not intended as a guarantee for each load of instruments in a given sterilization unit. The interval of BI testing is set by a variety of agencies and may vary for each jurisdiction. Following the regulations for each workplace location is critical to ensure safety.

⁂ CASE APPLICATION 7-2.2

Sterilization Monitoring Records

Records on the sterilizer used indicated that the unit routinely passed a weekly BI test, so it was presumed that the error was operator generated and not caused by an equipment malfunction.

Instrument processing

After all dental procedures are performed, instruments and equipment must be reprocessed for future use.* At this point, items have been contaminated and must be handled safely until they are disinfected or sterilized.

Transporting Contaminated Items

The first step in contaminated transfer is to gather all items and use appropriate ECs and WPCs to prevent exposure or injury during the transfer of items to the reprocessing area. WPCs may include the use of utility gloves (PPE), hard-sided transport bins, and instrument cassettes (EC). Care must be taken not to create further contamination of workspaces and to prevent injury from any sharp items (WPC).

Cleaning Instruments

Cleaning is the first step in decontaminating reusable instruments and should precede all disinfection and sterilization processes. Cleaning involves removal of debris as well as bioburden. Removal of debris and contamination is achieved either by scrubbing with a surfactant, detergent, and water, or by an automated process (e.g., ultrasonic cleaner or instrument washer or washer-disinfector). The CDC recommends using automated equipment, which can be safer and more efficient than manually cleaning contaminated instruments, and it can increase productivity, improve cleaning effectiveness, and decrease worker exposure to blood and body fluids.[19] Presoaking or scrubbing of instruments is not recommended and not necessary prior to using automated methods After cleaning, instruments should be inspected prior to packaging for sterilization to ensure removal of all visible debris. Cleaned instruments are still considered potentially contaminated. DHCP should use appropriate PPE and safe-work practices to prevent exposure and sharps injuries.

> ### Note
> Clean reusable critical and semi-critical patient care items prior to sterilization.[19,85,95]

Packaging Instruments for Sterilization

Selecting appropriate packaging for the method of sterilization used is another important step.[81,95] A number of pouches, wrapping types, and cassettes are available to manage dental instruments. These may be constructed of paper or plastic and some of cloth. Cassettes are an excellent means to reduce possible injury during the handling of sharp instruments throughout the reprocessing cycle. Pouches and wrapping material to accommodate a variety of cassette sizes are also available. Reviewing the manufacturer's instructions for each sterilization unit is necessary to ensure that appropriate wrapping materials are used. Selecting packaging materials that integrate sterilization monitoring processes can assist in an overall monitoring program.

---

*References 3, 19, 26, 59, 76, 77, 81.

To monitor and retrieve packs, every pack that is sterilized should be labeled with a control number to indicate the sterilizer used, the cycle or load number, the date of sterilization, and an expiration date (if time limits are placed). Resterilization packs and trays are necessary when contamination is expected or evident.

✦ CASE APPLICATION 7-2.3

Sterilization Monitoring Tracking

In following up on this pack, the student discovered that the batch number was used to determine the group of instruments that were processed together. This number describes another level of monitoring and tracking. The information was used to determine that two groups of instruments had been distributed without indicating that appropriate sterilization had taken place.

Sterilization

> *Note*
>
> Any item that *can* be sterilized *must* be sterilized.*
>
> *References 26, 43, 47, 59, 81.

The critical factors[81] used to develop SOPs may include the method of sterilization to be used, appropriate packaging materials and methods, appropriate storage and handling of the package, appropriate environmental controls, cleanliness, appropriate sterilization methods, and appropriate inventory control. The goal is to achieve sterilization of instruments and critical items in a safe and effective manner for DHCP and the patient.

Loading the sterilizer in a way that allows for the appropriate physical criteria to be met and maintained throughout the cycle is critical to successful load sterilization. Instruments should be loosely packed, avoiding excess wrapping material and refraining from overloading the sterilizer chamber. Room must be available for the heat, steam, and chemicals to circulate around and through the packs with maximal penetration to the instruments.

Although no one universal standard for sterilization is recommended, any sterilizer used in health care must be FDA-cleared as a medical device for this purpose. Therefore each dental healthcare facility is responsible for its own assessment of the needs and the environment for sterilization at the point of use and for the proper operation of the unit selected.

Storage of Sterilized Items

Care should be taken in the storage of sterilized items because improper handling and storage can compromise the integrity of the package. If any packaging is damaged, then the contents

> *Storage Care*
>
> Storing sterilized packs of instruments should ensure that packages are not crushed or punctured by items in the bags, which will compromise sterility.[81]

should be considered contaminated or nonsterile. Instruments must be repackaged and resterilized if any sign of damage to the wrapping is apparent. All items should be stored in a clean,

dry area that allows the oldest packs to be used first. Both open- and closed-shelving systems can be used, and ideally items should be protected from dust. Instruments may be stored as sterile tray setups, as groups, or individually wrapped. Evidence must appear on the wrapping, such as autoclave tape or color indicator, that the correct temperature was achieved in the sterilization cycle.

Research has defined the length of time sterile goods can be stored and still be considered sterile to range from as short as 1 week to indefinitely.[81] A number of factors can affect this determination, including the wrapping material used, the manner of handling, the use of cassettes for sharp instruments, and the conditions for storage.

Managing sharp items and related injury

Numerous risks exist for DHCP to become injured by a sharp object. All DHCP *must* routinely apply WPCs and ECs to reduce the handling of contaminated sharp objects, including reusable items (e.g., instruments) and disposable items (e.g., needles, burs, wires, matrix bands). Careful transport, cleaning, and disposal practices are required. All sharp items should

> *Prevention*
>
> Additional information for developing a safety program and for identifying and evaluating safer dental devices is available at http://www.cdc.gov/OralHealth/infectioncontrol/forms.htm (forms for screening and evaluating safer dental devices) and at http://www.cdc.gov/niosh/topics/bbp (state legislation on needlestick safety).

be handled with the utmost care. Using utility gloves, transport bins, and instrument cassettes provides protection when DHCP recycle instruments.

Recapping needles should be performed only with the use of a recapping device (e.g., EC) or a one-handed scoop technique (e.g., WPC) (Figure 7-15). Two-handed needle recapping without a protective device is not permitted. The recapping device should be prepared before the needle is unsheathed.

After use, the needle is removed from the syringe with the sheath in place, the exposed sharp end is placed over the opening of the sharps container, and the sheath-covered needle is placed into the container. Needles should *never* be bent or broken after use (i.e., the *no-handling* approach). Current revisions to OSHA regulations include an increased focus and emphasis on the use of ECs to prevent sharps-related injuries for healthcare employees. Because of the potential serious outcome of percutaneous injury, WPCs and ECs should be strictly followed. As soon as possible after use, sharp items must be removed from the treatment area and placed into an appropriate puncture-proof, leak-proof container. Items to be placed in the sharps container are shown in Box 7-4. Sharp objects must never be forced into an over-filled container (see Figure 7-15, *B*).

An injury involving a potential exposure to human body fluid or materials contaminated with body substances (e.g., needle stick, splash to mucous membranes or nonintact skin) should be reported as soon as possible to the practice's designated infection control officer.

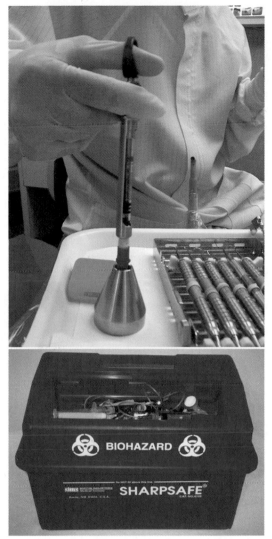

FIGURE 7-15
A, WPC for recapping needles. **B,** Overfilled sharps container.

BOX 7-4

ITEMS TO BE PLACED IN SHARPS CONTAINER

Used and unused anesthetic carpules (unless other containers are designated for glass carpules)
Anesthetic needles
Other syringe needles

Worn-out burs
Broken instruments
Instrument tips
Any other sharp items that may injure individuals handling waste

Postexposure Management

Postexposure evaluation and follow-up are managed by a designated staff member, and appropriate measures will be determined by the attending healthcare provider.* Postexposure follow-up may include blood tests, a medically indicated

*References 14, 19, 30, 74, 78.

Instrument Decontamination at Chairside

What is the risk to the dental hygienist in wiping a contaminated instrument free of visible debris with a gauze sponge (via a pinching motion) during a procedure, then returning directly to the mouth? This process could be repeated numerous times during a scaling appointment without the hygienist giving it a second thought.

If the instrument were both sharp and contaminated with a significant mass of blood and debris (i.e., adhered to the blade of the curet), then a puncture or small tear to the glove that could possibly break the skin would potentially expose DHCP to infectious agents.

Distinct Care Modifications

During the management of occupational blood exposures, the effectiveness of postexposure medication is related to the length of time between exposure and the administration of medical attention. Postexposure plans (PEPs) may vary slightly among medical facilities. Obtaining the latest postexposure recommendations from the CDC will provide the information required to develop a clinical protocol.

Provide immediate care to the exposure site:
- Wash wounds and skin with soap and water.
- Flush mucous membranes with water.
- Render first aid as appropriate to injury.
- Transport to medical facility for postexposure care.

prophylaxis, counseling, and an evaluation of subsequent reported illnesses.[17]

Preparation for the possible event of an injury is important for its timely management. Guidelines and protocols are available from the CDC,[19] OSHA,[78] and ADA.

Laboratory procedures

As with instrument processing and handling of x-ray films, items removed from the immediate treatment area must also be properly handled to prevent cross-contamination,[3] including all materials and appliances that require handling for laboratory work, cleaning, or repair. These items must be disinfected before they are transported from the office. In addition, all appliances and materials being returned from the laboratory must be disinfected and rinsed before they are inserted into the patient's mouth, including removable prostheses and appliances and any instruments (e.g., spatulas, laboratory knives, acrylic burs and stones, carvers) contaminated during the laboratory phase of treatment. All impression and treatment trays must be sterilized or discarded (if disposable) after use.

Impression and bite registration materials vary in their compatibility with disinfection agents. The manufacturer's instructions must always be consulted to ensure that the impression is not damaged. Both biohazardous and chemical risks are present in the management of impressions, and DHCP should use appropriate PPE.

When removable appliances are polished with an office dental lathe, WPCs should again be used to eliminate cross-contamination from the pumice or rag wheel or both. PPE to protect the eyes is also indicated.

Waste management

7-7
7-8

The classification of waste generated in the dental environment is based on the potential risk to humans and the environment during the disposal, transport, and treatment of the waste.[3,19,43,62,69]

Categories of Waste
- Physical
- Biohazardous
- Chemical

General waste does not pose any significant risk; infectious (biohazardous) waste and toxic (chemical) waste pose possible or definite risks. Biohazardous waste is identified as either sharps or saturated absorbent material that is *dripping* with blood or saliva.

Relevant waste categories that are regulated include items referred to as *sharps,* which includes used and unused needles, local anesthetic needles and carpules, and instruments and broken glass; human tissues and foreign bodies, which include teeth removed during surgery; blood-contaminated items that when compressed release blood; or OPIMs, including saliva. Sharps should be disposed of in an appropriate biohazard-labeled, puncture-resistant, leak-proof sharps container.

All waste generated during treatment should be considered contaminated and therefore potentially infectious. Biohazardous waste is to be segregated at the point of generation during treatment into designated containers—biohazard bag—in the treatment room and then appropriately disposed of in the facility's main waste receptacle after completion of treatment. Materials placed in this bag include but are not limited to soaked or blood-contaminated cotton rolls, gauze, cotton pellets, and similar items.

Each facility should consult its local governing agency for rules and regulations about collection, storage, transport, and treatment of biohazardous and toxic waste from a healthcare facility. Regulations vary, and strict adherence to local regulations is required.

The overall health and safety of each patient and DHCP is in the hands of each employee. A commitment to sound practices based on inherent risk and science are necessary for the health of all involved.

References

1. American Academy of Pediatrics (AAP) Childhood Immunization Support Program (CISP): *Varicella immunization* [Internet], Elk Grove Village, Ill, 2006. [http://www.cispimmunize.org].
2. American Dental Association: Dental unit waterlines: approaching the year 2000, *J Am Dent Assoc* 130:1653-1664, 1999.
3. American Dental Association: Infection control recommendations for the dental office and the dental laboratory, *J Am Dent Assoc* 127(5):672-680, 1996.
4. American Dental Association: *Statement on backflow prevention and the dental office,* ADA position statement, Chicago, 1996, ADA.
5. American Dental Association: *Statement on dental unit waterlines,* Chicago, 1995, ADA.
6. Atlas et al: *Legionella* contamination of dental-unit waters, *Appl Environ Microbiol* 61:1208-1213, 1995.
7. Bednarsh HS, Eklund KJ: *Dental staff health and safety training,* Brunswick, Me, 1999, InVision.
8. Bednarsh HS, Eklund KJ: CDC issues final TB guidelines, *Access* 10(5):6-13, 1995.
9. Bednarsh HS, Eklund KJ, Mills S: Check your dental unit water IQ, *Dent Assist* 65(6):9-10, 1996.
10. Benenson AS: *Control of communicable diseases in man,* ed 15, Washington, DC, 1990, American Public Health Association.
11. Bentley CD, Burkhart NW, Crawford JJ: Evaluating spatter and aerosol contamination during dental procedures, *J Am Dent Assoc* 125(5):579-584, 1994.
12. Bernstein DE, de Medina MD: *Hepatitis viruses,* Deerfield Beach, Fla, 1998, Health Studies Institute.
13. Blanco C et al: Latex allergy: clinical features and cross-reactivity with fruits, *Ann Allergy* 73:309-314, 1994.
14. Bolyard EA et al: Guideline for infection control in health care personnel 1998, *Am J Infect Control* 26:289-354, 1998.
15. Carmichael CG et al: *HIV/AIDS: what health professionals need to know,* Miami, 1996, Health Studies Institute.
16. Centers for Disease Control and Prevention: *Fact sheet: Basic information about SARS* [Internet], Atlanta, 2005, CDC [http://www.cdc.gov/ncidod/sars/factsheet.htm]
16a. Centers for Disease Control and Infection: Guidelines for preventing the transmission of M. tuberculosis in healthcare settings, *MMWR* 54(RR-12):1-141, 2005.
17. Centers for Disease Control and Prevention: Updated US Public Health Service Guidelines for management of occupational exposure to HIV and recommendations for post exposure prophylaxis, *MMWR* 54(RR-9):1-17, 2005
18. Centers for Disease Control and Prevention: *West Nile virus: treatment information and guidance for clinicians* [Internet], Atlanta, 2004, CDC, [http://www.cdc.gov/ncidod/dvbid/westnile/clinicians/treatment.htm].
19. Centers for Disease Control and Prevention: Guidelines for infection-control in dental health-care settings—2003, *MMWR CDC Surveill Summ* 52(RR-17):1-66, 2003.
20. Centers for Disease Control and Prevention: *Infection control in dentistry—airborne* [Internet], Atlanta, 1999, CDC [http://www.cdc.gov].
21. Centers for Disease Control and Prevention: *Infection control in dentistry—bloodborne* [Internet], Atlanta, 1999, CDC [http://www.cdc.gov].
22. Centers for Disease Control and Prevention: *Infection control in dentistry—waterborne* [Internet], Atlanta, 1999, CDC [http://www.cdc.gov].
23. Centers for Disease Control and Prevention: Guidelines for preventing the transmission of *Mycobacterium tuberculosis* in health-care facilities, 1994. *MMWR CDC Surveill Summ* 43(RR-13):1-132, 1994.
24. Centers for Disease Control and Prevention: Prevention and control of influenza. Part I. Vaccines, *MMWR CDC Surveill Summ* 43(RR-9):1-13, 1994.
25. Centers for Disease Control and Prevention: Prevention and control of influenza. Part II. Antiviral agents—recommendations of ACIP, *MMWR CDC Surveill Summ* 43(RR-15):1-10, 1994.
26. Centers for Disease Control and Prevention: *Practical infection control in the dental office,* Atlanta, 1993, CDC.
27. Centers for Disease Control and Prevention: Recommendations of the Advisory Committee on Immunization Practices: use of vaccines and immune globulins for persons with altered immunocompetence, *MMWR CDC Surveill Summ* 42(RR-4):1-17, 1993.
28. Ceisel RJ et al: Evaluating chemical inactivation of viral agents in handpiece splatter, *J Am Dent Assoc* 126(2):197-202, 1995.
29. Challacombe SJ, Fernandes LL: Detecting *Legionella pneumophila* in water systems: a comparison of various dental units, *J Am Dent Assoc* 126(5):603-608, 1995.

30. Chenoweth CE, Gobetti JP: Postexposure chemoprophylaxis for occupational exposure to HIV in the dental office, *J Am Dent Assoc* 128(8):1135-1139, 1997.

31. Christensen GJ: Using rubber dams to boost quality, quantity of restorative services, *J Am Dent Assoc* 125:81-82, 1994.

32. Cleveland JL et al: Risk and prevention of hepatitis C virus infection: implications for dentistry, *J Am Dent Assoc* 130:641-647, 1999.

33. Cleveland JL et al: Hepatitis B vaccination and infection among U.S. dentists, 1983-1992, *J Am Dent Assoc* 127(9):1385-1390, 1996.

34. Cleveland JL et al: TB infection control recommendations from the CDC, 1994: considerations for dentistry, *J Am Dent Assoc* 126(5):593-599, 1995.

35. Columbia University Department of Medical Informatics: *Tuberculosis resources* [Internet], New York, NY, 1999, The University [http://www.cpmc.columbia.edu/tbcpp.html].

36. Columbia University Department of Medical Informatics, TB resources: *About tuberculosis* [Internet], New York, 1999, The University [http://www.cpmc.edu/tbcpp/abouttb.html].

37. Columbia University Department of Medical Informatics, TB resources: *Preventing tuberculosis* [Internet], New York, 1999, The University [http://www.cpmc.columbia.edu/tbcpp/prevent.html].

38. Columbia University Department of Medical Informatics, TB resources: *TB: getting cured* [Internet], New York, 1999, The University [http://www.cpmc.columbia.edu/tbcpp/tbcure.html].

39. Columbia University Department of Medical Informatics, TB resources: *The tuberculin skin test* [Internet], New York, 1999, The University [http://www.cpmc.columbia.edu/tbcpp/skintest.html].

40. Cottone JA, Terezhalmy GT, Molinari JA: *Practical infection control in dentistry*, ed 2, Media, Penn, 1996, Williams & Wilkins.

41. Diagnosis: latex allergy! Now what? *Latex Allergy News* I(1), 1999 (entire issue).

42. Eleazer PD et al: A chemical treatment regimen to reduce bacterial contamination in dental waterlines, *J Am Dent Assoc* 128:617-623, 1997.

43. Environmental management and pollution prevention: a guide for dental programs. Adapted from Local Hazardous Waste Management Program of King County: *Waste management guidelines for King County dental offices*, King County, Wash, 1993, The Program.

44. Falcons KJ, O'Fee PD: Latex allergy: implications for oral health care professionals, *J Dent Hyg* 72(3):25-32, 1998.

45. Fons MP et al: Multiple herpes viruses in saliva of HIV-infected individuals, *J Am Dent Assoc* 125(6):713-719, 1994.

46. Gillcrist JA: Hepatitis viruses A, B, C, D, E, and G: implications for dental personnel, *J Am Dent Assoc* 130:509-520, 1999.

47. Goodman HS, Carpenter RD, Cox MR: Sterilization of dental instruments and devices: an update, *Am J Infect Control* 22(2):90-94, 1994.

48. The Hepatitis Information Network: *Epidemiology & natural history of hepatitis B* [Internet], Schering, Canada, 1998, HepNet [http://www.hepnet.com/boca/seef2.html].

49. The Hepatitis Information Network: *Epidemiology and natural history of hepatitis C, virus infection hepatitis C* [Internet], Schering, Canada, 1998, HepNet [http://www.hepnet.com/boca/epidem.html].

50. The Hepatitis Information Network: *Hepatitis A: Hepatitis A—what is it?* [Internet], Schering, Canada, 1998, HepNet [http://www.hepnet.com/hepa/hepafact.html].

51. The Hepatitis Information Network: *Hepatitis A, D, E, & G* [Internet], Schering, Canada, 1998, HepNet [http://www.hepnet.com/update14.html].

52. The Hepatitis Information Network: *Hepatitis D: the hepatitis D virus* [Internet], Schering, Canada, 1998, HepNet [http://www.hepnet.com/hepd/wormhdv.html].

53. The Hepatitis Information Network: *Hepatitis G press release: hepatitis G* [Internet], Schering, Canada, 1998, HepNet [http://www.hepnet.com/hepg/hepg1.html].

54. The Hepatitis Information Network: *HepNews press release: hepatitis A deadly in hepatitis C sufferers* [Internet], Schering, Canada, 1998, HepNet [http://www.hepnet.com/hepc/news12898.html].

55. The Hepatitis Information Network: *HepNews press release: new report on hepatitis C epidemic indicates time is now to stop killer disease* [Internet], Schering, Canada, 1998, HepNet [http://www.hepnet.com/hepc/news31698.html].

56. Huntley DE, Campbell J: Bacterial contamination of scrub jackets during dental hygiene procedures, *J Dent Hyg* 72:3:19-23, 1998.

57. Journal of the American Medical Association, JAMA HIV/AIDS Information Center: *Treatment center—secondary prevention recommendations* [Internet], Chicago, 1999, AMA [http://www. ama-assn.org/special/hiv/treatmnt/guide/rr4719/rr4719j.html].

58. Karpay RI et al: Validation of an in-office dental unit water monitoring technique, *J Am Dent Assoc* 129:207-211, 1998.

59. Kolstad RA: The emergence of load-oriented sterilization, *J Am Dent Assoc* 125:51-54, 1994.

60. Larson EL: APIC guideline for handwashing and antisepsis in healthcare settings, *Am J Infect Control* 23:251-269, 1995.

61. Merchant VA: An update on herpes viruses, *J Calif Dent Assoc* 24(1):38-46, 1996.

62. Metro King County Hazardous Waste Management Program: *Disinfectants and cleaners* [Internet], Seattle, 1999, King County, [http://www.metrokc.gov/hazwaste/yb/disinfectant.html].

63. Miller CH, Palenik CJ: *Infection control and management of hazardous materials for the dental team*, St Louis, 1998, Mosby.

64. Molinari JA: Practical infection control for the 1990s: applying science to government regulations, *J Am Dent Assoc* 125(9):1189-1197, 1994.

65. Murdoch-Kinch CA et al: Comparison of dental water quality management procedures, *J Am Dent Assoc* 128(9):1235-1243, 1997.

66. Nisengard RJ, Newman MG: *Oral microbiology and immunology*, Philadelphia, 1994, WB Saunders.

67. Organization for Safety and Asepsis Procedures: *Organization for safety and asepsis procedures infection control in dentistry guidelines*, Annapolis, Md, 1997, OSAP.

68. OSAP Monthly Focus: *1999 in review: infection control highlights & headlines from the past year*, Annapolis, Md, 1999, OSAP.

69. OSAP Monthly Focus: *Dental office waste management*, Annapolis, Md, 1998, OSAP.

70. OSAP Monthly Focus: *Emerging diseases with an impact on dentistry*, Annapolis, Md, 1999, OSAP.

71. OSAP Monthly Focus: *Environmental surface disinfection*, Annapolis, Md, 1998, OSAP.

72. OSAP Monthly Focus: *Hand asepsis*, Annapolis, Md, 1998, OSAP.

73. OSAP Monthly Focus: *Latex-associated allergies & conditions*, Annapolis, Md, 1998, OSAP.

74. OSAP Monthly Focus: *Postexposure prophylaxis: CDC issues recommendations for healthcare workers exposed to HIV*, Annapolis, Md, 1998, OSAP.

75. OSAP Position Papers: *Dental unit waterlines*, Annapolis, Md, January 1997, OSAP.

76. OSAP Position Papers: *Instrument processing*, Annapolis, Md, January 1997, OSAP.

77. OSAP Position Papers: *Percutaneous injury*, Annapolis, Md, January 1997, OSAP.

78. Occupational Safety and Health Administration: *OSHA regulations: bloodborne pathogens*. Final rule. Federal Register, 29 CFR. Part

1910.1030. 56(235):64175-82, Washington, DC, December 6, 1992, OSHA.

79. Occupational Safety and Health Administration: *Personal protective equipment for general industry.* Final rule. Federal Register, 29 CFR. Part 1910.132. 59(66):16334-16364, Washington, DC, April 6, 1994, OSHA.

80. Recommended clinical guidelines for infection control in dental education institutions, *J Dent Educ* 55(9):621-630, 1991.

81. Reichert M, Young JH: *Sterilization technology for the health care facility,* ed 2, Gaithersburg Md, 1997, Aspen.

82. Rhode J: Ambidextrous gloves—can they contribute to carpal tunnel syndrome? *Dent Today* 9(5):1-2, 1990.

83. Runnells RR: *Infection control in the wet finger environment,* Salt Lake City, 1984, Publishers Press.

84. Rutala WA: APIC guideline for selection and use of disinfectants, *Am J Infect Control* 24:313-342, 1996.

85. Rutala WA: *Chemical germicides in health care, International Symposium,* Washington, DC, May 1994, Association for Professionals in Infection Control and Epidemiology.

86. Sanchez E, Macdonald G: Decontaminating dental instruments: testing the effectiveness of selected methods, *J Am Dent Assoc* 126(3):359-362, 1995.

87. Shulman ST, Phair JP, Sommers HM: *The biologic & clinical basis of infectious diseases,* Philadelphia, 1992, WB Saunders.

88. Slavkin HC: The A, B, C, D, and E of viral hepatitis, *J Am Dent Assoc* 127(11):1667-1670, 1996.

89. Slavkin HC: Infection and immunity, *J Am Dent Assoc* 127(12):1792-1796, 1996.

90. Solomon ES: Curriculum guidelines for the dental care management of patients with bloodborne infectious diseases, *J Dent Educ* 55:9:609-619, 1991.

91. Spaulding EH: Chemical disinfection of medical and surgical materials. In Lawrence CA, Block SS, eds: *Disinfection, sterilization, and preservation,* Philadelphia, 1968, Lea & Febiger.

92. Sussman GL, Beezhold DH: Allergy to latex rubber, *Ann Intern Med* 122:43-46, 1995.

93. *Using Millipore samplers in dental settings,* Millipore Technical Brief, TB094, Bedford, Mass, 1998, Millipore.

94. Westlund R, Kim HH, Schulman J: *Tuberculosis resurgent,* Miami, 1995, Health Studies Institute.

95. Willett NP, White RR, Rosen S: *Essential dental microbiology,* Norwalk, Conn, 1991, Appleton & Lange.

96. Williams JF et al: Assessing microbial contamination of dental unit waterlines: prevalence, intensity and microbiological characteristics, *J Am Dent Assoc* 124:59-65, 1993.

97. Williams HN et al: Assessing microbial contamination in clean water dental units and compliance with disinfection protocol, *J Am Dent Assoc* 125(9):1205-1211, 1994.

98. Williams HN, Baer ML, Kelley JI: Contribution of biofilm bacteria to the contamination of the dental unit water supply, *J Am Dent Assoc* 126(9):1255-1260, 1995.

Positioning and Prevention of Operator Injury

Susan J. Daniel • Patricia J. Nunn • Rebecca M. Barry •
William Woodall

INSIGHT

Learning and adapting ergonomic positioning and practices is critical for physical comfort, proper muscle tone, and reduction of musculoskeletal challenges of the dental hygienist. The benefits of good posture and performance logic positioning during dental hygiene procedures are fundamental to establishing and maintaining musculoskeletal health.

CASE STUDY 8-1 — Musculoskeletal Problems Resulting from Equipment

Suzanne Wong is a dental hygienist who graduated from dental hygiene school 2 years ago. While in school, Suzanne learned that good ergonomics would be important to her continuing career as a dental hygienist. She can recall Professor Bowers giving an interesting lecture on ergonomics, as well as the faculty recommending protective postures as students began preclinical laboratory sessions and practiced instrumentation techniques on one another. She also remembers later that faculty members sometimes told her to "watch her posture" as she was seeing patients in the school clinic.

As soon as Suzanne began to see patients with more severe and complex needs in her senior clinic, she became so focused on their needs that she forgot to focus on prevention—not with respect to her patient's oral healthcare needs but in relation to her own physical well-being. It began as a compromise in patient positioning to avoid violating the patient's personal space as she carried out treatment modalities. Then Suzanne began to avoid asking patients to adjust their position because it was simply easier and faster to adjust her own posture. Suzanne even began to believe that she could see better and do what she needed to do more easily in the nonergonomic positions she adopted. Unfortunately, the faculty at Suzanne's dental hygiene program mentioned her posture only infrequently; consequently, she continued to develop bad postural habits.

Currently, Suzanne works 4 days a week in a dental practice that she loves: the people, the environment, but especially the patients

seem perfect! Suzanne is one of two full-time dental hygienists and is the newest dental hygienist in the dental practice. Although her employer plans to build a new facility in the future to accommodate her growing practice, at present Suzanne works in the "extra" treatment room, originally set up for denture "try-ins" and emergency patient screenings. This smaller room restricts free movement of equipment and personnel. Access to the suction and air/water syringe requires stretching across the patient; reaching the instrument tray requires Suzanne to stretch and twist each time she changes instruments. The operator's stool is a surplus secretarial chair from the front office and has seen better days.

Now in her second year of dental hygiene practice, Suzanne is experiencing significant discomfort both at work and at home. The discomfort begins with headaches that are increasing in frequency and severity. She is also beginning to suffer a burning and stiffness that she describes as an achy feeling in her upper back just under her right shoulder blade that is now developing into an almost constant nagging pain that involves both her upper and lower back. Recently, Suzanne is experiencing tingling and numbness in her little and ring fingers of her left hand, followed by the same feelings in her right hand. Pain in her right thumb and wrist follows the tingling and numbness. Suzanne vividly remembers the lecture about carpal tunnel, and she is seriously contemplating a new and different professional career.

KEY TERMS

annulus fibrosus	kyphosis	operator positioning	supine position
biocentric technique	ligaments	patient positioning	synovial joints
diopter magnification	lordosis	performance logic positioning	telescopic loupes
ergonomics	musculoskeletal disorders	postural syndrome	thoracic outlet syndrome
eye loupes	neutral position	proprioceptive	work-related musculoskeletal
facet joint	nucleus pulposus	repetitive strain injury	disorder
fiber optics	Occupational Safety and Health	semisupine position	
herniated (slipped) disc	Administration		

LEARNING OUTCOMES

After reading this chapter the student will be able to:

1. Develop an appreciation for evidence-based knowledge of ergonomics in the dental environment.
2. Understand the relationship among correct operator posture and positioning, patient and equipment positioning, and musculoskeletal problems.
3. Describe the physical changes that occur from repetitive strain injuries.
4. Demonstrate correct operator, patient, and equipment positioning for maximal efficiency and minimal risk of developing musculoskeletal problems.

5. Compare, contrast, and evaluate alternative operator and patient positions.
6. Correct improper positioning by recognizing cues that indicate that an aspect of positioning is incorrect.
7. Develop an awareness of new technology that may reduce operator stress and fatigue and promote optimal performance.
8. Incorporate preventive exercises into instrumentation procedures.
9. Perform preventive exercises throughout the workday and at home.
10. Apply correct operator, patient, and equipment positioning for maximal efficiency for ultrasonic scaling.

8-1
8-2

Ergonomics Associated with Dental Hygiene Practice

Prevention

Without good posture, overall health and efficiency can become so compromised that many long-term effects are experienced.

In the long term, poor posture can affect the musculoskeletal system, as well as other body systems that include digestion, elimination, and breathing. A dental hygienist who consistently jeopardizes his or her posture may often experience inexplicable fatigue and may be unable to work efficiently or unable to enjoy recreational activities. In fact, the individual eventually may be unable to move normally without experiencing pain. Bad posture can contribute to the majority of neck and back pain experienced by clinicians.

Learning and practicing good posture at work and at play should begin immediately. Regardless of the stage of professional development, whether first-year student or a seasoned practitioner, it is never too early or too late to learn the ergonomic principles that can contribute to a long-lasting, pain-free

Prevention

Proper positioning is critical for the dental hygienist's physical longevity in the practice of dental hygiene.

way to practice with more energy, less stress, and less fatigue. The benefits of good posture may be among the best kept secrets of successful dental hygiene practice!

The practice of dental hygiene requires the operator to perform intricate tasks in a relatively small area with limited visibility. Consequently, the practitioner often assumes that an uncomfortable posture (e.g., leaning forward, dropping the head, rolling the shoulders forward to improve visibility), projecting the arms away from the body, and remaining in a static position for a long time are all necessary to do a good job.

Dental literature first mentions **musculoskeletal disorders** (MSDs) associated with dentistry in the late 1950s and 1960s. However, MSDs related to the practice of dental hygiene were scarcely documented before the early 1980s. Numerous studies over the last 20 years identify MSDs as a common occupational complaint of dental hygienists, even temporarily or permanently compromising the hygienist's ability to work.* These complaints range from neck, shoulder, and back problems to carpal tunnel and thoracic outlet syndromes, all of which affect dental hygiene students, recent graduates, and experienced hygienists. One study on dental students followed dental students for 4 years and found female students experienced greater pain than male students and that the intensity of pain increased as students progressed through the curriculum.[28] Although early recognition of these problems is important, developing postural habits that promote prevention is even better.

---

*References 1, 10, 12, 17, 22, 23, 32.

Developing Musculoskeletal Problems

It appears that Suzanne may be joining the unnecessary and unfortunate silent exodus of dental hygienists who love what they do but hurt so badly that they are willing to give up their professional careers and move into another. What a horrific and preventable scenario! Suzanne and similar colleagues are experiencing a condition that goes by several names that are used synonymously: *cumulative trauma disorder* (CTD), **repetitive strain injury** (RSI), and **work-related musculoskeletal disorder** (WMSD).

The situation described in Case Study 8-1 occurred often before extensive knowledge of ergonomics, RSIs, and CTDs was widely known by those in the dental hygiene profession; however, disorders still develop when practitioners compromise themselves while providing patient care. This case also illustrates another common problem in Suzanne's and her employer's failure to recognize immediately the consequences of a poorly designed workspace. Perhaps, too, like many healthy and fit young people, Suzanne held the common belief that she knew what was acceptable for her own body and that somehow *her* body was immune to musculoskeletal problems.

Musculoskeletal Problems

DEFINITIONS

RSIs are defined as follows[18]:

. . . cumulative trauma disorders resulting from prolonged repetitive, forceful, or awkward movements. These movements result in damage to the muscles, tendons, and nerves. RSI[s] are referred to as repetitive stress injuries, CTDs, repetitive motion disorders, occupational overuse injuries, and [WMSDs].

The dental professional is at risk for developing RSIs for the following three reasons:

- Repetition of tasks performed
- Awkward postures during work
- High force needed to perform a task (high workforce)[36]

Other contributing factors include the following:

- Static or sustained positions
- Insufficient rest breaks
- Vibrations
- High pressures
- Poor tool and workstation design
- Poor-fitting equipment
- Poor worker fitness level

Complaints and injuries do not suddenly appear, nor are they visible conditions that can be outwardly or readily seen. They occur as a result of repetitive (chronic) movements and are noticed only after the nerves and tendons become inflamed and painful.

Note

Whether referred to as RSI, CTD, or WMSD, musculoskeletal pain and problems (especially in the lower back, neck, and shoulder area), carpal tunnel syndrome, and thoracic outlet syndrome are occupational hazards in the dental hygiene profession.*

*References 1, 10, 12, 22, 24.

Box 8-1 briefly describes two common musculoskeletal conditions and their symptoms. (See Treatment and Exercises later in this chapter, which addresses musculoskeletal conditions in greater detail.)

HISTORY OF INJURY PREVALENCE AND PREVENTION GUIDELINES

The **Occupational Safety and Health Administration** (OSHA) establishes guidelines to protect workers. Significant changes have occurred in the clinical dental environment to protect employees from diseases (see Chapter 7).

In 1999, CTD accounted for 34% of all lost workday injuries and illnesses in the United States, with business costs exceeding $15 billion in workers' compensation each year.[23] It is estimated that millions of dollars are lost in income due to CTDs.[24] The lost workdays and the rising costs of workers' compensation resulted in the development of an ergonomic standard for workers in general industry by OSHA. Individual states are also developing their own form of ergonomic standards designed to prevent WMSD. OSHA defines **ergonomics** as follows[23]:

. . . the science of fitting the job to the worker. When there is a mismatch between the physical requirements of the job and the physical capacity of the worker, WMSD can result.

OSHA also recognizes that individuals who repeatedly perform the same tasks, sustain awkward working positions, use a great deal of force, repeatedly lift heavy objects, or have a combination of these risk factors are most likely to develop WMSDs.

OSHA's ergonomics program standard was issued on November 14, 2000, and took effect on January 16, 2001. Congress, acting under the authority of the Congressional Review Act of 1996, filed a joint resolution disapproving OSHA's ergonomic standard. President George W. Bush on March 20, 2001, signed the joint resolution, stating:

The safety and health of our nation's workforce is a priority for my administration. Together we will pursue a comprehensive approach to ergonomics that addresses the concerns surrounding the ergonomics rule repealed today. We will work with the Congress, the business community, and our nation's workers to address this important issue.

This information is available in its entirety at the following web address: http://www.osha-slc.gov.

In a news release issued in April 2004, Secretary of Labor Elaine L. Chao outlined a number of ergonomic principles that urge an approach based on prevention. The principles include or are based on prevention, sound science, incentives, flexibility, feasibility, and clarity. This information also is available at http://www.osha.gov/SLTC/ergonomics.

Note

Although dental hygiene is not specifically identified as a job in the once proposed ergonomic standard, dental hygienists are exposed to five of the six ergonomic risk factors listed in the document.

BOX 8-1

CARPAL TUNNEL SYNDROME AND THORACIC OUTLET SYNDROME

Carpal Tunnel Syndrome

Description: Carpal tunnel syndrome[24] is a form of peripheral neuropathy leading to compression of the median nerve between the forearm flexor muscle tendons and the transverse superficial carpal ligament. This syndrome is more prominent in women and occurs more frequently after 40 years of age.

Symptoms: Pain, numbness, or pins-and-needles sensation in the thumb, index, and middle fingers (may even include ring finger) and on the radial side of the hand may occur. Symptoms may also involve the wrist, forearm, and shoulder. Pain begins slowly and may progress to a constant sensation. The affected individual may state that the pain is usually worse at night and that daily activities are limited because of the increased weakness or clumsiness or both of the involved hand.

Causes: The syndrome can result from compression or vascular insufficiency of the median nerve at the carpal tunnel. Possible causes for the compression or vascular insufficiency include cumulative trauma, overuse injury, and physiologic disorders or structural changes. In dentistry, it may result from flexion or overextension of the wrist. Systemic conditions that have been associated with carpal tunnel syndrome include thyroid disorders and arthritis.

Thoracic Outlet Syndrome

Description: Thoracic outlet syndrome is a combination of symptoms marked with paresthesias and pain that slowly appear in the shoulder, neck, arm, or hand and extend to the anterior portion of the chest wall. Onset occurs between 35 and 55 years of age and is observed more frequently in women.

Symptoms: The affected individual may experience fatigue after overhead arm activities, pins-and-needles sensation in the affected arm, and muscle spasms in the shoulder and neck areas.

Causes: Cause is undetermined but may be compression of the brachial plexus, axillary artery, and subclavian vessels. In dentistry, thoracic outlet syndrome can be a result of dropping the head too far forward (forward flexion) and rounding (slumping) of the shoulders or working with the arms above the waist level or both.

Examples of musculoskeletal disorders, according to OSHA, are injuries or disorders to nerves, ligaments, muscles, tendons, joints, cartilage, and spinal discs.

Because of the increased awareness and diagnosis of these conditions, the terms *ergonomics, RSI, CTD, WMSD, carpal tunnel syndrome,* and **thoracic outlet syndrome** are now common in the dental literature.

ADDITIONAL CONSIDERATIONS

Although dental hygiene programs provide fundamental instructions for students regarding proper **operator positioning** and **patient positioning,** many do not offer additional information on ergonomics.[3] Frequently, practitioners and faculty members have engrained practice habits that are not in keeping with good ergonomic practice and, when focusing on patient needs, revert to old habits. The emphasis on good ergonomic practice taught early in the students' preclinical education often gets lost once students begin to focus on meeting the needs of real patients. True ergonomic practice for students, educators, and practitioners seems to be neglected in concern for the patient. Attention to and awareness of new approaches in instrumentation techniques, new technology, and positioning associated with such techniques and technology is needed to reduce stress and fatigue. Interestingly, the dental hygienist, whose mission it is to prevent one disease, may inadvertently cause another disease by failing to practice prevention in his or her own life!

Each person has a different body structure and a unique threshold to various activities and tasks. Furthermore, systemic diseases, such as diabetes, may mimic or contribute to RSI.[13] Practitioners should be aware of the signs and symptoms common to RSI; if they begin to experience any of them, then they should seek diagnosis and care as soon as possible to prevent further injury. Although information is available in the medical and dental literature and on the Internet, the prudent practitioner will seek diagnosis and subsequent treatment from the appropriate healthcare professional rather than gambling on losing the ability to practice. The following sections describe normal anatomy—changes that can occur as a result of improper operator, patient, and equipment positioning; and appropriate operator, patient, and equipment positioning. Dental hygiene students should develop and maintain these good postural habits early in their clinical education.

Normal Anatomy and Anatomical Changes

An understanding of the musculoskeletal prevention of the RSI of the neck and back that most often affects dental hygienists requires familiarity with the anatomy of the area. The spine is a dynamic structure made up of many small units. It is not a static structure designed to be a simple rigid post; rather, it is designed to move. Joints between each of the 25 vertebrae make up the moveable segments of the spine. These joints have similar characteristics to other **synovial joints** throughout the body and must be treated as such. Each vertebra stacks on top of another with an intervertebral disc found between the bodies of adjacent vertebrae. The spine, when in proper static alignment, has three normal curves. In the cervical and lumbar regions, the normal orientation of the curves is called **lordosis.** This means that the convex side of the curve is anterior, whereas the concave side of the curve is posterior. In the thoracic region the curve is oriented exactly opposite of the cervical and lumbar curves and is referred to as **kyphosis**

(Figures 8-1 and 8-2). The most common postural abnormalities found at the spine involve decreases in cervical and lumbar lordosis and increases in the thoracic kyphosis, or, in common terms, *slouching* (Figure 8-3). Positioning of the spine that maintains the normal curves, called **neutral position,** creates little stress on soft tissues and joints. However, when the normal curves are lost, either through increase or decrease in the curves, the soft tissues (e.g., muscles, **ligaments**) have more stress applied to them. Too much stress continually applied to these soft tissues may result in painful RSI.

The intervertebral discs are similar to a jelly donut (Figure 8-4). The *gelatinous* center is the **nucleus pulposus,** and the outer layer is the **annulus fibrosus.** These discs are designed to rest between the vertebral bodies of adjacent vertebrae with the spine in its normal alignment. If the curves of the spine are changed significantly, then one side of the disc will be compressed and the other side will be stretched (Figure 8-5). If these forces are placed on the disc for long periods, then eventually the disc can become damaged. Although many different classifications of disc injury exist, in general a torn or stretched annulus can allow the nucleus pulposus to move out and compress a spinal nerve root (Figure 8-6). This **herniated** (or **slipped**) **disc** can cause radiating pain into the person's arm or leg.

Pain can originate from various soft tissues in the spine. These include ligaments, muscles, intervertebral discs, and the spinal **facet joint** itself. Identifying the cause of the pain is more important than the tissue from which the pain originates.[6] The two most common nontraumatic causes of pain originating from the spine are the following:

1. Significant limitation of movement of the joints, as found with immobilization
2. Abnormal stressing of the structures in and around the spine through overuse in an abnormal pattern[14,15]

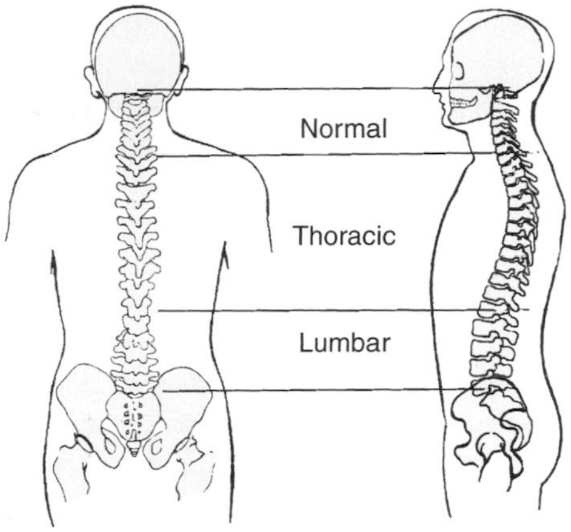

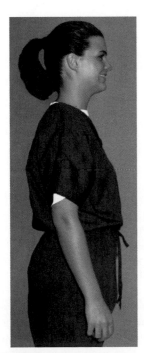

FIGURE 8-1
Skeletal view of spine.

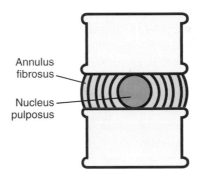

FIGURE 8-4
Vertebral disc.

FIGURE 8-2
View of standing posture.

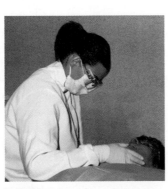

FIGURE 8-3
Operator slouching chairside.

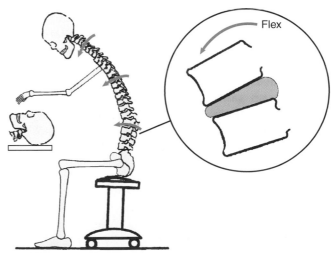

FIGURE 8-5
Anteriorly compressed disc with posterior stretch.

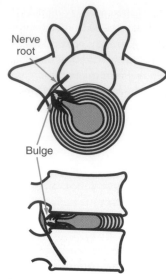

FIGURE 8-6
Bulging, compressed disc.

The dental hygienist must understand the cause of pain to prevent or, if injury occurs, treat the problem.

The first and simplest cause of pain can be from tissue that is of normal length but is maintained in a stretched position for a significant period. *Immobilization* is caused by poor posture. For example, stretching the finger into extreme extension and holding it (Figure 8-7) may not hurt immediately, but if that position or *posture* is maintained long enough, then pain will occur. In the McKenzie system of classifications, this extreme extension is referred to as a **postural syndrome.**[14] Slouching forward over a table reading or writing, an almost daily occurrence for most people, eventually results in pain or discomfort in the neck and back (Figure 8-8). Preventing pain of this origin involves simply sitting with the back in the neutral position. When working for extended periods, periodically stretching backward may also be helpful. (See Treatment and Exercises later in this chapter, which covers treatment for postural syndrome in greater detail.)

> ### Prevention
> A dental hygienist who maintains poor posture at work and at home may develop mobility problems.

The postural syndrome may progress in severity. Complete immobilization, such as that occurring to an extremity that has been placed in a cast, can lead to adaptive shortening of tissues. The tissue does not cause pain when it is left in its shortened state; however, stretching this shortened tissue will cause pain.

Poor posture results in tissues around the spine becoming shortened and tight. When the individual then attempts movements that stretch the tight structures, as found with an attempt to return to a more normal posture, pain results. In the McKenzie system of classifications, this is referred to as a

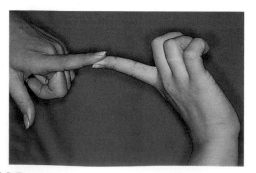

FIGURE 8-7
Finger stretched into extreme extension.

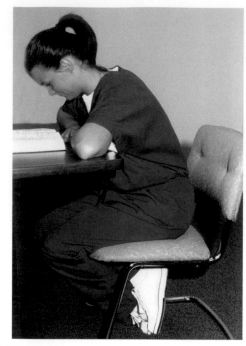

FIGURE 8-8
Student slouched while reading.

dysfunction syndrome.[14] Individuals with dysfunction syndrome experience pain when attempts are made to return to normal posture, making the individual less likely to correct poor postures. This vicious circle makes this problem difficult to treat.

When poor posture becomes typical for an individual, the normal mechanics of the spine become affected. Ligaments and joint capsules are stretched, and muscles have to work overtime to attempt to overcome the poor posture. All these effects may lead to RSI and pain. At this point, medical intervention is often necessary to improve the condition, which results in missed time from work and money spent for medical treatment.

If left untreated, a dysfunction syndrome can progress to a more severe state, known as a *derangement syndrome.*[17] Actual tearing of tissues can occur in this syndrome. For example, the annulus fibrosus tears, allowing the nucleus pulposus to press against a spinal nerve root. This stage requires medical intervention and may produce chronic effects.

> ### Note
> As a prevention specialist, the dental hygienist should make every effort to learn and practice protective posture to avoid injury in the first place.

The progressively severe and degenerative continuum from postural to dysfunction to derangement syndromes makes treatment difficult. Early recognition and treatment can prevent progression to the next step in the continuum.

Positioning

8-3

Maximizing efforts to maintain proper operator, patient, and equipment positions reduces the risks for musculoskeletal problems. Good postural habits help prevent these postural syndromes. However, dental hygiene students and even experienced practitioners strive to achieve optimal access to the oral cavity by frequently assuming awkward positions, such as twisting, bending, or leaning over the patient. Fortunately, faculty members and clinical instructors may correct students' improper postural positions. Conversely, practitioners' posture habits are usually unobserved. One pilot study supports the concept that graduates do not practice what is taught. Fewer than one half of the respondents practice the principles of proper body mechanics as taught during their clinical education, and 63% of the reported pain is attributed to dental hygiene practice.[9]

Breaking bad habits requires approximately 21 days of conscientious effort; therefore, learning and practicing techniques correctly the first time is more efficient and less stressful.[25]

Performance logic positioning (PLP) places the operator's spine in a neutral position, resulting in better posture and less fatigue to the operator. The use of magnification loupes has been shown to improve visibility and posture.[5,7] Changing the way in which operator positioning has been taught is one strategy for addressing the WMSD associated with clinical dental hygiene.[35] To encourage the development of good posture and proper techniques while performing clinical dental hygiene, PLP combined with the use of magnification loupes can provide the ideal combination for obtaining and maintaining appropriate posture during clinical procedures. The evidence suggests that PLP can reduce WMSD; therefore this positioning technique is presented first, followed by other positioning techniques.

OPERATOR CHAIR

An understanding of any operator position requires having a well-designed operator chair. Ideally, the operator's chair should have an adjustable backrest, lumbar support, a reasonable and easily adjustable height range, and a five-wheeled, high-quality base.[25,27] Adjustable armrests are also recommended.[21,25]

Dentists probably use adjustable armrests more than do dental hygienists (Figure 8-9). However, dental hygienists must consider the benefits of armrests in the reduction of muscle fatigue. The main benefit of an operator armrest is in the increased operator arm stability and the reduction of muscle activity in the upper trapezius (i.e., muscle between the neck and shoulder). This muscle helps suspend the shoulder girdle to the trunk and is typically irritated with postural syndromes. When properly used, forearm rests can reduce up to 12% of body weight stress on the spine.[27] Reducing the strain essentially reduces the cumulative fatigue currently experienced by dental hygienists. In addition to the operator chair armrests, one researcher recently devised a horseshoe-shaped cushion that is adapted to the patient's headrest.[27] This cushion provides additional support to the operator's wrist and forearm, thus decreasing the strain placed on these areas.

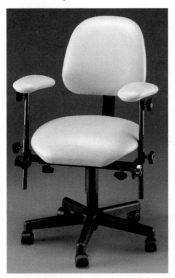

FIGURE 8-9
Chair with armrests.

CASE APPLICATION 8-1.2

Proper Operator Positioning
In the case study, Suzanne began using the front-office secretarial chair rather than a properly designed operator chair. Using this chair caused her to develop poor postural habits to access areas within the oral cavity.

A reference point for describing operator positioning while working on a patient is to consider locations on the patient's head as a clock face with the chin representing 6 o'clock, the top of the head 12 o'clock, the right ear 9 o'clock, the left ear 3 o'clock, and so on. The operator positioning technique the hygienist uses will be associated with hours or zones on the clock. Using this guide, the operator's working positions for operator positioning techniques can be described.

PERFORMANCE LOGIC POSITIONING
Operator
The PLP uses **proprioceptive** self-derivation of balanced reference posture to determine the operator's chair height, optimal posture, and position described in Boxes 8-2 and 8-3.

The performance logic (PL) concept developed by Dr. Daryl Beach consists of the following basic beliefs[8]:
- Each individual has the "innate capability to self-determine an optimal posture and position for the perception and control of fine motor activity."
- This optimal position can be readily reproduced.
- This self-determined posture and position is basically the same for each person performing similar tasks.

To determine the correct height of the operator chair, the head of the fibula on the side of the leg should be located (Figure 8-10). The correct position can be found by placing a hand on the side of the knee and feeling for the junction between the head of the fibula and the lateral femoral condyle. The head of the fibula is at this joint line. The height of the seat should be adjusted to ensure that the top of the seat cushion is level with the top of the head of the fibula or no lower than the middle of the fibula. Thighs will have a slightly downward incline rather than being parallel with the floor.

According to one source, PL[29]:

. . . allows an individual to logically derive the most natural method for the practice of dentistry. Following the principles of [PL], one can use

BOX 8-2

PROPRIOCEPTIVE SELF-DERIVATION METHOD OF BALANCED REFERENCE POSTURE

This exercise may be conducted in the following two ways:
1. Students work individually as the instructor reads the protocol to the class.
2. Students work in pairs and read the protocol to each other as they progress through the exercise.
   Equipment needed: Adjustable operator stool

Protocol

1. Set the *seat* of the stool at the *lowest* possible position.
2. Sit on the stool with *buttocks well supported* and *feet flat on the floor.* Let *arms hang freely* at the *sides,* except when adjusting the stool height. Keep *eyes closed* throughout the exercise and concentrate on how the *body feels.*
3. Gradually *raise the stool* and continue to raise and lower the stool until the height that feels the most stable and comfortable is reached. Readjust if necessary after a few seconds until the best height is attained. If the stool is impinging on the thighs, then sliding forward on the stool may be desired. Readjust the height again, if necessary. Now the *optimal seating height* is obtained.
4. Remember to allow the *arms* to *hang loosely at the sides* and to *keep the eyes closed.*
5. Take several deep breaths and *relax.* Try to be completely at ease.
6. Move the upper body forward and backward, lean to each side, twist if desired, and sense the many options available for upper body positioning. Finally, decide on the preferred *position* of the *upper body* to self-maintain a stable, comfortable, and natural upper body posture. Once the preferred position has been found, assume and maintain that position.
7. Now, follow the same steps with the head and decide on the preferred *position* of the *head* to self-maintain a stable, comfortable, and natural head position. Once the preferred position has been found, assume and maintain that head position.
8. Become *proprioceptively aware* of the *body posture selected to this point.* If possible, choose to sit in this manner as tasks are performed. Choosing to alter this *stable, comfortable, and natural posture* would be unlikely.

9. Think of the *thumb and index finger* of each hand. With the arms hanging loosely at the sides, *touch* the thumb and index finger together.
10. Making every effort not to alter the posture that has been established and keeping the eyes closed, *bring the thumbs and index fingers* of the two hands *together* at a point in front; that is, the preferred position to thread a needle. At this time, this position cannot be seen. Once this point has been found, assume and maintain it.
11. Without moving the head or hands, *open the eyes* and try to see the point at which the two index fingers make contact. At this time, the quality of the image seen should not be a concern, only whether the point can be seen. If the needle can be theoretically threaded, then maintain this position.
12. If this point cannot be seen or if it can be seen with only great and unacceptable discomfort, then consider whether another preferred position should be assumed to make it possible to see the point or to see the point with reasonable comfort. If *tilting the head* slightly downward is preferred, then do so until the point of index finger contact can be seen. If *moving the hands* and relocating the point of index finger contact is preferred, then do so until the point can be seen. If the preference is to *do both,* then do so. Once the option has been selected, maintain this position.
13. The point at which the needle can be threaded is called the *optimal control point.*
14. Once the *natural proprioceptive inclinations* have been satisfied, visual acuity problems may then improve with the use of corrective eyewear.

Alternative Method to Determine Seat Height

The following method is not as accurate as steps 1 through 3 of the previous list, but it is an acceptable alternative:
1. Identify the *head of the fibula* on the side of the lower leg. It is the uppermost bone of the lower leg, located approximately at the level of the lower half of the kneecap.
2. Set the height of the *seat* of the operator stool to the level of the midpoint of the head of the fibula.

From Schoen DH, Dean MC: *Contemporary periodontal instrumentation,* Philadelphia, 1996, WB Saunders.

BOX 8-3

CHARACTERISTICS OF BALANCED REFERENCE POSTURE

1. Position head in the least strained position vertically and horizontally.
2. Shoulders should feel loose, hanging free vertically.
3. Upper *arms* should feel loose, hanging free vertically.
4. Lower *arms* in the least strained position vertically and horizontally, in line with the palms.
5. Wrists should be neither flexed nor extended.
6. Position hands near the level of the apex of the heart, palms vertical, fingers relaxed and flexed, and index fingers near the median plane.

7. Hold back straight and erect.
8. Buttocks weight should be evenly distributed.
9. Position thighs clear and free of distracting contacts, separated and unstrained, front of thighs sloping downward from trunk to knees.
10. Legs should be clear and free of distracting contacts.
11. Position feet clear and free of distracting contacts.

From Schoen DH, Dean MC: *Contemporary periodontal instrumentation,* Philadelphia, 1996, WB Saunders.

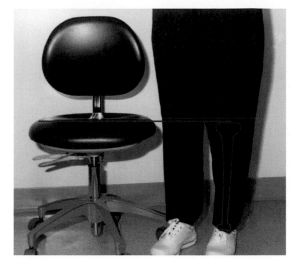

FIGURE 8-10
Determining operator chair height.

proprioceptive self-awareness to determine the most effective, stress-free process for performing dental procedures; design an optimal human-centered setting for dental practice; provide the highest quality of oral care; and increase productivity and profitability.

Furthermore, the World Health Organization (WHO) cited the importance of PL and stated the following[29]:

. . . oral health can be improved and the cost of equipment reduced if the workplaces are designed to ensure optimum performance . . . the [PL] approach may be considered as a pointer to the future.

The PL concept is relatively new in dental hygiene education. The benefits and limitations of the implementation of PL were studied among students at Vancouver Community College.[34] According to the report:

. . . participants indicated the greatest benefits were increased operator comfort and performance and decreased operator fatigue, muscle strain, and back/neck/shoulder discomfort.

Improved time management, instrument accessibility and control, enhanced intraoral fulcrums, increased patient comfort, less frequent headaches, and augmented indirect vision skills were other reported benefits. Both students and faculty members agreed on the major benefits derived from the PL approach. When asked to compare traditional operator and patient positioning with the PL approach, experienced clinicians indicated that PL "definitely" improves the ideal alignment of forces during stroke activation and decreases operator strain and fatigue. No discernible differences occurred between faculty and student responses, although faculty members provided more detailed information. Limitations were largely focused on equipment features and the patients' acceptance of the **supine position.** (Box 8-4 lists the benefits of using PLP.)

In PLP, the operator works within the range of a 10 o'clock to a 12:30 position for the right-handed operator or a 2 o'clock to an 11:30 position for the left-handed operator.[30] In Table 8-1, PL operator positions have been translated into the clock positions traditionally used by clinicians.

Using PLP can maintain the wrist in a neutral position. Long-term research is needed to determine whether PLP eliminates or reduces the musculoskeletal complaints repeatedly experienced and documented by dental hygienists.

Patient

Patients are placed in the supine position with the top of the head at the upper edge of the headrest. With PLP the operator position determines the optimal control point; the patient's mouth is at the height of the optimal control point. This point is between waist and heart level; thus the operator's hands and elbows form an angle of slightly less than 90 degrees.

To access certain areas of the mouth and with the patient in a supine position, the patient must move his or her head as requested by the operator:

* Positioned straight up
* Turned slightly to the right
* Turned further to the right (far right) almost on the ear
* Turned slightly to the left
* Turned further to the left (far left) almost on the ear

The patient's maxillary plane should parallel the upper body of the operator. Rucker and Boyd suggest that the relationship of the maxilla to the operator's body posture is usually parallel to the operator's spine.[29] These authorities further state that this relationship remains the same regardless of where the operator is sitting or the site of treatment and suggest that operators use the maxilla as a gauge to control posture. However, they also state the following:

. . . conscientious control of the patient's maxillary plane does not guarantee good postural balance for the operator, but lack of control of the patient's maxillary plane is certain to cause poor postures.

Enhancing Visibility
Magnification

Two ways to increase visibility are to move closer to the object or to magnify it. Without magnification, students and practitioners typically bend forward to "see well." As previously discussed, bending forward is an improper posture; therefore magnification is the best option. The use of **eye loupes** (for magnification) in dentistry has gradually increased. Common use of eye loupes for dental hygienists is likely to follow. A

BOX 8-4

REPORTED BENEFITS OF USING PERFORMANCE LOGIC POSITIONING

* Increased operator comfort and performance
* Decreased fatigue; muscle strain; back, neck, and shoulder discomfort
* Improved time management
* Increased accessibility and control
* Enhanced intraoral fulcrum
* Increased patient comfort
* Less frequent headaches
* Augmented indirect vision skills

Table 8-1	Proprioceptive and Self-Derivation–Based Performance Logic Instrumentation Positions for Operator and Patient Equated to Clock Positions	

AREA	OPERATOR POSITIONING	PATIENT'S HEAD POSITION*
Right-Handed Operator		
Maxillary right facial	10 o'clock	Straight to slightly to patient's left
Maxillary anterior facial	11 to 12 o'clock	Slightly to patient's right[†]
Maxillary left facial	11 to 12 o'clock	Slightly to patient's right to far right
Maxillary right lingual	11 o'clock	Far right
Maxillary anterior lingual	11 to 12 o'clock	Slightly to patient's right[†]
Maxillary left lingual	12 o'clock	Slightly to patient's right to far right
Mandibular left facial	11 o'clock	Far right
Mandibular anterior facial	12 o'clock	Straight to slightly to patient's right[†]
Mandibular right facial	10 o'clock[‡]	Slightly to patient's left
Mandibular left lingual	10 o'clock	Slightly to patient's left
Mandibular anterior lingual	12 o'clock	Slightly to patient's right[†]
Mandibular right lingual	12 o'clock	Far right
Left-Handed Operator		
Maxillary right facial	1 to 2 o'clock	Slightly to patient's left
Maxillary anterior facial	1 to 2 o'clock	Slightly to patient's left[†]
Maxillary left facial	2 o'clock	Straight to slightly to patient's right
Maxillary right lingual	12 o'clock	Slightly to patient's left to far left
Maxillary anterior lingual	1 o'clock	Far left[†]
Maxillary left lingual	1 to 2 o'clock	Far left (toward operator)
Mandibular left facial	Approximately 1 to 2 o'clock	Slightly to patient's right (toward operator)
Mandibular anterior facial	12 o'clock	Straight to slightly to patient's right (toward operator)[†]
Mandibular right facial	1 o'clock	Far left
Mandibular left lingual	11 to 12 o'clock	Far left
Mandibular anterior lingual	12 o'clock	Slightly to patient's left
Mandibular right lingual	1 to 2 o'clock	Slightly to patient's left

*Patient positioned supine for maxillary and mandibular arches for left- and right-handed operator.
[†]Operator may ask patient to move the head toward and away from operator as operator moves from canine to canine.
[‡]Clock position changed from that depicted in Schoen and Dean's *Instrumentation* text,[30] which demonstrates the position at approximately 12 o'clock, with patient's head slightly to the right. At this position, reaching the area is extremely difficult.

leading manufacturer of magnification systems estimates that 15% to 20% of the dental hygiene programs have already begun requiring the purchase of eye loupes for clinical practice.[2]

Two types of magnification systems are used in dentistry: (1) single-lens and (2) multilens.[11] For clinical use, the single-lens magnifier system is probably not the best choice in the selection of a magnification system for clinical practice. The single-lens produces **diopter magnification,** which restricts the operator's working distance to a set length. With this restricted working distance, maintaining focus is difficult because the operator has limited range and opportunity for movement. This places the operator in a restricted position and posture, which could increase poor posture and back and neck pain.

The multilens (**telescopic loupes**) is the better choice for magnification. These loupes improve posture and optical performance. The models currently available use Galilean optics, which are preferred in dentistry because of the relatively wide-field depth that is maintained as the magnification increases. In dentistry, a magnification power of 2× to 3.5× is recommended.[29] Strassler states that a periodontist may use a 2× to

2.5× magnification power; general dentists and dental hygienists may use 2× for scaling and root-planing procedures.[33] In the previously mentioned study by Sunell and Maschak completed at Vancouver Community College, the dental hygiene faculty and students used 2.5× magnification.[34] The range for dental hygienists would appear to be 2× or 2.5×. These power levels offer a greater field depth than those needed by oral surgeons and endodontists[31] (Figure 8-11).

A learning curve is required for the operator to become confident and comfortable using eye loupes. In addition, an accurate measurement of the operator's working distance must be determined before selecting the proper magnification power. When the operator requires prescriptive lenses, the same prescription must be added to the magnification system. One study reported 81% of the dental hygiene students became comfortable with magnification 2.6× within 1 to 2 days. In addition, 95% of the students indicated their vision was clearer; the vast majority reported improved clinical performance and all reported improved posture.[5] To further illustrate the benefits of eye loupes, the Vancouver study, which used the PL

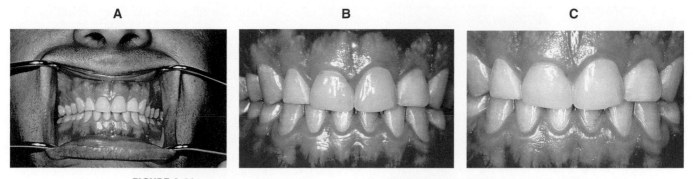

FIGURE 8-11
A, Normal view, no magnification. **B,** Magnification 2×. **C,** Magnification 2.5×.

approach to positioning, also incorporated the use of eye loupes into its program.[34] Participating faculty members and students reported a decrease in neck, back, and shoulder complaints; an increase in visual acuity; reduced eye strain; and minimal need for exaggerated forward head flexion. An additional benefit to the eye loupes was demonstrated in radiographic interpretation. Cost, the time involved in learning to adapt, and the inability to view the patient's facial expressions easily were identified as drawbacks to their use.

Eyestrain can be a concern for dental hygienists. Additional illumination is available on loupes, enhancing visibility even more than with magnification alone (Figure 8-12). Overall, the use of eye loupes improves posture by eliminating the need to bend closer (Figure 8-13).

Dental light

Proper lighting is a critical component in patient care. Although the use of **fiber optics** in dentistry has produced advances, its use in dental hygiene is limited. The overhead light remains indispensable, and proper placement is necessary to allow the hygienist to maintain an ergonomically correct position. Two primary dental lighting systems are available:

1. Light fixed in a ceiling-mounted track
2. Dental light attached to a pole connected to the patient's chair

In PLP the dental light is seldom readjusted once it has been positioned. After the patient has been seated in the supine position, the dental light is positioned to direct the beam down onto the patient's mouth. When the patient's head is straight and the mouth is open, the mouth will be illuminated. As with access to all areas of the patient's mouth, the patient must be directed to turn his or her head to enable the light to be on the working area. Asking the patient to turn the head will ensure that the working area is illuminated with only minor adjustments.

TRADITIONAL POSITIONING

Operator

The simplest method used to determine the correct height of the operator chair is for the operator to sit with the feet flat on the floor and elevate or lower the chair seat until the thigh is either parallel to the floor or until the hips are slightly higher than the knees. At the correct height the operator should be able to sit tall in the chair with legs separated, thighs parallel to the floor, and feet flat on the floor. The operator's back should be against the chair back so that the lumbar region (small of back) is supported (Figure 8-14). Operators should be properly seated in the chair before attempting to position themselves or their patients correctly.

The operator's eyes should be approximately 14 to 16 inches from the patient's oral cavity.[20] The shoulders should be relaxed and not elevated. To help maintain the shoulders at the

> *Note*
> Incorrect determination of the height of the operator's chair may adversely affect other aspects of erect positioning.

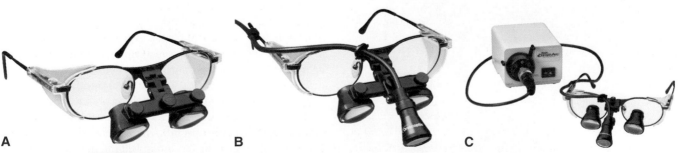

FIGURE 8-12
A, HiRes loupes (flip-up). **B,** HiRes loupe with a Zeon LumenArc light source. **C,** Light transformer unit, HiRes loupes (through the lens). (Courtesy Orascoptic, Middleton, Wisc.)

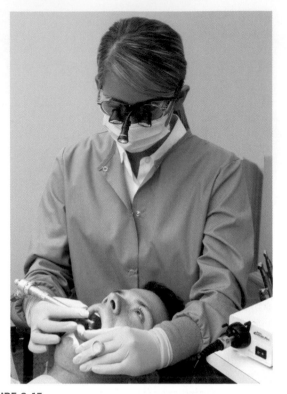

FIGURE 8-13
Hygienist working with HiRes loupes and a Zeon LumenArc light. (Courtesy Orascoptic, Middleton, Wisc.)

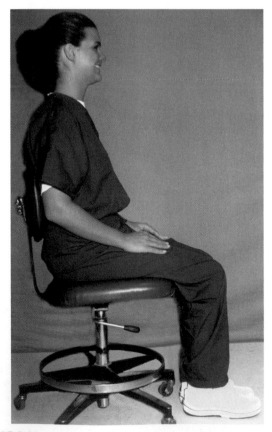

FIGURE 8-14
Correct sitting posture.

appropriate height, the elbows should be approximately even with the occlusal plane and held close to the body. Ideally, the operator's hands should be kept level with the elbows.[33]

Raised shoulder and arm postures contribute to neck and shoulder complaints. To illustrate this point, readers should lift their shoulders as they raise their elbows to shoulder height and hold that position as the next section is read. Readers will begin to experience neck and shoulder fatigue or strain after a short time. Keeping the shoulders up or elbows out or elevated during all-day treatment of patients will eventually contribute to damaging neck and shoulder strain. Again, once the clinician is focused on patient needs, ignoring the signals that the body is sending is easy.

Patient

Dental hygienists should remember that the patient's head is moveable. Although practicing hygienists typically work 8 hours each day, a patient is usually in the dental chair for only 1 to 1½ hours and certainly not every day. Therefore hygienists should place the patient in the correct position and request that the patient move his or her head accordingly, rather than constantly assume awkward positions to avoid inconveniencing the patient.

After the operator is correctly seated in the operator chair, the patient should be positioned. In the traditional working position, the patient is placed in a supine position, with the dental chair back nearly parallel to the floor. In the supine position, the patient's feet and head are on the same plane. The chair back, however, may be raised approximately 20 degrees (**semisupine position**) to accommodate medically compromised patients. With the traditional working position, the semisupine position may be used to treat the mandibular arch.[20] The height of the patient's chair off the floor should be determined by the height of the operator's elbows.[19] To test the proper chair height, the operator folds the arms across the waist. The tip of the patient's nose should be lower than the operator's elbow level position (Figure 8-15).

Dental Light

In traditional positioning, the dental light is readjusted for visibility in the maxillary and mandibular arches. When the dental hygienist is working in the mandibular arch, the patient is in a semisupine position and the light is directly above the patient's head, with the beam directed downward into the oral cavity. For the hygienist to view the maxillary arch, the light should be directly above the patient's chest, with the beam directed into the patient's oral cavity on an angle (tilted slightly upward). To maximize illumination, the light should always be at arm's length (approximately 36 inches). Positioning the light closer lessens the illumination.

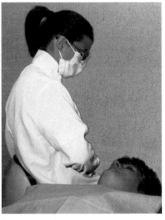

FIGURE 8-15
Test for correct patient chair height.

ALTERNATIVE WORKING POSITIONS

Authorities recommended that the operator should maintain the *neutral position* throughout daily activities for optimal musculoskeletal health.[20] In the neutral position an appendage is not moved away or directed toward the body's midline, including no turning or twisting (Box 8-5). To help maintain this neutral position, the operator is encouraged to imagine a steel pole connecting the hips (pole parallel to floor) with each end bolted to the chair.[20] This position limits or restricts the operator from twisting and helps maintain the pelvic movement forward and backward. Using the PLP assists the hygienist in maintaining the neutral position.

Clinicians also use and recommend the **biocentric technique** of positioning (Box 8-6).* The biocentric technique uses the 7 o'clock, 9 o'clock, and 12 o'clock positions.[16]

OPERATOR POSITIONING DURING INSTRUMENTATION PROCEDURES

The simplest way to maintain protective operator positioning is to remember three simple rules:

1. *Keep the spine in the neutral position.* Periodically, the clinician should consciously take a posture check. If he or she is out of neutral, then the cause should be determined. Is it due to patient body or head position? Where is the operator in relation to the area of instrumentation? Did the operator simply get lazy and revert to old poor postural habits? Once identified, every effort should be made to correct the cause and return the posture to the neutral position.

2. *Face the area of instrumentation.* Facing the operator's work is accomplished by ensuring that the body is in neutral posture and that the operator's buttocks, chest, and head are parallel to the area of instrumentation without any twisting or bending of the body away from the neutral position. Facing the operator's work may require changing the position of the operator stool or having the patient turn his or her head until parallelism is reached.

3. *Keep shoulders down.* The operator should make certain that the shoulders are relaxed and down. As clinicians become engrossed in their work, stress tends to cause them to lift one or both shoulders in the air. The stress that this movement causes to the muscles and ligaments may not be evident until significant pain ensues. During the deliberate posture check, the clinician should locate where his or her shoulders are—in case they are somewhere between where they should be and close to the ears—and relax them before they protest via pain and headaches!

---

*References 4, 8, 16, 30, 34.

Positioning for Powered Instrumentation

These three simple rules for instrumentation can certainly be applied to powered or manual instrumentation with equal success; however, some prefer the following alternative method:

When performing powered scaling, the operator should be seated in the operator's chair in the same manner as when performing manual instrumentation—in the 12 o'clock position. When in this position, the top of the patient's head is at the top of the chair, which allows the operator close access to the dentition and face-forward positioning, minimizing strain to the operator's head and neck, similar to the PLP. The water spray from a powered scaling instrument requires the hygienist to use indirect vision in most areas of the mouth. PLP is the most efficient patient and operator positioning when using powered instruments.

Unlike manual scalers, which have single, one-directional cutting edges, any side of the powered instrument insert or tip is capable of removing calculus deposits and plaque biofilm. This feature allows the operator to change positions only once.

- Seated in the 12 o'clock position, sextants 2, 3, 4, and 5 and the palatal aspects of sextant 1 and the lingual aspects of sextant 6 can be reached by asking the patient to turn his or her head to either the left or right.
- Seated from the 11 o'clock to the 9 o'clock position, the facial surfaces of sextants 1 and 6 can be reached and, if it is necessary, additional instrumentation of sextant 3 from the palatal and mandibular anteriors can be accessed.

Using a Hygoformic (Pulpdent Corporation of America, Brookline, Mass.) or a Tipadilly system (Pelton & Crane, Charlotte, N.C.) allows for water control during the procedure.

- Placement of the Hygoformic saliva ejector in the left mandibular vestibule controls water in sextants 2, 3, 4, and 5. With the patient's head turned slightly to the left, the water flows in that direction.
- Placement of the saliva ejector in the right mandibular vestibule controls water while the hygienist is working on the palatal aspects of sextant 1 and the lingual aspects of sextant 6. The patient's head is turned slightly to the right.

This efficient water control requires only one movement of the operator, patient, and saliva ejector.

POSITION OF DENTAL EQUIPMENT

The instrument tray, hand pieces, suction, and air/water syringe should be reasonably accessible and as close to the operator as possible to avoid excessive bending and twisting. Approximately 20 inches is a reasonable working distance for equipment.[25] This distance enhances good posture. Hand piece tubing should be straight, not coiled, and have a smooth outer surface.[26] Straight tubing decreases the force and grasp strength required to pull and detangle the coil. A smooth outer surface is also more easily disinfected.

The dental hygienist profession is constantly looking for new and more ergonomically designed offerings from instrument and equipment companies. Hand pieces are available that do not place undue stress on the muscles of the hand and forearm. The wider base in the ergonomically designed hand piece allows it to rest in the palm of the hand and, thus, be used in a more natural, relaxed position. In addition, the wider base allows the fingers to grip the hand piece with less stress and strain. Similarly, powered instrument inserts and tips are designed to alleviate hand fatigue with a larger diameter and cushioned grip, which rotates easily in the hands and fingers of the clinician, resulting in less fatigue and stress throughout the procedure.

✦ CASE APPLICATION 8-1.3

Inappropriate Operator Chair

The use of the front-office chair as an operator chair and the inaccessibility of the dental equipment were the two contributing factors to Suzanne's musculoskeletal problems.

RECOGNITION OF ERRORS IN POSITIONING

The following section provides five problems and the cues students should be aware of to help recognize incorrect positioning of operator or patient. Identifying corrections to the following situations may help the student more readily recognize the problem:

1. *Problem:* An operator has to move the dental light sideways because a shadow is being cast in the oral cavity.
   Solution: The student's position or the patient's head position should be corrected. Rarely, if ever, is moving the dental light sideways a correct light adjustment.
2. *Problem:* A student knows she is holding the instrument correctly and has the correct working end but finds herself unable to adapt the cutting edge to the surface or activate the working or exploratory stroke.
   Solution: When the student faces this situation, she should stop the procedure and self-assess the positions of both the patient and the operator rather than assume an awkward position.
3. *Problem:* The student operator's body is at 9 o'clock, and the chair back is at 11 o'clock. The operator, intent on his work, moves to a different area of the oral cavity without moving the operator chair and consequently adapts his body to reach the area.
   Solution: The student needs to move the operator chair as he works to maintain proper posture.
4. *Problem:* The student becomes fatigued and begins to slouch in the chair with legs either extended or crossed.
   Solution: When the student realizes this has occurred, she needs to stretch and incorporate the exercises described in the next section, Treatment and Exercises. Slouching in the chair creates an enormous amount of extra force on the shoulder and neck area, thus exacerbating fatigue.
5. *Problem:* The student never truly learns to use the dental mirror for indirect vision. Failure to use indirect vision

results in the student assuming an awkward position to gain visual access and places the operator and patient at unnecessary risk. The operator has compromised posture, and the subsequent poor visibility may result in tissue laceration.

Solution: The student should take every opportunity during the educational process to practice and develop the skills required to master indirect vision. An exercise that may help students develop this skill is to practice tracing an object while looking in a hand mirror. Using a red and blue pencil to trace the object will reveal how closely the student's tracing comes to the original object.

Treatment and Exercises

Good posture is key to good health. To both prevent and treat the common musculoskeletal RSI reported by dental hygienists, good posture habits must be reinforced. Poor posture is actually a bad habit. How can injuries be prevented when the activities of the job potentially require the use of poor posture on a routine basis? Poor posture cannot always be avoided during the practice of dental hygiene. However, dental hygienists should minimize the total time poor posture is maintained.

What postures are good and poor? Generally, good posture includes the head being held back over the shoulders. The shoulders should be back and not rounded forward. When the hands are in use, the elbows should be held as close to the side as possible, for as much of the time as possible. As stated earlier, the dental hygienist should sit squarely on the chair with the lumbar spine in a normal amount of lordosis and touching the backrest of the seat. The thighs should be parallel to the floor, and the feet should be flat on the floor (see Figure 8-14). Too many poor postures exist to name them all, but most involve some degree of forward flexion. In other words, when the hygienist leans forward and down, the head strains forward, the body moves to the edge of the seat, and the lumbar spine slumps. The list could go on forever. The importance of maintaining good, correct posture whenever possible cannot be overstated; but, what does a hygienist do when it is impossible to maintain good posture?

> ### Prevention
> Because poor postures cannot be completely avoided during the practice of dental hygiene, hygienists must do as much as possible in their personal lifestyles to minimize the possibility of developing an RSI.

Hygienists must break up the time spent in a poor posture position that they are forced to endure in their work. For example, if a hygienist is in a poor posture while performing a procedure, then the hygienist can change the poor posture while changing position or reaching for a different instrument (Figure 8-16). Specific postural exercises that can be performed chairside during these short breaks in treatment are described in the next section, Types of Exercises. These postural exercises prevent extended periods of self-imposed immobilization.

The dental hygienist benefits from periodic breaks from patient treatment, but anyone who has been involved in patient

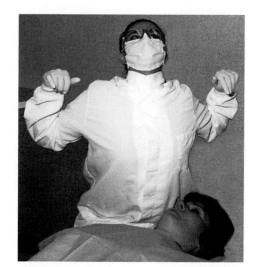

FIGURE 8-16
Operator stretching chairside.

care realizes that breaks are not always possible. However, discontinuing poor posture at chairside is always possible during patient treatment.

Keeping good postures and spinal mobility while not at work, taking part in aerobic and cardiovascular exercise programs, and not smoking helps accomplish good posture and a healthful lifestyle. Limiting activities that are similar to those tasks performed as dental hygienists (e.g., needlework) helps minimize exposure to continual poor posture.

The most important aspect of these lifestyle changes is posture and spinal mobility away from work. While at work, every hygienist is going to have some postural syndrome symptoms as described; therefore they must limit these poor postures while away from work. If they do not, they will progress to the dysfunction syndrome more quickly. Good postures while away from work include maintaining good posture while driving, watching television, reading, and all other activities of daily living (Figure 8-17). Although good posture cannot be maintained all the time, the hygienist does not want poor posture to become typical.

The optimal lifestyle includes sessions three to four times a week for 30 to 60 minutes of continual exercise at a target heart rate of 70%

> ### Prevention
> An exercise program that targets the hygienist's cardiovascular system can be a tremendous help in the prevention of musculoskeletal RSIs.

of individual maximum heart rate. Exercising at a level lower than this is still beneficial; for example, exercising only once a week or at heart rates lower than 70% of an individual's maximum is better than no exercise.

Although the problems associated with the use of tobacco and nicotine are becoming common knowledge, many people may not be aware of the effect of nicotine on the capillary blood supply to the structures of the spine. Nicotine can inhibit blood flow to tissues, altering tissue response to injury—another reason to avoid using tobacco products.

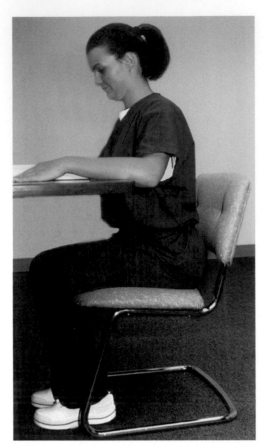

FIGURE 8-17
Student reading with good posture.

TYPES OF EXERCISES

Exercises used to treat and prevent musculoskeletal RSI can be divided into three main groups: (1) postural, (2) stretching, and (3) strengthening. Postural and stretching exercises are by far the most important in the prevention of musculoskeletal RSI.

Postural Exercises

The four main postural exercises are neck retraction, neck extension, shoulder retraction, and low back extension. Attempting to slide the head back over the shoulders without extending the face upward is neck retraction. When performed correctly, the head does not tilt; it simply slides straight back, correcting the forward head posture (Figure 8-18).

Neck extension involves a simple upward look as far as the head can reach (Figure 8-19). Neck retraction must be performed before neck extension is attempted. If neck extension is attempted before the forward head is corrected, the individual ends up with the *turtle* posture in the cervical spine (Figure 8-20). This hyperextension is not healthy for the cervical spine.

Shoulder retraction is performed when the shoulders are brought back and an attempt is made to pinch the shoulder blades together (Figure 8-21). This simple exercise breaks the habit of forward shoulders. A combination of neck retraction and shoulder retraction can be performed when the individual lies supine on the floor with a small towel roll placed at the base of the skull (Figure 8-22). The individual can lie in this position for 10 to 15 minutes and let gravity pull the neck and shoulders into retraction. This combination exercise is good after a long day of patient care.

Low back extension can be accomplished by placement of the hands on the low back, followed by a backward leaning (Figure 8-23); this exercise can be performed standing or sitting. It helps reverse the effects of the forward slumped posture.

These simple postural exercises can be incorporated into daily activities. They can be easily performed chairside during patient care during movement from one position to another or during changing of instruments. Many individuals perform some of these movements periodically throughout the day without even thinking about it. These descriptions allow the hygienist to perform the exercises in the most correct manner possible.

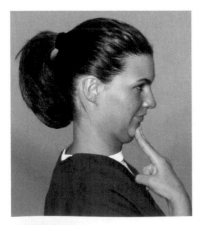

FIGURE 8-18
Neck retraction.

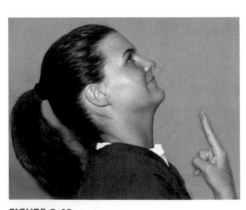

FIGURE 8-19
Neck retraction and extension. Retraction occurs first, followed by extension from a retracted position.

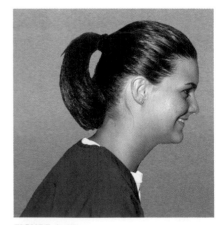

FIGURE 8-20
Turtle posture.

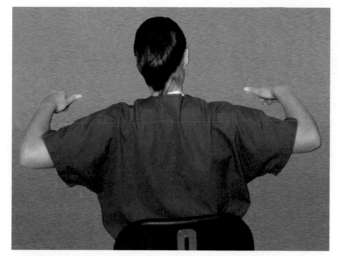

FIGURE 8-21
Shoulders back.

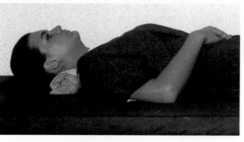

FIGURE 8-22
Operator lying on table with towel roll.

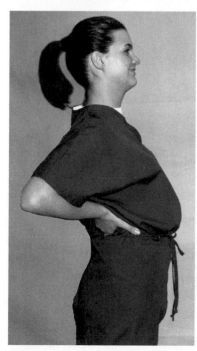

FIGURE 8-23
Operator leaning backward.

Stretching Exercises

With any stretching exercises, all stretches should be performed slowly and held for at least 10 seconds. Stretching when the tissues are warm is ideal, such as after exercise or a hot shower. The neck is the first area to address. It should be stretched into lateral flexion to both sides, rotated to both sides, and stretched into forward flexion (Figure 8-24). The stretching exercises should not cause a lasting increase in symptoms of pain. If stretching causes pain to increase or to become more persistent, the exercise should be discontinued and medical evaluation should be sought.

> *Note*
> Specific stretching exercises should be performed to address muscles that can become tight if poor postures are maintained.

The anterior aspect of the shoulder is the next area to stretch. A corner stretch (Figure 8-25) is the simplest, most effective exercise for this region. The stretch should be felt across the front of the shoulders into the chest. This important exercise helps stretch out muscles that have become tight during the maintenance of a rounded shoulders posture.

Strengthening Exercises

Developing strength in the neck, back, and shoulder musculature does not *automatically* cause better posture. It will, however, help place the individual in a better posture. As previously stated, posture is a habit.

> *Note*
> Developing strength in certain muscles helps an individual develop good postural habits.

Strengthening exercises begin with isometric exercises for the neck, performed by pushing the head into the hands without letting the head move. This movement should be held for a count of five, and five repetitions of each exercise should be performed (Figure 8-26). The next exercise involves extension of the shoulder and retraction of the scapulae. It can be accomplished with resistance from an outside source, such as weights or elastic band (Figure 8-27), or with resistance from the person's body weight (Figure 8-28). In a gym these exercises might be described as *bar pull-downs*, *rowing exercises*, or *shoulder extension*. A key to this exercise involves pinching the shoulder blades together (scapular retraction) as the shoulders are extended. Other shoulder exercises include military press, bench press, and shoulder depression. The lower back can be addressed by exercises that strengthen the abdominal muscles. Sit-ups or crunches (Figure 8-29) accomplish this, but care must be taken with these exercises. The individual performing the exercise should not pull on the neck while performing the exercise. This unnecessarily stresses the neck and makes the exercise less efficient. In addition, the exercise should be performed without the feet being held down by someone or something else. Readers may benefit from joining a gym or fitness center and from receiving instruction in the proper performance of all exercises. A trained professional can help determine appropriate weights and resistance and the number of repetitions to ensure that the exercise program is performed in the safest and most efficient manner possible.

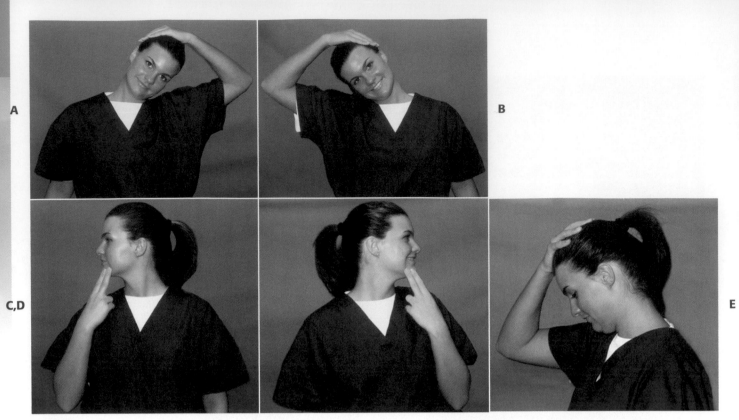

FIGURE 8-24
A, Left lateral flexion. **B,** Right lateral flexion. **C,** Right lateral rotation. **D,** Left lateral rotation. **E,** Forward flexion.

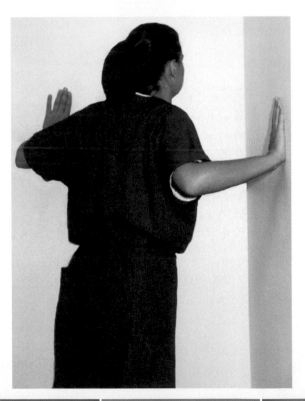

FIGURE 8-25
Corner stretch.

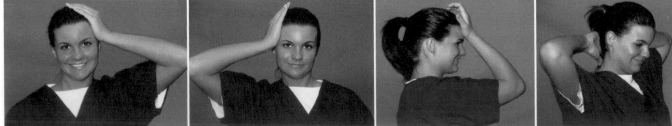

FIGURE 8-26
Isometric exercises.

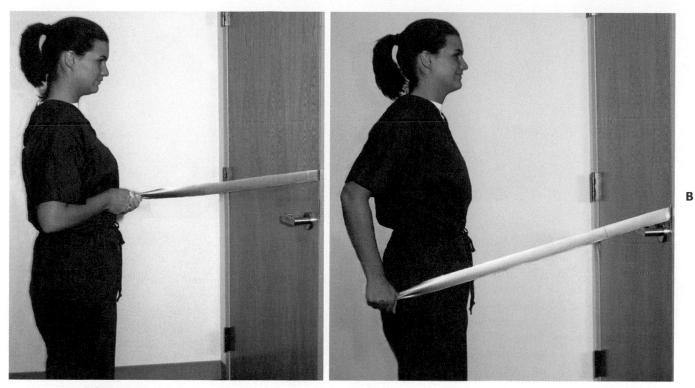

FIGURE 8-27
Clinician pulling elastic band. **A,** Bilateral shoulder extension and scapular retraction. **B,** Single-shoulder extension.

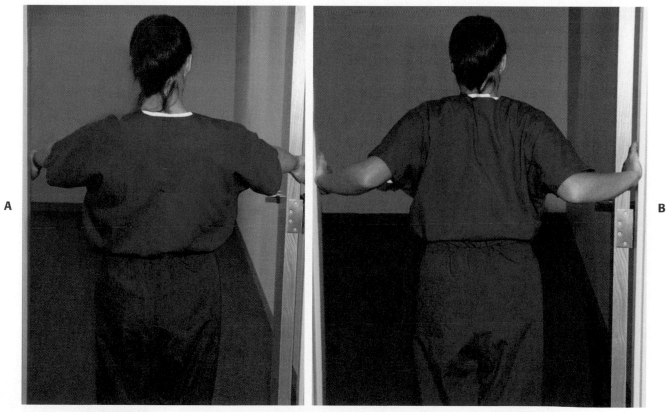

FIGURE 8-28
Clinician pulling in the doorframe. **A,** Beginning position. **B,** Ending position.

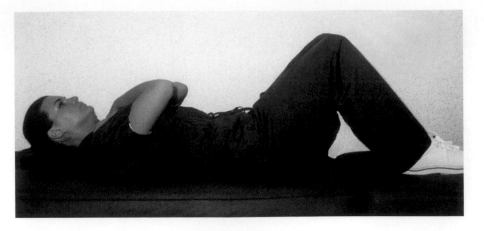

FIGURE 8-29
Clinician performing crunches.

The clinician in the photographs in this chapter is not wearing personal protective equipment to ensure that posture and positioning examples are more easily visualized.

References

1. Barry RM, Woodall WR, Mahan JM: Postural changes in dental hygienists: four year longitudinal study, *J Dent Hyg* 66(3):147-150, 1992.
2. Baudo TV: Personal communication, March 2000, Surgitel Systems.
3. Beach JC, DeBiase CB: Assessment of ergonomic education in dental hygiene curricula, *J Dent Educ* 62(6):421-425, 1998.
4. Belenky MM: Human-centered ergonomics: proprioceptive pathway to occupational health and peak performance in dental practice. In Murphy DC, ed: *Ergonomics and the dental care worker,* Washington, DC, 1998, American Public Health Association.
5. Branson BG et al: Effect of magnification lenses on student operator posture, *J Dent Educ* 68(3):384-389, 2004.
6. Caillet R: *Soft tissue pain and disability,* ed 2, Philadelphia, 1988, FA Davis.
7. Christensen GJ: Magnification in dentistry: useful tool or another gimmick? *J Am Dent Assoc* 134(12):1647-1650, 2004.
8. Colangelo G, Belenky MM: Performance logic: a key to improving dental practice, *J Dent Pract Adm* 7(4):173-177, 1990.
9. Dean MC et al: Back, neck, and shoulder pain: results of a pilot study, *J Dent Educ* 61(2):229, 1997.
10. Gravois S, Stringer RB: Survey of occupational health hazards in dental hygiene, *Dent Hyg* 54:518-523, 1980.
11. Kanca J, Jordan PG: Magnification systems in clinical dentistry, *J Can Dent Assoc* 61(10):851-856, 1995.
12. Macdonald G: Hazards in dental workplace, *Dent Hyg* 61:212-218, 1987.
13. Marxhausen P: *Computer related repetitive strain injuries* [Internet], 2000, http://www.engr.unl.edu.
14. McKenzie R: *The lumbar spine: mechanical diagnosis and treatment,* Waikanae, New Zealand, 1981, Spinal Publications New Zealand.
15. McKenzie R: *Treat your own back,* Waikanae, New Zealand, 1997, Spinal Publications New Zealand.
16. Meador HL: The biocentric technique: a guide to avoiding occupational pain, *J Dent Hyg* 67(1):38-51, 1993.
17. Miller DL: An investigation into attrition of dental hygienists from the work force, *J Dent Hyg* 65:25-31, 1991.
18. Nainzadeh N et al: Repetitive strain injury (cumulative trauma disorder): causes and treatment, *Mt Sinai J Med* 66(3):192-196, 1999.
19. Nield-Gehrig JS, Houseman GA: *Fundamentals of periodontal instrumentation,* ed 3, Baltimore, 1996, Williams & Wilkins.
20. Nunn P: Posture for dental hygiene practice. In Murphy DC, ed: *Ergonomics and the dental care worker,* Washington, DC, 1998, American Public Health Association.
21. Oberg T: Ergonomic evaluation and construction of a reference workplace in dental hygiene: a case study, *J Dent Hyg* 67(5):262-267, 1993.
22. Oberg T, Oberg U: Musculoskeletal complaints in dental hygiene: a survey study from a Swedish county, *J Dent Hyg* 67(5):257-261, 1993.
23. Occupational Safety and Health Administration: *Ergonomics* [Internet], 1999, http://www.osha-sla.gov.
24. Osborn JB et al: Musculoskeletal pain among Minnesota dental hygienists, *J Dent Hyg* 64:132-138, 1989.
25. Pollack R: Dento-ergonomics: the key to energy-saving performance, *J Calif Dent Assoc* 24(4):63-68, 1996.
26. Pollack R: The ergo factor: the most common equipment and design flaws and how to avoid them, *Dent Today* 15(1):112-113, 120-121, 1996.
27. Pollack-Simon R: Beware of your chair: sitting down is not enough! *Dent Today* 15(9):78, 80-81, 1996.
28. Rising DW et al: Reports of body pain in a dental student population, *J Am Dent Assoc* 136(1):81-86, 2005.
29. Rucker LM, Boyd MA: Optimizing dental operatory working environments. In Murphy DC, ed: *Ergonomics and the dental care worker,* Washington, DC, 1998, American Public Health Association.
30. Schoen D, Dean MC: *Contemporary periodontal instrumentation,* Philadelphia, 1996, WB Saunders.
31. Shugars D et al: Musculoskeletal pain among general dentists, *Gen Dent* 35(4):272-276, 1987.
32. Stockstill JW et al: Prevalence of upper extremity neuropathy in a clinical dentist population, *J Am Dent Assoc* 124:67-72, 1993.
33. Strassler HE et al: Enhanced visualization during dental practice using magnification systems, *Compendium* 19(6):595-596, 600, 602, 604, 606, 608, 610, 1998.
34. Sunell S, Maschak L: Positioning for clinical dental hygiene care preventing back, neck, and shoulder pain, *Probe* 30(6):218-219, 1996.
35. Valachi B, Valachi K: Preventing musculoskeletal disorders in clinical dentistry: strategies to address the mechanisms leading to musculoskeletal disorders, *J Am Dent Assoc* 134(12):1604-1612, 2003.
36. Wolny K, Shaw L, Verougstraete S: Repetitive strain injuries in dentistry, *Ont Dent* 76(2):13-19, 1999.

Instrument Design and Principles of Instrumentation

Mary Kaye Scaramucci

INSIGHT

Dental instruments are a basic component of intraoral evaluation and treatment. Complete knowledge and understanding of dental instruments and their design, function, and clinical applications make up the foundation of successful treatment outcomes. This complete understanding affords the clinician the critical thinking skills necessary to adapt appropriately and use successfully any dental instrument.

✳ CASE STUDY 9-1 | Instrument Selection Evaluation

Cassidy, a first-year dental hygiene student, is preparing for her first official patient in clinic. She has studied and has been tested on all of the instruments in her kit and is anxious to use every instrument.

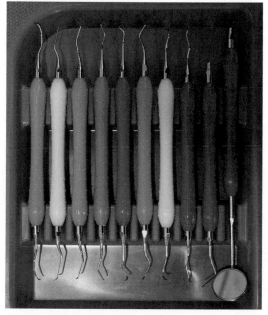

Courtesy Dentsply International, York, Pa.

KEY TERMS

area-specific curet	handle	powered
burnished calculus	knurled	instruments
calculus	lateral pressure	shank
circumferential	lateral sides	sickles
cross-section	long axis	tactile sensitivity
curets	oblique	terminal shank
cutting edge	parallel	tip
explorers	periodontal	toe
face	debridement	universal
files	perpendicular	vertical
fulcrum		working end

LEARNING OUTCOMES

After reading this chapter the student will be able to:

1. Identify instruments by classification, design name, and design number.
2. Describe the function of each part of any instrument.
3. Analyze each principle step by step as it relates to instrumentation.
4. Select the appropriate instrument design based on the periodontal condition.
5. Demonstrate correct principles of instrumentation in preclinical and clinical sessions.
6. Compare and contrast the powered instrument design and principles of use with hand instruments in periodontal debridement.

Evolution of Instruments

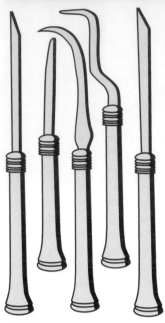

FIGURE 9-1
Pierre Fauchard's design for scaling instruments (1728).

Instruments for **calculus** removal have been in existence as early as the twelfth century. An Arabian physician wrote about the formation of calculus and described and illustrated various instruments that would remove it. He invented 14 scalers and recommended a thorough cleaning of the teeth.[1]

In 1728, Pierre Fauchard of France was compelled to invent his own set of instruments because "most of the instruments used for cleaning the teeth seem to me very unsuitable and even clumsy."[1] His instruments consisted of a rebbet chisel, parrot's bill, graver with three faces, small knife, and Z-shaped hook (Figure 9-1).

James Snell of London published a guide to scaling in 1832, which unequivocally recommended instruments with special design features for specific tooth surfaces. Snell was noted for his belief that using a different instrument for the right and left sides of the mouth was a *new method* for calculus removal.

From that point, instruments designed for the detection and removal of calculus deposits have evolved into various modern-day instruments: **curets, sickles, files,** hoes, **explorers,** periodontal probes, and **powered instruments.** Instrument design is dependent on the type of deposit to be removed and specific tooth surfaces. Designers of instruments over the years attempted to develop those that are easy to use, conform well to the tooth surface, and function effectively. The goal of instrumentation, however, has changed significantly. No longer is the goal to have glassy, smooth root surfaces but rather the removal of plaque biofilm from the root surface, which can be accomplished with either hand or powered instruments.

The novice clinician benefits from understanding the relationship of instrument design to **periodontal debridement** techniques. Understanding the specific design features of contemporary instruments affords the clinician the critical thinking skills necessary to adapt appropriately and use successfully any instrument.

Parts of the Instrument

To follow the principles of instrumentation in an effective manner, the clinician must be thoroughly familiar with specific terminology that identifies the standard parts of the instrument. All dental instruments consist of three parts: the **handle, shank,** and **working end** (Figure 9-2). Each instrument has specific design features that help the clinician determine its proper use.

HANDLE

Handles on manual instruments vary in weight, diameter, and texture. The handles can be narrow and solid or wide and hollow (Figure 9-3). Narrow handles are normally heavier in weight, whereas wide handles are lighter in weight. To prevent finger fatigue and to ease the instrumentation skills of the novice clinician, wide, hollow handles are the instruments of choice. First graders learning to write use pencils as round and large as a pretzel rod. The size of the pencil makes it easier to hold and use. The writing skills do not change as the pencil size shrinks. The same occurs with perfecting dental hygiene skills.

Hollow handles offer the additional advantage of being more efficient at transmitting tactile sensations. Because much of the instrumentation is below the gingival margin and is therefore not visible, the clinician must rely on vibrations transmitted from the instrument to discern the topography of the root surface. When an instrument is drawn over a calculus deposit, varying degrees of vibrations are transmitted to the instrument handle, which, in turn, are felt in the hand of the clinician. This sensation is similar to the vibrations felt in the steering wheel when a car drives over a speed bump or on a gravel road. This sensation is known as **tactile sensitivity** and is a critical component of instrumentation.

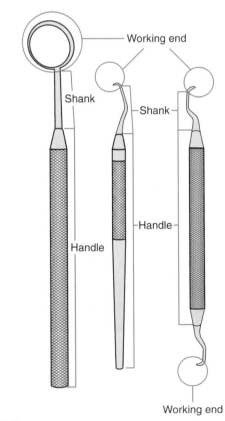

FIGURE 9-2
Instrument parts. *Handle* is used to grasp instrument. *Shank* connects the handle and the working end and permits adaptation of the working end to the tooth surface. *Working end* does the work of the instrument.

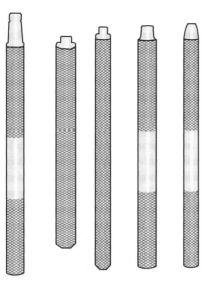

FIGURE 9-3
Instrument handles. Handles are available in a variety of shapes and styles. The following factors should be considered in the selection of instrument handles: *Weight:* Hollow handles increase tactile sensitivity and minimize operator fatigue. *Diameter:* Large handles maximize control and encourage a lighter grasp. *Serration:* Knurled handles enhance control by providing a positive gripping surface.

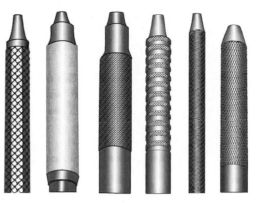

FIGURE 9-4
Handle serration (knurling). Handle serrations vary from manufacturer to manufacturer. Some designs offer better control than others.

The surface texture of the handle can be **knurled** or smooth (Figure 9-4). The amount and type of texture helps provide a firm grasp of the instrument and prevents slipping, particularly in a wet environment. Knurling can vary from manufacturer to manufacturer. However, the *waffle iron* pattern provides the best grasp and control.[3]

The handle of an ultrasonic instrument is actually the round receptacle (hand piece) into which the **tip** or insert slides. Water flows through the hand piece to cool the tip. The ultrasonic handle is not designed to facilitate transmission of tactile sensations.

SHANK

The shank is located at the end of the handle, between the handle and the working end, and varies in diameter, curvature, and length. The design features of the instrument shank reflect its intended use. Shanks with a thick diameter are considered rigid in nature and therefore are capable of removing heavy calculus deposits. If the diameter of a shank is thin, then the design is considered flexible for the removal of light calculus. Thin, flexible shanks also increase tactile sensitivity for the clinician. The curvature of the shank is defined as the bends that deviate from the **long axis** of the handle (Figure 9-5). The curvature of the shank determines the area where the instrument can be used. Shanks containing many deviations from the long axis are used in treatment areas with restricted access, such as posterior teeth. Shanks with few or no deviations are used in treatment areas with easy access, such as anterior teeth.

The length of the shank is measured by the first bend away from the handle to the beginning of the working end; this measurement determines the area of use (Figure 9-6). Long shanks (Figure 9-7, *A*) are used in restricted areas, whereas short

shanks (Figure 9-7, *B*) are used in unrestricted treatment areas. The **terminal shank** is that portion of the shank closest to the working end (see Figure 9-6). The terminal shank serves as an important visual cue for the clinician to determine whether the correct working end has been chosen. The general rule is the terminal shank is **parallel** to the long axis of the tooth. The functional shank can be short, long, or moderate in length. Moderate-to-long functional shanks are needed to reach the tooth or root surfaces of difficult access, such as posterior teeth. Short functional shanks are used to reach the tooth or root surfaces of easy access, such as anterior teeth.

The shank on a powered instrument insert or tip is specific to each manufacturer. Because the power to remove the deposit is converted electrical energy, the shank on a tip is comparatively rigid. Tips are either straight for anterior teeth and posterior teeth where adaptable or contraangled or curved for posterior teeth.

WORKING END

The working end of the instrument is that portion of the instrument that comes in contact with the tooth and performs the intended task. The working end of the manual instrument can be wirelike or rod-shaped or a blade. Instruments can have one working end, termed *single-ended instruments,* or two working ends, termed *double-ended instruments* (Figure 9-8). Double-ended instruments can be paired or unpaired. Paired working ends (see Figure 9-8, *C*) are mirror images of each other and perform the same function in opposite areas of the mouth. For example, one working end can be used on the facial surfaces of the maxillary right quadrant, and the same end can be used on the lingual surfaces of the left quadrant. Double-ended instruments provide the best efficiency and motion economy because for every double-ended instrument used, the clinician needs two single-ended instruments to complete the same task. Unpaired working ends (see Figure 9-8, *A*) are not mirror images and do not always perform the same function. However, unpaired working ends are useful, depending on the type of instrument at each end. Many unpaired instruments are double-ended based on their function. Instruments such as

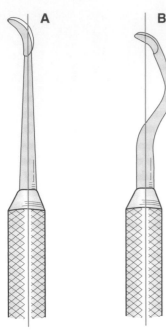

FIGURE 9-5
To determine whether an instrument shank is straight or curved, the clinician should hold the instrument so that the tip or the toe of the working end is facing the clinician. A straight shank is one that has no bends that deviate from the long axis of the shank. A curved shank has one or more bends that deviate from the long axis of the shank. **A,** Straight shank. **B,** Curved shank.

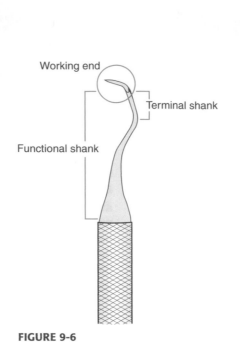

FIGURE 9-6
Instrument shank. Terminal shanks extend between the blade and the first bend. Functional shanks extend from the working end to the handle.

FIGURE 9-7
Functional shank length extends from the working end to the shank bend closest to the instrument handle. **A,** Long functional shank. **B,** Short functional shank.

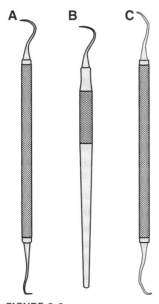

FIGURE 9-8
A and **C,** Double-ended instrument. **B,** Single-ended instrument. The working ends can be unpaired **(A)** or paired **(C).**

explorers and probes (Figure 9-9) may be combined because they are considered examination instruments.

The actual parts of the working end vary with each instrument. Some working ends are wirelike or rod-shaped with a sharp or blunt point (see Figure 9-9), whereas others have a blade, **face, lateral sides,** back, and **toe** (see Figure 9-8). Explorers and probes are wirelike or rod-shaped, forming a sharp or blunt point at the end. The side or tip of these instruments is adapted to the tooth surface during instrumentation. The working ends of scaling instruments are slightly more integral. The face and lateral sides join to form a blade or **cutting edge.** Some instruments have two cutting edges, whereas others have only one. The toe of the working end can be rounded or pointed. The back of the working end is op-

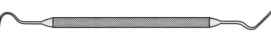

FIGURE 9-9
Unpaired double-ended instrument. One working end is a probe and the other is an explorer. Collectively, this instrument is considered an instrument of examination.

posite the face and may be rounded or pointed depending on the instrument classification (Figure 9-10). Identifying and understanding the intricate working ends of instruments is vital to proper instrumentation skills and preservation of the original shape and design of each instrument during sharpening.

The working end of a powered instrument insert or tip may vary in the cross-sectional design, depending on the manufacturer and conversion of energy to motion. No cutting edges exist on powered instrument inserts or tips.

✹ CASE APPLICATION 9-1.1

Working-End Design

Cassidy must first complete the examination of her patient. Looking at the instruments in her kit (or the instruments in the school's instrument kit), which instruments have a working end designed for examination and which instruments have a working end designed for scaling?

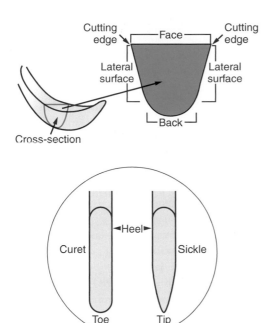

FIGURE 9-10
Working end (blade) is made of several components: face, lateral surfaces, cutting edge, and back. A blade that ends with a rounded toe is classified as a *curet*. A blade that ends with a pointed tip is classified as a *sickle*.

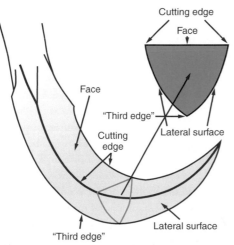

FIGURE 9-11
The sickle scaler has two cutting edges. Lateral surfaces join to form a pointed back (sharp one-third edge) that should be dulled to reduce possible tissue trauma. The face of the instrument is the surface between the two blades that converges to form a point.

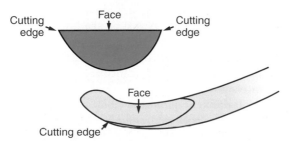

FIGURE 9-12
The universal curet has a rounded back and toe that enhances its use in subgingival areas. This back and toe are less likely to cause inadvertent trauma than the sharp-edged back and pointed toe of the sickle.

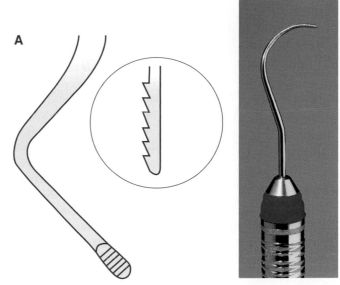

FIGURE 9-13
A, Files are composed of a series of parallel blades on a flat working head. Heavy files have a few large blades, whereas fine files have many small blades. **B,** The DiamondTec file has a 360-degree diamond coated working end. (Part B is courtesy Hu-Friedy Manufacturing Company Inc., Germany.)

Instrument Identification

Instrument identification is divided into three components:
1. Classification
2. Design name
3. Design number

CLASSIFICATION

The shape of the working end of the instrument determines instrument classification. Scaling instruments are classified as follows:

- Sickles
  - Pointed toe and pointed back
  - Triangular in cross-section (Figure 9-11)
  - Removes heavy supragingival calculus deposits
- Curets
  - Rounded toe and rounded back
  - Semicircular working end in cross-section (Figure 9-12)
  - May be supragingivally and subgingivally used to remove fine calculus deposits
  - Used particularly in root planing
- Files
  - Rounded or rectangular working end with multiple cutting edges (Figure 9-13)
  - Excellent for crushing large tenacious calculus deposits
- Hoes
  - Beveled working end (Figure 9-14)
  - Designed to remove supragingival calculus
- Chisels
  - Beveled working end (see Figure 9-14)
  - Designed to remove supragingival calculus

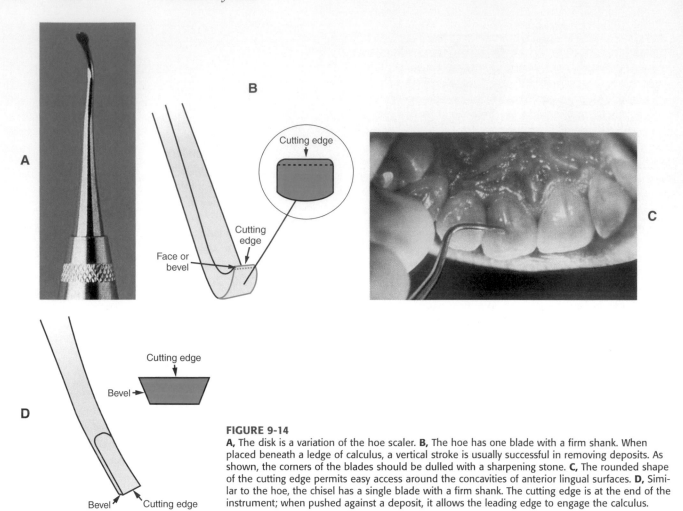

FIGURE 9-14
A, The disk is a variation of the hoe scaler. **B,** The hoe has one blade with a firm shank. When placed beneath a ledge of calculus, a vertical stroke is usually successful in removing deposits. As shown, the corners of the blades should be dulled with a sharpening stone. **C,** The rounded shape of the cutting edge permits easy access around the concavities of anterior lingual surfaces. **D,** Similar to the hoe, the chisel has a single blade with a firm shank. The cutting edge is at the end of the instrument; when pushed against a deposit, it allows the leading edge to engage the calculus.

- Powered instruments (See Chapter 31 for more information.)
  - Universal in design
  - Used supragingivally or subgingivally to remove any type of deposit (The design of the insert or tip will determine whether the use is subgingival or supragingival, the type of deposit to be removed, and the location within the mouth.)

Examination instruments are classified as mirrors, explorers, and probes (Box 9-1):

- Explorers
  - Fine, wirelike working end with a sharp point
  - Circular in cross-section (Figure 9-15)
  - Vary in shape and size
  - Designed for maximum tactile sensitivity
- Probes
  - Rodlike, blunted working end delineated in millimeter markings
  - Circular or rectangular in cross-section (Figure 9-16)
  - Instruments of measurement

BOX 9-1

INSTRUMENT CLASSIFICATION

Scaling	Hoes	Mirrors
Sickles	Chisels	Explorers
Curets	Ultrasonic	Probes
Files	Examination	

DESIGN NAME

The design name is usually located on the instrument handle and is typically based on the name of the inventor or the academic institution from at which the instrument was designed. For example, *Gracey curets* are named for Clayton Gracey, a dentist who invented the original series of 14 single-ended, area-specific instruments in the late 1940s. A team of educators from the University of North Carolina developed the UNC-15 probe, and the EXD 11/12 was developed at Old Dominion University. The design name often provides information about the instrument's origins or design elements to assist in its classification (Figure 9-17).

The primary purpose of the mirror is to see oral structures that cannot be seen directly without compromising operator positioning. This technique is known as *indirect vision,* and the reflected image is reversed in the mirror. Indirect vision is essential for instrumentation in the maxillary right palatal aspect (left palatal for the left-handed operator) and the palatal aspects of anterior teeth.

Indirect Vision

Constant practice is required to become competent in viewing oral structures through the mirror.

Note

Dental mirror uses include the following:
- Indirect vision
- Retraction
- Illumination
- Transillumination

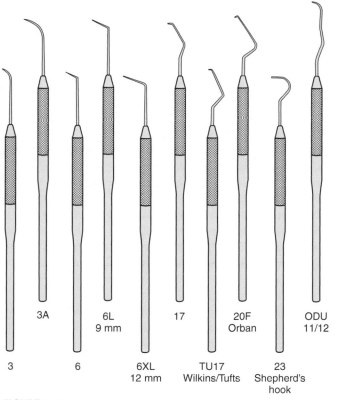

FIGURE 9-15
Explorers used to detect dental caries and examine teeth for calculus and other irregularities are available in a variety of shapes and sizes.

DESIGN NUMBER

The design number, also located on the handle, helps describe specific instruments of choice. The Gracey series consists of numerous instruments, and specific numbers identify each instrument (Figure 9-18). The series consists of the Gracey 1/2, 3/4, 5/6, and so on up to the Gracey 17/18. As a general rule, low-numbered instruments are designed for easy access areas, such as anterior teeth, and high-numbered instruments are designed for difficult-to-reach areas or posterior teeth.

On the other hand, a design number that represents the millimeter markings identifies probes. The earlier reference to the UNC-15 probe indicates that the millimeter markings of this probe are incremented to 15 mm (and greater). Other probes, such as the PCP-10 or PCP-12, indicate a 10-mm or 12-mm increment, respectively.

DESIGN FEATURES OF SPECIFIC INSTRUMENTS

Dental Mirrors

The dental mirror is used as a supplement to enhance access to instrumentation. Dental mirrors have four uses:

1. Indirect vision
2. Retraction
3. Indirect illumination
4. Transillumination

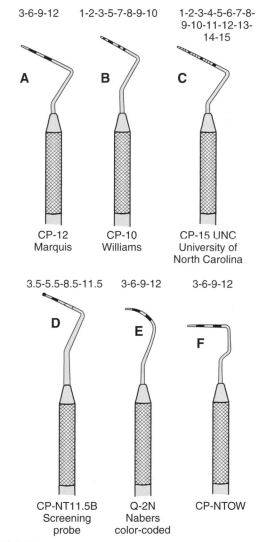

FIGURE 9-16
A, Marquis color-coded probe with 3-6-9-12 mm markings. **B,** Williams probe with 1-2-3-5-7-8-9-10 mm markings. **C,** UNC-15 probe with 1-2-3-4-5-6-7-8-9-10-11-12-13-14-15 mm markings. **D,** PSR screening probe with 3.5-5.5-8.5-11.5 mm markings. A guide accompanies this probe to assist with periodontal assessment. **E,** Nabers probe with 3-6-9-12 mm markings. This probe is ideal for measurement of molar furcations. **F,** Novatech probe with 3-6-9-12 mm markings. The angular-shaped shank is noted. This probe provides easy access and reading of probing depths in the posterior area.

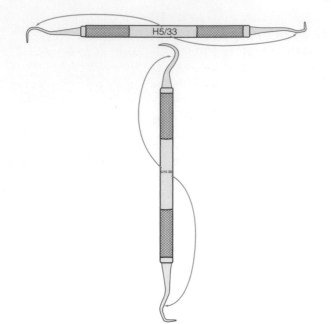

FIGURE 9-17
Instrument markings. When the design name and number are labeled along the length of the handle, the number closest to each working end identifies it. If the design name and number are labeled around the instrument handle, then the first number (on the left) identifies the working end at the top and the second number identifies the working end at the bottom of the handle.

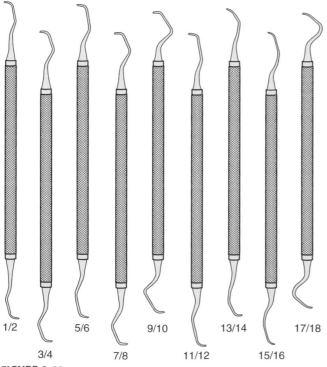

1/2   5/6   9/10   13/14   17/18
   3/4   7/8   11/12   15/16

FIGURE 9-18
Gracey curets provide a variety of shank designs to facilitate access to all areas of the dentition. Each instrument is specific to the area. The design of the working end is well suited for removal of fine deposits in subgingival areas. The original series consisted of 14 instruments.

The mirror is also used to retract tissue to enhance visibility with direct vision. The cheeks and tongue can be gently moved by the face of the mirror to enhance visibility. Illumination allows the clinician to use the mirror as a spotlight to reflect light from the dental light onto a specific area of the mouth. This technique works best in the maxillary left palatal aspect (right palatal for the left-handed operator).

Transillumination seemingly makes the tooth transparent. This technique is useful in the anterior sextants and consists of placing the mirror behind the teeth and directing the dental light **perpendicular** to the long axis of the teeth. Variations in density from the presence of calculus and dental caries become apparent (see Chapter 17).

Mirrors can be one-sided or two-sided. A two-sided mirror permits the clinician to observe a visible image on either side. The two-sided mirror is preferred because the clinician can retract and simultaneously use it for indirect vision. The following three types of mirror faces exist:

1. *Plane or flat surface mirror:* Has a reflecting surface on the back of the mirror lens and may produce a double image.
2. *Concave surface mirror:* Produces a magnified image that may be distorted.
3. *Front surface mirror:* Has the reflecting surface on the front of the lens that eliminates the double image, producing a clear image.
   - Is the mirror of choice for dental hygiene procedures.
   - Can be easily scratched.
   - Care should be taken to protect the mirror during the removal of bioburden and the sterilization process.

> ### *Prevention*
> Care of dental mirrors includes the following:
> - Mirrors should not be placed in the ultrasonic cleaner, where other instruments can bump against the face of the mirror, causing scratches.
> - The mirror face should also be wrapped in gauze before sterilizing to prevent scratching.

Explorers

Explorers are considered instruments of evaluation and are used to examine the tooth and root surface for the presence of the following:
- Dental caries
- Calculus
- Surface irregularities such as the cementoenamel junction
- Deficient or overhanging margins of restorations

The design features of explorers include a fine, wirelike working end; sharp point; and circular **cross-section.** The shape of the explorer can vary in design from a Shepherd's hook, right angle, pigtail, to contraangle (see Figure 9-15).

Periodontal Probes

Similar to the explorer, the periodontal probe is an instrument of evaluation and cannot be used to remove calculus. Probes are used to perform the following:

- Measure sulcus depth
- Determine sulcus topography
- Measure the amount of attached gingiva
- Identify gingival bleeding
- Measure the size of lesions
- Aid in calculus detection and identification of root morphologic characteristics

The design features of periodontal probes include a rod-shaped working end and a smooth, blunted point. The probe is round or rectangular in cross-section and marked in millimeters (see Figure 9-16). The millimeter markings can be color-coded with black markings that will not chip, flake, or fade with sterilizing.

Clinicians should know how the probe is calibrated because the millimeter markings may vary. Some probes are calibrated in increments of 3 mm (see Figure 9-16, *A*), whereas others are calibrated as 1-2-3-5-7-8-9-10 (see Figure 9-16, *B*). The UNC-15 is calibrated to 15 mm. This probe is calibrated as 1-2-3-4-5-6-7-8-9-10-11-12-13-14-15 (see Figure 9-16, *C*). A new screening-type probe has been developed with markings of 3.5-5.5-8.5-11.5 (see Figure 9-16, *D*). Two types of probes that vary in shape include the Nabers probe (see Figure 9-16, *E*), which is used to provide an accurate root furcation measurement, and the Novatech right-angle probe (see Figure 9-16, *F*), which is designed for easy adaptation in the posterior regions. (Table 9-1 offers a quick reference for use of examination instruments.)

Sickle Scalers

> ***Prevention***
> The pointed back and two straight cutting edges of the sickle in cross-section limit its use subgingivally because the gingival tissue may be traumatized.

Sickle scalers are designed for the removal of supragingival calculus deposits. The shank of these instruments can be straight for anterior teeth or contraangled for posterior teeth. The working end consists of two parallel cutting edges that join to form a pointed toe. The face of the blade may be flame-shaped or triangular, whereas the back is pointed or blunted (see Figure 9-11).[5]

Area-Specific Curets

Curets are used for subgingival calculus removal and root debridement. The original Gracey series consists of 14 single-ended instruments referred to as **area-specific curets** (Table 9-2). (See Figure 9-18, which shows all 18 as double-ended, designed for specific teeth and tooth surfaces.) Although two visible cutting edges are curved and join to form a rounded toe, only one edge is used for debridement. The unique feature of the Gracey curet is the offset face of the blade. The face of the blade is at a 60- to 70-degree angle to the shank, rendering one cutting edge lower than the other. When viewing the face of the working end with the terminal shank perpendicular to the floor, the clinician can see a lower and higher cutting edge (Figure 9-19). The lower cutting edge removes calculus. The pur-

pose of this offset angulation is to permit easy insertion below the gingival margin and adaptation to the tooth surface.

The working end of the Gracey curet may be styled small in overall size, known as the *mini Gracey curet*. The overall working end is approximately one half the length of the standard Gracey. The mini is designed to adapt to narrow pockets or furcations (Figure 9-20, *A*).

The Gracey curets used in the anterior region consist of slightly angled shanks, whereas those instruments used in the posterior region have multiple contraangled shanks. The long, flexible shanks are designed for superior access in difficult-to-reach areas with an increase in tactile conduction. Because of the limited ability of these Gracey curets to remove moderate-to-tenacious calculus deposits, the Gracey series has been designed with rigid shanks. Gracey curets with rigid shanks are

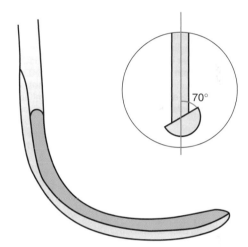

FIGURE 9-19
The offset relationship of the cutting edge of this Gracey curet is noted. One blade is lower than the other.

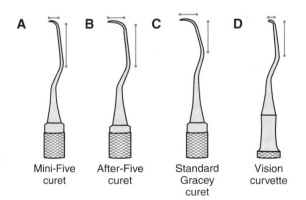

FIGURE 9-20
Comparison of area-specific curets. **A,** The Mini-Five curet has a long terminal shank and small working end. **B,** The After-Five curet has a long terminal shank and standard working end. **C,** The standard Gracey curet is shown. Compare the terminal shank and working end with the Mini- and After-Five curets. **D,** Vision curvette has a long shank with 5-mm and 10-mm markings and a 50% curved working end.

Table 9-1 — Areas for Examination Instrument Use

INSTRUMENT	AREA OF USE	SURFACE	TERMINAL SHANK	DESCRIPTION OF USE
Probe	Anterior teeth	All	Parallel with tooth surface	Insertion at distal line angle; light walking stroke into interproximal area; light walking stroke from distal across straight facial or lingual surfaces; light walking stroke from mesial line angle into interproximal area
	Premolars	All	Parallel with tooth surface	Insertion at distal line angle; light walking stroke into interproximal area; light walking stroke from distal across straight buccal or lingual surfaces; light walking stroke from mesial line angle into interproximal area
	Molars	All	Parallel with tooth surface	Insertion at distal line angle; light walking stroke into interproximal area; light walking stroke from distal across straight buccal or lingual surfaces; light walking stroke from mesial line angle into interproximal area
11/12 Explorer*	Anteriors	All	Parallel with long axis	Insertion at midline; light walking stroke into interproximal area
	Premolars	Distal	Parallel with long axis	Insertion at distal line angle; light walking stroke into interproximal area
		Straight buccal and lingual	Oblique	Insertion at distal line angle; light walking stroke to mesial angle
		Mesial	Parallel with long axis	Mesial line angle; light walking stroke into interproximal area
	Molars	Distal	Parallel with long axis	Insertion at distal line angle; light walking stroke into interproximal area
		Straight buccal and lingual	Oblique	Insertion at distal line angle; light walking stroke to mesial line angle
		Mesial	Parallel with long axis	Mesial line angle; light walking stroke into interproximal area

*During insertion and activation, the instrument tip or toe is pointed in the direction of the proximal surface toward which the instrument is moving.

Table 9-2 — Areas for Gracey Curet Use

GRACEY AREA-SPECIFIC CURET	AREA OF USE	SURFACES	TERMINAL SHANK	DESCRIPTION OF USE
1/2	Anterior teeth	All	Parallel with long axis	Insertion at midline; scaling into interproximal area
3/4	Anterior teeth	All	Parallel with long axis	Insertion at midline; scaling into interproximal area
5/6	Anterior teeth	All	Parallel with long axis	Insertion at midline; scaling into interproximal area
7/8	Premolars	All	Parallel with long axis	Insertion at midline; scaling into interproximal area
	Molars	Straight buccal and lingual	Oblique	Insertion at distal line angle; scaling to mesial line angle
9/10	Premolars	All	Parallel with long axis	Insertion at midline; scaling into interproximal area
	Molars	Straight buccal and lingual	Oblique	Insertion at distal line angle; scaling to mesial line angle
11/12	Premolars	Straight buccal and lingual	Oblique	Insertion at distal line angle; scaling to mesial line angle
		Mesial	Parallel with long axis	Mesial line angle; scaling into interproximal area
	Molars	Straight buccal and lingual	Oblique	Insertion at distal line angle; scaling to mesial line angle
		Mesial	Parallel with long axis	Mesial line angle; scaling into interproximal area
13/14	Premolars	Distal	Parallel with long axis	Insertion at distal line angle; scaling into interproximal area
	Molars	Distal	Parallel with long axis	Insertion at distal line angle; scaling into interproximal area
15/16	Premolars	Straight buccal and lingual	Oblique	Insertion at distal line angle; scaling to mesial line angle
		Mesial	Parallel with long axis	Mesial line angle; scaling into interproximal area
	Molars	Straight buccal and lingual	Oblique	Insertion at distal line angle; scaling to mesial line angle
		Mesial	Parallel with long axis	Mesial line angle; scaling into interproximal area
17/18	Premolars	Distal	Parallel with long axis	Insertion at distal line angle; scaling into interproximal area
	Molars	Distal	Parallel with long axis	Insertion at distal line angle; scaling into interproximal area

stronger and can remove more tenacious deposits; however, a slight reduction in tactile sensitivity results.

The After-Five Gracey curet offers yet another unique style. The After-Five curet has a terminal shank that has been redesigned to be 3 mm longer than the standard curet (Figure 9-20, *B*). This design feature affords access to deep periodontal pockets and root surfaces of 5 mm and greater. Many times, the After-Five feature is coupled with the mini–working end to create an instrument that can reach the base of a deep, narrow periodontal pocket.

Various innovations have resulted in several contemporary redesigns of the original Gracey series. The Gracey mesial-distal curets (11/14 and 12/13) are a combination of the instrument used on the facial and mesial surfaces and the distal surfaces of posterior teeth. This feature allows the clinician to complete a posterior sextant with one instrument as opposed to the combination of the 13/14 and 11/12. Another pattern design mimics the 11/12, in which the shank has accentuated contraangled bends, and the cutting edge is positioned to reach the mesial surfaces of posterior teeth and is known as the Gracey 15/16. The Gracey 17/18 is an accentuated version of the 13/14, improving access to the distal posterior surfaces.

The Vision curvette series (Figure 9-21) has long shanks with 5- and 10-mm shank markings and a 50% shorter, curved working end. These instruments exhibit improved adaptation into furcations and deep periodontal pockets. Finally, the Turgeon Modified Gracey series is designed with a different cross-section of the blade angulation (Figure 9-22), providing a sharper cutting edge that is easier to sharpen. The blades are also narrow for easy subgingival insertion.

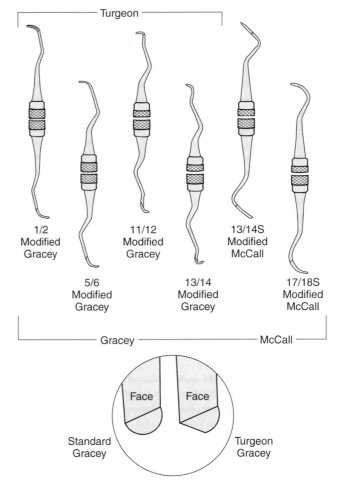

FIGURE 9-22
Turgeon modified Gracey curets. The angulation of a standard Gracey curet versus the Turgeon Gracey curet is noted.

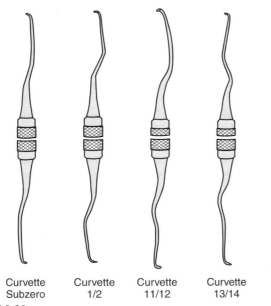

FIGURE 9-21
Vision curvettes. Curvette Subzero has a long shank that reaches deep into the sulcus, adapting to the facial and lingual root surface. Curvette 1/2 is recommended for anterior and premolar surfaces, as well as interproximal areas. Curvette 11/12 is designed for mesial surfaces of molars with improved adaptation into furcations. Curvette 13/14 is for distal surfaces of molars with improved adaptation into furcations.

Universal Curets

Universal curets have a variety of styles and patterns. However, they all possess basic design features representative of all universal curets. The **universal** design permits adaptation to all tooth surfaces of the anterior and posterior regions alike, without changing instruments. The working end consists of two parallel and straight cutting edges that join to form a rounded toe (see Figure 9-12). Both cutting edges are used for calculus removal and root debridement. The face of the blade is at a 90-degree angle to the shank. Universal curets require great care to ensure that the opposite cutting edge is not engaged to remove the pocket lining adjacent to the root surface. The Langer curets are unique types of universal instruments (Figure 9-23). These instruments have the shank design of a Gracey curet with a universal cutting edge design. They feature a series of working ends such as L1/2 for mandibular posterior teeth, L3/4 for maxillary posterior teeth, L5/6 for maxillary and mandibular anterior teeth, and L17/18 for maxillary and mandibular posterior teeth. The Langer series can also be obtained with a rigid or After-Five shank and a mini–working end.

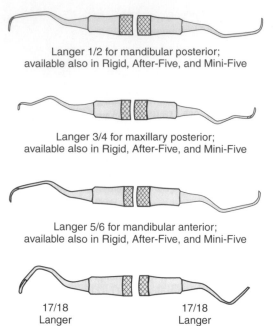

Langer 1/2 for mandibular posterior;
available also in Rigid, After-Five, and Mini-Five

Langer 3/4 for maxillary posterior;
available also in Rigid, After-Five, and Mini-Five

Langer 5/6 for mandibular anterior;
available also in Rigid, After-Five, and Mini-Five

17/18
Langer

17/18
Langer
Rigid

Langer 17/18 for maxillary and mandibular posterior

FIGURE 9-23
Langer curets combine the features of the Gracey and universal curets. The Langer has two cutting edges similar to the universal curet and the shank design of the Gracey curet. The Langer series consists of the 1/2, 3/4, 5/6, and 17/18. The series can be modified as Rigid, After-Five, or Mini-Five.

Hoes

The hoe scaler (see Figure 9-14, *A*) is designed to remove ledges of calculus and heavy stain from the facial, lingual, and palatal surfaces of teeth. The face of the blade joins the beveled toe to form one straight cutting edge. This face of the blade is at a 99- to 100-degree angle to the instrument shank, whereas the toe has a 45-degree bevel. Hoes consist of straight or contraangled shanks. The straight shank is designed for anterior teeth, and the contraangled shank is designed for posterior teeth. The hoe is activated with a pull stroke.

The disk scaler (see Figure 9-14, *B*) is a variation of a hoe scaler. The working end is disk shaped, and the cutting edge surrounds the entire working end. The rigid terminal shank and acute angulation of the working end enables the use of a pull stroke in all directions along the anterior lingual surfaces for efficient stain and calculus removal[5] (see Figure 9-14, *C*).

Chisels

Chisels (see Figure 9-14, *D*) are designed to break apart bridges of supragingival calculus deposits between teeth, particularly in the anterior region. Like hoes, chisels have one straight cutting edge and a beveled toe. The blade is slightly curved to enhance adaptation around tooth surfaces and is positioned at a 45-degree angle to the face of the working end. Chisels have straight or curved shanks and are activated with a push stroke.

Files

Periodontal files are used to crush large pieces of tenacious subgingival calculus. The working ends are either oval or rectangular in shape, containing multiple rows of straight cutting edges (see Figure 9-13, *A*). Files have straight or contraangled shanks and are activated with a pull stroke. Table 9-3 identifies areas of use for all scaling instruments.

The DiamondTec File Scaler is an innovative file design (see Figure 9-13, *B*) that is shaped like a Nabers probe. The working end has a 360-degree diamond coating that never needs sharpening. The diamond files are designed for definitive scaling in furcations and root depressions. This file is activated with a push-pull motion.

Powered Instruments

Powered instruments were introduced to dentistry in the early 1950s for the removal of decay in cavity preparations. With the advent of the high-speed hand piece, the powered scaler was no longer needed for its original purpose. In the late 1950s the powered scaler was used for heavy supragingival calculus removal. Along with the evolution in design, additional benefits soon were realized; currently, the most common use by far of this instrument is in periodontal debridement for calculus and plaque biofilm removal.

Each powered scaler consists of the following:
- Control box or dental unit
- Hand piece
- Selection of specifically designed inserts or tips
- Associated hoses
- Foot-activated pedal

The hand piece is filled with water through the depression of the foot pedal, and the selected insert or tip is placed into the hand piece. The insert or tip is then *tuned* by manipulating the power setting and water flow until a fine, mistlike spray is achieved when the insert or tip is activated.

The powered scaler uses electrical energy that is converted to mechanical energy, and the cycles per second depend on the type of mechanical energy conversion and the specific equipment. The insert or tip in most units vibrates at least 28,000 times per second. When the working end of the insert is placed on a deposit, the deposit virtually implodes as the vibrating force destroys the crystal structure of calculus. Use of the powered scalers requires specific techniques, cautions, and awareness of contraindications (see Chapter 31).

⚡ **CASE APPLICATION 9-1.2**

Instrument Design Identification

Looking at Cassidy's instrument kit (or the instruments in the school's instrument kit in the figure in Case Study 9-1), which instruments are sickle scalers, which instruments are universal curets, which instruments are area-specific curets, and which instruments are powered inserts?

Table 9-3   Areas of Use for Periodontal Instrumentation

INSTRUMENT	AREA OF USE	SURFACE	TERMINAL SHANK	DESCRIPTION OF USE
Anterior Sickle*	Anterior teeth	All	Parallel with long axis	Placement at midline; scaling into interproximal area
Posterior Sickle*	Premolars	Distal	Parallel with long axis	Placement at distal line angle; scaling into interproximal area
		Mesial	Parallel with long axis	Placement at mesial line angle; scaling into interproximal area
	Molars	Distal	Parallel with long axis	Placement at distal line angle; scaling into interproximal area
		Mesial	Parallel with long axis	Placement at mesial line angle; scaling into interproximal area
Universal Curet*	Anteriors	All	Oblique	Insertion at midline; scaling into interproximal area
	Premolars	Distal	Parallel with long axis	Insertion at distal line angle; scaling into interproximal area
		Straight buccal and lingual	Oblique	Insertion at distal line angle; scaling to mesial line angle
		Mesial	Parallel with long axis	Mesial line angle; scaling into interproximal area
	Molars	Distal	Parallel with long axis	Insertion at distal line angle; scaling into interproximal area
		Straight buccal and lingual	Oblique	Insertion at distal line angle; scaling to mesial line angle
		Mesial	Parallel with long axis	Mesial line angle; scaling into interproximal area
Hoe	Anteriors	Straight buccal and lingual	Parallel with long axis	No insertion; placement is coronal to gingival margin; stroke pulled downward toward incisal surface
	Premolars	Straight buccal and lingual	Parallel with long axis	No insertion; placement is coronal to gingival margin; stroke pulled toward occlusal surface
	Molars	Straight buccal and lingual	Parallel with long axis	No insertion; placement is coronal to gingival margin; stroke pulled toward occlusal surface
Disk	Anteriors	Straight lingual	Parallel with long axis	No insertion; placement is coronal to gingival margin; stroke pulled in all directions
Chisel	Anteriors	Interproximal area	Perpendicular with long axis	No insertion; stroke pushed from facial to lingual surface
File	Anteriors	Straight facial and lingual	Parallel with long axis	Insertion apical to deposit; stroke pulled toward incisal surface
	Premolars	Straight buccal and lingual	Parallel with long axis	Insertion apical to deposit; stroke pulled toward occlusal surface
	Molars	Straight buccal and lingual	Parallel with long axis	Insertion apical to deposit; stroke pulled toward occlusal surface

*During insertion and activation, the instrument tip or toe is pointed in the direction of the proximal surface toward which the instrument is moving.

Fundamentals of Instrumentation

INSTRUMENT GRASP

Understanding the design features of basic instruments is necessary to apply principles of instrumentation. These principles describe the relationship of the instrument to the hand and to the tooth or root surface. The fundamentals of instrumentation include the following (Box 9-2):

- Grasp
- Insertion
- Fulcrum
- Angulation
- Adaptation
- Activation

Instrument grasp describes how the clinician holds the instrument. The two grasps used during dental hygiene care are (1) the modified pen grasp and (2) the palm grasp. The palm grasp has limited usage: to hold and use the air/water syringe or tuck the mirror away when not in use. With the palm grasp the syringe or instrument is held in the palm of the dominant hand, and the fingers are wrapped around the handle. The thumb is free to activate the air and water buttons or to provide leverage on the shank of an instrument (Figure 9-24).

The modified pen grasp is a variation of the pen grasp (Figure 9-25). Students should notice the placement of the thumb, index finger, and middle finger. Whereas a pen grasp varies from person to person, the

BOX 9-2

FUNDAMENTALS OF INSTRUMENTATION

1. Grasp
2. Fulcrum
3. Adaptation
4. Insertion
5. Angulation
6. Activation

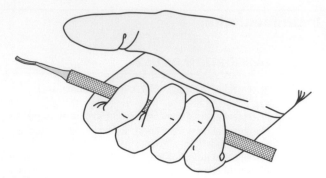

FIGURE 9-24
Palm grasp. The instrument handle is held in the palm grasp by cupped index, middle, ring, and pinky fingers.

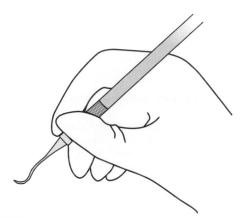

FIGURE 9-25
Typical pen grasp. The thumb and index finger grasp the handle. The middle finger supports the instrument from underneath. The pen grasp varies from person to person.

modified pen grasp requires that all clinicians hold the instrument in a similar manner.

The modified pen grasp offers the following three advantages:

- Control of the instrument
- Prevention of finger fatigue
- Increase in tactile sensitivity

Note

Patient and operator positioning can affect appropriate implementation of the principles. When the application of the principles is difficult after *instrument grasp,* patient and operator positioning should be checked.

The instrument is held in the dominant hand with the pads of the index finger and thumb opposite each other on the handle closest to the working end. The thumb and index finger are not touching, thereby creating a tripod effect with the middle finger placed along the shank of the instrument. This tripod effect balances the instrument in the clinician's hand to provide stability and control. Keeping the index finger and thumb separated allows the clinician to roll the instrument between these digits with ease and control. The thumb is either straight or slightly bent in a **C** shape, whereas the index finger is straight from the fingertip to the second joint. The index finger bends at the second joint, and the instrument handle rests somewhere between the second and third joints.

The side pad near the fingernail of the middle finger is against the shank and serves to guide the instrument. The middle finger also bends at the second joint and should not be used to apply pressure to the instrument. The middle and ring fingers always should remain in contact somewhere along the length of either finger. This contact ensures proper wrist motion and limits the amount of finger motion to activate the instrument (Figure 9-26).

Concerning Grasp

If the index finger bends at the first joint, its grasp will cause a loss of wrist motion and power for scaling.

FULCRUM

The pad, specifically the tip of the ring finger of the dominant hand, serves as the fulcrum finger (Figure 9-27). When activating the instrument, the clinician exerts downward pressure on the fulcrum finger and slightly squeezes the instrument with the index finger and thumb to increase stability and control

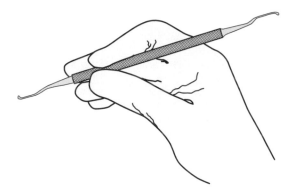

FIGURE 9-26
Modified pen grasp. Both the first and second fingers hold the handle, opposed by the thumb. The third finger is in position to rest on the tooth to create stability and to act as a finger rest to move the instrument and hand as a unit.

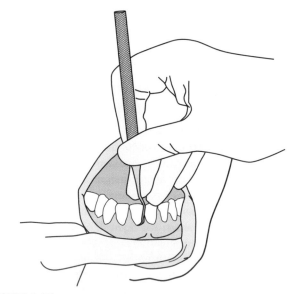

FIGURE 9-27
The finger rest in the modified pen grasp is intraorally on a solid tooth surface in the same arch and as close as possible to the working area.

during scaling while not causing patient discomfort. A lazy fulcrum in which the clinician uses the middle of the pad can hinder the maneuverability or pivot the fulcrum finger, thereby limiting the ability to adapt, angle, and activate the instrument properly. General guidelines for an appropriate fulcrum include the placement of the ring finger on solid tooth surface, in the same arch, and close to the work area.

The fulcrum finger serves as a pivot point for instrument adaptation and activation. This action of the fulcrum finger and wrist is what is needed to activate the instrument.

Auxiliary Fulcrums

Although the conventional intraoral fulcrum may be the only

fulcrum permitted during skill development, a variety of auxiliary fulcrums deviate from the general intraoral fulcrums. Auxiliary fulcrums are necessary during certain circumstances that may prohibit the use of intraoral fulcrums. The advantages include the following:

- Enhances access to the treatment area.
- Improves instrument-to-tooth angulation.
- Increases power because of the wider range of motion in the wrist, hand, and arm.

Serious disadvantages include the following:

- Lack of stability and control occurs, which is offered with the traditional intraoral fulcrum.
- Risk of patient or operator injury is present.

These fulcrums should be practiced and used only after the traditional intraoral fulcrum has been mastered. Auxiliary fulcrums build on the skills learned with the intraoral fulcrum.

The traditional intraoral fulcrum includes the following four variations:

- Cross-arch (Figure 9-28)
  - Requires a finger placement on solid tooth structure.
  - Although the placement is in the same arch, it is in the opposite quadrant of instrumentation.
- Opposite-arch (Figure 9-29)
  - Placement of the finger rest is in the opposite arch of instrumentation.
    - *Example:* Clinician uses instruments on the mandibular anterior sextant while a finger rests on the maxillary anterior sextant.
- Finger-on-finger (Figure 9-30)
  - Follows the general principles of a finger rest in the same arch and close to the working area, but actual placement of the fulcrum finger is on the finger of the nondominant hand.

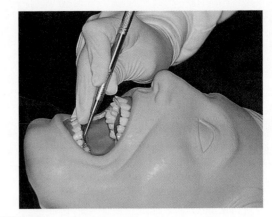

FIGURE 9-28
Intraoral cross-arch fulcrum. The clinician fulcrums in quadrant four to instrument in quadrant three. A cross-arch fulcrum permits greater movement of the hand and instrument as a unit, thereby increasing lateral pressure.

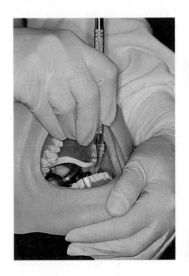

FIGURE 9-29
Intraoral opposite-arch fulcrum. The clinician fulcrums in the maxillary arch to perform instrumentation in the mandibular arch. Similar to the cross-arch fulcrum, this alternative fulcrum provides greater movement and pressure.

- Works best in the maxillary right quadrant (left quadrant for the left-handed clinician) during instrumentation of the buccal surfaces and in the mandibular anterior facial sextant.
  - *Maxillary right quadrant:* Index finger of the nondominant hand serves to retract the cheek and is placed in the occlusal surfaces of the posterior teeth. The index finger also serves as a finger rest for instrumentation (Figure 9-30, *A*).
  - *Mandibular region:* Index finger of the nondominant hand is placed in the vestibule and retracts the lower lip. The index finger is used again as a rest for the fulcrum finger (Figure 9-30, *B*).
- Reinforced (Figure 9-31)
  - Allows the clinician to exert more pressure on scaling.
  - Requires caution to prevent the instrument from breaking or injury to the patient.

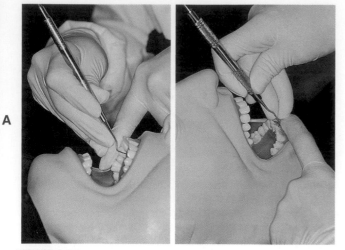

A

B

FIGURE 9-30
Intraoral finger-on-finger fulcrum is also referred to as the *built-up fulcrum.* It can be used in the maxillary posterior **(A)** or mandibular anterior area **(B).** This fulcrum permits superior instrument-to-tooth angulation.

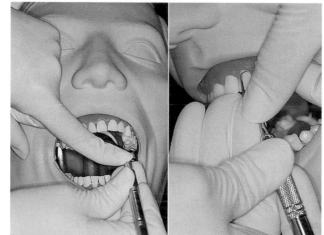

A

B

FIGURE 9-31
Intraoral reinforced fulcrum. By placing a finger **(A)** or thumb **(B)** near the end of the shank closest to the handle, lateral pressure is increased.

- Follows all principles of a finger rest in the same arch, on solid tooth surface, and as close to the working area as possible.
  - Addition of the thumb or index finger of the nondominant hand is placed on the shank of the instrument.
  - Pressure is gently exerted by the index finger (Figure 9-31, *A*) or thumb (Figure 9-31, *B*) to increase lateral pressure on the instrument to remove the deposit.
  - This technique is ideal in the maxillary left lingual quadrant (right lingual for left-handed clinicians).
    - Works best with rigid instruments.

Extraoral fulcrums can help the clinician establish the correct instrument for tooth angulation. The extraoral fulcrum (Figure 9-32) is ideal in the maxillary posterior region, where instrument angulation may be challenging. When using an extraoral fulcrum on the maxillary right facial quadrant (left facial for the left-handed operator), the clinician places the back of the hand against the patient's chin with the nail sides of the middle and ring fingers gently pressing against the face. The clinician's palm is facing up. Instrumentation on the left maxillary facial quadrant (right facial for the left-handed operator) requires a modified palm-down approach. This time, the pads of the middle and ring fingers are placed against the chin while light pressure is exerted against the face (Figure 9-33).

The use of powered instruments can require auxiliary finger rests. Lateral pressure is not applied when using powered instruments. Intraoral fulcrums that provide more stability when lateral pressure is needed are not required.

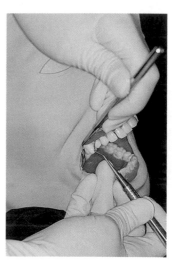

B

FIGURE 9-32
Extraoral fulcrum. By using an extraoral fulcrum, the clinician has the opportunity to increase motion and stroke power. The fulcrum on the maxillary right requires a palm-up approach.

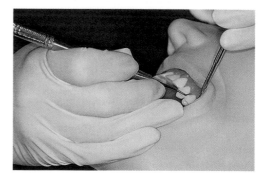

FIGURE 9-33
The extraoral fulcrum on the maxillary left is approached with a modified palm-down approach.

ADAPTATION

Adaptation is the third principle of instrumentation.

Proper adaptation of the instrument to the tooth surface means placement of the lower one third to two thirds of the instrument working

> **Note**
> Adaptation is defined as the relationship between the instrument and the tooth surface that is maintained during instrumentation.

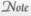

end (Figure 9-34), specifically the lower one third of the cutting edge of scaling instruments or the side tip of the explorer and probe, against the tooth. The goal is to keep the side tip or lower one third of the cutting edge or working end against the tooth surface at all times, while the terminal shank is maintained parallel to the long axis of the tooth.

Adaptation of the instrument varies as the instrument is activated and moved around the tooth. The size and shape of individual tooth surfaces dictate how much of the working end is adapted to the tooth surface.

Clinicians can adapt the instrument by rolling the handle between the index finger and thumb and pivoting on the fulcrum finger. Another aspect of appropriate adaptation is the initial placement of the lower one third of the instrument on a specific area of the tooth. The tooth surface location varies from

instrument to instrument but is usually at the mesial or distal line angles of posterior teeth and the midline of anterior teeth.

The powered instrument is adapted in much the same way as hand instruments. The point of the instrument is never adapted directly on the tooth surface.

ANGULATION FOR INSERTION AND ACTIVATION

Angulation is the fourth principle of instrumentation (Figure 9-35).

Instruments used subgingivally must be inserted before activation. Initial angulation to insert an instrument to the base of the sulcus should be as close as possible to 0 degrees.

This angulation requires the face of the blade to be against the tooth surface. To achieve this position, the clinician tilts the instrument handle as close to the tooth surface as possible, permitting easy insertion with the toe third of the working end beneath the gingival margin and preventing injury to the hard and soft tissues. Once the insertion angle is accomplished, various angles are established, depending on the type of stroke applied. If the clinician is beginning an exploratory or examination stroke, then the angle should be approximately 5 degrees so that the cutting edge of scaling instruments is not engaged against the tooth surface.

If the working stroke is a scaling stroke for calculus removal, then the angulation will be closer to but less than 90 degrees. This angulation affords the clinician the greatest opportunity to engage the hard deposit. If the working stroke is for root planing, then the angulation will lessen to 60 to 80 degrees. A smaller angulation smoothes the root surface and does not cut or gouge the root, which is the goal of root planing. As a general rule, proper angulation is established when the terminal shank of the instrument is parallel to the long axis of the tooth. This position is accomplished by tilting of the instrument handle slightly from the tooth after the instrument is inserted. Special care should be taken around line angles and proximal surfaces when instruments have two cutting edges. Care must be taken to disengage the cutting edge adjacent to the gingival sulcus. To disengage this cutting edge, the terminal shank should be tilted toward the proximal tooth surface that is being scaled.

The tip of powered instruments is inserted gently beneath the gingiva, adapted to the tooth surface, and activated. The tip also can be placed supragingivally, then gently guided subgingivally as the tip is activated. The tip never remains for more than a second in any given location because energy from the number of vibrations or cycles per second generated by the tip may cause heat and result in tooth damage and sensitivity.

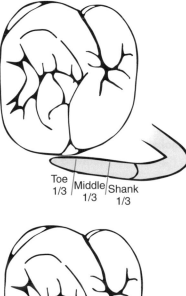

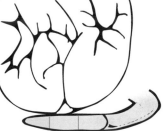

Toe 1/3 | Middle 1/3 | Shank 1/3

FIGURE 9-34
The toe one third of the cutting edge should be adapted to the tooth surface. When adapting the toe one third, the middle and heel thirds are not touching the tooth surface. These surfaces are rotated away from the tooth. When the middle or heel one third is adapted to the tooth surface, the toe one third is not against the tooth, which would result in trauma to the gingiva.

ACTIVATION

9-3

Activation is divided into exploratory strokes and working strokes. Exploratory strokes are used to detect calculus and root irregularities. These strokes are used intermittently with scaling

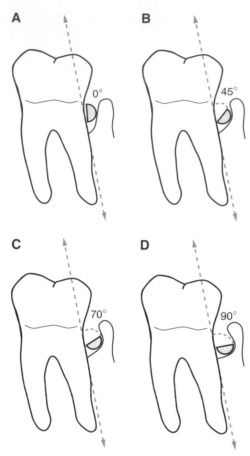

FIGURE 9-35
Angulation. **A,** Insertion angle of close to 0 degrees is ideal for initial blade placement before activation. **B,** A 45-degree cutting edge to tooth angulation is too close to remove calculus effectively (with burnishing most likely to occur). **C,** A 70-degree cutting edge to tooth angulation is ideal for debridement. **D,** A 90-degree cutting edge to tooth angulation is too open with the potential of damage to the adjacent tissue. The terminal shank is noted as the cutting edge to the tooth angle is increased.

> **Note**
> Instrument activation is defined as a single unbroken movement made by an instrument.

> **Lateral Pressure**
> The pressure the clinician exerts on the instrument with the thumb and index finger while pushing with the fulcrum finger determines the firmness of the instrument grasp, known as **lateral pressure,** which varies with the type of stroke used.

instruments or continually with explorers and probes. Exploratory strokes are light and long, covering the entire root surface. Work-scaling strokes for calculus removal are firm, short, and controlled, whereas root-planing strokes are not as firm and are longer. Scaling strokes are used on the enamel and root surface for the removal of plaque biofilm and calculus, and root-planing strokes are used only on the root surface for debridement of residual calculus deposits and for the removal of plaque biofilm and endotoxins.

Root-planing strokes are designed to smooth the root surface and follow scaling strokes. The instrument grasp is light when exploratory strokes are used, a bit firmer for root-planing strokes, and very firm for scaling strokes.

Proper pressure is necessary to ensure that calculus is efficiently removed without removing an excess amount of cementum and dentin.

Calculus should not be removed in layers because it burnishes the deposit into the root surface. **Burnished calculus** is difficult to remove and can prevent complete tissue healing.

Stroke direction in relationship to the long axis of the tooth can be **vertical, oblique,** or horizontal. Vertical and oblique strokes are predominantly used with vertical strokes frequently used on the proximal surfaces of

> **Note**
> If too much pressure is used, then the root surface can become gouged. If too little pressure is used, then the instrument will slide over the calculus deposit.

the tooth or root and oblique strokes used mainly on facial and lingual surfaces of the tooth or root (Figure 9-36). The toe one third of the instrument is adapted to the tooth surface, and the instrument is pulled by the action of the lateral movement of the wrist and forearm rock. Certain circumstances require a horizontal (circumferential) stroke direction. Some mandibular anterior teeth are extremely narrow, prohibiting proper adaptation of the instrument working end (Figure 9-37). These strokes are also used on line angles of posterior teeth because of the lack of proper adaptability (Figure 9-38). **Circumferential** strokes must be used with care to prevent damage to the epithelial

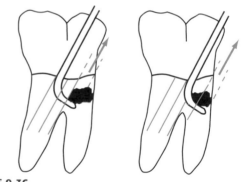

FIGURE 9-36
Once the cutting edge is engaged at the proper angle to the tooth, vertical or oblique overlapping strokes can be used for debridement.

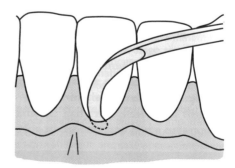

FIGURE 9-37
Debridement strokes in a horizontal (circumferential) direction are used in areas where vertical or oblique strokes are ineffective. Horizontal strokes work well on the facial and lingual surfaces of mandibular anterior teeth because of their narrow shape.

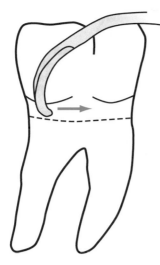

FIGURE 9-38
Strokes in a horizontal direction also are used on line angles of posterior teeth.

attachment. To accomplish this stroke, the toe is inserted into the sulcus at a 90-degree angle to the epithelium. Short, controlled strokes are used in a horizontal direction. This stroke direction requires more finger motion than wrist and forearm motion and should be used in limited situations.

Various types of strokes are used with different instruments. A pull stroke is the common stroke type used for scaling instruments to remove calculus, although some instruments require the push stroke for calculus removal. A combined push-pull stroke that is equally light in pressure is used with the explorer in an exploratory stroke around the tooth. The walking stroke is used with the periodontal probe to walk the instrument along the junctional epithelium.

Stroke, or instrument movement, with a powered instrument consists of short, rapid instrument movement against the surface being debrided. Lateral pressure is not needed, and the instrument is never held in one place for more than 1 second—usually less than a full second.

TYPES OF STROKES

Exploratory, scaling, and root-planing strokes are used intermittently throughout the procedure with manual instruments. Strokes are not differentiated when a powered instrument is used. Initial instrument insertion and adaptation with manual instruments are exploratory in nature with a light grasp. Once calculus is detected, the grasp becomes firm, and the working stroke is activated. Clinicians can achieve a firm grasp by squeezing the instrument between the thumb, index and middle fingers while pushing down on the fulcrum finger. Stroke activation occurs with the lateral movement of the wrist and forearm with an occasional pivot of the fulcrum finger. The working stroke is either vertical or oblique in a coronal direction.

Calculus is easier to remove in segments rather than in an attempt to remove the entire deposit at once or to shave it in layers. Once the calculus is identified by location and size, the deposit should be mentally divided into sections. The goal is to remove the entire deposit one section at a time (a process known as *channel* or *zone scaling*)[3,4] (see Figure 9-36). This technique is critical in the interproximal area. The toe one third of the cutting edge is directed beneath the contact area and interdental papilla to provide complete coverage of the proximal tooth surface. Overlapping the scaling strokes on the proximal surfaces occurs from the facial and lingual aspects during instrumentation.

When the working stroke is completed, the clinician uses an exploratory stroke to determine the texture of the root and to ensure complete calculus removal. If the entire deposit is removed and the root surface feels rough, then the clinician initiates root-planing strokes. These strokes require a firm grasp that is not as firm as the scaling grasp. The root-planing stroke is activated by the same means as the scaling stroke; however, the strokes are more numerous, longer, push-pull, and lighter in nature than the scaling stroke. Once all zones of the root surface have been scaled and/or root-planed, and the clinician determines the root is smooth, the next tooth is treated in a similar pattern.

Certain situations occur when the exploratory stroke is the only necessary stroke on a tooth surface. If the clinician uses a scaling instrument to explore a tooth surface for calculus and finds none, then the scaling stroke is not needed. Subgingival surfaces of all teeth should be approached in some way. Scaling instruments should be used with an exploratory stroke or a combination of exploratory, scaling, and root-planing strokes. When only exploratory strokes are used, the clinician is removing plaque biofilm from the gingival sulcus to disrupt plaque biofilm that may have formed between appointments. This instrumentation is the minimal amount required for all patients.

References

1. Glenner RA: Scaler, *Bull Hist Dent* 38(1):31-33, 1990.
2. Hoi D, Barr A, Loomer P, et al: The effects of finger rest positions on hand muscle load and pinch force in simulated dental hygiene work, *J Dent Educ* 69(4):453-460, 2005.
3. Nield-Gehrig JS: *Fundamentals of periodontal instrumentation*, ed 5, Philadelphia, 2004, Williams & Wilkins.
4. Pattison AM, Pattison GL: *Periodontal instrumentation*, ed 2, East Norwalk, Conn, 1992, Appleton & Lange.
5. Schmidt CR: Task analysis of the Nevi 1 and Nevi 2 periodontal instruments, *J Pract Hyg* 11(3):15-20, 2002.

Instrument Sharpening

Mary Kaye Scaramucci

INSIGHT

Instrument sharpening techniques, critical to successful instrumentation, are often learned early in the dental hygiene curriculum. Unfortunately, many dental hygiene students hold the misconception that they will never have to sharpen an instrument in private practice! Eventually, every dental hygienist realizes that maintaining sharp instruments will ultimately make hand-scaling procedures more effective and efficient. In 1908, G.V. Black recognized the effectiveness of sharp instruments; his thoughts are reinforced daily in dental hygiene practice. Simply stated, periodontal debridement cannot be accomplished with dull instruments. Learning proper sharpening techniques early and developing good, consistent sharpening procedures will keep instruments sharp and ready for the procedures to be performed.

CASE STUDY 10-1   Disadvantages of Using a Dull Instrument

A student is debriding quadrant 1 of a patient classified as a periodontal case type II. She is having difficulty removing calculus deposits from the distal surfaces of teeth #2 and #3. The student is correctly following the principles of instrumentation, yet the deposits cannot be removed. Further observation of the instrument under a bright light reveals a definite reflection of light along the cutting edge of the instrument.

KEY TERMS

acrylic test stick	burnished calculus	Mandrel-mounted stones	slow-speed hand piece
angles	cutting edge	parallel	sludge
Arkansas stone	honing machine	perpendicular	wire edges
beveled edges	India stone	rounded edges	

LEARNING OUTCOMES

After reading this chapter the student will be able to:

1. Value the need for sharp instruments and demonstrate sharpening as indicated by the criteria in this chapter.
2. Compare and contrast the various types of sharpening methods and equipment.
3. Compare and contrast the variety of handheld stones available for sharpening.
4. Explain the rationale in selecting particular sharpening stones.
5. Select an appropriate sharpening method for instrument design, and explain the rationale for the selection.
6. Debate the pros and cons of the sharpening techniques that remove metal from the lateral sides of the working end or from the face of the blade.
7. Explain the rationale used to learn the stationary instrument–moving stone technique over the moving instrument–stationary stone technique.
8. Explain the care and maintenance of all varieties of sharpening stones.
9. Demonstrate the steps used to sharpen each of the following instruments: sickles with flame-shaped cutting edges, sickles with straight cutting edges, Gracey curets, universal curets, hoe scalers, disk scalers, files, and explorers.

In 1908, G.V. Black said[13]:

> Nothing in the technical procedures of dental practice is more important than the care of the cutting edges of instruments. No man has ever yet become a good and efficient dentist until after he had learned to keep his cutting edges sharp.

This statement is as applicable today to the practice of dental hygiene as it was in 1908. It takes the clinician only a few strokes with a dull instrument to appreciate the clinical benefits of a well-maintained, properly sharpened dental instrument.

This chapter discusses the following:
- Goals of sharpening, with an explanation of the various sharpening devices available and equipment needed
- Importance of maintaining sharp instruments and the original designs
- Skills necessary to master the sharpening procedure

Sharpening dental instruments requires an understanding of the parts of the instrument, the **angles** of the working end, and precise principles of sharpening.

Goals for Maintenance of Sharp Instruments

Instrument sharpening is a critical component of the periodontal debridement process. Simply stated, periodontal debridement cannot be accomplished with dull instruments. The goals of instrument sharpening are the following:
- To produce a functionally sharp edge
- To preserve the shape (contour) of the instrument
- To maintain the useful life of the instrument

To achieve these goals, the clinician should have a precise understanding of the design features of each instrument before learning the sharpening technique. A review of instrument design in Chapter 9 is essential.

The union of the lateral side and face forms the cutting edge of a scaler and curet (Figure 10-1, *A*). The sharp cutting edge is the most exact meeting of the lateral side and face. Undesirable **wire edges** are unsupported metal fragments extending beyond the cutting edge from the lateral side or face of the blade. **Rounded edges** that began as sharp edges but are dulled through use or overuse are also undesirable, as are **beveled edges,** which are cutting edges created beneath the original cutting edge by improper stone-to-instrument placement.

Ideally, the internal angle formed by the juncture of the face and lateral sides is 85 degrees and should be maintained throughout the sharpening procedure. A deviation of the stone-to-instrument placement of only 5 degrees can alter the ideal internal angle, which renders the instrument less functional. Little room exists for error in the maintenance of an effective cutting edge.

The desired outcome of an accurate sharpening technique is to remove a minimal amount of metal from the instrument blade to reestablish the fine cutting edge while maintaining the original shape of the instrument.[18] Maintaining the original shape of the instrument is as important as maintaining a sharp edge. Volumes of research, care, and time are incorporated into the design of instruments to produce effective and safe instruments for debridement. To change the original shape of an instrument by a poor sharpening technique is to create an opportunity for ineffective treatment and potential harm to the patient.

Maintaining the sharpness of periodontal instruments has many advantages (Box 10-1). Properly sharpened instruments reduce operator fatigue, improve calculus removal, save time, enhance tactile sensitivity, and minimize patient discomfort. Sharp instruments improve

BOX 10-1

ADVANTAGES OF SHARP INSTRUMENTS

Improved tactile sensations
Increased efficiency of deposit removal
Less pressure required for deposit removal
Improved instrument control
Less root gouging
Decreased burnished calculus
Minimized patient discomfort

A

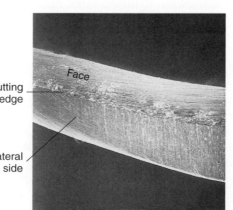

B

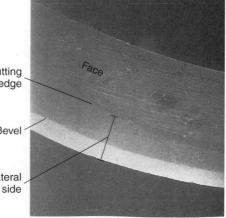

FIGURE 10-1
A, Scanning electron micrograph shows the junction of the face and lateral side of a curet, which forms the cutting edge. **B,** Scanning electron micrograph shows a bevel on the lateral side of the curet, resulting from incorrect sharpening technique.

the tactile sensations transmitted through the instrument, and the clinician's detection skills are increased because the instrument does not need to be held in a tight grasp. Scaling efficiency is increased because sharp instruments remove calculus easier by requiring fewer instrumentation strokes than needed with dull instruments. Sharp instruments save time and lessen operator fatigue. Less pressure is required with sharp instruments, which improves control of the instrument and decreases the likelihood of gouging a root surface.

✸ CASE APPLICATION 10-1.1

Problems Removing Deposits
The student was having difficulty removing deposits. What other problems was this student likely to experience?

In addition, sharp instruments decrease the probability of burnishing calculus by *biting* into the deposit and not shaving over it. **Burnished calculus** is calculus that is not completely removed, most often because of a dull or improperly sharpened instrument. When a deposit is smoothed but not completely removed, it continues to harbor plaque biofilm and builds new calculus more readily. Burnished calculus is many times more difficult to detect and remove than nonburnished deposits.

Most importantly, sharp instruments minimize patient discomfort. When dull instruments are used, the operator grasp is tighter and more lateral pressure is applied to the tooth surface. This increase in pressure is uncomfortable to the patient and makes the clinician seem heavy handed. The tighter grasp also makes it easier for the instrument to slip off the tooth surface, increasing the likelihood of trauma to the surrounding tissue.[15] The clinician cannot hope to attain clinical excellence without mastering the skill of instrument sharpening.

Sharpening Needs

Unlike other equipment maintenance procedures, no standard timeline exists for instrument sharpening. The clinician cannot set a specific schedule of instrument sharpening; for example, every Monday morning.

Considerations as to the best time to sharpen instruments include the number of patients scheduled for the day, frequency of use, degree of patient difficulty, and type of procedure to be completed. To lessen the chance of contamination with nonsterile instruments, sharpening should occur after sterilization.

> *Note*
>
> Instruments should be sharpened before every scaling and root-planing procedure or whenever the instruments become dull during treatment.

Dulling of the fine, sharp edge is a normal outcome of scaling and root planing. Approximately 15 working strokes produce a slightly rounded cutting edge, whereas 45 strokes create a very rounded cutting edge.[2,5] Ideally, instruments should be sharpened at the first sign of dullness.[7,19-21]

Manufacturers are now producing instruments that stay sharper longer. Newer stainless steel alloys and heat treatment processes create a more durable edge that can maintain sharpness for up to 3 to 4 months. Diamond coated technolgoy is another type of instrument that maintains a sharp edge for years. These instruments cannot be resharpened and, therefore, must be replaced.

Testing Sharpness

A sharp cutting edge appears as a line having no shape or width. A dull cutting edge has a wide, rounded shape. When light is directed on a dull cutting edge, it reflects the light and appears shiny.

> *Note*
>
> The relative sharpness of an instrument can be determined by a visual or tactile test.

✸ CASE APPLICATION 10-1.2

Sharpness of Cutting Edge
The cutting edge of the student's instrument reflected light. A sharp cutting edge having no width cannot reflect light and has a lackluster appearance (Figure 10-2, *A*; see also Figure 10-1, *A*).

The tactile test for sharpness uses an **acrylic test stick.** The instrument is held in the dominant hand with a modified pen grasp while the test rod is held in the nondominant hand. A fulcrum should be established either on top of the test stick or on the side (Figure 10-3). Following the principles of instrumentation for activation, the clinician should press the cutting edge of an instrument into the stick. If the instrument catches or cuts making a *pinging sound* into the acrylic, the instrument is sharp. When the instrument glides over the stick, the instrument is considered dull. Care must be taken to examine or test the entire length of the cutting edge to ensure sharpness.

Sharpening Technique

The sharpening technique uses the grinding of a coarse stone against the instrument to create a sharp edge. The following three different hand-sharpening methods result in sharp instruments:

1. Reducing the face of the blade
2. Reducing the lateral surface to create a sharp edge through movement of a sharpening stone against a stationary cutting edge
3. Moving the instrument against a stationary sharpening stone

The first method, reducing the face of the blade, creates a weaker instrument that will, in turn, break more readily.* Either the stationary stone or the stationary instrument method of sharpening produces a wire edge that may interfere with the

---

*References 2, 6-8, 13.

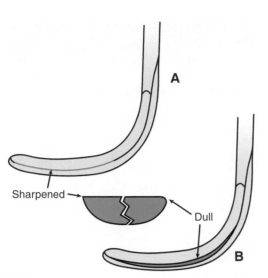

FIGURE 10-2
A, A sharp cutting edge does not reflect light. **B,** A dull cutting edge appears as a bright area at the junction of the face and lateral surface.

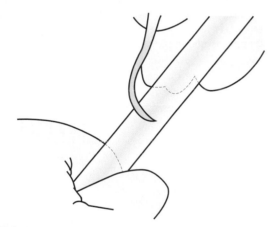

FIGURE 10-3
Acrylic test stick is used through the application of light pressure against the stick with the instrument at its working angle.

sharp edge of the blade. Researchers indicate that the direction of the wire edge may have a profound effect on the quality of sharpness.[1,2,4]

Wire edges are unsupported metal fragments that extend beyond the cutting edge from the lateral side or the face of the blade. They are termed *functional* or *nonfunctional*. Studies have indicated that when the wire edge is **parallel** to the scaling direction, the edge is considered functional. A functional wire edge does not gouge into the tooth surface; it *digs in* to the tooth deposit. Therefore it helps remove accretions and does not damage the tooth. Grinding against the lateral sides produces functional wire edges.[1,2,4]

A nonfunctional wire edge is a metal fragment that is **perpendicular** to the scaling direction and is produced when the instrument is sharpened from the face of the blade. Nonfunctional wire edges produce gouging on the root surface and do

not aid in the removal of accretions from the tooth,[1,2,4] thus establishing a second reason for sharpening the lateral surfaces of an instrument.

Devices Used to Sharpen Instruments
MECHANICAL

A **honing machine** is an example of a mechanical sharpening device. This bench-type piece of equipment follows the principles of instrument preservation. Specially designed honing disks are mounted on top of the machine, and a sharpening guide positions the instrument according to the instrument classification. The stones are mechanically rotated as the working end is pressed against the stone. The disk rotates up to a powerful 7000 rpm. This device removes metal from the face of the blade, and the clinician controls the pressure.

The honing machine rapidly sharpens instruments, thus saving time. However, if the clinician is inexperienced and not confident in instrument positioning and the application of pressure, then the instrument can be quickly ruined. In addition, although sharpening guides assist with the proper angulation of instrument to stone, the device sharpens so quickly that the gentle curve of the Gracey or the flame shape of some sickles is lost.

A battery-operated device (Figure 10-4) using ceramic stones is another example of a mechanical sharpening apparatus. This sharpener contains an instrument guide channel and vertical backstop to control the blade angulation. A template is provided to sharpen sickles and universal curets and a separate template is available to sharpen Gracey curets. In addition, it has a toe guide to maintain the roundness of curet toes. Although this device removes metal from the lateral side of the working end, the clinician must be careful in maintaining the contour of curved working ends.

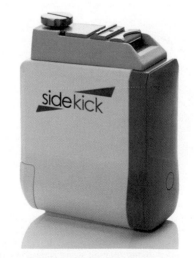

FIGURE 10-4
Battery-operated sharpening device, which removes metal from the lateral side of the blade. (Courtesy Hu-Friedy Manufacturing Company Inc., Chicago.)

MOUNTED STONES

Mandrel-mounted stones (Figure 10-5) are used with a **slow-speed hand piece.** The attached stones are cylindrical in shape with either a flat or a cone-shaped end. Most common mounted stones are **Arkansas stone** and Ruby stone. The rotating stone should be larger than the diameter of the instrument blade to be sharpened. While the hand piece is activated at a slow speed, the stone is passed over the face of the blade to sharpen both cutting edges at once. This method requires stabilization of the instrument in one hand and the hand piece in the other. Again, if the clinician is inexperienced with the application of pressure, then too much of the face of the blade might be quickly removed, rendering the instrument useless.

HANDHELD STONES

Handheld stones are a common tool for instrument sharpening. These stones are available in a variety of shapes and materials. Stones can be rectangular and flat, rectangular and wedge-shaped, or cylindrical (Figure 10-6). Although no one stone shape is superior, the flat stone is ideal for the moving instrument technique and the cylindrical stone is efficient in removing wire edges. The wedge-shaped stone contains a rounded side that can be used like the cylindrical stone to remove wire edges, thus serving as an all-purpose stone. Newer designs include a channel-shaped stone system (Figure 10-7). These stones are designed with a trough in which the instrument is placed and then moved through the trough. The channel-shaped system has been shown to produce a smoother cutting edge with fewer wire edges.[10]

Stone types vary from natural, quarried from natural mineral deposits (Arkansas stone), to synthetic (manufactured). Texture varies from fine to medium to coarse. Selection of type and texture is based on the extent to which the cutting edge needs sharpening or recontouring. Sharpening stones are made

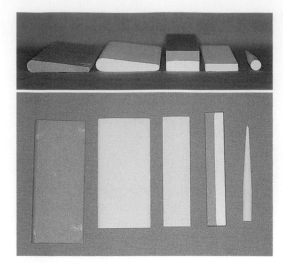
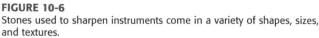

FIGURE 10-6
Stones used to sharpen instruments come in a variety of shapes, sizes, and textures.

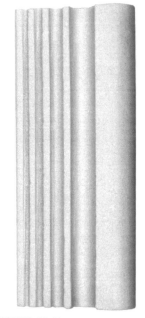

FIGURE 10-7
A channel-shaped stone contains a trough in which the instrument is placed for sharpening. (Courtesy Hu-Friedy Manufacturing Company Inc., Chicago.)

of abrasive particles that are harder than the surface of the instrument to be sharpened. Coarse stones have large particles and quickly remove metal from the instrument. Fine stones have small particles and remove less material from the instrument. If instruments are excessively dull or require a great deal of recontouring, then a coarse stone (**India stone**) is recommended. A fine or medium (Arkansas) stone is preferred for routine sharpening and instrument finishing and has been shown to produce a quality edge.[11] A chart that compares sharpening stones helps in selecting the appropriate stone (Table 10-1).

Stone Care

Stones should be lubricated as specified by the manufacturer before use. Stones require either water or oil as a lubricant, and the two lubricants should never be interchanged.[7] The lubricant is used to reduce heat resulting from friction, to prevent metal particles from embedding in the stone, and to prevent dryness.[3,7] Cleaning the stone should also be based on the manufacturer's guidelines, especially with an artificial stone. Natural stones can be cleaned with soap and water or abrasive emery

> *Note*
> Handheld stones require care to maintain their longevity.

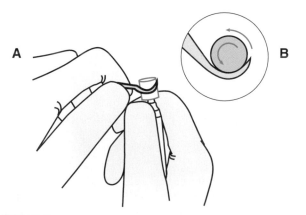

FIGURE 10-5
Mandrel-mounted stones. **A,** A mounted stone with a diameter appropriate for the curved blade to be sharpened is positioned across the face for even sharpening of the cutting edges. **B,** With low speed to minimize heat production, the rotating stone is passed along the face of the instrument. Near the toe, the stone is moved upward to prevent flattening of a curved instrument.

Table 10-1	Sharpening Stone Comparison Chart				
NAME	**ORIGIN**	**METHOD**	**LUBRICANT**	**TEXTURE**	**APPLICATION**
Arkansas Stone	Natural	Unmounted, mounted, or rotary	Oil	Fine	Routine sharpening and finishing
India Stone	Synthetic	Unmounted	Water or oil	Medium	Sharpening of excessively dull instruments or those requiring recontouring
Ceramic Stone	Synthetic	Unmounted	Water or dry	Fine	Routine sharpening and finishing
Composition Stone	Synthetic	Mounted	Water	Coarse	Reshaping of excessively worn instruments

Courtesy Hu-Friedy Manufacturing Company, Inc., Chicago.

paper. Sharpening stones should be cleaned, properly packaged, and sterilized with every use. Stones lubricated with oil should be wrapped in a gauze square to absorb excess oil during sterilization. Some manufacturers require lubrication before sterilization. To maintain the useful life of the stone, sharpening should not be limited to one area of the stone. Using the entire stone's surface can prevent grooves from forming in the stone.

Workstation and Equipment

Ideal conditions for a sharpening workstation include a firm countertop to support the instruments and a light source such as the dental light or a high-intensity lamp. A magnifying glass is helpful to observe wire edges, but it is not necessary. An armamentarium for instrument sharpening should consist of the following (Figure 10-8):

- Fine stone
- Medium-to-coarse stone
- Conical stone
- Sharpening file for sharpening periodontal files
- Gauze for removing **sludge,** which is debris created by metal particles and lubricant during sharpening
- Personal protective equipment (PPE), including eye protection, mask, and examination gloves

Ideally, instruments should be sharpened when sterile, before the beginning of the appointment. When sharpening is necessary during patient treatment, all sharpening armamentaria must be sterile. In addition, sharpening should always be completed with the appropriate work-practice controls in place, including PPE, a solid work surface, and an appropriate light source (Box 10-2).

Note

Sharpening should be performed at the first sign of dullness, which means a sharpening workstation needs to be incorporated into the dental hygiene treatment room.

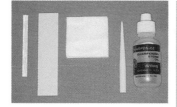

FIGURE 10-8
Supplies used for instrument sharpening *(left to right):* Cylindrical sharpening stone, rectangular Arkansas stone, cotton gauze, acrylic test stick, and lubricating oil.

BOX 10-2

SHARPENING ARMAMENTARIUM

Light source
Stable work surface
Magnification
Sharpening stones
Test stick or rod
Gauze
PPE (e.g., eye protection, examination gloves, mask)

Manual Sharpening Methods

Two methods of instrument sharpening with handheld stones can be used. In the first method of manual sharpening, the sharpening stone is placed in a stationary position and the instrument is moved across the surface of the stone. In the second method, the instrument is held in a stationary position and the sharpening stone is moved against the instrument. Although these techniques vary significantly in visibility and control, both methods require skill, visual acuity, control, and precision to master. Researchers have discovered that when students use the stationary instrument–moving stone method, effective sharpening is accomplished.[8] This method permits the clinician to see the shape of the face of the blade, an important feature because the method reduces the width of the instrument blade. Therefore instruments can be more evenly contoured to provide a better fit subgingivally without significantly reducing the instrument strength.[5] The following text discusses the stationary instrument–moving stone technique.

Note

Two methods of instrument sharpening with handheld stones can be used.

10-1 to 10-4

STATIONARY INSTRUMENT–MOVING STONE TECHNIQUE

The following steps are useful for sharpening:

- *Select* the appropriate stone for the type of instrument to be used and the degree of dullness.
- *Lubricate* the stone, based on the manufacturer's suggestions. Apply small drops of oil or water, and rub it into the flat surfaces of the stone.
- *Grasp* the instrument to be sharpened in a palm grasp or modified pen grasp with the nondominant hand, and place the hand against the countertop (Figure 10-9).
- *Rest* the hand holding the instrument on the tabletop and the instrument handle against the edge of the countertop (Figure 10-10). If the instrument is not stabilized against

a hard stationary surface, then it may move slightly during the sharpening process, and the stone will not be correctly or consistently drawn across the blade.

- *Point* the toe of the instrument toward the clinician, and place the face of the blade parallel to the floor. The instrument should be held low enough for the clinician to be able to look down on the face to visualize the contour (Figure 10-11).
- *Hold* the stone in the dominant hand. If a wedge-shaped stone is being used, then the wedge should be directed toward the clinician. The stone can be held in two ways; both require the stone to be held lengthwise. Method 1 involves grasping of the stone at either end with the thumb on top and the fingers on the bottom (Figure 10-12). Method 2 is similar to a palm grasp in which the stone is grasped near the bottom (see Figure 10-10, *A*). If a rectangular flat stone is used, then it can be grasped from the sides (see Figure 10-10, *A).*

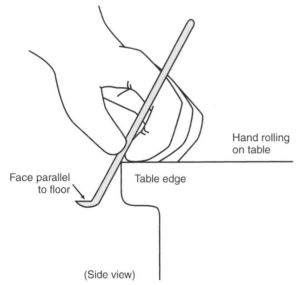

FIGURE 10-9
While the hand is braced against the tabletop, the instrument handle is secured against the edge of the tabletop.

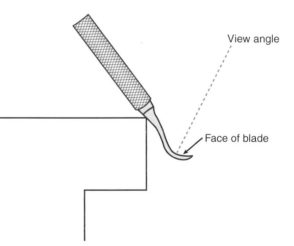

FIGURE 10-11
Through bracing of the instrument against the edge of the tabletop, the instrument is positioned for a clear view of the face of the blade.

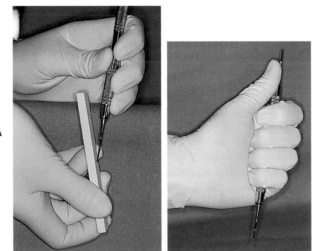

FIGURE 10-10
A, Instrument is held in the nondominant hand. This grasp is the modified pen grasp with the bottom of the hand braced against the tabletop. **B,** Instrument is held in the nondominant hand with a palm grasp. Again, the hand should be braced against the tabletop.

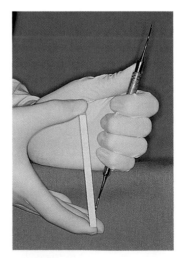

FIGURE 10-12
The stone is grasped in the dominant hand in a palm grasp with the thumb on the top and the fingers on the bottom.

- *Position* the stone on the lateral side of the instrument, near the heel of the working end at a 90-degree angle to the face of the blade (Figure 10-13).
- *Move* the stone from the 90-degree position to 100 to 110 degrees (Figure 10-14).
- *Begin* the sharpening motion on a downstroke, moving the stone down and up while maintaining the 100- to 110-degree angulation. The downstroke should consist of firm pressure, whereas the upstroke should be lighter.
- *Continue* the down-up motion, following the contour of the cutting edge until the toe is reached (Figure 10-15).
- *Stop* the sharpening procedure on a downstroke to reduce the chance of creating a wire edge.
- *Reposition* the stone on the lateral side of the opposite cutting edge of the instrument near the heel at a 90-degree angle (Figure 10-16).
- *Move* the stone away to a 100- to 110-degree angle from the face of the blade.

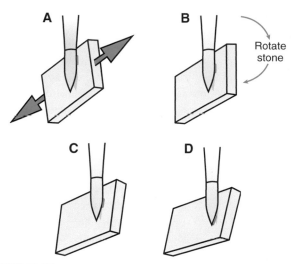

FIGURE 10-15
A, Beginning at the heel of the working end, the stone is inched around the cutting edge, following the contour (**B** and **C**). **D,** The sharpening stroke is completed on a downstroke when the stone is placed against the toe of the working end.

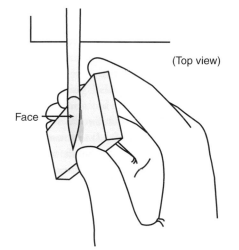

FIGURE 10-13
If the stone is not wedge shaped, then it can be grasped in a modified palm grasp with the thumb on the lateral surface toward clinician and the fingers on the opposite lateral surface.

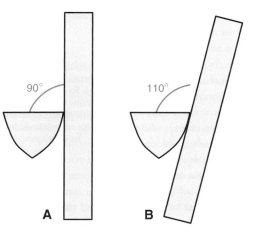

FIGURE 10-14
A, Stone at initial placement set-up at 90 degrees to the face of the blade. **B,** Stone at sharpening activation placement of 110 degrees to the face of the blade.

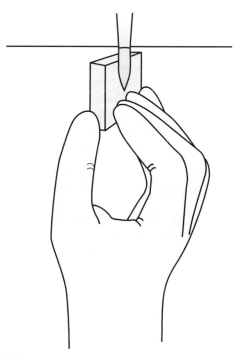

FIGURE 10-16
Grasping the stone in the dominant hand, the clinician positions it against the heel of the left side of the working end.

- *Follow* the sharpening steps as previously described to sharpen the opposite cutting edge.
- When sharpening is completed, *examine* the cutting edge for wire edges. Wire edges, whether functional or nonfunctional, should be removed because they do not wholly contribute to the cutting ability of the instrument.
- To remove a wire edge, use a conical-shaped stone. *Gently stroke* the stone along the face of the blade, maintaining a minimal amount of pressure (Figure 10-17).

- During the sharpening process, *observe* for a layer of sludge. Sludge occurs as a mixture of the lubricant and metal shavings accumulates on the face of the blade as the stone is drawn across the cutting edge. The appearance of sludge indicates that the correct stone-to–cutting edge angle is being maintained.[14]
- *Wipe* the sludge from the instrument, using a gauze square.
- *Test* the instrument for sharpness, using an acrylic test stick or visual inspection.

Many students who are beginning to learn the sharpening technique have difficulty visualizing the stone-to-instrument angles necessary for proper sharpening. Because sharpening must be precise to maintain the contour and cutting edge of scaling instruments, an angle guide may be helpful to students. Research has indicated that angle guides enhance the clinician's ability for precise sharpening.[9]

> **Note**
> The entire procedure should include approximately four to five stroke sequences, and the down-up movement of the stone should be ½ to 1 inch in length.

Many commercial angle guides are available; however, a guide can be made with a note card and protractor:

- Draw a 90-degree vertical line in the middle of a 3- × 5-inch note card.
- With a protractor, draw another line to the left of the center line to represent 110 degrees and another line to the right of the center to represent 110 degrees.
- The center line is used for instrument placement and initial stone placement; the right and left angle lines represent stone angulation for sharpening. The face of the working end should be perpendicular to the center line.
- The guide can be taped to the front edge of the countertop, or it can be folded over the edge to serve as a guide. A piece of masking tape can be placed on either side of the 110-degree line to further enhance stone positioning[9] (Figure 10-18). In addition, the guide can be laminated and disinfected for use during patient treatment.

Specific Instruments

Chapter 9 reviews the basic design of each instrument.

SICKLES

Sickle scalers have two cutting edges and a pointed tip. The shape and contour of the face of the blade and cutting edges should be examined. The majority of sickles have a flame-shaped contour, which means the cutting edges are not straight but gently curved from heel to toe. However, some sickles, particularly those called *jacquettes,* may be triangular in contour. When sickle scalers are flame shaped, the entire cutting edge cannot be placed against the sharpening stone. The stone should be positioned at the heel portion of the working end and then rotated along the cutting edge until the stone is flat against the side of the tip (see Figure 10-15). If the sickle is triangular in design with straight cutting edges, then the entire cutting edge can be sharpened at one time; in other words, the stone can be placed along the entire cutting edge, and the instrument can be sharpened all at once. Box 10-3 shows the steps necessary to sharpen sickle scalers.

> **Note**
> A helpful tip for stone movement along the cutting edge is to place a 1-inch-diameter dot with a pencil in the middle of the stone. When the stone is positioned against the heel of the instrument, the dot should be against the heel. As the stone is moved forward, the dot always should remain in contact with the cutting edge (Figure 10-19).

AREA-SPECIFIC CURETS

Area-specific curets, such as the Gracey curets, have two edges and a rounded toe; however, only one cutting edge is used for instrumentation. When the terminal shank of a Gracey curet is perpendicular to the floor, the face of the blade is angled or *offset* from the shank to create upper and lower cutting edges. This offset cutting edge gives the Gracey curets area-specific use. The most important step in sharpening these curets is to determine the correct cutting

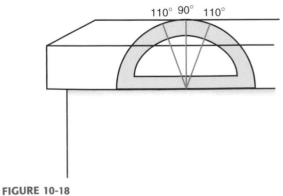

FIGURE 10-17
Tapered cylindrical stone is applied to the facial surface of the instrument to help remove wire edges.

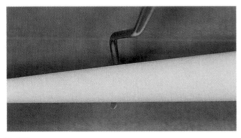

110° 90° 110°

FIGURE 10-18
An angle guide can assist the beginner in precise instrument-to-stone placement.

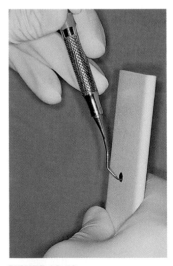

FIGURE 10-19
A dot can be applied to the center of the stone as a guide during the rotation of the stone along the cutting edge. As the stone moves forward, the dot is kept against the cutting edge.

BOX 10-3

TECHNIQUE USED TO SHARPEN SICKLE SCALERS

Flame-Shaped Sickle

1. Position the instrument in the nondominant hand.
2. Place the instrument handle against the countertop with the face of the blade parallel to the floor.
3. Place the sharpening stone in the dominant hand, and position it against the heel of the surface.
4. Angle the stone at 90 degrees to the face of the blade.
5. Move the stone away from the cutting edge to obtain a 110-degree angle to the face of the blade.
6. Activate the stone in a downward stroke that is ½ to 1 inch in length.
7. Follow the curvature of the blade with the sharpening stroke while using slight overlapping strokes.
8. Complete sharpening action on a downward stroke when the toe portion is flat against the stone.
9. Sharpen the opposite cutting edge in the same manner.
10. Clear wire edges with conical stone, and remove sludge with gauze.
11. Check instrument sharpness.

Triangular Sickle

1. Position the instrument in the nondominant hand.
2. Place the instrument handle against the countertop with the face of the blade parallel to the floor.
3. Place the sharpening stone in the dominant hand, and position it flat from heel to toe against the entire cutting surface.
4. Angle the stone at 90 degrees to the face of the blade.
5. Move the stone away from the cutting edge to obtain a 110-degree angle to the face of the blade.
6. Activate the stone in a downward stroke that is ½ to 1 inch in length.
7. Complete the sharpening action on a downstroke.
8. Sharpen the opposite cutting edge in the same manner.
9. Clear wire edges with conical stone, and remove sludge with gauze.
10. Check instrument sharpness.
11. Complete sharpening action on a downstroke when the side of the toe is flat against the stone.
12. Sharpen the opposite cutting edge in the same manner.
13. Clear wire edges with conical stone, and remove sludge with gauze.
14. Check instrument sharpness.

edge to be sharpened. The cutting edge used in instrumentation is the lower cutting edge. The upper edge is called the *nonworking edge* or the *trailing edge.* To position the instrument correctly for sharpening, the face of the blade must be placed parallel to the floor. The clinician should examine the angle of the face when the terminal shank is perpendicular to the floor and then determine whether the handle should be moved to the right or to the left to make the face of the blade parallel to the floor.

The sharpening stone should be placed at the heel of the blade and rotated along the cutting edge until the stone contacts the line angle of the toe (Figure 10-20). Placing a dot on the sharpening stone, a helpful tip with sickles, also may be used as a guide with the Gracey curet.

Occasional sharpening of the toe maintains the overall shape of the Gracey curet. Instead of stopping on a downstroke at the line angle of the toe, the clinician should continue the sharpening stroke, increasing the angle of the stone 15 to 25 degrees from the face of the blade as it is moved around the toe. The sharpening process is stopped on a downstroke once the line angle of the opposite side of the toe is reached (Figure 10-21). Pressure around the toe should be light because only the shape is being maintained; a cutting edge is not being created. Box 10-4 lists the steps used to sharpen area-specific curets.

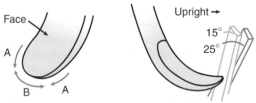

FIGURE 10-21
Sharpening the toe. The clinician lightly sharpens the toe by moving the stone around the corner of the toe. As the tip of the toe is reached, the stone-to-face angle is increased from 15 to 25 degrees.

UNIVERSAL CURETS

Universal curets have two usable and parallel cutting edges and a rounded toe. Unlike Gracey curets, both cutting edges of the universal curets must be sharpened. The cutting edges are straight from heel to toe; therefore the entire cutting edge can be placed against the sharpening stone (Figure 10-22). When rounding the toe, the clinician should lift the stone away from the heel of the blade and begin rotating around the toe (see

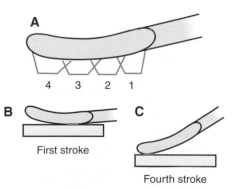

FIGURE 10-20
A, Four different adaptations of the stone are necessary to sharpen the entire surface. **B,** First stroke should start at the heel of the blade. **C,** Last stroke should end at the toe.

BOX 10-4

TECHNIQUE USED TO SHARPEN AREA-SPECIFIC CURETS

1. Position the instrument in the nondominant hand.
2. Place the instrument handle against the countertop with the face of the blade parallel to the floor. (The handle of the instrument must be angled to the right or left.)
3. Place the stone in the dominant hand, and position it against the heel of the blade at a 90-degree angle to the face of the blade; the anterior portion of the stone will not be in contact with the instrument.
4. Angle the stone away from the cutting edge to obtain a 110-degree angle to the face of the blade.
5. Use light pressure, beginning at the heel of the instrument, and activate the stone in a downstroke ½ to 1 inch in length.
6. Rotate the stone along its vertical axis as the stone is moved from heel to toe.
7. Follow the curvature of the blade with the sharpening stroke, while using slight overlapping strokes.
8. Complete sharpening action on a downstroke when the stone contacts the line angle of the toe.
9. Round the toe from the cutting edge every fourth or fifth sharpening.
10. Clear wire edges with conical stone, and remove sludge with gauze.
11. Check instrument sharpness.

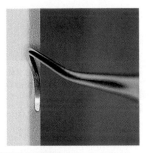

FIGURE 10-22
The stone is positioned at a 90-degree angle to the face of the blade with complete contact from the heel to the toe.

Figure 10-21). The toe of the universal curet must be rounded from both cutting edges. Rounding should stop at the toe-line angle opposite the cutting edge being sharpened. The steps necessary to sharpen the universal curet are outlined in Box 10-5.

A helpful tip that helps maintain instrument-to-stone contact is to draw a 1-inch vertical line with a pencil down the middle of the stone. The line is placed against the instrument to ensure that it is positioned in the middle of the working end. As the stone is moved up and down against the working end, the line should remain positioned in the center (Figure 10-23).

HOES

Hoe scalers have one straight cutting edge and a beveled toe. (The toe is flat and angled from the cutting edge.) When a hoe scaler is sharpened, the stone is placed on a countertop and the hoe is pulled across the stone. The instrument is held in the dominant hand with a modified pen grasp and a finger resting on the stone. The beveled working end should be placed flat against the stone with the handle of the instrument at an angle approximately 70 degrees to the stone and the working end at an angle approximately 45 degrees to the stone (Figure 10-24). The instrument is gently and evenly pulled across the length of the stone two to three times. Pressure should be exerted on the pull stroke. The instrument should be lifted from the stone at the conclusion of the pull stroke and placed on the stone again to perform another pull stroke. At the conclusion of the sharpening procedure, the stone is pulled over the corner angles to round the

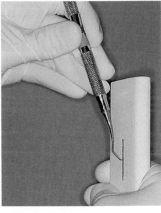

FIGURE 10-23
A straight line can be drawn down the center of the stone to serve as a guide for the universal curet. By keeping the line in contact with the cutting edge during sharpening, the clinician maintains correct stone-to-instrument contact.

BOX 10-5

TECHNIQUE USED TO SHARPEN UNIVERSAL CURETS

1. Position the instrument in the nondominant hand.
2. Place the instrument handle against the countertop with the face of the blade parallel to the floor.
3. Place the stone in the dominant hand, and position it against the entire length of the cutting edge of the instrument at a 90-degree angle to the face of the blade.
4. Move the stone away from the cutting edge to obtain a 110-degree angle to the face of the blade.
5. Using light pressure along the entire length of the cutting edge, activate the stone in a downstroke that is ½ to 1 inch in length.
6. Continue with downstrokes and upstrokes without moving the stone forward.
7. Complete sharpening action on a downstroke.
8. Sharpen the opposite cutting edge in the same manner.
9. Round the toe from both cutting edges once every fourth or fifth sharpening event.
10. Clear wire edges with conical stone, and remove sludge with gauze.
11. Check instrument sharpness.

sharp corners (Figure 10-25). The steps necessary to sharpen a hoe are listed in Box 10-6.

Because the disk has a cutting edge around the circumference of the working end, it needs to be sharpened with a special channel-shaped stone. The heel of the disk is placed at one end of the trough with the back against the wall. The disk is rotated on its axis to the opposite side as it is pulled through the trough in a pendulum-like action (Figure 10-26). This procedure is repeated as necessary to create a sharp edge.

FILES

Periodontal files are unique in that they have several cutting edges. A special sharpening file is needed to sharpen the rows of cutting edges on the file's working surface.[17] Figure 10-27 shows the technique used to sharpen a periodontal file. The sharpening file is placed in each of the V shapes formed by two cutting edges. The sharpening file is drawn back and forth across the edge of each row while the file is maintained within

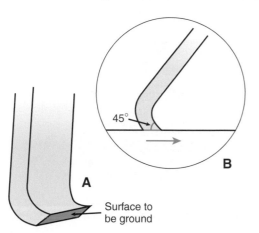

Figure 10-24
Sharpening hoe. **A,** The beveled toe is the surface to be ground. **B,** The bevel is placed flat against the stone. To maintain the angle of the bevel, the handle-to-stone angle should be approximately 70 degrees.

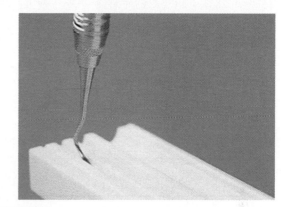

FIGURE 10-26
The disk is sharpened in a circumferential direction following a pendulum motion.

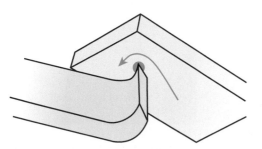

FIGURE 10-25
To round the corners of the hoe scaler, a flat stone is drawn over each end of the cutting edge with a gentle rolling motion.

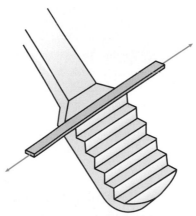

FIGURE 10-27
The tang file is positioned parallel along the entire length of the cutting edge. Each edge is individually sharpened.

BOX 10-6

TECHNIQUE USED TO SHARPEN HOES

1. Place the stone flat on the countertop.
2. Hold the instrument in the dominant hand, using the modified pen grasp with a finger rest on the stone.
3. Position the bevel flat against the stone. (The handle should be at an angle of approximately 70 degrees from the stone.)
4. Pull the hoe across the length of the stone two to three times, maintaining the 70-degree angle with the finger rest.
5. To round the corners, hold the stone in the dominant hand and the instrument in the nondominant hand with the beveled toe facing away.
6. Round the corner closest to the stone by pulling the stone over the corner angles from heel to toe.
7. Turn the instrument around so that the bevel is toward the clinician, and sharpen the opposite corner in the same manner by pulling the stone over the corner angle from heel to toe.
8. Remove sludge with gauze.
9. Check instrument sharpness.
10. Check for dullness at the corners by determining whether the corners glide over the test stick.

the area between the cutting edges. The clinician then moves the sharpening file to the next area and continues the process of sharpening the next cutting edge.

CHISELS

Although chisels are seldom used in modern instrumentation techniques, sharpening of the chisel is necessary to maintain a sharp cutting edge for the instrument's occasional use. Figure 10-28 demonstrates the technique used to sharpen a chisel. The stone is stationary, and the chisel bevel is placed on the stone and drawn across the stone to sharpen the cutting edge.

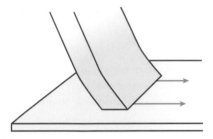

FIGURE 10-28
The chisel is adapted to the stone in the same manner as the hoe. An increase in the angle of the shank to the stone is noted. The handle is positioned at an 80-degree angle to the stone.

EXPLORERS

Explorers are sharpened to produce a sharper point or to recontour the working tip. Considering the current recommendations for detection of carious lesions, the need for a pinpoint on an explorer for caries detection is questionable (see Chapter 17). However, maintaining a sharp pinpoint aids in the detection of root surface irregularities and calculus deposits. To sharpen an explorer the clinician places the side of the tip against the stationary stone and, using light pressure, moves the instrument against the stone, away from the tip. The explorer tip is rotated slightly, and the process is repeated until all sides have been sharpened.

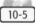

Common Technique Errors

> *Note*
>
> If the exact principles are not followed, then the shape and contour can be destroyed, rendering the instrument unusable.

The goal in instrument sharpening is to maintain the shape and contour of an instrument and, at the same time, to create a sharp cutting edge.

Common technique errors include the following:

- Sharpening beyond the pointed toe of a sickle shortens the overall length of the instrument (Figure 10-29).
- Flame-shaped or curved cutting edges can be flattened if the stone is not rotated along the cutting edge to maintain the correct contour (Figure 10-30).
- When the stone is not placed at the heel of the instrument, when the last downstroke is made with excess pressure, or when a longer-than-normal downstroke is made, gouging can occur along the cutting edge, creating an uneven edge (Figure 10-31).

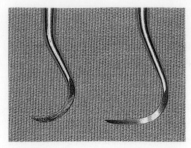

FIGURE 10-29
Sharpening can easily shorten sickle scalers, which changes the balance of the instrument.

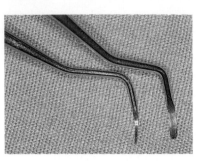

FIGURE 10-30
Poor contour of curet blades. The most common error in sharpening Gracey curets is failing to follow the contour of the cutting edge and sharpening a small portion of the edge with each downstroke. The contoured cutting edge loses its shape and becomes a straight cutting edge that no longer adapts to the root surface.

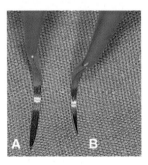

FIGURE 10-31
Sharpening was not started at the heel of the blade. Sickle blades must be sharpened entirely from heel to toe to preserve the contoured blade design. **A,** A new sickle with a distinct contour. **B,** A sickle blade that has been thinned at the center; its contoured shape is lost.

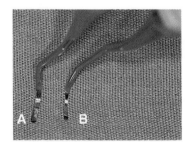

FIGURE 10-32
Rounding the toe of curets too often or not often enough. Universal curets can easily be thinned at the working end if the toe of the blade is not rounded. Many curets lose the rounded toe and look like sickles with pointed toes. **A,** New universal curet. **B,** Curet that has been thinned with a pointed toe.

- Rounding the toe of a curet too often or with too much pressure can shorten the overall length of the working end (Figure 10-32).

All these technique errors can render an instrument ineffective.

Care and Maintenance of a Sharpened Instrument

Unnecessary dullness of instruments is preventable. Instruments should not be overly crowded in an ultrasonic bath before sterilization because they can become dulled when instruments bump against each other.[19] Stainless steel instruments may be sterilized with saturated steam (250° F), chemical vapor (270° F), or dry heat (340° F) without dulling the cutting edges. However, saturated steam sterilization has a negative effect on carbon-steel instruments.[13]

When following the principles of instrumentation near the margin of an amalgam restoration or fabricated crown, the clinician should be aware that nicking the cutting edge or at least creating a dulling effect may easily occur on the instrument. Instruments that have become thin from continuous sharpening and use should be discarded to prevent breakage during debridement[16] (see Figures 10-31 and 10-32).

Instrument sharpening is an important procedure to maintain the usefulness of instruments and to remove deposits effectively from the teeth. Ideally, sharpening should be performed at the first sign of dullness. If the clinician is always prepared to sharpen instruments by keeping a sterile stone and test stick available during all patient treatment, then sharpening can be performed quickly and effectively.

References

1. Antonini CJ et al: Scanning electron microscope study of scalers, *J Periodontol* 48(1):45-48, 1977.
2. Balevi B: Engineering specifics of the periodontal curet's cutting edge, *J Periodontol* 67(4):374-378, 1996.
3. Claney P: Sharpening hand cutting instruments, *Dent Assist* 55(6):23-24, 1986.
4. Clark SM, Ueno H: An examination of periodontal curettes: an SEM study, *Gen Dent* 38(1):14-16, 1990.
5. Green E: *Sharpening curets and sickle scalers,* ed 2, Berkeley, 1972, Praxis.
6. Huang CC, Tseng CC: Effect of different sharpening stones on periodontal curettes evaluated by scanning electron microscopy, *J Formos Med Assoc* 90(8):782-787, 1991.
7. Hu-Friedy Department of Education: *Smarten up, sharpen up,* ed 2, Chicago, 1982, Hu-Friedy.
8. Marquam BJ: Strategies to improve instrument sharpening, *Dent Hyg* 62(7):334-338, 1988.
9. Mazzone DM: Quantitative evaluation of scaling instrument contour and sharpening techniques [master's thesis], Ann Arbor, Mich, 1983, University of Michigan.
10. Moses O et al: Scanning electron microscope evaluation of two methods of resharpening periodontal curets: a comparative study, *J Periodontol* 74(7):1032-1037, 2003.
11. Murray GH et al: The effects of two sharpening methods on the strength of a periodontal scaling instrument, *J Periodontol* 55(7):410-413, 1984.
12. Paquette OE, Levin MP: The sharpening of scaling instruments: I—an examination of principles, *J Periodontol* 48(3):163-168, 1977.
13. Paquette OE, Levin MP: The sharpening of scaling instruments: II—a preferred technique, *J Periodontol* 48(3):169-172, 1977.
14. Parkes RB, Kolstad RA: Effects of sterilization on periodontal instruments, *J Periodontol* 53(7):434-438, 1982.
15. Pattison AM, Pattison GL: *Periodontal instrumentation,* ed 2, East Norwalk, Conn, 1992, Appleton & Lange.
16. Perry DA et al: *Techniques and theory of periodontal instrumentation,* Philadelphia, 1990, WB Saunders.
17. Schoen DH, Dean MC: *Contemporary periodontal instrumentation,* Philadelphia, 1996, WB Saunders.
18. Smith BA et al: The effect of sharpening stones upon curet surface roughness, *Quintessence Int* 18(9):603-613, 1987.
19. Wilkins EM: *Clinical practice of the dental hygienist,* ed 9, Philadelphia, 2005, Lippincott Williams & Wilkins.
20. Woodall IR: *Comprehensive dental hygiene care,* ed 4, St Louis, 1993, Mosby.
21. Zimmer SE: Instrument sharpening—sickle scalers and curettes, *Dent Hyg* 52(1):21-24, 1978.

CHAPTER

11

Life Stages

Victoria C. Vick • Maria Perno Goldie • Kenneth Shay

INSIGHT

Each patient has age-dependent needs that a clinician should take into account in assessment, treatment, and oral health instruction. These age-dependent variables can take on many forms, from physical to psychologic to physiologic, as well as combinations of all three forms. The clinician must be aware and alert to the implications these variables have on treatment and treatment outcomes.

✦ CASE STUDY 11-1 — Appreciating Lifestyle Changes to Build Rapport and Guide Treatment

Yolanda is the dental hygienist for a suburban general dental practice. Bridgette Tremaile, a patient new to the area and a stylish woman in her middle 40s, is her first patient of the day. Mrs. Tremaile has a nicely maintained dentition with a few older amalgams that may need replacement, several small interproximal anterior composites that are beginning to discolor, and a three-unit porcelain bridge replacing tooth #19. Probing interproximally causes some slight bleeding and mild marginal edema, but her mouth is nearly plaque free. Mrs. Tremaile also has some light intrinsic staining near the cervicals of her incisors, which a review of her health history suggests most likely is due to tetracycline prescribed for her as a child. Yolanda focuses much of her patient education time on flossing and then calls the dentist's attention to the deteriorating restorations, the cervical staining, and the gingivitis. The dentist completes the examination; recommends an onlay, two composites, and a computer synthesis of the way in which her anterior teeth would appear with veneers; and makes another appointment for Mrs. Tremaile for the next week.

At the second appointment, Mrs. Tremaile brings her 15-year-old daughter, Georgette, for a cleaning and examination. When the mother has been seated, Yolanda stops in to say hello. Mrs. Tremaile confesses that she has not really gotten into the habit of flossing yet. With her permission, Yolanda evaluates her gingival tissues and notes a complete absence of inflammation and no bleeding on probing. Puzzled, Yolanda notes these observations in the chart and turns her attention to Georgette, who is chewing gum and seems angry. Georgette answers questions in monosyllables and makes no eye contact. When the examination begins, she constantly turns her head away to clear her throat, swallow, or lick her lips. Her hair and clothes are unclean, and she has mild facial acne.

Yolanda notices that Georgette is wearing a soccer ball pendant and asks her whether she plays, and if so, which position. She responds that she is a goalkeeper and wants to play but has not been able to find an appropriate team since the family moved to "this stupid dump of a town." Yolanda tells Georgette that she was a goalkeeper in college and now referees on weekends and would be glad to put Georgette into contact with several teams in the area. Georgette's attitude improves immediately as she and Yolanda discuss their common interest, and the appointment proceeds smoothly. On examination Georgette has a full adult dentition with the exception of third molars, as well as abundant plaque biofilm and significant gingivitis except in the anterior facial areas. Dental caries are developing in occlusal and buccal pits of all first molars. Her edematous tissues have created some pseudopocketing. After the prophylaxis, which Georgette clearly finds uncomfortable, Yolanda focuses her educational efforts on diet, the importance of oral health to overall health and appearance, and proper brushing technique.

Approximately 6 weeks later, Mrs. Tremaile returns for her appointment with the dentist. Yolanda sees that Georgette has accompanied her and chats with the teen briefly in the reception area. She appears radiant and excitedly relates that one of the teams Yolanda suggested selected her as first-string goalkeeper, and she explains that the team has won both games in which she has played. Georgette also mentions that she has been trying to put to use some of the dietary tips Yolanda suggested during their last appointment.

As Yolanda sets up the treatment room, she sees the girl's mother in the dentist's treatment room. Yolanda greets the woman and inquires about the flossing; she responds that she has been doing it daily, as part of a deal with her daughter to get them both into the habit. Yolanda glances at the woman's mouth and is surprised and a little dismayed that she has a fairly notable marginal gingivitis. As Yolanda leaves the room, the patient asks, "Why do you suppose my mouth always seems more sensitive right before my period?" Yolanda then realizes that much of the soft tissue inflammation she has observed previously was probably caused by hormonal factors.

After answering the woman's question, Yolanda proceeds to the treatment room and momentarily thinks that she must be hallucinating; her first impression is that the girl's mother is in the chair now. After a moment of confusion, she realizes that this patient, who although quite youthful looking, is obviously of a more advanced age and is Georgette's *grandmother,* Simone Bouvoir. She is a widow in her 70s who has been invited to live with her daughter's family while she works on a graduate degree in Russian literature at the local university. Despite her extremely youthful appearance, her health history reveals that she is being treated for non–insulin-dependent diabetes mellitus (NIDDM), hypertension, glaucoma, and hypothyroidism.

Before the examination, Mrs. Bouvoir removes the remains of a mint from her mouth. She has upper and lower partial dentures that are clean, but they are causing stomatitis in the bearing tissues. She has generalized gingival recession and many open gingival embrasures. Mrs. Bouvoir also has several crowns, and most of her teeth have at least one if not more than one restoration. The large amalgam covering most of the tooth's surface on tooth #14 appears to have a large carious lesion. Although her plaque biofilm control in most areas is fairly good, her mouth seems dry; most of the abutment teeth have a thick coating of adherent plaque biofilm, and the tooth structure beneath the plaque in the cervical areas feels sticky. Yolanda focuses her educational efforts on the use of an interproximal brush, acid attacks, and the importance of fluoride, and she begins periodontal debridement procedures in the upper right quadrant. Later, when the dentist has completed the intraoral examination, Yolanda overhears Mrs. Bouvoir deferring endodontics on tooth #14 in favor of extraction and modification of the upper partial.

KEY TERMS

anticipatory guidance   biopsychosocial   intervention   prevention

LEARNING OUTCOMES

After reading this chapter the student will be able to:

1. Institute anticipatory guidance principles of health outcomes with patients in each life stage.
2. Identify specific patient needs, as identified for each life stage.
3. Develop patient relationships based on the knowledge of issues relative to each life stage of patients.
4. Understand the relationship between the biological and psychosocial aspects of patient care.
5. Explain the menstrual cycle process.
6. Discuss the relationship of hormonal changes to systemic and oral health.
7. Apply issues specific to the various life stages to the development of preventive and therapeutic interventions.

Life Stages

This chapter discusses life stages in terms of the dual role of psychology and physiology on physical well-being. This approach uses a **biopsychosocial** model rather than the biomedical model, acknowledging the complex interaction of biological and individual psychologic and social factors that mediate health and illness (Box 11-1).[20,52,65]

PHYSICAL-PHYSIOLOGIC CHARACTERISTICS

The first of these is the group of *physical-physiologic* components, which largely affect the diagnostic and therapeutic role of the dental hygienist. Physical-physiologic components include the following:

- Anatomical characteristics
- Number and condition of teeth
- Restorations and prostheses
- Soft tissue characteristics and bony support
- Size and condition of the dental pulp
- Accessibility of the teeth
- Pathologic findings
- Oral diseases
- Systemic conditions that affect oral health (including hormonal changes and imbalances)
- Systemic conditions that might be exacerbated by oral conditions
- Physiologic factors
- Tissue response
- Pulpal response
- Manual dexterity
- Sensory abilities
- Salivary flow
- Airway protection
- Homeostatic mechanisms

BOX 11-1

CHARACTERISTICS OF THE BIOPSYCHOSOCIAL MODEL

Physical-Physiologic Characteristics
- Anatomical characteristics of the teeth and soft and hard tissues, and accessibility of the teeth
- Pathologic findings (oral and systemic)
- Physiologic factors (tissue and pulpal response, manual dexterity, salivary flow, sensory abilities)

Psychosocial-Behavioral Characteristics
- Patient's perception of self in relation to family and society
- Perceived locus of control
- Learning and concentration ability
- Life circumstances

Although physical-physiologic factors largely influence diagnosis and therapy, they also may affect education and motivation, such as when disease (or medication taken to control disease) plays a significant role in other health conditions of the patient.*

PSYCHOSOCIAL-BEHAVIORAL CHARACTERISTICS

The second group of components is the *psychosocial-behavioral* factors, which largely influence the educational and motivational efforts of the dental hygienist.

Psychologic-behavioral factors include the following:
- Patient's perception of self relative to family and to society
- Patient's perceived locus of control
- Patient's learning ability
- Patient's concentration ability
- Patient's life circumstances[†]

Often the degree to which dental disease can affect a patient's life is not broadly considered. Many oral conditions may undermine self-image and self-esteem, discourage social interaction, and be significant chronic stressors.[52] They also may lead or contribute to other health issues, such as heart disease, diabetes, and pre-term and/or low–birth-weight babies, and interfere with vital functions, such as food selection, chewing, and swallowing.[‡]

The strong connection between oral health and a person's overall well-being emphasizes the importance of the dental hygienist's interaction with patients on many psychosocial-behavioral levels, including the following:

- Attitude
- Health beliefs
- Motivating factors
- Living situation
- Previous dental experiences

Just as physical-physiologic factors demonstrate some crossover, psychosocial-behavioral factors may in turn affect diagnosis and therapy. For example, a psychiatric disorder influences oral health (e.g., bulimia, which fosters tooth destruction through regurgitation; or depression, which can impair oral hygiene), or fear of dental procedures impairs communication or otherwise interferes with the provision of care.[§]

ANTICIPATORY GUIDANCE

Before initiating care, the clinician should anticipate the best ways to approach a patient through identification of particular patient characteristics. **Anticipatory guidance** is useful in dentistry to help the clinician predict patient needs and plan an educational approach to best meet those needs.[47,64] Anticipatory guidance is information given to children and families to promote health.[32] For example, characteristic physical and psychologic findings are encountered in patients at certain stages of life. Certainly every person is unique, and being a particular age does not guarantee possession of all of the characteristics typically associated with that age. However, familiarity with these characteristics allows recognition of physical findings that are not ordinary. Communication also benefits from an understanding of how different stages of life are likely to feature certain behaviors and attitudes. As the dental hygienist develops a more informed relationship with a patient, the initial age-indexed approach evolves to accommodate individual differences.

Dental hygiene practice demands application of diagnostic-therapeutic skills and educational-motivational skills. These skills are used in a different manner according to each patient, because every patient differs in the following:

- Dentition
- Manual dexterity
- Health behaviors and attitudes
- Learning ability
- Language skills

The patient's age helps explain many of these characteristics. In each dental appointment the dental hygienist is with a patient for only a short time, although the interactions may occur repeatedly over a number of years or even decades.

> *Prevention*
>
> The challenge for the dental hygienist is to discern as much about a patient as quickly as possible—health, habits, learning ability—to identify quickly what to watch for, what to provide, what to teach, and how to communicate with the patient most effectively. In part, a set of factors generally associated with different life stages helps the clinician determine how to proceed.

Early Childhood (In Utero to 6 Years)

This life stage is characterized by profound change and energy. Early childhood begins with the unborn baby and encompasses the infant, the toddler, and finally the preschool

---

*References 22, 24, 27, 46, 60, 74.
†References 8, 16, 22, 23, 28, 30, 42, 44, 62.
‡References 7, 22, 26, 27, 41, 43, 50, 52, 61, 73.
§References 8, 21, 23, 34, 59.

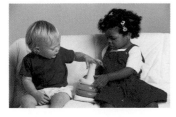

and school-age child (Table 11-1).

The growth rate in the first 6 months of life is faster than it will be at any other time during an individual's life. The human infant's weight doubles during the first 3 months after birth, and it triples within the first year. If growth continued at the rate typical of the first 6 months, then the average 10-year-old child would be 100 feet tall and weigh approximately 240,000 tons (based on computations for the data at 6 months of life).[31]

PHYSICAL-PHYSIOLOGIC CHARACTERISTICS

Physiologically, growth is most pronounced during early childhood. Long bones continue to grow and are responsible for energy and stature; the facial features become more defined. Along with skeletal development, the child's musculature and motor skills develop equally quickly. Infants and children show remarkable and rapid progress in the development of their motor skills, and by the end of the first year most infants are able to crawl, stand up, and take their first steps.[30,31] Walking, running, and climbing skills develop by the late toddler stage.[30,31] Eye-hand coordination develops and allows them to examine and manipulate objects. Practical skills such as self-dressing and self-feeding are developed during the toddler stage. Improved motor skills and coordination during preschool years allow them to become more independent. At this stage children may begin to brush their teeth; however, they still require assistance to ensure they have thoroughly cleaned their teeth.[13]

Numerous texts devoted to the child's physiologic development and written in lay terms are particularly useful for parents and caregivers to anticipate the physiologic stages from neonatal to age 5 years. (See suggested agencies and web sites on the Evolve site.)

> ### *Pregnancy*
> Heavy maternal smoking during pregnancy may lead to delayed tooth formation. Children exposed to cigarette smoke from both parents exhibited up to a 35% reduction in tooth maturation.[45]
> Another example of such influence is the adverse effect of a mother's calcium deficiency on the development of fetal bones and teeth.

DENTAL CONSIDERATIONS

Although not immediately apparent, care is an essential antecedent to a lifetime of dental health. Teeth begin to develop in utero, early in the gestational process. The teeth are affected by environmental factors (e.g., nutrition, maternal health, medications taken during pregnancy) and maternal lifestyle choices (e.g., alcohol consumption, smoking, illegal drug use), which can profoundly affect the developing baby.*

*References 7, 9, 35, 48, 52.

Table 11-1	Early Childhood Characteristics		
AGE	**ANATOMICAL CHARACTERISTICS**	**PATHOLOGIC CHARACTERISTICS**	**PHYSIOLOGIC CHARACTERISTICS**
Prenatal	Primary teeth begin forming in the fourteenth week of pregnancy.	Illness and medications taken during pregnancy can affect tooth formation.	Enamel formation begins in utero.
Birth to 6 Months	Eruption of the first primary tooth may occur by the age of 6 months.	Decreased birth weight increases prevalence of enamel defects.	Permanent teeth begin forming 3 to 4 months after a baby's birth.
6 Months to 12 Months	By the age of 1 year, a baby may have four to eight primary teeth.	Medication taken for chronic use or periodic use may affect oral health.	Caregiver should begin infant oral hygiene with the eruption of the first tooth.
12 Months to 18 Months	By the age of 18 months, a child may have 12 primary teeth.	Dental visits should begin. Infants sleeping with a bottle are at increased risk for tooth decay.	Weaning to a cup by the age of 1 year is desirable. Walking begins, as does the possibility of trauma.
18 Months to 2 Years	By the age of 2, 16 primary teeth may be present.	Weaning from pacifier or finger-sucking habits should begin.	Self-feeding is established, and a great variety of foods are enjoyed.
2 Years to 3 Years	All 20 primary teeth should be present.	Dental visits should occur every 6 months.	Fluoride adequacy should be evaluated.
3 Years to 6 Years	All 20 primary teeth should be present.	Dental visits should occur every 6 months.	

Maternal periodontal disease may increase relative risk for preterm or spontaneous preterm births.[32] Furthermore, periodontal disease progression during pregnancy might be a predictor of the more severe adverse pregnancy outcome of very preterm birth, independently of traditional obstetric, periodontal, and social domain risk factors.[49]

The importance of the provision of proper prenatal dental education by the dental hygienist cannot be overstated.*

---

*References 7, 9, 35, 40, 45, 47, 48, 52, 64.

Low–Birth–Weight Infants

Low–birth-weight infants are more likely to suffer from developmental disturbances of enamel mineralization.[40] The enamel mineralization of the primary incisors starts at 4 months of gestation (followed in sequence by the other primary teeth) and is complete at about 1 year of age. Increased prevalence of disturbances in enamel mineralization has been observed in children born preterm, in those who have experienced severe asphyxia, and in children of mothers with diabetes.

Distinct Care Modifications

Colonization of *Streptococcus mutans* can be delayed if the mother rinses with chlorhexidine daily or chews xylitol-containing chewing gum daily (in the appropriate amounts), from the sixth month of pregnancy until the child is 6 months of age.[10]

Birth to 6 Years

During the first developmental years, parents play a critical role in setting direction for the child's future oral health. Figure 11-1 shows a complete primary dentition.

Patient Education Opportunity

The dental hygienist must communicate the concept of "keeping teeth for a lifetime" to parents or primary caregivers[13] to ensure a positive effect on the future dental health of the child.

Educating children in oral hygiene behaviors must be coordinated with each child's ability both to comprehend the information and to perform the particular task required.[31] Providing education and anticipatory guidance for parents concerning sources of adequate fluoride, normal-abnormal oral development, sucking habits (thumb or pacifier), bottle use, tooth eruption, tooth cleaning, injury **prevention,** and overall dietary habits sets the foundation for a lifetime of good oral health.†

Dental caries is the most commonly experienced oral disease in children at this life stage. In spite of success with the inclusion of fluoride in many public water systems and the use of fluoridated dentifrice in this country, much progress is yet to be made. The incidence of dental caries in certain populations still poses a significant public health problem. A dental hygienist's focused attention to a patient's diet, access to adequate fluoride, oral hygiene habits, and caregiver attitude toward the impor-

---

†References 1, 13, 21, 38, 45, 48, 52, 64.
‡References 13, 14, 20, 21, 35, 45, 48, 64.

---

tance of dental health is essential to his or her **intervention** for the prevention of dental caries, and these concerns should be components of every child's dental visits.‡

Although many children today remain free of dental cries because of fluoridated water and dentifrice, one group of children is not so fortunate. Those children have a tremendous amount of decay at an early age. This decay is initiated when a bottle of cariogenic liquid such as milk or sweetened juice is given to a child to encourage sleep or to quiet the child. The liquid simply "pools" around the teeth. This produces a constant acidic assault to the enamel and promotes rampant decay. This condition is referred to as *early childhood*

Prevention

The dental hygienist may help prevent dental caries through patient education and anticipatory guidance with a child's parents or caregiver.

Note

The American Academy of Pediatric Dentistry recommends that first dental consultations occur shortly after eruption of the first tooth or no later than 1 year of age.

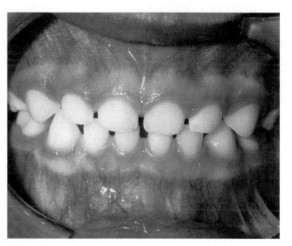

FIGURE 11-1
Primary dentition in health.

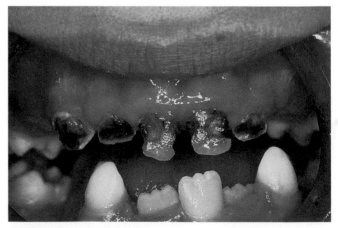

FIGURE 11-2
Early childhood caries (ECC). (From Cawson RA, Odell EW: *Cawson's essentials of oral pathology and oral medicine,* ed 7, London, 2002, Churchill Livingstone.)

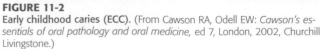

caries (ECC) (Figure 11-2). An estimated 5% to 10% of all children experience some degree of ECC. Some populations, such as Native Americans, are affected to a much larger degree.[21,45,48,52]

Children are more likely than adults to contract acute diseases such as influenza, measles, colds, and other common childhood conditions. Although chronic conditions are not likely to pose a threat to the development of the dentition, an acute episode of high fever or pharmacologic intervention could adversely affect tooth development.[11,21,35,48] An additional challenge for the dental hygienist is to be observant; the clinical signs of some childhood diseases first manifest in the oral environment (e.g., measles).

PSYCHOLOGIC-BEHAVIORAL CHARACTERISTICS

Much of the psychologic and behavioral energy in this life stage is devoted to the concept of self and how the self fits into the world.[31] Each child relates to the environment in a unique way. For example, one 2-year-old child is outgoing, cannot wait for a dental visit, is proud of her teeth, and is eager to please. Another child of the same age is fearful, will not leave the safety of his parents' arms, and will not or cannot cooperate during a dental examination. Although generalizations on psychologic-behavioral aspects of any age may be misleading, they set the stage for anticipatory guidance in medicine and dentistry.[31,64]

This particular age group of children poses several challenges to both the clinician and the caregiver in terms of oral care. Their personalities, attention spans, and motor skills undergo enormous change. Some children immediately accept having their teeth brushed, whereas others struggle with having someone else brush their teeth. Balancing a toddler's physical ability and emotional maturity during toothbrushing before bedtime may be challenging for any parent.

Nonnutritive Sucking

One of an infant's natural reflexes is sucking. Most young children have an emotional need for sucking beyond what is required to attain nourishment. This instinctual behavior is calming and is an important step in the development of self-regulation and emotional control.

However, at some point nonnutritive sucking may become a problem. Constant and intense sucking may damage the primary and permanent dentition and the jaw.

The constant sucking action continuing into the early years creates constant muscular pressure inward that can cause movement of structures medially. Although initial support for the nonnutritive sucking habit and the emotional benefits it provides is appropriate during early childhood, weaning must occur at the appropriate time (between the ages of 2 and 4 years, prior to the eruption of the first permanent teeth). Parents should be involved in identification of the best approach to help their child discontinue the nonnutritive sucking habit without causing undue stress to the child.[45]

> **Prevention**
> Nonnutritive sucking becomes a problem when constant and intense sucking damages the primary and permanent dentition, as well as the jaw.

11-2

Later Childhood (7 to 12 Years)

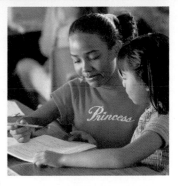

As children continue to grow physically and mature emotionally, they become more secure in independent activities. Children at this age begin to demonstrate their individuality and general behavior patterns. During this period of change, girls and boys tend to diverge in gender role acceptance; this period is often referred to as the *initiation of puberty*.

PHYSICAL-PHYSIOLOGIC CHARACTERISTICS

During the later childhood years, growth and development continues: the human face begins another phase of maturity; jaw growth continues; and a child of this life stage has more teeth than at any other stage (considering both the primary and the developing permanent dentitions) (Figure 11-3, Table 11-2).

Later childhood is a time for the dental hygienist to pay close attention to the size, location, and alignment of newly erupted teeth, as well as to the space allocated to the anticipated permanent teeth. Occlusal problems may be identified, and early intervention can assist with future orthodontic needs (Figure 11-4; see Chapter 37).

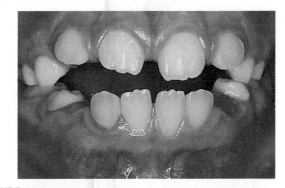

FIGURE 11-3
Transitional dentition.

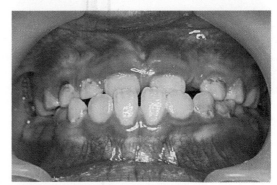

FIGURE 11-4
Mixed dentition with occlusal problems in need of orthodontic intervention. (From Nanda R: *Biomechanics and esthetic strategies in clinical orthodontics*, St Louis, 2005, Saunders.)

Table 11-2	Later Childhood Characteristics		
AGE	ANATOMICAL CHARACTERISTICS	PATHOLOGIC CHARACTERISTICS	PHYSIOLOGIC CHARACTERISTICS
7 Years to 9 Years	First permanent teeth begin to erupt around the age of 6.	Sealants on first molars aid in decay prevention.	Independent and active children are at risk for oral trauma.
10 Years to 12 Years	This is the "ugly duckling" stage of mixed dentition.	Increased plaque biofilm formation may occur in children afraid to brush loose teeth.	Early orthodontic intervention or space retainers may be necessary.

Later childhood is a dynamic period of physical growth, sexual maturation, and hormonal changes leading to adolescence. Female sex hormones include estrogen and progesterone. Estrogens are responsible for cyclical changes in the vaginal epithelium and endometrium of the uterus, as well as for the development of female sex characteristics. Hormonal fluctuations are evident at the onset of puberty or adolescence, when the girl begins to develop sex organs and secondary sex characteristics, and she begins menstruating and ovulating. A natural pattern of estrogen and progesterone levels occurs throughout the woman's reproductive life (Figures 11-5 and 11-6).

During the menstrual cycle, estrogen levels peak at ovulation and decrease during the second half of the cycle. Progesterone is responsible for changes in the endometrium in preparation for implantation of the fertilized egg and the development of the placenta and mammary glands. If fertilization does not occur, then the hormones cause a shedding of the uterine lining, which is called the *menses*. This cycle lasts 28 days, with variation from 22 to 34 days. Progesterone levels remain stable until after ovulation occurs.

Boys also go through a wide range of hormonal changes that often leave them confused and frustrated. The male hormone testosterone begins to reach higher levels, and boys begin to notice facial hair growth, lowering of the voice, and a change in how they relate to girls. This change takes place over a period of years, and that age range can vary widely. This change continues into the late teens and early twenties.

DENTAL CONSIDERATIONS

During this developmental stage the dental hygienist should provide education and anticipatory guidance to the child and parents concerning fluoride supplements, sealants, tooth exfoliation and eruption, oral hygiene, dietary habits, and injury prevention.[1] This life stage provides many opportunities for oral trauma.[18,21,29] Whether the child is involved in organized sports or simply riding a bicycle, the risk of orofacial trauma increases. In fact, accidents are the leading cause of death in children aged 1 to 14 years.

The child should be included in the discussion of anticipated consequences of good or poor oral care habits, because children should become responsible for their own oral health. Although they will certainly still need the influence and guidance of a primary caregiver, children should be developing the coordination, motor skills, and motivation to effectively brush and floss their own teeth at this age.[13,14]

Although many children in the United States enjoy excellent oral health, some experience a high level of disease. The dichotomy of adequate access to dental care is identified in the Surgeon General's *Report on Oral Health in America*, which has found a disproportionate number of economically disadvantaged and minority children receiving inadequate,

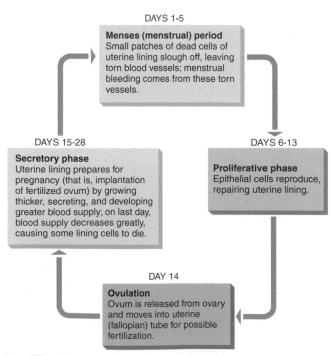

FIGURE 11-5
The 28-day menstrual cycle. (Modified from Thibodeau GA, Patton KT: *The human body in health and disease,* ed 3, St Louis, 2002, Mosby.)

Prevention

If a child develops an interest in a contact sport, then prevention of orofacial trauma becomes increasingly important. The use of a mouthguard in a contact sport is fundamental to the safety of the sport, as is wearing a protective helmet, whether playing baseball, riding a bike, or rollerblading. (See Chapter 39 for content on prevention of trauma and use of mouthguards.)

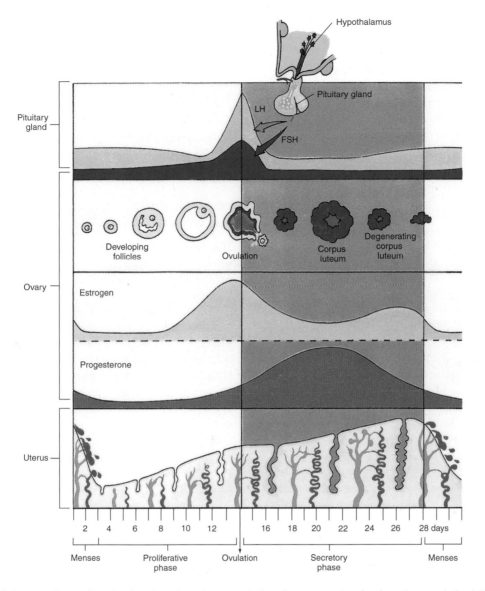

FIGURE 11-6
Interrelationship of pituitary, ovarian, and uterine functions throughout a typical 28-day menstrual cycle. Sharp increase in luteinizing hormone *(LH)* causes ovulation, whereas lower levels of progesterone initiate menstruation. *FSH,* Follicle-stimulating hormone. (From Thibodeau GA, Patton KT: *The human body in health and disease,* ed 3, St Louis, 2002, Mosby.)

if any, dental care.[52] If left untreated, oral diseases frequently lead to serious general health problems and significant pain. These children experience persistent pain, the inability to eat comfortably, and embarrassment in front of their peers.[54] These same children may be uncomfortable with dentistry later in life. When children from families who are socioeconomically challenged gain access to dental care, the dental hygienist's role as educator and role model becomes even more important. These children do not have the benefit of routine visits, and the time spent with them may influence their dental behaviors for a lifetime.

Because some children, especially female children, mature faster than others, these precocious individuals must be counseled about the hormonal changes that will occur. The next section, Adolescence to Young Adulthood, provides more specific information on this topic.

PSYCHOLOGIC-BEHAVIORAL CHARACTERISTICS

This life stage continues the exploration in the understanding of the concept of self. Peers begin to exert a major influence in behaviors and, for the most part, children of this and the next life stage spend more time outside the home than in it. Children begin to understand and use simple logic as they gain an understanding of relational concepts.[28,31] The clinician should understand these constructs before assuming responsibility for children's oral care. This is also an appropriate time to

> **Patient Education Opportunity**
> A child with even a modest improvement in oral hygiene responds to praise and the acknowledgment of accomplishment by trying to achieve even better results for the next visit. The dental hygienist may provide positive feedback that enhances the child's self-confidence and sense of competence (both integral to this developmental stage).

provide substance abuse counseling (e.g., smoking, smokeless tobacco), as well as counseling on intraoral and perioral piercing.[4]

A bright, healthy smile at this age often sets the tone for a child's social interaction. During these developmental years, a child's social skills evolve. A smile marred by decayed or damaged teeth or halitosis may lead to ridicule and rejection by peers. Children of this age are seeking approval and guidance; the dental hygienist can best provide oral health instruction by considering those needs.

The dental hygienist can support the child's sense of accomplishment and competency by saying, "I am proud of the way have you been keeping your back teeth much cleaner since your last visit." Emphasizing even minimal improvement fosters additional progress.

Adolescence to Young Adulthood (13 to 20 Years)

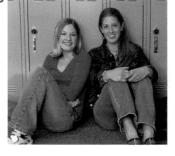

Adolescence is clearly a period of transition from the dependence of childhood to the independence of adulthood. It may be characterized in terms of sexual maturity, identity development, and a period of social transition into adulthood. This group is often identified as defiant, lazy, and egocentric. However, they are experiencing such significant change that even they do not necessarily understand their behavior.[16,28,31]

PHYSICAL-PHYSIOLOGIC CHARACTERISTICS

Adolescence can be defined in strictly biological terms (Table 11-3). Puberty and all associated physical changes may occur between the ages of 9 and 17 years. The pituitary gland is responsible for the control of the production of estrogens (from the ovaries in female adolescents) and androgens (from the testes in male adolescents). These hormones, responsible for the development of sex organs, continue to have a profound physical and emotional influence during this life stage. Physically, both male and female adolescents experience accelerated growth, height, weight, and muscle mass. Because of the pattern in growth spurts, adolescents may appear clumsy and awkward. Lack of physical coordination may become an issue and may affect self-esteem. Dermatologic changes, including acne, are often evident in this life stage and may cause immense concern in teens.[16,21,28,53]

DENTAL CONSIDERATIONS

This age group of patients presents clinicians with particular challenges to oral health care.[21,50] A significant number of adolescents are fortunate enough to have benefited from fluoridated water and dentifrice, and they often have not experienced any dental caries activity. However, adolescent patients need to understand the importance of good oral hygiene relative to plaque biofilm control and their periodontal health, regardless of whether they have experienced a dental caries problem. Some adolescents have no dental caries but have poor plaque biofilm control. Although age is on their side, over time they will likely experience gingival problems and possibly periodontal deterioration.

Contributing to periodontal diseases in this age group are the abundant sex hormones circulating in the bloodstream. Female adolescents are particularly sensitive, because they have high levels of circulating estrogen and progesterone. Because oral tissue has many receptors for these hormones, oral tissue will most likely be affected as hormone levels rise and fall (Figure 11-7).

Effects produced by these hormones include the following:
- Increased vascularity, leading to increased redness, edema, and bleeding on probing

Table 11-3	Adolescent and Young Adult Characteristics		
AGE	ANATOMICAL CHARACTERISTICS	PATHOLOGIC CHARACTERISTICS	PHYSIOLOGIC CHARACTERISTICS
13 Years to 14 Years	The period of mixed dentition continues. Most primary teeth are shed.	The beginning of hormonal changes may increase gingival problems. Frequent snacking and an unbalanced diet may increase dental caries risk. Bulimics are at risk for rampant dental caries because of increased acid.	The patient has the physical skills and proper dentition to master flossing. Bulimia and anorexia may manifest.
14 Years to 16 Years	Dentition consists of permanent teeth.	Hormonal changes may increase gingival problems. Frequent snacking and an unbalanced diet may increase dental caries risk. Bulimics are at risk for rampant dental caries because of increased acid.	The use of tobacco products may begin.
17 Years to 18 Years	Wisdom teeth may erupt.	Oral irritation occurs with tobacco use.	

- Decreased cell-mediated immunity, leading to an increase in subgingival bacteria, particularly *Provotella intermedia*.

Increased efficacy and frequency of self-care is vital during this life phase.

In women, researchers have reported hemorrhagic lesions associated with premenstruation, as well as an increase in gingival exudates and increased tooth mobility during the menstrual cycle.[54]

Pain scores were reported higher during premenstruation compared with postmenstruation scores. The clinical implications (although small [findings should not be generalized]) indicate that a clinician may consider scheduling nonsurgical visits after a woman's menstrual cycle to provide a more comfortable experience.[54]

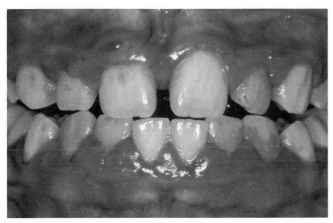

FIGURE 11-7
Puberty-associated gingivitis.

⭐ **CASE APPLICATION 11-1.1**

Gingival Sensitivity

In the case study at the beginning of the chapter, Mrs. Tremaile asks why her gingival tissue is more sensitive before her period. What could be the reason for the sensitivity and marginal inflammation?

The practice of anticipatory guidance with this group of patients is sometimes difficult but rewarding to the clinician. Although education regarding the importance of oral health to overall health may seem to fall on deaf ears, these patients are usually receptive to a clinician's true interest in their well-being.[39]

As with the earlier age groups, this life stage is also an appropriate time to provide substance abuse counseling (e.g., smoking, smokeless tobacco), as well as counseling on intraoral and perioral piercing.[4]

If the patient has commenced menstruation and is of child-bearing age, then ascertaining oral contraceptive (OC) use is advisable. Because this can be a sensitive subject, the patient's privacy should be protected.

One oral condition that becomes more apparent during adolescence is malocclusion. Malocclusion is not considered a disease as much as a condition or variation from proper alignment of the teeth and jaw. Many minor malocclusions have little or no effect on the patient's oral or general health and may not need treatment. However, some malocclusions can be disfiguring and can affect chewing and speaking. Cases involving craniofacial disturbances such as missing or unerupted teeth or severely malformed palates require treatment to maintain health and function. Many malocclusions are treated primarily for esthetic reasons.

Careful consideration is critical when making any decision about orthodontic treatment. Families must consider risk factors and the potential benefits and costs involved in the treatment of malocclusion. One significant psychologic benefit often achieved through orthodontic treatment is an enhanced self-image, which may have a profound positive effect on an adolescent's life. (See Chapter 37 for content on recognition of the need for orthodontics and orthodontic procedures.)

> *Patient Education Opportunity*
> Advising women using OCs that a possible reduction in efficacy of oral steroid contraceptives could occur during antibiotic therapy is also recommended. Patients should use additional forms of contraception during short-term antibiotic use.[5]

PHYSIOLOGIC-BEHAVIORAL CHARACTERISTICS

The adolescent focus is once again on the self. They seek, enjoy, and respond well to attention. Adolescents are physically maturing but not yet considered adults. Many inflated emotions result from their efforts to seek independence, which are often complicated by the conflicted state of fear of breaking or distancing the parental attachment. The quest for independence is accomplished by the questioning of authority figures, especially parents, and an increase in respect from adults outside the family circle.[31] These years are rarely easy ones for teens or their parents.

Adolescent patients require the clinician to be an educator, an observer, and a good communicator. Each of these patients has priorities, needs, and interests and is trying to establish a unique lifestyle. The clinician must consider each of these variables when deciding what information each patient needs.

Cognitively the adolescent begins to think less concretely and to understand and use some abstract thought constructs. This higher level of thinking allows adolescents to begin self-assessment and the development of their own identities. Some teenagers experience great experimentation in the determination of their values, beliefs, and attitudes.

However, others seem to move quietly into this period, feeling quite comfortable with childhood experiences and having little need to question or change their sense of self. Experimentation may also extend to the use of alcohol and drugs for those

✦ CASE APPLICATION 11-1.2

Communicating with the Adolescent

In Case Study 11-1 the dental hygienist's sensitivity to the 15-year-old patient's needs and life circumstances provided the basis for a patient-clinician relationship that resulted in improved oral hygiene and overall well-being. The dental hygienist realized a common interest with the patient, which led to the patient improving her attitude toward and responsibility for her oral hygiene needs. That sensitivity also gave the patient confidence in other aspects of her life. The rewards of clinical practice often extend beyond the clinical setting.

trying to find a sense of self—the feeling of importance and acceptance. Seeking identification with adult role models is a manner in which many teenagers begin to build their own identities.[28,31] (See Case Study 11-1.)

Issues concerning body appearance begin to manifest at this age as concerns over clothing and possessions begin to play a major role in identity and self-esteem. The dental hygienist needs to be observant for signs of abuse. (See Chapter 39 for more on this topic.)

Prevention

The pressure from peers or parents may produce psychologic problems in the form of eating disorders. Purging behavior of those with eating disorders may result in dental problems because the acid produced by repeated vomiting dissolves the enamel of teeth. The teeth may have a dull, chalky enamel surface. Often the lingual and palatal surfaces appear eroded, and restorations appear raised from the tooth (called *floating amalgams*). An oral examination indicating disordered eating should result in a frank discussion with the patient and a referral to the appropriate healthcare professional. (Disordered eating is covered in Chapter 45.)

Bulimia is a psychologic problem that should be approached from a medical-dental team perspective. The psychiatrist or other mental health professional needs to be aware of and involved in the progress or deterioration of the patient's oral health as it relates to the patient's recovery from this eating disorder.[2,21,59]

Early Adulthood (21 to 39 Years)

The changes that occur during the adult years may not seem as dramatic as those typified in childhood and adolescence, but they are just as real (Table 11-4). The transition from adolescence to adulthood is marked by the independent choices one makes. The sense of identity that one creates as an adolescent is put to use. Psychologic and social adjustments must be made for marriage, parenthood, and career choice. Although young adulthood is a season of excitement and opportunity in the identification of a person's place in life, this period also is stressful because many life-defining choices are made.[31,43]

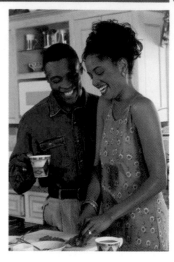

PHYSICAL-PHYSIOLOGIC CHARACTERISTICS

In terms of physical status of adulthood, the 20s and 30s usually are seen as the peak of physical health, although the occurrence of chronic diseases later in life is often influenced by lifestyle decisions made during these years. Health, generally taken for granted as a child and adolescent, may become a concern for the first time.

Table 11-4	Adulthood Characteristics		
AGE	**ANATOMICAL CHARACTERISTICS**	**PATHOLOGIC CHARACTERISTICS**	**PHYSIOLOGIC CHARACTERISTICS**
20 Years to 40 Years	Natural adult dentition has developed.	Gingival inflammation may occur (resulting from inadequate plaque biofilm control). Dental caries may occur because of changes in diet and poor plaque biofilm control. Periodontitis may occur. For women, pregnancy gingivitis may occur.	Overall health is affected by lifestyle choices. Periodontitis may be causal factor in low–birth-weight infants. Hormonal changes resulting from pregnancy may occur.
41 Years to 60 Years	Natural adult dentition has developed.	Periodontitis leading to loss of alveolar bone may occur. Gingival bleeding and periodontitis in response to what might otherwise be acceptable plaque biofilm levels may occur (onset of bone loss is often rapid). Periodontitis may occur.	For women, menopause begins. Osteoporosis may begin. Non–insulin-dependent diabetes mellitus (NIDDM) may be seen. An increased risk of cardiovascular disease or stroke exists.

Prevention

The effect of oral health on general health has been the focus of a significant body of research that has identified several systemic diseases exacerbated by oral disease.* In terms of anticipatory guidance, this may be a powerful and important motivator for adults.

*References 12, 26, 41, 43, 52, 61, 73-75.

DENTAL CONSIDERATIONS

Dentally, the focus for these patients is often on the maintenance of a level of oral health acquired through childhood and adolescence.[36,52,62] Some individuals may experience a pronounced increase in dental caries as they leave home and begin making their own decisions in areas affecting oral health, such as nutrition and selection of self-care products. Those in this age group should make appropriate changes to deal with the onset of potential new dental caries activity. They may be surprised and perhaps question the presence of cavities.

Although this may be a rude awakening to adulthood, the topic is better addressed sooner rather than later. The dental hygienist must be tactful in the presentation of this information to avoid offending the patient and damaging the clinician-patient relationship, which is so important to the long-term receptiveness to oral care by the patient. The clinician may need to ask patients to relate major life changes when taking their histories, because that information may be helpful in assessment of changes in the patients' dental caries activities. Patients cope with their change in health status by learning logical reasons for caries development and actions to reduce or eliminate the caries activity.

Patient Education Opportunity

During this life stage many women may start families, making oral care of expectant mothers and unborn children relevant issues. The dental hygienist can expect to educate pregnant women on oral health, preconception and postconception issues, and the effect of certain lifestyle choices on the oral health of the baby.

Pregnant women and those taking OCs experience significant hormonal changes. These changes can result in oral manifestations such as hormonal gingivitis, an important topic for oral care education. The relative proportion of the *Bacteroides* species, implicated in periodontitis, is increased fifty-fivefold in pregnant women and sixteenfold in women taking OCs over the control group. When circulating sex hormones are high, clinicians see a shift in bacteria from those that cause gingivitis to those that cause periodontitis. Both hormones (estrogen and progesterone) have been shown to be a substitute for naphthoquinone, which is an essential growth factor for the *Bacteroides* species and *Prevotella intermedia*. In addition, the bacteria and the lipopolysaccharide (LPS) elicit a host response, including production of cytokines and proinflammatory mediators, which contribute to the negative tissue response. Synthesis of prostaglandins (mediators of inflammation) is high during pregnancy, and researchers believe that progesterone functions as an immunosuppressant in the gingival tissues of pregnant women. This can be observed clinically in an exaggerated appearance of inflammation. Progesterone-induced inhibition of collagenase, superimposed on vascular changes, is considered the cause of pregnancy granulomas. This results in the accumulation of collagen within the connective tissue, sometimes caus-ing these tumorlike growths[3] (Figure 11-8). As mentioned previously, the antibiotic and OC interaction must be discussed.

This is a period of great receptivity to medical-dental knowledge, because expectant parents generally seek and appreciate information regarding health changes during this very important period of their lives. An expectant woman should not fear damage to her teeth during pregnancy if she maintains adequate care and gets the necessary vitamins and minerals for both herself and her unborn child. Gingivitis has been reported in 30% to 75% of all pregnant women. Clinically the gingival tissues appear bright red and edematous at the marginal gingiva and interdental papilla, with an increased tendency to bleed. The woman who uses OCs will experience hormonal imbalances similar to those in pregnancy. The hormones contained in OCs act to inhibit the release of the ovum from the ovary, thereby preventing fertilization.

Young adults who needed orthodontic intervention during adolescence but did not receive treatment may have that orthodontic treatment performed at this time. Patients of this age are beginning to realize the importance of their teeth from an esthetic standpoint and as an important element of their general health. The esthetic appearance of their teeth is indeed important to their overall oral health.

Patient Education Opportunity

Dispelling myths such as "you lose one tooth for every child you have" is another aspect in the education of the patient in this life stage.

Explaining the relationship between gingivitis during pregnancy and its effects on fetal development (e.g., preterm low birth weight) can significantly elevate the importance of oral self-care during this phase of adult life.[50]

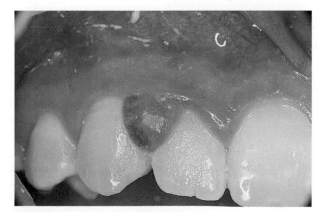

FIGURE 11-8
Pregnancy-associated pyogenic granuloma.

PSYCHOLOGIC-BEHAVIORAL CHARACTERISTICS

Patient Education Opportunity

Interest in one's oral condition can be used to the dental hygienist's advantage as a powerful motivational strategy. Health promotion theory indicates that people are often more willing to comply with health instruction if an esthetic benefit is involved than they would be if they were to gain only the health benefit.[8,37] For example, an overweight patient with diabetes wants to lose weight. Although a health benefit exists in weight loss, often a change in appearance is the real motivator behind the change in eating and exercise habits. This knowledge of health promotion theory allows the dental hygienist to present oral care information or treatment options to patients in terms that are relevant to their needs and desires—and beyond immediate oral health benefits.

This life stage is one of great transition and personal development.[17,28] Individuals begin to define themselves and build their futures. Interest in one's oral condition includes a strong interest in presentation in social environments.

Young adults are developing buying habits, even health habits, and they are often influenced by advertising and the entertainment industry. In today's commercial environment, ignoring advertisements when purchasing oral care products is difficult. These patients look to their oral healthcare professional for guidance in making appropriate decisions regarding their oral care regimen and specific products. Counseling provided to these patients strongly influences their current and future oral health habits.

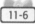

Mature Adulthood (40 to 60 Years)

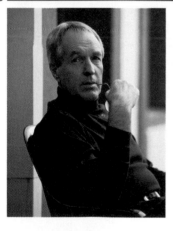

As the middle years of adulthood approach, many people feel settled. They have chosen their lifestyles and have established their places in the societal framework. However, this is also a time of reexamination of one's accomplishments and life situation. During this period, children generally leave home and start families of their own; for some, careers are winding down. Thus a period of apparent peacefulness is also laden with significant, stressful life changes. During this phase of life the reality of aging and a sense of finality begin to become apparent. Before reaching this age, people often have a sense that they are invincible and that life and its possibilities are limitless.[28]

A trend apparent in this age group is the increasing role assumed as a caregiver. Individuals at this life stage may have to care for aging parents, adult children who have returned home, or grandchildren.[52] They have become known as the *sandwich generation,* because they may be caring for children and parents at the same time. As life expectancies continue to increase,

parents may spend fewer years caring for their children than they do caring for their aging parents.

PHYSICAL-PHYSIOLOGIC CHARACTERISTICS

During middle age, people often begin to notice specific changes about themselves that, until this point, they thought happened only to other people. People begin to notice gray hair, thinning hair, a tendency to gain weight more easily, and physical inability to do the things they had done when they were younger. These physiologic changes occur in different time frames for many reasons, such as familial traits, lifestyle choices (e.g., exercise, lack of exercise), nutrition, stress, smoking, obesity, and alcohol abuse.[28,52] Given the myriad of possible interactions between these multiple factors, each patient must be evaluated individually and not in the context of general health amid an entire pool of patients.[75]

Numerous physiologic changes occur during this life stage that have an effect on oral health, or conversely, many oral conditions may affect other aspects of physiologic health.[41,52] A patient's understanding of the significance of oral health to overall health is extremely important. Initially the link of periodontal disease to systemic diseases was thought to be unidirectional, but growing evidence shows that the relationship may be bidirectional.[22,61]

As women approach midlife, estrogen and progesterone levels decrease, resulting in hormonal imbalances. Various symptoms such as irregular menstrual cycles and "hot flashes" are reflective of the changing hormone levels during perimenopause. Once a woman reaches menopause, the menses stops. Postmenopause is the period when the woman has reached the end of her reproductive cycle. Some women choose hormone replacement therapy (HRT) or estrogen replacement therapy (ERT) to control symptoms such as vaginal dryness, hot flashes, and increased urinary frequency. However, since the release of the results of the Women's Health Initiative Study, fewer women are taking oral hormones because of their potential deleterious effects. These effects include (but are not limited to) increased risk of breast cancer, heart disease, and stroke. Having lower levels of circulating sex hormones causes systemic and oral symptoms such as osteoporosis, xerostomia, and alterations in taste sensation.[76]

Patient Education Opportunity

Research connecting oral health to cardiovascular disease, stroke, diabetes, and other systemic conditions is emerging.* Case-control and cross-sectional studies indicate that periodontitis is correlated with a twofold increase in the risk for cardiovascular disease.[26] These interrelationships may prove extremely important in the development of appropriate intervention and prevention strategies from both the dental and the medical outcomes perspective.[75]

*References 12, 22, 26, 41, 43, 61, 73.

DENTAL CONSIDERATIONS

The oral health of patients in this group increases in complexity. As they age, mature adults begin to experience the onset of various chronic conditions. These conditions, or often the therapies used to treat them, may have significant effect on the oral tissues. For example, the onset of diabetes in someone with previously excellent plaque biofilm control may result in significant bleeding. This occurrence may frighten the patient, and the clinician should consider this in treatment planning and observation.

These patients must be educated (i.e., provided with anticipatory guidance) regarding the etiology of the gingival bleeding and the associated precautions needed to control it. Medications for chronic conditions may cause xerostomia, and subsequently root caries may pose a problem for this age group (Figure 11-9).

This group often tries to downplay the importance of their changing health conditions, so thoroughness is critical in updates of the medical-psychologic (life status) histories at each visit. Any significant change should be noted. This change may be the onset of diabetes; the addition of medication for hypertension; or a significant psychosocial change such as a divorce, children leaving for school, or older parents no longer able to care for themselves. These changes should be considered as potential factors in oral disease and its treatment and prevention.[36,52]

> **Note**
>
> As more of these patients present with complex medical and psychologic issues, the importance of the use of a biopsychosocial model in assessment of their needs becomes even greater.

Female Patients

During this time frame most women experience perimenopause and menopause. With the accompanying decline of estrogen, women are more susceptible to osteoporosis (i.e., reduced bone density), which also may affect the dental alveolar structure. Loss of dental alveolar bone that often may accompany osteoporosis is usually completely unexpected by the patient (Figure 11-10). The effect of reduced estrogen levels on bone density must be considered as a potential contributing factor in the onset of periodontal disease.[27,51]

Because women are taking fewer hormones since the release of the Women's Health Initiative Study, many have turned to the bisphosphonate family of drugs for bone loss prevention and treatment. This class of compounds is also used in the treatment of cancer and other medical conditions. One study shows that women using risedronate therapy show significantly less plaque biofilm accumulation, less gingival inflammation,

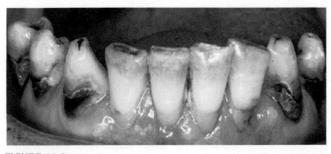

FIGURE 11-9
Permanent dentition with root caries. (From Sapp JP, Eversole LR, Wysocki GP: *Contemporary oral and maxillofacial pathology,* ed 2, St Louis, 2004, Mosby.)

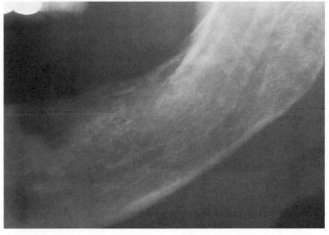

FIGURE 11-10
Osteoporosis of the mandible.

lower probing depths, less periodontal attachment loss, and greater alveolar bone levels. These observations suggest that risedronate therapy may play a beneficial role in periodontal status.[58] The side effects of bisphosphonate therapy are generally mild, but severe esophageal reactions have been reported with alendronate.[68] Consequently, its use is not recommended for patients with a history of upper GI complaints.

As more scientific evidence is accumulated about the effects of this family of drugs, there is evidence of osteonecrosis of the jaw with patients on chronic bisphosphonate therapy.[65] The potent intravenous bisphosphonates, pamidronate (Aredia; Novartis Pharmaceuticals Corp., East Hanover, NJ) and zoledronic acid (Zometa; Novartis Pharmaceuticals Corp.), are typically administered monthly in patients with metastatic bone disease. Except for ibandronate (Boniva; Hoffmann-LaRoche, Nutley, NY), all of the other bisphosphonates approved for the treatment of osteoporosis are dosed orally on a daily or weekly schedule. Only Fosamax, Actonel, and Boniva are nitrogen-containing oral bisphosphonates, and are most likely to cause osteonecrosis of the jaw.[63a]

The development of bisphosphonate-related osteonecrotic lesions of the jaw (BRONJ) is a clinical problem where spontaneous exposure of alveolar bone occurs, or much worse, the patient presenting for routine dental extractions or periodontal curettage develops an area of necrotic bone that does not respond to conservative treatment or surgical management.[63a] In 2003 and 2004, oral and maxillofacial surgeons were the first clinicians to recognize and report cases of non-healing exposed, necrotic bone in the maxillofacial region in patients treated with IV bisphosphonates.[4a] These compounds localize to bone and inhibit osteoclast-mediated bone resorption. Since bisphosphonates are not metabolized, high concentrations are maintained within bone for a long time; the exact duration remains unknown at this time.

> **Note**
>
> The following factors are thought to be risk factors for BRONJ:
> * Corticosteroid therapy
> * Diabetes
> * Tobacco/alcohol use
> * Poor oral hygiene
> * Chemotherapeutic drugs

Patients may be considered to have BRONJ if all of the following characteristics are present:[4a]

- Current or previous treatment with a bisphosphonate
- Exposed, nectronic bone in the maxillofacial region that has persisted for more than eight weeks
- No history of radiation therapy to the jaws.

Management strategies for patients treated with bisphosphonates for prevention of BRONJ include a thorough oral examination and removal of any unsalvageable teeth; and completion of all invasive oral procedures *prior to treatment with a IV bisphosphonate*. The treatment objectives for patients with an established diagnosis of BRONJ are to eliminate pain, control infection of the soft and hard tissue, and minimize the progression or occurrence of bone necrosis. Surgical treatment should be delayed if possible; if areas of necrotic bone are a constant source of soft tissue irritation, these areas should be removed or recontoured without exposure of additional bone.[35a]

Male Patients

Male patients during this stage of life can develop prostate problems. Prostate cancer is the most common form of cancer among American men aged 50 and older. In high-risk groups, such as blacks and those with a family history of prostate cancer, it is the most common form of cancer in men 45 and older. Men in this age group should have a prostate-specific antigen (PSA) blood test and a digital rectal examination once a year.[56]

Problems with the prostate can exhibit the following presentations:

- *Prostatitis:* Inflammation of the prostate gland that can be classified as acute bacterial prostatitis, chronic bacterial prostatitis, or nonbacterial prostatitis
- *Benign prostatic hyperplasia (BPH):* Enlargement of the prostate that begins to squeeze the urethra resulting in difficulty urinating
- *Prostate cancer:* Form of cancer that most often begins in the outer part of the prostate and does not cause any symptoms in the early stage

PSYCHOLOGIC-BEHAVIORAL CHARACTERISTICS

This life stage is accompanied by a lot of change, some related to growth opportunities and other changes that mark the onset of endings. These patients face the failure or fulfillment of their life's hopes and dreams. Change seems to mark each phase or life stage, and as with the others, change may be difficult. Clinicians should note such changes as divorce, job loss, death of a parent, or other significant events, if possible. The stress that accompanies such change can often bring about depression or anxiety,[28] both of which may affect oral health.[42] These topics are best not solicited from patients directly but rather with open-ended questions such as, "What's new in your life?" Patients are often grateful to have someone to whom they can confide some of life's changes; however, having patients initiate such a discussion is desirable.

People in this group are often self-conscious about their appearance and the fact they are growing older. The physical effects of aging become increasingly apparent.[28] Because society places such significance on youth and beauty, the aging process may be devastating to self-esteem. As a person matures the teeth tend to darken with age, which is just another visual sign of aging. Tooth whitening is relatively inexpensive, easy, painless, and quick. It provides patients with a more youthful smile that in turn can boost their self-confidence. Approaching the topic sometimes may be challenging; therefore information in the reception area and operatory is helpful. Patients who view whitening literature in the waiting room may ask about options for whitening, inviting a discussion of treatments that would meet the patient's needs. (See Chapter 36 for whitening and esthetic options.)

Cosmetic options to restore a more youthful smile range from cosmetic whitening with a peroxide-based product to more significant procedures, including veneers, replacement of amalgam restorations with composite materials, and porcelain crowns. The patient may feel more comfortable discussing these topics with the dental hygienist, at least initially, before consultation with the dentist. A patient's bright smile and enhanced self-esteem realized by appropriate counseling and treatment in the dental office is rewarding to the dental team.

The female patient approaching middle age is faced with hormonal changes inevitably brought about with the onset of menopause. These changes often present as alterations in emotions, because the hormonal changes may cause mood swings, depression, anxiety, and a general feeling of malaise.* Clinicians must be alert to these changes in addition to the potential physiologic changes mentioned earlier, and they must approach the patient in a calm and courteous manner.

These transitional years are filled with psychologic milestones that the clinician must consider in the determination of treatment plans and the provision of treatment. Awareness of and sensitivity to the major life changes people face may make a tremendous difference in the relationship that develops between patient and clinician. This relationship may be rewarding and enriching to both parties.

★ CASE APPLICATION 11-1.3

Discussing the Natural Dentition

In Case Study 11-1, what questions could Yolanda have asked Mrs. Bouvoir that might have provided an opportunity to discuss the value of retaining her natural teeth?

Late Adulthood (61 Years and Older)   11-7

Perhaps no age group is as encumbered with, and affected by, popular misconceptions as is the oldest segment of the population. Most of the popular lore about the last stages of life is based not on personal experience but on a variety of secondhand informa-

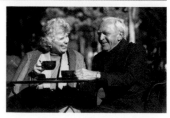

---

*References 17, 27, 28, 42, 53.

tion, usually derived from and later colored by personal interactions. Through much of the twentieth century, most Americans have learned and shared sets of unrealistic and likely inaccurate beliefs—termed *stereotypes*—about their elders. Some stereotypes are negative, including the following:

- Senile
- Toothless
- Ineffectual
- Inflexible
- Crabby
- Repetitive
- Deaf
- Self-centered
- Poor
- Helpless

Others stereotypes are positive but equally inaccurate when used to describe tens of millions of older adults:

- Sweet
- Energetic
- Generous
- Wise
- Funny
- Helpful
- Cute
- Selfless[28]

Both positive and negative stereotypes share a fundamental flaw; they do not account for individuality. Just as making sweeping generalizations about a group of children would be incorrect, asserting that the "children" sixty years later are all the same is ridiculous. Therefore dental hygienists should deliberately set aside culturally instilled stereotypes about patients older than the age of 60. This allows the dental hygienist to be attuned to the actual mix of physical-physiologic and psychologic-behavioral characteristics that is truly relevant to that patient (Table 11-5).

PHYSIOLOGIC CHARACTERISTICS

Chronic Disease

An older person unquestionably is more likely than a younger one to live with one or more chronic diseases, disabilities, or both. Unlike acute disease (e.g., influenza), which has a clearly defined beginning and ending, chronic diseases do not go away. The effects of chronic diseases such as hypertension, atherosclerosis, arthritis, periodontitis, and hearing loss are encountered more with advancing age, both because their pathophysiologies are cumulative (i.e., the physiologic changes that bring them about gradually accumulate over time) and because the changes are essentially irreversible.[25]

Many older individuals regularly take pain medications, such nonsteroidal antiinflammatory drugs (NSAIDs), to control arthritis. In April and July 2005, the U.S. Food and Drug Administration (FDA) issued letters to sponsors of all NSAIDs requesting that they make labeling changes to their products. These letters included recommended proposed labeling for both the prescription and the over-the-counter (OTC) NSAIDs, as well as a medication guide for the entire class of prescription products. cyclooxygenase-2 (COX-2) selective (which includes Bextra, Celebrex, and Vioxx) and nonselective NSAIDs were included. The letters also included a request that manufacturers revise the labeling (package insert) for their products to include a boxed warning that highlights the potential for increased risk of cardiovascular events and the well-described, serious, potentially life-threatening GI bleeding associated with their use. Vioxx and Bextra have been removed from the market. The Celebrex labeling will (in addition to the general labeling that will apply to all NSAIDs) also contain safety data from long-term treatment trials with celecoxib. (Refer to http://www.fda.gov/cder/drug/infopage/COX2/default.htm for more information.)

DENTAL CONSIDERATIONS

The effects of chronic disease on oral health and oral care are diverse. Arthritic changes may have significant effects on oral hygiene care: grasping and manipulation of oral hygiene devices can become painful, cumbersome, or impossible.[60] Declining visual acuity (particularly close up and in dim light) and hearing loss may impair the efficacy of patient instructions that are given verbally or in writing.

Table 11-5	Late Adulthood Characteristics		
AGE	**ANATOMICAL CHARACTERISTICS**	**PATHOLOGIC CHARACTERISTICS**	**PHYSIOLOGIC CHARACTERISTICS**
60 Years and Older	Natural adult dentition or partial to complete edentulism exists.	Root caries, recurrent root caries, gingivitis, and periodontitis may be seen.	It becomes more challenging for patients to practice adequate oral hygiene because of changes such as arthritis, dementia, poor eyesight, impaired coordination, and decreased grip strength.
		Periodontitis correlated with tooth loss and predisposition to candidiasis may be seen.	Non–insulin-dependent diabetes mellitus (NIDDM) may be seen.
		Recurrent decay, gingivitis, and halitosis may be seen.	Lowered salivary flow because of medications or disease may be seen.
		Gingival hyperplasia may be seen.	Calcium channel blockers may be used for cardiovascular disease and hypertension.
		Oral cancer (mainly in men) may be seen.	Impaired salivary flow and taste perception may be seen, as well as impaired oral intake and difficulty chewing and swallowing.

Diabetes, which affects nearly 10% of older Americans, interferes with the management of periodontal disease, is strongly correlated with tooth loss, and predisposes the patient to candidiasis.[74] Individuals with congestive heart failure may need to remain in an upright position during care to avoid experiencing pulmonary distress. Cognitive impairment resulting from past cerebrovascular disease or progressive dementia (most commonly Alzheimer's disease) often interferes with the provision and quality of daily care and may affect patient cooperation during dental appointments.[70,72]

Increasing prevalence of chronic disease customarily leads to increasing use of medications to slow disease progression, to minimize the effect of disease on function and comfort, or to do both.[25] Most medications commonly prescribed to older patients have the capacity to bring about significant oral health consequences.* Salivary hypofunction is a potential consequence of nearly 80% of the 200 most commonly prescribed medications. Absence of an adequate supply of properly constituted saliva increases intraoral acidity and raises bacterial counts, thereby fostering gingivitis, dental caries, and halitosis. Several of the calcium channel blockers, prescribed for cardiovascular disease and hypertension, cause a gingival hyperplasia in a quarter to a third of those ingesting the drugs. Cyclosporin, indispensable for preventing graft rejection in patients who have received an organ transplant (e.g., kidney, heart, liver), causes similar challenging periodontal effects. A wide variety of medications, including diuretics, beta blockers (for hypertension), and antineoplastic chemotherapy agents, are known to cause painful oral ulcerations.

Oral diseases in advanced age are the same as the maladies of younger adults, although their presentations may be distinctive. With advancing age, dental caries is more likely to be recurrent, and root areas of the teeth are more intensely affected. Tooth loss affects individuals at all ages; however, in older individuals, tooth loss is more likely to result in multitooth edentulous spans and even fully edentulous arches.[35,68,69]

Periodontal disease in older adults generally presents as loss of attachment, recession, and exposed root areas, rather than as deep and suppurating pockets (Figure 11-11). The reason for the different clinical presentations is because teeth susceptible to the more destructive forms of the disease are more likely to have been lost by advanced age. Teeth still present in later life stages are more likely to show signs of prior attachment loss that has fallen short of causing exfoliation. Oral cancer is most prevalent in individuals (mostly men) in their 50s and 60s, but it actually declines in prevalence by age 70 and beyond.[70]

Although chronic diseases are more common in elderly persons, aging must not be confused with disease. Everyone ages, but not everyone is afflicted with a particular disease—true even when the disease is common, such as arthritis in elderly individuals or gingivitis in those with one or more natural teeth. Most commonly held (but inaccurate) expectations about older individuals are in fact disease changes, rather than changes because of the aging process itself. Deafness, confusion, dry mouth, tooth loss, stiffness, and curvature of the spine are physiologic states that, although more common in older persons, are in fact the result of identifiable causes that are independent of the aging process.

The aging process is universal, progressive (i.e., the changes are additive over time), and irreversible. Unlike the causes of many diseases, the causative agent in the aging process (i.e., time) cannot be modified or eliminated. The exact mechanisms of aging are still being identified, but their effects are expressed at all levels in the organism.

The aggregate result of various age-related changes is frailty—impaired ability to recover from physiologic stress. Persons of advanced age often display high levels of function and health within the circumstances in which they customarily function, but their apparent robustness must not be confused with the resiliency of youth. People of advanced age and excellent health may slip on the ice or trip over a rug in the home. When they do, their slower reflexes are more likely to result in a fall, the fall more likely to result in a fracture, and the fracture more likely to result in extended hospitalization and isolation than would occur in a younger person.

Oral health in young adults is generally not thought to be a critical factor in overall wellness, except in extreme cases of neglect or those who are immunocompromised. However, in an older individual who may remain healthy only as long as his or her diet remains undisturbed, social relationships are not impaired, and one or more implanted prosthetic devices remain uninfected, oral health may be a life-or-death matter. Preventive dentistry in advanced age is not merely cosmetic or discretionary but a rational and cost-effective method for ensuring that a problem-prone yet essential body system remains healthy and functional.[70,72]

Aging in the Oral Cavity

Age-related changes in the oral cavity are difficult to separate from changes resulting from disease and environment, but they may have significant effect on oral healthcare behaviors. The most familiar age change concerns the gradual but steady deposition of secondary dentin on the walls of pulp chambers. Dental caries or prior restoration of a tooth stimulates a similar change, as do severe intraoral temperature swings. Pulps of

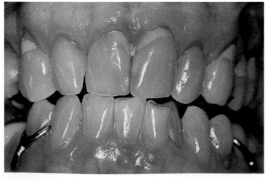

FIGURE 11-11
Permanent dentition with periodontal concerns.

*References 11, 15, 24, 25, 33, 58, 70, 71.

older teeth are smaller, resulting in a diminished need for blood supply and a consequent decline in nerve supply. Patients become less aware of unexpected sensitivity to sweets or other helpful reminders for dental attention and are more tolerant of fractured but asymptomatic teeth. Thus patients who are accustomed to waiting until they perceive a need for dental care before they arrange for appointments may become infrequent but high-need consumers of dental care.

Because of pulpal insensitivity, older patients tend to be more tolerant of oral care that would be intolerable without local anesthetic in younger patients (although diversity of psychologic overlays of the dental experience and of pain perception makes this generalization far from universal).[23,28,46]

PSYCHOLOGIC-BEHAVIORAL CHARACTERISTICS

Diversity within the aged population is not limited to physical characteristics. Socioeconomic differences throughout life, educational and vocational opportunities, early experiences with healthcare providers, cultural beliefs about health and the dentition, and exposure to societal attitudes about the role of the aged are different for each older person and have combined in each case to result in the emergence of a unique—and everchanging—individual. Yet through all this diversity are some generalizations that can be made and should be kept in mind when working with persons of advanced age.

The first generalization concerns changes in the perceived importance and ultimate fate of the natural dentition. Persons born around the beginning of the twentieth century most likely went through childhood and the appearance of the permanent dentition without having ever received dental care other than possibly extractions. Restorations and preventive care were unknown to the vast majority of Americans until later in the twentieth century. Total tooth loss by a person's 20s or 30s or even earlier, was much more common in those born in the first two decades of the twentieth century than those born in the 1920s and 1930s. Many of the latter group benefited in early adulthood from the growing number of bettertrained and more accessible dentists, resulting in a higher degree of tooth retention in early adulthood. The children born in the 1940s, 1950s, and early 1960s, known in popular culture as the Baby Boomers, include millions of Americans who have been exposed to fluoridated drinking water and dentifrice since birth.

Exposure to growing levels of oral health awareness, rising sophistication, and improvement of dental materials have raised most older Americans' expectations of their dentitions and of the dental profession. Members of the two oldest groups of Americans (ages 70 to 90 and older) who retain some teeth may believe their dentition has lasted longer than they would ever have thought possible; therefore they are somewhat resigned to deterioration to the edentulous state.

A second generalization concerns the relationship between a health provider and an older person. Until the late 1960s, most adults deferred to their physicians' and dentists' opinions. Patients believed, or behaved as if they believed, that clinicians knew what was in each patient's best interests and would act accordingly. Most patients knew little about their conditions or treatments other than what they were told. Today the public generally knows, or wants to know, all about health care.

Persons of advanced age are far more likely than their younger counterparts to maintain an unshakable faith in their providers and to give less legitimacy to their own concerns and questions. Dentists and dental hygienists are trained to empower patients by listening to and addressing their concerns and remaining open to alternatives that the patients suggest. They may inadvertently offend patients who habitually have no desire to be part of the clinical decision process and are disinterested or even frankly annoyed to hear details about their health or treatment. In addition, clinicians who expect older patients to be perfectly open with them because the patients have been given ample opportunities to voice concerns or ask for clarifications may be puzzled when home care instructions are not followed, to the point of compromising care. Dentists and dental hygienists caring for older patients must be mindful of this disparity in expectations and should take extra efforts to elicit information or repeat important instructions for patients who may not accept their right to be part of the clinical process.

A third generalization relates to the earlier discussion concerning aging and disease and to the immediately preceding point about communication. Older persons—particularly men—are notorious underreporters of symptoms. The customary explanation for underreporting problems is belief that pain, poor vision, or loose teeth accompany old age. This belief reduces the likelihood of older patients raising these issues with a physician, optometrist, or dentist and increases the likelihood of accepting and trying to adjust to these conditions. Oral healthcare providers must be alert for clues that the older patient is just accepting something that represents a treatable, unhealthful oral state, such as a new crown that is "just a little high" or an endodontically treated tooth that continues to hurt. This may be avoided by educating the patient about what sensations should be expected from a treatment and in particular which sensations mandate professional attention.

A fourth generalization deals with the respect accorded a patient of advanced age.[6] Healthcare providers display one or both of the following inappropriate behaviors when confronted with a debilitated older person in the company of a relative or caregiver who is younger or otherwise more robust.[19] The first behavior is to become engaged with the accompanying person in a dialog regarding the patient. This individual may be more prompt or appropriate in responding or may initiate responses even when questions are directed toward the patient. However, unless the patient indicates a preference otherwise, the healthcare provider should not allow discussion with the third party to supersede interaction with the patient. To do otherwise is to indicate that the patient is inadequate, incompetent, or otherwise diminished relative to the others present.

The second inappropriate behavior a healthcare professional may display is to call patients by their first names. When older

Note

Older individuals who have been exposed to preventive and restorative dental care throughout their lifetimes are more likely to continue such habits and practices into seniority and to take actions to preserve their dentitions.

individuals become dependent, a tendency exists to begin to treat them like children, such as speaking for them, reinterpreting their statements, and minimizing their complaints. Addressing a total stranger, who may be the retired president of a *Fortune 500* company or the chairperson of the board of a foundation, by first name can unconsciously but effectively deprive the patient of identity and self-respect. Until a patient of advanced age has specifically requested to be called by his or her first name, that person should be addressed by an appropriate title (e.g., Mr. Smith, Mrs. Jones).

The fifth important generalization is that patients of any age are still capable of learning new tasks, as long as their cognitive abilities are not impaired by disease. Abundant research published in the educational and psychologic literature has demonstrated repeatedly that learning ability is not impaired by age alone. Older learners may require a greater number of repeated exposures to the new material, may have visual or auditory impairments that require special efforts on the part of the instructor, or may need to have their own knowledge on an issue validated before incorporating new material. However, they will learn, and once having learned they may actually retain and apply the new material to a greater degree than they could when they were younger. "You can't teach an old dog new tricks" is an untrue adage. Teachers of "new tricks" must realize the shortcoming of delivering a message in a set fashion instead of adjusting the message to best suit a particular learner. When the specific needs of the cognitively unimpaired older person are identified and addressed, learning proceeds with excellent results.

The biopsychosocial model provides a framework for addressing variations among people at each life stage and how these facets affect health and disease. Understanding the characteristics associated with each life stage will assist the dental hygienist and others in providing age-appropriate diagnoses, education, prevention, and interventions.

References

1. Adair SM: Overview of the history and current status of fluoride supplementation schedules, *J Public Health Dent* 59(4):252-258, 1999.
2. Altshuler B: Anorexia nervosa and bulimia—a review for the dental hygienist, *J Dent Hyg* 10:466-471, 1986.
3. Amar S, Chung KM: Influence of hormonal variation on the periodontium in women, *J Periodontol 2000* 6:79-87, 1994.
4. American Academy of Pediatric Dentistry (AAPD): Clinical guideline on periodicity of examination, preventive dental services, anticipatory guidance, and oral treatment for children, *Pediatr Dent* 25(7):12, 2003.
4a. American Association of Oral and Maxillofacial Surgeons: Position paper on bisphosphonate-related osteonecrosis of the jaws. Approved by the Board of Trustees September 25, 2006. http://www.aaoms.org/docs/position_papers/osteonecrosis.pdf
5. American Dental Association Report: Antibiotic interference with oral contraceptives, *J Am Dent Assoc* 133:880, 2002.
6. Atchison KA, Anderson RM: Demonstrating successful aging using the international collaborative study for oral health outcomes, *J Public Health Dent* 60(4):282-288, 2000.
7. Barnett R, Shusterman S: Fetal alcohol syndrome: review of literature and report of cases, *J Am Dent Assoc* 111(10):591-593, 1985.
8. Ben-Sira Z: Eclectic incentives for health behavior: an additional perspective on health-oriented behavior change, *Health Educ Res* 6:211-229, 1991.
9. Bergner L, Susser MW: Low birth weight and prenatal nutrition: an interpretive review, *Pediatrics* 46(6):946-966, 1970.
10. Brambilla E et al: Caries prevention during pregnancy: results of a 30-month study, *J Am Dent Assoc* 129(7):871-877, 1998.
11. Burket LW et al: *Burket's oral medicine diagnosis and treatment,* ed 9, Philadelphia, 1994, JB Lippincott.
12. Casamassimo PS: Relationships between oral and systemic health, *Pediatr Clin North Am* 47(5):1149-1157, 2000.
13. Charonko CV, BeBiase CB: Dental health for children: an adult responsibility, *J Pract Nurs* 34:45-54, 1984.
14. Christen JA, Christen AG: Behavioral considerations in preventive dentistry: six lessons learned from the past, *J Indiana Dent Assoc* 66(4):17-21, 1987.
15. Ciancio S: *American dental association guide to dental therapeutics,* Chicago, 1998, ADA Publishing.
16. Compas BE et al: Coping with stress during childhood and adolescence: problems, progress, and potential in theory and research, *Psychol Bull* 127(1):87-127, 2001.
17. Donahue EM et al: The divided self: concurrent and longitudinal effects of psychological adjustment and social roles on self-concept differentiation, *J Pers Soc Psychol* 64(5):834-846, 1993.
18. Everett MS: Mouth protectors, *J Dent Hyg* 56:27-33,1982.
19. Eyison J et al: A comparative study of the attitude of dental students towards the elderly, *Eur J Prosthodont Restor Dent* 1(2):87-90,1992.
20. Feldman RS: *Understanding psychology,* ed 4, New York, 1996, McGraw-Hill.
21. Finkbeiner BL, Johnson CS: *Mosby's comprehensive dental assisting—a clinical approach,* St Louis, 1995, Mosby.
22. Fowler EB, Breault LG, Cuenin MF: Periodontal disease and its association with systemic disease, *Mil Med* 166(1):85-89, 2001.
23. Friedlander AH et al: Dental management of the geriatric patient with major depression, *Spec Care Dentist* 13(6):249-253, 1993.
24. Gage TW, Pickett FA: *Mosby's dental drug reference,* ed 5, St Louis, 2001, Mosby.
25. Ganong WF: *Review of medical physiology,* ed 13, East Norwalk, Conn, 1987, Appleton & Lange.
26. Genco RJ: Periodontal disease and the risk for myocardial infarction and cardiovascular disease, *Cardiovasc Rev Rep* 19(3):34-40, 1998.
27. Genco RJ, Grossi SG: Is estrogen deficiency a risk factor for periodontal disease? *Compend Contin Educ Dent* 19(suppl 22):23-30, 1998.
28. Gerow JR: *Psychology: an introduction,* ed 3, New York, 1992, Harper Collins.
29. Going RE, Loehman RE, Chan MS: Mouthguard materials: their physical and mechanical properties, *J Am Dent Assoc* 89:132-138, 1974.
30. Health and Human Services: *Health United States report,* ed 20 [Internet], Washington, DC, 1995, HHS [http://www.os.dhhs.gov].
31. Hetherington EM, Parke RD: *Child psychology: a contemporary viewpoint,* ed 4, New York, 1993, McGraw-Hill.
32. Holt K, Barzel H: *Open wide,* National Maternal and Child Oral Health Resource Center, Washington DC, 2006, Georgetown University (OHRC).

33. Jenkins GM: *The physiology and biochemistry of the mouth,* ed 4, Oxford, England, 1978, Blackwell Scientific Publications.

34. Johnson DL, Rue VM: The bulimic dental patient: recognition and recommendations, *J Dent Hyg* 8:372-377, 1985.

35. Johnson NW: *Dental caries markers of high and low risk groups and individuals,* Cambridge, 1991, Cambridge University Press.

35a. Kademani D et al: Primary surgical therapy for osteonecrosis of the jaw secondary to bisphosphonate therapy. *Mayo Clin Proc* 81:1100-03, 2006.

36. Kiyak HA: Successful aging: implications for oral health, *J Public Health Dent* 60(4):276-281, 2000.

37. Levine RA, Shanaman RH: Translating clinical outcomes to patient value: an evidence-based treatment approach, *Int J Periodontics Restorative Dent* 15(2):187-200, 1995.

38. Levy GF: A survey of preschool oral health education programs, *Public Health* 44(1):10-18, 1984.

39. Linn EL: Teenagers' attitudes, knowledge, and behaviors related to oral health, *J Am Dent Assoc* 92:946-951,1976.

40. Mellander M et al: Mineralization defects in deciduous teeth of low birth weight infants, *Acta Paediatr Scand* 71:727-733, 1982.

41. Meurman JH: Dental infections and general health, *Quintessence Int* 28(12):807-811, 1997.

42. Miller L: Depression in middle age patient, *Encephale* 18(4):507-510, 1992.

43. Miller LS et al: The relationship between reduction in periodontal inflammation and diabetes control: a report of 9 cases, *J Periodontol* 63(10):843-848, 1992.

44. Moss ME et al: Exploratory case-control analysis of psychosocial factors and adult periodontitis, *J Periodontol* 67:1060-1069, 1996.

45. Moss SJ: Preventive techniques in infant dental care, *Nurse Pract* 7:37-48, 1988.

46. Niessen LC, Gibson G: Aging and oral health for the 21st century, *Gen Dent* 48(5):544-549, 2000.

47. Nowak AJ, Casamassimo PS: Using anticipatory guidance to provide early dental intervention, *J Am Dent Assoc* 126(8):1156-1163, 1995.

48. Nowak AJ, Warren JJ: Infant oral health and oral habits, *Pediatr Clin North Am* 47(5):1043-1066, 2000.

49. Offenbacher S, Boggess K, Murtha A: Progressive periodontal disease and risk of very preterm delivery, *Obstet Gynecol* 107:29-36, 2006.

50. Offenbacher S, Katz V, Fertik G: Periodontal infection as a possible risk factor for preterm low birth weight, *J Periodontol* 67(suppl):1103-1113, 1996.

51. *Oral health for women* [Internet], East Setauket, NY, 2005, aboutsmiles.com [http://www.aboutsmiles.com].

52. *Oral health in America: a report of the surgeon general,* Washington, DC, 2000, Department of Health and Human Services.

53. O'Rourke T, Smith BJ, Nolte AE: Health risk attitudes, beliefs and behaviors of students grades 7-12, *J Sch Health* 54(5):210-214, 1984.

54. Özçaka Ö, Biçakç N, Köse T: Effect of the menstrual cycle on pain experience associated with periodontal therapy. Randomized, pilot study, *J Clin Periodontol* 32:1170-1174, 2005.

55. Palomo L, Bissada N, Liu J: Periodontal assessment of postmenopausal women receiving risedronate, *Menopause* 12(6):685-690, November/December 2005.

56. *Prostate cancer* [Internet], 2006, Prostate.com/LupronDepot (leuprolide acetate for depot suspension) [http://www.prostate.com/prostatecancer].

57. Raber-Durlacher JE, van Steenbergen TJ, Vander Vellen U: Experimental gingivitis during pregnancy and postpartum clinical endocrinological and microbiological aspects, *J Clin Periodontol* 21(8):549-558, 1994.

58. Remick RA, Blashberg B: Clinical aspects of xerostomia, *J Clin Psychiatry* 44(2):63-65, 1983.

59. Renshaw DC: Dentists and bulimia-anorexia nervosa, *Pa Dent J (Harrisb)* 52(4):20-21, 1985.

60. Risheim H, Kjarheim V, Arneberg P: Improvement of oral hygiene in patients with rheumatoid arthritis, *Scand J Dent Res* 100:172-175, 1992.

61. Rose LF, Steinberg BJ, Minsk L: The relationship between periodontal disease and systemic conditions, *Compend Contin Educ Dent* 21(10A):870-877, 2000.

62. Ruel-Kellerman M: What are the psychosocial factors involved in motivating individuals to retain their teeth? Dreams and facts, *Int Dent J* 34:105-109, 1984.

63. Ruggiero SL et al: Osteonecrosis of the jaws associated with the use of bisphosphonates: a review of 63 cases, *J Oral Maxillofac Surg* 62(5):527-534, 2004.

63a. Salmassy D: Fosamax: bad to the bone? *Modern Hygienist* 3:7, July 2007.

64. Sanchez OM, Childers NK: Anticipatory guidance in infant oral health: rationale and recommendations, *Am Fam Physician* 61(1):115-120, 2000.

65. Saunders RP: What is health promotion? *Health Educ* 19(5):14-18,1998.

66. Schnitzer T, Bone HG, Crepaldi G: Preventing bone loss in space, *ASGSB Bull 18(2)*:57, 2005.

67. Schnitzer T, Bone HG, Crepaldi G: Therapeutic equivalence of alendronate 70 mg once weekly and alendronate 10 mg daily in treatment of osteoporosis. Alendronate once weekly study group, *Aging (Milano)* 12(1):13-21, 2000.

68. Shay K: Restorative considerations in the dental treatment of the older patient, *Gen Dent* 48(5):550-554, 2000.

69. Shay K: Root caries in the elderly: an update for the next century, *J Indiana Dent Assoc* 76(4):37, 39-43, 1998.

70. Shay K: Identifying the needs of the elderly dental patient: the geriatric dental assessment, *Dent Clin North Am* 38(3):499-523, 1994.

71. Shay K, Reuhlar MR, Renner RP: Oropharyngeal candidosis in the older patient, *J Am Geriatr Soc* 45(7):863-870, 1997.

72. Shay K, Ship JA: The importance of oral health in the older patient, *J Am Geriatr Soc* 43(12):1414-1422,1995.

73. Shlossman M et al: Type 2 diabetes mellitus and periodontal disease, *J Am Dent Assoc* 121(4):532-536, 1990.

74. Taylor GW, Loesche WJ, Terpenning MS: Impact of oral diseases on systemic health in the elderly: diabetes mellitus and aspiration pneumonia, *J Public Health Dent* 60(4):313-320, 2000.

75. Vick VC, Harfst SA: The oral risk assessment and early intervention system—a clinician's tool for integrating the bio-psychosocial risk into oral disease interventions, *Compend Contin Educ Dent,* 21(30 suppl):57-62, 2000.

76. Wassertheil-Smoller S et al: Effect of estrogen plus progestin on stroke in postmenopausal women: the Women's Health Initiative: a randomized trial, *JAMA* 289:2673-2684, 2003.

Comprehensive Health History

Samuel Paul Nesbit • Karen K. Tiwana •

Ralph Howard Leonard, Jr.

INSIGHT

The dental hygienist must be aware of the implications of systemic diseases and illness to prevent harm to patients and to provide safe and effective care. Studying the diseases associated with each organ system, knowing signs, and recognizing symptoms will aid in developing a professional approach to oral health care. Obtaining, accurately recording, and evaluating a comprehensive health history will help ensure successful treatment outcomes.

✡ CASE STUDY 12-1 | Significance of a Thorough Health History

The dental hygienist greets a 58-year-old black male patient, Stanley Belzak, in the reception room. He is obese and is seated on the edge of the chair and leaning forward, resting on his walking cane. When the hygienist calls his name, Mr. Belzak strains to stand and is unsteady. After a few seconds he begins to stand upright and walk. His gait is slow and unsteady, despite the use of a cane.

Once in the dental treatment room, his transition into the dental chair is slow and labored. After being seated in the dental chair, he requires a few moments to "catch his breath." To sit back in the chair, Mr. Belzak requires assistance in elevating his lower legs onto the dental chair.

A review of Mr. Belzak's health history reveals the following:
- *Age 42:* Mr. Belzak was diagnosed with non–insulin-dependent diabetes mellitus (NIDDM), treated with glipizide (Glucotrol) 15 mg once a day and metformin (Glucophage) 1000 mg twice a day. He states that he checks his blood sugar daily with a Dextrostix and that his fasting blood sugar is usually about 180+ mg/dl.
- *Age 45:* He was diagnosed with **chronic obstructive pulmonary disease** (COPD), high blood pressure, and **atrial arrhythmia.** Mr. Belzak states that his initial blood pressure before medication was 190/112 mm Hg. The hypertension is being treated with an angiotensin-converting enzyme (ACE) inhibitor (Accupril [quinapril] 40 mg twice a day), a diuretic (furosemide 60 mg/day), and a potassium supplement (K-Dur 8 mEq Extencaps [two Extencaps twice a day]). Mr. Belzak's atrial dysrhythmia resulted in multiple **transient ischemic attacks** (TIAs), and he is presently being managed with digoxin (Lanoxin) (0.125 mg/day) and warfarin (Coumadin) (alternating doses of 5 mg and 2.5 mg). His last international normalized ratio (INR) was 2.5.

- *Age 55:* A physical examination revealed an enlarged prostate gland. The prostate-specific antigen (PSA) was within the normal range. His physicians decided to evaluate annually; no medications were prescribed at this time.
- *Age 56:* Mr. Belzak was diagnosed with angina pectoris. This condition is being managed with nifedipine (Adalat) (20 mg three times a day). At the time of diagnosis, the physician detected a heart murmur (HM). An echocardiogram revealed a stenotic aortic valve. In addition to the existing COPD, Mr. Belzak is now experiencing congestive heart failure (CHF).
- *Allergies:* Mr. Belzak states that he is allergic to penicillin and sulfonamides.
- *Social history:* Mr. Belzak's **social history** includes the fact that he is a widower. (His wife died 2 years ago.) He has two grown children, a son and daughter, and he lives at home alone. He smokes two packs of cigarettes per day now (one pack per day until his spouse died). He has smoked for at least 40 years (40+ pack years). He states that he has tried to quit on numerous occasions using the gum and patch, but they did not work. His alcohol consumption is minimal (less than three drinks per week). The chance of this patient experiencing a mild to moderate form of depression should be considered.
- *General:* Mr. Belzak states that he is supposed to see his physician every 3 months, but he has not seen her regularly since his spouse died. His medications have been refilled by a telephone call to the physician's office.

Mr. Belzak's dental status consists of the following findings:
- *Dental caries:* Interproximal enamel lesions, root caries, and Class V lesions in every sextant

✴ CASE STUDY 12-1 Significance of a Thorough Health History—cont'd

- *Periodontal disease:* Gingival recession, increased probing depths with spontaneous bleeding, overt marginal inflammation, generalized edematous gingival tissue, with the mandibular buccal area exhibiting a pronounced hypertrophy
- *Missing teeth:* Numerous teeth are missing in the maxilla and mandible. To replace the missing teeth in the maxilla, Mr. Belzak wears a removable partial denture. He states that he has a partial denture for the bottom teeth, but because it does not fit well, he does not wear it.
- *Oral soft tissues:*

  Palate—A generalized whitish appearance is present, with numerous elevated areas with a red center (**nicotinic stomatitis**). The palatal tissue below the framework of the partial denture is bright red.

  Buccal mucosa—Generalized atrophic in appearance, with the presence of ulcerative lesions, with a white, lacelike pattern in the posterior mandibular regions.

Lips—The patient complains that the lips feel swollen. **Angular cheilitis** is present.

- *General comments:* Mr. Belzak states that he brushes his teeth twice a day. He uses whatever toothpaste is on sale. He does not use a mouthrinse; he does not floss or scrape his tongue. He states that his mouth feels dry, and he has to drink fluids often during the day to keep his mouth moist. A clinical assessment determines that no saliva is pooling in the floor of the mouth, and the buccal mucosa does not appear to have a saliva layer.

The dental hygienist should mentally review the office emergency protocol.

The dental hygienist must encourage this patient to see his physician and perhaps make a follow-up phone call a week or so later to determine whether he has done so. This attempted phone call should be noted in the patient's dental chart.

KEY TERMS

Addison's disease	dysuria	hypothyroidism	rheumatic heart disease
adrenocorticotropic hormone	edema	international normalized ratio	scleroderma
angina pectoris	endogenous	ketoacidosis	Sjögren's syndrome
angular cheilitis	epistaxis	lupus	social history
atrial arrhythmia	exogenous	myasthenia gravis	teratogens
chancre	fainting (syncope)	myocardial infarction	thrombocytopenia
chronic obstructive pulmonary disease	family history	nicotinic stomatitis	tinnitus
	fibromyalgia	parathyroid hormone	transient ischemic attacks
comprehensive health history	gall stones	paresis	trigeminal neuralgia (cranial nerve V)
congestive heart failure	Health Insurance Portability and Accountability Act	pellagra	
Crohn's disease		pernicious anemia	tuberculosis
Cushing's disease (primary aldosteronism)	hematuria	polycythemia	type 2 herpes
	hepatitis	polydipsia	upper respiratory infection
diabetes mellitus	hypertension	polyuria	vasovagal syncope
dyspnea	hyperthyroidism	ptosis	ventricular fibrillation

LEARNING OUTCOMES

After reading this chapter the student will be able to:

1. Identify the essential components of a comprehensive patient health history.
2. List the parts of each component of the health history.
3. Recognize the importance of each component of the health history to the acquisition of an accurate health database.
4. Analyze verbal and written patient responses to the health questionnaire to anticipate and initiate the needed modifications in the treatment plan.
5. Analyze verbal and written patient responses to the health questionnaire to recognize when a medical or dental consultation is warranted.

Role and Importance of the Patient History

The patient history is the most basic and (arguably) most important element of each encounter that the dental hygienist will have with a patient. Patient history is an essential part of the practice of dentistry, dental hygiene, and all healthcare professions. In a responsible professional practice, the patient history is touched on at each patient visit and covered in greater depth at each periodic visit. Taking the patient's history is the first step in the treatment process, the continuum of care that begins with the following:

- Conducting the initial oral examination (including the patient history, clinical examination, radiographic imaging, and any diagnostic tests and consultations)

- Making a comprehensive diagnosis
- Planning care with informed consent
- Providing the planned comprehensive treatment
- Evaluating the need for long-term supportive care after the completion of the active phase of treatment

Without an accurate and complete patient history, all other parts of this continuum become suspect.

> **Note**
> The healthcare professional's ability to communicate with the patient at this encounter in a manner that builds trust and promotes open and honest dialog can have a significant effect on the accuracy and completeness of the information that is derived.

The patient history constitutes the *subjective* portion of the patient examination in two ways: (1) the history is derived exclusively from the patient (the subject), and (2) the information is, by necessity, filtered and interpreted by the patient (thus biased or subjective by its very nature). By contrast, the findings from the clinical examination, radiographic imaging, and diagnostic testing are performed and interpreted by the healthcare professional and are characterized as the *objective* portion of the examination.

The patient examination "constitutes the foundation not only for an intelligent approach to diagnosis, but also for the establishment of a successful patient/dentist (and/or hygienist) relationship."[6] The process of taking the patient history is, in most cases, the initial point of communication with the patient. Not only is this the first opportunity for the healthcare professional to assess the patient but also the patient's first opportunity to assess the healthcare professional's competence and compassion.

> **Note**
> At the most basic level, a patient who does not trust his or her care provider is less likely to return for treatment, to be on time for dental appointments, and to comply with home care recommendations.

How a patient history is taken can have a major effect on how well the patient will cooperate with the dental team and comply with professional recommendations.

Another significant benefit of the patient history is that it can impart to the dental team critical healthcare information. A complete patient history will reveal the following:

- Any oral concern or concerns that the patient may have
- Previously unrecognized oral or systemic disease
- Conditions that may modify or limit the nature or scope of dental treatment
- Medical conditions or problems that are likely to predispose the patient to having a medical emergency in the dental office

From a risk management perspective, the importance of having a thorough and complete patient history cannot be overemphasized. Poor record keeping and lack of a thorough patient history in particular often become a source of concern by State Boards of Dental Examiners when they are called on to investigate a complaint (for more information regarding legal and ethical considerations, see Chapter 3). Lack of documentation is rarely the original cause of the complaint, but it may surface as a compelling issue during the review of the patient record.

A thorough patient history is a benchmark for professional competence. Ideal documentation is often the single most effective strategy to use in trying to avoid malpractice litigation. When a case is litigated, good documentation can be instrumental in helping the dental team to defend themselves successfully. Even in cases that are resolved with a judgment that is unfavorable to the dentist or hygienist, damages can be minimized when the documentation meets or exceeds the standard of care.

Formatting Options for the Patient History

Historically, the interviewer has had three general formats from which to select when deriving the patient history:

1. Open-ended
2. Closed
3. Combination

OPEN-ENDED FORMAT

In the open-ended format, the care provider asks the patient a series of preprescribed questions and records the findings on a blank sheet of paper. If the patient responds positively to any of the questions, then additional questions are posed to elicit the relative importance of the issue and ferret out any implications to dental treatment. This process is aptly described as a "branching tree" process. Inherent in this process is the expectation that the dentist or hygienist has a complete working knowledge of a complete array of medical problems and their implications.

Certainly this is an ideal mode of interviewing from a communication perspective—because the patient and care provider are engaged in dialog throughout the process. This format is often used in oral and maxillofacial surgery settings and hospital dentistry settings, as well as when delivering care to patients with complex medical histories such as a geriatric population.

CLOSED-ENDED FORMAT

The closed-ended format uses a completely self-contained medical history questionnaire, whereby the patient responds to a lengthy and detailed series of written medical (and dental) questions. Dialog with the patient is not a required element. The prototype of a closed-format questionnaire has been the Cornell Medical Index. With the advent of artificial intelligence, having a complete summary of the findings with interpretation of the significance of each condition prepared exclusively by computer analysis is now possible—leaving the care provider out of the primary role of interviewer. When the patient completes the questionnaire accurately, the derived information can be extremely detailed and complete, saving the practitioner considerable chair time.

However, significant disadvantages to this format exist. Because of the length of the questionnaire and the detail of the questions, many patient who do not have a high level of education may not be able to negotiate it successfully or may become bored and dismiss the process altogether. Some of the questions may seem overly intrusive and irrelevant to the patient—thereby reducing the compliance and accuracy of the instrument.

Perhaps most importantly, this format does little to enhance the communication process. At a time when many patients are already feeling that health care is being delivered in an unfeeling, bureaucratic, and impersonal manner, this does not enhance a positive image of dentistry.

COMBINATION FORMAT

Most general dental offices use the third mode of capturing the patient history—a combination format. (See Figure 12-1; forms are also located on the Evolve web site.)

In this venue the patient is asked to "check off" *yes*, *no*, or *don't know* responses to a series of major medical and dental problems or complaints on a written (or computer screen) questionnaire. After the patient has completed the form and signed to attest accuracy, the dental provider reviews the responses and asks appropriate follow-up questions to determine the significance of each positive response. In this mode the patient is responsible for the initial written responses, but dialog between the provider and patient is necessary. A key element in this process is that the dental care provider is responsible for the assessment and analysis of the medical and dental history information. This combination of patient-driven and practitioner-driven activities has the advantage of being a relatively efficient process that can be very accurate and complete and still preserve the positive aspects of open conversation with the patient.

In the past the patient has generally completed the patient history using paper and pencil. Although this continues to be the standard in many dental practices, many more options are now available. Some offices have made the same questionnaire available online for the patient to complete at home or on arrival in the office. Some dental offices have developed a user-friendly kiosk format so that patients can use a touch screen on their arrival. Asking the patients to bring any medications with them and giving them a preview of the questionnaire can further speed the process.

Some practices will have a staff person enter the patient's responses into the computer. For patients who are illiterate or unable to negotiate a computer format, this may be a necessity.

Prevention

Whether it be a paper or electronic venue, when using the combination format described previously, the dental care provider is responsible for reviewing the responses with the patient, assessing the significance of all positive responses, and determining any implications that the general and oral healthcare history may have on how dental care is to be delivered.

University of Dental Health Care	Patient Name: _____
Anytown, USA	Record No.: _____
Department of Dental Hygiene	Birth Date: _____ / _____ / _____

HEALTH HISTORY QUESTIONNAIRE

Directions to the patient: The following information about your health history is very important for us to provide you with the best possible dental hygiene services safely. Incorrect information may be dangerous to your health. All questions must be answered completely and accurately. If you don't understand a question, or are unsure of the answer, or want to discuss it with the dentist/or faculty, circle its number or letter. This Health History Questionnaire will become a part of your dental treatment record and will be considered confidential information.

HEALTH HISTORY

Are you under the care of a physician? Yes No Don't Know
Reason for last visit? _____
Date of last physical examination _____
Physicians   Name _____ Phone _____
                    Address _____

                    Name _____ Phone _____
                    Address _____

Have you had any serious illness, operation or been hospitalized in the past 5 years? If so, explain
_____

How long has it been since you've seen a dentist?   Within past 3 months
Within 3 months to 1 year   Within 1—3 years   Over 3 years

Reason for **last** visit? _____

Reason for **this** visit? _____

GENERAL

1. Are you in good health? Yes No Don't Know

2. Has there been any change in your health in the last year? Yes No Don't Know
   If yes, explain _____

3. Have you ever been hospitalized or had major surgery? Yes No Don't Know
   If yes, explain _____

4. Have you had an allergic reaction to any of the following?
   Any medication (list) _____
   Latex _____
   Metals _____
   Iodine _____
   Foods _____
   Other (list) _____

5. Have you ever had or been treated by a physician for:
   Tumors or growths   Yes No Don't Know
   Cancer   Yes No Don't Know
   If yes, list type, treatment, year _____
   X-ray treatments   Yes No Don't Know
   Chemotherapy   Yes No Don't Know

6. Do you use or have you ever used recreational drugs? Yes No Don't Know

7. Do you use tobacco in any form?   Yes No Don't Know
   If yes,
   Cigarette   Amount per day _____
   Cigar   Amount per day _____
   Pipe   Amount per day _____
   Chew/Dip/Spit   Amount per day _____

8. Have you quit using tobacco?   Yes No Don't Know
   If yes,   Within the last year   1–5 years   Longer than 5 years

9. How often do you use alcoholic beverages?
   ___ Never
   ___ Special occasions
   ___ A few times a month
   ___ A few times a week
   ___ Daily   Amount per day _____
   Have you quit using alcohol?   Length of time abstaining _____

10. For women,
    Are you pregnant or do you think you may be pregnant? Yes No Don't Know

    Are you currently taking birth control pills? Yes No Don't Know

    Are you nursing?   Yes No Don't Know

    Are you menopausal or perimenopausal?   Yes No Don't Know

MEDICATIONS

11. Are you taking any of the following medications?
    If yes to any, please list drug name and dosage
    a. Antibiotics or sulfa drugs   Yes No Don't Know
       If yes, list _____

    b. Anticoagulants (blood thinners)   Yes No Don't Know
       If yes, list _____

    c. High/low blood pressure medications   Yes No Don't Know
       If yes, list _____

    d. Cortisone / Steroids   Yes No Don't Know
       If yes, list _____

    e. Tranquilizers/Sedatives   Yes No Don't Know
       If yes, list _____

FIGURE 12-1
Sample health history questionnaire.

Continued

f. Antihistamines   Yes   No   Don't Know
If yes, list: _____

g. Aspirin   Yes   No   Don't Know
If yes, list: _____

h. Insulin, or diabetes medications   Yes   No   Don't Know
If yes, list: _____

i. Digitalis or heart medications   Yes   No   Don't Know
If yes, list: _____

j. Nitroglycerine   Yes   No   Don't Know
If yes, list: _____

k. Hormones   Yes   No   Don't Know
If yes, list: _____

l. Pain medications   Yes   No   Don't Know
If yes, list: _____

m. Thyroid medication   Yes   No   Don't Know
If yes, list: _____

n. Vitamins, calcium, iron   Yes   No   Don't Know
If yes, list: _____

o. Any inhaler delivered medication   Yes   No   Don't Know
If yes, list: _____

p. Any other medications not listed above   Yes   No   Don't Know
If yes, list: _____

Have you ever been treated by a physician for:

SKIN

12. Itching, dermatitis, or eczema?   Yes   No   Don't Know

13. Psoriasis, seborrhea, or other skin disease?   Yes   No   Don't Know

14. Pigmentation problems?   Yes   No   Don't Know

15. Skin cancer, moles, or melanoma?   Yes   No   Don't Know

16. Allergies/adverse reactions to latex, medication, or metals?   Yes   No   Don't Know

MUSCULOSKELTAL

17. Stiff or swollen joints, arthritis, or rheumatism?   Yes   No   Don't Know

18. Lupus, polymyositis, scleroderma, Sjögren's syndrome?   Yes   No   Don't Know

19. Muscle weakness, pain, or fibromyalgia?   Yes   No   Don't Know

20. Bone deformity?   Yes   No   Don't Know

21. Prosthetic joints?   Yes   No   Don't Know
Has your physician recommended premedication?   Yes   No   Don't Know
If yes, type and dosage _____

EYES

22. Double vision?   Yes   No   Don't Know

23. Drooping eyelids?   Yes   No   Don't Know

24. Glaucoma?   Yes   No   Don't Know

25. Cataracts?   Yes   No   Don't Know

EARS, NOSE, THROAT

26. Hearing loss, tinnitis, hearing aid, or vertigo?   Yes   No   Don't Know

27. Frequent nosebleeds?   Yes   No   Don't Know

28. Frequent sore throats, tonsillitis, or swollen glands?   Yes   No   Don't Know

29. Sinusitis or rhinitis?   Yes   No   Don't Know

30. Hoarseness?   Yes   No   Don't Know

31. Mouth ulcers, canker sores, fever blisters, or cold sores?   Yes   No   Don't Know

RESPIRATORY

32. Acute or chronic coughing?   Yes   No   Don't Know

33. Blood in sputum?   Yes   No   Don't Know

34. Wheezing or asthma?   Yes   No   Don't Know

35. Bronchitis or emphysema?   Yes   No   Don't Know

36. Tuberculosis?   Yes   No   Don't Know

37. Pneumonia?   Yes   No   Don't Know

CARDIOVASCULAR

38. Shortness of breath?   Yes   No   Don't Know

39. Fainting?   Yes   No   Don't Know

40. Pain or pressure in your chest or angina?   Yes   No   Don't Know

41. Swollen ankles?   Yes   No   Don't Know

42. High or low blood pressure or orthostatic hypotension?   Yes   No   Don't Know

43. Rheumatic fever or rheumatic heart disease?   Yes   No   Don't Know

44. Congenital heart disorder?   Yes   No   Don't Know

45. Heart murmur or mitral valve prolapse?   Yes   No   Don't Know
Has your physician recommended premedication?   Yes   No   Don't Know
If yes, type and dosage _____

46. Cardiac dysrhythmias, abnormal heartbeats/flutters?   Yes   No   Don't Know

47. Do you have a pacemaker or defibrillator?   Yes   No   Don't Know

48. Congestive heart failure?   Yes   No   Don't Know

49. History of endocarditis?   Yes   No   Don't Know

50. Damaged or artificial heart valves?   Yes   No   Don't Know
Has your physician recommended premedication?   Yes   No   Don't Know
If yes, type and dosage _____

51. Myocardial infarct or heart attack?   Yes   No   Don't Know

52. Arteriosclerosis or atherosclerosis?   Yes   No   Don't Know

53. Stroke or transient ischemic attacks?   Yes   No   Don't Know

GASTROINTESTINAL

54. Difficulty in swallowing (dysphasia)?   Yes   No   Don't Know

55. Abnormal pain and ulcers?   Yes   No   Don't Know

56. Gastroesophageal reflux?   Yes   No   Don't Know

57. Hepatitis?   Yes   No   Don't Know

GENITOURINARY

58. Difficulty or pain on urination (dysuria)?   Yes   No   Don't Know

59. Blood in urine (hematuria)?   Yes   No   Don't Know

60. Excessive urination (polyuria)?   Yes   No   Don't Know

61. Kidney infections or urinary calculi?   Yes   No   Don't Know

62. Sexually transmitted disease or venereal disease?   Yes   No   Don't Know

63. Renal or kidney dialysis?   Yes   No   Don't Know

ENDOCRINE

64. Thyroid gland problems?   Yes   No   Don't Know

65. Weight changes?   Yes   No   Don't Know

66. Diabetes mellitus?   Yes   No   Don't Know

67. Excessive thirst (polydipsia)?   Yes   No   Don't Know

68. Adrenal gland problems?   Yes   No   Don't Know

HEMATOPOIETIC

69. Do you bruise easily?   Yes   No   Don't Know

70. Excessive bleeding problems?   Yes   No   Don't Know

71. Have you ever had a blood transfusion?   Yes   No   Don't Know

72. Anemia or sickle cell?   Yes   No   Don't Know

73. Hemophilia?   Yes   No   Don't Know

74. Leukemia?   Yes   No   Don't Know

75. AIDS, AIDS-related condition, or HIV positive?   Yes   No   Don't Know

NEUROLOGIC

76. Frequent headaches?   Yes   No   Don't Know

77. Dizziness or fainting spells?   Yes   No   Don't Know

78. Epilepsy or seizures disorder?   Yes   No   Don't Know

79. Neuritis or neuralgia?   Yes   No   Don't Know

80. Paralysis or stroke?   Yes   No   Don't Know

81. Alzheimer's disease?   Yes   No   Don't Know

82. Muscular dystrophy?   Yes   No   Don't Know

83. Lyme disease?   Yes   No   Don't Know

84. Parkinson's disease?   Yes   No   Don't Know

PSYCHIATRIC

85. Nervousness?   Yes   No   Don't Know

86. Depression or bipolar disorder?   Yes   No   Don't Know

87. Any other mental health condition?   Yes   No   Don't Know

88. Are there any other diseases, conditions or problems regarding your health not listed above?   Yes   No   Don't Know

If yes, explain _____

FIGURE 12-1, cont'd

Signature of Patient:
I understand the need for these questions to be answered truthfully. To the best of my knowledge, the answers I have given are accurate. I also understand it is very important to report any changes or updates in my medical status. I give permission to the Department of Dental Hygiene to obtain from my physician any additional information regarding my medical history needed to provide me the best treatment possible.

Signature_____   Date_____

If you have completed this form for another person, please print your name and sign below along with your relationship to patient.

Print_____   Relationship_____

Signature_____   Date_____

Health History Update: On a regular basis the patient should be questioned about any medical history changes, date and comments notated along with signature.

Date	Comments	Signature of Patient and Dentist
____	_____	_____
____	_____	_____
____	_____	_____
____	_____	_____
____	_____	_____
____	_____	_____
____	_____	_____
____	_____	_____

FIGURE 12-1, cont'd

With electronic entry, efforts must be made to ensure accuracy of the recorded information. **Health Insurance Portability and Accountability Act** (HIPAA) regulations demand confidentiality. There must also be safeguards to ensure security of the system and a means of ensuring that the information once captured and verified by the patient cannot be altered. But with these considerations in mind, the inherent accuracy and legibility of an electronic database is a significant benefit.

The reader should also note that many offices use a separate, more abbreviated form for an urgent-care or acute-care patient. An example of such a form is found in Figure 12-2.

Process for Obtaining the History

The importance of using good communication skills in the practice of dental hygiene is discussed at length in Chapter 5. Strong communication skills are particularly important when the hygienist is taking the general and oral health history from a patient. The dental professional should do the following when attempting to establish a positive communication process with the patient:
- Create a physical environment that is comfortable, tasteful, and nonthreatening to the patient
- Evoke a positive, caring attitude
- Use a chair position and demonstrate body language that is open and receptive, yet professional
- Maintain appropriate eye contact
- Talk at a pace that fits the comfort and abilities of the patient
- Be sensitive to the patient's needs and expectations

Questions asked of the dental patient can generally be categorized as *direct*, *open ended*, or *leading*. Direct questions are answered with a simple yes-or-no response. No discussion is needed, and no interpretation or explanation is expected. An example of a direct question is, "Have you ever had a heart transplant?" By asking a series of direct questions, the interviewer can quickly, efficiently, and accurately establish a baseline of critical information.

An open-ended question requires a considered reply by the patient and needs—at a minimum—a phrase or, commonly, one or more sentences to convey the response. An example of an open-ended question is, "Please describe what your previous dental experience has been like." Open-ended questions are useful when the examiner seeks to determine the *quality* of an event, experience, or disease process (and not just whether something happened). As noted earlier, such questions and conversations can be an important means of opening dialog between the care provider and the patient. These questions can also help establish a level of trust in the relationship. It can take more time to ask open-ended questions, but the information derived is generally much richer and fuller. In most cases the interview process, and the questionnaire itself, will contain both direct and open-ended questions to maximize the benefits of both types.

ABBREVIATED PATIENT HEALTH HISTORY URGENT CARE SERVICE

PATIENT NAME:_____

RECORD NO.:_____

DIRECTIONS TO THE PATIENT: The following information about your health history is very important to provide you with safe dental care. Incorrect information may be dangerous to your health. Please ANSWER ALL QUESTIONS by circling the response most appropriate for you.

Name of your Physician or Place you receive medical care:_____

Physician's office phone:_____ Office address:_____

1. Are you in good health?.. Yes No Don't Know

2. Has there been any change in your health during the last year?................. Yes No Don't Know

3. Are you currently under the care of a physician for any condition?
   If yes, explain._____ Yes No Don't Know

4. Are you currently taking any medications of any kind?.................. Yes No Don't Know
   If yes, please list medicine(s), dosage, and reason for taking._____
   _____

5. Do you need to have antibiotic premedication before dental treatment?.......... Yes No Don't Know

6. Have you ever had any allergic or unusual reactions to dental anesthetic?........ Yes No Don't Know

7. Have you ever had excessive bleeding during dental treatment?.............. Yes No Don't Know

8. Have you ever had or been treated by a physician for any of the following conditions:
   a. Allergies, especially to medications .... Yes No Don't Know
   b. Asthma .... Yes No Don't Know
   c. Abnormal bleeding .... Yes No Don't Know
   d. Blood transfusion... Yes No Don't Know
   e. High blood pressure .... Yes No Don't Know
   f. Congenital heart defect or infective endocarditis................... Yes No Don't Know
   g. Heart disease or heart valve problems .... Yes No Don't Know
   h. Hepatitis.. Yes No Don't Know
   i. Epilepsy or seizures .... Yes No Don't Know
   j. Diabetes.. Yes No Don't Know
   k. Sexually transmitted diseases.................................. Yes No Don't Know
   l. AIDS, AIDS-related condition, or HIV positive .... Yes No Don't Know
   m. Psychologic or mental problems................................ Yes No Don't Know

9. Women–are you pregnant now?.................................. Yes No Don't Know

10. Explain any other condition or problem the dentist should know in order to provide you with safe
    dental care._____
    _____

SIGNATURE OF PATIENT: *I understand the need for these questions to be answered truthfully. To the best of my knowledge, the answers I have given are accurate.*

PERSON COMPLETING THIS FORM:

Signature_____ Date_____ Time_____

If other than patient, indicate relationship:_____

EXAMINING DENTIST'S COMMENTS AND SUMMARY OF SIGNIFICANT FINDINGS:

_____
_____
_____

Signature_____ Date_____ Time_____

FIGURE 12-2
Abbreviated patient health history for urgent care.

In general, leading (or loaded) questions are to be avoided in the interview process. A question such as "How many times per day do you brush your teeth?" is likely to generate an artificially high response by the patient, because many patients will assume from the wording of the question that "once a day is not enough," and "less than once a day must be bad." Some patients with a hypochondriacal personality, or those who tend to embellish the seriousness of their medical or dental experiences, may need to have questions phrased to them in a somewhat leading manner for the provider to sort out what is "ground truth."

An experienced practitioner who has already established rapport with a patient can use a leading question in a humorous or joking manner to help allay the patient's anxiety. However, this approach must be done with caution, because if the patient does not understand that the question is being asked in a lighthearted way, then it may undermine rather than enhance the provider-patient relationship.

A comprehensive patient history needs to be taken at the time of the initial oral examination. Verbally asking the patient whether any changes have occurred in the medical history is appropriate at each subsequent visit. In many professional settings, a formal (written) update of the original General and Oral Health History Questionnaire is performed at no longer than a 6-month interval, and the entire Questionnaire is repeated at no longer than a 3-year interval.

Elements of the Patient History

PATIENT IDENTIFICATION (BIOGRAPHIC DATA)

Baseline personal information is needed for any dental patient. At a minimum, this will include the patient's name, address, telephone number, and date of birth. The record also needs to include the physician's name, address, and phone number—in case the patient's physician needs to be consulted or in the event of a medical emergency while the patient is under the dental professional's care. If multiple medical specialists have seen the patient, then the clinician should obtain their names and contact information as well—especially for those specialists whose area of expertise is likely to have a direct bearing on the delivery of dental treatment (e.g., cardiology, pulmonology).

Whenever possible, recording the physician's fax number and e-mail address is helpful. Identification of an emergency contact party with contact phone number and address are also very useful in the event of an emergency in the dental office. Private offices and most dental clinics also routinely request dental insurance information and the identification of the responsible party (if other than the patient) who will be taking care of the patient's financial obligations. Gender is not an essential element on the patient record; however, it can be helpful because many medical and dental conditions exist that have a gender predilection (Table 12-1).

Similarly, race or ethnicity, occupation, and education level, although not required, can be helpful because many oral pathologic conditions exist that are more commonly found in specific ethnic groups (Table 12-2), or individuals of higher or lower

Table 12-1	Medical Conditions that Have a Significant Difference in Occurrence Rate Based on Gender

DISEASE	Gender FEMALE	Gender MALE
Thyroid dysfunction	X	
Thyroid carcinoma	X	
Cerebrovascular disease	X	
Rheumatoid arthritis	X	
Sjögren's syndrome	X	
Fibromyalgia	X	
Systemic lupus erythematosus (SLE)	X	
Temporomandibular joint (TMJ) dysfunction	X	
Oral carcinoma		X
Pharyngeal carcinoma		X
Laryngeal carcinoma		X
Human immunodeficiency virus (HIV)		X

Table 12-2	Medical Conditions that Have a Rate of Occurrence that Differs with Race or Ethnicity

DISEASES	BLACKS	HISPANICS	WHITES	ASIANS
Hypertension	X	X		
Stroke	X	X		
Heart failure	X	X		
Diabetes	X	X		
Heart disease	X	X		
Osteoporosis			X	X
Cystic fibrosis			X	

socioeconomic status. Knowing about a patient's education level can be useful as the dental care provider seeks to tailor patient information and home care instructions to meet a specific patient's level of understanding. These latter issues can also be useful in research endeavors that are commonly carried out in academic health centers. Obviously, use of the information must conform to HIPAA guidelines, institutional human subjects research guidelines, and internal review board approval.

Some patients are reluctant to divulge personal information and, of course, those wishes must be respected. The only exception is when refusal to reveal personal information to the dental care provider is determined to jeopardize the patient's health or safety.

Medical Condition Related to Age and Ethnic Group

Mr. Belzak is a 58-year-old black man. His age and ethnic group are prone to which medical conditions?

CHIEF CONCERN

Whether symptomatic or not, every patient has a chief concern. Simply put, the chief concern (sometimes referred to as the *chief complaint*) is the reason why the patient has come to the dental office. The concern may be a toothache or bleeding gums; it may be of an esthetic nature such as "I want whiter teeth," or it may be as innocuous as "I need a checkup and cleaning." The clinician may also find it helpful to ask about the concern in an open-ended question such as, "What brings you to see us today?"

The patient's chief concern should be recorded as a direct quote or (in the case of a lengthy concern) as a paraphrased note. This is particularly beneficial in two regards: (1) it captures the patient's perception of the problem, and (2) it often gives the dental care provider a perspective on the patient's awareness and level of understanding of dental and dental hygiene issues.

Asking about the patient's chief concern at the beginning of the patient interview has the dual benefit of suggesting to the patient that his or her concerns are important and that the dental team is taking them seriously; it also emphasizes to the provider issues that will need immediate or urgent or focused attention. Such an awareness on the part of the dental team is also very useful in drawing attention to specific issues that need to be addressed in the course of the remainder of the patient examination. The chief concern should be a primary focus to the dental team and serious efforts should be made to satisfy the patient's chief concern early in the treatment process.

History of Chief Concern

The history of the chief concern includes the background, chronology of events, and explanation of the circumstances that caused the chief concern. For a symptomatic concern such as dental pain, the history would typically include a description of the nature, intensity, location, and duration of the pain. Common questions include the following:

- "What makes it hurt (hot, cold, sweets, pressure)?"
- "How long does it last?"
- "Does it keep you awake at night?"
- "Do you take pain killers? If so, do they help?"
- "Do you have swelling or drainage?"
- "Do you have fever or swollen glands?"

For the patient without symptoms, investigating the history of the chief concern is still a useful exercise. For the patient who comes to the clinic simply because he or she is "overdue for a checkup," follow-up questions about the frequency and nature of previous dental treatment can be very revealing.

- Has the patient had periodic visits and prophylaxis, or has the patient had treatment only when he or she experienced discomfort or needed something to be fixed?
- What have the patient's previous dental experiences been like?
- Were they routine? Did the patient feel stressful and anxious?
- Was the patient satisfied with the treatment?

The history of the chief concern can be an important diagnostic tool—in some cases leading the dental team quickly and directly to a diagnosis of the chief concern. In other cases the history will alert the dental team to specific locations or issues of concern that will need further investigation, testing, or consultation. In many instances, the history will give invaluable clues into the motivation, interest, dental knowledge, and attitude of the patient. Patients who have a troubling history of dissatisfaction with multiple care providers can often be identified at this stage of the patient examination.

Health History

Mr. Belzak reports that he cannot chew well because he cannot wear his lower partial denture and he has to drink fluids all day to keep his mouth wet. What additional line of questions does the dental care provider need to explore to get a complete understanding of his needs?

GENERAL HEALTH HISTORY

The general health history includes four major components:

1. General medical history
2. Medication history
3. Family history
4. Review of organ systems

In many dental offices these components are collapsed into a single questionnaire that encompasses all aspects of the patient history; however, for purposes of illustration and clarity, they are dealt with separately in this chapter.

General Medical History

Included in the general medical history are broad issues that are relevant to the patient's past and present medical health. Classic questions include reference to any serious illnesses, hospitalizations, or operations; any current medical problems; any recent changes in general health; and any allergies. Some specific questions that are commonly included in the general medical history are as follows:

- Has the patient had any surgery?
- If so, when did it occur?
- What was the diagnosis?

- Were there any complications or subsequent problems?
- Was there any required follow-up treatment? What is the current status?
- Does the patient have allergies to anesthetics, antibiotics, other medications, specific foods, iodine, or latex? Does he or she have any seasonal allergies? (Here the interviewer will need to differentiate true allergic reactions from side effects or idiosyncratic reactions. The importance of a true allergy to a local anesthetic or medications commonly used in the practice of dentistry is self-evident. What is perhaps less obvious is the importance of a food or seasonal allergy that may predispose a patient to an allergic reaction to a medicament, latex, or other environmental agent in the dental operatory.)
- Does the patient have a history of generalized infections, communicable diseases, or immune-compromising conditions? (If the patient has an infectious disease, an immune-compromising condition, or both, then the dental team certainly needs to be aware of the problem so that appropriate measures can be taken to ensure that the patient's health will not be jeopardized by engaging in dental treatment without appropriate medical clearance and precaution.)
- Has the patient experienced a recent gain or loss of weight? (A change in the patient's body weight is often an indicator of a change in his or her homeostasis, caloric intake, or exercise level. Some changes are desirable and intentional, such as weight loss under a nutritionally supervised diet program or a physician-prescribed cardiovascular exercise program. Breast-feeding, trauma, infection, cancer, and metabolic disease can be causes of weight loss. Weight gain can result from a sedentary lifestyle or from a metabolic disease such as **hypothyroidism.** If the cause of the weight change is not readily apparent, then a physician's consultation is usually warranted before initiating dental treatment.)

Any or all of these issues may have an effect on the manner that dental treatment is planned or carried out. The clinician will need to determine what issues are relevant and what modification, if any, needs to be made to the dental plan of care.

Medication History

The dental hygienist should record any and all of the patient's current medications, the purpose for which the medication is being taken, the dose, and an indication of whether the patient is fully compliant in taking the medication. The medication register needs to include all herbal remedies, vitamins, birth control pills, over-the-counter (OTC) medications (most notably, aspirin, sleeping pills, cough syrup, antacids, antihistamines), and prescription medication (including those borrowed from friends and family members). The hygienist and the dental team have a responsibility to be sure that all the names of the medications are spelled correctly (a drug manual may be helpful in this regard) and understand the possible systemic side effects, the possible adverse oral effects, possible drug interactions, and

other implications that may relate to management of the patient's oral condition or the delivery of oral health care.

> ### ✦ CASE APPLICATION 12-1.3
>
> **Pharmacologic History**
> How would Mr. Belzak's medications be listed?

Family History

The primary purpose of the **family history** is to identify oral and general health problems that the patient may be predisposed to acquiring. Many oral and systemic conditions occurring with frequency in the general population have a known genetic cause. Most families will also be more likely to exhibit certain oral and systemic diseases because of the shared heritable and environmental influences. Identifying these conditions can be beneficial to the dental team as it seeks to understand the causes of current conditions, identify treatment modalities that are most effective to manage those conditions, and anticipate the future occurrence of oral or systemic disease. (Box 12-1 lists conditions for which familial predispositions exist.)

The family history also provides an opportunity to explore the patient's ethnic and cultural beliefs about health care and medicine. A common way to broach the general health concerns is with queries such as the following:

- "Do you have a family history of cancer, heart problems, or diabetes?"
- "Do you have any other family health problems?"

Culturally based attitudes toward diet, nutrition, disease, and general and oral health care may have a profound effect on the dental team's approach to educating the patient, as well as the nature of treatment that the patient is willing to accept and how oral health care can be delivered. The discussion of the family history is an opportune time to begin to identify cultural or family attitudes that will affect the delivery of dental care. A simple query about the dental experiences of other family members can be revealing and can also provide an entree into a broader discussion of family oral health values.

The patient's response to the dental professional's questions can reveal how he or she feels about the importance of "saving" the teeth. Some patients, because of family or cultural values, have no concept of preventive dental care in a contemporary American setting (or they may hold beliefs very different from the norm). In such cases, there needs to be a true dialog with the patient to begin to find some common ground on preventive issues and issues of oral health. As discussed in Chapter 5, when the dental professional feels that he or she knows the "one true way" that people should treat their teeth and believes that the patient simply needs to come over to the "correct side," then efforts to convince the patient to do so are almost certain to fail. In most cases this is a conversation that will need to be

---

BOX 12-1

CONDITIONS FOR WHICH FAMILIAL PREDISPOSITIONS EXIST

- Cancer*
- Cardiovascular problems*
- Diabetes*
- High blood pressure
- Allergies
- Asthma, stroke

- Epilepsy
- Arthritis
- Hemophilia
- Sickle cell anemia
- Chronic myelogenous leukemia (CML)

Oral heritable health problems can be explored by asking whether the patient has a history of the following:
- Orthodontic problems (crowded teeth)
- Clefts
- Unusual size, shape, appearance, or number of teeth

*Common conditions that are leading causes of death in the United States.

---

continued over many dental visits as the patient-provider relationship develops and mutual trust builds. When the hygienist and patient both enter into this conversation with an open mind, the opportunity for both to learn from the other has significant benefits for both parties, and likelihood that the patient's oral health will be improved is increased.

★ CASE APPLICATION 12-1.4

Family History

What bearing does Mr. Belzak's family history have to his case? Are there any health risks for his children?

Review of Organ Systems

The purpose of the review of systems (ROS) is to assess the patient's state of health and function with regard to each of the major body systems.[8] Usually accomplished through the open-ended format, the ROS is composed of a series of direct questions posed to the patient regarding symptoms, signs, and diseases related to each particular organ system. Each system is reviewed in sequence. Most **comprehensive health history** questionnaires do not include a distinct ROS. Rather, selected questions from the ROS are culled out and inserted into the questionnaire using a different organizing scheme. The great benefit to doing a specific ROS is that it provides a safety net, helping ensure that all pertinent medical information has been elicited from the patient. A standardized questionnaire may leave gaps in the information base. Especially when the process is hurried, the patient may choose to skip or ignore certain issues. Sometimes the patient will forget specific events in the health history. With the ROS, questions are asked in a different way and in a different context—thereby increasing the likelihood that the dental team will capture all the useful and necessary health information.

Another distinct advantage of using the ROS is that it can help the dental team identify previously undiagnosed medical conditions. Because many of the questions focus on signs, symptoms, and findings, the astute dental hygienist is able to recognize that the patient may have a significant medical condition and assist the patient in getting a diagnostic evaluation and appropriate medical treatment. Similarly, the ROS may reveal a direct

relationship of the oral signs and symptoms to a medical condition. Examples include severe oral ulcerations with **Crohn's disease,** glossodynia (burning tongue) with anemias, and increased dental caries incidence and candidiasis with patients receiving head and neck radiation therapy. The ROS is a particularly effective instrument to use with elderly patients, for patients with extensive medical problems, and for special-care patients.

Table 12-3 provides a list of clues obtained from the ROS, possible diagnoses, and dental implications.

The following is a typical ROS. Specific signs and symptoms of diseases most often associated with each system are located under the specific organ system. This information will better prepare the dental hygienist in providing safe, effective health care to each patient.

The dental hygienist prefaces the review of each system with a lead question; for example, "Have you ever experienced _____ _____?"

Skin (integument)

- Eczema, psoriasis, seborrhea
- Itching (pruritus), rash (dermatitis—contact or atopic)
- Pigmentations (vitiligo, ephelis, senile lentigo, nevi)

> *Functions of Skin*
> - Protection from infection and dehydration
> - Regulation of body temperature
> - Collection of sensory information

- Skin cancer (basal cell or squamous cell carcinoma, melanoma)
- Changes in appearance of moles (nevi), and age spots (lentigo)
- Conditions requiring systemic steroid (cortisone or prednisone) treatment

Itching, Dermatitis, and Eczema

A common cause of itching (pruritus) is psychogenic (i.e., a reaction to stress). Itching in the scalp area is often associated with a bitter taste and glossodynia. Itching without a visible rash may be the result of a drug reaction and may be caused by OTC drugs such as aspirin, or by prescribed drugs such as opiates, quinidine, penicillin, or other antibiotics. The clinician should ask patients exactly what their reactions were (adverse

Table 12-3	Clues from the Review of Systems (ROS)	
ROS CLUE	**POSSIBLE DIAGNOSES**	**DENTAL IMPLICATIONS**
Itching	Allergic reaction	Potential life-threatening reaction to anesthetics, drugs, or other agents used in dentistry
Rash on Face; Butterfly-Shaped Rash	Systemic lupus erythematosus (SLE)	Arthritis (difficulty in oral self-care; positioning in dental chair), immune compromised, organ involvement; often needs high doses of steroid to treat
Bulging Eyes, Agitation, and Feeling Hot	Hyperthyroidism	Potential *thyroid storm;* life-threatening crisis in dental chair
Cloudy Vision	Cataracts	Visual impairment may adversely effect oral self-care
Dizziness	Meniere's disease	May limit patient positioning; avoid rapid repositioning
Hearing Impairment	Aging	May impede communication; face the patient, increase volume, speak clearly
Frequent Nose Bleeds (Epistaxis); Black and Blue (Ecchymosis); Blood Blisters; Petechiae; Spontaneous Bleeding	Leukemia, platelet deficiency (thrombocytopenia), bleeding disorder (hemophilia/von Willebrand's disease), taking anticoagulant medication (warfarin [Coumadin]; aspirin)	Acute bleeding following scaling on dental surgical procedures
Painful Sinuses; Sinus Discharge (Pus)	Sinusitis	Sinus symptoms may be confused with pain of dental origin in maxillary posterior and vice-versa
Persistent Hoarseness, Sore Throat, or Difficulty Swallowing	Pharyngeal cancer	Needs referral to medical specialist (otolaryngologist); may limit dental treatment (see Chapter 48)
Blood in Sputum	Pulmonary infection, lung cancer, tuberculosis (TB)	Need referral to medical specialist (pulmonary or infectious disease) before providing dental treatment
Coughing, Wheezing, and Shortness of Breath	Asthma	Possible status asthmaticus; acute asthmatic episode in the dental chair
Fainting	Vasovagal syncope	Need anxiety control to decrease probability of future episodes of medical emergencies in the dental setting
Pain or Pressure in Chest	Angina or myocardial infarction (MI)	Need to prepare for medical emergency; reduced stress protocol; limit use of epinephrine
Swollen Ankles	**Congestive heart failure** (CHF)	Must follow stress reduction protocol[4a,4b]
Cardiac Pacemaker or Defibrillator	Cardiac arrhythmia	May contraindicate use of ultrasonic instrumentation; follow stress reduction protocol[4a,4b]
Sudden Onset of Inability to Speak, or Loss of Mobility on One Side of Face or Body (on Extremities)	Stroke or cerebrovascular accident (CVA)	Difficulty with communication, ambulation, oral self-care; bleeding due to anticoagulant therapy
Heartburn; Gastric Reflux	Gastroesophageal reflux disease (GERD)	Position patient semi-upright in the dental chair
Yellow Discoloration of Eyes, Skin, or Oral Mucosa	Jaundice (liver disease caused by viruses, bacteria, toxic substances, alcohol, or cancer)	Be aware of the inability to metabolize local anesthetics and other drugs; bleeding potential; risk for cancer

Continued

Table 12-3	Clues from the Review of Systems (ROS)—cont'd	
ROS CLUE	**POSSIBLE DIAGNOSES**	**DENTAL IMPLICATIONS**
Blood in Urine (Hematuria)	Chronic glomerulonephritis (CGN); kidney failure	Potential for infection, immune compromise, poor wound healing, bleeding during scaling; if on dialysis, may need antibiotic premedication and must avoid blood pressure cuff placement at site of shunt
Frequent Urination (Polyuria); Frequent Hunger (Polyphagia); Frequent Thirst (Polydipsia)	Diabetes mellitus (DM)	Need to prepare for medical emergency; if poorly controlled, poor wound healing, potential for infection; periodontal disease
Tired, Weak, Faint, Headaches, and Cold Intolerance	Anemia (iron deficiency)	Need laboratory tests and physical consult; if not treated, may cause altered taste (glossodynia) and beefy red burning tongue (glossopyrosis), delayed healing, and increased risk of infection; with good control, no restriction of dental treatment
Lightheadedness with Nausea, Anxiety, Tremors, and Difficulty Concentrating	Hypoglycemia	Potential medical emergency in the dental setting; can be triggered by dental anxiety
Immobility on One Side of the Face	Bell's palsy	Condition can be diagnosed and managed by the dental team; usually reversible
Slow Movement, Muscle Weakness, Imbalance, and Tremors	Parkinson's disease	Patient has difficulty taking care of dental prostheses and has difficulty with oral self-care
Avoidance of Dental Treatment; Fear of the Dentist	Dental anxiety	Can be a significant barrier to care, limiting both the nature and scope of dental treatment; may require sedation to manage it effectively

reaction versus anaphylaxis) and to describe the symptoms associated with the incident.

Itching may be localized (e.g., dermatitis). The most common inflammatory skin disease is eczematous dermatitis. The various types include primary contact dermatitis, allergic contact dermatitis, and atopic dermatitis. All three share the common presentation of a breakdown of the epidermis.

Pigmentations

Genetic factors. Vitiligo is an autosomal-dominant trait characterized by a localized or generalized hypomelanosis of the skin and hair. Vitiligo has a strong association with **Addison's disease, hyperthyroidism,** hypothyroidism, **pernicious anemia,** and alopecia areata.

Neurofibromatosis is a dominant trait characterized by café-au-lait spots. The presence of six or more spots with diameters greater than 1.5 cm is a strong indicator of the diagnosis of neurofibromatosis.

Peutz-Jeghers syndrome is a dominant trait characterized by the presence of mucocutaneous hypermelanosis on the lips and in the oral cavity. The importance of the oral finding is that this entity is associated with polyposis of the jejunum and ileum. The polyps are most often benign.

Metabolic and endocrine factors. Hemochromatosis is a familial disorder of iron metabolism that produces liver damage resulting in cirrhosis. Iron deposition in the pancreas and adrenal glands results in **diabetes mellitus** (DM) and hypoadrenalism. The skin becomes hyperpigmented (bronze).

Adrenal gland disorders resulting in the overproduction of **adrenocorticotropic hormone** (ACTH) and melanin-stimulating hormone (MSH) cause addisonian hyperpigmentation.

Nutritional factors. Kwashiorkor, decreased protein in the diet, causes the hair to change color to a brownish-red, then to gray. Sprue, or malabsorption in the small intestine, produces a brown pigmentation that can occur anywhere on the body. **Pellagra,** deficiency of niacin, has a cutaneous component that begins as erythematous-appearing skin and then progresses to a darker keratotic skin.

Chemical and physical factors. Progesterone, whether **endogenous** (resulting from pregnancy) or **exogenous** (resulting from birth control pills), may cause hyperpigmentation on the abdomen and forehead. This is known as *melasma* or *chloasma.*

Psoriasis and Seborrhea

Psoriasis is a common chronic disease characterized by dry, silvery, well-circumscribed plaques of various locations and sizes. A strong association exists with family history of psoriasis and reflects an autosomal-dominant inheritance. Seborrhea is an inflammatory scaling and involves the scalp and face. It appears as a dry or greasy diffuse scaling of the scalp with variable degrees of itching.

Skin Cancer and Malignant Melanoma

Moles may be small or large; flat or raised; smooth or hairy; flesh-colored, yellow-brown, or black. If a mole enlarges suddenly or becomes spotty in color, has an irregular border, or becomes painful and bleeds, then it must be excised. Approximately 40% to 50% of malignant melanomas arise from ordinary moles. The presence of color changes may be caused by actinic damage, a melanoma, basal cell carcinoma, keratoacanthoma, and squamous cell carcinoma.

Allergies and Adverse Reactions to Latex, Medications, and Metals

Many allergies to medications, metals, and latex are due to the body developing antibodies or sensitized lymphocytes that develop during a sensitization period after an initial exposure to a specific agent. A later exposure to the same agent (e.g., penicillin) may result in a severe sensitive reaction (e.g., itching, hives, vomiting) or a life-threatening reaction (e.g., anaphylaxis).

> ### ✺ CASE APPLICATION 12-1.5
>
> #### Symptoms of Disease
> Of what significance is Mr. Belzak's rash? What could be contributing to his report of swollen lips?

Extremities (musculoskeletal system)

- Stiff and swollen joints (rheumatoid arthritis or osteoarthritis; degenerative joint disease [DJD])
- Loss of mobility and function (lupus, multiple sclerosis, **scleroderma, Sjögren's syndrome**)
- Muscle weakness and pain (fibromyalgia, polymyositis)
- Bone weakness, fracture, pain (osteoporosis)
- Prosthetic joints
- Conditions requiring steroid therapy

> *Functions of Musculoskeletal System: Skeleton Provides Framework for the Body*
> - Bones produce blood cells in red marrow
> - Bones store calcium salts to be used by body
> - Bones protect delicate structures such as brain and spinal cord
> - Muscles and joints work together for movement
> - Muscles maintain posture
> - Muscles generate heat

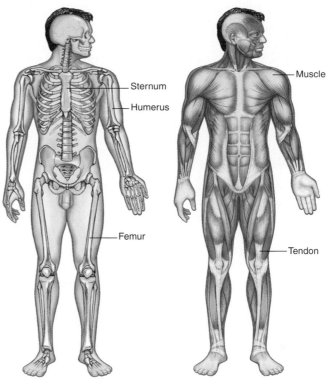

FIGURE 12-3
Overview of the musculoskeletal system. (From Thibodeau GA, Patton KT: *The human body in health and disease*, ed 4, St Louis, 2005, Mosby.)

See Figure 12-3 for a review of skeletal bones, muscles, and components of a joint. Muscles and bones of the head and neck are presented in Chapter 14.

Stiff and Swollen Joints, Arthritis, and Osteoporosis

Trauma, infection, metabolic disturbances, immunologic disturbances, and neoplasms may cause swollen painful joints. The patient experiences pain, swelling, stiffness, and decreased or limited motion in addition to redness and a feeling of warmth.

Two main forms of arthritis exist: (1) rheumatoid arthritis and (2) osteoarthritis. Rheumatoid arthritis is autoimmune in origin, has an earlier onset, and frequently involves multiple joints. Rheumatoid arthritis has a 3:1 female/male predilection and is much more likely to effect the temporomandibular joint (TMJ). Osteoarthritis is degenerative, more commonly effects older individuals, and primarily involves the load-bearing joints. Inflammation of the joints (evidenced by redness and a feeling of warmth) can occur with either type of arthritis but is always expected with rheumatoid arthritis. Osteoporosis is an increased porosity of the bone that places individuals at risk of hip and spinal vertebrae fractures.

> *Distinct Care Modifications*
> Oral self-care strategies must be evaluated carefully to accommodate any lack of manual dexterity. The patient may need additional support (neck or back padding) while in the dental chair and may become stiff or sore in a fixed position, necessitating periodic repositioning. Accommodations may need to be made to transport the patient to the office and assist the patient in getting to the operatory and into the dental chair.

Lupus, Polymyositis, Scleroderma, and Sjögren's Syndrome

Lupus is a chronic, progressive disease often presented as a butterfly-shaped face rash. Symptoms include photosensitivity, arthritis without deformities, oral and nasal ulcerations, and pericarditis. Polymyositis is a connective tissue disease characterized by dermatitis and **edema,** inflammation, and degeneration of the muscles. Scleroderma varies in progression and severity and is seen more in women than in men, causing diffuse fibrosis, degenerative changes, and vascular abnormalities in the skin, articular structures, and internal organs. Sjögren's syndrome occurs most frequently in postmenopausal women, causing severe dry mouth and keratoconjunctivitis; the syndrome is often related to rheumatoid arthritis (see Chapter 11).

Muscle Weakness, Pain, and Fibromyalgia

Ocular palsies are manifested by double vision (diplopia). Drooping of the eyelid **(ptosis)** may be an early sign of **myasthenia gravis.** Facial palsy (known as *Bell's palsy*) is the paralysis of the facial nerve. This condition is usually unilateral, and the patient is unable to smile, expose teeth, or close the eye on the affected side. **Fibromyalgia** is a nonspecific illness characterized by overall fatigue, muscle and joint pain, tenderness, and stiffness.

Bone Deformity and Fracture

Bone is a dynamic tissue that is constantly being repaired and remodeled throughout an individual's life. The calcium-to-phosphorus ratio is important in bone health. Any condition that alters the calcium-to-phosphorus ratio affects the integrity of the bone. **Parathyroid hormone** (PTH), calcitonin, vitamin D, and serum protein all affect the calcium-to-phosphorus ratio. Vitamin D affects the calcium and phosphorous absorption from the gastrointestinal (GI) tract. Serum protein is directly related to the amount of calcium and phosphorus bound to the albumen. Thus liver and GI tract problems may have a direct effect on the health of the skeletal tissue.

Prosthetic Joints

More than 400,000 total joint prostheses are placed annually. The prostheses replace both the hip and the knee. Pain is the main reason that the surgery is performed, and osteoarthritis is the major medical condition causing the joint pain.[1] For more information on prosthetic joints, see Hematogenous Prosthetic Joint Infection later in this chapter.

Eyes, ears, nose, and throat

- Visual problems (other than corrective lenses) such as glaucoma or cataracts
- Hearing loss, ringing in the ears **(tinnitus),** hearing aid, dizziness (vertigo)
- Frequent nosebleeds (see also under Hematopoietic System)
- Hoarseness
- Frequent sore throats, tonsillitis
- Sinusitis, rhinitis

> *Functions of the Eyes, Ears, Nose, and Throat*
> - Vision   • Sight
> - Smell   • Voice

- Trauma to the head or neck
- Mouth ulcers, canker sores, fever blisters, cold sores
- Stiffness in the neck (arthritis, spondylitis)
- Cysts, tumors, cancers of the mouth or throat

Figure 12-4 provides a review of ear and eye anatomy.

Double Vision

Double vision (diplopia) occurs when the points of the visual receptors are far apart and two images are formed. Other causes of double vision may occur in the cerebrum: trauma, cerebrovascular accident, or vascular abnormalities. Damage to the optic nerve also may cause double vision.

Drooping Eyelids

Drooping of the eyelid may be an early manifestation of myasthenia gravis. This also may occur with **paresis** of the third cranial nerve.

Glaucoma

Glaucoma is an elevation of the intraocular pressure and is the most common cause of blindness in many regions of the world. Chronic primary open-angle glaucoma is the most common type of glaucoma.[5] The canal of Schlemm is the site of the resistance to outflow of the aqueous material. An estimated 2% of the population has this type of glaucoma.

Cataracts

A cataract is a developmental or degenerative opacity of the lens. The classic symptom is a progressive painless loss of vision. The degree of vision loss depends on the location and the extent of the opacity. Pain may occur if the cataract swells and produces secondary glaucoma.

The dental hygienist must carefully evaluate oral self-care strategies to accommodate vision impairment.

Hearing Loss, Tinnitus, Hearing Aid, and Vertigo

Transient hearing loss may be caused by an acute or chronic external otitis. Hearing loss also may be caused by a malformed auditory organ anatomy, impaired transmission of the sound waves via the eighth cranial nerve, or both.

Tinnitus is a ringing in the ears and is a subjective phenomenon. Approximately 90% of the population has reported tinnitus at one time or another. Salicylates and quinine drugs are notorious for causing tinnitus.

Patients with hearing deficits, regardless of whether they use hearing aids, may require the dental hygienist to speak louder and face the patient during interactions.

Patients with vertigo may feel they are moving in space with a loss of equilibrium.

Frequent Nosebleeds (Epistaxis)

The most common cause of **epistaxis** (nosebleed) is the tearing of Kiesselbach's plexus as a result of nose picking. Epistaxis also may occur as a normal finding during an **upper respiratory infection** (URI) or may be a sign of **hypertension,** a bleeding diathesis (clotting deficiency, **thrombocytopenia,** or **polycythemia**), nasal tumors, or Osler-Rendu-Weber disease (hereditary hemorrhagic telangiectasia [HHT]).

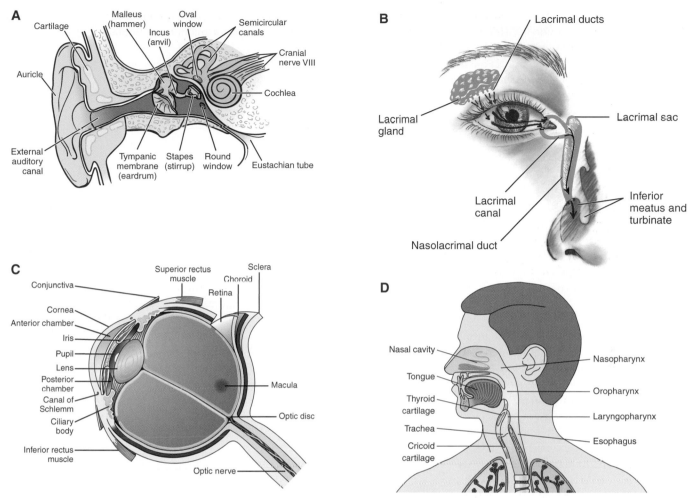

FIGURE 12-4
Review of parts of the ears **(A)**, eyes **(B** and **C)**, and nose and throat **(D)**. (**A, C,** and **D** from Copstead-Kirkhorn LC, Banasik JL: *Pathophysiology,* ed 3, Philadelphia, 2005, Saunders; **B** from Jarvis C: *Physical examination and health assessment,* ed 4, Philadelphia, 2004, WB Saunders.)

Frequent Sore Throat (Pharyngitis) and Tonsillitis

Sore throat is the most common manifestation of pharyngitis. Two thirds of all cases of pharyngitis are due to viral URIs. Serious complications of a bacterial pharyngitis are peritonsillar cellulitis or abscess. Carcinoma of the tonsillar tissue, although rare, is the second most common tumor of the superior airway. Signs of a tonsillar carcinoma include reports of pain in one enlarged tonsil with no signs or symptoms of an infection.

Tonsillitis is an infection of the tonsils, usually resulting from viral or streptococcal infections.

Sinusitis and Rhinitis

The most common predisposing factor for acute sinusitis is a viral URI. This leads to blockage of draining of the paranasal sinuses and the development of pain, tenderness, and low-grade fever. The maxillary sinus is the most common sinus infection, characterized by pain, swelling, and tenderness in the anterior portions of the maxilla and infraorbital regions; infection in the frontal sinus is characterized by pain over the forehead; ethmoid sinus infection is characterized by pain in the upper lateral areas of the nose; and sphenoid sinus infection is characterized by pain and tenderness over the vertex of the skull, mastoid bones, and the occipital portion of the head.

Rhinitis (runny nose), the most frequent URI, is characterized by edema and nasal discharge and obstruction and vasodilation of the nasal mucous membrane.

Hoarseness

Hoarseness is a change in the character of the voice most commonly resulting from a local laryngeal infection. Hoarseness may be caused by exophytic lesions such as papillomas and tumors and disorders of the structures around the upper airway (e.g., edema or tumors of the esophagus). Uncomplicated hoarseness resulting from benign local factors is of short duration; however, persistence of symptoms of hoarseness longer than 2 to 3 weeks warrants a direct examination by an otolaryngologist.

Mouth Ulcers

Oral ulcers associated with pain are a common reason the patient seeks dental treatment. These ulcers may be the result of trauma, viral and bacterial infections, or autoimmune reactions.

Tobacco and Smokeless Tobacco Use

Tobacco use (all forms) is a major cause of illness and death. A movement in the healthcare profession is trying to establish tobacco assessment as the fifth vital sign (after blood pressure, pulse, temperature, and respiration). Dental hygienists may have a significant effect on education and cessation of tobacco with patients (see Chapter 29).

Respiratory system

> *Note*
>
> The primary function of the respiratory system is the exchange of air from the outside to the blood.

- Cough or wheezing
- Shortness of breath
- Blood in the sputum
- Asthma
- Bronchitis, emphysema, COPD
- Exposure to **tuberculosis** (TB)

Figure 12-5 provides a review of respiratory anatomy.

Cough

A cough is an explosive expiration of air that clears the tracheobronchial tree of secretions and foreign bodies. Inflammatory, chemical, or thermal stimulation of the cough may cause coughing receptors. Most commonly, acute episodes of coughing are due to viral or bacterial infections, whereas chronic cough is due to bronchitis (usually caused by cigarette smoking), pulmonary TB, or pulmonary neoplasms.

Blood in Sputum

Blood in the sputum is known as *hemoptysis*. Many diseases, such as lung carcinoma, a bronchial tumor or bronchiectasis, lobar pneumonia, lung infarction, and pulmonary edema, may cause hemoptysis.

Wheezing and Asthma

The classic triad of symptoms for asthma is coughing, wheezing, and **dyspnea.** Viral URIs, physical exertion, emotional excitement, and exposure to allergens can precipitate asthmatic attacks.

Asthma is a reversible lung disorder characterized by narrowing of the airways, resulting from bronchial constriction, edema, and inflammation of the bronchial mucosa.

Bronchitis and Emphysema

Bronchitis usually is associated with cigarette smoking, which results in bronchial irritation

> *Distinct Care Modifications*
>
> Smoking cessation should be encouraged in patients with bronchitis or emphysema. Often these patients cannot tolerate being in a supine position. The clinician should have supplemental oxygen available for use if the patient experiences shortness of breath (or if the patient's own portable oxygen supply becomes depleted).

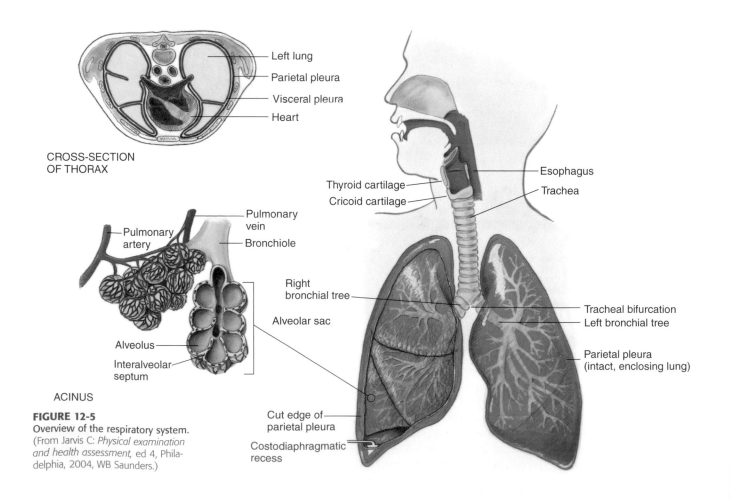

CROSS-SECTION OF THORAX
- Left lung
- Parietal pleura
- Visceral pleura
- Heart

ACINUS
- Pulmonary artery
- Pulmonary vein
- Bronchiole
- Alveolus
- Interalveolar septum

- Thyroid cartilage
- Cricoid cartilage
- Esophagus
- Trachea
- Right bronchial tree
- Alveolar sac
- Tracheal bifurcation
- Left bronchial tree
- Parietal pleura (intact, enclosing lung)
- Cut edge of parietal pleura
- Costodiaphragmatic recess

FIGURE 12-5
Overview of the respiratory system. (From Jarvis C: *Physical examination and health assessment,* ed 4, Philadelphia, 2004, WB Saunders.)

with increased production of mucus and structural changes in the bronchi that result in significant airway obstruction.

Emphysema is an enlargement and destruction of the alveolar tissues in the lungs. This is generally a predictable sequela of long-term cigarette use. COPD consists of both bronchitis and emphysema. Both of these conditions are preventable by not smoking or cessation of smoking. In advanced stages the patient often needs supplemental oxygen.

Exposure to Tuberculosis

TB is a disease caused by mycobacterium that are spread from person to person, or animal to person through the air. TB usually affects the lungs but can affect the brain, kidney, or spine. General symptoms of TB include feelings of weakness, weight loss, fever, a productive cough, and night sweats. In the past decade, the incidence of TB in both the United States and the world has increased. This is due to many factors, which include the increasing population and potential for disease transmission, the inability of public health authorities to identify and manage affected individuals, newer strains of *Mycobacterium tuberculosis* that are resistant to conventional drug therapy, and the increasing prevalence of immune-compromising conditions, such as acquired immunodeficiency syndrome (AIDS).

A distinction must be made between individuals who have the disease and those who have the infection. An individual who has the infection has been exposed to the organism and will exhibit a reactive tuberculin skin test (TST). The patient is not considered to be infectious, does not have any active lung lesions, and the sputum does not harbor any organisms. An individual in this state cannot transfer the organism to another person. An individual who has the disease has a positive TST, exhibits positive lung findings on clinical examination and chest radiographs, and has demonstrated organisms in the sputum. This individual can transfer the disease to other individuals up to the time that a negative sputum culture is evident (generally 2 to 3 weeks on multiple drug therapy; see Chapter 7).

DENTAL CONSIDERATIONS

A patient who has been exposed to TB but who does not have the active disease can be treated routinely. A patient who has been exposed to TB and who exhibits symptoms of the active disease (e.g., coughing with bloody sputum, weakness, shortness of breath) should be given a mask and be immediately referred to his or her physician or public health authority. Any patient with active communicable TB cannot be managed in a typical outpatient dental office and needs to be referred to a hospital or academic health center where administrative controls and environmental controls are in effect (and where personal respiratory protection is available for healthcare workers per Centers for Disease Control and Prevention [CDC] guidelines). After initial antibiotic treatment and a negative sputum culture, the patient can resume normal dental care; however, these patients should be monitored for recurrence of symptoms.

Pneumonia

In the older adult population, pneumonia may be fatal. This population must have a current pneumonia vaccination. Another population at risk is individuals who have had a splenectomy (removal of the spleen).

Cardiovascular system

- Shortness of breath
- Fainting (syncope)
- Angina or pain and pressure in the chest
- Swelling of the ankles
- High or low blood pressure
- Dizziness when getting up quickly (orthostatic hypotension)
- Need to use multiple pillows under the head at night (orthopnea)
- Endocarditis, congenital heart disorder
- Irregular heartbeat, flutter (arrhythmia)
- Prosthetic heart valves and inserts
- Heart attack (**myocardial infarction** [MI])
- Hardening of the arteries (arteriosclerosis, atherosclerosis), coronary artery disease (CAD), or congestive heart failure (CHF)
- Stroke (TIA)

Figure 12-6 provides a schematic of the cardiovascular system.

> **Note**
> The function of the cardiovascular system is to circulate blood to all parts of the body.

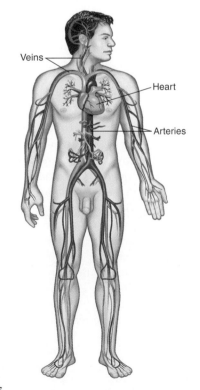

FIGURE 12-6
Overview of the circulatory system. (From Thibodeau GA, Patton KT: *The human body in health and disease*, ed 4, St Louis, 2005, Mosby.)

Shortness of Breath

Shortness of breath or abnormal awareness of breathing is a cardinal sign of disease of both the respiratory and the cardiovascular systems. An early manifestation of left ventricular heart failure is dyspnea (difficulty breathing) at rest or during the performance of a menial task. The dyspnea related to heart disease develops and progresses relatively quickly in comparison to dyspnea resulting from respiratory disease (COPD).

Fainting (Syncope)

Fainting (syncope) is a momentary loss of consciousness that may be caused by cardiovascular problems, arrhythmias, hyperventilation or neurologic or metabolic problems. **Vasovagal syncope** is usually precipitated by a physical or an emotional event.

Angina and Pain or Pressure in the Chest

Pain or pressure in the chest may be the sign of myocardial ischemia, which is a decrease in the oxygen supply in relation to the need for oxygen in the heart muscles. Atherosclerosis of the coronary arteries is the main cause of myocardial ischemia. Symptomatic myocardial ischemia is known as **angina pectoris.** The pain from an MI may be distinguished from angina pain in that the MI pain is more severe, of longer duration, and unresponsive to nitroglycerine.

Swelling of the Ankles

Swelling of the ankles may be a sign of right ventricular failure that results in systemic venous congestion and edema.

High or Low Blood Pressure and Orthostatic Hypotension

Arterial blood pressure must be maintained at adequate levels to provide perfusion of the capillary system. The blood pressure depends on the level of the preload (venous return), the afterload, and the myocardial contractile force.

Essential hypertension is the most common cause of elevated blood pressure, and this form of hypertension has a familial tendency. The elevated blood pressure may be manifested with an increase in the systolic pressure. An increased preload resulting from anemias, hyperthyroidism, aortic insufficiency, or a combination of these factors may cause this elevated pressure. A normal stroke volume that is pumped out into a noncompliant arteriosclerotic aorta also results in an elevated systolic pressure. The diastolic blood pressure is elevated when the afterload is increased as a result of an increased arteriolar resistance.

Hypertension, if untreated or poorly managed, results in secondary end-organ damage to the heart, kidney, and central nervous system. This significantly shortens the life span of the individual by 10 to 20 years.

Hypotension results from a decrease in the cardiac output or a decrease in the peripheral resistance. A fall in the blood pressure upon standing is known as *orthostatic hypotension* and is a common finding in older adults with atherosclerosis.

History of Endocarditis

Endocarditis is an infection of the endocardium characterized by an elevated temperature, presence of HMs, petechiae, anemia, emboli, and vegetations on the endocardium that result in heart valve damage, myocardial abscess, or aneurysm. Males are affected with endocarditis almost twice as often as females. The median age for the infection is in the 50s. Endocarditis of the right side of the heart is associated with cardiac diagnostic procedures and intravenous (IV) drug abuse. Cardiac surgeries have resulted in an increase of nosocomial endocarditis. An increase in the older adult population with calcific changes on the valve leaflets is another subset of IE patients.[5] IE, if untreated, is almost always fatal. When IE is treated, the morbidity and mortality varies according to the patient's age, severity of the disease, site of the infection, microorganism involved, and complications.

Oral bacteria introduced into the blood stream during invasive dental procedures have been implicated in some cases of IE. Because of that association and the potentially serious consequences of IE, the American Heart Association has developed guidelines for the prevention of endocarditis, which are applicable to the dental setting. Key elements of that policy are captured in this chapter. Medical conditions that are known to predispose patients to IE are summarized in Box 12-2. For patients who are at elevated risk for acquiring IE, the aggressive management of any oral infection—including periodontal disease—is imperative. Box 12-3 describes important management issues and treatment that need to be carried out by the dental team.

Box 12-2 also identifies those dental procedures that do and do not warrant antibiotic premedication in an individual who has been determined to be at risk for IE.

> ### Prevention
> The two conditions (endocarditis and hematogenous prosthetic joint infection) requiring special medical management have special national guidelines established through the work of the American Heart Association, the ADA, and the American Academy of Orthopedic Surgeons. Failure to comply with these guidelines may put a clinician at risk for malpractice litigation or sanction by dental licensure governing bodies.

> ### Note
> Once the patient is known to be at risk for IE, premedication with antibiotics should be considered before specific dental and dental hygiene procedures.

DENTAL CONSIDERATIONS

Patients who have an artificial heart valve, certain types of unrepaired congenital heart defects, or who have had IE are all considered to be at high risk for developing endocarditis. Therefore the American Heart Association recommends antimicrobial prophylaxis for these patients when undergoing invasive dental procedures[3] (see Boxes 12-2, 12-3, and Table 12-4).

Hematogenous Prosthetic Joint Infection

More than 400,000 total joint prostheses are placed annually in the United States. Pain is the main reason that the surgery is performed, and osteoarthritis is the major medical condition causing the joint pain. A small percentage of the patients who

---

BOX 12-2

CARDIAC CONDITIONS AND DENTAL PROCEDURES FOR WHICH THE AMERICAN HEART ASSOCIATION RECOMMENDS ANTIBIOTIC PROPHYLAXIS

Cardiac Conditions Associated with the Highest Risk of Adverse Outcome from Endocarditis
- Prosthetic cardiac valve
- Previous infective endocarditis (IE)
- Congenital heart disease (CHD)*
  - Unrepaired cyanotic CHD, including palliative shunts and conduits
  - Completely repaired congenital heart defect with prosthetic material or device, whether placed by surgery or by catheter intervention, during the first 6 months after the procedure†
  - Repaired CHD with residual defects at the site or adjacent to the site of a prosthetic patch or prosthetic device (which inhibit endothelialization)
- Cardiac transplantation recipients who develop cardiac valvulopathy

Dental Procedures for Which Endocarditis Prophylaxis is Recommended (Applies to Those Patients Who Have One or More of the Above Cardiac Conditions)
All dental procedures that involve manipulation of gingival tissue or the periapical region of teeth or perforation of the oral mucosa‡
See Table 12-4 for recommended prophylactic antibiotic regimens.

---

*Except for the conditions listed above, antibiotic prophylaxis is no longer recommended for any other form of CHD.
†Prophylaxis is recommended because endothelialization of prosthetic material occurs within 6 months after the procedure.
‡The following procedures and events do NOT need prophylaxis: routine anesthetic injections through noninfected tissue, taking dental radiographs, placement of removable prosthodontic or orthodontic appliances, adjustment of orthodontic appliances, placement of orthodontic brackets, shedding of deciduous teeth, and bleeding from trauma to the lips or oral mucosa.
Modified from Stefanac SJ, Nesbit SP: *Treatment Planning in Dentistry,* ed 2, St Louis, 2007, Mosby, p. 103.

BOX 12-3

PREVENTION PLAN FOR PATIENTS AT RISK FOR INFECTIVE ENDOCARDITIS (IE) OR HEMATOGENOUS TOTAL JOINT INFECTION (HTJI)

1. Determine the patient's risk for developing IE or HTJI.
2. Establish optimal oral health.
3. Maintain optimal oral health.
4. Schedule appointments for periodic oral examinations at optimal intervals.
5. Prevent or treat acute oral infections.
6. Prescribe and monitor antibiotic prophylaxis as appropriate based on the patient's medical risk status.

---

have a major joint replacement will fall prey to a deep joint infection, which may require revision surgery, an extended hospital stay, and the treatment of other potentially serious medical complications. For many years members of the medical and dental communities discussed whether the patient with a total joint prosthesis—hips and knees in particular—should receive antimicrobial prophylaxis before invasive dental procedures. In 1997 the ADA and American Academy of Orthopedic Surgeons jointly established guidelines regarding antibiotic prophylaxis for dental patients with total joint replacements. The Joint Advisory Statement affirms that the majority of total joint prostheses are not at risk for developing a late joint infection caused by a dental procedure.[1] However, for the first 2 years after joint replacement surgery, all patients should be premedicated using the same antibiotic regimen as recommended for the prevention of IE (see Table 12-4). After 2 years, premedication is limited to patients who have a total joint prosthesis and also have an immunocompromising disease (i.e., uncontrolled insulin-dependent diabetes mellitus [IDDM],

systemic lupus erythematosus (SLE), severe and symptomatic rheumatoid arthritis). These patients may benefit from antimicrobial prophylaxis (i.e., antibiotic premedication).

The trend today is to sharply curtail the use of antimicrobial agents in clinical situations in which no proven benefit exists. The potential for allergic reactions to the antibiotics, the increasing prevalence of antibiotic-resistant organisms, and the known risk for suprainfections in many patients taking repeated doses of antibiotics have also been part of the rationale for moving toward more conservative use of antibiotics. With respect to both the prevention of IE and the prevention of hematogenous total joint infection, the long-held axiom of "if in doubt, premedicate" is no longer a professionally reasonable or defensible course to take. Rather, a recommendation to the patient regarding the need for antibiotic premedication must weigh carefully the risks of premedicating versus not premedicating in light of the published guidelines, the patient's specific medical condition, and the dental team's estimation of the patient's risk with either course of action. The dental hygienist

Table 12-4	**Prophylactic Antibiotic Regimens for a Dental Procedure**		
SITUATION	**AGENT**	**ADULTS**	**CHILDREN**
Oral	Amoxicillin	2 g	50 mg/kg
Unable to Take Oral Medication	Ampicillin OR	2 g IM or IV	50 mg/kg IM or IV
	Cefazolin or ceftriaxone	1 g IM or IV	50 mg/kg IM or IV
Allergic to Penicillins or Ampicillin—Oral	Cephalexin*† OR	2 g	50 mg/kg
	Clindamycin OR	600 mg	20 mg/kg
	Azithromycin or clarithromycin	500 mg	15 mg/kg
Allergic to Penicillins or Ampicillin and Unable to Take Oral Medication	Cefazolin or ceftriazone† OR	1 g IM or IV	50 mg/kg IM or IV
	Clindamycin	600 mg IM or IV	20 mg/kg IM or IV

IM, intramuscular; IV, intravenous.
*Or other first-generation or second-generation oral cephalosporin in equivalent adult or pediatric dosage.
†Cephalosporins should not be used in an individual with a history of anaphylaxis, angioedema, or urticaria with penicillins or ampicillin.
Modified from Stefanac SJ, Nesbit SP: *Treatment Planning in Dentistry,* ed 2, St Louis, 2007, Mosby, p. 104.

must take a thorough and accurate patient history on which the dental team can base appropriate professional decisions.

Congenital Heart Disorder

The list of congenital heart disorders is lengthy. It includes aortic valve (stenosis and bicuspid), ventricular septal defects, coarctation of the aorta, patent ductus arteriosus, and tetralogy of Fallot. Patients with unrepaired cyanotic congenital heart disorders are considered to be at high risk for developing IE.

Heart Murmur

An HM results from vibrations of the heart valve leaflets as a result of turbulent blood flow through valves and chambers of the heart.[2] HMs may be classified by intensity of the sound ranging from grade I (barely audible) to grade VI (very loud and audible with the stethoscope not on the chest).

The discovery of HM requires careful assessment and diagnosis by the physician. HMs may be classified as either *innocent/ benign functional* or the *result of valvular abnormality.* Often a child, adolescent, or active young person is told that he or she has an HM; also pregnant women may experience a physiologic murmur. Most of the time this finding is due to strenuous myocardial contraction, which results in a stronger blood flow during systole and the movement of the blood from the large ventricle into the smaller sized aorta and blood vessels. In thin-chested young persons, the sound of the movement of the blood is easier

to hear. These findings are termed *innocent HMs* and are not a risk factor for the development of IE. Thus antimicrobial prophylaxis is not recommended for this type of HM.

The most commonly diagnosed form of HM is mitral valve prolapse (MVP), a developmental condition that is found in up to 15% of the population. Prior to 2007, certain types of heart murmurs (e.g., mitral valve prolapse with regurgitation) were generally believed to increase the patient's risk for developing IE and, therefore, warranted prophylactic antibiotic therapy prior to invasive dental procedures. In the 2007 AHA Guidelines for the Prevention of Endocarditis,[3] some congenital heart conditions (see Box 12-2) do warrant antibiotic prophylaxis prior to dental procedures where there will be tissue manipulation, but heart murmurs do not.

✦ CASE APPLICATION 12-1.6

Premedication

Which of the previously mentioned heart valve disorders does Mr. Belzak have? According to the American Heart Association, is premedication required for Mr. Belzak's condition?

Cardiac Arrhythmia, Abnormal Heartbeat, and Flutter

Normal heartbeats originate in the sinoatrial node. The impulse then enters the atrioventricular node and passes through the bundle of His into the left and right bundles. Any electrical deviations may result in abnormal heartbeats.

Pacemaker and Defibrillator

If the heart rate decreases significantly, then a pacemaker is inserted in the chest to restore a normal heart rate. Severe arrhythmias that result in disorganized ventricular contractions (**ventricular fibrillation**) may result in death if intervention (i.e., cardiopulmonary resuscitation [CPR]) is not implemented immediately. To prevent this life-threatening form of arrhythmia, defibrillators are implanted to "shock" the person back into a more stable heart rhythm.

Prosthetic Heart Valves and Inserts

Heart valves that become nonfunctional and result in serious cardiovascular problems are surgically replaced with prosthetic devices. The heart valve that most commonly has prosthetic replacement is the mitral valve, followed by the aortic valve. The presence of a prosthetic heart valve is a high-risk factor for developing IE and *must* be premedicated with an antimicrobial agent before dental procedures where there will be tissue manipulation. Prosthetic devices such as stents in the coronary vessels, Dacron graft material, and synthetic tube material placed in the major vessels do not place the individual at increased risk for developing IE. Therefore antimicrobial prophylaxis for dental procedures is not recommended[3] (see Boxes 12-2 and 12-3, Table 12-4).

Heart Attack or Myocardial Infarction

A heart attack or MI occurs when occlusion of one or more of the coronary arteries occurs and a portion of the heart muscle loses its blood supply resulting in cellular death (necrosis) in that portion of the heart. In some cases this series of events leads to cardiac arrest and death. In other cases it may result in permanent damage to the myocardium and thus a decreased capability of the heart to pump blood to the periphery. In the months after an MI the patient remains at increased risk for another MI or for arrhythmia.

If a patient gives a history of a heart attack, the clinician must determine the following:
- Date of the MI
- Degree of damage to heart tissue
- Present medications to manage the post-MI period
- Lifestyle modifications resulting from the MI
- Current health status

(See Boxes 12-2, 12-3, and Table 12-4 for premedication guidelines.)

Arteriosclerosis and Atherosclerosis

Arteriosclerosis is a generic term for a number of diseases in which the arterial wall becomes thickened and losses elasticity (e.g., in aging). Atherosclerosis begins with fat and plaque deposits in the smooth muscle of the arterial wall. If the deposits continue, then complete occlusion prevents blood flow in the arteries.

Congestive Heart Failure

With CHF the heart cannot adequately pump blood to the lungs (right-sided failure) or the rest of the organs, body, and periphery (left-sided failure). Common features include shortness of breath and swollen ankles with pitting edema. Fifty percent of persons with CHF will die within 5 years.

Stroke and Transient Ischemic Attack

Cerebral vascular accident or stroke is the most common cause of neurologic disability in developed countries. Most strokes are due to atherosclerosis and hypertension.

TIAs usually are due to cerebral emboli arising from plaques or atherosclerotic ulcers involving the carotid or ventricle arteries. TIAs are often recurrent and at times presage a stroke. Often TIAs are referred to as *ministrokes*. The plaques in the carotid artery may be visualized in a dental panoramic radiograph.

Gastrointestinal system

Complications of the gastrointestinal system include:
- Difficulty in swallowing (dysphasia)

- Abdominal pain, ulcers
- Acid stomach or heartburn (gastroesophageal reflux)
- Frequent indigestion, diarrhea, or constipation
- Bloody stools or black tarry stools
- Intestinal polyps or inflammation (diverticulitis, irritable bowel syndrome [IBS])
- Colon cancer
- Liver (**hepatitis**) or gallbladder problems (**gall stones**)

See Figure 12-7 for a review of the GI system.

Difficulty in Swallowing (Dysphagia)

Difficulty in swallowing (dysphagia) is a subjective symptom that may be caused by an emotional disturbance or a disease or dysfunction condition. Dysphagia is caused by a transport dysfunction of the musculature of the esophagus. Swallowing disorders may be caused by neuromuscular disorders (e.g., myasthenia gravis, bulbar palsy) or lesions (e.g., esophageal carcinoma, the strictures associated with progressive systemic sclerosis [scleroderma], Plummer-Vinson syndrome, and the disseminating candidiasis that can be found in AIDS). Patients who have xerostomia or who have had head and neck radiation therapy also have difficulty with swallowing.

Abdominal Pain and Ulcer

The area of pain in the abdomen is important in determining the cause of the pain. Pain in the right upper quadrant (RUQ) may be a sign of hepatitis (liver), cholecystitis (gallbladder), or carcinoma of the head of the pancreas. Pain in the left upper quadrant (LUQ) may be a sign of an enlarged spleen or inflammation or carcinoma of the tail of the pancreas. Pain in the lower right quadrant (LRQ) may be a sign of acute appendicitis or pneumonia in the lower right lung; pain in the lower left quadrant (LLQ) may be a sign of diverticulitis; and pain in the epigastric area may be a sign of acute pancreatitis.

Patients with a history of ulcers also have a distinct location and character of pain. Gastric ulcers produce a diffuse pain on the left side, whereas duodenal ulcers have pain localized to the right side with a focal area of tenderness. The cycle of pain for the duodenal ulcer is as follows:

Pain→Food→Relief→Pain

For the gastric ulcer the pain cycle is as follows:

Pain→Food→Increased pain

Gastroesophageal Reflux

Gastroesophageal reflux disease (GERD) is a reflux or regurgitation of gastric contents into the esophagus.

DENTAL CONSIDERATIONS

Patients with GERD should be kept in a semi-sitting position during dental treatment.

Genitourinary system

Complications of the genitourinary system include:
- Difficulty urinating, pain on urination

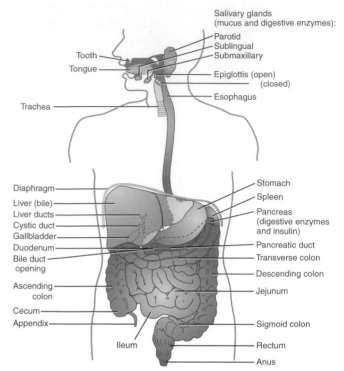

FIGURE 12-7
Gastrointestinal system. (From Mahan LE, Escott-Stump SK: *Krause's food, nutrition and diet therapy,* ed 11, St Louis, 2004, WB Saunders.)

- Blood in the urine
- Excessive urination
- Incontinence
- Kidney infections, kidney stones
- Kidney failure and renal dialysis (hemodialysis or peritoneal dialysis)

Figures 12-8 and 12-9 provide a review of the urinary system and the female and male reproductive systems, respectively.

> *Functions of the Genitourinary System*
> - Excretion
> - Regulation of blood volume, blood pressure, and electrolytes
> - Reproduction

Difficulty and Pain on Urination (Dysuria)

Dysuria may be a sign of prostate enlargement (hypertrophy or carcinoma), streptococcal glomerulonephritis, cystitis (bladder infection and inflammation), urethritis, pyelonephritis, gonorrhea, or a combination of these problems.

Blood in the Urine (Hematuria)

Hematuria, whether microscopic or overt, is a serious sign. Hematuria may be caused by severe hypertension (end-organ damage to the kidneys), acute glomerulonephritis, trauma, cystitis, gonorrhea, bladder carcinoma, or a toxic reaction to drugs.

Excessive Urination (Polyuria)

Four major medical disorders can cause **polyuria:**
1. DM
2. Diabetes insipidus

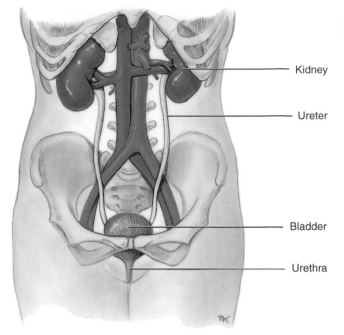

FIGURE 12-8
Urinary system. (From Applegate E: *The anatomy and physiology learning system,* ed 3, Philadelphia, 2006, WB Saunders.)

3. Acquired renal lesions
4. Psychogenic polydipsia

Kidney Infections and Urinary Calculi

Kidney infections may occur anywhere in the urinary tract. Infections in the lower urinary tract are known as *cystitis* and *urethritis* and are caused by colonic flora or gonococci. Infections of the upper urinary tract are known as *pyelitis* and *pyelonephritis.* Kidney infections are not to be confused with glomerulonephritis, which is an autoimmune response to a streptococcal infection.

Urinary calculi (stones) may occur anywhere in the urinary tract. They can cause pain, obstruction, and secondary infections. Approximately 1 in every 1000 adults requires hospitalization for kidney stones.

Renal or Kidney Failure and Dialysis

When the kidneys are no longer able to maintain body homeostasis because of kidney failure, the patient is treated by hemodialysis. Dialysis is a process during which the blood is removed from the patient, passed through membranes and filters to remove impurities, restored with electrolyte concentration, and then returned to the patient. Common medical complications with patients on renal dialysis include hypertension, uremia, anemia, clotting problems, and impaired immune response. This population tends to be at an increased risk for IE and viral hepatitis. These patients are also prone to depression and may become suicidal.

> *Distinct Care Modifications*
>
> For patients on a regular dialysis program, blood pressures should not be taken on the arm where the shunt or fistula has been placed.

Patients with kidney failure are subject to oral and systemic infection, and they have poor wound healing after invasive dental procedures. A physician's consult is recommended for any patient on hemodialysis. The physician can provide valuable information including the patient's condition and prognosis, risk for endocarditis, need for antibiotic pre-medication, drugs that need to be avoided (because of altered excretion, metabolism, or both), coagulation status, timing of dental appointments (usually same day as dialysis), and any limitations or contraindications to dental treatment. The blood pressure must be evaluated at each visit.

The dental team needs to recognize and manage ulcerations, oral infections, and candidiasis, should any of these present in the oral cavity. Extensive fixed prosthodontic reconstruction is generally not recommended. Meticulous oral self-care is especially important for these patients. Scaling and any procedures that manipulate the oral soft tissues must be done as atraumatically as possible.

Sexually Transmitted Diseases and Venereal Disease

Sexually transmitted diseases (STDs), such as gonorrhea and syphilis, remain a concern. Syphilis may have classic oral lesions. In the primary stage, a **chancre** may be present (teeming with infectious organisms); in the secondary stage, mucous patches and split papules may be present; and in the tertiary stage, a gumma and interstitial glossitis may be present. Genital herpes **(type 2 herpes)** and genital warts (condyloma acuminata) may be present in the oral cavity and in the genital mucosa (see Chapter 7).

Pregnancy

Pregnancy induces multiple physiologic and metabolic effects. Hormonal changes are responsible for alteration in the coagulation mechanism, the inflammatory response, and the patient's response to trauma and local irritants (in the mouth and elsewhere). The pregnant patient is susceptible to anemia, hypertension, postural hypotension, (reversible) HMs, and hyperglycemia or hypoglycemia. Risk of miscarriage and fetal susceptibility to birth defects is greatest in the first trimester. In the third trimester, the pregnant patient is most likely to experience physical discomfort and have circulatory problems, especially while in a supine position. Patient positioning will need to be modified for comfort and to prevent postural hypotension returning to the upright position.

The question of how best to manage the pregnant dental patient has sometimes been controversial. In general, the best time to perform elective dental treatment is in the second trimester. However, for each treatment decision,

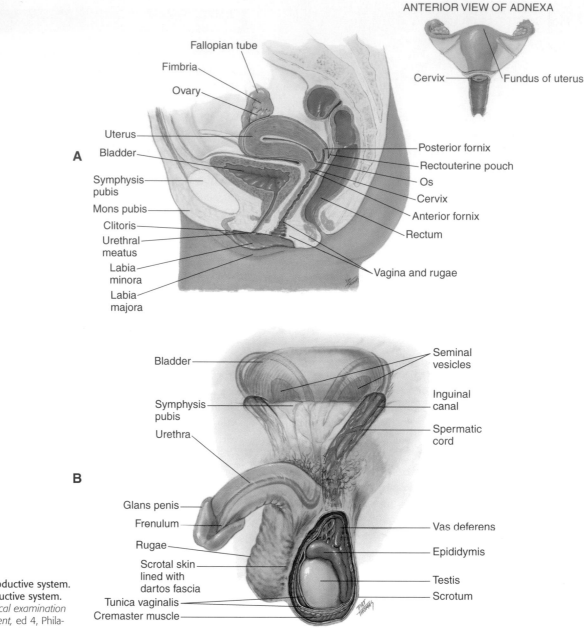

ANTERIOR VIEW OF ADNEXA

Cervix — Fundus of uterus

Fallopian tube
Fimbria
Ovary

A

Uterus
Bladder
Symphysis
pubis
Mons pubis
Clitoris
Urethral
meatus
Labia
minora
Labia
majora

Posterior fornix
Rectouterine pouch
Os
Cervix
Anterior fornix
Rectum

Vagina and rugae

B

Bladder
Symphysis
pubis
Urethra

Seminal
vesicles
Inguinal
canal
Spermatic
cord

Glans penis
Frenulum
Rugae
Scrotal skin
lined with
dartos fascia
Tunica vaginalis
Cremaster muscle

Vas deferens
Epididymis
Testis
Scrotum

FIGURE 12-9
A, The female reproductive system.
B, The male reproductive system.
(From Jarvis C: *Physical examination and health assessment,* ed 4, Philadelphia, 2004, WB Saunders, 2004.)

the benefits of doing the dental treatment must be weighed against the possible ill effects on both the pregnant patient and the fetus. In a non–high-risk pregnancy, any trimester is suitable for dental hygiene procedures. Given the minimal medical risk to the patient and the obvious health benefit of establishing and maintaining a healthy oral condition during pregnancy, the patient should be strongly encouraged to come into the office for any appropriate initial or supportive periodontal therapy. Establishing an effective oral self-care regimen is essential.

Emergency dental care should be provided whenever appropriate, because the benefits of eliminating oral disease and infection far outweigh the risks of using a local anesthetic and performing conservative acute-care dental treatment. In some cases, endodontic therapy is preferred

to extraction of a tooth, because the root canal treatment is less invasive.

Any radiographs indicated for the management of urgent dental needs should be taken. Elective diagnostic radiographic images can be taken with the consent of the patient after a full conversation of the relative risks and benefits of taking versus not taking the images.

In the unstable pregnant woman, oral self-care education should be stressed, and planned definitive dental procedures should be discussed with her physician. Prescribing medications for the pregnant patient should be done within guidelines set by the patient's obstetrician.

Patient education should include current concepts in the link between periodontal disease and preterm, low–birth-weight infants.

⭐ CASE APPLICATION 12-1.7

Genitourinary System History

What in Mr. Belzak's history pertains to the genitourinary system?

Prostate

Prostate cancer is a common malignancy in men older than age 50 years, and the incidence increases with each decade of life.[4] More than 210,000 new cases of adenocarcinoma of the prostate are diagnosed annually. Hormonal influences have been identified as a cause of adinocarcinomas.[4]

Endocrine system

> *Functions of the Endocrine System*
> • Regulation of hormones
> • Works with nervous system to control all other systems

Complications of the endocrine system include:
• Excessive thirst or hunger
• Listlessness or fatigue
• Agitation, excitability
• Difficulty sleeping
• Feeling too hot or too cold all the time
• Increase or decrease in weight
• Hot flashes or mood swings
• Diabetes, thyroid (hyperthyroidism or hypothyroidism), pituitary (pheochromocytoma), or adrenal problem (Cushing's syndrome, Addison's disease)
• Chronic use of steroid (prednisone) medication (cushinoid condition)

Figure 12-10 provides a review of the organs in the endocrine system.

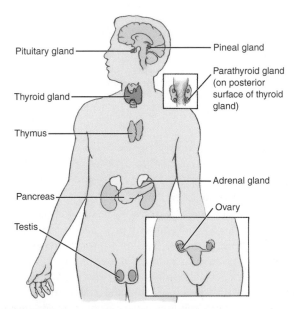

FIGURE 12-10
Parts of the endocrine system. (From Applegate E: *The anatomy and physiology learning system,* ed 3, Philadelphia, 2006, WB Saunders.)

Labels: Pituitary gland, Thyroid gland, Thymus, Pancreas, Testis, Pineal gland, Parathyroid gland (on posterior surface of thyroid gland), Adrenal gland, Ovary

Thyroid Gland Problems

When patients state they have or have had thyroid problems, the clinician must ascertain the nature of the problem and how the patient is managing it. Is the patient taking a synthetic thyroid medication? What is the dose? How often is the thyroid function evaluated? A patient who is obese or gaining weight and relates symptoms of fatigue, drowsiness, cold intolerance, and poor memory and who presents with physical signs including dry, coarse skin and hair, decreased heart rate, loss of the lateral one third of the eyebrow, and prolonged reflexes may have decreased thyroid gland activity (hypothyroidism). However, a patient who relates symptoms of headaches, diarrhea, increased appetite, weight loss, and heat intolerance, and whose physical signs include exophthalmia, increased heart rate, and dyspnea, may have increased thyroid gland activity (hyperthyroidism).

DENTAL CONSIDERATIONS

An undiagnosed hyperthyroid patient or a known hyperthyroid patient whose medical management has not been stabilized should not be given a dental local anesthetic agent with a vasoconstrictor (see Chapter 41).

Weight Change

In an adult, an increase in body weight may reflect an increase in adipose tissue or an accumulation of fluid. Obesity is the single most prevalent metabolic disorder in countries with an abundance of food. Obesity occurs when the caloric intake is greater than the energy requirement of the body for normal physical growth and maintenance. Increased fluid retention may be caused by excessive salt intake, excessive fluid intake, or a decreased sodium and water excretion. A decreased sodium and water excretion may indicate a cardiovascular, renal, hepatic, or adrenal problem. Weight gain resulting from increased fluid retention occurs in a short period of time (hours to days). Excessive loss of weight may be the first indication of a wasting disease such as HIV infection. Weight loss also is an ominous prognostic indicator of the progression of a malignancy (see Chapters 47 and 48).

Diabetes Mellitus

DM is the most prevalent of all endocrine disorders. The two major types of DM are (1) IDDM (type 1) and (2) NIDDM (type 2). IDDM is acquired at younger ages, in people with a thinner physique. Those with type 1 DM are prone to develop **ketoacidosis** and do not produce any insulin. NIDDM is typically acquired by obese individuals (60% to 90% of individuals

> **BOX 12-4**
>
> **SIGNS AND SYMPTOMS OF INSULIN-DEPENDENT DIABETES MELLITUS**
>
> Polydipsia
> Polyphagia
> Polyuria
> Increased weakness and fatigue
> Loss of weight

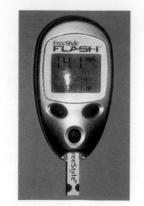

FIGURE 12-11
Freestyle Flash glucometer. Smallest amount of blood required.

BOX 12-5

SIGNS AND SYMPTOMS OF NON–INSULIN-DEPENDENT DIABETES MELLITUS

Blurred vision
Older than 40 years of age
Overweight
Numbness and tingling in extremities
Postural hypotension
Urination at night

BOX 12-6

LABORATORY TESTS FOR THE DIAGNOSIS OF DIABETES MELLITUS

Fasting blood glucose: Normal range 60 to 100 mg/dl
2-Hour postprandial: Abnormal greater than 200 mg/dl
Glycosylated hemoglobin: Normal range 3% to 6%

---

with NIDDM are obese), older than 40 years of age. Type 2 diabetics do produce some insulin and are less likely to have ketoacidosis. Their underlying physiologic problem is insufficient insulin production, an abnormality of insulin receptor activity, or both.[7] The vascular and metabolic changes caused by DM are pervasive and significant, potentially effecting multiple organ systems. Some of the more common and serious clinical effects include immune compromise, visual impairment, paresthesia, gangrene, hypertension, heart attack, and stroke.

An understanding of DM is important in dentistry because dental healthcare professionals are in a position to detect new cases and are also responsible for the treatment of patients who have the disease. The signs and symptoms suggestive of IDDM can be found in Box 12-4. Usual symptoms or profiles for those with NIDDM are shown in Box 12-5, and laboratory tests that help diagnose DM are provided in Box 12-6.

In-office monitoring for the evaluation of suspected patients with diabetes, or the evaluation of known patients with diabetes, can be accomplished with blood glucose meter systems (Figure 12-11). The patient's skin is punctured with a lancet device, and a drop of blood is placed on the test strip. The test result is displayed within 30 seconds. Box 12-7 outlines the criteria for diabetes.

DENTAL CONSIDERATIONS

For the dental team, the most common problem for this patient is insulin shock.

Generally, morning appointments are better suited for diabetic patients because they have more energy at that time, and their glucose and insulin levels are more likely to be in balance. A source of glucose that can be rapidly absorbed should be available in the dental office at all times (in case of a hypoglycemic attack). Common oral findings in the patient with diabetes are xerostomia—often resulting in an increased dental caries rate, candidiasis, impaired wound healing, and periodontal disease. The patient with diabetes who is well-managed with hypoglycemic agents does not appear to have any compromise in healing or combating infections.

BOX 12-7

CRITERIA FOR DIABETES

Normal
Fasting* blood glucose less than 110 mg/dl
2-Hour postprandial
Random plasma glucose less than 140 mg/dl
Impaired
Fasting blood glucose greater than 110 and less than 126 mg/dl
2-Hour postprandial
Random plasma glucose greater than 140 mg/dl and less than 200 mg/dl
Diabetes
Fasting blood glucose greater than 126 mg/dl
2-Hour postprandial
Random plasma glucose greater than 200 mg/dl

---

*Fasting refers to no food intake for 8 hours before the blood sample is taken.

Prevention
Prevention of insulin shock involves discussion with the patient of the importance of adequate food intake and an appropriate hypoglycemic agent. Patients should be monitored for signs of hypoglycemic shock during dental visits.

Adrenal Hyperfunction (Cushing's Syndrome) and Cushinoid Condition

Patients who have long-term exposure to high levels of catabolic steroids share similar features. If the steroid production is internally produced (endogenous), or it comes from external (exogenous) drug source such as prednisone, then common physical features arise including "buffalo hump," "moon facies," trunkal obesity, abdominal striae, and wasting of the extremities. The skin becomes thin and prone to ulceration. Bruising, ecchymosis, and the appearance of petechiae are common features. Steroids are a powerful and effective tool used to control the symptoms of many autoimmune, inflammatory, and dermatologic disorders. Unfortunately, when taken in therapeutic doses for an extended period, they also have very significant metabolic effects including the breakdown of body protein. As a result, many cushinoid patients develop an insulin-resistant form of diabetes. Especially relevant in the practice of dental hygiene are the decreased immune response, poor wound healing, and susceptibility to (oral) infection.

DENTAL CONSIDERATIONS

Cushinoid patients have suppressed adrenal gland function and therefore may lack the normal "fight or flight" response that occurs when an individual faces physical or emotional stress. With the stress of a dental procedure, the lack of cortisol production by the patient may precipitate an adrenal cortical crisis—a potentially life-threatening medical emergency. For this reason, the dental team should be aware of any systemic catabolic steroids that the patient may be taking or has taken in the last 2 years. Depending on the type of steroid (the relative potency can be highly variable), the daily dose, and the length of time the patient has taken the steroid, the dental team can determine whether the patient has compromised adrenal cortical output. The *rule of twos* is one commonly used guide for this purpose. If the patient is determined to be at risk for an adrenal cortical crisis, then additional steroids may be required—especially when the patient has significant dental anxiety, before surgical dental procedures (i.e., periodontal surgery, multiple extractions), or when infection is present. An excellent discussion of the rule of twos and the proper management of the cushinoid patient can be found in Malamed's *Medical Emergencies in the Dental Office* (Mosby, 2007).

A patient with a severe form of Cushing's syndrome or who has a debilitating disease such as severe arthritis, fibromyalgia, or SLE for which he or she is taking high levels of steroids is usually not a good candidate for comprehensive dental treatment. For these patients the emphasis should focus on pain control and maintenance therapy. Antibiotics may be indicated before invasive procedures given their poor wound healing and propensity to develop infection. The dental team needs to be prepared to treat oral ulcerations, infections, and stomatitis when they arise.

Excessive Thirst (Polydipsia)

Increased thirst (**polydipsia**) and increased urination (polyuria) should alert the clinician to the possibility of the presence of diabetes. This finding also may be present in the patient with **Cushing's disease (primary aldosteronism).**

Hematopoietic system

Complications of the hematopoietic system include:
- Easy bruising
- Excessive bleeding (but never needed a transfusion)
- Anemia (or sickle cell anemia)
- Hemophilia
- Leukemia

Easy Bruising

The presence of a bruise may be explained by eliciting a history of trauma, or it may be the sign of a vascular or platelet abnormality.

Excessive Bleeding

Bleeding is one of the most serious manifestations of a disease process. The presence of blood, whether from the gingival sulcus representing periodontal disease or in the form of hematuria or hemoptysis, should alert the clinician to pursue this concern. Excessive bleeding may be caused by the patient taking medications such as warfarin (Coumadin), aspirin, or nonsteroidal antiinflammatory drugs (NSAIDs), or it may represent a defect in that patient's hemostatic system. Box 12-8 lists laboratory tests for hemostasis.

Anemia and Sickle Cell Anemia

Anemia is a manifestation of an underlying disease process. Approximately 20% of females in the United States have iron-deficiency anemia. Anemia is a decrease in the oxygen-carrying capacity of the red blood cells (RBCs) and may be manifested as a decrease in the hemoglobin content or a decrease in the number of RBCs. The anemic patient is tired, weak, and faint, and he or she has headaches and is intolerant of cold. Oral findings in the anemic patient may range from no obvious changes in the oral tissues to the classic beefy red, bald tongue, and the subjective complaint of altered taste or glossodynia. These findings should alert the clinician to the possible presence of an anemic condition. Box 12-9 lists laboratory tests used to detect anemia.

Taking dietary replacement of either iron or folic acid can reverse iron- and folate-deficiency anemia. If vitamin B_{12} is the deficient factor, then vitamin B_{12} injections are required to treat this condition. An undiagnosed or untreated vitamin B_{12} deficiency (pernicious anemia) may result in irreversible degeneration of the spinal cord.

Sickle cell anemia is a chronic anemia in blacks, affecting 0.3% of blacks in the United States.[5] The sickle cell trait affects 8% to 13% of blacks and does not result in any signs or symptoms.[5] The anemia in sickle disease is severe. The RBC sickles or loses its shape and plugs up small vessels, causing swelling of the spleen and liver, thus severely compromising the immune system and placing the patient at risk for infection. A sickle cell event is extremely painful.

DENTAL CONSIDERATIONS

Radiographically the molar region may have a decreased trabecular pattern, characterized by a stepladder pattern.

BOX 12-8

LABORATORY TESTS FOR HEMOSTASIS

Vascular Phase

In this phase the endothelial cells that line the blood vessels restrict the blood cell elements to the vessel. If a defect in the vessel wall integrity exists, then blood cell elements may pass between the endothelial cells into the connective tissue. To evaluate the vessel integrity, place a blood pressure cuff in the normal position and inflate to 90 to 100 mm Hg. Leave the cuff at that pressure for 5 minutes. Then count the number of petechiae that occur within a circular area of 2.5 cm diameter (approximately 1 inch). This is called the *tourniquet test,* and a normal value is less than 10 petechiae.

Platelet Phase

If the vessel is damaged, platelets adhere to the exposed subendothelial tissues, continue to aggregate, and ultimately form a mechanical plug. Platelets can fail to form the plug if either a decrease in number or a decrease in activity occurs. Researchers report that aspirin and nonsteroidal antiinflammatory drugs (NSAIDs) alter the activity of the platelets; however, patients who take aspirin daily for cardiovascular benefit do not have bleeding times outside the normal range. Either Duke's or Ivy's method is used to determine the bleeding time. In Duke's method, a lancet cuts the earlobe; in Ivy's method, a lancet cuts the forearm. The cut is blotted every 30 seconds until bleeding stops.
- *Platelet count:* Normal 100,000 to 400,000 platelets per mm^3
- *Bleeding time:* Less than 5 minutes

Coagulation Phase

This phase can be initiated by either the extrinsic or intrinsic pathways. The extrinsic pathway is the first to be activated and is initiated by the action of the tissue thromboplastin in combination with calcium (factor IV) and factor VII. The intrinsic pathway is initiated by contact between the Hageman factor (factor XII) and the negatively charged endothelial surface. Several clotting factors require vitamin K for their production in the liver. Coumadin and other warfarin derivatives are similar in structure to the vitamin K–producing chemical factors but are nonfunctional in clotting activities. The **international normalized ratio** (INR) tests the extrinsic pathway, and the partial thromboplastin time (PTT) tests the intrinsic pathway. The INR is used to measure the effects of warfarin (Coumadin).*
- *INR:* 1.2 to 1.4
- *PTT:* 35 to 50 seconds

Fibrinolysis Phase

The fibrinolytic system is required to prevent the coagulation activity in areas far removed from the site of injury and also to dissolve the clot after it has served its hemostatic purpose. This process involves plasminogen that is converted to plasmin. The plasmin splits large and small pieces from the fibrin clot and stops the activity of the coagulation factors.*

*Data from Little JW et al: *Dental management of the medically compromised patient,* ed 7, St Louis, 2007, Mosby.

BOX 12-9

CHARACTERISTICS OF DIFFERENT FORMS OF ANEMIA

Hypochromic Microcytic Anemia
- Normal red blood cell (RBC) count
- Iron deficiency: Decreased mean corpuscular cell volume (MCV)
- Chronic blood loss: Decreased mean corpuscular hemoglobin concentration (MCHC), decreased hematocrit

Normochromic Normocytic Anemia
- Decreased RBC count
- Acute blood loss: Normal MCV

- Hemodialysis: Normal MCHC
- Hemolysis: Decreased hematocrit, decreased/increased reticulocyte count

Macrocytic (Megaloblastic) Anemia
- Normal RBC count
- Folate deficiency: Increased MCV
- Vitamin B$_{12}$ deficiency: Normal MCHC
- Chronic alcoholism: Decreased reticulocyte count

Hemophilia

This hereditary disorder results in a coagulation deficiency and initially presents in childhood. Hemophilia A (factor VIII deficiency) is the most common form. Genetically, hemophilia is transmitted to males and carried by females. Patients with hemophilia have factor VIII ranging from 1% to 25% of the norm. Regardless of the range, dental surgical procedures result in severe bleeding. Diagnosis of hemophilia A is based on a prolonged partial thromboplastin time (PTT) and a low factor VIII activity.[6]

DENTAL CONSIDERATIONS

Before invasive dental procedures, patients with hemophilia should have factor VIII replacement, and their factor VIII level should be 50% of normal or greater at the time of the dental surgical procedure. This disease is marked by hematoma formation, hemarthrosis, and bleeding after dental extractions.[6]

Leukemia

Leukemia is an increase in the number of immature cells of the white blood cell line. Leukemia may arise in either the granulocytic or lymphocytic line. Patients with leukemia commonly have generalized lymph node enlargement (lymphadenopathy) and are prone to numbness, burning, and tingling sensations (paresthesias). With the overproduction and overabundance of immature white cells, often a diminution of red cells (causing anemia) and platelets (causing thrombocytopenia) occurs. Consequently, the patient is often weak and lethargic and has poor coagulation. Commonly the immune response is impaired, and wound healing is a problem. Some forms of leukemia are now able to be treated very successfully, and the patient will recover and have a normal life expectancy. Unfortunately, other patients with aggressive forms of leukemia may have an early demise.

DENTAL CONSIDERATIONS

Acute forms of leukemia may have oral signs such as bleeding around the gingiva, leukemic infiltrates in the oral tissues, candidiasis, serious fungal infections (aspergillosis or mucormycoses), and debilitating viral infections. The patient's hematologist may ask the dental clinician for assistance in his or her efforts to control intraoral hemorrhage or to determine the cause of oral lesions (i.e., fungal, viral, graft versus host). If uncertainty exists about the patient's condition, diagnosis, prognosis, bleeding potential, need for antibiotic premedication, or medical restrictions on dental treatment, then a physician's consultation is warranted. During the active phase of the disease, dental treatment is usually limited to palliative and urgent care. The importance of maintaining the oral tissues in as healthy a state as possible cannot be overemphasized.

Hepatitis and Jaundice

Jaundice means a greenish-yellow color. A jaundiced condition manifested by a yellow discoloration of the skin, mucous membranes, and sclera is due to an increase in the bilirubin level in the blood. Bilirubin increases with an increased rate of destruction of RBCs, a decreased conjugation of the lipid-soluble bilirubin in the liver, a decreased rate of removal of the conjugated bilirubin via the bile duct into the small intestine, or a combination of these factors. Newborn infants may have jaundice.

Thus a history of jaundice is not necessarily synonymous with a history of hepatitis, an inflammation of the hepatocyte, or cells in the liver. Some causes are medications, toxic chemicals, alcohol, and viruses.

Causes of viral hepatitis are as follows (see Chapter 7 for more information):

- Hepatitis A: waterborne, food borne, fecal-oral route, no carrier state (vaccine available)
- Hepatitis B: blood borne, carrier state (vaccine available)
- Hepatitis C: blood borne, carrier state (no vaccine, variable clinical progression)
- Hepatitis D: blood borne (occurs only in presence of hepatitis B virus [HBV] infections; HBV vaccine effective)
- Hepatitis E: waterborne and food borne, fecal-oral route (no vaccine)
- Mononucleosis: Epstein-Barr virus (EBV), transmitted in saliva, no carrier state

DENTAL CONSIDERATIONS

The concern in dentistry is the transmission of viral hepatitis from a patient to the dental health care personnel (DHCP) or another patient. With the acceptance of universal precautions and the hepatitis B vaccine, the threat to the DHCP has been decreased significantly. However, clinicians should still thoroughly review the patient's medical history and attempt to identify the cause of jaundice or hepatitis (see Chapter 7).

Radiation and Chemotherapy

See Chapter 48 for information on this subject.

Human Immunodeficiency Virus and Acquired Immunodeficiency Syndrome

See Chapter 47 for information on this subject.

Neurologic system

Complications of the neurologic system include:

- Frequent headaches (tension, migraine, cluster, or other)
- Dizziness, fainting
- Tremors, shakes
- Muscle weakness or paralysis
- Balance problems
- Stroke, seizures, trauma to the head
- Neuritis, neuralgia
- Alzheimer's disease
- Multiple sclerosis, demyelinating disease
- Parkinson's disease

Figure 12-12 provides a review of spinal nerves and the autonomic nervous system innervation.

Chapter 44 provides more content on conditions and illnesses, as well as modifications to care for this organ system.

Frequent Headaches

Headaches along with fatigue, hunger, and thirst represent an individual's most frequent complaints of discomfort. A headache most often is the expression of minor tension or fatigue associated with the events of the day. However, if the individual is incapacitated by the headache and the headache is of a long duration, then the individual may have migraine headaches, or some underlying organic disease state may exist.

Dizziness and Fainting

Dizziness may be related to a hypoglycemic state, anemias, and disturbances in the vestibular component of the auditory nerve.

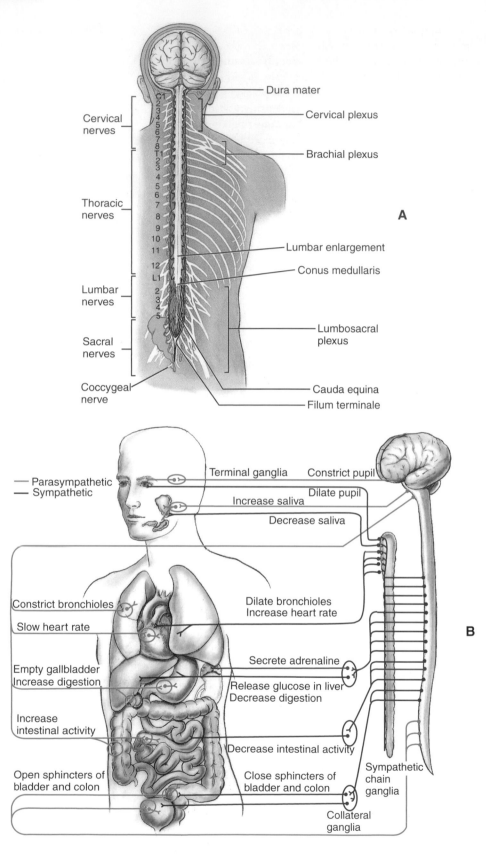

A

B

FIGURE 12-12
A, Spinal nerves. **B,** Innervation of the autonomic nervous system.
(From Applegate E: *The anatomy and physiology learning system,* ed 3, Philadelphia, 2006, WB Saunders.)

Fainting refers to a lack of strength with the sensation of impending loss of consciousness. Dizziness and fainting rarely appear when the patient is in the recumbent position (see also the section on the cardiovascular system).

Epilepsy (Seizure Disorders)

Epileptic attacks may occur at any time of day or night, and they occur regardless of the patient's position. With the classic grand mal seizure, the onset is sudden—an aura is present, the patient becomes unconscious, and tonic-clonic contractions begin. After the seizure terminates, the patient is confused, may have a headache, and is physically exhausted.

DENTAL CONSIDERATIONS

The dental team should confirm at each visit that a patient with a seizure disorder is taking his or her medication or medications as prescribed. If the patient does have a seizure during treatment, then the clinician must ensure that the patient does not injure himself or herself. If the patient is standing, then the team member should ease the patient to the floor and make sure that the head does not strike the floor or other hard object.

Patients with seizure disorders who are treated with phenytoin (Dilantin) may exhibit gingival enlargement.

Neuritis and Neuralgia

Neuralgias that affect the head and neck region are **trigeminal neuralgia (cranial nerve V)** and glossopharyngeal neuralgia (cranial nerve IX).

Paralysis

The most common head and neck paralysis is Bell's palsy. This is due to an inflammatory reaction in or around the nerve in the area of the stylomastoid foramen. Bell's palsy may be associated with DM, the postsequelae of a viral infection, or a recurrent herpes infection.

Alzheimer's Disease

Alzheimer's disease is a degenerative process with loss of cells in the cerebral cortex, resulting in memory loss. Behavior may be variable from childlike to angry and aggressive. A caretaker typically escorts the patient to the dental office. The clinician should maintain a close watch of these patients.

Muscular Dystrophy

This is an inherited progressive muscle disorder, characterized by wasting and atrophy of muscle.

Multiple Sclerosis and Demyelinating Disease

Multiple sclerosis is a slowly progressive central nervous system disorder. In the brain and spinal cord, patches of demyelination occur, resulting in multiple and varied neurologic symptoms and signs, usually with remissions and exacerbations.

Lyme Disease

Lyme disease is a tick-transmitted disorder that results in neurologic, cardiac, and joint problems.

Parkinson's Disease

Parkinson's disease is a degenerative central nervous system disorder characterized by slow movement, rigid muscles, tremors at rest, and inability to remain upright.

Psychiatric and psychologic problems

Emotional complications include:
- Nervousness
- Depression
- Other psychologic problems (bipolar disorder, schizophrenia, posttraumatic stress disorder)

Chapter 45 provides more specific content on illnesses associated with this system and modifications to care.

Nervousness

Many patients admit to being nervous or anxious about dental treatment. If this is in direct relation to a stressful event, then the nervousness is accepted as a normal response. However, if the nervousness is uncontrollable and accompanied by physical effects, then further evaluation may be necessary before any dental procedures are performed.

Depression and Bipolar Disorder

Depression is a recognized medical illness with multiple possible causes, and it can have many comorbid conditions. Bipolar disorder is characterized by intermittent cyclical periods of depression and mania typified by euphoria or grandiosity. A myriad of pharmacotherapeutic agents exist to treat these disorders. The dental team needs to be aware of the diagnosis and management strategies and have a good understanding of the level of control of the condition. The hygienist needs to accurately document any and all medications that the patient is taking and be familiar with the actions, side effects, and possible drug interactions—particularly with those agents that may be used in dentistry.

✪ CASE APPLICATION 12-1.8

Psychiatric or Psychologic Problem Inquiry

The clinician suspects that Mr. Belzak may suffer from depression. This means that he likely will have a much more difficult time in tobacco and substance cessation than someone who has not experienced depression.

DENTAL CONSIDERATIONS

The patient who suffers from clinical depression or bipolar disorder who is not being medically managed (or who has inadequate control of the depression) presents the dental team with a significant challenge. This patient is typically lethargic and unmotivated. Concern about oral health is low, and a lack of attention to oral self-care is seen. The patient may be reluctant to schedule visits for hygiene services; if appointments are made, then he or she may be tardy or absent. Motivating the patient is difficult; therefore dental treatment may need to be limited to the most basic services. With good control, the patient is usually a good candidate for full range of restorative and hygiene therapy; however, many of the antidepressant and antipsychotic medications cause xerostomia. Consequently, many of these patients suffer an increased rate of dental caries and recurrent dental caries, candidiasis, and inflammed tissues (stomatitis). Some medications, most notably the tricyclic antidepressants, can interact synergistically with epinephrine, causing a potential medical emergency in the dental office.

Bipolar disorder is having depression and elevated manic periods. Bipolar disorder has a younger age of onset between episodes and a higher rate of social dysfunction (see Chapter 45).

Results of inquiry

If the patient responds positively to any of the primary questions regarding the systems, then typical follow-up questions would be the following:

- Have you been told what is causing your symptoms (diagnosis)? If so, then what is it?
- What treatment have you had? Has it been effective?
- Are you taking medications for the condition? (The clinician should refer to the patient's drug history.)
- How well is your condition being controlled?
- What is the prognosis?

As this dialog is played out, the dental hygienist can decide which medical signs or symptoms need further evaluation and diagnosis, identify medical issues that need better management, and discover diseases and conditions that either predispose the patient to a medical emergency in the dental chair or may require modification to the way in which dental care is to be delivered. When the patient history, and in particular the ROS, reveals diseases, disorders, treatments, drug therapies, and oral sequelae with which the oral healthcare provider is not familiar, he or she should consult with the dentist, other healthcare provider, or one or more of the excellent on-line or printed textbooks listed at the end of this chapter. A medical compendium, or a dental textbook that focuses on oral medicine, dental management of medically compromised patients, or management of medical emergencies in the dental office, can be very helpful. Providing information on the wide array of medical problems

and the manner in which they can affect the provision of dental hygiene services is beyond the scope of this book.

ORAL HEALTH HISTORY

The patient's oral health history (also known as the *past dental history*) provides the dental hygienist with insight into the patient's awareness about oral health issues and the relative importance that the patient attaches to oral health and dental treatment. A review of the patient's oral health history includes an assessment of the following:

1. *The frequency of dental visits and oral prophylaxis (cleanings).* Did the patient return on a regularly scheduled frequency or use dental services infrequently? Were special circumstances (e.g., anxiety or a particular bad experience in the dental chair) affecting this behavior? This information reveals the patient's attitude toward oral health and gives some indication of the relative importance of preventive dental procedures to the patient.

2. *The reason for the past dental visits.* Were previous dental visits for episodic or emergency treatment only, or were they part of the patient's regular oral healthcare maintenance schedule? This information reveals the patient's knowledge about oral health and the importance of periodic visits (i.e., "checkup and cleaning"). Patients participating in a regular preventive program have a much greater appreciation of good oral health than do patients who seek oral care only when they have a problem. Patients who have had a reparative attitude toward dental care in the past are not necessarily locked into that mode indefinitely; however, to modify their behavior and their perspective, some candid conversation will need to occur to decipher and address real and perceived barriers to care. Only then can the patient be expected to adopt a more preventive or holistic approach to oral health care.

3. *Type of dental care provided in the past.*
   a. *Extractions.* Were the extractions part of orthodontic therapy, the result of unrestorable carious lesions, or caused by bone loss resulting from periodontal disease? Were the extractions performed because the patient could not afford the recommended treatment?
   b. *Periodontal therapy.* Does the patient have a past history of periodontal disease? Has the patient had periodontal surgery? Did the patient participate in a periodontal therapy maintenance regimen? How has the patient responded to the periodontal treatment? All of these questions help the clinician determine the severity and prognosis for the periodontal disease and the likelihood of success for different modalities of periodontal therapy.
   c. *Endodontic therapy.* Has the patient had root canal therapy? Was it successful? Has he or she had any subsequent problems? In general, a history of successful endodontic therapy suggests that the patient is interested in preserving the teeth and willing to put financial resources into that effort. Occasionally, a patient will report a negative experience with endodontic therapy or may have subse-

quently lost the tooth (caused by a vertical fracture) and have an aversion to doing any more root canal treatment.

  d. *Restorative dentistry.* Were the restorations placed as part of a comprehensive dental program, or were they placed as part of managing a dental emergency?

  e. *Prosthodontic treatment.* What type of prosthodontic treatment was performed? How long ago? Has the patient been satisfied with the dentures, appliances, or prostheses? Is the patient interested in improving or replacing the prosthesis (perhaps with implants)?

  f. *Treatment for TMJ problems.* Does the patient have a history of TMJ disease? How has the TMJ disease been treated in the past? How successful was the past treatment? A prior history of a TMJ disease is a definite risk indicator for future TMJ diseases.

  g. *Orthodontic treatment.* Has the patient had braces? If so, then for how long? Was it comprehensive or limited tooth movement? Was it successful? Is the patient wearing a retainer? Successful completion of comprehensive orthodontic therapy is suggestive of a patient with a high esthetic consciousness and usually is consistent with a strong preventive attitude. In short, most orthodontic patients want to "protect their investment." Orthodontic therapy can leave the patient with some negative outcomes including dental caries, blunted roots, loss of periodontal support, and tooth mobility.

4. *Oral home care practices.* What is included in the patient's current oral self-care regimen? Were these procedures recommended by the dental health professional? Were any self-care recommendations made in the past but not followed? A neutral and effective way to phrase an initial question to the patient is, "Tell me what you do to take care of your teeth and gums." This information helps the clinician to understand what is being done currently and what has been effective in the past. It also helps the dental hygienist to begin a discussion with the patient about possible future oral care strategies.

If the patient is determined to be at high or moderate risk for dental caries, then the clinician should ask about the patient's fluoride history: Has the patient lived in a community with optimally fluoridated water? If so, for how long? What about during childhood? Does the patient use a fluoridated toothpaste? Fluoridated mouthrinse? Other forms of fluoride? This information can be very useful as the dental team develops and implements a dental caries control strategy to meet the patient's specific needs.

PSYCHOSOCIAL HISTORY (PERSONAL HISTORY, HABITS, SOCIAL HISTORY)

The psychosocial history includes a variety of nonmedical issues that may have an effect on the dental plan of care. Included in this review are dietary issues and various habits in which the patient may participate (sometimes collectively referred to as a *personal history*), as well as social issues that may affect the patient's ability to attend dental appointments, comply with therapeutic recommendations, and pay for dental services. Delving into the psychosocial history, when done in a sensitive and professional manner, can also help the interviewer "connect" with the patient. By understanding and responding empathetically to life issues that are significant to the patient, the dentist, hygienist, and other team members will be more effective in relating to the patient ultimately and more successful in assisting the patient with his or her oral health needs.

Following are common issues that are appropriate to raise in the psychosocial history.

Tobacco Use

Does the patient use any tobacco products? Has he or she used any in the past? If so, then an effort should be made to quantify the use history. A convenient way to quantify cigarette use is with a pack-year history. To determine the patient's pack-year history, the clinician multiplies the number of packs smoked per day by the number of years the patient has smoked. The deleterious systemic and oral effects of tobacco use are well documented. (See suggested agencies and web sites on the Evolve site and also Chapter 29.)

Alcohol Consumption

Daily alcohol intake should also be quantified. Patients with a known history of alcohol abuse or who admit to frequent binge drinking or high levels of daily alcohol consumption are at risk for multiple medical problems including oral cancer and bleeding diathesis. Patients with alcoholic liver disease often have an altered tolerance for analgesics and anesthetics, and they suffer from poor wound healing, malnutrition, and ineffective oral home care. The uncontrolled alcoholic patient often exhibits undesirable behaviors such as being tardy or absent for dental appointments, not paying for dental treatment, and noncompliance with professional instructions. If a patient is a recovering alcoholic, then the clinician must avoid suggesting alcohol-containing preparations, such as commercial mouthwashes.

Recreational Drug Use

Asking about the use of illicit substances is often difficult for dental healthcare providers. However, doing this is appropriate and necessary. Significant oral effects can occur with substance use and abuse. Some systemic effects can be debilitating and potentially life-threatening. For example, a patient who ingests cocaine shortly before a dental appointment is at risk for a cardiovascular crisis if the dentist or dental hygienist administers a local anesthetic. Substance abusing patients are also prone to exhibiting uncooperative or noncompliant behavior patterns.

Dietary Intake

The oral and systemic effects of chronic malnutrition are significant. Investigating the nutritional intake of the patient is within the purview of dental practice and appropriate for the dental team. A simple way to quickly get a perspective on this issue is to ask, "What is your typical diet like over the course of a day?" Most patients are aware of qualitative (if not quantitative) deficiencies in their diet. Often the patient will volunteer, "I eat too much junk food," or "I do not get enough fruits and vegetables." Even such a brief conversation may be enough for the hygienist to make some recommendations about how the patient may improve his or her diet. In some cases, use of a 3- or 5-day diet history can be an effective means of identifying more subtle deficiencies and making more strategic recommendations for improvement. Chapter 19 provides more information on dietary and nutritional assessment.

Acid and Refined Sugar Exposures

Acidic foods and beverages are the primary cause of dental erosion. Citrus fruits such as lemons and limes, as well as tomatoes, strawberries, and vinegar are all known culprits. Individuals who consume large amounts of carbonated beverages—especially diet sodas—are particularly at risk. Determining whether the acidic agents are "sipped" or consumed quickly is important. Rinsing the mouth immediately after an acid insult is helpful to provide clearance and raise the pH on the tooth surface. Brushing immediately after an acid exposure may compound the effect of the dental erosion. Both acidic substances and refined carbohydrates are known to be cariogenic. Questioning patients about the nature and frequency of ingestion of any sweets is appropriate, especially for those patients who are at risk for dental caries. Patients with an active dental caries need to be counseled about the relationship between a refined carbohydrate diet and the cause of dental caries, and they should be given suggestions on dietary modification.

Clenching or Bruxing

Does the patient clench or grind his or her teeth? Does he or she have any symptoms? Has the patient ever sought professional help? Taken any medications? Used a bite splint or night guard? If so, then was it effective?

Other Parafunctional Habits

Does the patient give a history of mouth breathing or biting objects (e.g., pencils, pipe stems, chicken bones)? Does the patient chew ice? Bite the fingernails? Does he or she have any other deleterious oral habits? How were the parafunctional habits managed, and what was the success of the treatment?

Functional Assessment

For frail older adults and special-needs patients, asking whether they can perform a complete array of activities of daily living (ADLs) unassisted is appropriate. Individuals who need the help getting to the dental office or who need assistance with oral self-care will require special management by the dental team.

Occupation and Hobbies

Asking the patient about his or her work, interests, and hobbies is a good way to build rapport and make a connection that can be a source of conversation over the years of an extended professional relationship. Delving into these issues also can give the dentist or the hygienist insight into sources of stress and exposure to toxic substances that can cause various forms of oral pathology, as well as carcinogens or **teratogens** (which promote the development of cancer).

Cultural Background

Cultural attitudes about oral health and disease and dental treatment can significantly modify a patient's expectations, his or her willingness to accept proposed treatment, or both. If cultural issues were not explored in the family history, then addressing them during the psychosocial history is appropriate.

Available Transportation

Patients who need to use public transportation, or who depend on a family member or friend for transportation to the dental office, may have limited access to dental care. The dental team needs to be aware of such limitations when establishing the length, number, and timing of appointments.

Available Time

Because of their work schedule, a child, or elder care responsibilities, some patients may have severe limitations on their availability for dental treatment. The dental hygienist needs to be aware of these issues and may need to be very creative and flexible in accommodating some patients' schedules. Lacking this insight, the dental provider may erroneously come to the conclusion that the patient "is not motivated" or "does not value dental treatment."

Anxieties, Stresses, or Patient Concerns Unrelated to Dental Treatment

The recent death of a loved one, divorce, relocation to a new area, beginning a new job, job loss, or a recent marriage—any of these major life events may cause stress for the patient. Stress is a major causative factor in the expression of many oral and systemic diseases and conditions. Dealing with stressful events can be a distraction that limits the patient's attention to oral self-care and dampens his or her enthusiasm for dental treatment. Dealing with these issues may also have a financial effect and thereby limit the resources available to pay for dental and hygiene services.

Patient Desires and Expectations for Treatment if Other than the Chief Concern

This is an ideal opportunity to investigate whether the patient has any previously undisclosed concerns about or desire for dental treatment.

Financial Means

Does the patient have the financial resources to cover the cost of the proposed treatment? Does the patient have concerns in this regard? Does the patient need financial assistance to be able to engage in the dental treatment? If so, then what are some options? Does the dental team need to assist the patient in finding financial support? A candid discussion of these issues is needed, because it may affect both the nature and the scope of the dental treatment plan.

Other Information

At the conclusion of obtaining the patient history, the clinician should ask the patient, "Is there anything else that you think is important for us to know?" At this point a high level of rapport and trust usually has been established, and the patient is willing to divulge to the hygienist and the dental team any previously undisclosed pertinent information.

Once the information is collected, important tasks remain. The DHCP is now responsible for the analysis and documentation of the findings from the comprehensive health history. This process merges into the medical referral and management of medical issues that will affect the dental and dental hygiene treatment of the patient. These aspects of planning care constitute the systemic phase of the dental treatment plan. The parts of this process are as follows:

- The DHCP should differentiate findings that are benign and noncontributory from those that are significant.
- All significant positive findings should be documented. Often the dental record has (at the end of the medical-dental health history questionnaire) a designated location to record a summary of the findings that may have an effect on dental treatment. Most patient records also have a cover sheet—a medical problem list—which records such findings. Summary notes and a medical problems list can be recorded electronically or can be handwritten by the dentist or dental hygienist. Potentially life-threatening conditions are typically flagged as an *ALERT* in a bright motif in a prominent location in the dental record.

- If the patient has symptoms that are unexplained or suggest that the patient has a new or different medical problem, the patient should be referred to the appropriate physician or medical specialist for evaluation and treatment.
- Similarly, if the review of the history leads the DHCP to believe that the patient's condition or disease is not being adequately controlled, then a referral back to the patient's care provider is warranted.
- When medical conditions are identified that may necessitate limitation, modification, or contraindication of the dental treatment—but uncertainly exists about the extent of the effect—a consultation with the patient's physician should be obtained.
- As all medical diagnoses are pursued, consultations obtained, and medical conditions treated or stabilized—the dental team can construct a comprehensive dental plan of care that includes any appropriate modification to accommodate the patient's medical conditions.
- As a mode of categorizing the patient's relative medical risk to receive dental treatment, many practitioners use the American Society of Anesthesiologists' (ASA) classification system. This system is based on a four-class designation as described in Table 12-5.

In general, ASA I patients can undergo a complete range of dental services with no restriction whatsoever. ASA II patients may need minor modification or precaution but are generally not restricted as to the scope or duration of treatment. ASA III patients are expected to have significant restriction to the type of dental treatment, as well as the complexity and the duration of the therapy. ASA IV patients are usually limited to urgent services, and even those should be undertaken in a hospital setting where emergency resuscitation equipment and personnel are readily available.

Table 12-5	American Society of Anesthesiologists (ASA) Physical Status Classification with Examples	
CATEGORY	**DEFINITION**	**EXAMPLES**
ASA I	A normal healthy patient with no evidence of systemic disease	
ASA II	A patient with mild systemic disease or a significant health risk factor—The patient is able to walk up a flight of stairs or two level city blocks without difficulty.	Well-controlled diabetes, controlled hypertension, history of asthma, mild obesity, pregnancy, smoker, extreme anxiety or fear toward dentistry
ASA III	A patient with moderate to severe systemic disease that limits activity but is not incapacitating—The patient can walk up one flight of stairs or two level city blocks but stops at times because of distress.	Stable angina, postmyocardial infarction, poorly controlled hypertension, symptomatic respiratory disease, massive obesity
ASA IV	A patient with severe systemic disease that is life-threatening—The patient is unable to walk up a flight of stairs or two level city blocks and is in distress at rest.	Unstable angina, liver failure, severe congestive heart failure, or end-stage renal disease

From Stefanac SJ, Nesbit SP: *Treatment planning in dentistry,* ed 2, St Louis, 2007, Mosby.

Conclusion

Obtaining a comprehensive health history on every new patient is a pivotal and indispensable part of any contemporary dental or dental hygiene practice. Collecting and recording a thorough, accurate, and complete history on each patient is essential if the hygienist is to be able to provide treatment in a safe manner, anticipate possible medical emergencies, and properly monitor the patient's medical condition while under the clinic's care. A dental hygienist fills a key role as part of the patient's healthcare team, and he or she is in a unique position to help diagnose previously unrecognized diseases, assist the patient in getting medical treatment for unstable conditions, and ensure that dental treatment will be provided with minimal medical risk. A well-done health history is the starting point for a trusting and rewarding long-term patient-hygienist therapeutic relationship. In its absence, seeds are sown for patient distrust, medical mismanagement, and legal risk and vulnerability.

References

1. Advisory statement: Antibiotic prophylaxis for dental patients with total joint replacements, *J Am Dent Assoc* 128:1004-1008, 1997.
2. American Heart Association: *Cardiovascular disease in dental practice,* Pub No 71-0009, Dallas, 1991, The Association.
3. American Heart Association: Wilson W, et al: Prevention of Infective Endocarditis. Guidelines from the American Heart Association. *Circulation:* published online before print April 19, 2007. Available at: http://circ.ahajournals.org/cgi/reprint/CIRCULATIONAHA.106.183095v1.
4. Greenlee RT et al: Cancer statistics, 2001, *CA Cancer J Clin* 51(1):15-36, 2001.
4a. Little JW et al: *Dental management of the medically compromised patient,* ed 7, St Louis, 2008, Mosby.
4b. Malamed SF: *Medical emergencies in the dental office,* ed 6, St Louis, 2007, Mosby.
5. *The Merck manual of diagnosis and therapy,* ed 17, Internet edition provided by Medical Services, USMEDSA, USHH, 1999-2005 by Merck & Co. Available at http://www.merck.com/mrkshared/mmanual/home.jsp. Accessed Sept 2006.
6. Redding SW, Montgomery M: *Dentistry in systemic disease: diagnostic and therapeutic approach to patient management,* Portland, 1990, JBK Publishing.
7. Ship JA, Mohammed AR: *Clinician's guide to oral health in geriatric patients,* Baltimore, 1999, American Academy of Oral Medicine.
8. Taybos GM, Terezhalmy GT, Pelleu GB: Assessing patients' health status with the Navy dental health questionnaire, *US Navy Med* 2:24-31, 1983.

Drug-Induced Adverse Oral Events

Ann Eshenaur Spolarich • JoAnn R. Gurenlian

INSIGHT

13-1
to
13-4

Dental hygienists treat many patients who are taking medications. Invariably, they encounter issues related to drugs and their use, including drug indications, adverse events, drug interactions, and factors affecting adherence. Additionally, managing oral side effects of medications remains an ongoing challenge for dental hygienists. The ability to evaluate these issues, accurately assess the patient's status, and plan for medication-related prevention and treatment interventions is an essential part of the dental hygiene process of care.

CASE STUDY 13-1 Erythema Multiforme

A 65-year-old white man, Harry Liebowitz, is scheduled for his 6-month supportive care appointment. He states that his mouth is sore and that this soreness has been present for almost the past 6 months.

The hygienist reviews Mr. Liebowitz's medical history and finds the following medical problems and medications:
- Hypertension—Lopressor (metoprolol)
- Elevated cholesterol—Lopid (gemfibrozil)
- Rheumatoid arthritis—Naprosyn (naproxen), Darvocet-N100 (propoxyphene with acetaminophen), aspirin (acetylsalicylic acid [ASA])
- Gastrointestinal disturbance—Zantac (ranitidine)

Mr. Liebowitz's social history is negative. He states that he has never used any tobacco products and does not consume alcoholic beverages.

The clinical examination reveals the following:
- Buccal mucosa—Bilateral; diffuse white lacy mucosal lesions over erythematous mucosa, and focal areas of ulcerations on the left side (6 mm × 8 mm)
- Tongue—A 8-mm × 20-mm area of white lacy lesions over erythematous tissue with ulcerations (6 mm × 10 mm) on the left side of tongue (in the middle to posterior third on the ventrolateral surface)

The overall oral cancer screening examination does not reveal any abnormal findings except the documented lesion on the tongue. This is a high-risk area for oral cancer. Additional follow-up questioning of the patient and biopsy is indicated.

KEY TERMS

angioedema
candidiasis

dysgeusia
gingival hyperplasia

lichenoid drug reaction
medication list

pharmacologic history reviews
xerostomia

LEARNING OUTCOMES

After reading this chapter the student will be able to:
1. Conduct a thorough pharmacologic history review to determine whether the patient's medication use has the potential to cause adverse oral events.
2. Assess the patient's medication list to identify those medications associated with adverse oral side effects.
3. Identify strategies used to prevent or treat medication-induced adverse oral events.
4. Confidently discuss the relationship of the patient's chief complaint, oral presentation, and medications with the patient, the patient's physician, and the dentist.

All dental hygienists treat patients who are taking medications and inevitably encounter issues related to specific drugs and their use, including drug indications, adverse drug events, drug interactions, and factors affecting adherence.[69] To manage these issues as they arise in practice, dental hygienists must possess a sound knowledge and understanding of pharmacology and drug therapy.[67] The ability to evaluate these issues is necessary to accurately assess the patient's status, as well as to plan for medication-related prevention and treatment interventions for inclusion in the dental hygiene process of care.

Dental hygienists are often the first to learn about drugs taken by patients while they are conducting comprehensive health history and **pharmacologic history reviews.** The pharmacologic history is a series of questions used to assess how the patient's medication use may potentially affect the process of care (Box 13-1).[72] The pharmacologic history provides extensive information about a patient's current medical status, as well as important clues regarding changes in disease status, compliance with suggested health recommendations, and orientation toward health and wellness.[71] Information obtained through the pharmacologic history is used to determine the risks associated with treating medicated patients. The **medication list,** including a record of all drug names, doses, and prescribed regimens for use, is the first part of the pharmacologic history review and is compiled for each patient before initiating treatment. Patients should also be questioned regarding their use of over-the-counter (OTC) medications, including naturopathic products, herbal remedies, and vitamin and mineral supplements, all of which are included in the medication list.

Drugs are chemicals that act selectively on biological systems to diagnose, prevent, and treat disease, as well as to prevent pregnancy.[87] The pharmacotherapeutics, or study of these selective effects, are known for all drugs approved for use in humans, including both prescription and OTC medications. The effects of these drugs may be beneficial, dangerous, or both, depending on their indications and use. Drugs will always affect the health and well-being of the person who is taking them. Differences in body composition, age, metabolism, and systemic condition may affect drug actions; unfortunately the effects are not always known or predictable.[67,87]

All drugs have the potential to cause adverse or harmful effects that are either related or unrelated to the principal action of the drug. Harmful effects that are directly related to the drug action are predictable and occur as a consequence of that action. For example, increased gingival bleeding during instrumentation is often seen in patients taking warfarin, because of the anticoagulant action of the drug. These effects are reversible when the drug is discontinued. Harmful effects that are unrelated to the principal action of the drug are rare; often they produce unusual and unpredictable responses, such as anaphylaxis. Harmful effects also include toxicity reactions in which drug-reactive metabolites formed during metabolism cause cellular damage; drug hypersensitivity reactions in which the drug (or its metabolites) triggers the immune system; and drug interactions, which can either increase or decrease the amount of active drug in the circulation.[69,87]

All drugs produce side effects, which occur for one of two reasons. A drug may produce an exaggerated effect on its target tissue when given at its correct dose (this side effect is simply an extension of the therapeutic effect of the drug). In other cases the drug may affect a nontarget tissue, which produces an effect that is different from the intended outcome. This is typically the mechanism for adverse oral side effects of medication use. The U.S. Food and Drug Administration (FDA) requires the reporting of all known side effects for all medications, including the percentage of the population affected, which can be found in published reference texts.[69] Side effects can also occur if the patient is not managing medications correctly, such as failing to understand or comply with instructions, self-medicating, and undermedicating or overmedicating. Helping patients comply with their medication use is an important role for the dental hygienist.[68]

Managing oral side effects caused by medication use is an ongoing challenge for dental hygienists. Oral side effects cause patient discomfort and interfere with the patient's ability to chew, swallow, and digest food. Often a patient loses interest in eating or makes poor food choices, which can significantly affect nutritional status. This is especially problematic in those patients undergoing treatment for cancer. Some oral side effects contribute to the risk for oral trauma, whereas others contribute to infection, pain, and possible tooth loss. Dental hygienists need to accurately diagnose these oral conditions to recommend the appropriate treatment interventions. Timely recognition and professional interventions are necessary to improve the patient's comfort level and ability to function.[69] Common oral signs and symptoms associated with adverse drug reactions are summarized in Box 13-2.

BOX 13-1

PHARMACOLOGIC HISTORY

1. Why is the patient taking this medication?
2. Are symptoms reported by the patient caused by the conditions for which the patient is being treated or are they possible side effects of the drug or drugs?
3. What are the adverse effects of this drug?
4. Do these findings suggest a problem with drug dose?
5. Are there potential drug interactions?
6. How is this patient managing medications?
7. Will any oral side effects of the medication require dental hygiene intervention?
8. Given these findings and all other information, what are the risks of treating this patient?

From Spolarich AE, Gurenlian JR: Deductive reasoning with pharmacology: a prescription for quality patient care, *Comp Cont Ed Oral Hyg* 1:3-9, 1994.

ORAL SIGNS AND SYMPTOMS ASSOCIATED WITH ADVERSE DRUG REACTIONS

Angioedema

Atrophic mucosa

Candidiasis

Cough

Dental caries

Dysgeusia

Dysphagia

Erythema multiforme

Gingival bleeding

Gingival hyperplasia

Glossodynia glossitis

Hairy tongue

Increased gag reflex

Increased periodontal disease progression

Infection

Lichenoid drug reaction

Mouth or jaw discomfort

Mouth ulcerations or stomatitis

Oral paresthesia

Reflux or hyperacidity

Tooth disorder

Vomiting

Xerostomia

Xerostomia

SIGNS AND SYMPTOMS

Xerostomia has been described as a symptom that acts like a disease[21] and is the most commonly occurring drug-related adverse oral event. Xerostomia, by definition, is the "subjective feeling of oral dryness" and is the result of hypofunction of the salivary glands.[73] The perception of a dry mouth is not enough to actually diagnose salivary gland function, because salivary output must decrease by approximately 50% before the patient will experience the symptom of dryness.[12] Xerostomia can manifest as either a quantity change (reduced volume and flow), quality change (change in viscosity or natural defensive properties), or both.

Saliva serves a vital role in maintaining the homeostasis of the oral cavity, and it serves as the first enzyme in the process of digestion. Saliva acts as a normal lubricant, protecting the mucous membranes from trauma and ulceration, preventing the penetration of toxins and carcinogens, and facilitating soft tissue repair. Lubrication aids in the breakdown of food substances, preparation of the food bolus for swallowing, and digestion. Mucin glycoproteins keep the oral mucous membranes hydrated and pliable, and they maintain soft tissue integrity. Salivary immunologic and nonimmunologic processes, coupled with antimicrobial processes, protect the oral tissues from microbial colonization on hard and soft tissues, as well as help reduce oral infections. Salivary buffers maintain oral pH (combating the acid attacks of fermented sugars, food substances, and cariogenic bacteria), protecting the teeth from demineralization, dental caries, and dentinal hypersensitivity. Pellicle formation and salivary electrolytes further protect the teeth by promoting remineralization of early enamel lesions by calcium and phosphate.[38,45] Any alterations in these natural properties of saliva will result in an imbalance of the oral environment, leading to a variety of oral complications. Therefore patients with medication-induced xerostomia will have a variety of signs and symptoms that reflect changes in the normal characteristics and properties of natural saliva.[45,69]

Xerostomic patients will have increased risk for dental caries, especially on exposed root surfaces, at or underneath crown margins, and in root furcations. Incipient lesions appear along the gingival margin, and areas of decalcification may be evident on cusp tips. Without intervention, these lesions can invade all surfaces of the tooth. Increased erosion and abrasion are also apparent in xerostomic patients, which facilitates plaque biofilm accumulation, root caries formation, gingival inflammation, recession, and dentinal hypersensitivity.[20,40,45,86] Gingival disease will appear; if already present, then it may increase in extent and severity.[70] Xerostomia also places the patient at risk for opportunistic infections, especially fungal infections caused by *Candida* species. Parotid saliva contains peptides that have antifungal properties against *Candida albicans,* and the loss of this copious, serous saliva often leads to chronic, recurrent fungal infections.[56] Salivary mucosal antibodies are protective against a variety of viruses, and salivary mucins protect the oral mucous membranes from herpes simplex virus and human immunodeficiency virus (HIV).[28,34] The most common viruses encountered in dentistry include primary herpes simplex, recurrent herpes simplex (herpes labialis), herpes zoster, and HIV. Increased viral infections are a risk in xerostomic patients.[69] Proteolytic enzymes produced by bacteria can alter oral mucosal integrity and cause ulcerations.[45]

Ulcerations that are of nonviral origin, mucositis, and stomatitis are known painful side effects of many medications, especially drugs used for chemotherapy. Ulcerations may also develop from trauma caused by friction of the oral tissues against denture clasps, appliances, and edges of worn or defective restorations. Loss of lubrication also contributes to patients accidentally biting themselves while talking and chewing, causing aphthous ulcers to form. The lips may appear dry, cracked, and bleeding. The tongue may also appear fissured and sore. The mucous membranes will be dry and friable to the touch. In patients with extremely dry mouths, a gloved finger or mouth mirror will stick to the mucosa; when removed, it may peel the top layer of epithelium away, causing residual soreness and discomfort. The loss of saliva may affect taste sensation and may heighten sensitivity to spicy or highly seasoned foods. Difficulties encountered with eating (because of the loss of lubrication, taste alteration, and risk for trauma and pain from friction and biting) all decrease the enjoyment of eating and may alter the patient's food choices and compromise his or her nutritional intake[45,69,80] (Box 13-3).

ETIOLOGY

Although not caused by aging, xerostomia is most frequently reported among the elderly. Although salivary flow does decline somewhat with age, the perception of xerostomia is most likely related to the patient's compromised health because of systemic diseases or the medications used to manage those diseases.[21] Older patients also have more chronic diseases, including heart disease, diabetes, and depression; therefore they take more

BOX 13-3

ORAL SIGNS AND SYMPTOMS ASSOCIATED WITH DRUG-INDUCED XEROSTOMIA

Angular cheilitis
Cemental abrasion on exposed root surfaces
Dental caries
Dentinal hypersensitivity
Difficulty speaking, chewing, swallowing
Difficulty wearing dentures or appliances
Dry, cracked, bleeding lips

Enamel demineralization
Enamel erosion
Fissured, sore tongue
Friable oral mucosa
Increased gingivitis and periodontal infection
Increased viral infections
Opportunistic infections
Oral ulcerations/stomatitis
Taste alteration

BOX 13-4

DRUG CLASSES THAT PRODUCE NEURAL EFFECTS ON THE SALIVARY GLANDS

The following are examples of anticholinergic drugs that reduce the volume of serous saliva:
- Antidepressants
- Antiemetics
- Antihistamines
- Antihypertensives
- Antiparkinsonian drugs
- Antipsychotics
- Antispasmodics
    The following are examples of sympathomimetic drugs that produce a viscous, mucinous saliva:
- Amphetamines
- Appetite suppressants
- Bronchodilators
- Decongestants

Adapted from Sreebny LM, Schwartz SS: A reference guide to drugs and dry mouth, *Gerodontology* 14:33-47, 1997; Porter SR, Scully C, Hegarty AM: An update of the etiology and management of xerostomia, *Oral Surg Oral Med Oral Pathol Oral Radiol Endod* 97:28-46, 2004; Nähri TO, Meurman JH, Ainamo A: Xerostomia and hyposalivation: causes, consequences and treatment in the elderly, *Drugs Aging* 15:103-116, 1999.

medications, many of which cause xerostomia as a side effect.[46,70] More than 500 medications cause xerostomia, and the severity of the xerostomia complaint increases among the elderly because of a synergistic effect that occurs when taking multiple medications.[57,74] Because xerostomia can have both salivary and nonsalivary etiologies, the dental hygienist must conduct a thorough health history evaluation to assist with determining the true cause of the symptoms.[26,71]

The most common cause of medication-induced xerostomia is alteration of the neural pathways that stimulate salivary gland secretion.[51] Stimulation of the parasympathetic nerves (cholinergic action) produces an increased fluid volume of serous saliva. Stimulation by the sympathetic nerves (sympathomimetic action) produces less volume and more viscous saliva.[38,57] Thus anticholinergic drugs reduce the volume of serous saliva, and sympathomimetic drugs produce a more viscous, mucinous saliva with less volume.[26,51,57] Drugs can also produce neural effects on the higher centers of the brain, most notably by producing inhibitory effects on the salivary nuclei.[74] Drug classes that produce these neural effects are summarized in Box 13-4.

Drugs can also produce xerostomia by nonneural mechanisms. Inhaled medications may produce a sensation of dryness from their topical effects without actually altering flow rate.[74] Clinicians hypothesize that antihypertensive medications cause xerostomia as a result of decreased fluid volume because of the loss of electrolytes from increased urination and dehydration.[4] Finally, drugs can also compromise salivary flow rate by producing vasoconstriction in the salivary glands.[74]

Prevention

Dental professionals can work with their patients' physicians to reduce chronic medication-induced xerostomia. A patient may be switched to another medication (if possible) that produces less xerostomia. Dosing regimens may be altered so that the peak plasma levels of the drug do not correspond to the time of day when patients experience maximum dryness, such as nighttime. Doses may be split into smaller quantities and ingested more frequently to allow for natural periods of salivary stimulation (e.g., chewing during mealtimes) to counteract dryness.[74]

ASSOCIATED SYSTEMIC DRUGS

The drug categories shown in Box 13-5 are associated with causing xerostomia.[82]

BOX 13-5

DRUG CLASSES ASSOCIATED WITH CAUSING XEROSTOMIA

Antiacne agents
Antianxiety agents
Anticholinergics/antispasmodics
Anticonvulsants
Antidepressants
Antidiarrheals
Antiemetics
Antihistamines
Antihypertensives
Antiinflammatory analgesics

Antinauseants
Antiparkinsonian agents
Antipsychotics
Anorexiants
Bronchodilators
Decongestants
Diuretics
Muscle relaxants
Narcotic analgesics
Sedatives

From *USP DI volume I: drug information for the health care professional*, ed 24, Englewood, Colo, 2004, Micromedex.

MANAGEMENT

Given the numerous oral sequelae of drug-induced xerostomia, the dental hygienist must learn to develop individualized treatment plans that address the unique needs of each patient. Many dental drugs are available for use to treat the common infections associated with this chronic condition. Dental hygienists are encouraged to consult a dental drug reference guide to review a selection of available medications and to confirm the appropriate indications for use, as well as contraindications, dosing regimens, and any special instructions to give to the patient before initiating treatment. Many of these medications are also available OTC, and patients can be given the appropriate instructions during the dental hygiene appointment for purchasing and using these products at home. Recommendations for product selection should be based on sound, documented evidence of product safety and efficacy, FDA approval, and approval by the American Dental Association (ADA) Council on Scientific Affairs, when appropriate. Dental hygiene

interventions for addressing oral complications caused by drug-induced xerostomia are summarized in Table 13-1.

The FDA has approved two medications for the treatment of xerostomia: (1) pilocarpine (Salagen) and (2) cevimeline (Evoxac). These drugs are cholinergic agonists that produce parasympathetic stimulation of the exocrine glands to increase serous secretions. These medications are not approved for the treatment of drug-induced xerostomia; pilocarpine is approved for use in patients undergoing head and neck radiation and in patients with Sjögren's syndrome. Cevimeline is approved for use in patients with Sjögren's syndrome only. These medications increase secretions from all glands—a distinct advantage for patients with Sjögren's syndrome.[26,27] However, increased sweating is the most common unwanted side effect. Caution

Table 13-1	Dental Hygiene Interventions for Addressing Oral Complications Associated with Drug-Induced Xerostomia
ORAL COMPLICATION	**DENTAL HYGIENE INTERVENTIONS**
Dental Caries, Demineralization	• In-office fluoride treatment–tray technique, rinses, varnish • Prescription home fluoride therapy–dentifrices or gels using brush or trays • Chlorhexidine rinses • Bicarbonate-containing dentifrices for home use • Xylitol–gum, mints • Recaldent chewing gum
Dentinal Hypersensitivity	• In-office desensitization treatment • In-office fluoride treatment–tray technique, varnish • Potassium nitrate with sodium fluoride/stannous fluoride dentifrices for home use
Salivary Stimulation/Replacement	• Cholinergic agonist medications–pilocarpine (Salagen) or cevimeline (Evoxac) • Artificial salivary substitutes • Frequent water ingestion to maintain hydration • Sugarless gum • Sugarless mints
Gingivitis/Periodontal Disease	• Antimicrobial mouthrinses • Antimicrobial dentifrice–triclosan • Antiseptic mouthrinses–chlorhexidine or essential-oil mouthrinse • Power-assisted devices • Oral irrigation • Host modulation therapies • Mechanical plaque biofilm removal
Fungal Infections	• Topical antifungal therapy • Systemic antifungal therapy–caution with multiple drug interactions; risk for liver toxicity • Replace all oral hygiene devices • Treat all dentures and appliances • Antiseptic mouthrinses for long-term prevention
Viral Infections	• Topical antiviral medications • Systemic antiviral medications • Topical anesthetics as needed • Increase fluid intake • Vitamin supplements as needed • Adequate rest

From Spolarich AE: Managing the side effects of medications, *J Dent Hyg* 74:57-69, 2000.

Continued

ORAL COMPLICATION	DENTAL HYGIENE INTERVENTIONS

Table 13-1 **Dental Hygiene Interventions for Addressing Oral Complications Associated with Drug-Induced Xerostomia—cont'd**

Pain and Ulceration
- Topical anesthetics—over the counter (OTC) (benzocaine, tetracaine, liquid Benadryl)
- Topical anesthetics—prescription lidocaine rinse
- Coating agents mixed with liquid Benadryl—Kaopectate, Maalox, Mylanta
- Evaluate for vitamin deficiencies—iron, folic acid, or vitamin B_{12}
- Sulfonated phenolic agents to cauterize lesions
- Antiseptic mouthrinses for long-term prevention
- Prescription amlexanox paste (Aphthasol)
- Prescription triamcinolone acetate dental paste (Kenalog in Orabase 0.1%)
- OTC adhesives with benzocaine
- Avoid citrus, acidic, and spicy foods if ulcerations are present

Nutrition
- Reduce intake of acidic beverages
- Reduce time teeth are exposed to starches and sugars
- Avoid spicy, acidic, and citrus foods if ulcerations are present

Smoking
- Recommend and promote smoking cessation
- Behavioral modification therapy using multidisciplinary approach
- Nicotine replacement therapy

Mechanical Plaque Biofilm Removal
- Power-assisted devices
- Oral irrigation
- Interdental cleaning

must be used when prescribing these medications to patients with cardiovascular disease, chronic respiratory conditions, and kidney disease. These medications are contraindicated in patients with uncontrolled asthma, angle-closure (narrow angle) glaucoma, and liver disease.[27,71]

Salivary Gland Stimulators

Throughout the chapter, *Rx* is used to indicate the prescription, *Disp* is used to indicate to dispense, and *Sig* is the direction for the patient on dosing. Drug and dosing information for salivary gland stimulators[88] is as follows:

Rx: Pilocarpine hydrochloride 5-mg tablets
Disp: 90 tablets
Sig: Take one to two tablets three to four times per day, not to exceed 30 mg per day.
Refills × _____ (determined by treatment provider)
or
Rx: Cevimeline 30-mg capsules
Disp: 90 capsules
Sig: Take one capsule three times per day, not to exceed three capsules per day.
Refills × _____ (determined by treatment provider)

Dental Caries Prevention

Drug and dosing information for dental caries prevention[88] is as follows:

Rx: Stannous fluoride gel 0.4%
Disp: 4.3 oz
Sig: Place 5 to 10 drops in a custom tray and insert in mouth for 5 minutes daily; do not swallow.

and
Rx: Chlorhexidine gluconate 0.12%
Disp: 480 ml (one bottle)
Sig: Rinse with 20 ml for 30 seconds two times a day; do not swallow.

Candidiasis

SIGNS AND SYMPTOMS

Fungal infections vary in appearance and surfaces affected. Acute pseudomembranous, atrophic, and hyperplastic forms of fungal infections are associated with drug-induced xerostomia. Fungus is also associated with denture stomatitis and symptomatic geographic tongue. Typically, fungal infections appear as a white pseudomembrane overlying bright-red tissues, although they may also be erythematous or hyperplastic in appearance.[20] This is commonly seen on the palate underneath the denture of an elderly patient with chronic xerostomia. Patches of candidiasis can occur on any mucosal surface; however, the palatal mucosa and dorsum of the tongue are most typically affected.[45,86] The tongue may also appear red, fissured, and sore.[31] Previously, this appearance of candidiasis was known as *antibiotic stomatitis* or *antibiotic glossitis* because of its association with antibiotic therapy for acute infections.[58] Angular cheilitis, often associated with vitamin deficiency, is actually a fungal infection with a bacterial coinfection in the majority of cases and is a classic clinical finding in xerostomic patients. Angular cheilitis is a chronic complaint in patients with a loss of facial vertical dimension, such as patients with a history of stroke, facial paralysis, or ill-filling dentures, because the fungal organisms in the saliva pool around the folds of skin in the corners of the mouth.[20,69]

ETIOLOGY

Candidiasis is the most common opportunistic fungal infection of the oral cavity and is caused by an overgrowth of the organism *Candida albicans* (Figures 13-1 and 13-2). The candida organism is a commensal organism found on the skin, as well as in the gastrointestinal and genitourinary tracts. *C. albicans* exists in a symbiotic relationship with *Lactobacillus acidophilus*. In the healthy patient, the intact epithelium with a competent immune system results in the maintenance of the normal microbial flora and this symbiotic relationship.[19,25,49]

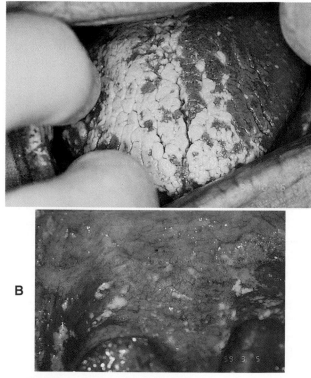

A

B

FIGURE 13-1
Candidiasis. **A,** 60-year-old woman with erosive lichen planus (ELP). Present medications are hormone replacement therapy (estrogen and progesterone) and topical corticosteroids for the treatment of ELP. Pseudomembranous form of candidiasis on the dorsum of the tongue. **B,** Junction of the hard and soft palate.

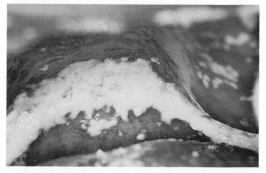

FIGURE 13-2
Candidiasis. Combination of pseudomembranous form of candidiasis and the atrophic form. This is an elderly woman who has asthma and uses a corticosteroid inhalant three to four times daily.

C. albicans is of weak pathogenicity and requires local or systemic predisposing factors to produce a diseased state.

Immunosuppression, endocrinopathies, anemias, nutritional deficiencies, medications, malignancies and their therapies, dental prostheses, epithelial alterations, age, poor oral hygiene, xerostomia, and a history of smoking are factors that may enable *C. albicans* to become opportunistic and lead to tissue penetration and infection.[19,25,49]

ASSOCIATED SYSTEMIC DRUGS

The medications associated with the development of candidiasis are systemic antibiotics, topical and systemic corticosteroids, hormones, cytotoxic drugs, and medications that cause xerostomia. The tetracyclines (TCNs) suppress the endogenous microflora that inhibit *Candida* species growth. The glucocorticoids suppress the nonspecific inflammatory response and cell-mediated immunity. Cytotoxic (methotrexate and cyclophosphamide) and immunosuppressive (azathioprine) drugs cause a decrease in the number of neutrophils and suppress cell-mediated immunity. Drugs that cause xerostomia decrease the production of saliva and reduce protective salivary immunoglobulin A (IgA) and histidine-rich peptides, resulting in an overgrowth of fungal organisms.[56]

TREATMENT

Treatment of candidiasis is a twofold process: identifying the predisposing factors and treating the local infection. Fungal infections are treated topically or systemically, depending on the extent and severity of the condition. Azole antifungals are systemic medications used to treat chronic, extensive mucocutaneous candidiasis. Polyene antifungals are topical medications that are used to treat local candidiasis.[50,69] Combination products that contain both an antifungal agent and a corticosteroid are used to treat the fungal infection and the inflammation of angular cheilitis.

The efficacy of topical antifungal therapy depends on contact with the tissues; thus topical agents come in a variety of delivery forms, including liquids, pastilles, and troches. Liquid swish-and-swallow preparations are also available and are especially helpful when the fungal infection covers a large surface area or extends into the upper oropharynx. Liquids can also be used to treat dentures and oral appliances by submerging or soaking. Caution must be used when prescribing the systemic antifungals, given their multiple drug interactions with commonly prescribed medications and the emergence of resistant fungal organisms after repeated exposure to these drugs. Infection with a resistant fungal organism can be life-threatening to immunocompromised patients; thus dental hygienists should consider systemic medication "reserve" drugs to treat those fungal infections that do

Prevention

Removable oral appliances and dentures can be treated with a 1:1 disinfectant solution of hydrogen peroxide and water during treatment of superficial fungal infections, to prevent reinfection of the oral tissues. All oral hygiene devices contaminated with fungal organisms should be thrown away and replaced.[49]

not adequately respond to topical therapy. Antifungal medications should be used for a minimum of 48 hours after the disappearance of clinical signs and symptoms, with a reevaluation scheduled after 14 days of therapy. A second period of treatment may be required for severe infections.[50,69]

Topical Antifungal Agents

Drug and dosing information for topical antifungal agents[88] is as follows:

> Rx: Nystatin (Mycostatin) oral suspension, 100,000 U/ml
> Disp: 60 ml
> Sig: Use 1 teaspoonful four to five times per day; rinse and hold in mouth as long as possible before swallowing or spitting out (2 minutes); do not eat or drink for 30 minutes after application.
> Refills × _____ (determined by treatment provider)

or

> Rx: Nystatin (Mycostatin) pastilles, 200,000 U
> Disp: 70 pastilles
> Sig: Dissolve one pastille in the mouth until gone, four to five times per day for 14 days.

or

> Rx: Clotrimazole troches (Mycelex), 10 mg
> Disp: 70 troches
> Sig: Dissolve one troche in the mouth five times per day for 14 days.

or

> Rx: Nystatin (Mycostatin) ointment
> Disp: 15-g tube
> Sig: Apply liberally to affected areas four to five times per day; do not eat or drink for 30 minutes after application.

Systemic Antifungal Agents

Drug and dosing information for systemic antifungal agents[88] is as follows:

> Rx: Ketoconazole (Nizoral) 200-mg tablets
> Disp: 10 tablets
> Sig: Take one tablet daily for 10 days.

or

> Rx: Fluconazole (Diflucan) 100-mg tablets
> Disp: 15 tablets
> Sig: Take two tablets on the first day and one tablet for 10 to 14 days.

Erythema Multiforme

HISTORY

In 1866, Dr. Ferdinand von Hebra, in his treatise *On Diseases of the Skin*, wrote about "erythema exsudativum multiforme."[83] He is credited with originating the term *erythema multiforme* (EM). The characteristics of EM as described by von Hebra were an acute, self-limiting, mild skin disease characterized by skin lesions, located primarily on the extremities and by a tendency for recurrences. In 1922, Drs. Stevens and Johnson described an acute febrile illness with skin lesions resembling EM, an associated stomatitis, and a severe conjunctivitis with visual impairment.[76] By the early 1940s this severe form of EM was universally known as *Stevens-Johnson syndrome*. In 1950, Thomas developed the terms *EM minor* (to describe the mild cutaneous form that von Hebra discussed) and *EM major* (to describe the severe mucocutaneous form that Stevens and Johnson characterized).[35]

EPIDEMIOLOGIC FINDINGS

EM occurs in young, healthy individuals, predominantly in men. Most cases occur in the 20- to 40-year-old age group, but about 20% occur in children and adolescents. The annual incidence of EM is estimated to be 0.01% to 1.0%. The rate of recurring EM cases is 22% to 37%.[35] Patients experiencing recurrences tend to have them in the spring or autumn.

SIGNS AND SYMPTOMS

The initial symptoms of EM include the nonspecific complaints of fever, malaise, headache, sore throat, rhinorrhea, and cough. These symptoms appear to be more common in major EM than minor EM. The cutaneous lesion is a round, erythematous macule that becomes papular and progresses to the classic *iris, target,* or *bull's-eye* appearance with a central area of necrosis. The oral mucosa is involved in 25% to 60% of the cases. The oral lesions begin as erythematous areas with edema that quickly progresses to large erosive lesions with a pseudomembranous surface. Hemorrhagic crusting of the vermilion border of the lips is common. The oral involvement in EM major is severe and may result in extensive tissue damage and morbidity. EM major has a more prolonged course consistent with the severe mucocutaneous destruction of the mouth, eyes, esophagus, and genitalia.

EM major has frequent complications. The most common complications involve the eye. Visual impairment resulting from keratitis or conjunctival scarring associated with the disease has been reported in 10% of the cases. Pneumonia has been reported in 30% of the cases and death in 5% of the cases. The gastrointestinal tract may be affected with esophagitis and strictures.

Another rare variant of EM major, toxic epidermal necrolysis (TEN) causes diffuse necrosis and sloughing of cutaneous and mucosal epithelial surfaces. The clinical presentation is similar to that of a person who has been badly scalded or burned. TEN tends to occur in older individuals and has a female predilection. It heals in 2 to 4 weeks, oral lesions take longer, and significant ocular damage may occur. TEN is fatal in 30% to 35% of patients.[42,60]

EM minor usually lasts 2 to 4 weeks from onset to healing. EM minor is a benign illness without any complications. The main concern may be difficulty with eating and drinking, which leads to dehydration.[35]

ETIOLOGY

The cause of EM is unknown; however, a hypersensitivity reaction is suspected. In approximately half of the cases, precipitating or triggering factors can be identified. Generally these factors can be attributed to infections or drugs. Other triggering factors include malignancy, vaccination, autoimmune disease, radiotherapy, or gastrointestinal conditions.[54,60,88]

ASSOCIATED SYSTEMIC DRUGS

Sulfa antibiotics are the most common drug class associated with EM, as are the sulfonylurea oral hypoglycemic agents used to treat type 2 diabetes.[43] Systemic drugs associated with EM are listed in Table 13-2.[35]

Table 13-2	Systemic Drugs Associated with Erythema Multiforme
CATEGORY	**AGENTS**
Antimicrobial Agents	Sulfonamides, penicillins, TCN, chloramphenicol, isoniazid, rifampin, clindamycin, dapsone, TMP-SMZ
Oral Hypoglycemic Agents	Diabinese (chlorpropamide), Glucotrol (glipizide)
Chemotherapeutic Agents	Alkylating agents, MTX
NSAIDs	Aspirin, ibuprofen, fenoprofen, sulindac, Relafen (nabumetone), Daypro (oxaprozin)
Hormones	Estrogen
Anticonvulsant Drugs	Carbamazepine, trimethadione, ethosuximide, Depakote (divalproex), Dilantin (phenytoin)
Opioid Analgesic Agents	Codeine
Antianxiety Agents	Meprobamate
Muscle Relaxants	Quinine
Cardiovascular Agents	Diuretics: furosemide Vasodilator: minoxidil ACE inhibitors: Vasotec (enalapril)
Antiinflammatory Agents	Glucocorticoids
H₂ Antagonist Agents	Cimetidine
Antihelminth Agents	Thiabendazole
Antigout Agents	Allopurinol

From Huff JC, Weston WL, Tonnesen MG: Erythema multiforme: a review of characteristics, diagnostic criteria, and causes, *J Am Acad Dermatol* 8(6):763-75, 1983.
ACE, Angiotensin-converting enzyme; *MTX*, methotrexate; *NSAIDs*, nonsteroidal antiinflammatory drugs; *TCN*, tetracycline; *TMP-SMZ*, trimethoprim-sulfamethoxazole.

PRECIPITATING FACTORS

The literature identifies three EM syndromes: (1) herpes associated, (2) mycoplasma associated, and (3) drug associated.

Herpes-Associated Erythema Multiforme

The association of herpes virus infections and EM has been recognized for more than 100 years. The proportion of EM cases ranges from 15% to 63%. This form of EM usually affects young adults and occurs 1 to 3 weeks after the recurrent herpetic infection. Herpes-associated EM generally is in the form of EM minor. The pathogenesis for this form of EM is thought to be either a hypersensitivity reaction to the virus or an inadequate immune response to the recurrent infection[35] (Figures 13-3 and 13-4).

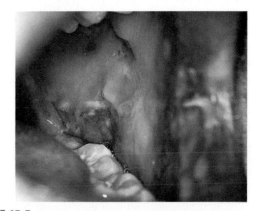

FIGURE 13-3
Erythema multiforme (EM). Diffuse ulcerations on the left buccal mucosa and retromolar pad areas.

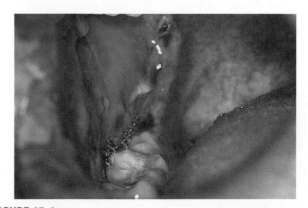

FIGURE 13-4
Erythema multiforme (EM). Diffuse ulcerations on the right buccal mucosa and retromolar pad areas.

Mycoplasma-Associated Erythema Multiforme

A clear association exists between EM and *Mycoplasma pneumoniae* infections. This form of EM occurs primarily in children and young adults, follows a severe respiratory infection with *M. pneumoniae*, and resembles EM major.[35]

Drug-Associated Erythema Multiforme

The best documented drug-associated EM is related to sulfonamides and more recently trimethoprim-sulfamethoxazole (TMP-SMZ) preparations (Table 13-3). The EM occurs usually 7 to 14 days after drug therapy and appears as EM major. Drug-associated EM most likely represents a hypersensitivity reaction to the drug.[35]

TREATMENT

The treatment by the dental healthcare team is based on the severity of intraoral mucosal lesions, the level of pain, and the degree of difficulty in eating, drinking, and swallowing. The patient with EM major (Stevens-Johnson syndrome) may require hospitalization to ensure adequate hydration and treatment of secondary infections.

The treatment for EM minor remains controversial. For adults, systemic corticosteroid therapy rapidly relieves the oral symptoms, hastens the healing of the intraoral tissues, and has few adverse effects. In addition to the systemic corticosteroid therapy, topical analgesic agents such as diphenhydramine elixir (Benadryl) or 2% viscous lidocaine may be prescribed as rinses to decrease the oral pain locally. Topical steroid rinses such as dexamethasone elixir (0.5 mg/5 ml) may supplement the effects of the systemic corticosteroids.[81]

An important part of treatment is determination of the precipitating factor. If the precipitating factor is a pharmacotherapeutic agent, then this agent should not be prescribed for that patient. If the precipitating factor is a recurrent herpetic infection, then suppressive antiviral therapy, such as acyclovir therapy, can prevent recurrences and may be necessary before initiating steroid therapy.[54]

Topical Analgesic Agents

Drug and dosing information for topical analgesic agents[88] is as follows:

Rx: Diphenhydramine hydrochloride (Benadryl) syrup 12.5 mg/5 ml

Disp: 4-oz bottle

Sig: Rinse with 1 teaspoonful for 2 minutes before meals and swallow.

or

Rx: Lidocaine hydrochloride (Xylocaine) viscous 2%

Disp: 450-ml bottle

Sig: Rinse with 1 tablespoon four times per day for 2 minutes and spit out.

Topical Steroids

Drug and dosing information for topical steroids[88] is as follows:

Rx: Dexamethasone elixir (Decadron) 0.5 mg/5 ml

Disp: 100-ml bottle

Sig: Rinse with 1 teaspoonful for 2 minutes four times per day; do not swallow.

Systemic Steroids

Drug and dosing information for systemic steroids[88] is as follows:

Rx: Prednisone 5 mg

Disp: 60 tablets

Sig: Take four tablets in morning with food and four tablets at noon with food for 4 days; then decrease the total number of tablets by one each day until down to zero.

Lichenoid Drug Reaction

SIGNS AND SYMPTOMS

A **lichenoid drug reaction** results in the appearance of oral lesions that resemble lichen planus. The lesions are located on the posterior buccal mucosa and exhibit a central erythematous area with a surrounding zone of radiating white striae. Patients state that the lesions are painful. The designation of a lichenoid drug reaction is based on the temporal relationship by which the individual takes the medication and then subsequently develops the oral lesion. Both lichen planus and lichenoid reactions are thought to represent a delayed hypersensitivity reaction. The cells of the oral mucosa are exposed to an antigenic challenge that initiates interactions, resulting in both the clinical and the histologic appearance of a lichen planus type of lesion[14,17,65] (Figures 13-5 and 13-6).

Table 13-3	Drugs Linked to Minor and Major Erythema Multiforme
CATEGORY	**AGENTS**
Cardiovascular Agents	Vasotec
Anticonvulsants	Dilantin, Depakote
NSAIDs	Relafen, Daypro
Antibiotic Agents	TMP-SMZ
Antigout Agents	Allopurinol

NSAIDs, Nonsteroidal antiinflammatory drugs; *TMP-SMZ,* trimethoprim-sulfamethoxazole.

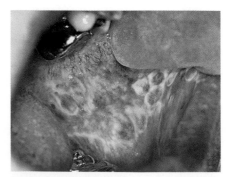

FIGURE 13-5
Lichenoid drug reaction. Left buccal mucosa with Wickham's striae on an erythematous tissue and focal areas of ulcerations.

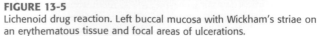

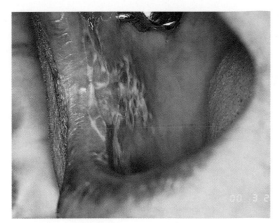

FIGURE 13-6
Lichenoid drug reaction. Right buccal mucosa with Wickham's striae on an erythematous tissue.

HISTOLOGIC FINDINGS

Indirect immunofluorescence for IgG may demonstrate a distinctive pattern, termed *strings of pearls,* along the cell membrane of the basal cell layer of the stratified squamous epithelium. This technique may be helpful in evaluating oral lichenoid drug reaction lesions.[54]

ASSOCIATED SYSTEMIC DRUGS

The drugs most commonly associated with lichenoid lesions are levamisole (Levantine) for colon cancer, quinidine drugs, thiazide diuretics, methyldopa, and photographic dyes.[22,43] Systemic drugs associated with lichenoid reactions are listed in Table 13-4.

Table 13-4	Systemic Drugs Associated with Lichenoid Drug Reactions
CATEGORY	**AGENTS**
Analgesic Agents	NSAIDs, propoxyphene/acetaminophen, acetaminophen/codeine
Antianxiety Drugs	Benzodiazepines
Anticonvulsant Drugs	Depakote (divalproex)
Cardiovascular Agents	β-Adrenergic blockers, angiotensin II antagonists, calcium channel blockers, cardiac glycoside, diuretics, potassium supplements
Gastric Acid Secretion Inhibitors	H₂ antagonists
Hormone Replacement	Thyroid hormone, insulin, sulfonylureas, metformin, oral contraceptives, estrogen, progesterone
Uricosuric Agents	Allopurinol

H₂, Histmaine 2; *NSAIDs,* nonsteroidal antiinflammatory drugs.

⭐ CASE APPLICATION 13-1.1

Pharmacologic Considerations

Mr. Liebowitz is taking a beta blocker (Lopressor), analgesic agents (nonsteroidal antiinflammatory drugs [NSAIDs]: naprosyn propoxyphene compound), and an H₂ antagonist (Zantac). Each of these drugs has been implicated in causing lichenoid drug reactions.

TREATMENT

The treatment for a lichenoid drug reaction is to eliminate the causative agent, if possible. If the medication cannot be stopped or an adequate substitution cannot be found, then the oral signs and symptoms can be managed through initial use of topical corticosteroids. The type of corticosteroid therapy is determined by the extent of the lesion. If the lichenoid reaction is localized to a few areas of the oral mucosa, then the topical steroid agents placed on the affected mucosa four times a day result in a decrease of the signs and symptoms. If the lichenoid reaction is generalized, then rinsing with a teaspoonful of dexamethasone elixir (0.5 mg/5 ml) for 2 minutes four times per day can reduce the erythema and the pain. Systemic corticosteroid therapy is indicated when the lichenoid reaction has not responded to the topical therapy or when the reaction is generalized with severe ulcerations. Oral candidiasis may occur in patients using steroids. These patients should be monitored for the presence of oral candidiasis. Patients with a history of developing candidal infections while using steroids or antibiotics are considered to be candidal carriers and should be prescribed antifungal therapy.[81]

Topical Steroid Agents

Drug and dosing information for topical steroid agents[88] is as follows:

> Rx: Fluocinonide ointment (Lidex) 0.05% (mix with equal parts of Orabase)
> Disp: 30 g total
> Sig: Apply a thin layer to oral lesions four to six times per day.

or

> Rx: Triamcinolone acetonide (Kenalog) in Orabase 0.1%
> Disp: 5-g tube
> Sig: Apply a thin film to the lesion after each meal and at bedtime.

or

> Rx: Dexamethasone elixir (Decadron) 0.5 mg/5 ml
> Disp: 100 ml
> Sig: Rinse with 1 teaspoonful for 2 minutes four times per day; do not swallow.

High-Potency Topical Steroid Agents

Drug and dosing information for high-potency topical steroid agents[88] is as follows:

> Rx: Clobetasol propionate cream (Temovate) 0.05%
> Disp: 15-g tube
> Sig: Apply locally four to six times per day.

Gingival Hyperplasia

ETIOLOGY

Anticonvulsant drugs, calcium channel blockers, and cyclosporine are the most common medications associated with gingival enlargement, or **gingival hyperplasia**.[7,8]

CLINICAL HISTORY

The gingival enlargement usually occurs within 1 to 3 months after initiation of drug therapy. Drug-induced gingival enlargement may be localized or generalized and range from mild changes to severe enlargement of marginal and papillary tissues. The maxillary and mandibular anterior gingival tissues are most affected. Enlargement of the labial gingiva is seen more frequently than enlargement of the lingual gingiva or edentulous areas. The affected tissues may appear as fibrotic, pebbly papillae that can coalesce as the enlargement worsens. In severe cases, function may be affected.[7,8]

MECHANISM FOR GINGIVAL ENLARGEMENT

Many theories have been postulated to explain the drug-induced gingival enlargement. Studies of phenytoin-induced gingival hyperplasia have demonstrated that gingival macrophages exposed to phenytoin secrete increased amounts of platelet-derived growth factor-B, and that phenytoin regulates secretion of the proinflammatory cytokine interleukin-1β (IL-1β) in inflamed tissues. Furthermore, phenytoin may stimulate osteoblast proliferation, leading to bone formation. Phenytoin-induced gingival enlargement is often associated with poor oral hygiene. Increased dental plaque biofilm increases accumulation of inflammatory cells such as monocytes and macrophages. Patients taking calcium channel blockers, most notably, nifedipine, have also demonstrated inflammatory type of enlargement resembling phenytoin-induced gingival enlargement. Although the exact mechanism of cyclosporine gingival enlargement is not fully known, dose-related, plaque biofilm associated, and direct effects on cellular targets are likely components in the pathogenesis of this disease.[8,13,37,52,77]

HISTOLOGIC FINDINGS

The histologic appearance is similar for phenytoin, calcium channel blockers, and cyclosporine. A chronic inflammatory infiltrate is seen with an increased formation of collagen and fibroblasts.

ASSOCIATED SYSTEMIC DRUGS

Phenytoin (Dilantin) is prescribed for the prevention of seizures (grand mal, status epilepticus, and absence seizures) and also may be used to manage trigeminal neuralgia. Gingival enlargement is seen in approximately 50% of the patients taking phenytoin, and the enlargement is more common in children and adolescents. The severity of the enlargement is directly proportional to the drug dose, the plasma drug level, and the patient's oral hygiene habits.[2] Other anticonvulsant agents have been reported to cause gingival hyperplasia, although the incidence is rare.[3,41,78]

Anticonvulsants that have been reported to cause gingival enlargement (Figures 13-7 and 13-8) are listed in Table 13-5.

Calcium channel blockers are used to manage hypertension, angina pectoris, cardiac arrhythmias, and for the prevention of vasospastic angina (Prinzmetal's angina). This class of drugs causes relaxation and dilation of the coronary arteries, reduced peripheral resistance, decreased myocardial oxygen consumption, as well as decreased atrioventricular conduction, heart rate, and blood pressure. Ten calcium channel blockers have been approved for use in the United States—seven of which have been reported to cause gingival hyperplasia. Most reports in the literature are case reports, with few patients affected. Nifedipine has the highest incidence of gingival

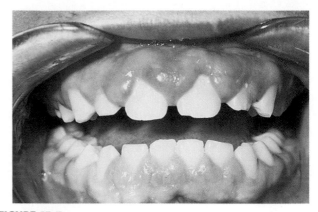

FIGURE 13-7
Example of gingival hyperplasia resulting from Dilantin therapy for the treatment of seizure disorders.

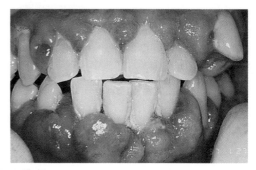

FIGURE 13-8
Example of gingival hyperplasia resulting from the patient taking nifedipine (Procardia) for the treatment of hypertension.

Table 13-5	Selected Anticonvulsant Agents Reported to Cause Gingival Enlargement
GENERIC NAME	**BRAND NAME**
Phenytoin	Dilantin, Phenytek
Valproic Acid	Depakote, Depacon, Depakene
Vigabatrin	Sabril

hyperplasia, with approximately 30% of users affected.[5,23,53,75] Diltiazem and verapamil have also been implicated, but with an extremely low incidence.[47] One case report has described gingival overgrowth in a patient taking felodipine.[44] Amlodipine, the newest drug in this class, has an incidence of less than 1%.[39] No factors exist that allow the clinician to predict which individuals will develop gingival enlargement.[79] The prevalence rate for gingival enlargement ranges from 6.3% to 43.6%.[18,53,66] Selected calcium channel blockers reported to cause gingival enlargement are listed in Table 13-6.

Table 13-6	Selected Calcium Channel Blockers Reported to Cause Gingival Enlargement
GENERIC NAME	**BRAND NAME**
Amlodipine	Norvasc
Diltiazem	Cardizem, Dilacor
Felodipine	Plendil
Isradipine	DynaCirc
Nifedipine	Procardia, Adalat
Nitrendipine	Baypress (not approved in the United States)
Verapamil	Calan, Isoptin, Verelan

Cyclosporine is an immunosuppressant medication used in the treatment of autoimmune disorders and to prevent rejection of solid organ transplants and bone marrow transplants. Cyclosporine has increased the 5-year survival rate from 50% to 96%, but this medication is not without side effects. Some of the side effects are nephrotoxicity, hepatotoxicity, lymphoma, hypertension, and gingival enlargement. The gingival enlargement occurs in approximately 25% of the patients taking cyclosporine.[33]

MANAGEMENT AND TREATMENT

Poor oral hygiene is a risk factor directly correlated with the severity of the gingival enlargement. At every dental appointment, the dental hygienist must debride the dentition and reinforce oral hygiene procedures. Ultrasonic debridement with an antimicrobial rinse could be beneficial in reducing bacterial counts. The use of an antimicrobial aftercare mouthrinse such as 0.2% chlorhexidine gluconate (Peridex, PerioGard) or an OTC essential-oil mouthrinse (e.g., Listerine) may be of benefit by reducing the plaque biofilm–forming bacteria and the resultant inflammation. Surgical excision of the enlarged gingiva may be necessary for the most severe cases; however, the enlargement may recur.

The clinical effects of the calcium channel blocker on the gingiva are usually reversible. In consultation with the patient's physician, substitution of the offending drug for a similar drug

may reduce or even prevent the gingival enlargement.[85] Discontinuing the offending drug often results in marked improvement within 1 week and a complete resolution within 8 weeks. Patients taking cyclosporine do not have an acceptable alternative immunosuppressive agent. A reduction in the dose of cyclosporine may prove somewhat beneficial in reducing the gingival enlargement in some patients.[11] In some cases, substituting tacrolimus for cyclosporine may be considered because drug-induced gingival hyperplasia is uncommon with this medication. However, tacrolimus and cyclosporine each have specific indications for use.[8]

Patient Educational Opportunity

The patient should be shown where drug-induced gingival overgrowth is located in his or her mouth. The dental hygienist should explain that although oral hygiene cannot prevent the lesion from occurring, excellent plaque biofilm control can limit the extent and severity of the lesion. The hygienist should also help the patient select the appropriate oral hygiene aids to clean the enlarged tissue.

Antimicrobial Rinse

Drug and dosing information for antimicrobial rinse[88] is as follows:

Rx: Chlorhexidine gluconate 0.12%
Disp: One bottle
Sig: Rinse with 20 ml for 30 seconds two times per day; do not swallow.

Dysgeusia

SIGNS AND SYMPTOMS

Dysgeusia is a distortion in one's ability to taste. Taste is the perception of saltiness, bitterness, sourness, and sweetness by the tongue. Taste is influenced by the texture of the food and the sense of smell. More than 2 million people in the United States have complaints of taste and smell abnormalities. Taste complaints are more frequently noted in elderly women and significantly alter quality of life. The inability to taste decreases the ability to identify foods, and to recognize the flavors of foods, and, ultimately, it may result in both nutritional and psychologic disorders.[9]

ANATOMY

The taste buds are located in the tongue, and taste receptors are located in the soft palate, epiglottis, pharynx, and larynx. Each taste bud is composed of 50 to 150 modified neuroepithelial cells that are renewed every 10 to 14 days.[32] The mushroom-shaped fungiform papillae (200 to 400) appear red and are located on the dorsum of the tongue. Each fungiform papilla contains two to five taste buds. The circumvallate papilla (8 to 12) are located on the dorsum of the tongue in a V-shaped line that separates the anterior two thirds from the posterior one third of the tongue; each papilla contains 250 taste buds. The foliate papillae contain 1300 taste buds and appear as vertical folds on the posterior lateral aspect of the tongue. The soft palate contains 400 taste buds.[10] The chorda tympani branch of the facial nerve (cranial nerve VII) innervates the fungiform papillae; the glossopharyngeal nerve (cranial nerve IX) innervates the posterior foliate and circumvallate papillae. The superior laryngeal branch of the vagus nerve (cranial nerve X) innervates the epiglottis and esophagus.

An evaluation of the patient who complains of altered taste perception must include a comprehensive medical history that details a complete listing of medications (prescription and OTC). The dental hygienist must question the patient regarding current and past medical conditions, such as diabetes mellitus, thyroid gland dysfunction, and radiation therapy. Sinusitis and recent viral upper respiratory infections should be ruled out as possible causes of the altered taste. Central nervous system neoplasms, migraine headaches, Bell's palsy, or herpes zoster may also be factors associated with dysgeusia. Local causes of dysgeusia include periodontal or dental abscesses, candidiasis, gingivitis, and periodontitis.[54] The onset and duration of the taste disorders should be determined in an attempt to correlate the onset with medications, changes in medications, and medical conditions.

ASSOCIATED SYSTEMIC DRUGS

More than 250 medications have been reported to cause alterations in taste and smell.[29] These drugs may be excreted in the saliva and the gingival crevicular fluid and may modify the taste. Saliva is important in dissolving and transporting tastants to receptors in the taste buds and taste receptors. Drugs that decrease the salivary flow concentrate the electrolytes in saliva, resulting in a salty or metallic taste. In addition, drugs that decrease the turnover rate of the taste receptors may result in an altered taste perception[1,62,63] (Box 13-6).

Oral Pigmentation

ETIOLOGY

TCN antimicrobial agents may cause abnormal pigmentation of the teeth. TCN is a broad-spectrum, bacteriostatic antibiotic often prescribed for acne vulgaris and ear infections. The systemic ingestion of TCN causes irreversible yellow-brown intrinsic staining in the developing teeth and bones. This type of staining is seen in the gingival third of the affected teeth and results from the deposition of a TCN-calcium orthophosphate complex during tooth development. This staining is directly proportional to the age at drug exposure, the dose, and the duration of the drug therapy[55,58] (Figures 13-9 and 13-10).

Minocycline is a semisynthetic TCN with additional antiinflammatory properties. Minocycline is used to treat acne vulgaris and rheumatoid arthritis. Minocycline also is associated with pigmentation of the teeth, bone, sclera, nails, and soft tissues.[36,48] Unlike TCN, which affects the developing teeth and bones, minocycline staining may occur after the teeth are fully developed and erupted. Minocycline is a fat-soluble drug with great penetration into the soft tissues and calcified tissues. It concentrates in the saliva at 30% to 65% of the serum concentration. The pigmentation of the developed dentition may be produced by the incorporation of minocycline complexes from

BOX 13-6
DRUGS THAT ALTER TASTE

Alcohol detoxification agents
Alzheimer's medications
Analgesics (nonsteroidal antiinflammatory drugs [NSAIDs])
Anesthetics (general and local)
Anorexiants
Antacids
Antianxiety agents
Antiarthritics
Anticholinergics
Anticonvulsants
Antidepressants
Antidiabetics (oral hypoglycemics)
Antidiarrheals
Antiemetics
Antifungals
Antigout medications
Antihistamine (H₁) antagonists
Antihistamine (H₂) antagonists
Antihyperlipidemics
Antiinfectives
Antiinflammatory/antiarthritics
Antimigraine agents
Antiparkinsonian agents
Antipsychotics
Antithyroid medications
Antivirals
Anxiolytics/sedatives
Asthma preventives
Bronchodilators
Calcium-affecting drugs
Cancer chemotherapeutics
Cardiovascular medications
Central nervous system (CNS) stimulants
Decongestants
Diuretics
Gall stone solubilization agents
Glucocorticoids
Hemorrheologics
Immunomodulators
Immunosuppressants
Irritable bowel syndrome (IBS) medications
Methylxanthines
Nicotine replacement drugs
Ophthalmics
Proton pump inhibitors
Retinoids, systemic
Salivary stimulants
Skeletal muscle relaxants
Vitamins

From Gage TW, Pickett FA: *Mosby's dental drug reference,* ed 7, St Louis, 2005, Elsevier.

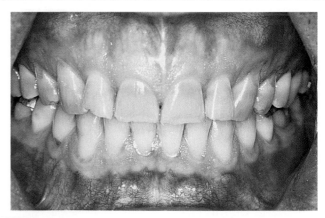

FIGURE 13-9
Oral pigmentation. Tetracycline (TCN) staining of the dentition. This patient was treated with a TCN medication during infancy.

the pulp into the dentin and from demineralization of the enamel and the subsequent oxidation of the drug from the saliva and gingival crevicular fluid. The pigmentation is green-gray or blue-gray and is seen in the middle and incisal third of the crown. The gingival one third is spared. Minocycline pigmentation is irreversible.[85] The incidence of minocycline-induced pigmentation in the facial bones is reported to be 10%

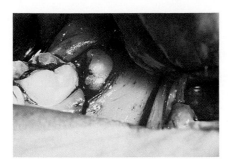

FIGURE 13-10
Oral pigmentation. Tetracycline (TCN) staining of the bone. Because the bone is a dynamic tissue and is constantly remodeling, the uptake of TCN in the bone may occur at any age when a person is exposed to the drug.

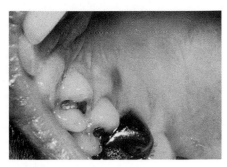

FIGURE 13-11
Oral pigmentation. This is a 34-year-old white woman with a medical history of lupus erythematosus. In addition to taking a corticosteroid, she is taking Plaquenil (hydroxychloroquine) to treat the arthritic component of her lupus.

in a study of patients who took oral minocycline for more than 1 year and increased to 20% if the drug was taken for 4 or more years.[15]

Other drugs that have been reported to cause oral pigmentation include the antimalarial agents (i.e., chloroquine, hydroxychloroquine, quinacrine [Atabrine]) and the antiretroviral drugs (e.g., zidovudine)[30] (Figure 13-11).

Hairy Tongue

SIGNS AND SYMPTOMS

Hairy tongue is a benign condition that results from elongation, hyperkeratinization, and retardation of the normal rate of desquamation of the filiform papillae. Hairy tongue is confined to the middorsal part of the tongue anterior to the circumvallate papillae. The increased length of the filiform papillae produces a matted appearance that may be black, brown, or yellow. The color may be related to chromogenic bacteria or exogenous pigments from food, beverages, or tobacco products.[61] Candidiasis may also be present (Figure 13-12).

Predisposing factors for the development of hairy tongue include poor oral hygiene, tobacco use, oxidizing mouthrinses (e.g., hydrogen peroxide), antibiotics, xerostomia, overgrowth of fungal or bacterial organisms, and radiation therapy.[24] This condition is found in approximately 0.5% of adults.[6]

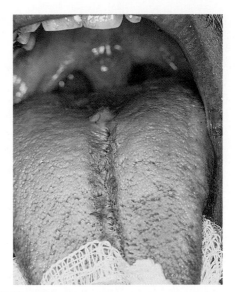

FIGURE 13-12
Hairy tongue in a white man in his late twenties. This patient gives a history of one to two packs of cigarettes per day for the past 8 years and heavy consumption of coffee during the day.

ASSOCIATED SYSTEMIC DRUGS

Drugs associated with hairy tongue include penicillins, broad-spectrum antibiotics, TCNs, phenothiazines, griseofulvin, and corticosteroids.[16]

TREATMENT

Treatment of hairy tongue involves eliminating predisposing factors such as tobacco, antibiotics, or mouthrinses and encouraging excellent oral hygiene. Cleansing the tongue with a toothbrush or tongue scraper will promote desquamation of the hyperkeratotic papillae. For individuals who have undergone radiotherapy, brushing the tongue and use of a 1% solution of podophyllum resin with thorough rinsing may be helpful. Educating the patient that this condition is benign and that the tongue will return to normal with proper oral hygiene is important. If candidiasis is present, then that condition must be treated with antifungal therapy.

Angioedema

SIGNS AND SYMPTOMS

Angioedema is a condition that features an acute onset of swelling in the skin, soft tissues, and subcutaneous and submucosal tissues of the head and neck. Angioedema may appear as a painless, nonpitting edema of the face, cheeks, eyelids, lips, tongue, floor of the mouth, soft palate, uvula, and pharynx. The edema is often mild with a quick onset but may progress to laryngeal edema and death. Angioedema may be idiopathic, secondary to foods, food additives, trauma, medications, or a deficiency of the C1 esterase enzyme[16] (Figure 13-13). Reactions to drugs and anesthetic agents may occur within or around the oral cavity. The reaction is usually rapid, occurring quickly after exposure to the antigen. The lesion is painless,

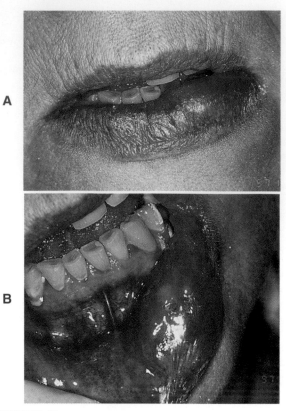

FIGURE 13-13
Angioneurotic edema. **A,** Swelling on the lower left lip of a white woman. This swelling occurred shortly after the completion of a dental restorative procedure on tooth #19 performed using the rubber dam. This patient was not sensitive to latex. **B,** Intraoral view of the same individual.

with soft tissue swelling, and it may itch or burn. The lesion persists from 1 to 3 days; then it should begin to resolve spontaneously.[43]

ASSOCIATED SYSTEMIC DRUGS

Drugs that have been implicated in angioedema are penicillins, aspirin, NSAIDs, propranolol, cimetidine, angiotensin-converting enzyme (ACE) inhibitors, and angiotensin II receptor antagonists.[16]

HISTOLOGIC FINDINGS

The hereditary form of angioedema is a rare autosomal-dominant trait that features the C1 esterase inhibitor deficiency.[16] The nonhereditary form features an immunoglobulin E (IgE)-mediated hypersensitivity reaction with mast cell degranulation and the release of histamine. This reaction may occur secondary to the administration of drugs. ACE inhibitors have been reported in the literature to cause angioedema. These drugs are prescribed to treat essential and renovascular hypertension and congestive heart failure. This class of drugs prevents the conversion of angiotensin I to angiotensin II, which is a potent vasoconstrictor. The ACE inhibitors also inhibit an enzyme that degrades bradykinin, a vasoactive substance that promotes vasodilation and fluid accumulation. The overall incidence of angioedema secondary to ACE inhibitors is 0.1% to 0.2%.[64] Most cases occur very shortly after the drug is administered (i.e., within 48 hours).[59]

TREATMENT

Treatment consists of identification of the primary causative factor. Oral antihistamines (diphenhydramine [Benadryl]) should be given for a period of 1 to 3 days.[43] Diphenhydramine hydrochloride 25-mg capsules are available OTC. The patient is instructed to take two tablets (50 mg) every 4 hours orally for 1 to 3 days, until the swelling resolves. Length of treatment is determined by the practitioner.[43] If antihistamines do not control the swelling, or if laryngeal involvement occurs, then epinephrine should be administered intramuscularly. If this treatment is unsuccessful, then intravenous corticosteroids and antihistamines should be administered. When angioedema is associated with ACE inhibitors, all types of ACE inhibitors should be avoided in the future.[54]

References

1. Ackerman BH, Kasbekar N: Disturbances of taste and smell induced by drugs, *Pharmacotherapy* 17(3):482-496, 1997.
2. Addy V et al: Risk factors in phenytoin-induced gingival hyperplasia, *J Periodontol* 54(6):373-377, 1983.
3. Anderson H, Rapley J, Williams D: Gingival overgrowth with valproic acid: a case report, *J Dent Child* 64:294-297, 1997.
4. Atkinson JC et al: Effects of furosemide on the oral cavity, *Gerodontology* 8:23-26, 1989.
5. Barclay S et al: The incidence and severity of nifedipine-induced gingival overgrowth, *J Clin Periodontol* 19:311-314, 1992.
6. Bouquot JE, Gundlach K: Odd tongues: prevalence of common tongue lesions in 23,616 white Americans over 35 years of age, *Quintessence Int* 17(1):719-730, 1986.
7. Bradfeldt GW: Phenytoin hyperplasia found in edentulous patients, *J Am Dent Assoc* 123:61-64, 1992.
8. Ciancio SG, Mealey BL, Rose LF: Medications impacting the periodontium. In Rose LF et al: *Periodontics: medicine, surgery, and implants,* St Louis, 2004, Elsevier.
9. Cowart BJ et al: Clinical disorders of smell and taste, *Occup Med* 12(3):465-481, 1997.
10. Cullen MM, Leopold DA: Disorders of taste and smell, *Med Clin North Am* 83(1):57-74, 1999.
11. Daly C: Resolution of cyclosporine A-induced gingival enlargement following reduction in CsA dosage, *J Clin Periodontol* 19:143-145, 1992.
12. Dawes C: Physiologic factors affecting salivary flow rate, oral sugar clearance, and the sensation of dry mouth in man, *J Dent Res* 66(spec issue):648-653, 1987.
13. Dill RE et al: Phenytoin increases gene expression for platelet-derived growth factor B chain in macrophages and monocytes, *J Periodontol* 64:169-173, 1993.
14. Duffey D, Eversole LR, Abemayor E: Oral lichen planus and its association with squamous cell carcinoma: an update on pathogenesis and treatment implications, *Laryngoscope* 106:357-362, 1996.
15. Eisen DE: Minocycline-induced oral pigmentation, *Lancet* 349:400, 1997.
16. Eisen DE, Lynch DP: *The mouth: diagnosis and treatment,* St Louis, 1997, Mosby.

17. Eisenberg E: Clinicopathologic patterns of oral lichen planus, *Oral Maxillofac Surg Clin North Am* 6(3):445-463, 1994.

18. Ellis JS et al: Prevalence of gingival overgrowth induced by calcium channel blockers: a community-based study, *J Periodontol* 70(1):63-67, 1999.

19. Epstein JB, Polsky B: Oropharyngeal candidiasis: a review of its clinical spectrum and current therapies, *Clin Ther* 20(1):40-57, 1998.

20. Epstein JB, Scully C: The role of saliva in oral health and the causes and effects of xerostomia, *J Can Dent Assoc* 58:217-221, 1992.

21. Ettinger RL: Review: xerostomia—a symptom which acts like a disease, *Age Ageing* 25:409-412, 1996.

22. Eversole LR: Allergic stomatitis, *J Oral Med* 34:93-102, 1979.

23. Fattore L et al: Gingival hyperplasia: a side effect of nifedipine and diltiazem, *Spec Care Dent* 11:107-109, 1991.

24. Flaitz CM: Diseases of the mouth. In Rakel R, ed: *Conn's current therapy 2002*, ed 54, Philadelphia, 2002, WB Saunders.

25. Fotos PG, Lilly JP: Clinical management of oral and perioral candidiasis, *Dermatol Clin* 14(2):273-280, 1996.

26. Fox PC: Differentiation of dry mouth etiology, *Adv Dent Res* 10:13-16, 1996.

27. Fox PC: Salivary enhancement therapies, *Caries Res* 38:241-246, 2004.

28. Fox PC et al: Saliva inhibits HIV-1 infectivity, *J Am Dent Assoc* 116:635-637, 1988.

29. Gage TW, Pickett FA: *Mosby's dental drug reference*, ed 7, St Louis, 2005, Elsevier.

30. Giansanti JS et al: Oral mucosal pigmentation resulting from antimalarial therapy, *Oral Surg* 31(1):66-69, 1971.

31. Glass BJ: Drug-induced xerostomia as a cause of glossodynia, *Ear Nose Throat J* 68:776-781, 1989.

32. Guyton AC, Hall JE: *Textbook of medical physiology*, ed 10, Philadelphia, 2000, WB Saunders.

33. Hassell TM, Hefti AF: Drug-induced gingival overgrowth: old problem, new problem, *Crit Rev Oral Biol Med* 2(1):103-137, 1991.

34. Heineman HS, Greenberg MS: Cell protective effect of human saliva specific for herpes simplex virus, *Arch Oral Biol* 25:257-261, 1980.

35. Huff JC, Weston WL, Tonnesen MG: Erythema multiforme: a review of characteristics, diagnostic criteria, and causes, *J Am Acad Dermatol* 8(6):763-775, 1883.

36. Hung P, Caldwell JB, James WD: Minocycline-induced hyperpigmentation, *J Fam Pract* 40:183-185, 1995.

37. Iacopino AM et al: Phenytoin and cyclosporine A specifically regulate macrophage phenotype expression of platelet-derived growth factor and interleukin-1 in vitro and in vivo: possible molecular mechanism of drug-induced gingival hyperplasia, *J Periodontol* 68:73-83, 1997.

38. Jensen SB et al: Xerostomia and hypofunction of the salivary glands in cancer therapy, *Support Care Cancer* 11:207-225, 2003.

39. Jorgensen MG: Prevalence of amlodipine-related gingival hyperplasia, *J Periodontol* 68:676-678, 1997.

40. Karmiol M, Walsh RF: Dental caries after radiotherapy of the oral regions, *J Am Dent Assoc* 91:838-845, 1975.

41. Katz J et al: Vigabatrin-induced gingival overgrowth, *J Clin Periodontol* 24:180-182, 1997.

42. Kumar V, Abbas AK, Fausto N: *Robbins and Cotran pathologic basis of disease*, ed 7, Philadelphia, 2005, Elsevier.

43. Little JW et al: Allergy. In *Dental management of the medically compromised patient*, St Louis, 2002, Mosby.

44. Lombardi T et al: Felodipine-induced gingival hyperplasia: a clinical and histologic study, *J Oral Pathol Med* 20:89-92, 1991.

45. Mandel ID: The role of saliva in maintaining oral homeostasis, *J Am Dent Assoc* 119:298-304, 1989.

46. Miller CS et al: Documenting medication use in adult dental patients: 1987-1991, *J Am Dent Assoc* 123:41-8, 1992.

47. Miller CS, Damm DD: Incidence of verapamil-induced gingival hyperplasia in a dental population, *J Periodontol* 63:453-456, 1992.

48. Morrow GL, Abbott RL: Minocycline-induced scleral, dental, and dermal pigmentation, *Am J Ophthalmol* 125(3):396-397, 1998.

49. Muzyka BC, Glick M: A review of oral fungal infections and appropriate therapy, *J Am Dent Assoc* 126:63-72, 1995.

50. Muzyka BC, Somerman M: Antifungal and antiviral agents. In Ciancio SC, ed: *ADA guide to dental therapeutics*, ed 2, Chicago, 2000, ADA Publishing.

51. Nähri TO, Meurman JH, Ainamo A: Xerostomia and hyposalivation: causes, consequences and treatment in the elderly, *Drugs Aging* 15:103-116, 1999.

52. Nakade O, Baylink DJ, Lau K-HW: Phenytoin at micromolar concentration is an osteogenic agent for human-mandibular-derived bone cells in vitro, *J Dent Res* 74(1):331-337, 1995.

53. Nery EB et al: Prevalence of nifedipine-induced gingival hyperplasia, *J Periodontol* 66:572-578, 1995.

54. Neville BW et al: *Oral & maxillofacial pathology*, ed 2, Philadelphia, 2002, WB Saunders.

55. Parks ET: Lesions associated with drug reactions, *Dermatol Clin* 14(2):327-337,1996.

56. Pollock JJ et al: Fungistatic and fungicidal activity of the human parotid salivary histidine-rich polypeptides on *Candida albicans, Infect Immun* 44:702-707, 1984.

57. Porter SR, Scully C, Hegarty AM: An update of the etiology and management of xerostomia, *Oral Surg Oral Med Oral Pathol Oral Radiol Endod* 97:28-46, 2004.

58. Regezi JA, Sciubba JJ, Jordan RCK: *Oral pathology: clinical pathologic correlations,* ed 4, St Louis, 2003, WB Saunders.

59. Roberts JR, Wuerz RC: Clinical characteristics of angiotensin-converting enzyme inhibitor-induced angioedema, *Ann Emerg Med* 20(5):555-558, 1991.

60. Sapp JP, Eversole LR, Wysocki GP: *Contemporary oral and maxillofacial pathology*, ed 2, St Louis, 2004, Mosby.

61. Sartii GM et al: Black hairy tongue, *Am Fam Physician* 41(6): 1751-1755,1990.

62. Schiffman SS: Taste and smell disease, *N Engl J Med* 308: 1275-1279, 1337-1343, 1983.

63. Scott AE: Clinical characteristics of taste and smell disorders, *Ear Nose Throat J* 68:297-315, 1989.

64. Sharma PK, Yium JJ: Angioedema associated with angiotensin II receptor antagonist losartan, *South Med J* 90(5):552-553, 1997.

65. Shiohara T, Modya N, Nagashima M: The lichenoid tissue reaction, *Int J Dermatol* 27(6):365-373, 1988.

66. Silverstein LH et al: Medication-induced gingival enlargement: a clinical review, *Gen Dent* 45:371-376, 1997.

67. Spolarich AE: Understanding pharmacology: the pharmacologic history, *Access* 9:33-35, 1995.

68. Spolarich AE: Understanding pharmacology: medication management, *Access* 10:28-30, 1996.

69. Spolarich AE: Managing the side effects of medications, *J Dent Hyg* 74:57-69, 2000.

70. Spolarich AE: Getting to the bottom of dry mouth, *Dimens Dent Hyg* 4:22-24, 2005.

71. Spolarich AE: Medication use and xerostomia, *Dimens Dent Hyg* 7:22-24, 2005.

72. Spolarich AE, Gurenlian JR: Deductive reasoning with pharmacology: a prescription for quality patient care, *Comp Cont Ed Oral Hyg* 1:3-9, 1994.

73. Sreebny LM: Dry mouth and salivary gland hypofunction. I. Diagnosis, *Compendium Cont Educ Dent* 9:569-578, 1988.

74. Sreebny LM, Schwartz SS: A reference guide to drugs and dry mouth, ed 2, *Gerodontology* 14:33-47, 1997.

75. Steele RM, Schuna AA, Schreiber RT: Calcium antagonist-induced gingival hyperplasia, *Ann Intern Med* 120:663-664, 1994.

76. Stevens AM, Johnson FC: A new eruptive fever associated with stomatitis and ophthalmia, *Am J Dis Child* 24:526-533, 1922.

77. Stinnett E, Rodu B, Grizzle WE: New developments in understanding phenytoin-induced gingival hyperplasia, *J Am Dent Assoc* 114(6):814-816, 1987.

78. Syrjanen S, Syrjanen K: Hyperplastic gingivitis in a child receiving sodium valproate treatment, *Proc Finn Dent Soc* 75:95-98, 1979.

79. Tam IM, Wandres DL: Calcium channel blockers and gingival hyperplasia, *Ann Pharmacother* 2:213-214, 1992.

80. Taybos GM: Xerostomia—common complaint and challenging dental management problem, *J Mich Dent Assoc* 54(3):24-25, 1998.

81. Terézhalmy GT, Batizy LG: *Urgent care in the dental office,* Carol Stream, Ill, 1998, Quintessence Int.

82. USP DI volume I: drug information for the health care professional, ed 24, Englewood, Colo, 2004, Micromedex Inc.

83. von Hebra F (Fagge CH, translator): *On diseases of the skin including the exanthemata,* London, 1866, New Sydenhour Society.

84. Westbrook P et al: Regression of nifedipine-induced gingival hyperplasia following switch to a same class calcium channel blocker, isradipine, *J Periodontol* 68:645-650, 1997.

85. Wolfe ID, Reichmister J: Minocycline hyperpigmentation: skin, tooth, nail, and bone involvement, *Cutis* 33:457-458, 1984.

86. Wright WE: Management of oral sequelae, *J Dent Res* 66(spec issue):699-702, 1987.

87. Wynn RL: General principles of drug action. In Holroyd SV, Wynn RL, Requa-Clark B, eds: *Clinical pharmacology in dental practice,* ed 4, St Louis, 1988, Mosby.

88. Wynn RL, Meiller TF, Crossley HL: *Drug information handbook for dentistry,* ed 10, Hudson, Ohio, 2005, Lexi-Comp Inc.

Physical and Extraoral Examination

Karen K. Tiwana • Ralph Howard Leonard, Jr. •
Samuel Paul Nesbit

INSIGHT

The dental hygienist is in an excellent position to assist in the diagnosis of pathologic systemic conditions. Recognition of normal anatomy and physiologic function, normal variations, and the early signs and symptoms of disease is important. These observations lead to a diagnosis and proper treatment.

✦ CASE STUDY 14-1   Examination Process

Fadi Jabir has returned for his supportive care appointment. He has not been to the dental office in 18 months. While the dental hygienist reviews his health history, Mr. Jabir reports having been diagnosed with prostate cancer shortly after his last visit and that he has had surgery and chemotherapy. He states that his physician gave him a clean bill of health at his last medical visit 4 months ago. While performing the extraoral examination, the hygienist notes enlarged lymph nodes in the subclavicular area.

KEY TERMS

aspiration	external auditory meatus	parotid glands	submandibular glands
auscultation	lymph nodes	percussion	temporomandibular joint
bruits	muscles	salivary glands	thyroid gland
crepitus	palpation	sublingual glands	visual inspection

LEARNING OUTCOMES

After reading this chapter the student will be able to:

1. Perform a thorough extraoral examination, identifying structures and abnormalities during the examination.
2. Take patients' vital signs according to techniques presented in the chapter.
3. Evaluate readings obtained when taking vital signs and identify whether precautions or consultations are needed before the performance of dental hygiene care.

This chapter provides information to the dental hygiene student to enable proficient performance of the head and neck (head, eyes, ears, nose, and throat [HEENT]) examination and an in-depth assessment of the dental patient's vital signs. This information is limited to the extraoral portion of the HEENT examination. The intraoral examination is discussed in Chapter 15.

The techniques used to perform the HEENT examination include inspection, palpation, olfaction, auscultation, percussion, diascopy, and aspiration. The structures to be examined include the facial and neck skeleton, **muscles,** glands, blood vessels, and skin. The vital signs to be reviewed include blood pressure, pulse rate, temperature, and respiration.

The thorough HEENT examination and assessment of the vital signs reveals any deviations from normal. The most important concept to grasp is that the dental hygienist must be comprehensive in evaluating *all* the essential information and findings and must recognize *any* variations from normal. Follow-up monitoring, additional diagnostic evaluations, consultations, or referrals must then be planned accordingly. Regular performance of these techniques makes the comprehensive examination an efficient process. This process leads to an accurate determination of any pathologic or infectious process in the head and neck region. A thorough evaluation of the patient's vital signs may reflect disease beyond the head and neck region.

This chapter also presents a review of the vital signs and the anatomical structures in the head and neck, as well as the techniques by which to examine them.

Physical Evaluation

The recognition of variations from a normal health status is crucial for two major reasons. First, this observation may identify medical or dental conditions that are undiagnosed. Second, the observation may determine the status of the identified conditions that may place patients at risk for serious complications from the dental treatment.

The thorough, comprehensive examination facilitates recognition of medical problems; the need to modify or defer treatment; or the need to refer the patient to the appropriate healthcare provider. The clinician should not discount the importance of the comprehensive examination for every patient, lest something significant, serious, or even disastrous go unrecognized.

The dental health of the patient is the primary focus of the dental hygienist's attention. However, before the examination of the oral cavity, the clinician must see the dental patient as a whole human being. Medical diseases may present a serious threat to the patient's life. Attention to serious medical conditions supersedes any routine dental treatment. Recognizing the patient with a serious medical condition (e.g., hypertension, diabetes mellitus) and making the proper referral may save a life. Modifying dental treatment to prevent a medical emergency (e.g., stroke, heart attack) or serious medical condition (e.g., infectious endocarditis [IE], bleeding) is the responsibility of everyone in the healthcare field.

Principles and Techniques of Physical Evaluation

Illness is the interaction of a particular disease process with an individual patient. Subjective sensations resulting from the disease that are reported by the patient are called *symptoms. Signs* of illness are objective findings that the clinician observes (see Chapter 12). The comprehensive examination must be performed in a systematic, standardized manner to avoid missing any signs or symptoms of an infection or medical problem.

> *Prevention*
>
> Detection of illness depends on the determination and accurate interpretation of the symptoms and signs; therefore it relies principally on the knowledge, training, and skill of the clinician.
>
> To paraphrase Sir William Osler, what the mind does not know, the eyes cannot see. The examination process begins the moment the dental hygienist meets the patient and continues throughout the appointment.

GENERAL PHYSICAL OBSERVATIONS

General physical observations begin the minute the dental hygienist encounters the patient. By carefully observing the patient in the reception room and in the treatment room, as well as at all times during the appointment, the dental hygienist may detect variations from normal or a disease process in the patient. General physical observations are shown in Box 14-1.

Body type, stature, and symmetry are related to hereditary characteristics. These characteristics also may reflect endocrine or metabolic problems. Variations from normal gait, mobility, and posture may reflect a musculoskeletal or inflammatory connective tissue disorder or a central nervous system (CNS) disturbance. The patient's mental activity and communicability may be related to CNS problems, psychologic problems, or general physical debilitation. The patient's nutritional status should also be appraised. Obese and underweight patients usually have a host of medical problems, some of which may be undiagnosed. Evaluation of each patient should include an appraisal of symmetry in the head and neck region. Color of the skin may reveal liver disease (jaundice), cardiovascular disease

---

BOX 14-1

GENERAL PHYSICAL OBSERVATIONS

Stature	Hair
Body type	Extremities
Symmetry	Sexual characteristics
Gait	Responses
Mobility	Function
Posture	Cleanliness, personal hygiene,
Color	dress
Skin	Odor

From Halstead C et al: *Physical evaluation of the dental patient,* St Louis, 1982, Mosby.

(cyanosis), bleeding disorders (petechiae, red; anemia, pallor), or infections. Characteristics of the distribution of body hair, such as alopecia (i.e., sparse or loss of hair) or hirsutism (i.e., excessive body hair), or hyperpigmentation of the skin and excessive secondary sexual characteristics (e.g., gynecomastia) may indicate endocrine (hormonal—hyperthyroidism, pituitary, or adrenal), CNS, or drug problems.

Examination of the extremities may reveal changes in the color of the skin, presence of bleeding or bruising, arthritic changes in the wrist and fingers, clubbing of the fingertips, or cyanosis of the nail beds. All of these findings may indicate a serious medical problem. The hygienist should look for masses, pigmentation, hair texture and distribution, scars, and lesions. *Lesion* is defined as an abnormal structural change. With respect to a differential diagnosis, the hygienist should look for location, size, shape, morphology, and color.

PRINCIPLES OF CLINICAL EXAMINATION FOR THE HEAD AND NECK

The basic techniques of diagnosis are visual inspection, palpation, olfaction, auscultation, percussion, diascopy, and aspiration. These techniques are used every time an examination is performed.

Visual Inspection

Visual inspection is a systematic, standardized observation of a set of criteria performed in an orderly manner to ensure completeness and accuracy of the examination. The clinician performs a visual inspection of the head (skull), the skin, mucosa, eyes, ears, and other anatomical structures in the head and neck.[3,4] It begins when first meeting the patient and becomes more detailed as the dental appointment proceeds. Visual inspection includes evaluation of bilateral symmetry—the comparison of the anatomy on one side of the head, face, and neck to the opposite side. Most normal anatomical structures are bilaterally symmetrical. If a structure of the head, face, or neck appears different on one side than the other, then this may indicate some pathologic process. When performing a visual inspection, anatomical structures must not be obstructed with items such as clothing, cosmetics, or eyeglasses. Additionally, excellent lighting is needed to properly perform a visual inspection.

Palpation

14-1 to 14-3

Palpation is used to determine the size, texture, consistency, symmetry, firmness, fluctuance, temperature, and other qualities evaluated by the sense of touch. Often a structure cannot be adequately evaluated simply by inspection. The structure must be palpated to determine its true nature. Palpation may be accomplished by using both hands, comparing one side of the head, face, and neck with the other in terms of texture, size, and consistency. This is called *bimanual palpation*. This palpation technique is particularly helpful when examining the floor of the mouth and the **temporomandibular joint** (TMJ).

In certain cases, unilateral palpation may be used to assess anatomical structures. With unilateral palpation, one anatomical structure is pressed against another to assess the contents of that

area. In some areas, bidigital palpation (two fingers) may be necessary, as in the floor of the mouth. Bidigital compressions are used when examining lymph nodes of the lips and buccal mucosal tissue. Findings discerned through palpation include but are not limited to induration, texture (rough or smooth), consistency of tissue, and presence of muscles and their size. Additionally, involvement of skin, organs, elevated temperature, and enlarged nodes must be evaluated. Lymph nodes may be easily detected with a circular motion performed during compression.

Students should note the method of palpation used for examination of each structure.

Olfaction

Some odors can be associated with certain conditions such as poor hygiene, smoking, alcohol use, periodontal disease, necrotizing ulcerative gingivitis (NUG), rhinitis, sinusitis, tonsillitis, bronchitis, metabolic disorders, lung abscesses, and gastrointestinal disorders.

Auscultation

Auscultation is listening to sounds. This may indicate to the dental hygienist whether the structure being evaluated is normal. Auscultation may be performed by listening with the unaided ear or with the assistance of a stethoscope. For example, the clinician may use auscultation to listen to the TMJ for **crepitus** or popping, to measure the blood pressure, and to assess for the presence of **bruits** in the carotid artery.[3,4]

Percussion

Percussion is performed by tapping on a structure, usually with the fingers, hand, or an instrument. This evaluation may help the dental hygienist determine whether a structure is sensitive and the relative density of the structure (solid, hollow, or fluid filled). Percussion may elicit pain or discomfort, especially in areas of inflammation associated with sinusitis, pulpitis, or periodontal disease. Examples for which percussion is used include the examination of muscles, bones, and teeth.[3,4]

Diascopy

Diascopy is the examination technique in which the dental hygienist compresses tissue with a glass slide. This examination technique is used to determine whether a reddish or bluish lesion is vascular. The glass slide is pressed evenly over the lesion. If the lesion is vascular, then it blanches on diascopy and returns to its original color when the pressure is released. If the lesion does not blanch, then the color may be the result of some other cause such as amalgam tattoo, nevi, or pigmentation.

Aspiration

Aspiration is the removal of fluid from a body cavity. The area aspirated may be a soft tissue lesion or a lesion central in bone. A purulent aspirate indicates an inflammatory or infectious process; yellow, straw-colored fluid is consistent with a cyst; a predominance of blood indicates a vascular lesion, such as hemangioma; little or no aspirate may indicate a traumatic bone cyst or air embolism.

HEAD AND NECK EXAMINATION

The head and neck examination begins when meeting the patient in the reception room and continues while reviewing his or her medical history and performing the clinical examination. The general physical characteristics of habitus, such as body symmetry, posture, stature, skin color, and texture, and anatomical landmarks of the head and neck are evaluated by inspection. In addition to visual inspection, palpation is used to evaluate anatomical structures such as lymph nodes, muscles, and glands. When conducting a head and neck examination, the hygienist should do the following:

- Begin at the base of the skull, evaluating the occipital and nuchal lymph nodes and trapezius muscle (Figure 14-1).
- Continue down the sternocleidomastoid muscle, evaluating the cervical and jugular lymph nodes and palpating the carotid artery (Figure 14-2).
- Move laterally along the clavicles, palpating the supraclavicular lymph nodes (Figure 14-3).
- Return to the sternum and palpate upward in the midline of the neck, evaluating the thyroid, cricoid cartilage, and submental lymph nodes (Figures 14-4 and 14-5).

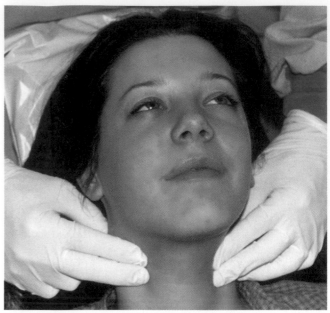

FIGURE 14-2
Inspection and bimanual, bidigital palpation. *Anatomical landmarks:* Sternum, clavicles. *Structures:* Supraclavicular lymph nodes. *Instructions:* The clinician proceeds laterally along the clavicles, pressing down into the supraclavicular triangle and the top of the clavicles, using bidigital circular compression until the trapezius muscle is reached.

- With bimanual, bidigital palpation, evaluate the gland, muscles, and lymph nodes associated with the mandible and floor of the mouth (Figure 14-6).
- Finally, palpate the parotid glands, auricular lymph nodes, masseter and temporalis muscles, and TMJ (Figure 14-7).

As depicted in the figures, once completed, all lymph nodes, muscles, glands, blood vessels, skeletal components, and the TMJ will be evaluated in a logical sequence.

Prevention

Although the approach taken to examine and evaluate patients varies among clinicians, it must be consistent from patient to patient so as not to overlook any area or aspect of concern.

Patient Educational Opportunity

The hygienist should review and describe the extraoral examination technique with the patient, pointing out by name the structure being evaluated, how the area is evaluated, how it should feel when normal, and the presence of any abnormalities. Encourage patient self-examination.

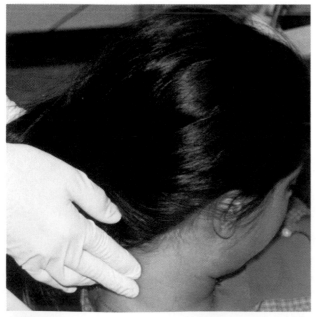

FIGURE 14-1
Bimanual palpation. *Anatomical landmarks:* Cervical vertebrae, base of skull. *Structures:* Lymph nodes (nuchal, occipital), trapezius muscle, skin. *Instructions:* The clinician proceeds bilaterally up the cervical spine, palpating for lymph nodes.

The dental clinician must be able to differentiate between normal and abnormal anatomy, as well as recognize normal variations. Common abnormal findings in the examination of the head and neck are listed in Box 14-2.

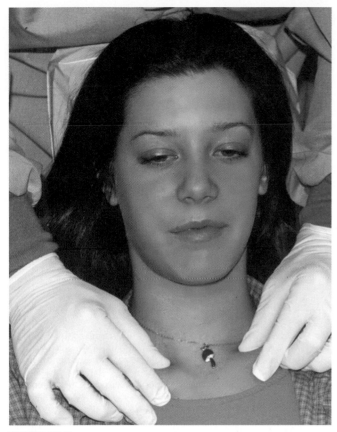

FIGURE 14-3
Bimanual, bidigital, circular compression for nodes. *Anatomical landmarks:* Sternocleidomastoid muscle, trachea. *Structures:* Lymph nodes (jugulodigastric, anterior cervical, accessory, posterior [cervical], carotid artery, jugular vein, skin. *Instructions:* The clinician palpates the anterior aspect of the sternocleidomastoid muscle. The cervical and jugular lymph nodes and the vessels may be detected by palpating the tissue medial to the sternocleidomastoid muscle. The carotid artery (pulse) is palpated here. The clinician palpates the posterior aspect of the sterno-cleidomastoid muscle (accessory and posterior cervical lymph nodes) down to the insertion of the trapezius muscle and then moves posterior to the cervical spine.

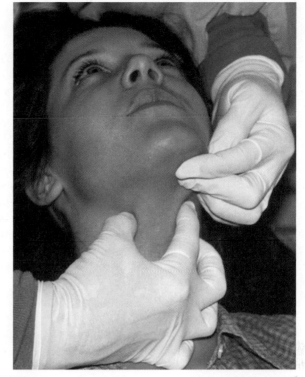

FIGURE 14-4
Palpation. *Anatomical landmarks:* Tracheal rings, cricoid cartilage, thyroid cartilage, hyoid bone, mental protuberance. *Structures:* Thyroid gland, submental lymph nodes. *Instructions:* The clinician returns to the sternum and palpates upward in the midline of the neck. The thyroid gland is palpated with the use of bidigital compression. The clinician proceeds upward and palpates the cricoid cartilage and submental lymph nodes.

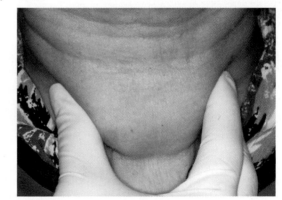

FIGURE 14-5
Enlarged thyroid gland tissue (i.e., goiter).

- Skeletal (bones and cartilage)
- Muscles
- Lymph nodes
- Glands
- TMJ
- Blood vessels

BOX 14-2

COMMON ABNORMAL FINDINGS: HEAD AND NECK

Lymphadenopathy	Dermoid cyst
Hypertrophy of the	Sebaceous cyst
salivary glands	Epidermal cyst
Thyroid hyperplasia or neoplasia	Sialadenitis, sialadenopathy
(including adenoma,	Lipoma
carcinoma, or goiter)	

Data from Bricker S, Langlais R, Miller C: *Oral diagnosis, oral medicine and treatment planning,* Philadelphia, 1994, Lea & Febiger; Coleman G, Nelson J: *Principles of oral diagnosis,* St Louis, 1992, Mosby.

COMPONENTS OF THE HEAD, EYES, EARS, NOSE, AND THROAT EVALUATION

The following are components of the HEENT evaluation, which should be evaluated during the clinical examination:

Head and Face

The skeletal structures of the head and face develop through a complex series of events. The growth process depends on many factors that must occur properly for normal anatomy

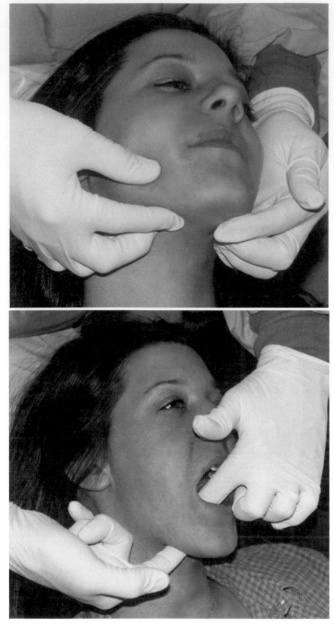

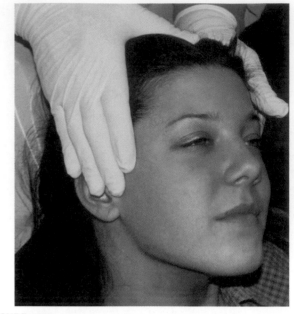

FIGURE 14-7
Bimanual palpation. *Anatomical landmarks:* Ear, temporomandibular joint (TMJ). *Structures:* Lymph nodes, parotid gland, TMJ, skin. *Instructions:* The clinician moves to the ears and palpates the posterior auricular lymph nodes and the anterior auricular nodes. The hands are moved upward, and the temporalis muscles are palpated while the patient goes through mandibular excursions. Move the hands down to the cheek palpating the masseter muscle and ask patient to clench the teeth. Check for symmetry.

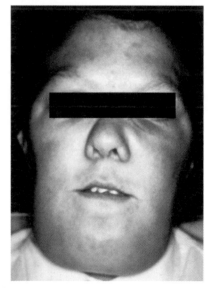

FIGURE 14-6
Bimanual, bidigital palpation. *Anatomical landmarks:* Mandible, floor of the mouth. *Structures:* Mylohyoid muscle, submandibular salivary gland, submandibular lymph nodes. *Instructions:* The clinician palpates under the chin and along the mandible. With one digit compressing the floor of the mouth and another digit placed medially to the inferior border of the mandible, the clinician palpates the submandibular gland and the submandibular lymph nodes.

FIGURE 14-8
Acromegaly resulting from a pituitary dysfunction.

and physiologic function. Variations in skull size and shape may be caused by developmental defects, endocrine or metabolic problems, nutritional disorders, or systemic disease. Enlargements of the skull or facial bones may indicate an acquired disease such as pituitary dysfunction (e.g., acromegaly; Figure 14-8) or an autoimmune connective tissue disease (e.g., Paget's disease). Malignant or benign conditions may affect the size, shape, and symmetry of the head and face; therefore any swellings in the facial structures must be evaluated.

Anatomical landmarks are important to every clinical examination. The landmarks in the head and face area are the malar or zygomatic areas, temporal portions of the skull, tragus of the ears, ala of the nose, philtrum of the lip, forehead, and orbits. An evaluation of the patient's skin is an important component of the examination. Any presence of erythema (i.e., redness), hyperkeratinization (i.e., thickened, white scaly skin), petechiae (i.e., ruptured capillaries), ecchymosis or purpura (i.e., bruises), angiomas, icterus (i.e., yellow, jaundice), or cyanosis (i.e., blue, hypoxia) should be noted and evaluated. The previous examples are indications of systemic conditions that may indicate serious medical problems, such as bleeding, infections, rheumatic disease, liver dysfunction, and cardiovascular problems. Hair thickness and distribution may indicate hormonal alterations. Alopecia (i.e., hair loss) may be a sign of hyperthyroidism, syphilis, or neurologic or psychologic problems. Hirsutism (i.e., excessive hair growth) may indicate endocrine or other systemic problems.[1,2]

Eyes, Ears, and Nose

The eyes may be the main indicator of systemic disease, such as hyperthyroidism, diabetes, liver disease, CNS disturbances, or infectious diseases. The eyes must be inspected to determine whether they are normal in size, shape, and position. Deviations from normal, such as ptosis (i.e., drooping eyelids), nystagmus (i.e., rapid, involuntary eyeball movements), hypertelorism, unusually dilated pupils (cranial nerve II or III damage), blue sclera (scleroderma), jaundice (yellow conjunctiva-liver disease), bacterial and viral infections (conjunctivitis), blepharitis (i.e., inflamed eyelids), keratoconjunctivitis sicca (i.e., dry eyes), retinopathy (diabetes), or exophthalmos (hyperthyroidism) may indicate an underlying medical problem. The examination of the dental patient's ear is limited to the **external auditory meatus** and the preauricular and postauricular areas. The examination of the skin of the ear and nose is performed with the same examination criteria as for the head and face.[3,4,6]

Lymph Nodes

Within the boundaries of the head and neck lie hundreds of **lymph nodes** (Box 14-3), which are among the most important structures of the head and neck. The lymphatic system's major function is to monitor the body's immune system. If infectious organisms or foreign material enter the body and pose a threat of disease, then the lymph system activates to remove them. Macrophages engulf bacteria, viruses, and other pathogenic agents. The cellular immune system activates the lymphocytes to neutralize the pathogens. The lymph system removes the pathogens from the body.

During infections the lymph nodes become engorged with immune components, dead cells, and pathogens. The lymph nodes become enlarged and can be palpated. If infections or malignancies are anywhere in the head and neck, then the lymph nodes in that anatomical location become enlarged. Lymph nodes may become enlarged during viral infections as influenza, herpes, mononucleosis, human immunodeficiency virus (HIV), chickenpox, colds, and upper respiratory infections

---

BOX 14-3

LYMPH NODE GROUPS OF THE HEAD AND NECK AND AREAS OF DRAINAGE

Submental: Tip of tongue, anterior floor of mouth, lower incisors, anterior lower gingiva, midlower lip

Submandibular: Salivary glands; lips; anterior nose; frontal, maxillary, and ethmoid sinuses; buccal mucosa; gingiva; teeth (except lower incisors); anterior palate; soft palate; anterior two thirds of tongue

Infrahyoid: Thyroid, larynx, trachea, and part of the pharynx

Pretracheal: Thyroid, larynx, trachea, and part of the pharynx

Medial and lateral lower deep cervical: Receive lymph drainage from the submental and submandibular lymph nodes; drainage for the base of the tongue and sublingual region

Medial and lateral upper deep cervical: Receive lymph drainage from the submental and submandibular lymph nodes

Occipital: Skin of posterior scalp

Inferior upper deep cervical: Receive lymph drainage from the submental and submandibular lymph nodes; drainage for the base of the tongue and sublingual region

Nuchal: Skin of back of neck, other nodes

Posterior auricular: Skin of scalp and neck, ear

Anterior auricular: Ear, skin of face and neck

Not Shown on Diagram

Superficial parotid: Lateral and frontal scalp, ears, eyelids

Deep parotid: Parotid gland, orbit, eyes, conjunctiva

Buccal: Median eyelids, mucous membranes of nose and cheek

Mandibular: Mucous membranes of nose and cheek

Jugulodigastric: Tongue, floor of mouth, lips

Internal jugular: Pharynx, larynx, tonsils, soft palate, tongue

Superficial cervical: Parotid and ear region, angle of the mandible

Spinal accessory: Occipital, nuchal, retroauricular nodes

Supraclavicular: Posterior triangle of neck, spinal accessory nodes, most other nodes

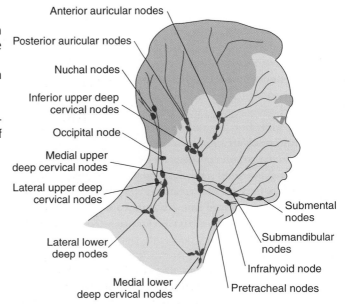

Anterior auricular nodes

Posterior auricular nodes

Nuchal nodes

Inferior upper deep cervical nodes

Occipital node

Medial upper deep cervical nodes

Lateral upper deep cervical nodes

Lateral lower deep nodes

Medial lower deep cervical nodes

Submental nodes

Submandibular nodes

Infrahyoid node

Pretracheal nodes

(URIs). They may also signal bacterial infections, tuberculosis (TB), sinusitis, and fungal infections. Chronic conditions and malignancies also cause lymph node enlargements. Cancer may invade the lymphatic system, in which case the prognosis for survival becomes much more grave. The enlargement of lymph nodes in the head and neck signal important changes that must be recognized by the astute health professional.[3,4,6]

The lymph nodes of the head and neck include the submandibular, submental, parotid, preauricular, postauricular, deep cervical, occipital, supraclavicular, and the nodes associated with the sternocleidomastoid muscle. Lymph node areas are listed in Box 14-3. All lymph nodes should be evaluated for size, mobility, attachment to surrounding tissue, and tenderness.

✦ CASE APPLICATION 14-1.1

Enlarged Lymph Nodes
The hygienist noted enlarged subclavicular lymph nodes. Given Mr. Jabir's history, what questions might the hygienist ask?

Muscles

Several muscle groups, including the muscles of mastication, are found in the head and neck region (Figure 14-9). The muscles in the neck include the sternocleidomastoid, digastrics, omohyoid, and trapezius. These muscles function in mastication, swallowing, positioning, and turning the head. The temporalis, buccinator, masseter, and pterygoid muscles are responsible for mastication and facial expression. Muscle abnormalities are most commonly detected by observing pain on palpation, changes in the muscle texture or consistency, or a change in head position or facial expression. Muscles that are enlarged, painful, tender, firm, or cramping (or a combination of these symptoms) may indicate infection, neoplasia, dysfunction, autoimmune inflammatory connective tissue diseases, metabolic or endocrine disorders, or emotional-psychologic disturbances.[3,4]

Blood Vessels

The head and neck region has an extensive network of blood vessels. The major blood vessels in the neck are the common carotid artery, which branches into the internal and external carotid arteries, and the jugular vein. With advancing atherosclerosis and cardiovascular disease, edema and engorgement of these blood vessels may occur. Many blood vessels are in the face, paraoral structures, eyes, nose, and skin. The blood vessels may become dilated, ruptured, or aneurysmal, resulting in the clinical appearance of petechiae, telangiectasias, angiomas, purpura, hematomas, and ecchymoses. This may indicate the presence of a serious hematologic abnormality, a bleeding problem, or both.[3,4,6]

Bones and Cartilage

Thyroid cartilage, cricoid cartilage, and the tracheal rings are found in the anterior median part of the neck. The cartilage structures provide support and protection to critical structures in the neck. They protect the thyroid gland, the major blood vessels, and the trachea. The hyoid (free-floating bone) is responsible for swallowing[6] (see Figure 14-10).

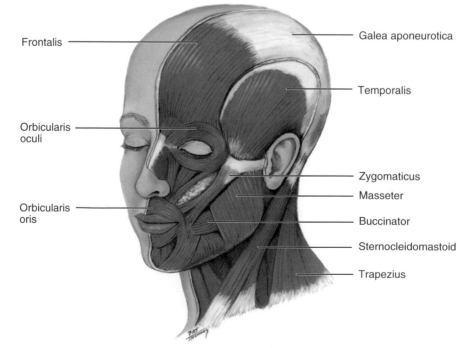

Frontalis

Orbicularis oculi

Orbicularis oris

Galea aponeurotica

Temporalis

Zygomaticus

Masseter

Buccinator

Sternocleidomastoid

Trapezius

FIGURE 14-9
Muscles of the head and neck. (From Applegate E: *The anatomy and physiology learning system,* ed 3, Philadelphia, 2006, Saunders.)

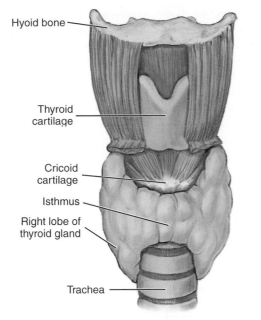

FIGURE 14-10
Thyroid gland in relation to other structures overlying the trachea. (From Fehrenbach MJ, Herring SW: *Illustrated anatomy of the head and neck*, ed 3, St Louis, 2006, Saunders.)

Thyroid

A thorough examination of the neck is vital. Figure 14-10 shows the position of the thyroid in relation to other structures overlying the trachea. The thyroid consists of two lobes, one located on each side of the midline of the neck. The **thyroid gland** produces hormones that regulate the body's metabolic activities. When abnormalities in tissue development, growth, or hormonal (pituitary) regulation are present, the thyroid tissue may become enlarged. Clinically, this enlargement may be detectable as a goiter (see Figure 14-5). Enlarged thyroid gland tissue may be clinically significant in identifying the patient with hyperthyroidism or hypothyroidism. The patient with hyperthyroidism may be at risk for cardiovascular problems (i.e., hypertension, arrhythmia). The thyroid is examined by palpating the structure on each side of the neck using two fingers along the muscle border and pressing lightly on the trachea (see Figure 14-4). Ask the patient to swallow to determine whether the thyroid gland moves easily up and down during swallowing. The thyroid cartilage should also move left and right when gently moved across the trachea.

While examining the thyroid, the hygienist should check for symmetry, size, and abnormalities such as nodules. Adenoma is a neoplasia of the thyroid gland, and early detection of this malignant neoplasm is critical.[3,4,6]

Other abnormalities that appear in the neck are cysts (i.e., thyroglossal duct cyst, brachial cleft cyst, dermoid cyst, sebaceous cyst, epidermal cyst), muscle problems, tumors, and blood vessel abnormalities such as bruits from atherosclerosis of the carotid arteries. The thorough neck examination can reveal these potentially serious conditions (see Figures 14-2 and 14-4).

Salivary Glands

Salivary glands that are infected, obstructed, or undergo neoplastic changes may become firm and enlarged. The major salivary glands are the paired **submandibular glands** and **parotid glands** (Figure 14-11). These glands produce more than 90% of all saliva. The **sublingual glands** and minor salivary glands are small and contribute only about 7% to 8% of saliva. The submandibular glands are located in the posterior part of the mandible and below the floor of the mouth (mylohyoid muscle). These glands are easily palpated even when normal. The ducts of the submandibular glands (Wharton's) exit lingual to the anterior mandibular incisors. The parotid glands are the largest glands and are located on the side of the face anterior to the ear. The ducts of the parotid glands (Stensen's) are located on the superior portion of the buccal mucosa adjacent to the second maxillary molars.[6] The salivary glands or their ducts may become enlarged and painful as a result of a bacterial (*Staphylococcus* or *Streptococcus* organisms) or viral infection. Chronic enlargement of salivary glands may also signal the presence of a neoplasm. Lymphoma, leukemia, adenoid cystic carcinoma, mucoepidermoid carcinoma, and other malignancies may affect the salivary glands. The salivary glands may undergo inflammatory changes as a result of systemic diseases such as Sjögren's syndrome, sicca syndrome, systemic lupus erythematosus (SLE), diabetes mellitus, liver disease, and HIV. Salivary gland enlargement may be the result of nutritional deficiencies, chronic alcoholism, or therapy with certain drugs. Sialoliths (calculi or stones) may develop in the ductal system of the salivary glands and cause obstruction. Often the sialoliths can be palpated in the duct, and the gland is enlarged and painful. Any pronounced, prolonged abnormalities of the salivary glands require close monitoring, follow-up, or referral[3,4] (see Figure 14-6).

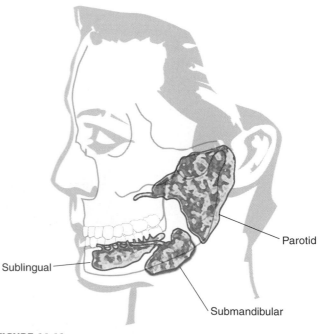

FIGURE 14-11
Major salivary glands.

Temporomandibular Joint

The TMJ is found just in front of the ear and can be seen in Figure 14-12. The TMJ may be examined by palpation and auscultation (Figures 14-13 and 14-14; see also Figure 14-7). Palpating with the index finger, index and middle finger over the head of the condyle, or a finger just inside the external auditory meatus allows the dental hygienist to evaluate the function of the TMJ. Auscultation for joint sounds may be accomplished by listening with the unaided ear or with a stethoscope placed over the TMJ (see Figure 14-14).

Anatomically, the TMJ is the articulation between the condyle and the mandible and the squamous portion of the temporal bone. The condyle is elliptically shaped; the articular surface of the temporal bone is composed of the concave articular fossa and the convex articular eminence. The meniscus (articular disc) is fibrous, biconcave, and smooth. It separates the condyle and the temporal bone (see Figure 14-12).

Normal TMJ function occurs as two separate motions within the joint when the mouth opens. The first motion is a rotation around a horizontal axis through the condylar heads, and the second is translation. When the mouth opens, the condyles and meniscus move together as a unit anteriorly beneath the articular eminence. In the closed-mouth position, the thick posterior band of the meniscus lies immediately above the condyle.

TMJ dysfunction is most often caused by internal derangement of the joint in which the posterior band of the meniscus is anteriorly displaced in front of the condyle. Often the displaced posterior band returns to its normal position when the condyle reaches a certain point. This is termed *anterior displacement with reduction.* When the meniscus reduces, the patient will often feel a click or pop in the joint. When the meniscus remains anteriorly displaced at full-mouth opening, the condition is referred to as *anterior displacement without reduction.* These patients often cannot fully open their mouths. Grinding noises are often heard if a tear or perforation of the meniscus occurs.[7]

Should the patient report one or more of the symptoms in Box 14-4, it should be brought to the attention of the supervising dentist for further consultation. Further queries by the hygienist can be made regarding any previous surgical history of the joint, any past trauma to the TMJ, or whether the patient has been diagnosed with arthritis.

Treatment of TMJ pain and dysfunction is multifaceted. The first step is patient education. Myofascial pain is often the

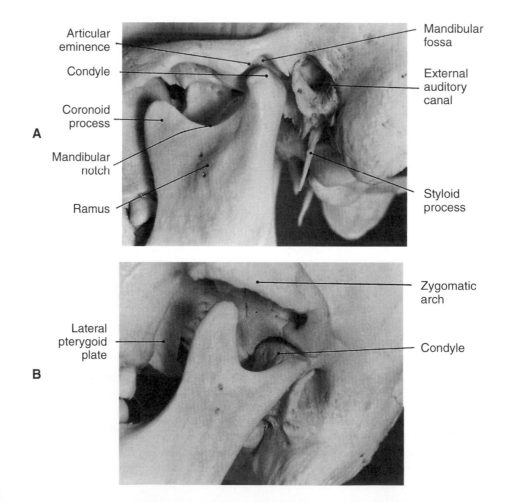

FIGURE 14-12
Anatomy of the temporomandibular joint. **A,** Relation of the condyle of the mandible to the glenoid fossa and the articular eminence of the temporal bone with the teeth in the intercuspal position. **B,** View of mandibular fossa and the infratemporal fossa. (From Ash MM, Nelson S: *Wheeler's dental anatomy, physiology and occlusion,* ed 8, St Louis, 2003, Saunders.)

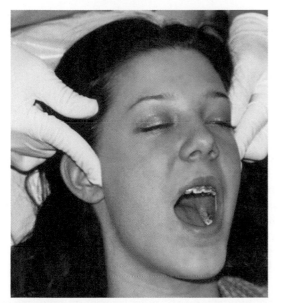

FIGURE 14-13
Palpation, bimanual auscultation. *Anatomical landmarks:* Temporomandibular joint (TMJ). *Structures:* TMJ. *Instructions:* The examination of the TMJ may be performed by palpation during mandibular excursions. This evaluation may be performed more accurately by using a stethoscope. The clinician uses movement of the fingers to examine the masseter muscles, the parotid gland, and the facial lymph nodes over the lateral aspect of the ramus of the mandible and palpation of the facial tissues (i.e., cheek).

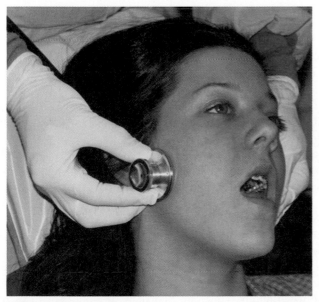

FIGURE 14-14
Temporomandibular joint examination.

result of parafunctional habits (e.g., nocturnal grinding and bruxism, daytime clenching of teeth) or muscular hyperactivity secondary to stress and anxiety. Patients can learn to reduce exposure to stressful situations through psychologic counseling. Stretching exercises at home or physical therapy are helpful in maintaining normal function. An aid to treatment is fabrication of a bite splint; these are specifically made to unload or reduce force placed directly on the TMJ area and can be worn by the patient during sleep. Four classes of medications are

useful in the treatment of TMJ disorders: (1) nonsteroidal antiinflammatory drugs (NSAIDs), (2) analgesics, (3) muscular relaxants, and (4) tricyclic antidepressants.[9] In more serious cases, referral to an oral and maxillofacial surgeon may be necessary for surgical intervention.

BOX 14-4

KEY DIAGNOSTIC QUESTIONS TO ASK THE PATIENT DURING THE TEMPOROMANDIBULAR JOINT EXAMINATION

Do you have or have you ever had the following:
- Pain on the lateral face?
- Mandibular dysfunction (limited opening <35 mm of interincisal opening or deviation on opening)?
- Joint sounds (clicking, popping, crepitus)?
- History of locking open or closed?
- History of frequent headaches (tension [not migraine])?

SUPPLEMENTAL DIAGNOSTIC AIDS

The HEENT examination is primarily one of screening for deviations from normal anatomy and physiologic function. The dental hygienist may not determine the definitive diagnosis based on the clinical examination; therefore additional diagnostic techniques and evaluations are required to obtain further diagnostic information. These adjunctive diagnostic aids are shown in Box 14-5.

BOX 14-5

ADJUNCTIVE DIAGNOSTIC AIDS

Radiographic imaging: Additional radiographs (e.g., Waters' projection, lateral skull), CT scans, MRI, videofluoroscopy, other tomograms, arthrograms, and sialograms
Laboratory tests: Blood tests, microbiological cultures, antibody tests, biopsy, and histologic examination
Special tests: Exfoliative cytology, DNA-PCR, ELISA, salivary function tests, and electromyography

---

CT, Computed tomography; *DNA-PCR,* deoxyribonucleic acid–polymerase chain reaction; *ELISA,* enzyme-linked immunosorbent assay; *MRI,* magnetic resonance imaging.

Vital Signs

Measurement of vital signs is an essential component of a patient's database. Physicians use vital signs to evaluate, diagnose, and treat their patients. The standardized assessment for vital signs consists of temperature, pulse rate, respiratory rate, and blood pressure. Vital signs should be taken on every new patient, at each periodic evaluation, and before administering any local anesthetic. Reasons to take vital signs include but are not limited to identifying patients with hypertension and providing a baseline in case a medical emergency arises during treatment.

14-7

TEMPERATURE

An elevated temperature is not an illness but simply how the body stimulates the immune system to defend against infection. To get an accurate temperature, the patient should not have smoked or consumed hot or cold beverages or food for at least 10 minutes before the placement of the oral thermometer. In addition, the patient should be resting, either sitting or lying down.[3,4,8]

Normal Temperature

Normal temperature is 98.6° F (37° C). The human body has a circadian rhythm with regard to body temperature. The temperature changes during the day, with lower readings in the morning and higher readings in the evening.

Hyperthermia

Body temperatures above normal are as follows:
- Slight—Normal to 101° F
- Moderate—101° to 103° F
- High—103° F or greater

The causes of elevation of body temperature are the following:
- Excessive exercise (increased metabolism)
- Infection
- Inflammatory diseases
- Hyperthyroidism (increased metabolic demand)
- Factitious causes (purposeful elevation of thermometer reading)

Hypothermia

Causes of hypothermia are the following:
- Hypothyroidism
- Certain viral infections
- Chronic debilitating diseases
- Excessive alcohol intake

14-8

PULSE

When taking the pulse, the clinician should ensure the patient is seated comfortably. The count should be for 60 seconds. In addition to the rate, the dental hygienist should also assess the rhythm and the force. The most commonly used site for taking the pulse is the radial artery; however, the facial artery and the carotid artery also may be used. The clinician should palpate with the pads of the fingers rather than the thumb.[3,4,8]

Pulse Rate
Normal
The rate varies with the activity, age, and the body's demand for oxygen. The pulse rate varies from 60 to 90 beats per minute in the normal adult and 80 to 120 beats per minute in the normal child. Well-trained athletes may have rates as low as 45 to 60 beats per minute. A rate of 100 beats per minute in the adult is considered to be the upper limit of normal in the relaxed, non-anxious state. Loss of consciousness may occur at fewer than 40 beats per minute. A rate of fewer than 60 beats per minute or more than 110 beats per minute in the adult dental patient with an unremarkable medical history should be investigated and referred.[3,4,8]

Sinus rhythm
Sinus rhythm is the beat of the normal heart with ventricular systoles equally separated in the series and with normal cardiac conduction originating in the sinoatrial (SA) node.

Sinus bradycardia
Sinus bradycardia occurs when the pulse rate is fewer than 60 beats per minute. This rate may be normal for some individuals or secondary to either (1) reduced metabolism from hypothermia, hypothyroidism, or hypoadrenalism or (2) cardiotonic agents or beta blockers.

Sinus tachycardia
Sinus tachycardia is defined as a pulse rate greater than 100 beats per minute. It may occur with any of the following conditions:
- Exercise
- Anxiety
- Hyperthyroidism
- Anemia
- Decreased blood volume
- Elevated temperature (5 to 10 beats per minute increase for every degree Fahrenheit increase in temperature)
- Heart disease

Pulse Rhythm

An even, regular force and rate is what is interpreted as *normal*. Regular rate and rhythm may be abbreviated as *rrr*.

Atrial fibrillation describes a total and complete irregularity of the pulse. In atrial fibrillation, the atria do not contract as units; different segments contract separately. Numerous stimuli arrive in complete disorder at the atrioventricular (AV) node. A small number of stimuli are transmitted to the ventricles at irregular intervals.

A 60-second examination of the pulse is mandatory to check for atrial fibrillation. Atrial fibrillation can result from the following: coronary heart disease, mitral stenosis, or hyperthyroidism.

Premature ventricular contractions (PVCs) are ectopic beats or systoles recognized as a pronounced pause in an otherwise normal rhythm. These are caused by an abnormal focus of electrical activity in the ventricles that triggers ventricular contraction. When the next normal impulse arising at the SA node arrives at the AV node, the ventricles are refractory and do not contract until the next impulse from the SA node.

Although PVCs are not significant in the healthy adult, they are significant when found in a patient with cardiovascular disease, such as coronary heart disease, congestive heart failure (CHF), valvular disease, or hypertension. Patients with a history of myocardial infarction (MI) who have five PVCs during a 60-second pulse examination should be urged to seek medical consultation.

RESPIRATION

14-9

The type, rate, and depth of breathing should be observed in the patient at rest. The patient has some control over respiration; therefore the rate should be determined without the patient's conscious knowledge, possibly while taking the pulse.[3,4,8]

Normal Respiration

The normal rate of respiration is 12 to 20 breaths per minute for the healthy adult, 24 to 28 for children, and 44 for infants. The rate should be equal and the rhythm should be regular. The rate, however, is affected by several factors, including the following:

- Age
- Gender
- High altitudes
- Exercise
- Elevated temperature (increases by 4 beats per minute for each degree Fahrenheit elevation)
- Metabolic acidosis and alkalosis
- Emotional stress
- Odors

Abnormalities in Respiratory Rate

Respiration in men is diaphragmatic, and the use of chest muscles indicates air hunger. In women, respiration is costal, and the use of the diaphragm could indicate air hunger (dyspnea or shortness of breath). Use of the accessory muscles (neck and shoulder) could indicate dyspnea associated with CHF, bronchial asthma, or emphysema. Pursing of the lips during expiration may be observed during expiration with emphysema. This action helps hold the collapsing smaller bronchi and bronchioles open.

Tachypnea, or rapid breathing, can be observed during excitement, stress, exercise, elevated temperature, or metabolic acidosis.

Dyspnea, or difficulty in breathing, can occur in CHF, congenital heart anomalies, emphysema, pneumonia, or TB. If dyspnea occurs when the patient is in the supine position, termed *orthopnea,* then the patient should be placed in an upright position for dental procedures.

Hyperventilation, or deep and rapid breathing, may be observed under emotional stress or diabetic ketoacidosis.

14-10 to 14-14

BLOOD PRESSURE

Prevention

Often referred to as the *silent killer,* high blood pressure usually has no symptoms. Opportunity to screen for hypertension is great, because patients seek dental care five times more often than medical care. Undiagnosed cases of hypertension may easily be referred for treatment.

In 1896, Riva-Rocci introduced a sphygmomanometer. In 1905, Korotkoff, with the use of the Riva-Rocci sphygmomanometer, introduced the auscultatory method for measuring systolic and diastolic blood pressures.[3-5,8] Taking and recording blood pressure is an important part of the examination procedure in dentistry.

The importance of early detection and early control of hypertension cannot be overlooked by either the clinician or the patient. Complications of CHF, angina pectoris, MI, cerebrovascular accident, and renal problems may be greatly reduced when blood pressure is appropriately regulated.

Guidelines for High Blood Pressure

In general, if an individual's blood pressure is consistently 140/90 mm Hg or higher, then the patient's pressure is considered high. For patients age 18 or older, Table 14-1 explains the American Heart Association's recommendations for actions to take based on initial blood pressure checks. High blood pressure is a major risk factor for stroke and heart disease in adults; however, high blood pressure can occur in children.

Prevention

The American Heart Association recommends that yearly blood pressure measurements be taken on children age 3 and older. Overweight children usually have higher blood pressure than those who are not overweight.

Parameters used to help determine whether a child has high blood pressure are age, gender, and height. Individuals, adults or children, who are classified as prehypertensive are at an increased risk for developing hypertension and need to adopt lifestyle modifications to help prevent strokes, heart attacks, and other ramifications of cardiovascular disease[1,10] (see Table 4-1).

Table 14-1	**Classification of Initial Blood Pressure Readings (mm Hg)** *	
CATEGORY	**SYSTOLIC/ DIASTOLIC BLOOD PRESSURE**	**RECOMMENDATIONS**
Normal	<120/<80	• Routine dental treatment
Prehypertension	120-139/80-89	• Routine dental treatment
Hypertension, Stage 1	140-159/90-99	• Routine dental treatment • Assess risk factors • Refer for consult with patient's physician
Hypertension, Stage 2	≥160/≥100	• Refer for consult with patient's physician

Data adapted from *Seventh report of the Joint National Committee on Prevention, Detection, Evaluation, and Treatment of High Blood Pressure (JNC 7),* NIH Publication No 03-5231 [Internet], Bethesda, Md, 2006, US Department of Health and Human Services [http://www.nhlbi.nih.gov].
*The recommendations provided may vary depending on past blood pressure readings, other cardiovascular risk factors, or the presence of other diseases. The clinician should recommend that the patient consult a physician for advice.

Hypertension

Common causes for secondary hypertension include renal artery stenosis and thrombosis, hyperaldosteronism, Cushing's disease, and coarctation of the aorta.

Hypotension

Conversely, hypotension may be the result of syncope, hypoadrenalism (Addison's disease), hypothyroidism, heart failure, anemias, or SLE.

Orthostatic hypotension

Orthostatic hypotension is syncope brought on by a sudden change from the horizontal position to the upright position or by prolonged standing (peripheral pooling). Occasionally, patients who stand up quickly after being reclined in a dental chair for a prolonged period of time experience orthostatic hypotension. The clinician should advise all patients to sit for just a minute, before standing, after a dental procedure.

> *Prevention*
>
> To prevent possible loss of consciousness in patients prone to orthostatic hypotension, small adjustments in chair positioning when moving the patient from the supine position to the upright position are required.

Patients at risk for orthostatic hypotension are those who take narcotics, tranquilizers, or antihypertensive agents, as well as those who suffer from diabetic neuropathy or Addison's disease.

Determination of Blood Pressure

The following procedure determines blood pressure:

1. The deflated cuff of the sphygmomanometer is placed on the patient's arm, which is held at heart level. The inflatable bladder of the cuff should be placed over the brachial artery; the lower edge of the cuff should be approximately 1 inch above the antecubital fossa.
2. The cuff is fastened evenly and snugly.
3. The stethoscope endpiece is placed over the brachial artery. The clinician locates and holds fingers on the radial pulse.
4. With the needle valve closed (air lock), the cuff is inflated until the radial pulse stops. The clinician notes the level of mercury. The dial is pumped 20 to 30 mm Hg beyond the point at which the radial pulse stopped. This is the maximum inflation level.
5. Using the endpiece of the stethoscope, the clinician listens for the first sound or tap as the air lock is slowly and gradually released. This is the systolic reading.
6. As air is continuously released from the cuff, the sound becomes louder, then gradually muffled, and disappears.
7. The number on the dial at the last distinct sound is the diastolic pressure reading.

Automatic blood pressure measuring devices are available to the medical and dental profession and to the general public. These devices have gained popularity because of their ease of use. They are usually contained in one unit and are good for patients with hearing loss, vision loss, and poor dexterity. The cuff may fit around the arm or wrist. Automatic devices can be used as a screening tool, but the mercury sphygmomanometers are more accurate and remain as the standard of care in measuring blood pressure.[2]

Referrals and Consultations

Often the knowledge and experience of the dental hygienist or other dental professional is not sufficient to allow for the determination of all possible definitive diagnoses or differential diagnoses. This is the point at which the astute professional realizes that additional expertise is needed and a consultation is in order. Consultation with a dental specialist (i.e., oral medicine, oral pathology, oral surgery) or physician (i.e., otolaryngologist, oncologist, dermatologist, internist) is mandated when the dental healthcare professional is uncertain of the significance of clinical findings. After the referral, the clinician should always follow up with the patient, the consultant, or both to determine the outcome and results of the referral.

References

1. American Heart Association: *High blood pressure in children, American Heart Association recommendations* [Internet], Dallas, 2007, American Heart Association [www.americanheart.org].
2. American Heart Association: *Home monitoring of high blood pressure* [Internet], Dallas, 2007, American Heart Association [www.americanheart.org].
3. Bricker S, Langlais R, Miller C: *Oral diagnosis, oral medicine, and treatment planning,* Philadelphia, 1994, Lea & Febiger.
4. Coleman G, Nelson J: *Principles of oral diagnosis,* St Louis, 1992, Mosby.
5. Glick M: New guidelines for prevention, detection, evaluation, and treatment of high blood pressure, *J Am Dent Assoc* 129:1588-1594, 1998.
6. Halstead C et al: *Physical evaluation of the dental patient,* St Louis, 1982, Mosby.
7. Liebgott B: *The anatomical basis of dentistry,* Toronto, 1986, BC Decker Inc.
8. Little JW et al: *Dental management of the medically compromised patient,* ed 6, St Louis, 2002, Mosby.
9. Peterson L et al: Contemporary oral and maxillofacial surgery, ed 4, St Louis, 2003, Mosby.
10. *Seventh report of the Joint National Committee on Prevention, Detection, Evaluation, and Treatment of High Blood Pressure (JNC 7),* NIH Publication No 03-5231 [Internet], Bethesda, Md, 2006, US Department of Health and Human Services [http://www.nhlbi.nih.gov].

Intraoral Examination

Alan W. Budenz • Douglas A. Young

INSIGHT

The dental hygienist must become familiar with the name, location, characteristics, and examination techniques of the intraoral anatomy.

Only with this knowledge will the dental hygienist be able to provide appropriate patient care.

✸ CASE STUDY 15-1   Thorough Intraoral and Extraoral Examination

Hilda Jorgensen, a 43-year-old Caucasian woman, recently moved into town and has come to the dental office for the first time, requesting a "routine checkup and appointment." She reports that she last visited a dental office approximately 2 years earlier, and her last appointment was for a routine dental cleaning. She is currently feeling no dental pain and is aware of no abnormalities. She states that she has received dental treatment on a relatively regular basis since childhood and has received "cleanings" and a number of fillings without incident.

KEY TERMS

ala
anterior
buccinator muscle
caliculus angularis
circumvallate papillae
diastema
dorsal surface
foramen cecum
Fordyce granules
frenum (frenulum)
fungiform papillae
incisive canal (nasopalatine canal)
incisive papilla (midline papilla)
inferior
labial fold
labial mucosa
lateral

leukoedema
linea alba
lingual frenulum
lingual tonsils
mandibular tori
maxillary tuberosity
medial
median lingual sulcus
median palatine raphe
median sulcus
mental labial fold (labiomental groove)
mucogingival
nasal septum (columella nasi)
nodule
oropharyngeal
oropharyngeal isthmus

palatine fovea
palatine raphe
palatine rugae
palatine tonsils
palatoglossal fold
palatoglossus muscle
palatopharyngeal fold
palatopharyngeal muscle
parotid papilla
pharyngeal
pharynx
philtrum
pillars of the fauces
plica sublingualis
posterior
pterygomandibular fold

pterygomandibular raphe
retromolar pad
Stensen's duct (parotid duct)
sublingual caruncle
sublingual fold
sublingual ridge
submandibular duct (Wharton's duct)
sulcus terminalis
superior
thyroglossal duct
uvula
ventral surface
vermilion border
vestibules
within normal limits

LEARNING OUTCOMES

After reading this chapter the student will be able to:

1. Identify the essential components of a comprehensive intraoral patient examination.
2. Recognize normal anatomical hard and soft tissue landmarks of the oral cavity.
3. Visually evaluate the integrity of the oral mucosa, noting any breaks that may exist and noting any irregularities in color or general appearance.
4. Determine tissue consistency (soft, firm, hard, nodular), tissue mobility (fixed, movable), and patient tenderness or discomfort using palpation and the sense of touch.
5. Assess anatomical bilateral symmetry for possible indications of underlying pathologic conditions.
6. Appropriately document both normal and abnormal findings.

Sequence and Documentation

A thorough examination of the oral cavity is an integral part of any comprehensive diagnostic sequence. The intraoral examination consists of observation; palpation; and evaluation of the lips and **labial mucosa,** the buccal mucosa and vestibular folds, the floor of the mouth, the tongue, the hard and soft palates, the oropharynx and **palatine tonsils,** the gingiva and periodontium, and the teeth. During the examination, visual emphasis should be on assessment of size, shape, color, and location; the sense of touch or palpation should emphasize the evaluation of consistency, texture, and patient discomfort. The goal of the intraoral examination is to evaluate the status of the various structures of the oral cavity and to detect any abnormalities apparent by sight and feel. This chapter discusses examination and evaluation of each of the aforementioned areas with the exceptions of the periodontium and the teeth, which are discussed in separate chapters later in this text.

Although careful inspection of all of the described intraoral regions is essential to a comprehensive intraoral examination, the sequence for this examination may be altered to suit individual preferences. The key for every dental healthcare provider is to develop a routine that is consistent and reproducible for every patient. A comprehensive intraoral examination should be performed at regular intervals for all active patients, examined by either the dentist or the dental hygienist, and for every new patient. The general recommendation is for an intraoral examination to be an integral part of a comprehensive assessment of new patients and at all subsequent supportive care appointments.

Lesion Description

15-2
to
15-4

Documentation of findings from the examination is also essential. All findings, both normal and abnormal, should be recorded in a consistent, clear, and specific manner in the chart record, either as part of the treatment record write-up or with a separate documentation form. A comprehensive head and neck physical examination documentation form should include the comprehensive intraoral examination (Figure 15-1). Normal findings are usually recorded as **within normal limits** (WNL), which recognizes that anatomical features may vary without being abnormal. Findings considered outside the range of normal should be carefully noted using the categories in Box 15-1. This is particularly important when no action is considered to be the judicious course or when referral to a specialist for consultation is necessary.

If a lesion is detected, the clinician should determine whether the lesion is elevated, flat, or depressed (Figures 15-2 through 15-6).

BOX 15-1

FINDINGS OUTSIDE THE RANGE OF NORMAL

Noted by the following:
- Color
- Texture
- Shape
- Size
- Mobility
- Location

Examination of the Lips and Labial Mucosa

15-5
to
15-7

ANATOMICAL LANDMARKS AND TOPOGRAPHY

The intraoral examination logically begins at the entrance to the oral cavity, the lips. The exposed red portion of the lips, the **vermilion border** or zone, forms a transition between the skin of the external lips and the moist mucous membrane of the internal labial mucosa and is therefore also referred to as the *transitional zone.* The vermilion border of the lips is a mucous membrane; however, it contains no mucous glands. Because of the unusual thinness of the mucosa, the underlying vascularity readily shows through to create the characteristic reddish color of the lips.

The mucocutaneous junction of the vermilion border with the skin of the external lips is generally quite distinct in young individuals but may become obscured with increasing age. The mucosa of the vermilion border may become thicker over time because of exposure to sun and other elements, and the normal light fissuring of this mucosa layer may become exaggerated and continuous with fissures and folds developing in the skin of the lips. The lower lip is more prone to these age-related changes than is the upper lip.

Several folds or sulci may crease the skin surrounding the lips. The upper lip is divided into two halves by a midline depression, a vertical groove called the **philtrum.** The philtrum extends from the base of the **nasal septum (columella nasi)** superiorly down to the upper lip inferiorly and ends in the center of the lip as a thickened area called the *tubercle of the lip.* At the corners of the mouth, also known as the commissures, the mesial **labial fold** starts at the junction of the upper and lower lips and extends down and out. Further to the side away from the oral opening, the **lateral** labial fold or sulcus runs roughly parallel to the mesial labial fold and extends up to its origin just lateral to the **ala** or wing of the nasal nostril. This fold is also known as the *nasolabial sulcus* or *groove.* The lower lip has a fold running parallel and just **inferior** to the mucocutaneous junction, the **mental labial fold (labiomental groove).**

The thick, pink labial mucosa that lines the internal surfaces of the lips may appear mildly lumpy or nodular on visual inspection. This appearance is due to the presence of numerous small mucous glands that keep the labial mucosal surface moist. These are called accessory *salivary glands* and are found just beneath the mucosal surface. In the midline, both the upper and lower lips have a flap of tissue called a **frenum** or **frenulum,** which attaches to the midline mucosa of the maxillary and mandibular alveolar processes. The size and tightness of these frenular attachments vary considerably among individuals. In some people the tension exerted by the frenular attachment or its extension up in between the teeth may be a contributing factor to **mucogingival** defects or to the creation of a space or **diastema** between the central incisor teeth. The upper labial frenum may frequently have a small bump or tag of tissue

HEAD AND NECK PHYSICAL EXAMINATION

GENERAL APPEARANCE & VITAL SIGNS: Blood pressure_____ /_____   Pulse/min_____   Date_____ /_____ /_____

Weight_____   Recall blood pressure_____ /_____   Pulse/min_____   Date_____ /_____ /_____

Height_____   Recall blood pressure_____ /_____   Pulse/min_____   Date_____ /_____ /_____

Recall blood pressure_____ /_____   Pulse/min_____   Date_____ /_____ /_____

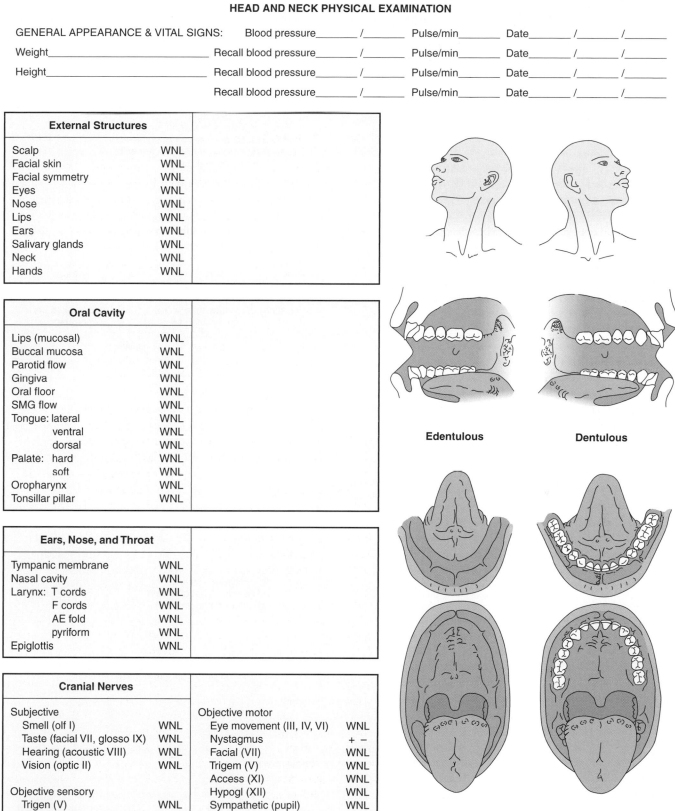

External Structures	
Scalp	WNL
Facial skin	WNL
Facial symmetry	WNL
Eyes	WNL
Nose	WNL
Lips	WNL
Ears	WNL
Salivary glands	WNL
Neck	WNL
Hands	WNL

Oral Cavity	
Lips (mucosal)	WNL
Buccal mucosa	WNL
Parotid flow	WNL
Gingiva	WNL
Oral floor	WNL
SMG flow	WNL
Tongue: lateral	WNL
ventral	WNL
dorsal	WNL
Palate: hard	WNL
soft	WNL
Oropharynx	WNL
Tonsillar pillar	WNL

Ears, Nose, and Throat	
Tympanic membrane	WNL
Nasal cavity	WNL
Larynx: T cords	WNL
F cords	WNL
AE fold	WNL
pyriform	WNL
Epiglottis	WNL

Edentulous   **Dentulous**

Cranial Nerves			
Subjective		Objective motor	
Smell (olf I)	WNL	Eye movement (III, IV, VI)	WNL
Taste (facial VII, glosso IX)	WNL	Nystagmus	+ −
Hearing (acoustic VIII)	WNL	Facial (VII)	WNL
Vision (optic II)	WNL	Trigem (V)	WNL
		Access (XI)	WNL
Objective sensory		Hypogl (XII)	WNL
Trigen (V)	WNL	Sympathetic (pupil)	WNL
Paresthesia	+ −		

FIGURE 15-1
Sample of a comprehensive head and neck physical examination documentation form. *SMG,* Submandibular gland.

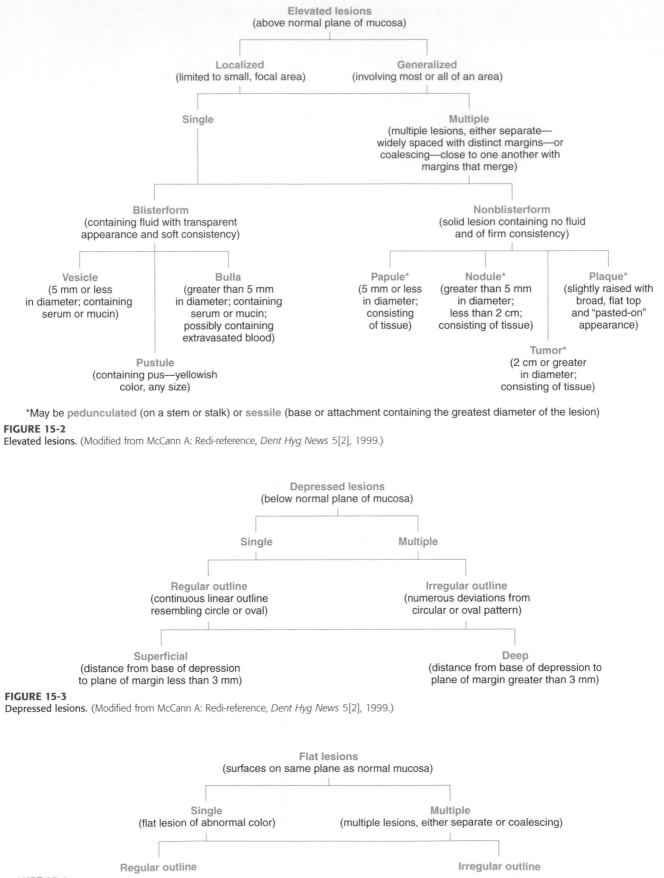

FIGURE 15-2
Elevated lesions. (Modified from McCann A: Redi-reference, *Dent Hyg News* 5[2], 1999.)

FIGURE 15-3
Depressed lesions. (Modified from McCann A: Redi-reference, *Dent Hyg News* 5[2], 1999.)

FIGURE 15-4
Flat lesions. (Modified from McCann A: Redi-reference, *Dent Hyg News* 5[2], 1999.)

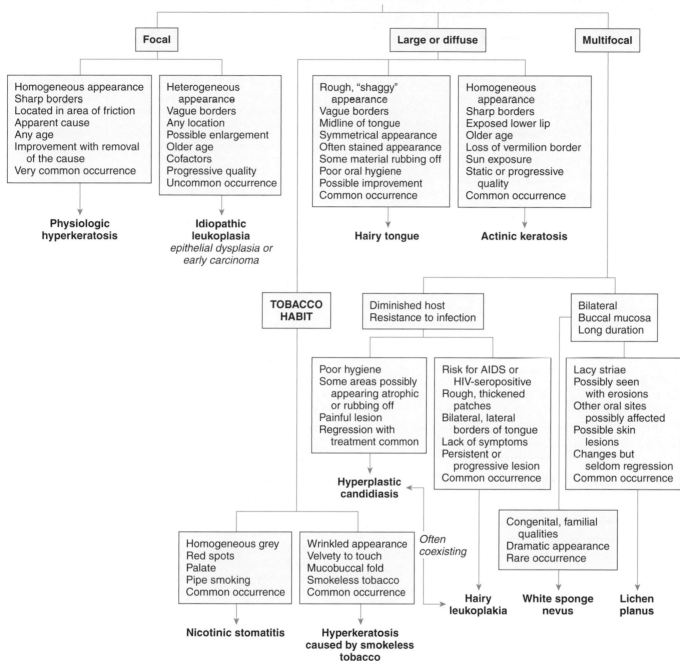

White oral lesions that are flat and do not rub off

Focal

Homogeneous appearance
Sharp borders
Located in area of friction
Apparent cause
Any age
Improvement with removal
of the cause
Very common occurrence

→ **Physiologic
hyperkeratosis**

Heterogeneous
appearance
Vague borders
Any location
Possible enlargement
Older age
Cofactors
Progressive quality
Uncommon occurrence

→ **Idiopathic
leukoplasia**
*epithelial dysplasia or
early carcinoma*

Large or diffuse

Rough, "shaggy"
appearance
Vague borders
Midline of tongue
Symmetrical appearance
Often stained appearance
Some material rubbing off
Poor oral hygiene
Possible improvement
Common occurrence

→ **Hairy tongue**

Homogeneous
appearance
Sharp borders
Exposed lower lip
Older age
Loss of vermilion border
Sun exposure
Static or progressive
quality
Common occurrence

→ **Actinic keratosis**

Multifocal

**TOBACCO
HABIT**

Diminished host
Resistance to infection

Bilateral
Buccal mucosa
Long duration

Poor hygiene
Some areas possibly
appearing atrophic
or rubbing off
Painful lesion
Regression with
treatment common

→ **Hyperplastic
candidiasis**

Risk for AIDS or
HIV-seropositive
Rough, thickened
patches
Bilateral, lateral
borders of tongue
Lack of symptoms
Persistent or
progressive lesion
Common occurrence

Lacy striae
Possibly seen
with erosions
Other oral sites
possibly affected
Possible skin
lesions
Changes but
seldom regression
Common occurrence

Homogeneous grey
Red spots
Palate
Pipe smoking
Common occurrence

→ **Nicotinic stomatitis**

Wrinkled appearance
Velvety to touch
Mucobuccal fold
Smokeless tobacco
Common occurrence

→ **Hyperkeratosis
caused by smokeless
tobacco**

*Often
coexisting*

Congenital, familial
qualities
Dramatic appearance
Rare occurrence

→ **Hairy
leukoplakia**

**White sponge
nevus**

**Lichen
planus**

FIGURE 15-5
White oral lesions. *AIDS,* Acquired immunodeficiency syndrome; *HIV,* human immunodeficiency virus. (Modified from Coleman GC, Nelson JF: *Principles of oral diagnosis,* St Louis, 1993, Mosby.)

along its free edge. Formation of these fibrous *polyps* on the frenum is thought to be the result of trauma.

EXAMINATION TECHNIQUE

Evaluation of the lips begins with observation of the patient at rest. The lips are normally in contact or slightly apart. The lip line, the level of the edge of the lip relative to the incisal edge of the teeth, should be observed and noted, both at rest and when

the patient smiles. Control of lip movements during speech and smiling also should be observed, and any abnormalities should be noted. Next, the vermilion borders of the lips are carefully examined. This examination is best performed through slight eversion of the lips manually to expose them fully to view. The vermilion border is then evaluated for consistency of color, texture, fissuring, and shape; again, any abnormalities should be precisely noted on the intraoral examination charting form. If

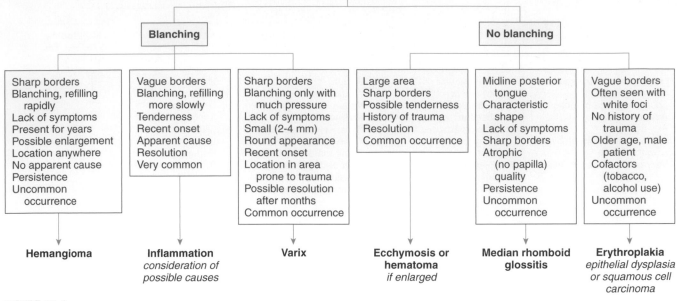

Isolated red lesions of the oral cavity

Blanching			No blanching		
Sharp borders Blanching, refilling rapidly Lack of symptoms Present for years Possible enlargement Location anywhere No apparent cause Persistence Uncommon occurrence	Vague borders Blanching, refilling more slowly Tenderness Recent onset Apparent cause Resolution Very common	Sharp borders Blanching only with much pressure Lack of symptoms Small (2-4 mm) Round appearance Recent onset Location in area prone to trauma Possible resolution after months Common occurrence	Large area Sharp borders Possible tenderness History of trauma Resolution Common occurrence	Midline posterior tongue Characteristic shape Lack of symptoms Sharp borders Atrophic (no papilla) quality Persistence Uncommon occurrence	Vague borders Often seen with white foci No history of trauma Older age, male patient Cofactors (tobacco, alcohol use) Uncommon occurrence
Hemangioma	**Inflammation** *consideration of possible causes*	**Varix**	**Ecchymosis or hematoma** *if enlarged*	**Median rhomboid glossitis**	**Erythroplakia** *epithelial dysplasia or squamous cell carcinoma*

FIGURE 15-6
Isolated red lesions. (Modified from Coleman GC, Nelson JF: *Principles of oral diagnosis,* St Louis, 1993, Mosby.)

the patient is wearing lipstick, then it should be thoroughly removed before the examination begins (Figure 15-7).

Continuing the examination with further eversion of the lips, the clinician gently squeezes the lips between the index finger and the thumb, which is called *bidigital palpation,* while the mucosal surfaces are carefully viewed. The mucosa should be intact to view and feel supple to the touch; the patient should feel no tenderness or discomfort. Any abnormalities to sight or feel should be recorded in detail. Secretion of the mucous glands of the lips may be checked through light drying of the mucous membrane, followed by a close watch for beads of saliva to form on the surface. By gently pulling the lips away from the teeth the clinician may observe the attachments of the labial frena, in addition to the vestibular reflection of the mucous membrane from the lips onto the alveolar processes of the

bones, maxilla or mandible, that support the teeth. The **vestibules** are the spaces lying between the lips or cheek and the gums of the teeth (Figure 15-8).

> ## ★ CASE APPLICATION 15-1.1
>
> ### Intraoral Examination
>
> Mrs. Jorgensen has mildly chapped lips (vermilion border), particularly on the lower lip. The skin around the lips is normal (WNL). The labial mucosa is uniformly moist with apparently normal salivary flow. Palpation of the lips reveals a slightly lumpy texture produced by the minor salivary glands. The labial frenula and vestibular reflections are also WNL. Figure 15-9 illustrates appropriate charting.

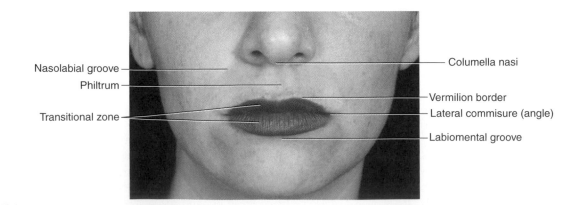

Nasolabial groove — Philtrum — Transitional zone — Columella nasi — Vermilion border — Lateral commisure (angle) — Labiomental groove

FIGURE 15-7
Anatomy of the external lip region. The patient's lipstick should be removed before the examination begins. (Modified from Liebgott B: *The anatomical basis of dentistry,* ed 2, St Louis, 2001, Mosby.)

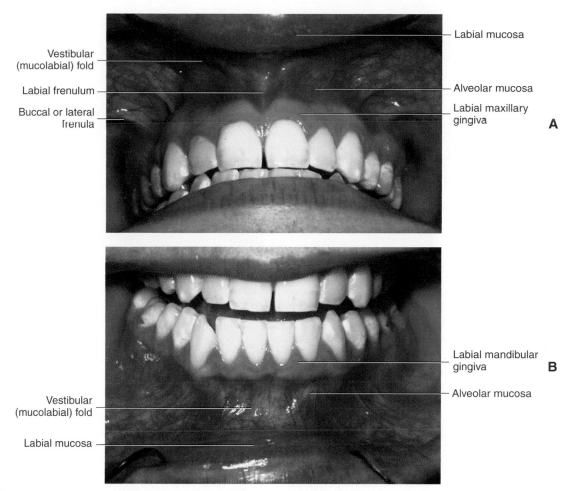

Labial mucosa

Vestibular (mucolabial) fold

Labial frenulum

Buccal or lateral frenula

Alveolar mucosa

Labial maxillary gingiva

A

Labial mandibular gingiva

B

Alveolar mucosa

Vestibular (mucolabial) fold

Labial mucosa

FIGURE 15-8
Everted lips exposing the vestibules and frenula. **A,** Maxilla. **B,** Mandible. (Modified from Liebgott B: *The anatomical basis of dentistry,* ed 2, St Louis, 2001, Mosby.)

External Structures		
Scalp	WNL	
Facial skin	WNL	
Facial symmetry	WNL	
Eyes	WNL	
Nose	WNL	
Lips	(WNL)	Mildly chapped lips
Ears	WNL	
Salivary glands	WNL	
Neck	WNL	
Hands	WNL	

Oral Cavity		
Lips (mucosal)	(WNL)	
Buccal mucosa	WNL	
Parotid flow	WNL	
Gingiva	WNL	
Oral floor	WNL	
SMG flow	WNL	
Tongue: lateral	WNL	
ventral	WNL	
dorsal	WNL	
Palate: hard	WNL	
soft	WNL	
Oropharynx	WNL	
Tonsillar pillar	WNL	

FIGURE 15-9
Appropriate chart documentation for examination of the lips and labial mucosa (mildly chapped lips).

Examination of the Buccal Mucosa and Vestibular Folds

15-8 to 15-12

ANATOMICAL LANDMARKS AND TOPOGRAPHY

The buccal mucosa is the internal lining of the cheek region. This mucous membrane often varies considerably in thickness from one area to another but is generally thick and pink like the labial mucosa with which it is continuous. Frequently, the occlusal plane of the teeth is marked on the mucosa of the cheek by a white line running **anterior** posteriorly. This line is produced by the buccal mucosa being pressed between the teeth during chewing by contraction of the **buccinator muscle** of the cheek. This constant mild abrasion of the cheek mucosa causes an increase in the keratin layer demarking the occlusal plane, forming a hyperkeratotic low ridge called the **linea alba** (Figure 15-10).

The linea alba ends anteriorly at the corner of the mouth, a site often further demarcated by a small, firm **nodule** called the **caliculus angularis.** An additional raised bump or papilla is found on the buccal mucosa opposite the maxillary second molar. A large duct draining secretions from the parotid gland into the oral cavity, named the **Stensen's duct** or **parotid duct,** opens onto the crest of this papilla and hence is named the

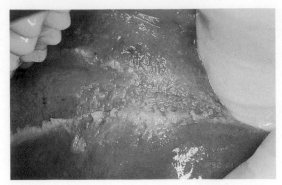

FIGURE 15-10
Buccal mucosa with a linea alba; above is the parotid papilla. (Courtesy Dr. Alice Curran, Jackson, Miss.)

parotid papilla. By lightly drying the papillae and the buccal mucosa, the clinician may check secretions from both the minor salivary glands of the cheek and the parotid gland.

Looking both superiorly and inferiorly into the vestibular folds or spaces of the cheek, the clinician observes additional frenular attachments. Called *lateral, labial,* or *buccal frenula,* these folds attach the buccal mucosa to the maxillary and mandibular alveolar processes in the area of the first premolar tooth in each quadrant (Figure 15-11). Frequently, small clusters of yellow nodules are found bilaterally in the mucosa of the buccal region and sometimes extend forward into the labial mucosa. These nodules, called **Fordyce granules,** are ectopic sebaceous glands that measure 1 mm or less in diameter, may be flat or slightly elevated, and are found in approximately 80% of adults. Fordyce granules are considered a variation of normal anatomy rather than a pathologic change (Figure 15-12). Another variation commonly observed is **leukoedema,** which appears as a filmy white, translucent surface of the mucous membrane. In this condition, the mucosa is often highly folded or wrinkled at rest, but the mucosal lining appears normal when the tissue is gently stretched taut. Leukoedema is most common in people with dark pigmented skin and is found in approximately 50% of white patients and up to 90% of black patients (Figure 15-13). Although this condition is considered a variation of normal, the dentist needs to differentiate leukoedema from a number of other conditions, some

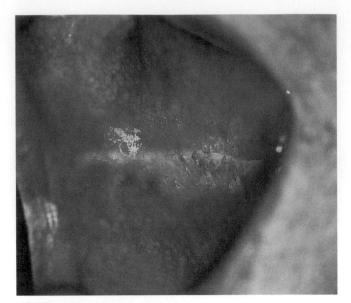

FIGURE 15-12
Fordyce granules. (Courtesy Dr. Alice Curran, Jackson, Miss.)

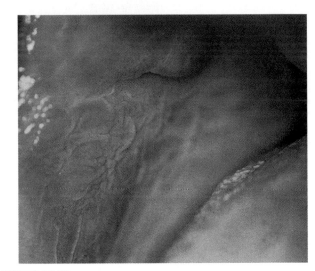

FIGURE 15-13
Leukoedema. (Courtesy Dr. Alice Curran, Jackson, Miss.)

pathologic in nature, which appear as white changes of the mucous membrane.

A low ridge or fold of tissue that extends from the crest of the mandible just behind the last molar tooth superiorly up to a point behind and slightly **medial** to the **maxillary tuberosity** defines the **posterior** boundary of the buccal mucosa. A tendinous band of tissue lying deep to the mucosal layer called the **pterygomandibular raphe** creates this ridge. The pterygomandibular raphe is the common origin for two muscles: (1) the buccinator muscle of the cheek, and (2) the **superior** constrictor muscle of the **pharynx.** This raphe is also an important landmark for administering local anesthetic injections to the lower jaw (Figure 15-14). Slightly distal to the origin of the **pterygomandibular fold** behind the last mandibular molar tooth is a dense pad of tissue called the **retromolar pad.**

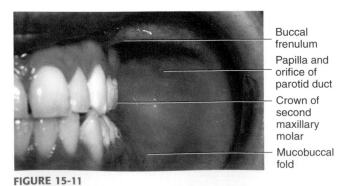

Buccal frenulum

Papilla and orifice of parotid duct

Crown of second maxillary molar

Mucobuccal fold

FIGURE 15-11
Buccal vestibules and frenula. (From Liebgott B: *The anatomical basis of dentistry,* ed 2, St Louis, 2001, Mosby.)

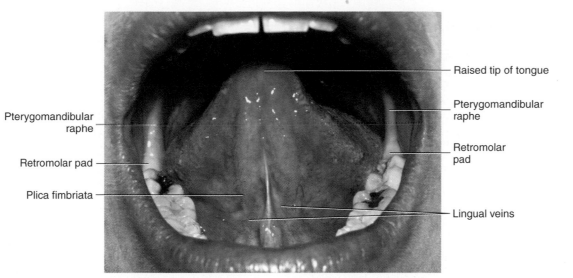

FIGURE 15-14
Ventral surface of the tongue shows pterygomandibular raphe, retromolar pad, plica fimbriata, tip of tongue, and lingual veins. (Modified from Liebgott B: *The anatomical basis of dentistry,* ed 2, St Louis, 2001, Mosby.)

EXAMINATION TECHNIQUE

The buccal mucosa can be best visualized when the patient opens the mouth wide but not completely open. Then a mouth mirror or the examiner's finger (or both) may be used to retract the cheek away from the teeth to expose clearly all of the buccal tissue. The patient's head should also be rotated toward and away from the examiner as needed to make both sides of the mouth clearly visible. Alternatively, a finger may be used to retract the cheek, and the mirror may be used to view the buccal tissue indirectly. Gauze should be used to dry the mucosal surface so that secretion of the accessory salivary glands of the cheek may be observed. Flow of saliva from the parotid gland should also be observed and is best stimulated through gentle stroking of the parotid region externally from posterior to anterior to "milk" secretions from the gland. The full extent of the buccal region should be palpated with either bidigital or bimanual palpation or a combination of the two techniques. Any abnormal findings should be carefully recorded and charted for size, color, shape, texture, mobility, and location.

★ CASE APPLICATION 15-1.2

Intraoral Examination: Buccal Mucosa

Mrs. Jorgensen's buccal mucosa is marked by bilateral linea alba, raised approximately 1 mm and ending just short of the corner of her mouth. Fordyce granules are present bilaterally, and each group of granules is 10 mm in diameter (see Figures 15-10 and 15-12). Palpation of the buccal mucosa again reveals a mildly lumpy texture resulting from the minor salivary glands, which are producing a moderately moist mucosal surface. The parotid papilla is bilaterally raised 2 mm and is 4 mm in diameter. After drying, watery (serous) saliva can be readily milked out of both papillae. The buccal frenula and vestibular folds are again WNL. Figure 15-15 illustrates charting of the buccal mucosa findings.

Examination of the Floor of the Mouth

15-13
15-14

ANATOMICAL LANDMARKS AND TOPOGRAPHY

Visually, the floor of the mouth is a narrow, horseshoe-shaped depression lying between the base of the tongue and the alveolar processes of the mandible. The mucous membrane covering the floor of the mouth is continuous with both the tongue and the mandible reflecting up off the floor onto these neighboring structures. A prominent landmark in the floor of the mouth is the midline **lingual frenulum,** connecting from the inferior aspect of the midline medial mandible back into the base and **ventral surface** of the tongue. On either side of the lingual frenulum is a small papilla, the **sublingual caruncle,** which holds the opening of a duct called the **submandibular duct** or **Wharton's duct,** draining from the submandibular gland (SMG), located posteriorly in the floor of the mouth and extending into the upper lateral superficial neck slightly below the inferior border of the mandible and onto the crest of the caruncle, anteriorly. Extending posteriorly from the caruncles (and following the curvature of the mandible) is an elevation of the floor of the mouth. This elevation is formed by the sublingual salivary glands and the pathway of the submandibular or Wharton's duct from the submandibular salivary glands. This elevation is called the **sublingual ridge** or **sublingual fold.** Along this fold are hairlike projections known as **plica sublingualis.** The sublingual salivary glands drain directly into the oral cavity through a series of short ducts (ducts of Rivinus) that open onto the top of this ridge (Figure 15-16).

EXAMINATION TECHNIQUE

The clinician may best view the floor of the mouth by asking the patient to lift the tongue up to the roof of the mouth and then using a mouth mirror to further retract the tongue away from the medial side of the mandible. The mucosa may be gently dried with gauze. The clinician may observe the

Oral Cavity		
Lips (mucosal)	WNL	
Buccal mucosa	WNL	Bilateral linea alba, raised 1 mm
Parotid flow	WNL	Fordyce granules, 10 mm diameter
Gingiva	WNL	Parotid papilla, raised 2 mm,
Oral floor	WNL	4 mm diameter
SMG flow	WNL	
Tongue: lateral	WNL	
ventral	WNL	
dorsal	WNL	
Palate: hard	WNL	
soft	WNL	
Oropharynx	WNL	
Tonsillar pillar	WNL	

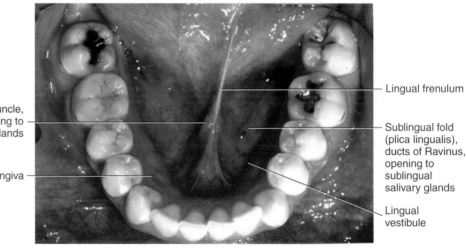

Edentulous   **Dentulous**

FIGURE 15-15
Appropriate chart documentation for the examination of the buccal mucosa and the vestibular folds (bilateral linea alba, raised 1 mm; Fordyce granules, grouping 10-mm diameter; parotid papilla, raised 2 mm, 4-mm diameter).

Sublingual papilla or caruncle, Wharton's ducts, opening to submandibular glands

Lingual gingiva

Lingual frenulum

Sublingual fold (plica lingualis), ducts of Ravinus, opening to sublingual salivary glands

Lingual vestibule

FIGURE 15-16
Features of the oral cavity. (Modified from Liebgott B: *The anatomical basis of dentistry*, ed 2, St Louis, 2001, Mosby.)

submandibular and sublingual salivary flow by milking the glands, stroking the skin just below the inferior border of the mandible from posterior to anterior. The floor of the mouth should be palpated with the index finger of one hand in the floor of the mouth and the opposite hand from outside of the mouth gently pressing up from medial to the inferior border of the lower jaw. Palpation is best started posteriorly from the submandibular region on one side, moving anteriorly through the submental region and around to the submandibular region of the opposite side. The index finger in the floor of the mouth is gradually moved around the base of the tongue. Gentle pressure is applied down to palpate structures between the two hands. SMG flow is noted on Figure 15-17 for Case Application 15-1.3.

The lingual aspect of the mandible also should be carefully palpated. Many patients reveal bony bumps or projections called **mandibular tori,** particularly in the premolar-to-cuspid area. These tori are benign bony overgrowths and should be noted and

carefully monitored for any changes over time. Such changes may or may not reflect development of pathologic processes.

Because the base of the tongue sits in the center of the floor of the mouth, it is normally examined in conjunction with the floor of the mouth. However, this portion of the examination is covered in the next section, which considers the tongue as a whole.

✺ CASE APPLICATION 15-1.3

Intraoral Examination: Floor of the Mouth

Mrs. Jorgensen's lingual frenulum has a 1-mm tissue tag slightly superior to her sublingual caruncles. Milking the submandibular salivary glands produces squirts of fluid from the submandibular ducts. Drying the floor of the mouth before palpation produces rapid flow from the sublingual salivary glands. The lingual vestibule and lingual gingiva appear normal. These findings are shown in Figure 15-17.

Oral Cavity	
Lips (mucosal)	WNL
Buccal mucosa	WNL
Parotid flow	WNL
Gingiva	(WNL)
Oral floor	(WNL)
SMG flow	(WNL)
Tongue: lateral	WNL
ventral	WNl
dorsal	WNL
Palate: hard	WNL
soft	WNL
Oropharynx	WNL
Tonsillar pillar	WNL

FIGURE 15-17
Appropriate chart documentation for examination of the floor of the mouth.

Examination of the Tongue

ANATOMICAL LANDMARKS AND TOPOGRAPHY

With the mouth wide open, the tongue fills the floor of the mouth with only the upper or dorsal surface of the tongue visible. The dorsum of the tongue is covered by mucous membrane, but unlike the smooth, moist mucosa observed throughout the rest of the oral cavity, the dorsal tongue appears rough. This rough surface is due to the presence of thousands of papillae projecting from the **dorsal surface.**

The most numerous of the papillae are the filiform papillae—small, spikelike projections covering most of the surface of the tongue. These papillae usually appear whitish in color because of an outer covering of keratin, which is constantly being sloughed from the tips of the papillae. The amount of keratin present varies considerably from one individual to another and also varies over time in any given individual because of diet and oral habits. The keratin may become stained by extrinsic factors such as coffee and smoking.

Prevention

Regular brushing of the dorsal surface of the tongue is recommended as part of proper oral hygiene, particularly to control potential halitosis.

The second most numerous type of papillae found on the dorsum of the tongue is called **fungiform papillae.** As the name suggests, these are small mushroom-shaped projections that are found scattered among the filiform papillae and are most commonly along the lateral border and tip of the tongue. Fungiform papillae are less keratinized compared with the filiform papillae and are therefore often reddish in color. In addition, the fungiform papillae contain taste buds in contrast to the filiform papillae. Posteriorly, at the junction of the horizontal body of the tongue and the vertical root of the tongue is a V-shaped groove with the apex directed posteriorly, termed the **sulcus terminalis.** Running parallel and slightly anterior to the sulcus terminalis is a row of 7 to 14 large and distinctive **circumvallate papillae.** Each circumvallate papilla is surrounded by a trough or crypt, into which numerous taste buds open.

The least prominent types of papillae found on the human tongue are the foliate papillae, sparsely scattered along the posterolateral borders of the tongue. These papillae are small, leaflike projections oriented in vertical ridges. They also contain taste buds.

From the anterior tip or apex of the tongue, the dorsum of the tongue is divided in half longitudinally by a midline depression, the **median lingual sulcus,** which varies in depth from one individual to another. The dorsal surface may be additionally indented by fissures generally oriented perpendicular to the **median sulcus.** These fissures may again be highly variable in number and depth from one individual to another. A common condition noted on the dorsum of the tongue is termed *wandering glossitis* or geographical tongue. The epithelium of the papillae is lost, and the dorsal surface becomes smooth in patches, resembling a topographic map. This condition can appear in irregular shapes and can change location, thus the term *wandering glossitis.* One final feature of the dorsum of the tongue is a small pit at the apex of the sulcus terminalis called the **foramen cecum** or blind opening, which marks the site of the former **thyroglossal duct.** This duct connects the thyroid gland to its site of origin from the base of the tongue (Figure 15-18).

The vertically oriented root or base of the tongue forms the anterior wall of the pharynx or throat as it drops away from the back of the oral cavity. This portion of the tongue is primarily composed of lymphoid tissue called the **lingual tonsils,** which produce a lumpy surface in this region. The lymphoid tissue may at times be mistaken for papillae or a pathologic process when it projects forward into the posterolateral body of the tongue. The body of the tongue is the anterior two thirds of the tongue and lies fully within the oral cavity (Figure 15-19).

The ventral surface of the tongue is a thin mucous membrane through which the vasculature is readily visible, particularly the large lingual veins. In older patients, these veins may become varicose, producing grapelike purplish masses under the tip of the tongue. The lingual frenulum reaches a variable distance up the ventral midline toward the tip of the tongue. Lateral to the lingual veins on each side is a low fold with fingerlike projections, which gives the folds the name *plica fimbriata* (Figure 15-20).

EXAMINATION TECHNIQUE

The dorsal and lateral surfaces of the tongue are best examined with the patient's mouth wide open and the tongue thrust forward. A piece of gauze is either wrapped or draped around the tip of the tongue, which enables the examiner to pull the tongue gently forward for better visualization. All surfaces of the tongue should be carefully viewed and then palpated as a finger is run firmly over the surfaces. Caution must be used in an examination of the posterior body and the root of the tongue to avoid stimulation of the patient's gag reflex. The clinician may best visualize the root of the tongue by pulling the tongue as far forward as possible and using a mouth mirror to look down at the root surface. Care must be taken not to stimulate the gag reflex of the soft palate or the **oropharyngeal** wall with the mirror. Use of a spray topical anesthetic may be helpful in visualizing this posterior region and is advised when

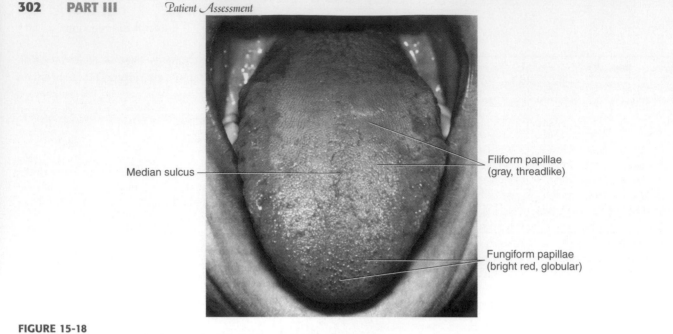

Median sulcus

Filiform papillae
(gray, threadlike)

Fungiform papillae
(bright red, globular)

FIGURE 15-18
Dorsum of the tongue. (Modified from Liebgott B: *The anatomical basis of dentistry,* ed 2, St Louis, 2001, Mosby.)

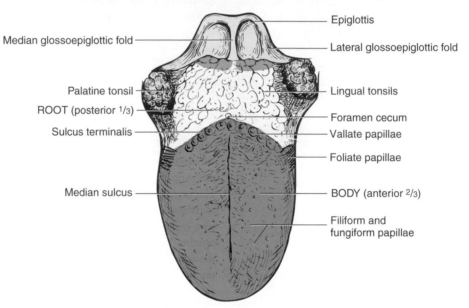

Epiglottis

Median glossoepiglottic fold

Lateral glossoepiglottic fold

Palatine tonsil

Lingual tonsils

ROOT (posterior 1/3)

Foramen cecum

Sulcus terminalis

Vallate papillae

Foliate papillae

Median sulcus

BODY (anterior 2/3)

Filiform and
fungiform papillae

FIGURE 15-19
Anatomical landmarks on the dorsum and root of the tongue. (Modified from Liebgott B: *The anatomical basis of dentistry,* ed 2, St Louis, 2001, Mosby.)

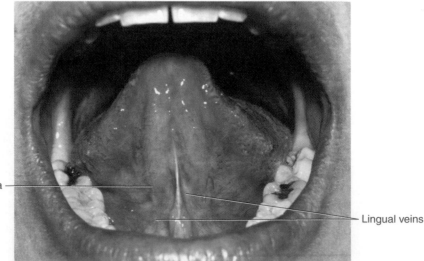

Plica fimbriata

Lingual veins

FIGURE 15-20
Ventral surface of the tongue. (Modified from Liebgott B: *The anatomical basis of dentistry,* ed 2, St Louis, 2001, Mosby.)

palpation of the root of the tongue is required for examination of suggested pathologic processes.

The ventral surface of the tongue may be readily viewed when the patient touches the tip of the tongue up to the front of the hard palate. A mouth mirror or fingertip also may be used to push the tongue first to one side and then to the other to view the lateral and posterior ventral surfaces of the tongue.

⟡ CASE APPLICATION 15-1.4

Intraoral Examination: Tongue

The dorsal surface of the tongue is mildly fissured and is light brown in the central area. On questioning, Mrs. Jorgensen reports that she drinks six to seven cups of coffee each day and does not brush her tongue. Palpation of the tongue is unremarkable, revealing a firm texture and a moist surface. Examination of the ventral surface of the tongue reveals normal lingual veins and a short frenulum. Figure 15-21 illustrates the findings of this portion of the examination.

Oral Cavity		
Lips (mucosal)	WNL	
Buccal mucosa	WNL	
Parotid flow	WNL	
Gingiva	WNL	
Oral floor	WNL	
SMG flow	(WNL)	
Tongue: lateral	WNL	
ventral	(WNL)	Short frenulum
dorsal	(WNL)	Mildly fissured, light brown
Palate: hard	WNL	
soft	WNL	
Oropharynx	WNL	
Tonsillar pillar	WNL	

FIGURE 15-21
Appropriate chart documentation for examination of the tongue (mildly fissured, light brown, short frenulum).

Examination of the Hard and Soft Palate

15-19 to 15-21

ANATOMICAL LANDMARKS AND TOPOGRAPHY

The roof of the mouth or the palate is composed of two subregions—the hard palate and the soft palate. The hard palate forms the anterior two thirds of the palatal region, lying between the alveolar processes of the two maxilla and supported by bony plates projecting horizontally to the midline from the maxilla and palatine bones (Figure 15-22). The soft palate is the posterior one third of the roof of the mouth and is formed by a group of small palatal muscles covered by a mucous membrane.

Anteriorly, the hard palate begins just lingual to the maxillary central incisor teeth. This area is distinguished by an **incisive papilla (midline papilla),** which overlies the **incisive canal (nasopalatine canal)** from the nasal cavity. Extending posteriorly from the incisive papilla is the midline **median palatine raphe,** which may be marked by a shallow depression or a low ridge created by the direct binding of the palatal mucosa to the underlying bony plates usually ending at the posterior extent of the hard palate, although it may extend further posteriorly into the soft palate. The anterior palate is also characterized by the **palatine rugae,** which are dense ridges of mucosa radiating roughly perpendicular to the **palatine raphe** slightly posterior to the incisive papilla. The mucosal covering of the hard palate is generally thicker than the mucosa observed throughout the rest of the oral cavity as a result of an increase in the keratin layer, which acts as a protective coating against the abrasive forces of mastication. Such heavily keratinized mucosa is termed *masticatory mucosa* and is a lighter shade of pink than nonmasticatory mucosa because the underlying blood vessels do not show through as clearly. Excessive bony growth at the midline of the palate, termed *torus palatinus* (similar to mandibular tori), is also common.

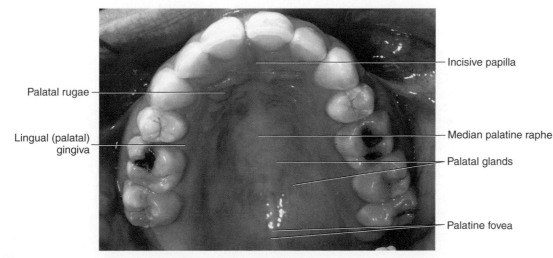

FIGURE 15-22
Hard palate. (Modified from Liebgott B: *The anatomical basis of dentistry,* ed 2, St Louis, 2001, Mosby.)

The junction of the hard palate posteriorly with the soft palate is indistinct at rest, but this junction can be easily delineated as the appropriately named vibrating line when the patient says "ahh." Slightly anterior to the *vibrating line* and on either side of the midline may be two small depressions known as the **palatine fovea,** which are formed by the common openings of two groupings of minor salivary glands. Laterally, the mucosa of the hard palate is continuous with that of the lingual alveolar processes (see Figure 15-22).

Posteriorly, the soft palate forms a flap hinged off the back edge of the hard palate that separates the oral cavity from the nasal cavity. The flap is generally rounded posteriorly until the midline is approached. At the midline the soft palate has a posterior projection of variable length and width called the **uvula.** The mucosa of the soft palate is thinner than that of the hard palate because of a decrease of the keratin layer and is therefore redder in color than the hard palate (Figure 15-23). The soft palate may appear inflamed when a patient experiences a cold, cough, or allergy. The mucosa of both the hard and the soft palates has numerous openings of small, accessory salivary glands, which may give the palates a dotted appearance.

EXAMINATION TECHNIQUE

The hard and soft palates can be best visualized when the patient's head is tilted back as the patient lies in a supine position with the mouth wide open. A mouth mirror is recommended to facilitate complete examination of the entire palatal region. In addition, asking the patient to say "ahh" as the examiner gently depresses the tongue may prove helpful. The hard palate can be easily palpated with a single finger. The mucosa is tightly bound down to bone along the palatine raphe but becomes increasingly resilient as palpation is directed out laterally because of increasing glandular and adipose tissues.

> *Prevention*
> Palpation should be continued onto the soft palate very cautiously because of the probable stimulation of the patient's gag reflex.

⬧ CASE APPLICATION 15-1.5

Intraoral Examination: Hard and Soft Palate

Examination of the hard palate reveals a flat, erythematous lesion in the right anterior quadrant measuring 3 mm wide by 5 mm long oriented parallel to the long axis of the palate. Mrs. Jorgensen reports that she burned the roof of her mouth eating pizza approximately 4 days ago. The hard palate is firm and moist on palpation. The soft palate is normal on visual examination. Figure 15-24 illustrates findings for the hard and soft palates.

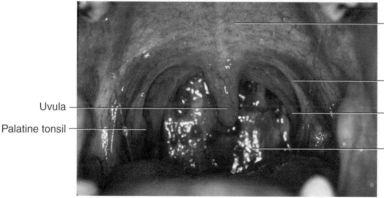

Uvula
Palatine tonsil

Soft palate

Palatoglossal (anterior) arch or fold

Palatopharyngeal (posterior) arch or fold

Posterior wall of pharynx

FIGURE 15-23
Soft palate. (Modified from Liebgott B: *The anatomical basis of dentistry,* ed 2, St Louis, 2001, Mosby.)

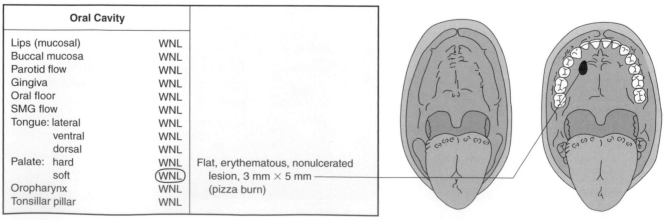

Oral Cavity		
Lips (mucosal)	WNL	
Buccal mucosa	WNL	
Parotid flow	WNL	
Gingiva	WNL	
Oral floor	WNL	
SMG flow	WNL	
Tongue: lateral	WNL	
ventral	WNL	
dorsal	WNL	
Palate: hard	WNL	Flat, erythematous, nonulcerated
soft	(WNL)	lesion, 3 mm × 5 mm
Oropharynx	WNL	(pizza burn)
Tonsillar pillar	WNL	

FIGURE 15-24
Appropriate chart documentation for examination of the hard and soft palates (flat, erythematous, nonulcerated lesion, 3 mm (5 mm [pizza burn]).

Examination of the Oropharynx and Palatine Tonsils

ANATOMICAL LANDMARKS AND TOPOGRAPHY

The opening from the oral cavity into the posteriorly located oropharynx is termed the *fauces* of the oral cavity or the **oropharyngeal isthmus.** The oropharynx is demarcated from the oral cavity by a tissue ridge running from the side of the soft palate superiorly down to the posterior lateral edge of the tongue. The **palatoglossus muscle** forms this ridge, hence its name, the **palatoglossal fold.** The palatoglossal fold also defines the anterior boundary of the palatine tonsillar bed, a depression of the lateral oropharyngeal wall containing the palatine tonsil. The posterior boundary of the tonsillar bed is the **palatopharyngeal fold** formed by the **palatopharyngeal muscle,** which extends from the lateral edge of the soft palate down to the larynx. The two folds are also referred to as the **pillars of the fauces.** The anterior pillar is the palatoglossal fold, and the posterior pillar of the fauces is the palatopharyngeal fold.

The palatine tonsillar tissue found lying between the pillars may vary considerably in size, from small, barely discernible lymphoid aggregates to masses large enough to essentially obscure the posterior **pharyngeal** wall, provided they were not removed by tonsillectomy (see Figure 15-23). When visible, the posterior pharyngeal wall has a thin mucous membrane and a rich vascular bed, resulting in a deep red coloration. As previously noted, the lymphoid lingual tonsil of the root of the tongue forms the anterior wall of the pharynx.

EXAMINATION TECHNIQUE

Examination of this region is largely limited to visual inspection with the exception of cautious palpation of the anterior tonsillar pillar and possibly the tonsillar bed. A mouth mirror should be used with care not to stimulate the gag reflex. A spray topical anesthetic may prove helpful with particularly sensitive patients. The clinician usually obtains the best view of the throat by asking the patient to open wide and say "ahh." Sometimes the clinician may find it helpful to ask the patient to sit in a somewhat upright position so that the patient's tongue falls naturally against the floor of the mouth. This positioning permits the clinician better vision of the oropharynx. Retraction of the tongue forward or depression of the tongue often aids the clinician in visualizing the root of the patient's tongue.

⬧ CASE APPLICATION 15-1.6

Intraoral Examination: Oropharynx

The oropharynx appears normal, with a moderately red (vascular), moist mucosa. Mrs. Jorgensen still has her palatine tonsils. They exhibit normal mucosal coloration and lie low within the tonsillar beds. Figure 15-25 is an example of appropriate charting of this region.

Oral Cavity		
Lips (mucosal)	WNL	
Buccal mucosa	WNL	
Parotid flow	WNL	
Gingiva	WNL	
Oral floor	WNL	
SMG flow	WNL	
Tongue: lateral	WNL	
ventral	WNL	
dorsal	WNL	
Palate: hard	WNL	
soft	WNL	
Oropharynx	(WNL)	
Tonsillar pillar	(WNL)	Tonsil present

FIGURE 15-25
Appropriate chart documentation for examination of the oropharynx and the palatine tonsils (tonsil present).

A thorough intraoral examination may seem initially rather slow and cumbersome. However, as each healthcare practitioner develops a consistent routine for this important element of a comprehensive patient examination, both efficiency and accuracy of the examination will improve. The accurate documentation of any abnormalities found in the course of the examination is most important. This documentation forms the basis for subsequent treatment or for re-evaluation during future appointments. Figure 15-26 summarizes the findings of the intraoral examination of Mrs. Jorgensen.

HEAD AND NECK PHYSICAL EXAMINATION

GENERAL APPEARANCE & VITAL SIGNS: Blood pressure_____ /_____   Pulse/min_____   Date_____ /_____ /_____

Weight_____   Recall blood pressure_____ /_____   Pulse/min_____   Date_____ /_____ /_____

Height_____   Recall blood pressure_____ /_____   Pulse/min_____   Date_____ /_____ /_____

Recall blood pressure_____ /_____   Pulse/min_____   Date_____ /_____ /_____

External Structures		
Scalp	WNL	
Facial skin	WNL	
Facial symmetry	WNL	
Eyes	WNL	
Nose	WNL	
Lips	(WNL)	Mildly chapped lips
Ears	WNL	
Salivary glands	WNL	
Neck	WNL	
Hands	WNL	

Oral Cavity		
Lips (mucosal)	(WNL)	
Buccal mucosa	(WNL)	Bilateral linea alba, raised 1 mm
Parotid flow	(WNL)	Fordyce granules, 10 mm diameter
Gingiva	(WNL)	Parotid papilla, raised 2 mm,
Oral floor	(WNL)	4 mm diameter
SMG flow	(WNL)	
Tongue: lateral	WNL	
ventral	(WNL)	Short frenulum
dorsal	(WNL)	Mildly fissured, light brown
Palate: hard	WNL	Flat, erythematous, nonulcerated
soft	(WNL)	lesion, 3 mm × 5 mm
Oropharynx	(WNL)	(pizza burn)
Tonsillar pillar	(WNL)	Tonsil present

Ears, Nose, and Throat	
Tympanic membrane	WNL
Nasal cavity	WNL
Larynx: T cords	WNL
F cords	WNL
AE fold	WNL
pyriform	WNL
Epiglottis	WNL

Cranial Nerves			
Subjective		Objective motor	
Smell (olf I)	WNL	Eye movement (III, IV, VI)	WNL
Taste (facial VII, glosso IX)	WNL	Nystagmus	+ −
Hearing (acoustic VIII)	WNL	Facial (VII)	WNL
Vision (optic II)	WNL	Trigem (V)	WNL
		Access (XI)	WNL
Objective sensory		Hypogl (XII)	WNL
Trigen (V)	WNL	Sympathetic (pupil)	WNL
Paresthesia	+ −		

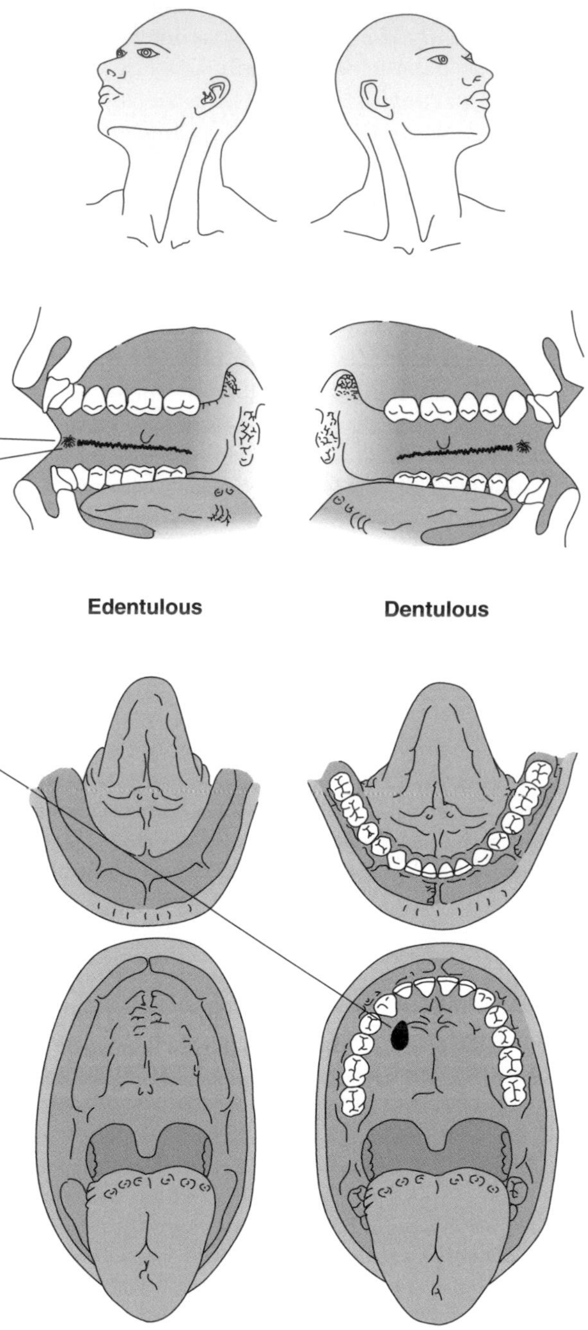

Edentulous   **Dentulous**

FIGURE 15-26
Summary of charted findings for Case Study 15-1.

Periodontal Examination

Francis G. Serio

INSIGHT

The dental hygienist is uniquely educated to perform a comprehensive periodontal examination and is frequently referred to as the periodontal co-therapist on the oral healthcare team.

✦ CASE STUDY 16-1   Completing the Periodontal Examination

Mollie Bozenski is a well-developed, well-nourished, 57-year-old white woman. She is 5 feet, 5 inches tall and weighs 160 pounds. She reports a history of mitral valve prolapse with no regurgitation or audible murmur. She is allergic to penicillin and tetanus toxoid. Her medications include propranolol (Inderal), furosemide (Lasix), potassium, and two aspirin per day. She reports eating a balanced diet.

Mrs. Bozenski's clinical examination reveals generalized accumulations of plaque biofilm and calculus. She has generalized severe marginal erythema and edema. Plaque biofilm or calculus is present on 89% of tooth surfaces. Probings range from 1 to more than 10 mm; 98% of the sites bleed on probing. She has several irregular restorative margins. She has noticed an increase in the spacing between her maxillary right and left central incisors.

Clinical photographs, a complete periodontal charting, and a full-mouth series of radiographs are included (Figure 16-1 on page 309; also see Figure 16-13).

KEY TERMS

abfraction lesions	dentoalveolar (dentoperiosteal)	interdental papillae	periodontium
acellular cementum	fibers	interradicular fibers	principal fibers
alveolar bone proper	dentogingival fibers	junctional epithelium	proteoglycans
alveolar crestal fibers	edema	keratinized	quiescence
alveolar mucosa	embrasure	Koch's postulates	radiolucent
anatomical crown	enamel	labial mucosa	radiopaque
ankylosed	endosteum	lamina densa	recession
apical fibers	epithelium	lamina lucida	Sharpey's fibers
attached gingiva	erythema	lamina propria	specific plaque (or qualitative)
attachment apparatus	free (marginal) gingiva	loss of attachment	hypothesis
basal lamina	free gingival groove	materia alba	stippling
bifurcations	free gingival margin	melanocytes	stratified squamous
biologic width	fremitus	mobility	stratum basale
bone	frena	mucogingival junction	stratum corneum
bruxism	furcation	necrotizing ulcerative gingivitis	stratum granulosum
buccal mucosa	gingiva	nonkeratinized	stratum spinosum
calculus	gingival sulcus	nonspecific plaque hypothesis	subgingival
cellular cementum	gingivitis	nucleic acid probes	sulcular epithelium
cementum	glycosaminoglycans	oblique fibers	supporting alveolar bone
circular fibers	ground substance	osteoblasts	suppuration
clinical crown	hemidesmosomal attachment	pellicle	supragingival
connective tissue	horizontal fibers	periodontal ligament	transseptal fibers
darkfield microscopy	immunoassays	periodontitis	trifurcations
dentin	indices		

LEARNING OUTCOMES

After reading this chapter the student will be able to:

1. Describe the roles of plaque biofilm and other local etiologic factors in periodontal diseases.
2. Identify the components of a periodontal assessment, their appearance in health and disease, and their significance.
3. Chart an involved periodontal condition, using the correct charting notations.
4. Interpret the periodontal findings from a chart (i.e., correctly read a periodontal chart), and discuss the ramifications.
5. Explain the interrelationships and suggested interrelationships between periodontitis and systemic diseases as presently reported in the scientific literature.
6. Identify those patients who have periodontitis or those who are at risk for periodontitis.

The periodontal assessment is the first step in planning a patient's periodontal treatment. The patient must be examined, a list of diagnoses developed, and the treatment plan formulated to address each of the diagnoses. The periodontal assessment is completed after the extraoral and intraoral examinations and typically after the dental assessment. In this way, dental factors that may contribute to the patient's periodontal status, such as those in the following list, have already been identified:

- Missing teeth
- Dental caries
- Open contacts
- Faulty restorations
- Poor restorative margins
- Malpositioned teeth
- Anatomical variations
- Palatogingival grooves
- Cervical enamel projections
- Impacted or supernumerary teeth

Because the appearance of periodontal disease may vary widely, visual inspection of the **periodontium** is not sufficient. The use of instruments such as the mouth mirror, periodontal probe, explorer, **furcation** probe, fiber-optic wand, compressed air, and study models allows for the complete clinical examination of the periodontium. A full-mouth series of radiographs includes vertical bite-wings (discussed in Chapter 18) and provides information about the oral hard tissue: teeth, restorations (if present), and alveolar bone.

The periodontal examination and radiographs provide a *snapshot* of the patient's periodontal health. Although they are not a predictor of future disease activity, the examination and radiographs can provide an evaluation of risk factors for developing disease. Until a reliable predictor of future disease is developed, an accurate charting of periodontal findings remains critical to the assessment of the effectiveness of therapy and the progress of disease. Previous chartings and radiographs are helpful in the evaluation of the rate of periodontal destruction.

This chapter outlines periodontal anatomy and details the various components of the periodontal examination. Classification and descriptions of the periodontal diseases are discussed. Proper rationale, armamentarium, techniques, and clinical findings are presented.

Periodontal Anatomy

The structures in the mouth are composed of a variety of tissues. The six major dental-related types of tissue in the mouth are the following: (1) **epithelium,** (2) **connective tissue,** (3) **bone,** (4) **enamel,** (5) **dentin,** and (6) **cementum.** Blood vessels, nerve fibers, and lymphatic channels are also present. Epithelium acts as a protective covering for all of the soft tissues of the body. Connective tissue, with its collection of fibers, blood vessels, lymphatic channels, and nerves, is found subjacent to the epithelium. Epithelium and connective tissue act as the covering for the jawbones, as well as for other bones in the body. The teeth are made of enamel, dentin, and cementum. Enamel, the hardest substance in the body (90% calcified), covers the **anatomical crown.** Dentin constitutes the bulk of both the crown and the root of the tooth. Cementum, 45% by volume mineral, covers the surface of the root.

EPITHELIUM

Epithelial tissues differ in structure and function depending on their location. Most oral epithelium is **stratified squamous** and is either **keratinized** (gingival or masticatory mucosa of the palate) or **nonkeratinized** (alveolar mucosa, buccal, or oral mucosa). The epithelium has different layers or strata. These layers include the **stratum basale** (basal cell layer) and the **stratum spinosum, stratum granulosum,** and **stratum corneum** (outer layer). Keratin is the proteinaceous surface of the epithelium and is either orthokeratin (thicker with few cells) or parakeratin (thinner with some cells and nuclei evident; Figure 16-2). The keratin gives the **gingiva** its characteristic pink color. The heavier the keratin layer, usually the lighter the color of the tissue because the underlying blood vessels are more completely masked. The gingiva and other masticatory mucosa are covered by keratinized stratified squamous epithelium, whereas the **alveolar mucosa** and **buccal mucosa** are covered by nonkeratinized stratified squamous epithelium.

Anatomical Landmarks of the Periodontium

16-1

Several visible intraoral landmarks are associated with the periodontium (Greek *peri,* meaning *around,* and *odontos,* meaning *tooth;* Figures 16-3 and 16-4). These landmarks include the

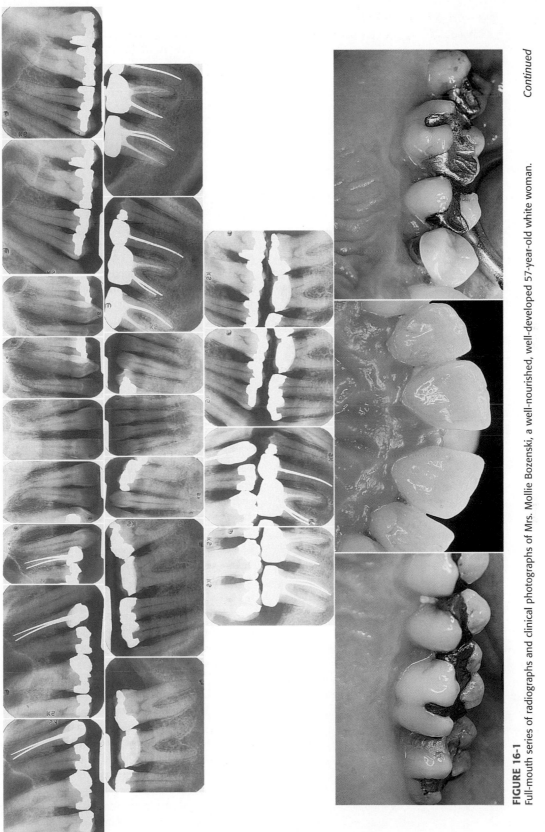

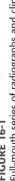

FIGURE 16-1
Full-mouth series of radiographs and clinical photographs of Mrs. Mollie Bozenski, a well-nourished, well-developed 57-year-old white woman.   *Continued*

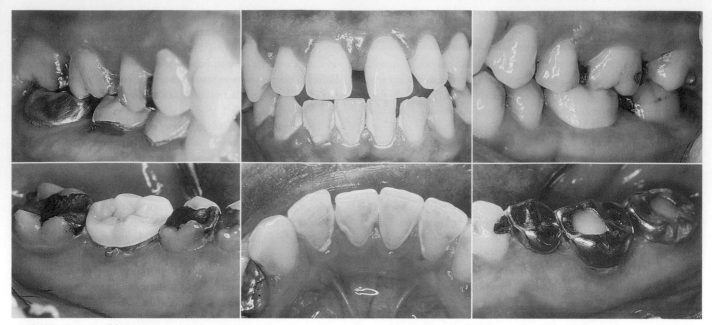

FIGURE 16-1, cont'd

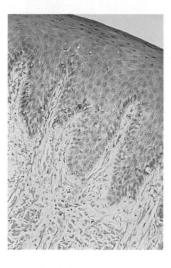

FIGURE 16-2
In this histologic section, the darker-stained epithelium is seen at right. It is covered with parakeratin. The connective tissue is below the rete pegs.

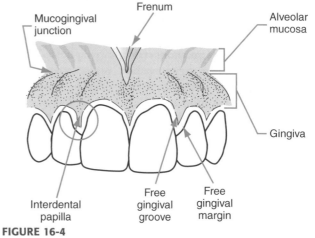

FIGURE 16-4
Normal visible landmarks of the periodontal tissues are identified.

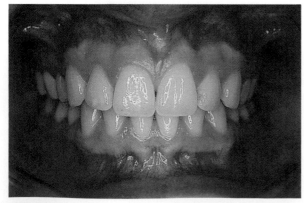

FIGURE 16-3
Normal, healthy periodontal tissues and dentition are shown. Anatomical landmarks are identified in Figure 16-4.

tooth crown, **free gingival margin, free gingival groove,** gingiva, **mucogingival junction,** alveolar mucosa, masticatory mucosa, and various frenula.

TOOTH AND GINGIVA INTERFACE

The portion of the tooth from the cementoenamel junction (CEJ) to the incisal-occlusal tip of the tooth is the anatomical crown. The **clinical crown** is that part of the anatomical crown visible in the oral cavity. The free gingival margin is the portion of the gingiva not attached to the tooth. In health, the free gingival margin is typically positioned on the anatomical crown of the tooth at the cervical portion. When **recession** has occurred, the free gingival margin may be located on the tooth root. The free gingival groove is a depression in the gingiva approximately 2 mm apical to the free gingival margin. The free gingival groove is thought to correspond to the base of the sulcus, but it is an imprecise landmark and often difficult to observe clinically.

GINGIVA

16-2 to 16-5

The gingiva is composed of the **free (marginal) gingiva** and the **attached gingiva.**[14,34] The boundaries of the free gingiva are the free gingival margin and the base of the sulcus. The boundaries of the attached gingiva are the base of the sulcus and the mucogingival junction. The mucogingival junction demarcates the gingiva from the alveolar mucosa. On the hard palate, the attached gingiva is continuous with the rest of the masticatory mucosa and is keratinized. The gingiva is covered with keratinized stratified squamous epithelium. This keratinization protects the gingiva from the forces of mastication and toothbrushing. The width of the gingiva varies by location from approximately 1 to 9 mm in width. It is generally narrowest on the facial surface of the mandibular canine and first premolar.[7,17]

The surface of the gingiva has a characteristic stippled appearance, similar to the surface of an orange. The intersection of epithelial rete ridges and the interspersing of connective tissue papillae from beneath the surface create this **stippling** effect. The intersecting ridges create the depression; the projecting connective tissue papillae cause the convexity[16] (Figure 16-5). **Melanocytes,** which are pigment-producing cells, are present in the stratum basale in all gingival epithelium. When melanin pigment is expressed, the gingiva has a brownish color ranging from faint to distinct. Pigmented gingiva is usually normal in dark-skinned individuals, although several diseases and the precipitation of heavy metals such as lead, mercury, and amalgam fillings also may cause gingival pigmentation.

The **interdental papillae** are the pyramidal gingiva found in the interproximal area **(embrasure)** between the teeth. A vertical interdental groove may be evident on the facial surface of the papilla. The **col,** a saddle-shaped depression in the gingival tissue just apical to the contact of adjacent teeth, connects the facial and lingual or palatal papillae. The col area is generally nonkeratinized and is susceptible to disease. When spaces exist between adjacent teeth, this interproximal tissue is keratinized.

Lamina propria is the connective tissue layer found beneath the epithelium. This layer is predominantly composed of type I collagen fibers, **ground substance,** and cells. In healthy

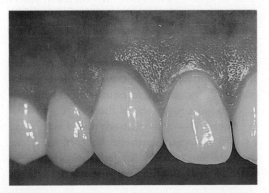

FIGURE 16-5
Stippling may be prominent in healthy gingival tissue, as shown here, or completely absent. Stippling alone is not a sign of health or disease.

individuals, fibroblasts are the predominant cell type with the presence of a small number of monocytes, macrophages, polymorphonuclear leukocytes, lymphocytes, plasma cells, and mast cells. Some types III and V collagen are also present. The proportion of the various cell types changes significantly in the presence of inflammation. The ground substance, which serves as a biological glue, consists of protein and carbohydrate complexes called **glycosaminoglycans** and **proteoglycans.**[30] Nerves, lymphatic channels, and blood vessels also are found in this connective tissue.

ALVEOLAR MUCOSA

Alveolar mucosa is covered with nonkeratinized stratified squamous epithelium. The alveolar mucosa is continuous with the **labial mucosa,** which makes up the inside lining of the lips, and the buccal mucosa, which lines the inside of the cheeks. The underlying connective tissue is thin with a vascular submucosal layer. The alveolar mucosa has a much redder appearance than the surrounding tissue because of the visibility of these blood vessels through the epithelium. It also contains a significant number of elastic fibers, which allows the alveolar mucosa to regain its shape after being stretched. **Frena** are attachments of the labial mucosa and buccal mucosa to the alveolar mucosa and gingiva.

Attachment Mechanisms

JUNCTIONAL EPITHELIUM

The **gingival sulcus** is a space bounded by the free gingival margin, tooth, and most coronal attachment of the **junctional epithelium.** The sulcus is lined by nonkeratinized stratified squamous **sulcular epithelium.** The base of the sulcus is formed by the attachment of the junctional epithelium, the most coronal attachment of gingiva to the tooth. The junctional epithelium is stratified with stratum basale and stratum spinosum–type cells; the cells approximating the tooth surface adhere to the tooth by a **hemidesmosomal attachment.** These hemidesmosomes may attach to the enamel, cementum, or dentin, or to a variety of restorative materials through the **pellicle** and **basal lamina.** The pellicle is a sticky substance composed primarily of proteins high in proline or hydroxyproline (or both) and mucopolysaccharides. The ultrastructure of the basal lamina includes a **lamina densa** (adherent to the enamel) and **lamina lucida** to which hemidesmosomes attach.[18,38] The junctional epithelium varies in thickness along the tooth. Over time, all epithelial structures undergo constant cell turnover and renewal. The turnover times vary for different types of oral epithelium in experimental animals, as follows:

5 to 6 days—palate, tongue, cheek
10 to 12 days—gingiva
1 to 6 days—junctional epithelium

GINGIVAL CONNECTIVE TISSUE FIBERS

The gingival connective tissue fibers (supracrestal connective tissue fibers) reinforce the epithelial attachment to the tooth and give tissue tone to the gingival papillae. These fibers insert into the cementum and are descriptively named for their position: **dentogingival fibers, dentoalveolar (dentoperiosteal) fibers, circular fibers,** and **transseptal fibers.** These dense fibers are predominantly type I collagen, although types III and V collagen are also present. These fibers hold the tissue firmly against the tooth surface and are embedded in the cementum or dentin of the tooth root. The transseptal fibers are often also classified as **principal fibers** of the **periodontal ligament.**

Connective Tissue

Numerous types of cells are found in healthy gingival connective tissue. Fibroblasts produce collagen and ground substance and are primarily responsible for the constant turnover of connective tissue fibers and maintaining the stability of this tissue. Small numbers of several types of inflammatory cells, including macrophages, polymorphonuclear leukocytes (neutrophils, polymorphonuclear neutrophils [PMNs]), lymphocytes, plasma cells, and mast cells, are also found. These cells dramatically increase in number when plaque biofilm induces the inflammatory response in gingival tissues.

The distance from the most coronal part of the junctional epithelium to the most apical extent of the gingival connective tissue fibers is called the **biologic width**[12] (Figure 16-6). This

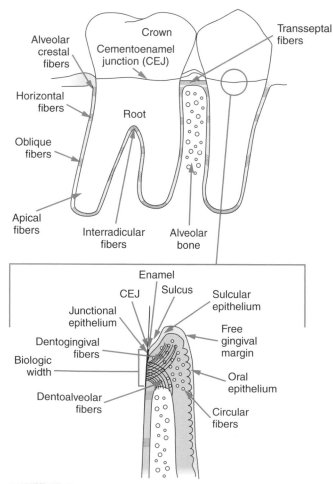

FIGURE 16-6
The various tissues and fibers of the gingiva and attachment apparatus are exhibited.

biologic width is relatively constant and averages approximately 2.04 mm. The body tries to maintain the biologic width. When restorative dentistry procedures compromise or injure the biologic width, the body may induce an inflammatory response to reestablish this dimension. This action may result in chronic inflammation even in a site relatively free of plaque biofilm.

Alveolar Bone

The **attachment apparatus** of the periodontium consists of the **alveolar bone proper,** which lines the tooth socket of the alveolar bone, the periodontal ligament, and the cementum that covers the tooth root. The alveolar bone proper is dense, lamellated or layered bone into which the **Sharpey's fibers** of the periodontal ligament insert. Sharpey's fibers are connective tissue fibers that insert into any calcified structure such as bone and cementum. The **supporting alveolar bone** surrounds the alveolar bone proper and supports the tooth sockets.[33] This bone consists of cortical bone on the outer surface, covering cancellous bone containing yellow or fatty marrow. A layer of tissue called the *periosteum* covers the surface of the bone. The outer layer of the periosteum is composed of dense fibrous connective tissue, and the inner (cambium) osteogenic layer contains **osteoblasts.** The lining of the inner surfaces of bone is called the **endosteum.** The endosteum contains both osteoblasts and osteoclasts responsible for the majority of bone remodeling throughout life. The crest of the alveolar bone follows the contours of the CEJ of each tooth and provides support for the overlying gingiva.

Periodontal Ligament

The periodontal ligament is the connective tissue attachment of the tooth to the alveolar bone proper.[5] The periodontal ligament maintains the biological activity of cementum and bone, supplies nutrients and removes wastes via the blood stream and lymphatic channels, is a source of undifferentiated mesenchymal cells necessary for periodontal regeneration, and provides support for the tooth in the alveolar bone. The periodontal ligament houses a reflex arc that automatically signals the mandible to open when a hard object is accidentally bitten. The principal fibers of the periodontal ligament are arranged into transseptal fibers, **alveolar crestal fibers, horizontal fibers, oblique fibers, apical fibers,** and **interradicular fibers.**[21] The transseptal fibers extend interproximally and are embedded in the cementum of adjacent teeth, coronal to the alveolar bone. Intact transseptal fibers may be found even when extensive destruction occurs to the attachment apparatus. The alveolar crestal fibers run from the cementum apical to the junctional epithelium and insert in the periosteum of the crest of the alveolar bone. The horizontal fibers extend from the tooth to the bone at right angles. The oblique fibers, which make up the largest group of principal fibers, run coronally from the tooth to the alveolar bone proper. These fibers provide the majority of support for the tooth and help the tooth resist displacement from apically applied forces. These forces are transferred from the tooth through the fibers into the alveolar bone proper. The apical fibers surround the apex of the tooth. The interradicular fibers are found extending between the roots of a multirooted tooth.

Cementum

The cementum consists of **acellular cementum,** located on the coronal third of the root surface, and **cellular cementum,** located more apically.[6] Cementum is approximately 45% to 50% inorganic hydroxyapatite; the rest is primarily collagen.

The principal fibers of the periodontal ligament insert into the cemental surfaces. Acellular cementum meets the CEJ in one of three ways. Approximately 60% to 65% of the time, the cementum extends onto the enamel surface. Approximately 30% of the time, the cementum butts against the CEJ, and in 5% to 10% of the cases, a gap exists between the cementum and the enamel (Figure 16-7).

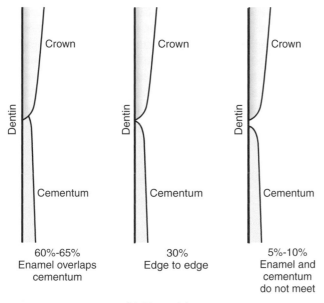

FIGURE 16-7
Cementum may overlap the enamel *(left)*, form a butt joint at the cementoenamel junction *(center)*, or leave a gap with the enamel *(right)*.

Cementum helps anchor the tooth in the alveolar bone proper by the insertion of Sharpey's fibers of the periodontal ligament. Cementum grows slowly, particularly at the apex of the tooth root, to compensate for tooth wear. This remodeling of cementum also permits continual rearrangement of the inserting fibers of the periodontal ligament. Cementum remodels at a significantly slower rate than does the corresponding alveolar bone proper.

Knowledge of the anatomy of the periodontium provides the necessary foundation for the assessment and evaluation of the periodontal status through the periodontal examination.

Components of the Periodontal Examination

The components of the periodontal examination are the following:

- Description of the visual characteristics of the gingiva:
  - Color
  - Contour
  - Consistency
  - Texture
- Periodontal pocket probe depths
- Measurement of the location of the free gingival margin and recession
- Calculation of attachment loss
- Measurement of keratinized or attached gingiva
- Detection of marginal and deep bleeding on probing
- Detection of **suppuration**
- Exploration of furcations
- Detection of **mobility**
- Detection of **fremitus**
- Assessment of plaque biofilm and calculus accumulations

⭐ **CASE APPLICATION 16-1.1**

Periodontal Assessment

As the components of a periodontal assessment are discussed in this text, Mrs. Bozenski's case should be referenced. Notes for each component should be made concerning this patient's condition.

GINGIVAL DESCRIPTION

Cardinal Signs of Inflammation

The five clinical signs indicative of the presence of inflammation are shown in Box 16-1. One or more of these signs of inflammation may be present in periodontal disease.

Color

Healthy gingiva has been described as being coral pink. Many individuals have natural melanin pigmentation. When gingival inflammation is present, the gingiva may appear erythematous (i.e., red, associated with acute symptoms) or cyanotic (i.e., purplish, associated with chronic conditions) or both. The **erythema** is due to the dilation of the capillaries within the gingival tissues. The cyanosis is a result of a decrease in the rate of blood flow through the gingival tissues (venous stasis). This color change may be exaggerated by a decrease in keratinization.

BOX 16-1

SIGNS OF INFLAMMATION

Erythema (redness, *rubor*)
Edema (swelling, *tumor*)
Heat (increased tissue temperature, *calor*)
Pain (*dolor*)
Loss of function (*functio laesa*)

16-6 to 16-8

Although tissue color is one indicator of health, color alone is not a good indicator of the presence or severity of disease. For example, the gingiva may maintain a pink color, which can signify health, even when significant inflammation exists deep in periodontal pockets. This condition is common when the gingiva is thick and fibrotic, such as when the patient is a heavy smoker. In addition, severe erythema can exist with both **gingivitis** and **periodontitis.**

> ### ✦ CASE APPLICATION 16-1.2
> #### Gingival Description: Color
> The color of Mrs. Bozenski's tissue should be noted.

Contour

Gingival thickness and contours have been classically described as thin and scalloped or thick and flat. In healthy individuals, the gingival margins follow the contours of the underlying alveolar bone and the CEJs of the teeth. In cases of disease, these contours change as a result of several factors. In the initial stages of inflammation, up to 70% of the connective tissue that constitutes the gingiva is destroyed. Accompanying **edema** (accumulation of extracellular fluid in the tissues) may contribute to changes in gingival contour. As the underlying alveolar bone is destroyed, the interproximal gingiva, particularly in the col area, may collapse. As attachment is lost, the gingiva may migrate apically along the root surface, causing recession and exposure of the root surface. In diseases such as **necrotizing ulcerative gingivitis** (NUG), the tips of the gingival papillae necrose or die, leaving a *punched out* or cratered appearance to the papillae.

Changes in gingival contour may also be noted in a marginal indentation called a *Stillman's cleft.* These V-shaped or slitlike areas of localized recession appear at the edge of the marginal gingiva but may extend to a depth of up to 6 mm.

A rimlike enlargement of the gingival margin, McCall's festoon, may also be observed. Referred to as *rolled* or *rounded* marginal gingiva, this gingival contour variation, although normal, may lead to plaque biofilm accumulation or entrapment, thus fostering inflammation.

The term *festooned gingiva* refers to rolled marginal gingiva on several adjacent teeth, usually noted on facial surfaces (Figure 16-8).

Consistency

As the gingival connective tissue is destroyed during the inflammatory process, gingiva loses its firmness and resiliency. The

> ### ✦ CASE APPLICATION 16-1.3
> #### Gingival Description: Contour
> The contour of Mrs. Bozenski's gingiva should be noted.

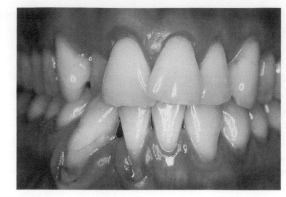

FIGURE 16-8
Festooned gingiva and gingival cleft are shown.

tissue becomes loose, and the papillae may be retractable, either with an instrument or puff of air. In healthy individuals, the attached gingiva is firmly bound down to the underlying tooth and bone.

> ### ✦ CASE APPLICATION 16-1.4
> #### Gingival Description: Consistency
> The consistency of Mrs. Bozenski's gingiva should be noted.

Texture

Stippling is the term used for the orange peel–like appearance of the gingiva. Histologically, stippling is formed by the intersection of epithelial rete ridges and the interspersing penetration of connective tissue papillae. In erythematous tissue, stippling may disappear, although it may be present in thick, fibrotic tissue, which is, nonetheless, diseased. Stippling is not an absolute sign of health and the absence of stippling is not necessarily a sign of disease.[3]

> ### ✦ CASE APPLICATION 16-1.5
> #### Gingival Description: Texture
> The texture of Mrs. Bozenski's gingiva should be described on the basis of clinical photographs.

DETERMINE THE PERIODONTAL POCKET DEPTHS

A periodontal pocket forms as the result of the apical migration of the junctional epithelium in the presence of disease from the CEJ. A calibrated periodontal probe must be used both to detect the pocket and to measure its depth. The periodontal probe consists of a handle connected to a tapered shank and the working end marked in millimeter increments, terminating in a blunt tip. Periodontal probes come in many designs and markings (Figure 16-9). One of the most common probes, the Michigan "O" probe, has Williams markings at 1-2-3-5-7-8-9-10 mm. The tip of the probe is approximately 0.48 mm in diameter. The World Health Organization (WHO) probe is used in determinations for the Community Periodontal Index of Treatment Needs (CPITN); it is also the probe type used in the Periodontal Screening and Recording (PSR) examination (Box 16-2). The WHO/CPITN/PSR probe has a small 0.5-mm ball at the tip and markings at 3.5-5.5-8.5-11.5 mm. This tip is useful for detecting **calculus** and measuring pockets. The WHO design with Williams markings is called the *Moffitt-Maryland probe* and is perhaps the most versatile manual probe available. The Novatech probe was designed with a different shaft angulation to facilitate reaching the distal areas of posterior teeth.

Probing measurements are made at six locations circumferentially around a tooth (Figure 16-10). Measurements are made on the mesiobuccal, midbuccal, distobuccal, mesiolingual, midlingual, and distolingual surfaces. The probe must be angled at approximately 10 degrees into the interproximal or col space to ensure an accurate reading. Periodontitis is predominantly an interproximal disease, and this angulation is necessary to place the tip of the probe beneath the contact area and into the col area. Care must be taken not to angle the probe excessively because doing so results in falsely high readings. Conversely, probing at the transitional line angle of the tooth results in shallow probe readings and missed detection of interproximal disease.

Many factors may influence the accuracy of probing measurements. These factors include probe design, probing force, probe angulation, location of the tooth in the mouth, presence of coronal or radicular calculus, presence of restorations, tissue sensitivity, and level of inflammation.

Pockets are measured by *gentle* placement of the tip of the probe into the sulcus or pocket until resistance is felt (Figure 16-11). Ideal probing force is approximately 20 to 25 grams of pressure, equivalent to pressing the periodontal probe into the finger pad of the thumb until it depresses approximately 2 mm (Figure 16-12). Studies have shown that probing force can range from 5 to 105 grams of force.[11] The tendency to probe more gently in the anterior region and more heavily in the molar areas leads to inaccurate measurements and patient discomfort. When performed correctly, periodontal probing should not be uncomfortable for the patient unless the gingiva is severely inflamed. Obviously, at increased probing forces, the periodontal examination may become uncomfortable for the patient.

When a clinician probes with 25 grams of force, a probe with a tip diameter of 0.5 mm will penetrate into the junctional epithelium in healthy tissue. In inflamed gingival tissues, this will result in the probe penetrating through the junctional epithelium and into the underlying connective tissue.[2,37] Therefore

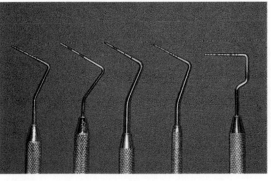

FIGURE 16-9
A variety of periodontal probes are available *(from left to right):* Williams, Marquis, PSR Screening, Moffitt-Maryland, and Novatech probes.

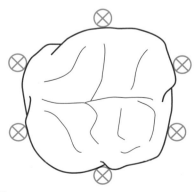

FIGURE 16-10
Each tooth should be examined with the periodontal probe at six positions. Bleeding on probing is also checked at these locations.

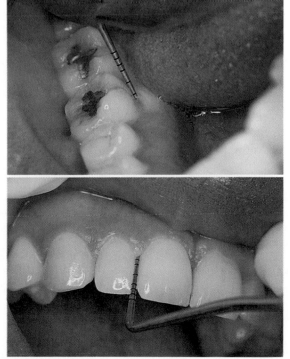

A

B

FIGURE 16-11
A, The proper position of the periodontal probe is within the sulcus.
B, Interproximal probing should be as close as possible to the contact with the probe at a 10-degree angle toward the center of the interproximal area.

BOX 16-2

PERIODONTAL SCREENING AND RECORDING

Periodontal Screening and Recording (PSR) is an early detection system designed by the American Dental Association and the American Academy of Periodontology to allow clinicians to streamline the documentation of an initial periodontal examination. Each tooth is examined at the usual six sites with the highest score in each sextant recorded. Treatment implications were developed, depending on the score obtained. The PSR probe with black markings extending from 3.5 mm to 5.5 mm and a 0.5 mm ball at the probe tip is used for this examination.

Code 0
The colored area of the probe remains completely visible (probing depth <3.5 mm in the deepest area of the sextant). No calculus or defective restorative margins exist. The tissue is healthy with no bleeding on probing (BOP).

Treatment Implications: Appropriate preventive care

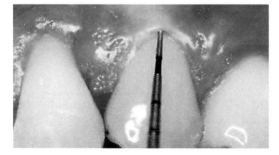

Code 1
The colored area of the probe remains completely visible in the deepest area of the sextant. No calculus or defective restorative margins exist. BOP is found.

Treatment Implications: Oral hygiene instructions (OHI) and appropriate therapy, including subgingival plaque biofilm removal

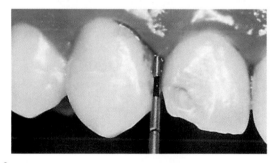

Code 2
Colored area of the probe remains completely visible in the deepest area of the sextant. Supragingival or subgingival calculus or defective restorative margins or both are found.

Treatment Implications: OHI and appropriate therapy including plaque biofilm and calculus removal

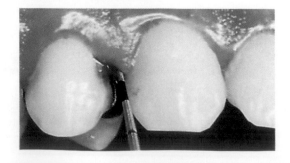

Code 3
The colored area of the probe remains partially visible (probing depth >3.5 mm but not more than 5.5 mm) in the deepest area of the sextant.

Treatment Implications: Comprehensive periodontal examination and charting of the affected segment including probing depths, mobility, gingival recession, mucogingival problems, furcation invasions, and radiographs of the area

If two or more sextants score Code 3, then a comprehensive full-mouth periodontal examination and charting is indicated.

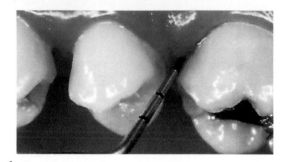

Code 4
The colored area of the probe completely disappears, signifying a pocket depth of >5.5 mm.

Treatment Implications: Full-mouth comprehensive periodontal examination and charting including probing depths, mobility, gingival recession, mucogingival problems, furcation invasions, and a full-mouth series of radiographs

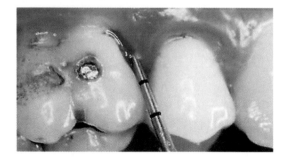

The asterisk symbol (*) should be added to any sextant score whenever findings indicate clinical abnormalities such as the following:

- Furcation invasion
- Mobility
- Mucogingival problems
- Recession extending 3.5 mm or greater

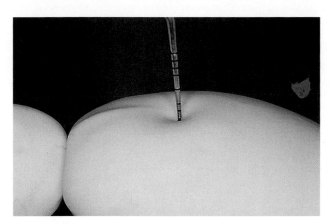

FIGURE 16-12
Probe force should be consistent at approximately 25 grams, similar to the displacement shown on this operator's thumb.

the clinical pocket depth is always greater than the histologic pocket depth (the measurement in a histologic section from the most coronal aspect of the junctional epithelium to the gingival margin).

Development of a consistent probing force and the use of the same style probe at each examination time point both lead to more reliable measurements. Using the same probe manufacturer also yields a more reliable result because manufacturer variations in probe design and tip diameter cause inconsistencies in probe measurements.

In health, probe depths normally range from 1 to 3 mm. Increased probing depths are an indication of either attachment loss or a coronal proliferation of gingival tissue, which forms a gingival pocket or pseudopocket. Human gingiva always has a probing depth of at least 1 mm, except for the first 10 days of healing after a gingivectomy surgical procedure. A measurement of 0 mm at any location or 1 mm interproximally must be rechecked for accuracy and is usually corrected by proper placement of the probe tip within the sulcus. Probe readings between whole numbers are always rounded up (e.g., 1.5 mm is recorded as 2 mm). Probing depths are recorded on a periodontal chart as a positive number (Figure 16-13).

CASE APPLICATION 16-1.6

Periodontal Charting

Mrs. Bozenski's periodontal charting should be reviewed, and the areas of probe depths greater than 4 mm should be noted.

LOCATE THE FREE GINGIVAL MARGIN IN RELATION TO THE CEMENTOENAMEL JUNCTION

Recession is defined as the apical migration of the free gingival margin from the CEJ of the tooth, resulting in exposure of the root surface. This recession may be associated with a periodontal pocket or may occur in areas where the probing depths are in the 1-to-3 mm range. The location of recession may be related to tooth anatomy and location in the arch and may be caused by

inflammatory periodontal disease or as a result of trauma induced by toothbrushing or other mechanical trauma.

Gingival recession may contribute to tooth sensitivity, root caries, or an unpleasant esthetic appearance. If the previously mentioned conditions are a concern for the patient or if the recession worsens over time, then surgical correction or stabilization of the recession is indicated. Recession in the presence of healthy tissue may be observed without immediate treatment.

Recession is measured in millimeters from the CEJ to the free gingival margin. Recession measurements are made in the same locations as pocket depth measurements. Sometimes, detecting a CEJ with subtle contours is difficult. A free gingival margin apical to the CEJ (recession) is recorded as a positive number. A free gingival margin coronal to the CEJ is recorded as a negative number. A free gingival margin at the CEJ is recorded as zero.

CASE APPLICATION 16-1.7

Periodontal Charting: Gingival Recession

Mrs. Bozenski's periodontal charting and clinical photographs should be reviewed for areas of gingival recession.

CALCULATE THE ATTACHMENT LOSS

Probing depth alone does not indicate the amount of periodontal destruction. Attachment loss occurs when the junctional epithelium migrates apically from the CEJ as a result of connective tissue and bone destruction. **Loss of attachment** (LOA), the distance between the CEJ and the base of the pocket, is the true clinical measure of the amount of destruction. LOA, or clinical attachment level (CAL), is calculated by adding the probing depth and the recession measurement. When the free gingival margin is coronal to the CEJ, the recession measurement is recorded as a negative number. Therefore in this situation the amount of attachment loss is *less than* the depth of the pocket.

The importance in the consideration of attachment loss and not just pocket depth may be illustrated as follows. If only probing depths are considered, then it would be logical that a 5-mm pocket would indicate more disease than a tooth with a 2-mm pocket. However, if the 5-mm pocket occurs on a tooth with a recession measurement of 0 mm, then the resulting LOA would be 5 mm. If the 2-mm pocket occurs on a tooth with 6 mm of recession, then the LOA would calculate to 8 mm (Figure 16-14).

CASE APPLICATION 16-1.8

Periodontal Charting: Clinical Attachment Level

The CAL readings on Mrs. Bozenski's chart should be noted, and the concept of CAL calculations should be confirmed.

University of Mississippi Medical Center

School of Dentistry Patient Record

PERIODONTAL STATUS

Patient Name:_____

Last   First   MI

Patient Account No:_____

GINGIVAL APPEARANCE

Color: _Red_

Consistency: _Soft, boggy_

Contour: _Swollen, cratered_

Mucogingival Considerations (tooth #s):

_____

PERIODONTAL SCREENING AND RECORDING (PSR) SCORING SYSTEM

Code 0: black completely visible; no calc., defect. marg., or bleeding

Code 1: black completely visible; no calc., defect. marg.; is bleeding

Code 2: black completely visible; is calc. or defect. marg.; is bleeding

Code 3: black partly visible—comp. perio. exam/chart sextant

Code 4: black completely disappears—comp. perio. exam/chart mouth

Sextant Score:

4	4	4
4	4	4

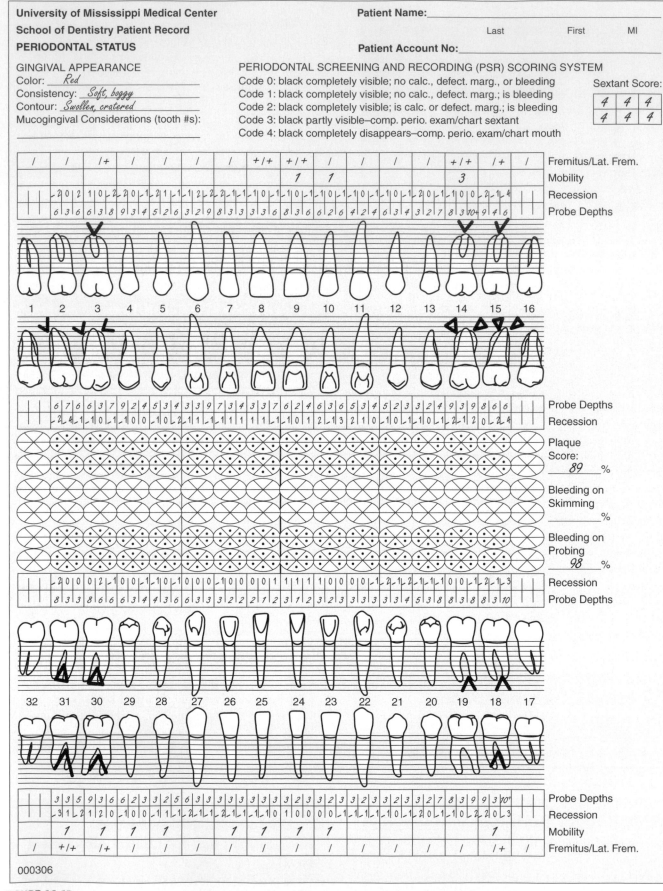

FIGURE 16-13

Example of a comprehensive periodontal chart is shown. Probe depths, recession, mobility, furcation involvement, bleeding on probing, bleeding on skimming, the plaque biofilm score, PSR score, and other information may be recorded in one place.

000306

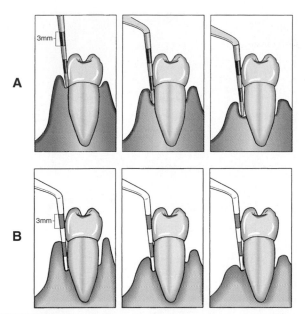

FIGURE 16-14
Probe depth alone does not tell the whole story. Deeper pockets with less recession may show less attachment loss than more shallow pockets with significant recession. **A,** 3-mm probing pocket depts related to different clinical attachment levels. Greater attachment loss indicates more periodontal destruction. **B,** Different probing pocket depths related to the *same* level of clinical attachment loss. Deeper probing pocket depths do not necessarily indicate more periodontal destruction.

DETERMINE AMOUNT OF KERATINIZED OR ATTACHED GINGIVA

Gingiva is divided into the free gingiva and attached gingiva. Free gingiva is demarcated from the free gingival margin to the base of the sulcus/pocket. The attached gingiva is that portion from the base of the sulcus/pocket to the mucogingival junction. Apical to the mucogingival junction is the alveolar mucosa. Often the color change between the gingiva and alveolar mucosa easily distinguishes the mucogingival junction. In situations in which the mucogingival junction is obscure or significant inflammation is present, the mucogingival junction may be found by placing a periodontal probe sideways against the alveolar mucosa and gently pushing the tissue in a coronal direction (Figure 16-15). The clinical mucogingival junction is located where the tissue folds. If the fold occurs at the free gingival margin of the tissue, then no keratinized tissue is present. In the absence of inflammation or progressive recession, it is possible for a tooth to have less than 1 mm of attached gingiva and maintain health.

DETECT MARGINAL AND DEEP BLEEDING ON PROBING

Bleeding is the primary sign of gingival inflammation, the importance of which cannot be overemphasized. Although not all gingival inflammation leads to periodontal destruction and LOA, all LOA begins as gingival inflammation or gingivitis. The amount of bleeding may range from sparse to severe. The amount of bleeding may be indicative of the level of inflammation in the tissues but does not necessarily correlate with the

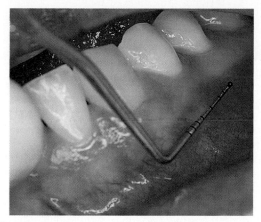

FIGURE 16-15
At times the mucogingival junction is not obvious but may be discerned by gentle pushing coronally with the side of the probe. The area of the tissue fold is the clinical mucogingival junction.

amount of attachment loss. Bleeding may be profuse with severe gingivitis or may be scant even though severe attachment loss has occurred. Bleeding may occur during gentle probing with a periodontal probe or other instrument, and it may occur when the patient eats, brushes, or flosses; it may also spontaneously occur. Bleeding, as evidenced by a *pink toothbrush,* may be the only indication to patients that something is wrong with their periodontal health. Unfortunately, many patients think that slight gingival bleeding while brushing is normal because bleeding has always occurred when they clean their teeth.

During the periodontal assessment, bleeding may be evaluated in two ways: (1) Bleeding on skimming, accomplished by gentle movement of the side of the probe between the free gingival margin and the tooth at a 45-degree angle, indicates the presence of marginal inflammation, primarily in the gingiva itself. (2) Bleeding stimulated when the probe is placed to the depth of the pocket indicates the presence of subgingival inflammation and the possibility of ongoing attachment loss. Minimal bleeding on skimming is not unusual, particularly in smokers, even in the presence of severe attachment loss with bleeding on probing. The gingiva in smokers is often thick and fibrotic, with a noticeable decrease in marginal inflammation. Clinically, the gingival tissues look healthy. Only careful examination can ascertain the extent of disease. The clinical appearance of gingiva is described as coral pink, but because of varying degrees of pigmentation, keratinization, and vascular blood supply, the gingiva may appear dark or even gray. Thus the gingiva of smokers may actually appear healthy. The detection of bleeding is especially important in the ongoing evaluation of the patient during maintenance appointments. More than 30% of the sites

---

⭐ **CASE APPLICATION 16-1.9**

Periodontal Charting: Bleeding Assessment

The areas of bleeding indicated on Mrs. Bozenski's chart should be noted. How do these areas correspond to tissue color, probe depths, and attachment loss?

that bleed when probed at four consecutive recall appointments are at risk for increased attachment loss.[24,25]

DETECT SUPPURATION

Suppuration is the formation or secretion of pus. *Pus* is a fluid product of inflammation consisting of leukocytes and the debris of dead cells and tissue elements liquefied by enzymatic breakdown. It is referred to as *exudate*. The presence of exudate is often but not always observed in periodontal inflammation. The presence or absence of exudate does not indicate the severity of disease; it may be present in gingivitis and absent in periodontitis. The amount of exudate is not related to pocket depth. Although the existence of an exudate or suppuration is noted in the periodontal charting, the clinical significance is unclear.

EXPLORE FURCATIONS

16-9 to 16-12

The point at which the root trunk on a multirooted tooth diverges to form more than one root is called a *furcation* or *furca*. In health, furcations are surrounded by alveolar bone and covered by the gingiva. In periodontal diseases, bone loss may progress to the level that results in exposure of the furcation in the oral cavity. Once a furcation becomes involved in the disease process, the possibility of a positive prognosis for that tooth decreases significantly. Furcation measurement is an estimate of the loss of bone support at the areas of root divergence. This reduced bone height is a significant problem for two reasons: (1) the tooth is less stable (possibly mobile), and (2) a furcation is a difficult area to clean for both the patient and the clinician. As the extent of furcation involvement increases, the prognosis for that particular tooth decreases.

Furcations between the two roots of the mandibular molars are referred to as **bifurcations** and are accessible from the buccal and lingual surfaces of the tooth. The bifurcation of the maxillary first premolar is accessible from the mesial and distal aspect. **Trifurcations** refer to the three furcations in maxillary molars.

As the name suggests, the buccal furcation is explored directly from the buccal surface of the tooth. Because the mesiobuccal root of maxillary molars is broad in the buccopalatal direction, the mesial furcation of these teeth may be reached only with the use of an approach on the palatal side of the tooth (Figure 16-16). The distal furcation may be approached from either the buccal or the palatal side, depending on the position of the tooth being examined and the adjacent tooth. The Nabers probe, a double-ended curved probe with or without 3-mm band markings, is the instrument used to explore furcations (Figure 16-17). The tip of the Nabers probe should be held as parallel as possible to the long axis of the tooth and the

⭐ **CASE APPLICATION 16-1.10**

Periodontal Charting: Detecting Furcation

Mrs. Bozenski's charting should be reviewed, and the teeth with furcation involvement should be identified. Is bleeding detected in these areas? If yes, then why?

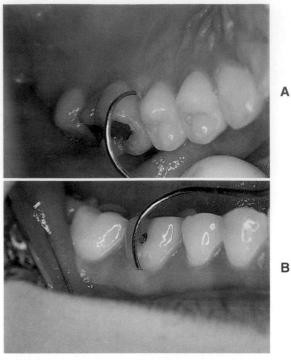

FIGURE 16-16
A, The mesial furcation of the maxillary first molar must be examined from a palatal approach because of the root anatomy. **B,** Mandibular molar furcations may be examined by direct approach of the furca with the instrument.

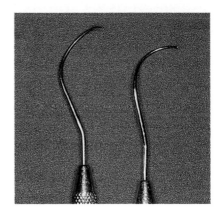

FIGURE 16-17
Furcation probes may be found using a Nabers probe with 3-mm markings *(right)* or without *(left)*.

furcation explored as the probe is moved with a horizontal walking stroke apically and laterally into the furca.

Classifications

Furcations are classified as Class I, II, III, or IV.[9] Class I furcations are incipient, and the Nabers probe penetrates the furcation entrance less than 3 mm. A Class II furca can be explored equal to or greater than 3 mm but not all the way through the furca. A Class III furca allows the probe tip to pass completely through the furcation opening (Figure 16-18). In a Class IV furca, the gingiva is receding, permitting visibility from facial to lingual. With the exception of Class I furcation involvement, bone loss in furcations is usually evident on posterior periapical and bite-wing radiographs (Table 16-1).

Table 16-1	**Grades of Furcation**		
DEGREE	**NAME**	**DESCRIPTION**	**CHARTING SYMBOL**
I	Incipient furcal lesion	Circumferential movement of the probe reveals slight V-shaped indentation (depression) <3 mm horizontally.	∧
II	Patent furcal invasion	Loss of bone extends horizontally underneath roof of furca ≥3 mm horizontally.	∇
III	Communicating furcal invasion	Furcation is open from both facial and lingual approaches (through and through) but covered by gingival tissue.	▲
IV	Clinically visible furcation	Furcation is through and through; loss of bone with furca is visible in the mouth.	◆

Data from Lindhe J, Nyman S: The effect of plaque control and surgical pocket elimination on the establishment and maintenance of periodontal health: a longitudinal study of periodontal therapy in cases of advanced disease, *J Clin Periodontol* 2:67, 1975; and Carranza FA Jr, Takei HH: Treatment of furcation involvement and combined periodontal–endodontic therapy. In Newman MG, Carranza FA Jr, Takei H, ed: *Carranza's clinical periodontology,* ed 9, Philadelphia, 2001, WB Saunders.

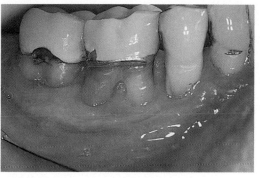

FIGURE 16-18
This patient has severe attachment loss resulting in a Class III furcation.

DETECT MOBILITY

16-13
16-14

Because of the soft periodontal ligament between the tooth and alveolar bone proper, teeth are naturally slightly mobile (physiologic mobility) unless they are **ankylosed** (fused to the bone) in the socket. Therefore tooth mobility is a concern only when it is excessive (1 degree or greater) or increasing. Possible causes of tooth mobility are listed in Box 16-3. When excessive occlusal or nonocclusal forces are applied to a tooth, the result may be a decrease in the density of the surrounding bone. Once the excessive force is relieved, the bone density returns to normal. The degree to which excessive or abnormal forces contribute to attachment loss in a periodontium stressed by inflammation is inconclusive.

Measurement of mobility is accomplished by placing the ends of the handles of two single-ended instruments on the buccal and lingual or palatal middle thirds of the tooth crown, followed by a gentle attempt to rock (move) the tooth in a buccolingual direction[32] (Figure 16-19). The clinician should examine the contact between the adjacent tooth to look for tooth movement. Movement is estimated in millimeters from 0 to 3 (Table 16-2). Vertical depressibility of the tooth is also examined by placing the side of the handle on the incisal or cuspal

BOX 16-3

POSSIBLE CAUSES OF ABNORMAL TOOTH MOBILITY

Attachment loss: Periodontal disease, periodontal surgery, orthodontic correction
Occlusal trauma: Malpositioned teeth, including teeth not in occlusion, clenching, bruxism
Inflammation: Periodontal or periapical, edematous gingival tissues
Diseases of the jaw: Cysts and benign and malignant tumors

edge of the tooth with gentle application of pressure in an apical direction. Mobility, particularly implant mobility, also may be electronically evaluated (the Periotest [Siemens AG, Bensheim, Germany]). Although getting an agreement on mobility patterns between two examiners is difficult, the relative mobility of one tooth compared with another is the key element in the assessment of mobility patterns. Although mobility is the movement of a tooth caused by the examiner, *fremitus* is the movement of teeth in function. Fremitus may be important when a patient has tooth pain or has had significant attachment loss.

The American Academy of Periodontology (AAP) has developed thirteen "Parameters of Care." These parameters are designed to assist clinicians in making decisions to provide appropriate services without sacrificing quality. The "Parameter on Comprehensive Periodontal Examination"[1] is summarized in Box 16-4. The complete parameters are available on the AAP web site at http://www.perio.org.

✦ CASE APPLICATION 16-1.11

Periodontal Charting: Mobility
Mrs. Bozenski's chart should be reviewed for notations of mobility. What other factors are identifiable with her case to cause mobility?

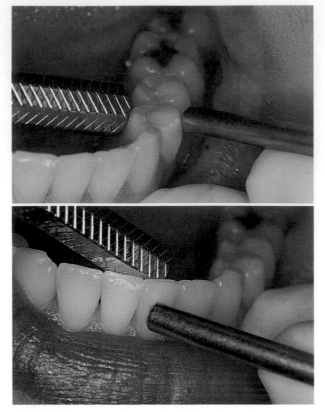

FIGURE 16-19
Mobility is detected with the blunt ends of two instruments, not with an instrument and finger.

BOX 16-4

PARAMETER ON COMPREHENSIVE PERIODONTAL EXAMINATION (AMERICAN ACADEMY OF PERIODONTOLOGY)[1]

- Medical history taken and evaluated.
- Dental history taken and evaluated.
- Extraoral structures examined and evaluated.
- Intraoral tissues and structures examined and evaluated.
- Teeth and their replacements examined and evaluated.
- Radiographs that are current and diagnostic should be used.
- Presence and distribution of plaque and calculus should be determined.
- Periodontal soft tissues should be examined and evaluated. Presence and types of exudates should be determined.
- Probing depths, attachment levels, and bleeding on probing should be evaluated.
- Mucogingival relationships should be evaluated.
- Presence, location, and extent of furcation invasions should be determined.
- Use of additional diagnostic aids may be warranted.
- All relevant clinical findings should be documented in the patient record.
- Referral to other healthcare providers should be made as appropriate.
- A diagnosis and treatment plan should be formulated and presented to the patient. (This parameter endorses the use of the PSR screening procedure when appropriate.)

Table 16-2	Tooth Mobility	
DEGREE	**DESCRIPTION**	**CHARTING SYMBOL**
1	Tooth moves 0.2 to 1 mm in horizontal direction.	1
2	Tooth moves >1 mm in horizontal direction.	2
3	Tooth is vertically depressible.	3

From Nyman S, Lindhe J: Examination of patients with periodontal disease. In Lindhe J et al, eds: *Clinical periodontology and implant dentistry,* ed 3, Munksgaard, Denmark, 1997, Copenhagen.

DETECT FREMITUS

Fremitus is tooth movement caused by occlusal forces or the ability of a patient to displace and traumatize his or her teeth. Unlike the measurement of mobility, where the clinician applies lateral or vertical pressure to a tooth and then measures the visible movement, the measurement of fremitus requires the patient to apply occlusal force by pressing/clinching the teeth together while the clinician feels for the vibratory pattern.

To measure fremitus, the clinician places a finger along the buccal or facial surfaces of the maxillary teeth (see Figure 16-20). As the patient taps his or her teeth together and grinds them in lateral and protrusive movements, the clinician will be able to feel teeth that are displaced and apply the following scale to the intensity of detected vibration or displacement:

Class I: Mild vibration or displacement
Class II: Easily detected vibration or displacement with no visible movement
Class III: Visible displacement

ASSESS PLAQUE BIOFILM AND CALCULUS ACCUMULATIONS

16-15

Deposits in the oral cavity include plaque biofilm, calculus, stain, and **materia alba.** These deposits may be found on the teeth, soft tissues, and restorative and prosthetic materials.

Plaque biofilm is a complex but organized collection of bacterial colonies. Although bacterial plaque biofilm is the primary etiology of periodontal diseases, the type of bacteria, the time the bacterial plaque biofilm is allowed to remain undisturbed on the teeth, and the host response to the bacteria are all critical factors for the risk of the initiation and progression of periodontal disease.[27,36]

At one time, periodontal diseases were thought to be degenerative in nature. As the general role that plaque biofilm plays

A   B   C

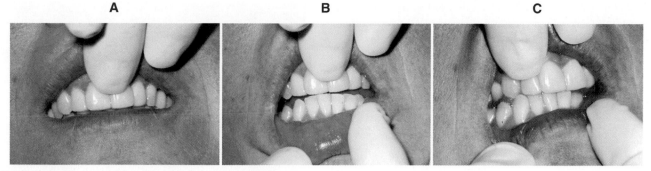

FIGURE 16-20
A, To feel vibratory patterns of teeth during occlusion, the clinician places a finger along the buccal or facial surfaces of the maxillary teeth. **B,** With edge-to-edge occlusion, placement of the finger can be made on the mandibular teeth. **C,** As the patient taps the teeth together and performs lateral and protrusive movements, the clinician will be able to feel teeth that are being displaced. (From Rose LF et al: *Periodontics: Medicine, Surgery, and Implants,* St Louis, 2004, Mosby.)

in inflammation became known, the **nonspecific plaque hypothesis,** or quantitative theory, was proposed. This theory stated that the composition of plaque biofilm was not important but that disease depended solely on the accumulation or presence of plaque biofilm on the teeth.[28] Current evidence supports the **specific plaque (or qualitative) hypothesis.** This hypothesis states that plaque biofilm composition may vary in the types and numbers of microbial organisms and that different microorganisms may cause different periodontal diseases. Additionally, periodontal disease activity exhibits bursts of activity, causing attachment loss, and periods of **quiescence,** during which attachment loss does not progress.

More than 400 species of bacteria have been isolated from human periodontal pockets. Only a relatively few of these bacteria are associated with periodontal disease. In health, plaque biofilm usually is composed of gram-positive, facultative aerobes that are not motile. The plaque biofilm is thin and stains pink with an erythrosin-disclosing dye. When plaque biofilm is not disturbed, plaque colonies continue to grow and mature; as bacteria die, the bacterial mass becomes thicker. The bacterial types shift to anaerobic cocci, filaments, rods, and spirochetes, and the microbes are generally more gram-negative, motile, and strictly anaerobic. Major components of the cell wall of gram-negative bacteria are lipopolysaccharides, an endotoxin. When a gram-negative bacterial cell dies, the endotoxin is released from the lipopolysaccharides layer, amplifying the inflammation process and promoting tissue damage and bone resorption.

Although several organisms closely associated with the initiation and progression of periodontal disease have been studied, **Koch's postulates** have yet to be satisfied for bacteria associated with either gingivitis or periodontitis. Koch's postulates[13] stipulate that the causative agent of disease must adhere to the following:

- Be routinely isolated from the diseased individual
- Be grown in pure culture in the laboratory
- Be able to produce a similar disease when inoculated into susceptible laboratory animals
- Be recovered from lesions in a diseased laboratory animal

Some researchers have theorized that Koch's postulates will

never be satisfied because of both the limitations of the postulates themselves and the nature of the periodontal diseases.[36] In 1979, other criteria were suggested that established an etiologic role of a microorganism in periodontal diseases.[35]

- Be associated with disease, as evident by increases in the number of organisms at the diseased site
- Be eliminated or decreased in sites that demonstrate resolution with treatment
- Demonstrate the stimulation of a host response
- Be capable of causing disease in experimental animal models
- Demonstrate virulence factors responsible for allowing the organism to cause destruction of the periodontal tissues in the host

Many of the microorganisms associated with periodontal disease, or periodontopathogens, are difficult to harvest and successfully culture. A partial list of suggested periodontal pathogens[36,39] is shown in Box 16-5.

How these bacteria relate to one another remains unclear. Is disease initiated by one bacterium and progression caused by another? Because these are mixed infections, does more than one species act together? What is the role of the host in the initiation and progression of disease? These and other research questions are the subject of continuous, ongoing dental research.

BOX 16-5

PERIODONTAL PATHOGENS

Actinobacillus actinomycetemcomitans
Campylobacter rectus
Eikenella corrodens
Fusobacterium nucleatum
Peptostreptococcus micros
Porphyromonas gingivalis
Prevotella intermedia
Streptococcus intermedius
Tannerella forsythensis (Bacteroides forsythus)
Treponema species

Plaque biofilm is typically not visible to the untrained eye unless significant accumulations are present. The trained eye can observe plaque biofilm by the dullness of the enamel surface and the lack of shine and reflection of light on the teeth (Figure 16-21). With the application of a disclosing solution or tablet, usually an erythrosin dye, plaque biofilm is easy to see (Figure 16-22). Plaque biofilm may be measured in several different ways: quantity, location on the tooth, or age of the plaque biofilm. However, of primary importance for periodontal reasons is the location of undisturbed bacterial plaque biofilm interproximally and along the gingival margin. Assisting patients in identifying and subsequently removing these plaque biofilm deposits is critical.

Calculus is a calcium and phosphate precipitate that firmly adheres to the tooth surface and dental prostheses (Figure 16-23). This hard, stonelike material consists of four crystal forms of calcium phosphate: hydroxyapatite (58%), octacalcium phosphate (21%), magnesium whitlockite (21%), and brushite (9%). Microscopically, calculus is a crystalline structure of approximately 70% to 90% inorganic and organic components. The primary crystalline form is hydroxyapatite with calcium phosphate the principle inorganic portion (75.9%). The variable number of calcium, phosphate, and hydroxyl groups distinguishes these forms of calculus.[8]

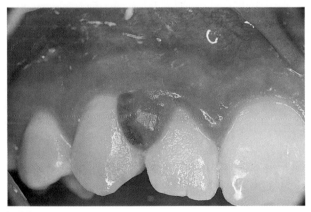

FIGURE 16-21
Unstained plaque biofilm may often leave a rough appearance on the tooth surface, as seen on the mesial surface of the lateral incisor, resulting in the enlarged gingival tissue.

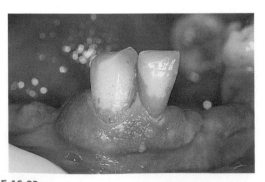

FIGURE 16-22
Dyes such as erythrosin allow good visualization of plaque biofilm.

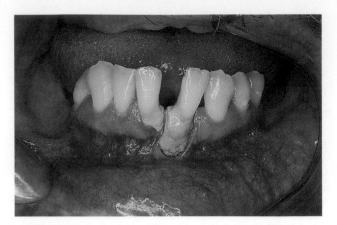

FIGURE 16-23
Left undisturbed, calculus may accumulate to a significant size.

Calculus attachment to the tooth surface has been described as one of the following four mechanisms[41]: (1) an organic pellicle, (2) penetration of calculus into cementum, (3) mechanical locking into surface irregularities, or (4) close adaptation of calculus to unaltered cementum. The attachment is often tenacious, particularly with calculus that has been present for a long time, and the calculus deposits may be difficult to remove with hand instrumentation. Powered instruments may be necessary to assist in removing long-standing calculus deposits.

Although calculus does not cause periodontal disease, it is considered a significant contributing factor to the disease because its surface provides excellent retention for bacterial plaque biofilm.[29] Therefore the periodontal assessment must yield an evaluation of the location and quantity of calculus to plan for professional removal and daily control of this deposit. Calculus is detected with the use of a fine-tined explorer or periodontal probe such as the PSR probe or Moffitt-Maryland probe, a good light, and compressed air. The instrument is held with a light grasp and guided along the tooth surface with the use of tactile sense to feel for irregularities in the smoothness of the crown or root. Radiographs may also be used in calculus detection; heavier interproximal deposits of calculus appear as opaque deposits on the tooth or root surface.

Supragingival (salivary) calculus deposits occur coronal to the gingival margin and are initially whitish or cream-colored until they absorb tobacco and food stains. Supragingival calculus is most frequently found opposite ducts to the major salivary glands, on the lingual surfaces of the mandibular anterior teeth adjacent to ducts from the submandibular glands, and on buccal surfaces of the maxillary posterior teeth adjacent to ducts from the parotid glands. As saliva pools in these areas, minerals from the saliva precipitate onto irregularities in the tooth surface, incorporating plaque biofilm contents into the calculus matrix.

As the name suggests, **subgingival** (serumal) calculus forms beneath the gingival margin (Figure 16-24). Mineral components precipitate from the gingival crevicular fluid to

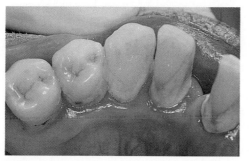

FIGURE 16-24
The light-appearing calculus is salivary calculus, whereas the dark calculus is serumal calculus. Serumal calculus starts in a subgingival location but may eventually be supragingival as a result of gingival recession.

calcify against the root surface, entrapping subgingival plaque biofilm as the deposit grows. Subgingival calculus is denser than supragingival calculus and may be located anywhere in the mouth apical to the margin of the gingiva. It can take the form of spicules, solid masses, or sheets of calculus and develops a dark stain from the blood pigment *hemosiderin*. Occasionally, subgingival calculus is close to the gingival margin and visible through the gingival tissue as a darkened spot on the tissue. When recession of the gingival margin occurs, which enables what was originally subgingival calculus to become visible, it may be referred to as *supragingival calculus,* even though the derivation and appearance are different from true supragingival calculus.

Indices

In clinical practice, **indices** are used to evaluate patient oral hygiene proficiency, gingival inflammation, and bleeding changes and to assist in patient education. Indices in periodontal assessment are categorized as bleeding, plaque biofilm, gingival, calculus, oral hygiene care, attachment levels, and other measurements of disease severity. As an alternative or in addition to the use of an index, clinicians may choose to draw the location of plaque or calculus deposits and record bleeding points on the periodontal chart as documentation and for use as a patient education tool.

When using a bleeding index, the clinician should distinguish whether the bleeding is from a gingival or a periodontal pocket because different procedures may be used to control inflammation in either pocket. Through appropriate self-care, patients can eliminate marginal gingival bleeding by mechanically controlling the plaque biofilm, but patients cannot reach the bacterial masses in deep pockets. To detect marginal bleeding, the periodontal probe is slid or swept circumferentially at a 45-degree angle, 2 to 3 mm along the inside of the gingival pocket. Bleeding on probing is detected during periodontal probing procedures. Stimulation of the papillary gingival areas with a soft wooden stick (e.g., Stim-U-Dent), dental floss, or probe may be used to obtain another measurement of interdental gingival bleeding.[31]

Bleeding may be recorded as a dichotomous event (present or absent) or given a score according to how quickly the bleeding appears, usually waiting 30 seconds or less before recording. Tobacco use has an adverse effect on the periodontium and an effect on bleeding scores. Bleeding scores of smokers have been shown to be both greater and lesser than the scores of nonsmokers. For this reason, bleeding indices should not be compared between smokers and nonsmokers[31] (Table 16-3).

The record of the quantity and location of plaque biofilm may serve as patient monitoring and patient educational tools. Again, however, clinicians must understand exactly what the index is measuring. Because the quantity of plaque biofilm does not equate well to the severity of disease, plaque biofilm indices are actually a measure of tooth-cleaning efficacy. The location of plaque biofilm rather than the quantity of plaque biofilm is emphasized in other plaque biofilm indices. Some indices record plaque biofilm only where it is in contact with gingiva, whereas other indices include plaque biofilm that occurs on any area of any tooth. Plaque biofilm indices may or may not use disclosing agents (Table 16-4).

Gingival indices usually include assessments of color, edema, contour, and bleeding. Clinical signs are generally obtained by inspections for color and contour and by the use of the probe to elicit edema or bleeding. Interpretation of color and contour criteria is more subjective than indices that score bleeding (Table 16-5).

Calculus indices are more frequently used in research studies and clinical trials involving anticalculus agents than they are in clinical practice. In patient care, the quantity and frequency of calculus accumulation is simply one indication of how frequently the patient needs professional debridement. Clinicians may choose to record calculus pictorially by drawing the location and shape of the calculus deposits on the chart rather than obtaining an index (Table 16-6).

Indices are also available that assess oral cleanliness or oral debris, often combining plaque biofilm, material alba, stain, and calculus into a single score. In patient care, the indices generally include all teeth and all tooth surfaces, unlike epidemiologic surveys in which only specified teeth or surfaces may be measured.

Periodontal indices attempt to measure the degree of periodontal destruction. The typical index in periodontal assessment is an historical record, one of past destruction or of current periodontal symptoms that are not predictive of the presence, severity, or future course of the infection (Table 16-7). Currently, evaluating attachment loss or gain is considered one of the most valid measurements of the status of periodontal disease. Although pocket or probing depths are usually obtained in indices of periodontal disease, pocket depth alone does not equate to attachment loss or necessarily to an unhealthy pocket. Periodontal indices provide only a record of previous destruction, not a prediction of the future course of the disease.

Table 16-3	**Bleeding Indices**			
NAME	**YEAR**	**AUTHORS**	**METHOD**	**SCALE**
Modified Sulcular Bleeding Index (mSBI)	1987	Mombelli et al[a]	Note bleeding on gentle probing.	Ordinal (0 to 3)
Interdental Bleeding Index	1985	Caton and Polson[b]	Insert wooden interdental cleaner interproximally facially 1 to 2 mm four times; observe for 15 seconds.	Dichotomous
Eastman Interdental Bleeding Index	1984	Abrams, Caton, and Polson[c]	Insert triangular wooden toothpick midinterproximally.	Dichotomous
Gingival Bleeding Time Index (BTI)	1981	Nowicki et al[d]	Slide probe back and forth against inner margin of gingiva; wait 15 seconds; may repeat once.	Ordinal (0 to 4)
Modified Papillary Bleeding Index (mPBI)	1980	Barnett, Ciancio, and Mather[e]	Add time to papillary bleeding index (PBI).	Ordinal (0 to 4)
Papillary Bleeding Score (PBS) Modified from PBI	1979	Loesche[f]	Insert Stim-U-Dent interproximally.	Ordinal (0 to 5)
Gingival Bleeding Index (GBI)	1975	Ainamo and Bay[g]	Perform circumferential stroke at gingival orifice; wait 10 seconds.	Dichotomous
GBI	1974	Carter and Barnes[h]	Slide unwaxed dental floss interproximally; wait up to 30 seconds.	Dichotomous
Gingival Sulcus Bleeding Index (SBI)	1971	Mühlemann and Son[i]	Perform sulcus probing on dry teeth.	Ordinal (0 to 5; score ≥2 on color if bleeding occurs)

[a]Mombelli A et al: The microbiota associated with successful or failing implants, *Oral Microbiol Immunol* 2:145, 1987.
[b]Caton JG, Polson AM: The interdental bleeding index: a simplified procedure for monitoring oral gingival health, *Compend Cont Educ Dent* 6(2):88, 1985.
[c]Abrams K, Caton J, Polson A: Histologic comparisons of interproximal gingival tissues related to the presence or absence of bleeding, *J Periodontol* 55:629, 1984.
[d]Nowicki D et al: The gingival bleeding time index, *J Periodontol* 52:260, 1981.
[e]Barnett M, Ciancio S, Mather M: The modified papillary bleeding index: comparison with gingival index during the resolution of gingivitis, *J Prev Dent* 6:135, 1980.
[f]Loesche WJ: Clinical and microbiological aspects of chemotherapeutic agents according to the specific plaque hypothesis, *J Dent Res* 58:2404, 1979.
[g]Ainamo J, Bay I: Problems and proposals for recording gingivitis and plaque, *Int Dent J* 25:229, 1975.
[h]Carter HG, Barnes GP: The gingival bleeding index, *J Periodontol* 45:801, 1974.
[i]Mühlemann HR, Son S: Gingival sulcus bleeding—a leading symptom in initial gingivitis, *Helv Odontol Acta* 15:107, 1971.

Dental Factors in Periodontal Disease Risk

Any condition in the patient that enhances the colonization of bacteria, increases the difficulty of plaque biofilm control, or alters the initiation or progression of disease should be considered a contributing factor to periodontal disease risk. These factors are listed in Box 16-6.

One type of anatomical variation is the palatogingival groove, which commonly appears on the lingual surface of the maxillary lateral incisor. This deep developmental groove extends apically from cingulum on the lingual aspect of the root (Figure 16-25).

BOX 16-6

PERIODONTAL DISEASE RISK FACTORS

Missing teeth	Anatomical variations
Dental caries	Palatogingival grooves
Open contacts	Cervicoenamel projections
Faulty restorations	Impacted or supernumerary teeth
Malpositioned teeth	Decreased salivary flow

Cervicoenamel projections occur in the furcations of mandibular molars, causing an abnormality in tissue attachment (Figure 16-26).

Table 16-4	Plaque Biofilm Indices			
NAME	**YEAR**	**AUTHORS**	**METHOD**	**AREA EVALUATED**
Distal Mesial Plaque Index (DMPI), Modified Navy (MN) Index	1987	Fischman et al[a]	Disclose.	Entire surface with more emphasis at proximal surfaces and a measure of quantity
Navy Plaque Index (Modified; MN)	1972	Elliott, Bowers, and Rovelstad[b]	Disclose. Score I (plaque biofilm present) for each of nine areas.	Nine divisions of tooth surface with more divisions at gingival margin
Plaque Control Record	1972	O'Leary, Drake, and Naylor[c]	Record presence of plaque biofilm to allow patient to visualize areas.	Four tooth surfaces of all teeth present
Turesky Modification of the Quigley-Hein Plaque Index	1970	Turesky, Gilmore, and Glickman[d]	Disclose.	Plaque biofilm assessment on facial and lingual surfaces of all teeth
Patient Hygiene Performance (PHP)	1968	Podshadley and Haley[e]	Disclose, and record presence or absence of plaque biofilm.	Teeth #3, #8, #14, #19, #24, and #30
Plaque Index (PI)	1964	Silness and Löe[f]	Dry teeth; use mouth mirror and explorer.	Gingival one third of tooth surfaces or tooth
Simplified Oral Hygiene Index (OHI-S)	1964	Greene and Vermillion[g]	Perform same as OHI with different teeth selected.	Facial surfaces of teeth #3, #8, #14, and #24, and lingual surfaces of #9 and #39
Quigley-Hein Plaque Index	1962	Quigley and Hein[h]	Disclose.	Surface scored from 0 to 5 with emphasis at gingival margin
Oral Hygiene Index; Debris Index; Calculus Index	1960	Greene and Vermillion[i]	Assess oral cleanliness by estimation of the mouth divided into six segments.	Tooth surface covered with debris or calculus or both

[a]Fischman S et al: Distal mesial plaque index: a technique for assessing dental plaque about the gingiva, *Dent Hyg* 61:404, 1987.
[b]Elliott JR, Bowers GM, Rovelstad GH III: Evaluation of an oral physiotherapy center in the reduction of bacterial plaque and periodontal disease, *J Periodontol* 43:221, 1972.
[c]O'Leary TJ, Drake RB, Naylor JE: The plaque control record, *J Periodontol* 43:38, 1972.
[d]Turesky S, Gilmore ND, Glickman I: Reduced plaque formation by the chloromethyl analogue of vitamin C, *J Periodontol* 41:41, 1970.
[e]Podshadley AG, Haley JVA: A method for evaluating oral hygiene performance, *Public Health Rep* 83:259, 1968.
[f]Silness J, Löe H: Periodontal disease in pregnancy. II. Correlation between oral hygiene and periodontal condition, *Acta Odontol Scand* 22:112, 1964.
[g]Greene JC, Vermillion JR: The simplified oral hygiene index, *J Am Dent Assoc* 68:7, 1964.
[h]Quigley GA, Hein JW: Comparative cleansing efficiency of manual and power brushing, *J Am Dent Assoc* 65:26, 1962.
[i]Greene JC, Vermillion JR: The oral hygiene index: a method for classifying oral hygiene status, *J Am Dent Assoc* 61:172, 1960.

Table 16-5	Gingival Indices		
NAME	**YEAR**	**AUTHORS**	**METHOD**
Gingival Index (GI)	1963	Löe and Silness*	Observe; perform circumferential stroke against soft tissue below gingival margin.
Papillary-Marginal-Attached Index (PMAI)	1947	Schour and Massler†	Observe; press probe against gingiva.

*Löe H, Silness J: Periodontal disease in pregnancy. I. Prevalence and severity, *Acta Odontol Scand* 21:533, 1963.
†Schour I, Massler M: Prevalence of gingivitis in various age groups, *J Am Dent Assoc* 35:475, 1947.

Table 16-6	Calculus Indices			
NAME		**YEAR**	**AUTHORS**	**METHOD**
Marginal Line Calculus Index (MLC-I)		1967	Mühlemann and Villa*	Divide tooth in half (mesial and distal); with air, visualize minute areas of supramarginal calculus next to gingiva on lingual four mandibular incisors.
Volpe-Manhold (V-M) Calculus Assessment		1965	Volpe, Manhold, and Hazen[†]	Measure with probe in three planes.
Calculus Index Simplified (CI-S), Part of Simplified Oral Hygiene Index (OHI-S)		1964	Greene and Vermillion[‡]	With an explorer, detect calculus on tooth surface or around cervical portion of tooth.
Calculus Surface Index		1961	Ennever, Sturzenberger, and Radike[§]	Use air, mirror, and explorer to detect calculus.

*Mühlemann HR, Villa PR: The marginal line calculus index, *Helv Odontol Acta* 11:175, 1967.
[†]Volpe AR, Manhold JH, Hazen SP: In vivo calculus assessment. Part I. A method and its examiner reproducibility, *J Periodontol* 36:292, 1965.
[‡]Greene JC, Vermillion JR: The simplified oral hygiene index, *J Am Dent Assoc* 68:7, 1964.
[§]Ennever J, Sturzenberger OP, Radike AW: The calculus surface index method for scoring clinical calculus studies, *J Periodontol* 32:54, 1961.

Table 16-7	Composite Periodontal Disease Indices			
NAME		**YEAR**	**AUTHORS**	**METHOD**
Periodontal Scoring and Recording (PSR) Index		1992	AAP, ADA[a]	This is an individual screening examination. Divide the mouth into six segments; record highest score according to four levels, including bleeding and probe depths.
Extent and Severity Index		1986	Carlos, Wolfe, and Kingman[b]	This index is for epidemiologic purposes. Estimate the attachment level from probe depths—14 sites in each of two contralateral quadrants.
Community Periodontal Index of Treatment Needs (CPITN)		1982	Ainamo et al[c]	This index is for epidemiologic purposes. Use O'Leary's sextants with specified index teeth or worst tooth, WHO probe, and 0 to 4 codes per sextant; evaluate bleeding, deposits, and pocket depth.
Periodontal Screening Examination		1967	O'Leary[d]	Divide mouth into six segments, and record highest score; score gingiva by color, contour, and consistency; score periodontium by mesiofacial line angle probe depth; score local irritants.
Periodontal Disease Index (PDI)		1967	Ramfjord[e]	Select the "Ramfjord" teeth (#3, #9, #12, #19, #25, and #28) and score for gingiva, attachment loss, calculus, and plaque biofilm.
Periodontal Index		1956	Russell[f]	Do not use probe; weight scores and combine gingival and periodontal status.

AAP, American Academy of Periodontology; *ADA*, American Dental Association; *WHO*, World Health Organization.
[a]American Academy of Periodontology and American Dental Association: *Periodontal screening and recording* (publication sponsored by Procter & Gamble), Cincinnati, 1992, Procter & Gamble.
[b]Carlos JP, Wolfe MD, Kingman A: The extent and severity index: a simple method for use in epidemiologic studies of periodontal disease, *J Clin Periodontol* 13:500, 1986.
[c]Ainamo J et al: Development of the World Health Organization (WHO) community periodontal index of treatment needs (CPTIN), *Int Dent J* 32:281, 1982.
[d]O'Leary TJ: The periodontal screening examination, *J Periodontol* 38:617, 1967.
[e]Ramfjord SP: The periodontal disease index (PDI), *J Periodontol* 38:602, 1967.
[f]Russell AL: A system of classification and scoring for prevalence surveys of periodontal disease, *J Dent Res* 35(3):350, 1956.

Both palatogingival grooves and cervicoenamel projections are considerably prone to plaque biofilm retention and are difficult to access by normal oral self-care measures.

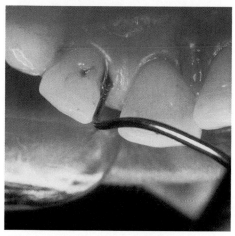

FIGURE 16-25
Palatogingival groove.

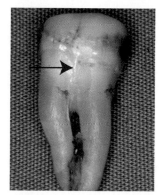

FIGURE 16-26
Cervicoenamel projection.

INTERPROXIMAL CONTACTS

Ideally, the interproximal surfaces of adjacent teeth contact each other at the heights of contour with the mesial surface of one tooth in contact with the distal surface of the adjacent tooth. The exception is the midline, where two mesial surfaces contact each other and the distal of the last tooth in the arch. The space apical to the contact area forms the gingival embrasure, a roughly pyramidal-shaped space filled with gingival papillae. When gingival recession is present, the gingival embrasure may be *open,* that is, no tissue filling the space. Table 16-8 classifies and describes gingival embrasure.

Any change in the character of an interproximal contact presents a greater challenge for plaque biofilm control. Contact areas that are too broad or too close to the gingiva or teeth not in contact all contribute to the accumulation of plaque biofilm and debris and food impaction. Missing and malpositioned teeth pose additional problems because surrounding teeth in the same arch and the opposing arch move into the space of the

Table 16-8	Classifications and Descriptions of Embrasures
CLASS	**DESCRIPTION**
I	Interdental papillae fill space between adjacent teeth in contact.
II	Interdental papillae are partially receded, resulting in small opening under contact.
III	Interdental papillae have completely receded, leaving triangular opening under contact.

Modified from Carranza FA, Newman MG: *Clinical periodontology,* ed 8, 1996, WB Saunders.

missing tooth. Thus the interproximal contacts of the teeth may move apart or shift to a different position over time, encouraging food impaction or tissue impingement.

★ CASE APPLICATION 16-1.12

Embrasure
What type of embrasure spaces does Mrs. Bozenski have?

RESTORATIVE MATERIALS

Restorations and prostheses must mimic the natural dentition as closely as possible to promote the maintenance of healthy gingiva. Conversely, faulty restorations may present the patient with areas that are exceptionally difficult to clean. Restorative materials with rough surfaces, overhangs, open or worn margins, or poorly contoured interproximal contacts result in plaque biofilm–retentive areas. Overcontoured or undercontoured restorations provide either too much or too little protection to the gingival embrasure area and may prevent normal physiologic cleansing (Figure 16-27).

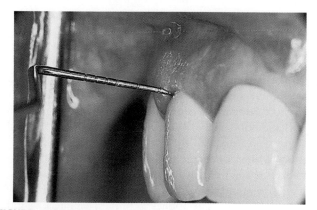

FIGURE 16-27
Overhanging restorations are harbingers for plaque biofilm accumulation and subsequent inflammation.

OTHER CONTRIBUTING FACTORS

Assessment of saliva, diet, and habits is also important to the quality and health of the periodontal tissues. Salivary flow is a major factor in normal physiologic oral cleansing. Individuals with reduced salivary flow, less than 1 ml/min, are prone to increased plaque biofilm retention and increased risk of dental caries. In addition, with less saliva available in the oral cavity, the protective mechanisms of the salivary components are reduced. Thus both quantity and quality of saliva should be evaluated with assessment of the periodontal condition.

Attention to the dietary choices of periodontal patients is important to ensure that the periodontal tissue receives adequate nourishment. Coenzymes such as vitamin C are necessary for the proper cross-linking of collagen to occur. Diet also influences plaque biofilm growth and retention. Additionally, some oral habits may be damaging to the oral cavity. Clenching and **bruxism** result in abnormal stress on the alveolar bone and may cause flexure of teeth, which results in root concavities called **abfraction lesions,** as well as accelerated wear of incisal edges, cusp tips, and occlusal surfaces. Incorrect brushing or incorrect use of auxiliary cleaning aids, such as toothpicks, may harm gingival tissues or root surfaces. Tobacco use is damaging to the periodontium. Particularly visible to the patient is the damage to the gingiva when smokeless tobacco quids are held in close proximity to gingival tissue, often resulting in areas of hyperkeratosis or gingival recession.

Examination and Evaluation of Dental Implants

For the patient with a dental implant, assessment of the periodontal health around it is an essential part of the periodontal examination. Examination of the surrounding tissue, implant mobility, the presence or absence of bleeding, alveolar bone height, patient comfort, and patient care of the implant are all part of the implant assessment. Inflammation may develop around an implant, similar to periodontal inflammation. A mobile implant is a failing implant.

Probing around implants may be somewhat different than examining natural teeth. Inadequate data exist on the relationship between osseointegration and probe depths, and occasional difficulties are encountered when probing around certain prosthetic devices attached to the implant. The gingiva is directly attached to the implant by a hemidesmosomal attachment of the junctional epithelium. The connective tissue forms a tight collar around the neck of the implant but is not directly attached to the implant fixture. Modification of assessment procedures is necessary to protect the implant surface,[26] usually titanium or hydroxyapatite, and the surrounding tissue. Any instrument used on or around implants must be plastic or graphite, not steel or metals other than titanium, to avoid altering the implant surface or the production of a galvanic reaction (Figure 16-28). This rule applies to probes, explorers, debridement instruments, rubber cup and air polishers, and personal oralcare devices.

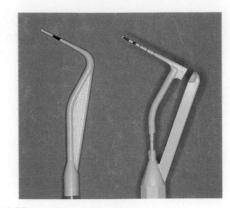

FIGURE 16-28
Plastic instruments, such as these probes, must be used around titanium implants.

Implant indices for plaque biofilm, gingival status, and bleeding have not been validated. The recommendation has been made that any periodontal index used for implants should be separate from the index used on teeth with roots. The appearance of the oral tissue next to the implant may differ, depending on whether the implant is surrounded by gingiva or alveolar mucosa. Careful inspection of the appearance of the implant and its surrounding tissue is necessary to observe cleanliness, deposit accumulation, erythema, bleeding, or the presence of suppuration. Regular intervals of radiographic assessment of alveolar bone levels are recommended when monitoring implant health.

Technology in the Periodontal Examination

Traditionally, periodontal examinations have been conducted using manual instruments. However, expanding technology has provided the clinician with automated methods of assessment and with additional diagnostic and monitoring tools. Some of these tests or assays are performed chairside, and some require laboratory analyses.[22,23] Although they are of scientific interest, many of these additional aids have yet to find a place in the everyday diagnosis of periodontal diseases and the prediction of disease activity.

One area of technology that has gained widespread acceptance is the use of the computerized or electronic dental record (EDR) and periodontal charting form. The paper periodontal chart may be reproduced in digital form with all clinical information stored electronically for immediate retrieval. The EDR allows for the collection of clinical data at different time points and the integration of digital radiographs and other digital clinical images of interest directly into the patient's EDR file. The recording process may be slow at first, but with practice, it becomes as fast as or faster than manual recording. Improvements in voice recognition software will soon allow for hands-free recording of clinical data with 99% accuracy.

IDENTIFYING INFLAMMATION

The PerioTemp (Abiodent, Inc., Danvers, Mass.) measures the sulcus temperature using an electronic probe. The theory of this instrument is based on the fact that inflamed tissue has a slightly higher temperature than healthy, uninflamed tissue. An elevated sulcus or pocket temperature may be an early sign of inflammation. Early gingival inflammation also may be evaluated, using the Periotron 8000 (Harco Electronics, Winnipeg, Manitoba, Canada), an instrument that measures the gingival crevicular fluid flow. Crevicular fluid flow is the first sign of clinical inflammation, increasing before either erythema or bleeding is evident in inflamed tissues.[10]

AUTOMATED PROBING SYSTEMS

Several automated probing systems are available that electronically record probe depths and can enter the readings into a computer file. Voice-activated recording systems are now a familiar tool in periodontal assessment. Advantages for these electronic, computerized assessment tools may be efficiency, improved infection control, and consistency in recording measurements. However, the clinician must properly use the measuring devices and understand the limitations of electronic measuring and recording. Some patients have reported increased discomfort of automated probing compared with manual probing.

IMAGING TECHNOLOGY

Improved methods of assessing bone loss or the progression of bone loss have been developed.[15] Using a copying process to provide greater contrast between structures, xeroradiography permits fine visualization of bone quality and density. Subtraction radiography converts radiographic images into digital images that, when superimposed, reveal minimal bone changes (bone loss as **radiolucent,** bone gain as **radiopaque**). Recently, the increasing use of digital radiologic techniques has allowed for improved imaging and detection of bone loss earlier than conventional radiographic techniques (see Chapter 18 for details).

A nuclear medicine method measures bone metabolism through means of a semiconductor radiation probe detector. A radiopharmaceutical agent is injected into a vein and then read by a semiconductor. A high degree of uptake by the bone may be predictive of future bone loss. These bone scans, visualizations predictive of bone loss, are more valuable than tests or radiographs that show the results of bone loss. As these tools for the evaluation and prediction of bone destruction improve, they should become part of the armamentarium for the prevention and control of periodontal diseases.

LABORATORY ASSAYS OF PERIODONTAL INFECTIONS

Clinical and radiographic examinations are essential methods of gathering assessment data to aid in the diagnosis of a periodontal condition. However, the ability to gather additional information via laboratory analysis is expanding. One of the earliest chairside procedures analyzing oral flora was the use of phase contrast or **darkfield microscopy** to identify the quantity, shapes, and motility of bacteria in the plaque biofilm. Placing a plaque sample on a slide and examining it has been used in the office as a patient educational and motivational tool and to assist in determining the age of the plaque biofilm by its morphologic characteristics and motility. However, neither type of microscopy can identify specific species of bacteria.[40]

Microbiologists are increasingly able to cultivate the anaerobic oral bacterial species and to associate these bacteria with certain types of periodontal diseases. Culturing permits the microbiologist to recover the widest range of bacterial species, which is an advantage because potential antibiotic use may then be more selective.

However, several problems exist with the cultivation of oral microorganisms. Culturing adequate samples from the diseased periodontal pocket is difficult because the bacteria may not survive the retrieval or transport process to the laboratory. Current culturing techniques do not always foster growth of highly sensitive periodontal pathogens. Culturing is also expensive and time-consuming. Finally, the bacteria that are isolated are only *presumed* to be those initiating or causing disease progression; their absolute role in periodontal disease has not been determined.

In addition to observing bacteria through the microscope or the culturing of oral microbes, other microbiologic assays are available. These include **immunoassays, nucleic acid probes,** and enzyme assays. Immunoassays use antibodies to detect bacterial antigens. Some types of immunoassays are available for use by clinicians in the office. The nucleic acid probe uses deoxyribonucleic acid (DNA) and occasionally ribonucleic acid (RNA) to hybridize the organism's genetic code and thus identify some species of oral microorganisms. DNA probes are available for many of the usual periodontopathogens, including *Actinobacillus actinomycetemcomitans, Tannerella forsythensis (Bacteroides forsythus), Campylobacter rectus, Eikenella corrodens, Fusobacterium nucleatum, Porphyromonas gingivalis, Prevotella intermedia,* and *Treponema denticola.*

Enzyme assays permit detection of enzymes the body may be producing to combat the effects of the periopathogenic organisms. Examples of the enzymes being studied are collagenase, elastase, beta-glucuronidase, and aspartate aminotransferase (AST). Although significant research has been conducted, these and other clinical assays have yet to find a place in routine periodontal care.[22]

Interleukin-1 (IL-1) is one of the many cytokines involved in the inflammatory process.[20] An association between a specific genotype of IL-1 and severe periodontal disease has been demonstrated.[19] A test has been developed, the PST (Medical Science Systems, Flagstaff, Ariz.), that can determine when a patient has this genotype that can produce as much as four times more IL-1 than other IL-1 genotypes. Although this test does not diagnose disease, it provides information to determine which patients have an increased susceptibility for the initiation and progression of disease. Based on computer models, patients with this specific IL-1 genotype who also smoke significantly increase their odds of developing severe periodontal disease. It has also been shown that patients of different ethnic and racial backgrounds show varying levels of IL-1 expression, rendering this test less useful than it might otherwise be.

Classification of Periodontal Disease

Periodontal disease is the result of predominantly gram-negative anaerobic microorganisms in a gingival pocket, thus stimulating an inflammatory response in the host. In patients susceptible to periodontal disease, this inflammation progresses from gingival inflammation into the attachment apparatus, causing destruction of connective tissue, apical migration of the junctional epithelium, and loss of bone surrounding the tooth. Left untreated, the ultimate fate is loss of a tooth or teeth.

In 1999 the Workshop on Classification of Periodontal Diseases and Conditions developed a new, comprehensive classification system for periodontal disease (Box 16-7).[4] Periodontal disease classifications are not age-dependent and are not based on the rate of progression. The extent of periodontal disease is

---

BOX 16-7

CLASSIFICATION OF PERIODONTAL DISEASES

I. *Gingival Diseases*
  A. Dental plaque biofilm–induced gingival diseases
    1. *Gingivitis associated with dental plaque biofilm only*
      a. Without other local contributing factors
      b. With local contributing factors (see VIII A)
    2. *Gingival diseases modified by systemic factors*
      a. Associated with the endocrine system
        i. Puberty-associated gingivitis
        ii. Menstrual cycle–associated gingivitis
        iii. Pregnancy-associated
          (1) Gingivitis
          (2) Pyogenic granuloma
        iv. Diabetes mellitus–associated gingivitis
      b. Associated with blood dyscrasias
        i. Leukemia-associated gingivitis
        ii. Other
    3. *Gingival diseases modified by medications*
      a. Drug-influenced gingival diseases
        i. Drug-induced gingival enlargements
        ii. Drug-influenced gingivitis
          (1) Oral contraceptive–associated gingivitis
          (2) Other
    4. *Gingival diseases modified by malnutrition*
      a. Ascorbic acid–deficiency gingivitis
      b. Other diseases
  B. Non–plaque biofilm–induced gingival lesions
    1. *Gingival lesions of specific bacterial origin*
      a. *Neisseria gonorrhea*–associated lesions
      b. *Treponema pallidum*–associated lesions
      c. Streptococcal species–associated lesions
      d. Other
    2. *Gingival diseases of viral origin*
      a. Herpes virus infections
        i. Primary herpetic gingivostomatitis
        ii. Recurrent oral herpes
        iii. Varicella-zoster infections
      b. Other diseases
    3. *Gingival diseases of fungal origin*
      a. *Candida* species infections
        i. Generalized gingival candidiasis
        ii. Linear gingival erythema

        iii. Histoplasmosis
        iv. Other
    4. *Gingival lesions of genetic origin*
      a. Hereditary gingival fibromatosis
      b. Other lesions
    5. *Gingival manifestations of systemic conditions*
      a. Mucocutaneous disorders
        i. Lichen planus
        ii. Pemphigoid
        iii. Pemphigus vulgaris
        iv. Erythema multiforme
        v. Lupus erythematosus
        vi. Drug-induced disorders
        vii. Other disorders
      b. Allergic reactions
        i. Dental restorative materials
          (1) Mercury
          (2) Nickel
          (3) Acrylic
          (4) Other materials
        ii. Reactions attributable to the following:
          (1) Toothpastes and dentifrices
          (2) Mouthrinses and mouthwashes
          (3) Chewing gum additives
          (4) Foods and additives
        iii. Other allergic responses
    6. *Traumatic lesions (factitious, iatrogenic, accidental)*
      a. Chemical injury
      b. Physical injury
      c. Thermal injury
    7. *Foreign body reactions*
    8. *Not otherwise specified*
II. *Chronic Periodontitis*
  A. Localized
  B. Generalized
III. *Aggressive Periodontitis*
  A. Localized
  B. Generalized

BOX 16-7

CLASSIFICATION OF PERIODONTAL DISEASES—CONT'D

IV. *Periodontitis as a Manifestation of Systemic Diseases*
A. Associated with hematologic disorders
  1. *Acquired neutropenia*
  2. *Leukemias*
  3. *Other*
B. Associated with genetic disorders
  1. *Familial and cyclic neutropenia*
  2. *Down syndrome*
  3. *Leukocyte adhesion deficiency syndromes*
  4. *Papillon-Lefèvre syndrome*
  5. *Chediak-Higashi syndrome*
  6. *Histiocytosis syndromes*
  7. *Glycogen storage disease*
  8. *Infantile genetic agranulocytosis*
  9. *Cohen syndrome*
  10. *Ehlers-Danlos syndrome (Types IV and VIII)*
  11. *Hypophosphatasia*
  12. *Other genetic disorders*
C. Not otherwise specified

V. *Necrotizing Periodontal Diseases*
A. Necrotizing ulcerative gingivitis
B. Necrotizing ulcerative periodontitis

VI. *Abscesses of the Periodontium*
A. Gingival abscess
B. Periodontal abscess
C. Pericoronal abscess

VII. *Periodontitis Associated with Endodontic Lesions*
A. Combined periodontal-endodontic lesions

VIII. *Developmental or Acquired Deformities or Conditions*
A. Localized tooth-related factors that modify or predispose to plaque biofilm–induced gingival diseases or periodontitis

  1. *Tooth anatomical factors*
  2. *Dental restorations and appliances*
  3. *Root fractures*
  4. *Cervical root resorption and cemental tears*
B. Mucogingival deformities and conditions around teeth
  1. *Gingival/soft tissue recession*
    a. Facial or lingual surfaces
    b. Interproximal (papillary)
  2. *Lack of keratinized gingiva*
  3. *Decreased vestibular depth*
  4. *Aberrant frenum/muscle position*
  5. *Gingival excess*
    a. Pseudopockets
    b. Inconsistent gingival margin
    c. Excessive gingival display
    d. Gingival enlargement (see "Gingival diseases modified by medications" and "Gingival lesions of genetic origin" sections)
  6. *Abnormal color*
C. Mucogingival deformities and conditions on edentulous ridges
  1. *Vertical or horizontal ridge deficiency or both*
  2. *Lack of gingival/keratinized tissue*
  3. *Gingival/soft tissue enlargement*
  4. *Aberrant frenum/muscle position*
  5. *Decreased vestibular depth*
  6. *Abnormal color*
D. Occlusal trauma
  1. *Primary occlusal trauma*
  2. *Secondary occlusal trauma*

Modified from Armitage GC: Development of a classification system for periodontal diseases and conditions. *Ann Periodontal* 1999, 4:1-6.

---

classified as *localized* when less than 30% of the existing sites are involved and *generalized* when more than 30% of those sites are involved. The severity of periodontal disease is based on CAL, with *slight* defined as 1 to 2 mm of CAL, *moderate* as 3 to 4 mm of CAL, and *severe* as 5 mm or more.[4]

Refractory is a term that can be applied to any classification of periodontal disease that is unresponsive to professional therapy and compliant patient self-care. The refractory classification is also applied to any specific disease category to further clarify the disease.[4]

Categories VI (abscesses of the periodontium), VII (periodontitis associated with endodontic lesions), and VIII (developmental or acquired deformities and conditions) represent specific and special diagnostic and treatment challenges within the scope of periodontics. Of these three categories, category VI is most likely to be used by the dental hygienist.[4]

It is important to understand that knowledge of periodontal diseases is continually changing through research and with the advent of new technology designed to assist in research. As re-searchers discover more about the etiology and treatment of disease, the current classification system will change.[4]

References

1. American Academy of Periodontology: Parameter on comprehensive periodontal examination, *J Periodontol* 71:847, 2000.
2. Anderson GB et al: Correlation of periodontal probe penetration and degree of inflammation, *Am J Dent* 4:177, 1991.
3. Armitage GC: (Clinical evaluation of periodontal diseases, *Periodontol 2000* 7:39, 1995.) The complete periodontal examination, *Periodontol 2000* 34:22, 2004.
4. Armitage GC: (Development of a classification system for periodontal diseases and conditions, *Ann Periodontal* 4:1, 1999.) Periodontal diagnoses and classification of periodontal diseases, *Periodontol 2000* 34:9, 2004.
5. Beersten W, McCullouch AG, Sodek J: The periodontal ligament: a unique, multifunctional connective tissue, *Periodontol 2000* 13:20, 1997.
6. Bosshardt DD, Selvig KA: Dental cementum: the dynamic covering of the root, *Periodontol 2000* 13:41, 1997.

7. Bowers GM: A study of the width of the attached gingival, *J Periodontol* 34:201, 1963.
8. Carranza FA Jr: Dental calculus. In Carranza FA Jr, Newman MG, eds: *Clinical periodontology*, ed 8, Philadelphia, 1996, WB Saunders.
9. Carranza FA Jr, Takei HH: Treatment of furcation involvement and combined periodontal-endodontic therapy. In Newman MG, Carranza FA Jr, Takei H, eds: *Carranza's clinical periodontology*, ed 9, Philadelphia, 2002, WB Saunders.
10. Caton J: Periodontal diagnosis and diagnostic aids. In Nevins M et al, eds: *Proceedings of the World Workshop in Clinical Periodontics*, Chicago, 1989, American Academy of Periodontology.
11. Freed HK, Gapper RL, Kallwarf KL: Evaluation of periodontal probing forces, *J Periodontol* 54:488, 1983.
12. Gargiulo AW, Wentz FM, Orban B: Dimensions and relations of the dentogingival junction in humans, *J Periodontol* 32:261, 1961.
13. Haake SK: Periodontal microbiology. In Newman MG, Carranza FA Jr, Takei H, eds: *Carranza's clinical periodontology*, ed 9, Philadelphia, 2002, WB Saunders.
14. Hassell T: Tissues and cells of the periodontium, *Periodontol 2000* 3:9, 1993.
15. Jeffcoat MK, Wang I-C, Reddy MS: (Radiographic diagnosis in periodontics, *Periodontol 2000* 7:54, 1995.) Mol A: Imaging methods in periodontology, *Periodontol 2000* 34:34, 2004.
16. Karring T, Loe H: The three-dimensional concept of the epithelium-connective tissue boundary of gingival, *Acta Odontol Scand* 28:917, 1970.
17. Kennedy J et al: A longitudinal evaluation of varying widths of attached gingival, *J Clin Periodontol* 12:667, 1985.
18. Kobayashi K, Rose G, Mahan C: Ultrastructure of the dento-epithelial junction, *J Periodontal Res* 11:313, 1976.
19. Kornman KS et al: The interleukin-1 genotype as a severity factor in adult periodontal disease, *J Clin Periodontol* 24:72, 1997.
20. Kornman KS, Page RC, Tonetti MS: The host response to the microbial challenge in periodontitis: assembling the players, *Periodontol 2000* 14:33, 1997.
21. Kvan E: Topography of principal fibers, *Scand J Dent Res* 6:282, 1973.
22. Lamster IB: In-office diagnostic tests and their role in supportive periodontal treatment, *Periodontol 2000* 12:49, 1996.
23. Lamster IB, Grbic JT: Diagnosis of periodontal disease based on analysis of the host response, *Periodontol 2000* 7:83, 1995.
24. Lang NP et al: Bleeding on probing: a predictor for the progression of periodontal disease, *J Clin Periodontol* 13:590, 1986.
25. Lang NP, Joss A, Tonetti MS: Monitoring disease during supportive periodontal treatment by bleeding on probing, *Periodontol 2000* 12:44, 1996.
26. Lang NP, Karring T, eds: *Proceedings of the 1st European workshop on periodontology*, London, 1994, Quintessence.
27. Lindhe J, Nyman S: The effect of plaque control and surgical pocket elimination on the establishment and maintenance of periodontal health. A longitudinal study of periodontal therapy in cases of advanced disease, *J Clin Periodontol* 2:67, 1975.
28. Loesche WJ: Chemotherapy of dental plaque infections, *Oral Sci Rev* 9:65, 1975.
29. Mandel ID, Gaffar A: Calculus revisited, *J Clin Periodontol* 13:249, 1986.
30. Mariotti A: The extracellular matrix of the periodontium: dynamic and interactive tissues, *Periodontol 2000* 3:39, 1993.
31. Newbrun E: Indices to measure gingival bleeding—a leading symptom in initial gingivitis, *Helv Odontol Acta* 15:107, 1971.
32. Nyman S, Lindhe J: Examination of patients with periodontal disease. In Lindhe J et al, eds: *Clinical periodontology and implant dentistry*, ed 3, Munksgaard, 1997, Copenhagen.
33. Saffar J-L, Lasfargues J-J, Cherruau M: Alveolar bone and the alveolar process: the socket that is never stable, *Periodontol 2000* 13:76, 1997.
34. Schroeder HE, Listgarten MA: The gingival tissues: the architecture of periodontal protection, *Periodontol 2000* 13:91, 1997.
35. Socransky S: Criteria for the infectious agents in dental caries and periodontal disease, *J Clin Periodontol* 6(7):16-21, 1979.
36. Socransky S: Microbiology of periodontal disease—present status and future considerations, *J Periodontol* 48:497, 1977.
37. Spray JR et al: Microscopic demonstration of the position of periodontal probes, *J Periodontol* 48:148, 1978.
38. Stern I: Current concepts of the dentogingival junction: the epithelial and connective tissue attachment to the tooth, *J Periodontol* 52:465, 1981.
39. Zambon JJ: Periodontal diseases: microbial factors, *Ann Periodontol* 1:879, 1996.
40. Zambon JJ, Haraszthy VI: The laboratory diagnosis of periodontal infections, *Periodontol 2000* 7:69, 1995.
41. Zander HA: The attachment of calculus to root surfaces, *J Periodontol* 24:16, 1953.

Hard Tissue Examination

Douglas A. Young • John D.B. Featherstone

INSIGHT

An accurate dental charting provides a picture of the patient's mouth with existing restorations; pathologic conditions; and other clinical information such as missing, rotated, and impacted teeth. This record is significant for future dental needs and for forensics for patient identification. The dental hygienist is often in a position to examine and record clinical findings and to update chartings periodically. Recognition of clinical conditions and knowledge of charting these conditions is essential for thorough patient documentation and treatment.

✷ CASE STUDY 17-1   Examination and Recording of Dental Findings

Miguel Cantara, a 37-year-old Hispanic man, has transferred his records to the dental office from his former dentist in another town. He reports that he is overdue for his usual 6-month checkup. His last appointment was for a routine cleaning and replacement of a cracked filling. Mr. Cantara says that he has received a variety of dental treatments since childhood and classifies his dental experiences as quite good. He says that he is unaware of any dental problems.

KEY TERMS

abfraction	crown fracture	gold onlay	recurrent (or secondary) caries
abrasion	cusp fracture	inactive caries	remineralization
active caries	demineralization	infected dentin	removable partial dentures
affected dentin	dental caries	overbite	root canal
Angle's classification	enamel flaking	overjet	sealant
approximal caries	enameloplasty	parafunction	sensitivity
arrested caries	erosion	partial gold crown	specificity
attrition	full gold crown	partially erupted teeth	tooth-colored restoration
bruxism	G.V. Black Caries Classification	periapical radiolucency	unerupted teeth
cavitation	System	porcelain fused to metal	wear facet
complete dentures	gold foil	porcelain jacket crown	white spot lesion
cracking	gold inlay		

LEARNING OUTCOMES

After reading this chapter the student will be able to:

1. Use a number of different comprehensive charting systems to assess the oral health of new patients and supportive care patients.
2. Be familiar with the different tooth-numbering systems.
3. Use proper infection control during performance of charting procedures.
4. Use the traditional G.V. Black Caries Classification System to chart existing conditions.
5. Be familiar with new classification systems for carious lesions.
6. Use different charting symbols that represent existing conditions, such as early carious lesions before cavitation, cavities requiring restoration, missing teeth, partially erupted teeth, malposed teeth, existing dental restorations, erosion, abrasion, attrition, abfraction, enamel cracking, and cusp fracture.
7. Define *dental caries* and related terms.
8. Recognize the signs of dental caries, including carious lesions, in varying stages of development.
9. Recognize the signs of arrested versus active carious lesions.
10. Recognize the signs of recurrent or secondary dental caries.
11. Recognize different stages of carious lesions and different dental restorations on a radiograph.
12. Classify occlusion with Angle's Classification System, measuring overbite and overjet and identifying the signs of occlusal trauma.

A proper hard tissue evaluation involves more than just accurate charting of those items visualized during the hard tissue examination; it also involves interpretation of this information and the making of useful clinical decisions. Many conditions can modify teeth. When a dental hard tissue evaluation is performed, a snapshot in time is gained, representing multiple events that could have modified tooth structure in either the recent or distant past. The purpose of hard tissue charting is to capture each snapshot in the chart records for legal, diagnostic, and clerical purposes.

During a hard tissue evaluation, the clinician also must be able to discern between currently active events and the results of history. Accurate dental charts can provide the clinician with a visual representation of every past examination completed on that patient—information that proves invaluable in the comparison and evaluation of many current concerns. In this chapter, comprehensive hard tissue charting of many conditions that modify teeth is reviewed, along with a brief summary of the information currently known about the condition. A brief introduction to occlusal analysis is presented, after which a significant portion of the chapter is dedicated to the detection of dental caries. The mechanism of dental caries and its management is covered in further detail in Chapter 25.

Why this emphasis on dental caries in a dental hygiene textbook? This is an exciting time in the dental profession, in which knowledge gained in dental caries research over the past 20 years is finally beginning to improve the clinical management of this disease. The information presented in this chapter is a review of the very latest information in the field, as well as a source of "new" knowledge for recent graduates. The newly evolving concepts of the way in which dental caries is managed in the United States is still in its infancy; however, a team approach is clearly required, representing a tremendous opportunity for the dental hygiene profession to participate as equally important members of the dental caries management team.

Comprehensive Hard Tissue Charting

[17-1 to 17-3]

Comprehensive charting should be an accurate and systematic representation of the dental hard tissues on the day of the clinical examination. The way and the order in which this process is accomplished depend on the clinician's preferences. Although no one correct way exists to complete the examination, the method selected should facilitate recording of findings. In that respect, completing the examination logically and consistently each time is important to ensure that all examinations are completed without omissions. Many clinicians prefer to start at tooth #1 and proceed to tooth #32 (i.e., the universal system of tooth numbering).

Types of Charting Forms

The manner in which information is recorded in the patient record is a decision that is made by the members of each individual practice. Although many chart formats exist, as well as countless ways in which to use them, no one "right" way exists. Instead, each office team may come up with its own variation of an existing technique. Therefore only a few of the most commonly used formats—such as anatomical, geometrical, and computer-assisted—are presented in this chapter.

ANATOMICAL CHARTING

Anatomical charting forms show the anatomy of each tooth in facial, occlusal, and lingual views, usually including the roots of the teeth, as seen in Figure 17-1. This chart form can record a specific part of the anatomy as it appears in the mouth, such as the distal pit of an upper first molar and specific areas on the roots.

GEOMETRICAL CHARTING

Geometrical charting forms use a box to represent each tooth, usually shown from a top or occlusal view only, of the facial, lingual, occlusal, mesial, and distal angles of each tooth, as seen in Figure 17-2. The same generic shape is used for each tooth

Baseline Clinical Examination and Re-Evaluation Record

University of the Pacific, School of Dentistry

Patient's Name: _____

Student's Name: _____

Baseline Date: _____ Re-eval Date: _____

Reviewed By (Faculty): _____

	1	2	3	4	5	6	7	8	9	10	11	12	13	14	15	16
Re-eval mobility																
Re-eval Probe																
Baseline Probe																

FACIAL — R — LINGUAL — L

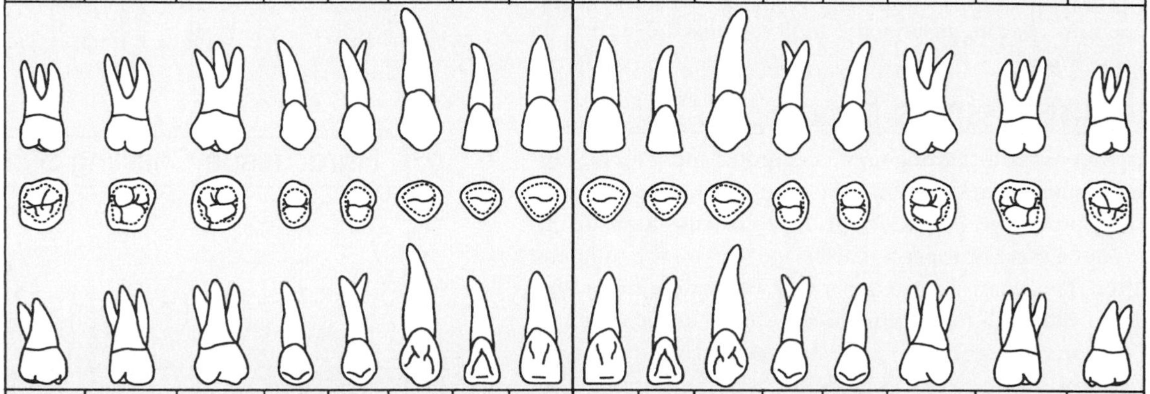

Baseline Probe																
Re-eval Probe																

Re-eval mobility																
Re-eval Probe																
Baseline Probe																

LINGUAL — R — FACIAL — L

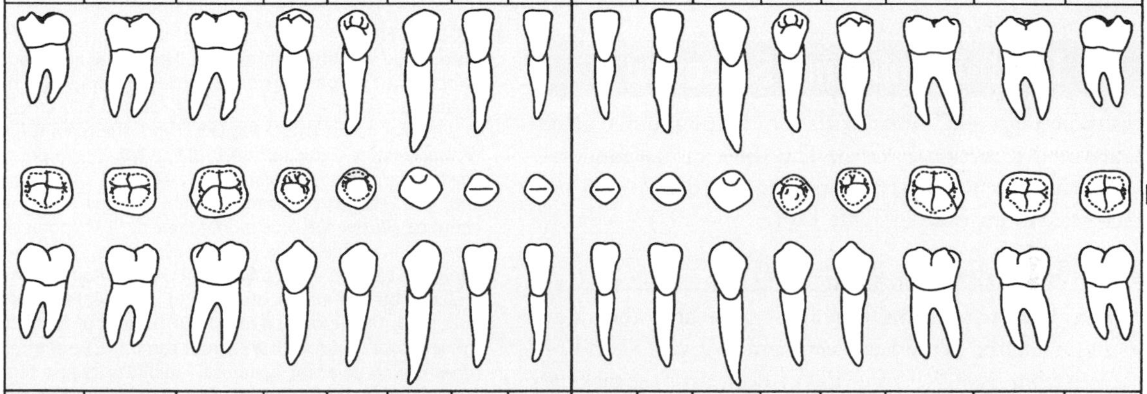

	32	31	30	29	28	27	26	25	24	23	22	21	20	19	18	17
Baseline Probe																
Re-eval Probe																

Initial Occlusal and TMJ Findings

CENTRIC RELATION:

Location: ☐ easy ☐ difficult ☐ impossible

TMJ discomfort to pressure ☐ none ☐ right ☐ left

Initial tooth contact: _____ vs. _____

CENTRIC RELATION-CENTRIC OCCLUSION DISCREPANCY:

Vertical slide _____ mm Forward slide _____ mm

Lateral slide ☐ right ☐ left _____ mm

CENTRIC OCCLUSION:

Canine classification (I,II,III) right _____ · left _____

Right canine vertical overlap _____ mm

Right canine functional horizontal overlap _____ mm

Left canine vertical overlap _____ mm

Left canine horizontal overlap _____ mm

Central incisor vertical overlap _____ mm

Central incisor functional horizontal overlap _____ mm

Wear facets: ☐ minimal ☐ moderate ☐ severe

CR TO CO	1	2	3	4	5	6	7	8	9	10	11	12	13	14	15	16
INTERFERENCES	32	31	30	29	28	27	26	25	24	23	22	21	20	19	18	17
RT.	1	2	3	4	5	6	7	8	9	10	11	12	13	14	15	16
LATERAL	32	31	30	29	28	27	26	25	24	23	22	21	20	19	18	17
LT.	1	2	3	4	5	6	7	8	9	10	11	12	13	14	15	16
LATERAL	32	31	30	29	28	27	26	25	24	23	22	21	20	19	18	17
PROTRUSIVE	1	2	3	4	5	6	7	8	9	10	11	12	13	14	15	16
	32	31	30	29	28	27	26	25	24	23	22	21	20	19	18	17

TEMPORO-MANDIBULAR JOINT:

Maximum opening _____ mm

Joint sounds during opening and closing: ☐ none ☐ right ☐ left

Joint sounds during excursions: ☐ none ☐ right ☐ left

History of TMJ treatment: ☐ yes ☐ no

Current joint pain: ☐ none ☐ right ☐ left

Plaque Index

TOOTH SURFACE	SCORE	
	Baseline	Re-eval
Facial 3		
Facial 8		
Facial 14		
Lingual 19		
Facial 24		
Lingual 10		
Plaque Index		

FIGURE 17-1

Anatomical charting form. (Courtesy University of the Pacific School of Dentistry, San Francisco.)

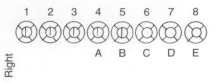

FIGURE 17-2
Geometrical charting form, right quadrant only. (Modified from Woodall IR: *Comprehensive dental hygiene care*, ed 4, St Louis, 1993, Mosby.)

and permits charting of primary, adult, or mixed dentition on the same form.

COMPUTER-ASSISTED CHARTING

Computer-assisted charting uses a computer and a dental software program to help increase the accuracy and speed of the charting procedure (Figure 17-3). The charting form in this case is not a piece of paper but an image seen on the computer monitor. The image format can either be anatomical or geometrical. Although the information is stored in the computer and supports the concept of *paperless* dental records, a neat and professional-looking color form can easily be printed when needed. The information is entered into the computer via a mouse or keyboard and is accomplished instantaneously, saving time. Many software programs offer voice recognition, making charting a one-person operation with improved infection control.

Tooth-Numbering Systems

Just as more than one format exists for charting, different systems are used to designate teeth. The three most common—the universal system, Palmer's notation, and the international system—are summarized in Table 17-1.

UNIVERSAL SYSTEM

The universal system, perhaps the most popular in the United States, numbers the permanent teeth from #1 to #32 and primary teeth from *A* to *T* (Figure 17-4). Tooth #1 is the maxillary right third molar, tooth #2 is the maxillary right second molar; this numbering format continues over to the maxillary left third molar, which is tooth #16. Numbering then continues to the mandibular left quadrant (where tooth #17 is the mandibular left third molar and tooth #18 is the mandibular left second molar), continuing to the lower right third molar, tooth #32. The same format is used for the primary dentition.

PALMER'S NOTATION

Palmer's notation numbers the permanent teeth (#1 through #8) and the primary teeth (*A* through *E*), always starting from the midline and working laterally. Therefore the central incisor

---

CASE APPLICATION 17-1.1

Charting a Fractured Restoration

Mr. Cantera reported having a "cracked" restoration repaired at this last dental visit. How would the cracked restoration be represented on a dental chart?

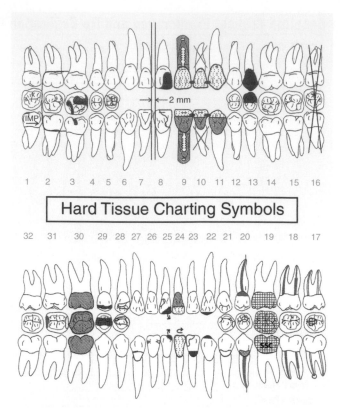

Hard Tissue Charting Symbols

FIGURE 17-3
Hard tissue charting symbols. **#1,** Horizontal impaction with tissue line *(black)*, IMP (impaction) on facial view *(black)*, and horizontal arrow indicating direction of impaction; **#3,** OL and MO amalgams *(solid blue)* and mesial defect *(red)*; **#5,** DO composite resin *(blue outline)* and O clinical fracture *(sawtooth red)*; **#7 to #8,** 2-mm diastema *(black parallel lines and distance in millimeters)*; **#8,** MIFL composite resin *(blue outline)* and F defect *(red)*; **#9,** implant *(slanted blue lines)*, transmucosal connector *(opposite blue slanted lines)*, PFM (porcelain fused to metal) crown with visible metal *(slanted blue lines)*, and porcelain *(blue stippling)* splinted to #10 *(solid blue)*; **#10,** missing root *(green or black X)*, replaced by PFM pontic attached to abutments 9 and 11 *(solid blue bar)*; **#11,** PFM crown; **#13,** MODF portion of tooth fractured *(red)*; **#16,** missing tooth *(black X)*; **#17,** root canal (RC) treatment in progress *(green)* with adjacent periapical radiolucency and temporary O filling *(red checkerboard)*; **#18,** occlusal pit defects *(red)* and RC treated plus post *(green)* [note: situation actually clinically impossible; no access opening filling present]; **#19,** temporary SCC (stainless steel crown) *(black)* *(red checkerboard)*; **#20,** O composite *(blue outline)*, F gold foil *(slanted blue lines)*, RC filling *(green)* with overextension *(green)*; **#21,** F composite *(blue outline)* and incipient dental caries seen only radiographically *(green outline)*; **#22,** I defect—attrition—*(red)*; **#23,** MIF comp *(blue outline)* and F defect—erosion or abfraction—*(red)*; **#24,** PFM as described previously, arrow *(black)* showing rotation; **#25,** DL composite resin *(blue outline)* and MIFL fracture *(red and black arrows)* indicating part of tooth missing; **#26,** radiographic findings (unconfirmed clinically) of M caries in enamel only *(green outline)* and D caries into dentin *(solid green)*; **#27,** F composite *(blue outline)* and clinically defective F margin *(red)*; **#28,** MO composite *(blue outline)* [note: outline extended too far on distally occlusal view]; **#29,** MOD alloy—same as amalgam—*(solid blue)*; **#30,** FVC—full veneer crown—*(blue slanted lines)*; and **#31,** M enamel caries—seen only radiographically *(green outline)*—and D caries into dentin *(solid green)*. Radiographic findings were transferred from radiographic diagnosis worksheet for teeth **#21, #26,** and **#31.**

is designated tooth #1, the lateral incisor tooth #2, the canine tooth #3, and the first premolar tooth #4. This numbering format continues to the third molar, which is always tooth #8. When the clinician faces the patient, the quadrant of the mouth is defined by a horizontal line representing the upper

Table 17-1	Summary of Tooth-Numbering Systems	
SYSTEM	**PERMANENT DENTITION**	**PRIMARY DENTITION**
Universal	A number (#1 to #32) designates each tooth.	A letter (*A* to *T*) designates each tooth.
International	Each tooth is designated by a quadrant number prefix (1 to 4) and tooth number suffix (1 to 8).	A number (5 to 8) designates a quadrant and 1 to 5 the tooth number.
Palmer's Notation	Each tooth is numbered (1 to 8) and positioned within intersecting axes to designate the quadrant.	Each tooth is lettered (*A* to *E*) and positioned within intersecting axes to designate the quadrant.

From Ash MM, Nelson SJ: *Wheeler's dental anatomy, physiology and occlusion,* ed 8, St Louis, 2003, Saunders.

arch above, the lower arch below, and a vertical line representing the midline. Both the number and the appropriate symbol designating the quadrant are always necessary, as is notation that the left quadrant is on the right and vice versa (Figure 17-5). For example, the permanent maxillary left central incisor is written as ⌊1, and the permanent mandibular left first bicuspid is ⌈4. An example of a primary mandibular right first molar is written as D⌉.

INTERNATIONAL SYSTEM

The international system (Figure 17-6) is numbered the same as Palmer's notation. However, instead of designating the quadrants by a symbol, a prefix number is used: 1 for the maxillary right, 2 for the maxillary left, 3 for the mandibular left, and 4 for the mandibular right. For example, the permanent maxillary right central incisor would be 11, and the permanent mandibular left first bicuspid would be 34. However, for the primary dentition the teeth are numbered 1 through 5 instead of with Palmer's notation (*A* through *E*). In addition, numbers 5 through 8 are used to designate the quadrants in the primary dentition (5 being the maxillary right, 6 the maxillary left, 7 the mandibular left, and 8 the mandibular right). Thus the primary mandibular right first molar is written as 84.

Infection Control

No matter which system is chosen to record the results of a hard tissue examination, proper infection control must be ensured.

As stated previously, the voice-recognition, computer-assisted software can eliminate

Prevention

When using paper forms, the clinician must never contaminate the pen or chart by touching them with a contaminated gloved hand. Trying to chart alone, even with overgloves, is extremely inefficient and is not recommended. A chairside assistant who prevents contamination of the operative field is invaluable during charting.

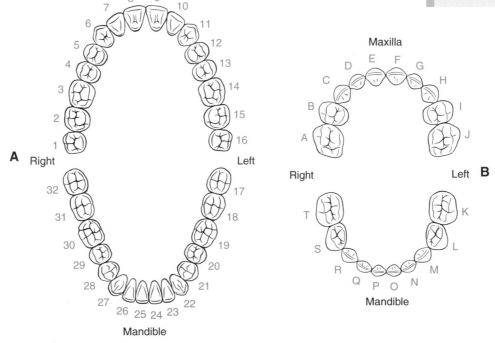

FIGURE 17-4
Universal numbering system for the permanent **(A)** and primary **(B)** dentition. (Modified from Finkbeiner BL, Finkbeiner CA: *Practice management for the dental team,* ed 6, St Louis, 2006, Mosby.)

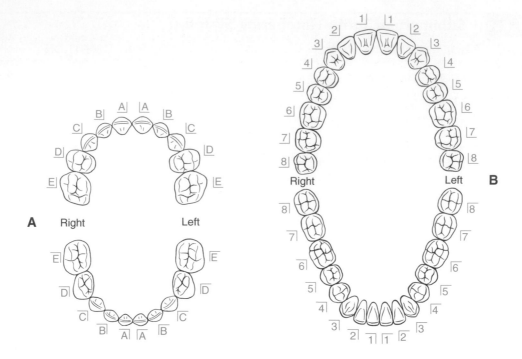

FIGURE 17-5
Palmer's notation system assigned to primary **(A)** and permanent **(B)** dentition. (Modified from Finkbeiner BL, Finkbeiner CA: *Practice management for the dental team*, ed 6, St Louis, 2006, Mosby.)

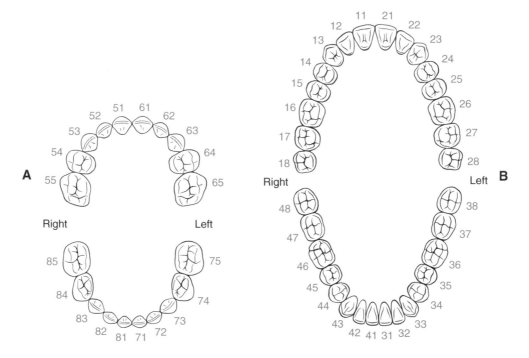

FIGURE 17-6
International system assigned to primary **(A)** and permanent **(B)** dentition. (Modified from Finkbeiner BL, Finkbeiner CA: *Practice management for the dental team*, ed 6, St Louis, 2006, Mosby; In Roberson TM, Heymann HO, Swift EJ: *Sturdevant's art and science of operative dentistry*, ed 5, St Louis, 2006, Mosby.)

cross-contamination concerns and, in many cases, can make charting a single-operator procedure. If single-operator charting is unavoidable and voice-recognition, computer-assisted software is not available, then a voice-activated tape recorder can be used to collect the data, leaving the actual charting to be completed later.

Classification Systems of Cavity Design

More than a century ago, Dr. G.V. Black developed a dental caries classification system (based on location of the carious lesion) and cavity preparation designs (based on restoration using the materials available in his time, such as amalgam).[32] Although material and preparation technologies have changed significantly in the last 100 years, the **G.V. Black Caries Classification System** and cavity designs still predominate and are discussed in the next section. The G.V. Black classification system (I through VI) based on lesion location is summarized in Table 17-2.

Although not yet in common use, new classification systems have been proposed[31] and are discussed later in the chapter in the section concerning new dental caries classification systems.

Charting Existing Conditions

Accurately charting existing hard tissue conditions is the most important task in charting, regardless of the chart format or numbering system selected. The information and the way in which the information is recorded may vary from practice to practice; room exists for customization, depending on office preferences. Therefore the following examples are meant to illustrate the concept rather than to be an all-inclusive formula.

When charting existing conditions, the clinician usually performs the following:

- Charts missing teeth first by crossing the teeth out with a vertical line or an *X* in black ink (This method helps to lessen the confusion, especially in mixed dentition.)
- Depicts **partially erupted teeth** by drawing a line to show the exposed part of the tooth
- Circles **unerupted teeth**
- Illustrates with arrows in the appropriate direction inclined, drifted, rotated, and supraerupted teeth
- Draws a double line noticeably between contact areas where a diastema is observed
- Draws brackets around teeth to mark **removable partial dentures** and **complete dentures**
- Draws outlines around restorations on the appropriate part of the tooth (The type of restorative material is keyed by either blue color, outlined versus filled, or with some kind of letter code.)

Examples of a letter-coded system are as follows:

- Amalgam (A)
- **Tooth-colored restoration** (TC)
- **Sealant** (SL)
- **Gold foil** (GF)
- **Gold inlay** (GI)
- **Gold onlay** (GO)
- **Partial gold crown** (3/4 GC)
- **Full gold crown** (FGC)
- **Porcelain fused to metal** (PFM)
- **Porcelain jacket crown** (PJC)
- Acrylic facing (AF)
- **Root canal** (RC)
- **Periapical radiolucency** (PAR)
- Stainless steel crown (SSC)
- Dental implant (DI)

Table 17-2	G.V. Black Caries Classification System	
CLASS	**DESCRIPTION**	**ILLUSTRATION**

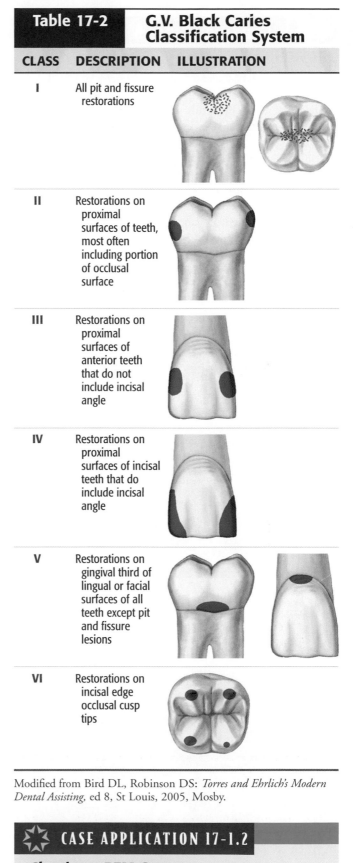

I	All pit and fissure restorations	
II	Restorations on proximal surfaces of teeth, most often including portion of occlusal surface	
III	Restorations on proximal surfaces of anterior teeth that do not include incisal angle	
IV	Restorations on proximal surfaces of incisal teeth that do include incisal angle	
V	Restorations on gingival third of lingual or facial surfaces of all teeth except pit and fissure lesions	
VI	Restorations on incisal edge occlusal cusp tips	

Modified from Bird DL, Robinson DS: *Torres and Ehrlich's Modern Dental Assisting,* ed 8, St Louis, 2005, Mosby.

✦ CASE APPLICATION 17-1.2

Charting a PFM Crown

Mr. Cantera had the "cracked" restoration repaired. The restoration was replaced with a porcelain fused to metal (PFM) crown. How would this be represented on a dental chart?

Other Conditions that Modify Teeth*

EROSION

Erosion (Figures 17-7 and 17-8) is the superficial loss of dental hard tissue because of a chemical process, usually resulting from nonbacterial acids. The acids that cause erosion may be either extrinsic or intrinsic. Extrinsic acids may include those found in foods and drinks, with examples including low-pH cola drinks, fruit juices, and wine. Some medications and vitamins are also acidic. Gastric acids coming from the stomach are intrinsic acids caused by chronic gastric reflux diseases or bulimia.

Because exposure to acid removes tooth mineral, erosion may very well potentiate abrasion, attrition, and abfraction (described in detail later in the chapter). Partial loss of enamel crystal surfaces or removal of dentin or cementum mineral makes the subsequent removal of mineral easier in the presence of acid.

---

*This section was written with significant contributions taken from Mount GJ, Hume WR: *Preservation and restoration of tooth structure,* St Louis, 1998, Mosby.

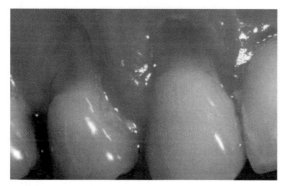

FIGURE 17-7
Severe erosion lesions. Teeth #13 and #14 show severe erosion, doubtless exacerbated by toothbrush abrasion. (From Mount GJ, Hume WR: *Preservation and restoration of tooth structure,* St Louis, 1998, Mosby.)

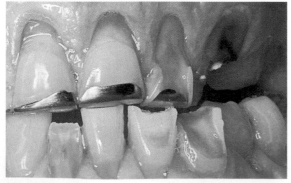

FIGURE 17-8
Severe erosion. Quadrant of teeth showing similar erosion to Figure 17-7 in addition to abrasion. (From Mount GJ, Hume WR: *Preservation and restoration of tooth structure,* St Louis, 1998, Mosby.)

DENTAL CONSIDERATIONS

Demineralization of dentin leaves collagen exposed to trauma; if this collagen is removed or damaged—by brushing teeth, for example—then it may no longer be present for remineralization, thus leading to permanent loss of tooth structure. Sources of acids in particular should be investigated when abrasion, attrition, and abfraction are evident.

ABRASION

Abrasion (Figures 17-9 to 17-11) is the wearing of tooth substance by exogenous material forced over the surface by incisive, masticatory, or teeth-cleaning functions. Exogenous material describes anything foreign to the tooth's substance, such as sand, grit, or foreign material found in food and includes the natural abrasive qualities of some foods, as well as any solid material held by or forced against the teeth. Therefore abrasion may occur during mastication or even during teeth cleaning. An abrasion area is generally not well defined and may manifest as a cusp tip or incisal edge that has been rounded, blunted, or worn flat and often exposes the dentin, causing a "scooped out" appearance that is softer and more porous than enamel. The location and extent of abrasive wear is influenced by such things as occlusion, diet, oral habits, age, loss of posterior teeth, and oral hygiene techniques.

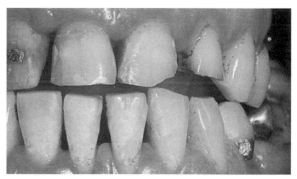

FIGURE 17-9
Abrasion on tooth #22 caused by many years of holding a pipe stem in this position. (From Mount GJ, Hume WR: *Preservation and restoration of tooth structure,* St Louis, 1998, Mosby.)

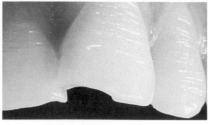

FIGURE 17-10
Abrasion on labial of maxillary anterior teeth. The horizontal, parallel scratch marks were caused by toothbrush abrasion. (From Mount GJ, Hume WR: *Preservation and restoration of tooth structure,* St Louis, 1998, Mosby.)

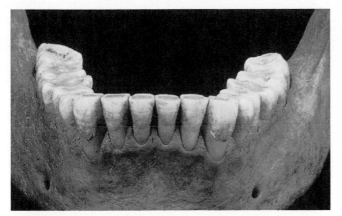

FIGURE 17-11
Abrasion pattern on ancient skull specimen. Reader should note the helicoidal wear pattern on posterior teeth, emphasizing the slope toward the tongue in the third molars. (From Mount GJ, Hume WR: *Preservation and restoration of tooth structure,* St Louis, 1998, Mosby.)

ATTRITION

Attrition (Figures 17-12 and 17-13) is tooth wear caused by tooth-to-tooth contact without the presence of exogenous material. Persistent tooth grinding is called **bruxism** or **parafunction.** The characteristic feature of occlusal attrition is the development of a **wear facet**—a flat, often shiny surface and with a

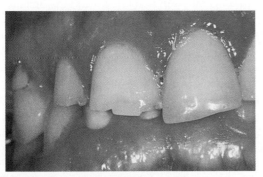

FIGURE 17-12
Attrition. Heavy attrition is evident on teeth #6, #7, and #8, as is enamel flaking. (From Mount GJ, Hume WR: *Preservation and restoration of tooth structure,* St Louis, 1998, Mosby.)

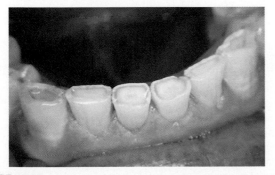

FIGURE 17-13
Attrition. One of the most common causes of this kind of wear is a deflective incline of the posterior teeth. (From Dawson PE: *Functional occlusion: from TMJ to smile design,* St Louis, 2007, Mosby.)

well-defined border. The distribution of facets is influenced by the occlusal morphology and the characteristic grinding pattern or patterns of the individual. Attrition facets may appear in seemingly impossible locations, such as the facial of a maxillary canine in a patient with Class I occlusion. Careful examination of these uniquely positioned attrition facets can reveal interesting (and occasionally damaging) patient habits that can produce temporomandibular (TMJ) dysfunction. In the presence of erosion, the facet may not appear shiny even if the bruxism is active. Facial pain and a stiff jaw (which may also have associated pain and tenderness in the TMJ) are symptoms that may indicate active tooth grinding.

ABFRACTION

Researchers believe that **abfraction** (Figure 17-14) is caused by excessive buccal or lingual occlusal load through either compression or tension in the cervical region of the tooth just above its bony support. The excess load may cause flexure of the tooth, with disintegration of the relatively brittle enamel or dentin in the cervical area. Such disintegration can add to erosion and abrasion, all of which can be contributing factors in so-called toothbrush abrasion.

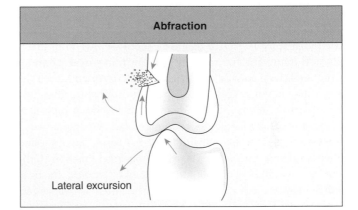

FIGURE 17-14
Affected dentin. *Abfraction* is a term used to describe flexure of a tooth under heavy occlusal (functional) load, which may lead to loss of tooth structure at the cementoenamel junction (CEJ). The process causes V-shaped (above) or saucer-shaped defects involving dentin and enamel. Abfraction probably accounts for erosion lesions for which no obvious explanation is evident. (Modified from Mount GJ, Hume WR: *Preservation and restoration of tooth structure,* St Louis, 1998, Mosby.)

Types of Tooth Fracture

ENAMEL FLAKING

Small amounts of enamel of various sizes may fracture from the incisal edges of anterior teeth or from the buccal or lingual edges of posterior teeth (**enamel flaking**)—possibly the result of unusual incisal or occlusal biting patterns and habits (Figure 17-15).

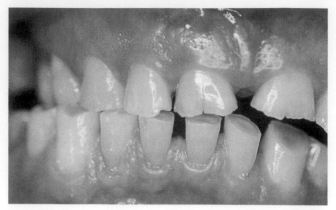

FIGURE 17-15
Enamel flaking. Forceful extreme mandibular movement from centric occlusion (CO) outward can cause the enamel flaking on the anteriors. (From Mount GJ, Hume WR: *Preservation and restoration of tooth structure,* St Louis, 1998, Mosby.)

CRACKING

Minor **cracking** in enamel is usually asymptomatic and requires no treatment. However, under heavy occlusal load, more significant cracks can involve the dentin. Cusp movement then is extremely painful because of hydraulic stimulation of odontoblast-sensory nerve receptors.

CUSP FRACTURE

If enough force is exerted against a tooth—either from direct physical trauma or as a result of parafunction—or if the tooth structure is weakened (often by restorative treatment), then the tooth may fracture. Cusps most prone to split and fail are the lingual cusps of mandibular molars and the facial or palatal cusps of maxillary first and second premolars. A common **cusp fracture** runs from the pulpal floor of an existing carious lesion downward and outward to the cementoenamel junction (CEJ) and is generally repairable. In contrast, a vertical fracture, which may sometimes involve the root, often is irreparable. Teeth under high occlusal load, such as endodontically treated posterior teeth, are also at increased risk because of loss of tooth structure, and the cusps of these teeth should be protected by a restoration, such as a crown or onlay.

CROWN FRACTURE

The crowns of anterior teeth are most at risk from direct trauma, with the main predisposing factors being the age of the patient and the tooth position. The highest incidence of **crown fracture** occurs in elementary school–age boys in anterior teeth. Mouthguards are useful in contact sports, but convincing children to use them in playgrounds is often difficult. (Chapter 39 provides more content on the use of mouthguards in athletics.)

Charting Dental Caries

At first glance, charting dental caries sounds very straightforward—simple tracing of the clinical dental caries on the chart (in red ink) as it appears in the mouth. In addition, to encourage a preclinical review of radiographs, some clinicians advocate the outlining of radiographic dental caries in green ink before the clinical examination begins. These areas (in green) remind the clinician to confirm the radiographic findings clinically, in which case the green outline may be filled in with red ink on the hard tissue chart.

Although this approach sounds simple to use, it contains many inherent pitfalls. Before a carious lesion can be recorded, it first must be detected in the mouth by the clinician. Unfortunately, different clinicians may detect and treat dental caries, even in the same patient, quite differently. In the last 20 years much has been learned about the disease, and as a result, new dental caries management techniques are emerging.[1-3] However, because changing treatment paradigms is far from instantaneous, early adopters and late adopters of new knowledge will always emerge—leading to differing opinions. Therefore dental professionals must review the current understanding of dental caries. The following sections focus on the definition and detection of dental caries. The mechanism of dental caries and its management is covered in detail in Chapter 25.

Defining Dental Caries and Related Terms

The term *dental caries,* along with its related terms, is often a source of confusion because the same term may be used differently depending on the person using it and the circumstance in which the term is used (Box 17-1). The realization that not all dental professionals agree on the true meaning of the term *dental caries* is sobering. The term is used to describe more than one concept. Understanding this fact can help the clinician and patient communicate more effectively.

Dental caries is an infectious disease caused by bacteria. The organisms involved include *mutans Streptococcus* and *Lactobacillus,* which produce acid when exposed to dietary fermentable carbohydrates. The acid then diffuses into the tooth, dissolves the tooth mineral (a chemical process known as **demineralization**), and is a result of the disease process. Demineralization can cause many changes in the tooth mineral, not all of which are visible to the naked eye (even with magnification). The term *dental caries* is used rather loosely by dental care

---

BOX 17-1

TERMS USED TO DESCRIBE THE RESULTS OF DENTAL CARIES

Active caries	Histologic gold standard
Approximal caries	Infected dentin
Brown spot lesion	Pit and fissure caries
Caries dye uptake	Polarized light microscopy
Cavitation	Radiographic caries
Clinical caries	Root caries
Demineralization	Soft dentin
Explorer stick	White spot lesion

providers and is frequently meant to describe the results of the demineralization process—a carious lesion—rather than the disease itself.

Clinicians' use of the term *caries* also may vary. For example, so-called contemporary clinicians who use new caries management techniques may use the term *caries* differently than their more traditional counterparts. The traditional clinician uses a surgical approach very similar to the way G.V. Black treated caries more than 100 years ago, in which the focus is on the treatment of carious lesions through removal of decay and placement of restorations. Carious lesions often are detected on a radiograph (i.e., radiographic caries) or in the clinical setting with visual and tactile methods (i.e., clinical caries). The patient then is periodically recalled, usually based on periodontal criteria, and more restorations are placed if new carious lesions are detected. Thus when the traditional clinician uses the term *caries,* it usually designates a carious lesion—or cavity—that needs to be restored rather than a disease that needs to be diagnosed.

Dental Considerations

Detection is not the same as diagnosis, because a disease is *diagnosed* and a carious lesion *detected.* This seemingly trivial point is the source of much confusion; when the term *caries* is used, of importance is whether it refers to the *disease* or the *lesion.*

The fact that the term *dental caries* may have different meanings, depending on whether a clinician or a researcher is using it, is also confusing. Researchers have the luxury of performing experiments in vitro (in the laboratory away from the patient's mouth) using specialized equipment and histologic techniques such as polarized light microscopy and microradiography, which describe ways to visualize the demineralized mineral in the laboratory. These research terms are sometimes referred to in the literature simply as *the histologic gold standard,* because they positively identify mineral loss and can be quantitative.

Because such laboratory techniques cannot be used clinically, the histologic terms are of little use to the clinician. In addition, mineral loss alone does not mean that the tooth needs restoration. Thus *caries* from a histologic or research perspective may not have the same meaning to a clinician. Whenever possible, clinical decisions should be based on scientific knowledge, which requires practitioners to read and understand the appropriate literature. However, if research terms are not defined in a way in which readers outside the field can understand easily, then the literature itself can be a source of confusion. Therefore authors must carefully define and explain the clinical relevance of the terms they use, and readers must be aware of the circumstance or perspective in which the authors are using those terms.

Even clinical terms such as *clinical caries, radiographic caries,* and *carious lesion* are considered vague, because they do not define the extent of the lesion in clinically relevant terms. Demineralization is a dynamic process occurring when the tooth is exposed to acid in the absence of protective factors, such as healthy saliva and fluoride. As stated previously, mere mineral loss does not always require surgical intervention. The earliest loss of mineral during the demineralization process is not visible to the naked eye. As more mineral is lost and the enamel becomes more porous, it produces optical changes in the enamel that appear first as a dull **white spot lesion.** The *dull* appearance often suggests that the lesion is in an active state of demineralization and is just one sign of something known as **active caries.** If the demineralization process can be halted or even reversed, then the dull appearance often turns shiny—one sign of **inactive caries** or **arrested caries.** This reversal of the demineralization process is called **remineralization** and is explained in more detail in Chapter 25.

White spot lesions often discolor with time, causing a brown spot lesion in the enamel (see the later section of this chapter concerning color changes in enamel). The exact mechanism for this occurrence is not yet known (discussed in Chapter 25). Again, if the surface of a white or brown spot lesion is smooth (noncavitated) and shiny, then the lesion is considered to be arrested or remineralized.

Dental Considerations

If an active carious lesion is allowed to progress, it eventually produces an actual hole, or **cavitation,** into or through the enamel; in the presence of surface cavitation, the control of plaque biofilm accumulation is no longer possible, representing a critical point in the process of diagnosis. Once the surface is cavitated, surgical intervention is required to restore a smooth surface that can be maintained free of plaque biofilm.

Accurate determination of the type and extent of the carious lesion is clinically important, because when carious lesions are detected at an early stage, clinicians may decide to use chemical rather than surgical restorative intervention. Chemical intervention treats the bacterial infection itself and preserves the natural tooth structure by helping the saliva remineralize the areas of early decay; this process is discussed in more detail in Chapter 25.

New Caries Classification Systems

The G.V. Black Caries Classification System has worked well for the past 100 years when only the standard Black cavity preparations were used. However, new knowledge of dental caries, coupled with an explosion in restorative material science, now allows nonsurgical treatment modalities and conservative cavity preparation designs. This new knowledge poses problems for the traditional G.V. Black Classification System. For example, no way exists to designate the size of the lesion or describe early lesions that are amenable to conservative treatment with the Black system. Two new classification systems consistent with conservative care are introduced in the following sections; however, neither conservative care nor the proposed classification systems can be considered a standard of care at the present time.

MOUNT AND HUME SYSTEM

Recently, a classification system has been suggested based on two simple parameters: (1) the location and (2) the size of a carious lesion.[31,32] The G.V. Black Classification System was designed to classify the cavities that had to be cut to eliminate a carious lesion, and it does not permit recognition of the size of the lesion at all. The system recently proposed by Mount and Hume is designed to recognize carious lesions beginning with the very earliest stage, in which remineralization is the indicated treatment rather than surgical intervention. It continues to classify the lesions as they become progressively larger without at any stage specifying a cavity design. This system is quite logical, because dental caries is found typically in only three sites on a tooth—(1) in pits and fissures, (2) at proximal contacts, and (3) on cervical surfaces. These three sites are consistent with the typical acid challenge patterns created by niches commonly colonized by the pathogens. In other words, plaque biofilm accumulates and is difficult to control below the floss contacts, on tooth roots, and in the pits and fissures of teeth. Lesions are treated differently depending on their location (site) and size, explaining the lack of specificity for cavity design.

- *Size 0 lesions* are those early signs of demineralization that may be noted as white spots on visible surfaces or early lesions at the contact areas identified in radiographs. Another example, the occlusal fissures on a newly erupted molar, may fit this classification if they are relatively deep and convoluted.
- *Size 1 lesions* are described as *minimal* but beyond the hope of remineralization treatment. Some cavitation is present, and therefore plaque biofilm control cannot be maintained. Some form of surgical intervention is required, but the cavity design should be based on the removal of only sufficient tooth structure to allow access to the dentin lesion, after which the cavity can be sealed with an adhesive restorative material.
- *Size 2 lesions* are described as *moderate*. That is, the cavity is beyond minimal, but adequate sound tooth structure remains to support the occlusion. The entire load will be borne by the restoration.
- *Size 3 lesions* have cavities that need to be enlarged, because the tooth structure is seriously weakened. The cavity design must be modified so that the restoration will take the entire occlusal load; otherwise one or more of the cusps is likely to split at the base.

- *Size 4 lesions* are described as *extensive,* with bulk failure or major breakdown of a cusp, requiring a cast or bonded final restoration.

Thus a #1.2 lesion in this classification system is really just a numeric way of indicating a medium-sized cavity in the occlusal-incisal surface of tooth relating to the fissure system. In the G.V. Black Classification System, this cavity would be a Class I, with a specific cavity preparation design prescribed for its restoration. The cavity design, incidentally, would require the removal of the entire fissure system, whether it was carious or not, because finishing an amalgam restoration within the fissures is impossible. In contrast with contemporary materials and techniques, a #1.2 lesion can be restored with an adhesive restorative material without the removal of all the fissures, because the restorative material can act as a fissure seal and a restoration (Table 17-3 and Figure 17-16).

COMPUTER-BASED SYSTEM

D.K. Benn and colleagues have suggested a computer-based classification system to help the clinician classify early and more advanced lesions; it also attempts to describe active versus inactive lesions.[4] In this system, several icons represent every possible clinical caries scenario and attempts to classify them by histologic lesion depth (as if the clinician could section the tooth in the laboratory to evaluate the depth of the lesion into enamel or dentin).

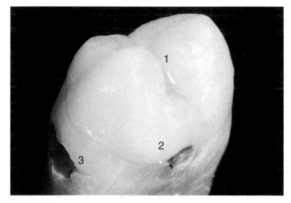

FIGURE 17-16
Three sites for dental caries. *1,* Pits and fissures on otherwise smooth surfaces; *2,* contact areas on the proximal surfaces of all teeth; *3,* cervical margins on the crown or exposed root surface of any tooth. (From Mount GJ, Hume WR: *Preservation and restoration of tooth structure,* St Louis, 1998, Mosby.)

Table 17-3	Cavity Classification			
SITE SIZE	**MINIMAL 1**	**MODERATE 2**	**ENLARGED 3**	**EXTENSIVE 4**
Pit/Fissure (1)	1.1	1.2	1.3	1.4
Contact Area (2)	2.1	2.2	2.3	2.4
Cervical Area (3)	3.1	3.2	3.3	3.4

The clinical caries classification is divided into the following:
- Sound
- White and brown spots on the surface
- Noncavitated pits and fissures
- Cavitations
- Noncavitated dentin caries
- Cavitated and noncavitated root caries (Figure 17-17)

Radiographic classification is divided into the following:
- No visible lesion (E0)
- A lesion in the outer half of the enamel (E1)
- A lesion in the inner half of the enamel (E2)

Similarly the dentin is divided into thirds, in which the following labels are used:
- A lesion in the outer third is labeled *D1*.
- A lesion in the middle third is labeled *D2*.
- A lesion in the inner third, including the pulp, is labeled *D3* (Figures 17-18 and 17-19).

The existing tooth condition is recorded on the electronic tooth chart when the appropriate icon is selected. In addition to the appropriate clinical and radiographic icons, the computer software automatically suggests a possible treatment for the charted condition (Figure 17-20).

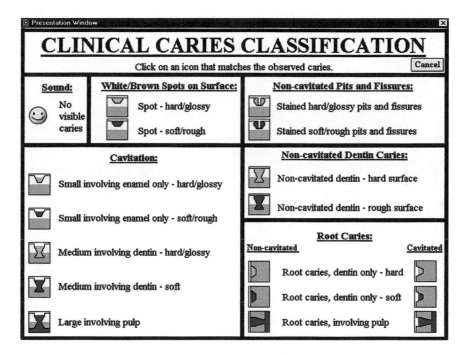

FIGURE 17-17
A set of pictorial computer icons represents different stages of lesion severity and activity from various anatomical sites. (From Benn DK et al: Practical approach to evidence-based management of caries, *J Am Coll Dent* 66[1]:27-35, 1999.)

RADIOGRAPHIC CLASSIFICATION

Click on an icon that best represents the observed radiographic depth:

E0 Healthy, no lesion visible (F1)

E1 Lesion in outer half of enamel (F2)

E2 Lesion in inner half of enamel but has not entered dentin (F3)

D1 Lesion in outer third of dentin (F4)

D2 Lesion in middle third of dentin (F5)

D3 Lesion in inner third of dentin (F6)

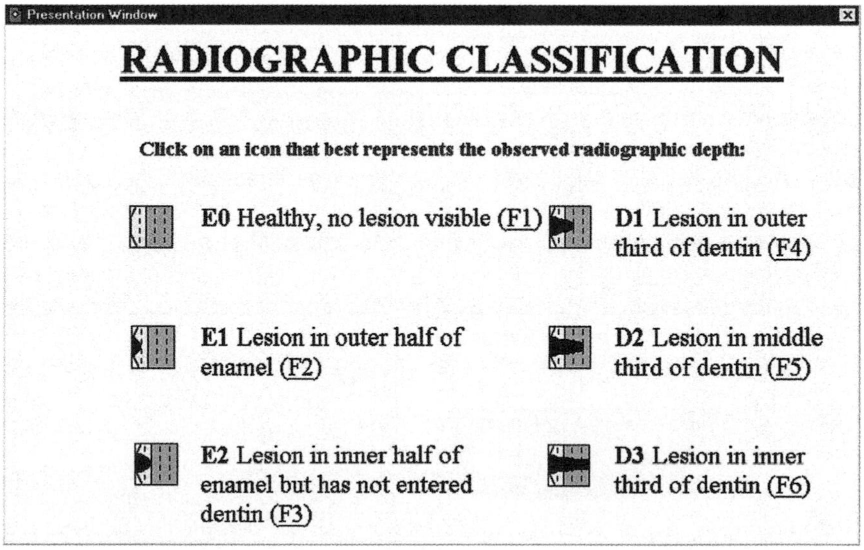

FIGURE 17-18
Radiographic caries classification. (From Benn DK et al: Practical approach to evidence-based management of caries, *J Am Coll Dent* 66[1]:27-35, 1999.)

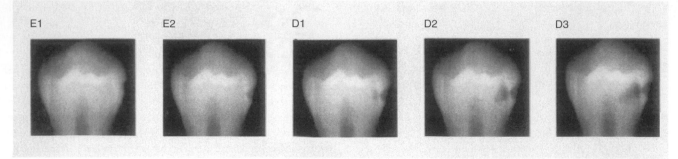

FIGURE 17-19
Examples of radiographic lesion classification. E0, Healthy, no lesion visible in enamel; *E1*, lesion in outer half of enamel; *E2*, lesion in inner half of enamel; *D1*, lesion in outer third of dentin; *D2*, lesion in middle third of dentin; *D3*, lesion in inner third of dentin. (From Benn DK et al: Practical approach to evidence-based management of caries, *J Am Coll Dent* 66[1]:27-35, 1999.)

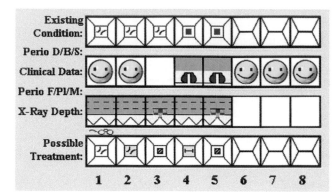

FIGURE 17-20
New dental caries tooth chart. (From Benn DK et al: Practical approach to evidence-based management of caries, *J Am Coll Dent* 66[1]:27-35, 1999.)

This suggested classification system has several advantages:
- It reminds the clinician to consider lesion severity and dental caries activity.
- It rapidly collects and records data with a simple click of the mouse.
- The software program automates the decision process, facilitating more consistent interexaminer agreement.

Although a step in the right direction, this system is not foolproof. One limiting factor is that the system assumes that the clinician can estimate the actual histologic lesion depth, which is questionable given today's crude diagnostic tools.

In summary, the preceding sections have presented two proposed classification systems to address the expanding knowledge in modern dental caries management. Perhaps more important than the discovery of an *ideal* classification system is the challenge to the dental community first to realize the need for new treatment modalities, then to explore new systems, and finally to implement them.

Current Methods of Dental Caries Detection

Any review of the literature on dental caries detection requires the definition of two commonly used terms—*sensitivity* and *specificity*. Simply put, **sensitivity** is the ability to correctly de-

tect a carious lesion that is truly carious, and **specificity** is the ability to correctly identify health, or an absence of carious lesions. Ideally a dental caries detection method would have both high sensitivity and specificity; however, in reality, the perfect detection tool or method has yet to be found.

VISUAL AND TACTILE METHODS

A typical conventional approach to dental caries management in the United States often begins with a careful tooth-by-tooth visual and tactile hard tissue examination. The main detection tools consist of a discriminating eye, conventional dental radiographs, and a sharp dental explorer. The clinician examines the tooth surfaces carefully by probing the sharp end of a dental explorer into any questionable areas of the tooth, such as white or brown spot lesions (see the later section of this chapter concerning color changes in enamel), pits and fissures, and marginal discrepancies (chips or gaps) in existing restorations. The test for dental caries, as described by Black in 1924 and Sturdevant in 1985,[6] is thought to be positive if the sharp explorer "sticks" when pressure is applied to the tip or has *tug back* on withdrawal. Because of the narrow tooth morphology in pit and fissure areas, these so-called conventional methods used to detect dental caries all may be inaccurate.[37]

DENTAL CONSIDERATIONS

Deep morphology of these areas can cause an explorer to stick or demonstrate tug back, not because the area is actually carious but because the sharp explorer has wedged in the narrow pit or fissure (a false-positive result). Conversely, narrow, deep anatomy of these areas may prevent the explorer from actually reaching the base of the pit or fissure, causing the clinician to miss an active carious lesion at the base (a false-negative result).

Given these facts, studies[29] showing that the use of a dental explorer does not improve detection of pit and fissure caries in comparison to a visual inspection alone are not surprising. In one study the percentage of correctly diagnosed teeth was only 42%, compared with a histologic gold standard method.[29] Such findings are consistent with other studies showing that only

Prevention

The dependence on the dental explorer is not only highly misleading (as in the pit and fissure areas) but also may be potentially harmful to the tooth,[19] especially on partially diminished smooth surfaces. Improper use of a sharp dental explorer during examination can adversely affect teeth[41] by damaging newly erupted teeth,[12] accelerating dental caries progression,[43] causing cavitations in previously noncavitated lesions,[45] and transmitting pathogens to a tooth not previously infected.[28]

20% to 40% of pit and fissure caries were correctly detected by visual techniques.[44]

The occlusal surface currently poses the greatest challenge for clinicians for four reasons. First, most of the incidence of dental caries today occurs on the occlusal surface.[29] Second, because of deep, narrow morphology the pits and fissures may be impossible to thoroughly clean and thus may act as a niche for bacterial growth.[14] Third, this morphology makes dental caries detection difficult, especially in early lesions in which a threat of the so-called hidden occlusal lesion exists. A hidden occlusal lesion describes an area in which a seemingly normal-appearing pit or fissure has an undetected lesion underneath that requires surgical intervention. Fourth and last, the deep morphology leaves the enamel layer extremely thin at the base of the fissure (Figure 17-21).

Pits and fissures now may be examined for visually undetectable dental caries with the DIAGNOdent (Figure 17-22), a device that detects and measures pathogenic bacterial byproducts in the subsurface lesion. The next method used to detect subsurface lesions is to perform an **enameloplasty** by opening the surface with a small dental bur and evaluating the underlying dental structure (Figure 17-23). This procedure requires removal of tooth structure and some form of restoration, regardless of whether a carious lesion is present.

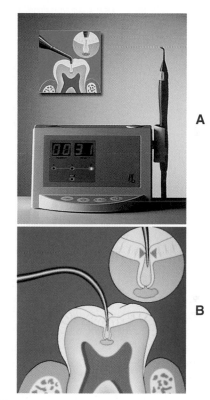

FIGURE 17-22
A, The DIAGNOdent used to detect subsurface carious lesions. **B,** The inability of the explorer to reach the extent of the subsurface lesion, making the DIAGNOdent preferable for dental caries detection. (Courtesy KaVo America Corporation, Lake Zurich, Ill.)

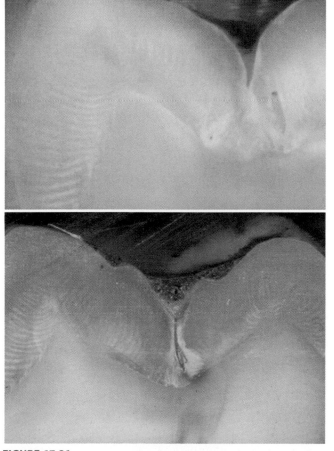

FIGURE 17-21
Anatomy of fissures. **A,** A simple, uncomplicated fissure that does not penetrate the full depth of the enamel. **B,** A more common anatomy in which the fissure has demineralized and the dentin is immediately involved. (From Mount GJ, Hume WR: *Preservation and restoration of tooth structure*, St Louis, 1998, Mosby.)

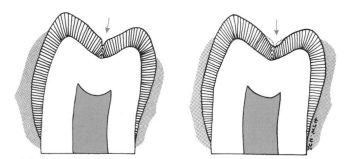

FIGURE 17-23
Enameloplasty. (From Roberson TM, Heymann HO, Smith EJ: *Sturdevant's art and science of operative dentistry*, ed 5, St Louis, 2006, Mosby.)

Recurrent (or Secondary) Caries

Recurrent (or secondary) caries refers to a new active lesion in relation to the margin of an existing restoration. These terms are always associated with a restoration placed as a result of a previous or primary acid attack. However, many so-called recurrent lesions occur on the tooth surface itself, clearly independent of the restoration, and actually represent a new primary attack called an *outer lesion*. In contrast, a carious lesion associated with a margin of a restoration between the restoration and the cavity wall is termed a *wall lesion*.[23] Interestingly, secondary caries is more likely to occur at the gingival margins than the occlusal margins (with 94% of amalgams and 62% of composites failing at the gingival floor of the restoration).[30] Thus amalgams rarely fail at occlusal margins, perhaps because of the self-sealing effects of the formed corrosion products. In

> ### Note
> Surgical intervention should be undertaken only in the presence of cavitated lesions (because of the inability to control plaque biofilm accumulation) and infected dentin, not necessarily ditching or staining.

fact, many experienced clinicians believe that marginal discrepancies (or a small explorer *catch* or *ditching* at the margin in the absence of dental caries) often are being misdiagnosed as secondary caries. Reports are that 75% of operative dentistry is involved in the replacement of existing restorations,[23] many of which may not be secondary caries at all.

Laboratory and histologic studies show a poor correlation between ditching and secondary caries.[22] A color change next to an amalgam restoration should be interpreted with caution because it may simply indicate corrosion products or the physical presence of the silver-colored restoration, rather than dental caries. Staining around tooth-colored restorations, either marginal staining or undermining staining, does not reliably predict soft dentin.[20] Using color change as the only guide would mean that many restorations would be replaced unnecessarily. Microbiological culturing of amalgam restorations shows that intact restorations and *narrow ditches* are minimally infected, requiring no intervention, whereas *wide ditches* are significantly more infected and should be replaced. In addition, findings indicate that color changes alone do not relate to infection and that only frank carious lesions at the margin constitute a reliable diagnosis of secondary caries.[19] Based on previously mentioned studies, one researcher defines a *wide ditch* as one into which the tip of a periodontal probe can fit.[22] Using a dull periodontal probe, a clinician can determine that narrow ditches and color changes alone should not trigger filling replacement, whereas wide ditches or frank carious outer lesions should be restored.[20]

The previous discussion applies to margins in enamel, and extreme caution should be used in any attempt to evaluate the gingival margins in cementum or dentin, where most secondary caries occurs.[30] These margins are often subgingival in cementum or dentin, making the areas difficult both to assess and to restore. More precise diagnostic criteria are necessary to help prevent clinical disagreement on secondary caries detection in these areas.

Color Changes in Enamel

One of the earliest signs of demineralization visible to the naked eye is the white spot lesion. The lesion appears white because the loss of mineral introduces porosities that change the refractive index compared with that of the surrounding translucent enamel. (This type of lesion is discussed further in Chapter 25; Figure 17-24). Often the white spot lesion turns brown, thus the term *brown spot lesion* (Figure 17-25). Dental professionals and researchers do not fully agree on the exact mechanism of this brown change. Many believe that the increased porosity causes exogenous proteins to diffuse and stain the area. One interesting note is that this white-to-brown color shift is most often a sign that the lesion already has remineralized and is resistant to dental caries. In fact, when remineralized in the presence of topical fluoride, this surface is more than likely fluorapatite and will resist future acid attacks, thus greatly decreasing the probability that a cavitation will occur at that particular site.

Perhaps more important than color in enamel is whether the surface is significantly cavitated. Cavitation through the enamel allows bacteria to enter the dentin, whereas an intact enamel surface layer does not allow the bacteria to penetrate the enamel and enter the dentin. The diffusion channels in enamel are too small to let bacteria in but are large enough to allow the entrance of small molecules, such as acid and fluoride. The

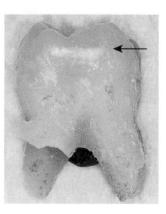

FIGURE 17-24
White spot lesion.

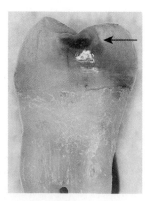

FIGURE 17-25
Brown spot lesion.

consequences of failure to remineralize an enamel lesion are usually not as severe as those related to failure to remineralize a dentinal lesion because of the differences in the rate of dental caries progression between the two tooth structures. In addition, enamel contains more mineral (85% by volume) than dentin (50% by volume), making remineralization more clinically practical in enamel.

Color Changes in Dentin and Cementum

AFFECTED VERSUS INFECTED DENTIN

Why do carious lesions sometimes stain dark or appear brown? This phenomenon may be the result of a combination of factors. Many researchers believe that the increase in porosity

caused by the demineralization of the dentin allows an ingress of exogenous stain, whereas others in the field believe the problem is caused by chromogenic bacteria.[18] More recently, the cause for the discoloration of carious dentin has been suggested to be a reaction between demineralized collagen and bacterially derived aldehydes or dietary sugars (or both).[26]

The affected layer, because of its increased porosity, is the area that often appears dark brown and can appear broader in rapidly advancing dental caries than in slowly advancing lesions.

ACTIVE VERSUS INACTIVE DENTAL CARIES

As stated previously, the use of color alone as an indicator of active dental caries is risky. Evaluating color changes on root surface cementum and dentin is often challenging and has more severe consequences. Compared with enamel, dentin is much more porous, with less mineral content. Dentin is susceptible to collagenase and is physically closer to the pulp. Many experienced clinicians have noticed that active dental caries is often normal in color or a very light brown. In contrast, inactive or arrested dental caries is dark brown to black in color. Microbiological studies have shown that the combination of optical criteria and conventional tactile sense in the clinical removal of dental caries (until the dentin is firm and hard) results in little to no infected dentin remaining.[21] Therefore the use of hardness and optical appearance as a clinical guide is more reliable than color alone.

The infected dentin feels soft to the touch, is often described as "mushy" or "leathery," and can be removed by careful use of large round burs in a slow-speed hand piece with spoon excavators. Cautious use of a specially formulated dental caries–indicating dye may help the novice clinician differentiate between affected and infected dentin (as long as the clinician understands that this method is not absolute). Dental caries–disclosing dyes are used in many dental schools to help students develop the tactile skills necessary to discern infected from affected dentin. Active lesions progress and lead to eventual cavitation, which can be seen radiographically, whereas inactive lesions do not progress and may appear smaller radiographically if remineralized. Again, this information should not encourage unrestrained use of dental radiographs.

Dental Caries–Indicating Dyes

Recently a number of dental caries–indicating products have become available on the market. First introduced in the early 1970s, these products consist of a dye in a carrier fluid. Once applied, the dye penetrates partially demineralized dentin because of the increased porosity. When carious dentin underlying carious enamel is exposed during a cavity preparation, the clinician can apply the dye solution to help judge the point at which all the carious dentin has been removed. The clinical goal of dental caries removal in dentin is to remove only the soft bacterial "infected" dentin, leaving partially demineralized affected dentin behind. Studies conducted in the early 1970s claimed that the dye did not stain noninfected dentin, and to this day the use of dental caries–indicating dye is met with enthusiasm based on these original studies.[13] However, subsequent studies since have shown that the dye stains demineralized areas of the dentin (not the bacteria itself) and also may stain noninfected dentin. An inherent danger of overremoval of tooth structure is present.[21] Because of this lack of specificity, such dyes are a very crude dental caries–detecting tool[24] and should not be used as the sole determining factor in clinical dental caries removal.

Detection with Dental Radiographs

Dental caries just under the floss contact between teeth is called *proximal* or **approximal caries** and is conventionally detected with dental bite-wing radiographs. Radiographic detection of dental caries consists of discerning whether radiolucent (dark) areas on the dental radiograph appear consistent with a carious lesion. Once a carious lesion is detected on the radiograph and preferably confirmed by the visual and tactile examination, the area is treatment-planned for surgical restorative treatment (often amalgam prepared to a G.V. Black outline form). After the restorative treatment is completed, the patient usually is recalled for a periodic oral examination. Ironically, this recall interval is based on the periodontal status of the patient, and recall criteria make little sense given that no direct biological relationship exists between periodontal disease and dental caries. At the recall appointment the patient again is examined for dental caries, and the process repeated if lesions are detected.

Conventional radiographic examination is the accepted standard used to detect proximal lesions and is a fairly crude but objective way to visualize the loss of mineral. Although the radiographic technique may be objective, the interpretation of the resulting image often is not. A common mistake is the assumption that the appropriate treatment for a radiolucent area on a radiograph is to "drill and fill." Studies have shown that demineralization measured in the laboratory with histologic techniques is more advanced than the information represented on the radiograph.[25] This one fact is grossly misinterpreted, leading many to believe that clinicians need to be more aggressive at surgically restoring small radiographic proximal lesions because they are actually much deeper than they appear on the radiograph. The interpretation error is in the failure to recognize that early demineralization often can be arrested and remineralized, especially if the surface layer of enamel is intact and noncavitated. In these cases the loss of mineral is most important to the diagnosis, as is the fact that the intact surface layer prevents bacteria from penetrating through the enamel into dentin. Although small molecules such as acid, calcium, and fluoride can diffuse into and from intact enamel, larger-sized bacteria cannot.

DENTAL CONSIDERATIONS

Thus when bacteria have not invaded or when little chance exists of invasion into the dentin, nonsurgical treatment modalities should be used. Dentin that has been invaded by bacteria is called *infected dentin,* and all such dentin should be surgically removed. Unfortunately, the conventional radiograph, which may qualitatively show areas where the mineral is less dense, does not show whether the surface is cavitated. Presently, needs exist for better quantitative dental caries detection tools and for modification of the drill-and-fill mentality concerning early lesions.

Until such time, dental professionals can apply some common rules of thumb based on laboratory studies and clinical experience. In many states the licensure board generally would reject a proximal lesion if the radiolucency did not touch or penetrate the dentinoenamel junction (DEJ). As it turns out, this description is comparable with the E2 or D1 histologic lesion described previously. This rule is a good clinical guide that can be used to evaluate proximal lesions on bite-wing radiographs until improved methods are perfected. Of course, many E2 and D1 lesions may not have cavitated, but the rule of thumb is an acceptable compromise until better quantitative detection methods are available.

> **Prevention**
> E1 lesions should be treated chemically to prevent cavitation.

Used properly, the bite-wing radiograph is a valuable tool to evaluate the proximal area. However, this radiographic method is less reliable in dental caries detection in the occlusal area, where, as mentioned previously, clinicians often have difficulty discerning pathologic processes. Therefore radiographs must be interpreted with great caution to prevent false-positive detections.[37,38]

In proximal lesions, minimal sound tissue is in the path of the x-rays, whereas the occlusal surface usually has a thick layer of sound hard tissue on either side, making detection in this area by conventional radiography difficult, unless the lesions are very large. Consequently, occlusal lesions are well advanced by the time they can be detected on a radiograph.[34] In 1995 a group of researchers[11] questioned routine use of radiographic examination for early occlusal lesions.[38] Computerized digital radiography is being used successfully in dental practice and subjects patients to less exposure from ionizing radiation; however, it still suffers from the same problems of basic physics and interpretation as described previously.

NEW ADVANCES IN DENTAL CARIES DETECTION

Recently, three commercial products have shown great promise in improving dental caries detection:

1. DIAGNOdent (KaVo, Lake Zurich, Ill.)
2. DiFOTI (digital fiber-optic transillumination; Electro-Sciences Inc. Irvington, NY.)
3. QLF (quantitative light-induced fluorescence; OMNII Oral Pharmaceuticals, West Palm Beach, Fla.)

DIAGNOdent

The DIAGNOdent is a lightweight, battery-operated detection device incorporating a solid-state diode laser that detects and measures fluorescence created by bacterial by-products that have diffused into porous subsurface lesions. The softening of enamel as the dental caries process continues makes it more porous and allows bacterial by-products, including chemicals called *porphyrins*, to soak into the lesion. Some of these chemicals interact with the red light–emitting fluorescent light in the near infrared that is detected by the DIAGNOdent—the higher the amount of porphyrin type chemical absorbed by the lesion, the larger the number that shows on the instrument output.[16,42,43] Specific wavelengths of light can excite fluorescence, and differences between sound and carious tissue can be detected indirectly as a measure of the porosity (but not as a direct measure of mineral loss). With the DIAGNOdent, a diode laser with a wavelength of 655 nm is used. This technique does not provide a two- or three-dimensional image showing the extent and severity of lesions for later comparison in the determination of a progression or reversal of the lesion; it simply gives a number from 0 to 100. If the number is more than 25, then the existence of a sizeable subsurface lesion is likely.

This device is commercially available to clinicians. Although a relatively new technology, the device is a valuable adjunct to conventional visual and tactile detection methods for lesions in the occlusal surface.

DiFOTI

The DiFOTI uses computer technology to interpret images captured by shining visible light on the tooth. Instead of ionizing radiation used in a bite-wing radiograph, a concentrated beam of visible light is shone on the tooth, and an image is captured via a mirror on the other side of the tooth. A real-time image is created through a computer system and is seen on a monitor. DiFOTI images detect only optical changes at or near the surface; the clinician must discern whether the optical changes are from demineralization or from other causes. Cracks can be visualized readily. Although very sensitive at picking up early surface changes, studies have yet to show that DiFOTI can be useful in assessing and monitoring lesion depth. A recent laboratory study showed that this technology cannot assess lesion depth; therefore it cannot be used as a substitute for radiography to decide whether to drill or fill these lesions.[46]

Qualitative Light-Induced Fluorescence

Recently, QLF technology has been introduced into the dental market for early dental caries detection and bacterial activity as the Inspektor Pro (OMNII Oral Pharmaceuticals). QLF works from the principle of light fluorescence. Blue light shines on the tooth, and the enamel is largely transparent to light at this wavelength. The underlying dentin fluoresces with blue light, and the green fluorescence passes back through the enamel. If a carious lesion exists in its path, then the light scatters and shows up as an area of little or no fluorescence. The Inspektor Pro can pick up this difference in contrast and produce an image that can be quantified and compared over time. Repositioning software is built into the system to enable lesions to be monitored over time. It can be used for the early detection of carious lesions and for monitoring of demineralization and remineralization of white spots by quantifying the mineral loss and the size of smooth surface lesions.[17] QLF is able to detect surface changes very early and shows great promise for tracking chemical treatments of early lesions over time. However, this technology has yet to demonstrate that it can give even an indirect measure of lesion depth.

At the time of this text's publication, all three devices are commercially available to clinicians. Although relatively new technologies, these devices represent valuable adjuncts to conventional detection methods. Only time will tell how much they will affect early dental caries detection.

DIFFERING VIEWS ON SURGICAL RESTORATIVE APPROACHES

Traditional G.V. Black cavity preparations are still being taught in U.S. dental schools, are used for state licensure examinations, and are the most predominant cavity forms used in private practice today. However, many clinicians believe these conventional treatment philosophies and a lack of aggressive preventive measures have contributed to the overpreparation of tooth structure. Currently, trends are emerging that look for opportunities to preserve tooth structure via prevention and conservative restorative procedures.[32] For example, growing evidence supports the idea that some conservative preparations, which remove much less tooth structure, are at least as retentive as the traditional G.V. Black cavity preparations.[10] The limitations of current detection techniques described previously have lead most traditional clinicians to watch questionable areas until they test positive with conventional detection techniques (i.e.,

an explorer stick or visible cavitation) or to restore early proximal radiographic lesions. However, some clinicians believe that watching pits and fissures can lead to large subsurface lesion progression, which can go undetected until preventive intervention is no longer possible. Still other clinicians believe that using these conventional management strategies, coupled with conventional Black preparation design, results in unnecessary loss of tooth structure. Given current knowledge, preventive sealants and new management protocols require further investigation.

Future Dental Caries Detection Technologies

Several alternative dental caries detection techniques are currently under investigation. Although some are being used clinically in certain countries, most have failed to surface in the United States. Because these methods are appearing in the research literature, each is introduced briefly in the following section.

CONDUCTANCE AND IMPEDANCE

Several approaches have been proposed to take advantage of the ability of water within teeth to conduct electricity because it contains dissolved minerals.[35] Carious tissue contains more water than sound tissue and therefore conducts electricity more readily. However, experiments using direct current (DC) conductance have been disappointing, demonstrating little discrimination between carious tissue and other noncarious porous tissue. Location of the lesion also is difficult to determine.

Electrical impedance may prove to be a relatively low-cost approach for the detection of occlusal dental caries and may help dental professionals decide whether to *open up* the tooth.[27,35,37,38] However, this method lacks two- or three-dimensional images of the lesion and produces no record of position or extent of the lesion.

> *Distinct Care Modifications*
> Electrical impedance measurements recently have shown considerable promise for lesion detection, demonstrating both high sensitivity and high specificity.

ULTRASOUND

Potentially, ultrasound may be used to provide images of carious lesions in all tooth surfaces; however, currently this methodology is unavailable for dental use because the resolution required is (for the present) beyond the scope of the technique.

FLUORESCENCE

Sound enamel produces an intrinsic fluorescence, the exact origin of which has yet to be explained. As the dental caries process continues, the alteration of sound enamel leads to changes in fluorescence, enabling observations to be made for potential dental caries detection.[16,39,40] Specific wavelengths of light can excite fluorescence, permitting detection of differences between sound and carious tissue. Although this technique has shown some promise for smooth surfaces and possibly for occlusal surfaces, it has not yet been perfected and requires more laboratory and clinical validation. This technique also does not provide a two- or three-dimensional image to show the extent and severity of lesions for later comparison to determine progression or reversal of the lesion.

OPTICAL COHERENCE TOMOGRAPHY

A new technique, optical coherence tomography (OCT), produces a tomographic image in two dimensions, showing the extent and potentially the severity of subsurface demineralization.[8,9] In the future it may also be possible to create three-dimensional images sufficiently quickly (because of improved computer technology and image-gathering systems). Near infrared light (usually approximately 1310 nm wavelength) is readily transmitted through sound enamel but is scattered by carious enamel. The back-scattered coherent light can be detected in contrast to the light scattered by the lesion to produce the tomographic image. OCT is in its early research stage and needs more development before it will be ready for clinical use. However, OCT shows great potential because of its ability to produce a permanent image that can record the position, severity, and extent of the lesion for future comparison. It will be especially useful for pit and fissure caries to detect lesions while they are still in enamel and to signal chemical intervention before drilling and filling is needed.

Occlusal Analysis

Occlusion is important to all aspects of dentistry at all ages. For example, in the primary dentition the clinician should check for adequate spacing between the deciduous teeth so that enough space remains to allow the permanent teeth to erupt properly. If crowding is present in primary or permanent dentition, then an orthodontic evaluation may be indicated. Each time a tooth is restored the dentist must consider the occlusion and the way in which the teeth will function (see Chapter 37 on occlusion). If such information is not considered, then the tooth may be restored with a tooth-to-tooth interference, and the patient may later develop headaches, jaw pain, or both,

which could indicate problems with the TMJ. These examples are just a few of the many demonstrating the important role of occlusion. A comprehensive review of occlusion is beyond the scope of this chapter, but a few basic observations should be recorded during the examination. The extraoral examination in Chapter 14 discusses the way to evaluate the TMJ and the muscles of mastication. The intraoral portion of the occlusal analysis is discussed briefly in the following text.

The basic information to record may include the patient's Angle's classification, overbite, overjet, maximum incisal opening (MIO), pathway of opening or closing, amount of movement from centric relation (CR) to centric occlusion (CO) (known as the *CR-CO shift*), initial contacts in CR, initial contacts in right and left lateral excursions, initial contacts in protrusive movements, and any signs of traumatic occlusion. These terms are defined in the following section, and Figure 17-26 summarizes one way to chart this information.

ANGLE'S CLASSIFICATION SYSTEM

In 1899, Dr. E.H. Angle developed **Angle's classification**—the traditional method used to identify occlusions that need orthodontic treatment. Originally this system used the position of the mesiobuccal (MB) cusp of the maxillary first molar in relationship to the buccal groove of the mandibular first molar.[42] Later, clinicians added the cuspid relationship as well. The ideal occlusion was defined as *Class I*, in which the MB cusp of the maxillary first molar is in line with the buccal groove of the mandibular first molar, as shown in Figure 17-27. *Class II* is defined as having the MB cusp of the maxillary first molar and the maxillary cuspid mesial to the mandibular landmarks. Class II can be subdivided further in to division 1 (anterior teeth flared) and division 2 (anterior teeth verted, or inclined, lingually), also illustrated in Figure 17-27. *Class III* is defined as the MB cusp of the maxillary first molar and the maxillary cuspid distal to the mandibular landmarks, as shown in Figure 17-27. Angle's classification system does have some drawbacks, however; it looks only at a few teeth to classify the entire mouth and is somewhat subjective in decisions about when the maxillary cusps are not in the ideal Class I relationship. If the cusp is

Initial Occlusal and TMJ Findings

CENTRIC RELATION:
Location: ☐ easy ☐ difficult ☐ impossible
TMJ discomfort to pressure ☐ none ☐ right ☐ left
Initial tooth contact: _____ vs. _____
CENTRIC RELATION-CENTRIC OCCLUSION DISCREPANCY:
Vertical slide _____ mm Forward slide _____ mm
Lateral slide ☐ right ☐ left _____ mm
CENTRIC OCCLUSION:
Canine classification (I,II,III) right _____ left _____
Right canine vertical overlap _____ mm
Right canine functional horizontal overlap _____ mm
Left canine vertical overlap _____ mm
Left canine horizontal overlap _____ mm
Central incisor vertical overlap _____ mm
Central incisor functional horizontal overlap _____ mm
Wear facets: ☐ minimal ☐ moderate ☐ severe

CR TO CO	1	2	3	4	5	6	7	8	9	10	11	12	13	14	15	16
INTERFERENCES	32	31	30	29	28	27	26	25	24	23	22	21	20	19	18	17
RT.	1	2	3	4	5	6	7	8	9	10	11	12	13	14	15	16
LATERAL	32	31	30	29	28	27	26	25	24	23	22	21	20	19	18	17
LT.	1	2	3	4	5	6	7	8	9	10	11	12	13	14	15	16
LATERAL	32	31	30	29	28	27	26	25	24	23	22	21	20	19	18	17
PROTRUSIVE	1	2	3	4	5	6	7	8	9	10	11	12	13	14	15	16
	32	31	30	29	28	27	26	25	24	23	22	21	20	19	18	17

TEMPORO-MANDIBULAR JOINT:
Maximum opening _____ mm
Joint sounds during opening and closing: ☐ none ☐ right ☐ left
Joint sounds during excursions: ☐ none ☐ right ☐ left
History of TMJ treatment: ☐ yes ☐ no
Current joint pain: ☐ none ☐ right ☐ left

FIGURE 17-26
Occlusal charting record. (Courtesy University of the Pacific School of Dentistry, San Francisco.)

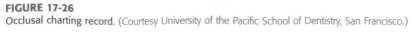

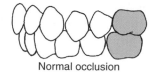
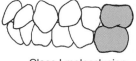

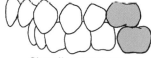
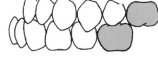

FIGURE 17-27
Normal occlusion and malocclusion classes as specified by Angle. This classification was quickly and widely adopted early in the twentieth century and is incorporated within all contemporary descriptive and classification schemes. (Modified from Proffit WR, Fields HW, Sarver DM: *Contemporary orthodontics,* ed 4, St Louis, 2007, Mosby.)

more than a half cusp from an ideal Class I, then this cusp is generally accepted as either a Class II or Class III, and even this determination is somewhat subjective.

OVERBITE AND OVERJET

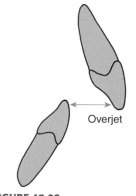

Overbite is the vertical distance that the maxillary anterior teeth overlap the mandibular anterior teeth when the teeth are fully occluded.[42]
Overjet is the horizontal distance measured from the labial or lingual surface (depending on clinician preference) of the maxillary incisors to the facial surface of the lower incisors when the teeth are fully occluded.[42] Figures 17-28 and 17-29 demonstrate the ways to measure overbite and overjet.

FIGURE 17-28
Overjet is defined as horizontal overlap of the incisors. (Modified from Proffit WR, Fields HW, Sarver DM: *Contemporary orthodontics,* ed 4, St Louis, 2007, Mosby.)

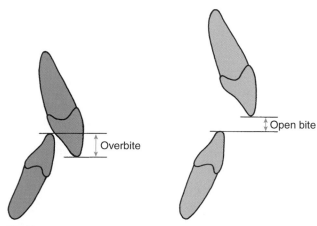

FIGURE 17-29
Overbite is defined as vertical overlap of the incisors. (Modified from Proffit WR, Fields HW, Sarver DM: *Contemporary orthodontics,* ed 4, St Louis, 2007, Mosby.)

MAXIMUM INCISAL OPENING

The MIO is measured from the incisal edges of the anterior teeth when the mandible is opened to its furthest extent (Figure 17-30).

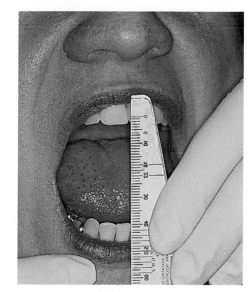

FIGURE 17-30
Maximum opening of patient's mandible is measured.

PATHWAY OF OPENING OR CLOSING

Ideally the midline path of opening and closing of the mandible follows a straight, or linear, path when viewed from the front of the patient. However, this path is not always the case, and deviations from it should be noted on the chart. Often the path the midline of the mandible takes an S-shape deviation to the right or left.

CENTRIC RELATION-CENTRIC OCCLUSION SHIFT

In its simplest definition, CR is the most retruded position of the mandible, and CO is the position of the mandible when the teeth are in maximum intercuspation.[33] The CR and CO are rarely in the same position, and often a shift or slide occurs from the CR to the CO position that can be estimated and recorded in the chart. A CO-CR shift by itself is not necessarily a pathologic condition.

INITIAL CONTACTS IN EXCURSIONS

A protrusive excursion occurs when the mandible moves from the CR or CO position anteriorly until the incisors are in the edge-to-edge position. Ideally when the teeth are in the protrusive position, the posterior teeth should no longer touch. A lateral excursion occurs when the mandible travels from the CO or CR to the right or left until the cuspids on that side are in the cusp-to-cusp position. In that position the teeth on the opposite side should not be in contact. Observing and recording in the chart which teeth touch during the performance of these different excursions can help discern between normal movements and those that may be considered pathologic interferences.

TRAUMATIC OCCLUSION

Occlusal trauma is a force capable of producing pathologic changes to the supporting periodontium. Two types of occlusal trauma exist: (1) primary occlusal trauma and (2) secondary occlusal trauma. Primary occlusal trauma occurs when excessive occlusal force is applied to a tooth with normal supporting structures. Secondary occlusal trauma occurs when normal occlusal forces cause trauma to the attachment apparatus of a tooth because of inadequate support structures. Occlusal trauma is not an inflammatory process, is not related to periodontal disease, and does not cause pocket formation.[5,7,15,47] A periodontally involved tooth may, however, be affected adversely by occlusal trauma. Many causes of occlusal trauma exist, including tooth position, oral habits, contacts with foreign objects, and iatrogenic causes.

References

1. Anderson MH, Bales DJ, Omnell K-A: Modern management of dental caries: the cutting edge is not the dental bur, *J Am Dent Assoc* 124:37-44, 1993.

2. Anusavice KJ: Efficacy of nonsurgical management of the initial caries lesion, *J Dent Educ* 61:895-905, 1997.

3. Anusavice KJ: Treatment regimens in preventive and restorative dentistry, *J Am Dent Assoc* 126(6):727-743, 1995.

4. Benn DK et al: Practical approach to evidence-based management of caries, *J Am Coll Dent* 66(1):27-35, 1999.

5. Carranza FA: *Glickman's clinical periodontology*, Philadelphia, 1979, WB Saunders.

6. Chan DC: Current methods and criteria for caries diagnosis in North America, *J Dent Educ* 57(6):422-427, 1993.

7. Chasen AI: Controversies in occlusion, *Dent Clin North Am* 34:1, 1990.

8. Colston BW et al: Imaging of hard- and soft-tissue structure in the oral cavity by optical coherence tomography, *Applied Optics* 37(16):3582-3585, 1998.

9. Colston BW et al: Non-invasive diagnosis of early caries with polarization sensitive optical tomography (PS-OCT). In Featherstone JDB, Rechmann P, Fried D, eds: *Proceedings of lasers in dentistry V,* Vol 3593, San Jose, Calif, January 24-25, 1999, The International Society for Optical Engineering.

10. Eakle WS et al: Mechanical retention versus bonding of amalgam and gallium alloy restorations, *J Prosthet Dent* 72(4):351-354, 1994.

11. Ekstrand KR et al: Relationship between external and histologic features of progressive stages of caries in the occlusal fossa, *Caries Res* 29(4):243-250, 1995.

12. Ekstrand KR, Ricketts DN, Kidd EA: Reproducibility and accuracy of three methods for assessment of demineralization depth of the occlusal surface: an in vitro examination, *Caries Res* 31(3):224-231, 1997.

13. Fusayama T, Terashima S: Differentiation of two layers of carious dentin by staining, *Bull Tokyo Med Dent Univ* 19(1):83-92, 1972.

14. Galil KA, Gwinnett AJ: Three-dimensional replicas of pits and fissures in human teeth: scanning electron microscopy study, *Arch Oral Biol* 20:493-495, 1975.

15. Goldman HC, Cohen DW: *Periodontal therapy,* St Louis, 1980, Mosby.

16. Hall AF et al: Dye-enhanced laser fluorescence method. In Stookey GK, ed: *Early detection of dental caries: proceedings of the 1st annual Indiana Conference,* Indianapolis, 1996, Indiana University.

17. Heinrich-Weltzien R et al: Quantitative light-induced fluorescence (QLF)—a potential method for the dental practitioner, *Quintessence Int* 34(3):181-188, 2003.

18. Kidd EA: Diagnosis of secondary caries. In Stookey GK, ed: *Early detection of dental caries: proceedings of the 1st annual Indiana conference,* Indianapolis, 1996, Indiana University.

19. Kidd EA: The diagnosis and management of the 'early' carious lesion in permanent teeth, *Dent Update* 11(2):69-70, 72-74, 76-78, 1984.

20. Kidd EA, Joyston-Bechal S, Beighton D: Marginal ditching and staining as a predictor of secondary caries around amalgam restorations: a clinical and microbiological study, *J Dent Res* 74(5):1206-1211, 1995.

21. Kidd EA, Joyston-Bechal S, Beighton D: The use of a caries detector dye during cavity preparation: a microbiological assessment, *Br Dent J* 174(7):245-248, 1993.

22. Kidd EA, O'Hara JW: The caries status of occlusal amalgam restorations with marginal defects, *J Dent Res* 69(6):1275-1277, 1990.

23. Kidd EA, Toffenetti F, Mjör IA: Secondary caries, *Int Dent J* 42(3):127-138, 1992.

24. Kidd EA et al: The use of a caries detector dye in cavity preparation, *Br Dent J* 167(4):132-134, 1989.

25. Kleier DJ, Hicks MJ, Flaitz CM: A comparison of Ultraspeed and Ektaspeed dental x-ray film: in vitro study of the radiographic and histologic appearance of interproximal lesions, *Quintessence Int* 18(9):623-631, 1987.

26. Kleter GA: Discoloration of dental carious lesions [review], *Arch Oral Biol* 43:629-632, 1998.

27. Levinkind M: Electrochemical impedance strategies for early caries detection. In Stookey GK, Beiswanger B, eds: *Indiana conference 1996: early detection of dental caries,* Indianapolis, 1996, Indiana University.

28. Loesche WJ, Svanberg ML, Pape HR: Intraoral transmission of *Streptococcus mutans* by a dental explorer, *J Dent Res* 58(8):765-770, 1979.

29. Lussi A: Validity of diagnostic and treatment decisions of fissure caries, *Caries Res* 25(4):296-303, 1991.

30. Mjör IA: Frequency of secondary caries at various anatomical locations, *Oper Dent* 10(3):88-92, 1985.

31. Mount GJ, Hume WR: A new cavity classification, *Aust Dent J* 43(3):153-159, 1998.

32. Mount GJ, Hume WR: *Preservation and restoration of tooth structure,* St Louis, 1998, Mosby.

33. Ramfjord SP, Ash MM: *Occlusion,* Philadelphia, 1983, WB Saunders.

34. Ricketts DN, Kidd EA, Beighton D: Operative and microbiological validation of visual, radiographic and electronic diagnosis of occlusal caries in non-cavitated teeth judged to be in need of operative care, *Br Dent J* 179(6):214-220, 1995.

35. Ricketts DN, Kidd EA, Wilson RF: The electronic diagnosis of caries in pits and fissures: site-specific stable conductance readings or cumulative resistance readings, *Caries Res* 31(2):119-124, 1997.

36. Ricketts D et al: Hidden caries: what is it? Does it exist? Does it matter? *Int Dent J* 47(5):259-265, 1997.

37. Ricketts DN et al: Histological validation of electrical resistance measurements in the diagnosis of occlusal caries, *Caries Res* 30(2):148-155, 1996.

38. Ricketts DN et al: Clinical and radiographic diagnosis of occlusal caries: a study in vitro, *J Oral Rehab* 22(1):15-20, 1995.

39. ten Bosch JJ: General aspects of optical methods in dentistry, *Adv Dent Res* 1(1):5-7, 1987.

40. ten Bosch JJ, Angmar-Mansson B: A review of quantitative methods for studies of mineral content of intra-oral incipient caries lesions, *J Dent Res* 70(1):2-14, 1991.

41. ten Cate JM, van Amcrongen JP: Caries diagnosis, conventional methods. In Stookey GK, ed: *Early detection of dental caries: proceedings of the 1st annual Indiana conference,* Indianapolis, 1996, Indiana University.

42. Thurow RC: *Atlas of orthodontic principles,* St Louis, 1977, Mosby.

43. van Dorp CS, Exterkate RA, ten Cate JM: The effect of dental probing on subsequent enamel demineralization, *ASDC J Dent Child* 55(5):343-347, 1988.

44. Wenzel A, Larsen MJ, Fejerskov O: Detection of occlusal caries without cavitation by visual inspection, film radiographs, xeroradiographs, and digitized radiographs, *Caries Res* 25(5):365-371, 1991.

45. Yassin OM: In vitro studies of the effect of a dental explorer on the formation of an artificial carious lesion, *ASDC J Dent Child* 62(2):111-117, 1995.

46. Young DA, Featherstone JD: Digital imaging fiber-optic transillumination, F-speed radiographic film and depth of approximal lesions, *J Am Dent Assoc* 136(12):1682-1687, 2005.

47. Zander HA, Polson AM: Present status of occlusion and occlusal therapy in periodontics, *J Periodontol* 43:540-544, 1977.

Radiographic Evaluation and Intraoral Photographic Imaging

Laura Jansen Howerton • W. Bruce Howerton, Jr.

INSIGHT

The dental hygienist should evaluate the patient before the dentist determines the appropriate radiographs to be ordered. Points to consider in this evaluation include the patient's medical and dental history, current chief complaint, previous radiographs, or other clinical information.

✪ CASE STUDY 18-1   Radiographic Overview

Mr. Janus has recently been promoted to vice president of his printing business. Taking on the new responsibilities has caused him to work longer hours and to neglect his personal care matters, including visits to his physician and dentist. His last visit to the dentist was nearly 2 years ago. Mr. Janus scheduled a dental appointment at his wife's urging, although he has been bothered by the appearance of what appears to be a cavity between teeth #9 and #10 (Figure 18-1). He also catches food in the mandibular right quadrant and has not been brushing or flossing regularly.

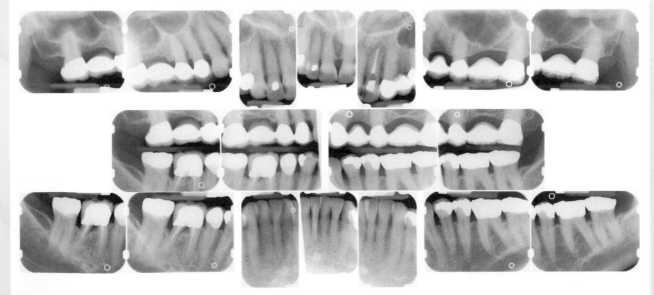

FIGURE 18-1
Diagnostic series of intraoral radiographs: bite-wings and periapical images.

✦ CASE STUDY 18-2   The Value of a Complete Series of Radiographs

Mrs. Kessler has arrived at her recall appointment nearly 30 minutes late. She requests that only four bite-wing radiographs be exposed at this appointment, even though the dentist had requested a complete series be taken. The hygienist tries to explain the importance of a more thorough radiographic examination, especially with the extensive dental history of this patient. However, Mrs. Kessler remains convinced that because of time constraints, her preference is to have prophylactic procedures begun and only four bite-wings exposed at this appointment. During instrumentation, Mrs. Kessler complains of sensitivity around teeth #19 and #30. Slight mobility is noted. Periodontal evaluation with a plastic, calibrated probe is completed and reveals increasing depths around #20 and #29 along with gingival bleeding, rolled margins, and inflammation. The patient is committed to flossing under the fixed bridges but admits avoiding the dental implants with the floss (Figure 18-2).

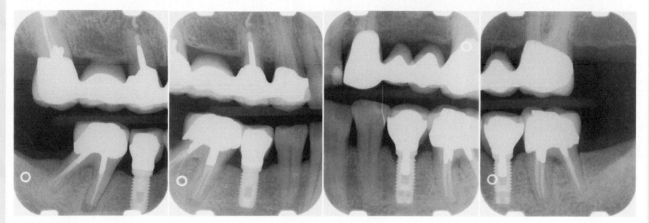

FIGURE 18-2
Four vertical bite-wing radiographs.

✦ CASE STUDY 18-3   Exposure Errors

The four bite-wing radiographs in this study exhibit several operator errors, resulting in films of poor quality. The first projection exposed on this patient was the left premolar bite-wing. After exposure, the dental hygienist realized that the x-ray machine was set to the wrong exposure setting; the setting was too low. The resultant film shows a light image that lacks contrast and therefore is nondiagnostic. The dental hygienist increased the time setting prior to exposing the left molar bite-wing but did not use proper horizontal angulation to open the contact areas. Therefore this image demonstrates overlap in the interproximal regions. The right premolar radiograph demonstrates good packet placement and angulation; however, the cone cut seen in the right molar radiograph nearly eliminates all information regarding the maxillary teeth (Figure 18-3).

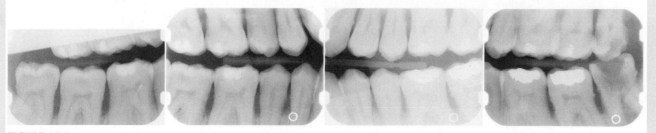

FIGURE 18-3
Four horizontal bite-wing radiographs.

✸ CASE STUDY 18-4   **Diagnostic Quality**

The parents of a 15-year-old boy were concerned when all of the child's permanent second molars had erupted, except for the maxillary left second molar. A panoramic image was exposed to determine the reason for the delayed eruption of tooth #15 (Figure 18-4, *A*). The clinician found that determining the cause of the delayed eruption from this alone, as well as the location of tooth #16, was difficult.

Through the use of cone-beam technology, the next two images were produced (Figure 18-4, *B* and *C*).

Figure 18-4, *B*, is a posterior coronal image of the area in question. A three-dimensional volume rendering of the maxilla and mandible seen from an inferior position is seen in Figure 18-4, *C*. Explanations of these can be found in the case applications in this chapter.

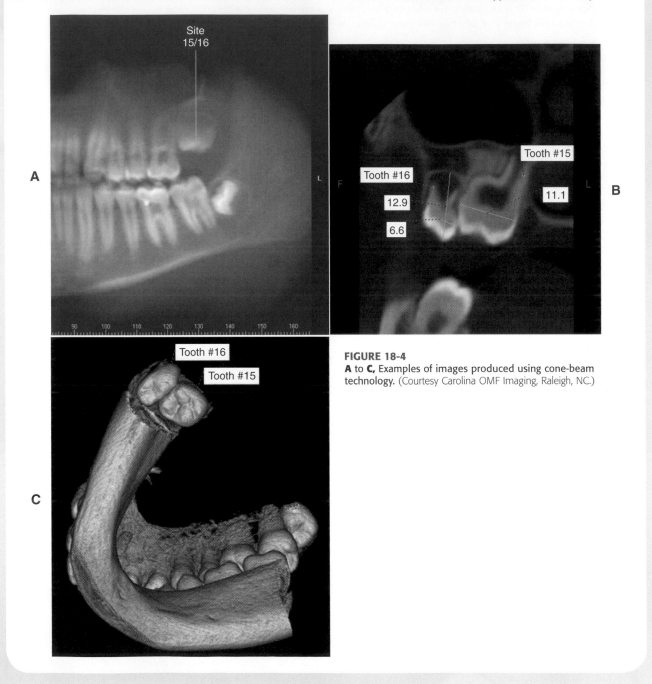

FIGURE 18-4
A to **C,** Examples of images produced using cone-beam technology. (Courtesy Carolina OMF Imaging, Raleigh, NC.)

✦ CASE STUDY 18-5 | Intraoral Images Enhance Treatment Acceptance

Sigorney Winston, a 45-year-old bank teller, comes into your clinical setting for the first time. As part of the patient interview, you learn that Ms. Winston has been told that she has periodontal disease but has not pursued treatment because she was not experiencing any pain. As part of the initial comprehensive examination, you take Ms. Winston on a video tour of her mouth. During this video tour, you recognize areas of the periodontium that exhibit disease.

KEY TERMS

ALARA principle	DICOM	panoramic image	storage phosphor imaging
analog format	digital format	periapical image	system
bite-wing image	digital radiography	pixel	vertical angulation
charge-coupled device	focal trough	sensor	vertical bite-wing radiographs
cone-beam imaging	horizontal angulation		

LEARNING OUTCOMES

After reading this chapter the student will be able to:

1. Establish the appropriate radiographic series for a given patient based on the guidelines for prescribing dental radiographs, including the ALARA (as low as reasonably achievable) principle.
2. List the various types of intraoral and extraoral radiographic projections and their uses.
3. Identify the factors that contribute to the poor diagnostic quality of radiographs.
4. Discuss the fundamentals of digital imaging and cone-beam technology.

5. Recognize and understand the use of intraoral photographic imaging (IPI) in dentistry.
6. Become familiar with the types of IPI equipment and accessories required for the documentation of intraoral anatomy.
7. Use radiographic imaging and IPI to gather assessment information and develop an appropriate care plan.

Computer technology has revolutionized the world. Dental offices are becoming *paperless healthcare providers,* as digital computer technology systems become critical. Digital systems are designed around the work flow of the dental practice, allowing practitioners to concentrate on what is important: delivering exceptional patient care.[10] The union of the digital age with the business aspects of clinical practice have allowed dental professionals to work faster, smarter, and more efficiently than in the past.[3] With the use of digital technology, two aspects that may be implemented into dental practice include digital radiography and intraoral photographic imaging (IPI). Digital and photographic imaging combines radiographic and clinical findings to present the information chairside. The purpose of this chapter is to discuss the ways digital imaging and intraoral photographs can be used together to generate a comprehensive dental hygiene treatment plan while delivering information for individualized patient education.

Importance of Radiographs: Selection Criteria

Dental radiographs are an important component of comprehensive patient care, and detection of disease is one of the most important uses of dental radiographs. The decision on whether or not to expose the patient to ionizing radiation should be based on the individual needs of the patient. Although guidelines have been developed for prescribing dental radiographs (Table 18-1), relying on similar patient protocols is discouraged. Patient selection criteria has been developed by an expert panel of dentists sponsored by the Public Health Service.[1] The

Table 18-1	**Guidelines for Prescribing Dental Radiographs***				
	Patient age and dental developmental stage				
TYPE OF ENCOUNTER	**CHILD WITH PRIMARY DENTITION (BEFORE ERUPTION OF FIRST PERMANENT TOOTH)**	**CHILD WITH TRANSITIONAL DENTITION (AFTER ERUPTION OF FIRST PERMANENT TOOTH)**	**ADOLESCENT WITH PERMANENT DENTITION (BEFORE ERUPTION OF THIRD MOLARS)**	**ADULT, DENTATE OR PARTIALLY EDENTULOUS**	**ADULT, EDENTULOUS**
New Patient[†] Being Evaluated for Dental Diseases and Dental Development	Individualized radiographic examination consisting of selected periapical/occlusal views or posterior bite-wings (or both) if proximal surfaces cannot be visualized or probed (Patients without evidence of disease and with open proximal contacts may not require a radiographic examination at this time.)	Individualized radiographic examination consisting of posterior bite-wings with panoramic examination or posterior bite-wings and selected periapical images	Individualized radiographic examination consisting of posterior bite-wings with panoramic examination or posterior bite-wings and selected periapical images (A full-mouth intraoral radiographic examination is preferred when the patient has clinical evidence of generalized dental disease or a history of extensive dental treatment.)		Individualized radiographic examination based on clinical signs and symptoms
Recall Patient[†] with Clinical Caries or at Increased Risk for Caries[‡]	Posterior bite-wing examination at 6- to 12-month intervals if proximal surfaces cannot be examined visually or with a probe			Posterior bite-wing examination at 6- to 18-month intervals	Not applicable
Recall Patient[†] with No Clinical Caries and Not at Increased Risk for Caries[‡]	Posterior bite-wing examination at 12- to 24-month intervals if proximal surfaces cannot be examined visually or with a probe		Posterior bite-wing examination at 18- to 36-month intervals	Posterior bite-wing examination at 24- to 36-month intervals	Not applicable
Recall Patient[†] with Periodontal Disease	Clinical judgment as to the need for and type of radiographic images for the evaluation of periodontal disease (Imaging may consist of, but is not limited to, selected bite-wing or periapical images [or both] of areas where periodontal disease [other than nonspecific gingivitis] can be identified clinically.)				Not applicable
Patient for Monitoring of Growth and Development	Clinical judgment as to need for and type of radiographic images for evaluation or monitoring (or both) of dentofacial growth and development		Clinical judgment as to need for and type of radiographic images for evaluation, monitoring, or both of dentofacial growth and development; panoramic or periapical examination to assess developing third molars	Usually not indicated	

Table 18-1	**Guidelines for Prescribing Dental Radiographs*—cont'd**				
	Patient age and dental developmental stage				
TYPE OF ENCOUNTER	**CHILD WITH PRIMARY DENTITION (BEFORE ERUPTION OF FIRST PERMANENT TOOTH)**	**CHILD WITH TRANSITIONAL DENTITION (AFTER ERUPTION OF FIRST PERMANENT TOOTH)**	**ADOLESCENT WITH PERMANENT DENTITION (BEFORE ERUPTION OF THIRD MOLARS)**	**ADULT, DENTATE OR PARTIALLY EDENTULOUS**	**ADULT, EDENTULOUS**
Patient with Other Circumstances Including, but Not Limited To, Proposed or Existing Implants, Pathologic Conditions, Restorative and Endodontic Needs, Treated Periodontal Disease, and Dental Caries Remineralization	Clinical judgment as to need for and type of radiographic images for evaluation, monitoring, or both in these circumstances				

*The recommendations in this chart are subject to clinical judgment and may not apply to every patient. These recommendations are to be used by dentists only after reviewing the patient's health history and completing a clinical examination. Because every precaution should be taken to minimize radiation exposure, protective thyroid collars and aprons should be used whenever possible. This practice is strongly recommended for children, women of childbearing age, and pregnant women.

†Clinical situations for which radiographs may be indicated include but are not limited to the following:

A. Positive historical findings
1. Previous periodontal or endodontic treatment
2. History of pain or trauma
3. Familial history of dental anomalies
4. Postoperative evaluation of healing
5. Remineralization monitoring
6. Presence of implants or evaluation for implant placement

B. Positive clinical signs and symptoms
1. Clinical evidence of periodontal disease
2. Large or deep restorations
3. Deep carious lesions
4. Malposed or clinically impacted teeth
5. Swelling
6. Evidence of dental and facial trauma
7. Mobility of teeth
8. Sinus tract (fistula)
9. Clinically suggested sinus pathologic findings
10. Growth abnormalities
11. Oral involvement in known or possible systemic disease
12. Positive neurologic findings in the head and neck
13. Evidence of foreign objects
14. Pain or dysfunction (or both) of the temporomandibular joint (TMJ)

15. Facial asymmetry
16. Abutment teeth for fixed or removable partial prosthesis
17. Unexplained bleeding
18. Unexplained sensitivity of teeth
19. Unusual eruption, spacing, or migration of teeth
20. Unusual tooth morphologic findings, calcification, or color
21. Unexplained absence of teeth
22. Clinical erosion

‡Factors increasing risk for dental caries may include but are not limited to the following:
1. High level of dental caries experience or demineralization
2. History of recurrent dental caries
3. High titers of cariogenic bacteria
4. Existing restoration or restorations of poor quality
5. Poor oral hygiene
6. Inadequate fluoride exposure
7. Prolonged nursing (bottle or breast)
8. Frequent high sucrose content in diet
9. Poor family dental health
10. Developmental or acquired enamel defects
11. Developmental or acquired disability
12. Xerostomia
13. Genetic abnormality of teeth
14. Many multisurface restorations
15. Chemotherapy or radiation therapy
16. Eating disorders
17. Drug and alcohol abuse
18. Irregular dental care

Modified from *Guidelines for prescribing dental radiographs*. Pub. No. N-80A. Rochester, NY, 1988, Eastman Kodak.

published guidelines are voluntary and are used solely as a decision-making aid for the dental practitioner. The information presented in Table 18-1 should be used in conjunction with a carefully recorded medical and dental history and a thorough clinical examination. The information in the clinical examination should include the patient history, previous radiographs, caries and periodontal risk assessment, and both the dental health needs and the general health needs of the patient.

Types of Intraoral and Extraoral Images

BITE-WING IMAGE

The **bite-wing image** examines the crowns of the maxillary and mandibular teeth with one intraoral projection. This image is particularly useful for examining the interproximal tooth surfaces; therefore the bite-wing is preferred to identify dental caries. Figure 18-5 demonstrates a diagnostic, properly positioned premolar bite-wing radiograph. Proper **horizontal angulation** allows for open contact areas to be seen on this radiograph, which assists in the diagnosis of the interproximal dental caries between the maxillary premolars. Bite-wings may be placed horizontally or vertically depending on the tissues needing evaluation.

★ CASE APPLICATION 18-2.1

Evaluation of Pathology on Vertical Bite-Wings

In Figure 18-2, vertical bone loss, especially around the dental implants, is evident, as is furcation involvement with teeth #19 and #30. The mesial root of tooth #30 demonstrates a widened periodontal ligament space with periapical radiolucency at the apex. Exposing **vertical bite-wing radiographs** (rather than horizontal placement) was a good choice for this patient, because more alveolar bone is visible. This patient, however, requires a full series of intraoral radiographs because of the concerns previously listed.

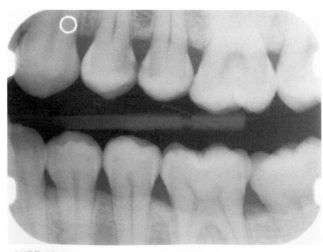

FIGURE 18-5
Diagnostic premolar bite-wing radiograph. Reader should note the interproximal dental caries seen between teeth #12 and #13.

PERIAPICAL IMAGE

A second type of intraoral projection is the **periapical image.** This image examines the entire tooth from crown to apex, as well as surrounding bone and supporting structures. The periapical projection is useful for detection of periodontal changes and periapical pathologic changes. The paralleling technique with beam-guiding devices is preferred when exposing periapical images, because this technique consistently produces images with dimensional accuracy. Figure 18-6 demonstrates a mandibular premolar periapical radiograph with proper **vertical angulation** and packet placement. A bite-wing radiograph alone would not have demonstrated the amount of bone loss revealed by this periapical image. The reader should note the amount and pattern of bone loss, along with the widened periodontal ligament space, which is usually an indicator of disease.

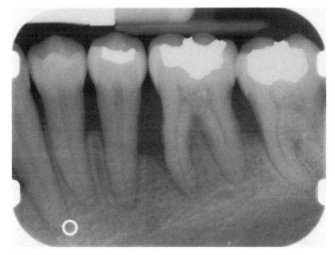

FIGURE 18-6
Mandibular premolar periapical radiograph. The amount of bone loss and the widened periodontal ligament space is exhibited.

★ CASE APPLICATION 18-1.1

Patient Appreciation for Dental Hygienist's Communication

During the exposure of the complete series of radiographs, the dental hygienist has time to discuss Mr. Janus's dental health. The hygienist mentions the money and time that Mr. Janus has already invested in his teeth, pointing out the numerous crowns, bridges, and other restorations, as well as the previous root-scaling procedures. The patient appreciates the dental hygienist's concern regarding his oral condition (see Figure 18-1).

PANORAMIC IMAGE

A panoramic radiograph is the most commonly exposed extraoral image. The **panoramic image** demonstrates a wide view of the maxilla, mandible, and surrounding structures on a single radiograph. The panoramic image is useful when a large area of the jaws require examination; however, this projection does not give the detail of an intraoral image. Figure 18-7 demonstrates a panoramic radiograph of a mixed dentition.

Prevention

The exposure of a full series of intraoral radiographs may be difficult for some patients because of the presence of a gag reflex. To prevent the stimulation of the gag reflex during radiographic procedures, the clinician should work from the anterior region to the posterior regions of the mouth on sensitive patients. Anterior projections are usually easier for the patient to tolerate and might give the patient some confidence to proceed with the more difficult posterior placements. The clinician should not lean the patient back in the chair; instead the patient's head should be supported (placing the occlusal plane parallel to the floor). The patient should be encouraged to breathe through the nose, and distraction should be used when needed. A cool drink of water may also suppress the sensory nerve endings.

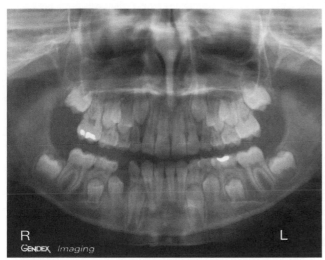

FIGURE 18-7
Panoramic radiograph revealing a mixed dentition.

Risk versus Benefit of Dental Radiographs

No matter how small the dose, x-rays are harmful to living tissues.[4,5] Biological damage results from radiographic exposure, and dental radiographs should be prescribed only when necessary. The *risk-versus-benefit* concept explains that the diagnostic information provided by the radiographic examination must override the potential harm from the ionizing radiation. When radiographs are properly prescribed, exposed, and processed, the benefit of detecting disease prevails over the risk of small doses of radiation the patient receives. Therefore all means of reducing excess radiation through patient protection must be accomplished. This includes following the *as low as reasonably achievable* principle, referred to as the **ALARA principle,** and keeping all exposures as low as reasonably achievable. Examples of good radiologic practice include the following:

- Use of the fastest image receptor compatible with the diagnostic task
- Collimation of the beam to the size of the receptor whenever possible

- Proper film exposure and processing techniques
- Use of leaded aprons and thyroid collars for all patients[8]

Two common clinical situations that require a radiographic examination include dental caries and periodontal disease. Because dental caries and periodontal disease may not always be visible during a clinical examination, these conditions may go unnoticed. Radiographs are exposed to benefit the patient for early intervention of disease before extensive treatment is needed. Thus the dental professional is saving the patient time and money while emphasizing the preventive aspect of dental radiography.

Many clinical situations exist in which radiographs may be indicated (see Table 18-1). Some of these include previous endodontic therapy, presence of implants, mobility of teeth, abutment teeth for fixed prostheses, and unexplained sensitivity of teeth.

Operator Technique

Operator technique is crucial to produce properly exposed radiographs. Incorrect horizontal or vertical angulation, cone cutting, improper packet placement, and errors during exposure and processing are technical problems that must be avoided to create radiographs of high diagnostic value. Because the dentist is ultimately responsible for the quality of radiographs produced in the office, the dental radiographer must be competent and knowledgeable in exposure and processing techniques.[8]

Note

When a radiograph is nondiagnostic, it must be retaken. Retakes expose the patient to unnecessary radiation and must be avoided.

★ CASE APPLICATION 18-3.1

Radiographic Findings

Other than the operator errors mentioned in Case Study 18-3, what other radiographic findings are present in Figure 18-3? This patient has much horizontal bone loss in the posterior regions of the mouth, which might lead the dental hygienist to expect the same type of bone loss in the anterior region. Many posterior teeth also demonstrate areas of radiopaque, deep, interproximal calculus. In addition, dental caries is evident on several of the teeth and appears to have penetrated the enamel, dentin, and pulp chambers.

Distinct Care Modifications

The production of diagnostic radiographs includes correct placement of the receptor over the appropriate teeth and tissues. Patients with bilateral mandibular tori may have a difficult time during radiographic procedures, especially those involving the mandibular premolar region. The patient may complain of the receptor "cutting" into the sensitive tissue surrounding the tori or feeling that not enough room is present to place the receptor correctly underneath the tongue or along the floor of the mouth.

Care should be used when placing the receptor between the torus and the tongue, and the clinician should try to avoid placing the receptor on the torus itself. Gentleness will help the patient know that the clinician understands the anatomical condition and is trying to make the procedure as comfortable as possible.

Although technique and processing errors are most commonly seen with intraoral images, these mistakes may also be present with extraoral films. Positioning the patient correctly into the panoramic machine, removing all radiodense materials from the head and neck region, and giving thorough instructions regarding the procedure involved during exposure are all important factors to accomplish during extraoral radiography. Figure 18-8 is an example of a panoramic radiograph in which the patient was placed anterior to the proper position; the teeth are anterior to the **focal trough.** Table 18-2 outlines common errors seen in panoramic radiography.

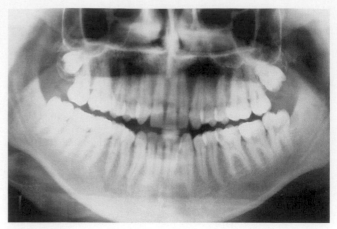

FIGURE 18-8
Example of a panoramic positioning error. Patient was positioned with the teeth anterior to the focal trough. The maxillary and mandibular anterior teeth appear thin and distorted, and the cervical spine is seen on the outer edges of the image.

Table 18-2	**Common Panoramic Errors**		
ERROR	**APPEARANCE**	**EXAMPLE**	**SOLUTION**
Patient's Chin Tipped Up; Frankfort Plane Positioned Upward	Hard palate superimposed over the maxillary teeth; a reverse smile line is apparent; loss of image quality in the maxillary anterior region		Position the patient so that the Frankfort plane is parallel with the floor
Patient's Chin Tipped Down; Frankfort Plane Positioned Downward	Mandibular incisors are blurred with a loss of image quality; the condyles may not appear on the image; an exaggerated smile line is apparent		Position the patient so that the Frankfort plane is parallel with the floor
Patient's Head Not Centered in Radiographic Machine	The ramus and posterior teeth will be unequally magnified		Position the patient so that the midsagittal plane is perpendicular to the floor

Panoramic images from Haring JI, Howerton LJ: *Dental radiography: principles and techniques,* ed 3, St Louis, 2006, Saunders.

Table 18-2	Common Panoramic Errors—cont'd			
ERROR	**APPEARANCE**	**EXAMPLE**		**SOLUTION**
Patient Not Standing or Sitting with a Straight Spine	Superimposition of the cervical spine will appear as a vertical radiopacity in the center of the image, obscuring information (*arrows*)			Position the patient so that the cervical spine is straight
Patient Not Placed into Focal Trough of Machine; Teeth Anterior to Focal Trough	The anterior teeth appear thin and out of focus on the image; the cervical spine is seen on the edges of the radiograph			Ensure that the patient is correctly positioned in the radiographic machine before exposure, with the teeth placed into the focal trough
Patient Not Placed into Focal Trough of Machine; Teeth Posterior to Focal Trough	The anterior teeth appear widened and out of focus; the condyles may not be evident on the image			Ensure that the patient is correctly positioned in the radiographic machine before exposure, with the teeth placed into the focal trough
Lead Apron Artifact Visible on Image	A cone-shaped radiopacity is visible in the middle of the image, obscuring information (*arrows*)			Place the lead apron low around the neck of the patient to avoid blocking the x-ray beam
Ghost Images Present on Radiograph	Ghost images appear when a metallic or radiodense object (e.g., jewelry, removable denture, hearing aid, eyeglasses) is not removed before the exposure of the image; obscures information (*arrows*)			Instruct the patient to remove all radiodense objects in the head and neck region before x-ray exposure

Digital Imaging

Since its introduction to dentistry in 1987, digital imaging has influenced the field of dental radiography significantly.[4] **Digital radiography** is a filmless system, meaning that no films or chemical processing is involved. Instead, a **sensor** is placed intraorally that captures the information. Shortly after the exposure, an image on a computer monitor is produced. Essential qualities of a digital-imaging system include the following:

- Properly exposed images
- Decrease in radiation dose to the patient
- Compatibility of the digital system with conventional radiographic machines
- Acquisition of the image occurring in a short time

The goal of digital radiography is to produce radiographic images with diagnostic quality in detection of dental disease, equal to that of conventional film. Digital radiographic images are produced in a **digital format** rather than **analog format** (or continuous information). Digital format refers to images in small electronic bits of information (referred to as *pixels*). Each **pixel,** or picture element, is arranged in a structured, ordered row and column, much different from the random arrangement of silver halide crystals present in film emulsion. Pixels represent levels of gray from 0 (black) to 255 (white), even though people cannot discriminate between 256 shades of gray (the human eye can differentiate only approximately 32 shades of gray).[13]

Computerized functions in clinical dentistry include appointment scheduling, procedure billing, and patient charting (see Chapter 49). These functions are integrated into seamless practice management software solutions, which must include integration of digital radiographic software. Paperless dental practices are becoming more popular; eventually most practices will use them.[13]

EQUIPMENT

The equipment needed for digital radiography includes the source of radiation, an intraoral sensor, and a computer.

Radiation Source

In most cases the source of radiation for digital imaging remains the office's conventional radiograph unit. However, the amount of radiation a patient receives using digital imaging is reduced by 50% to 80%, compared with traditional radiography. The reduction in radiation is the result of the sensitivity of the intraoral sensor. Digital imaging requires that the timer on the radiographic machine be calibrated for a lower radiation dose.

Intraoral Sensor

The intraoral sensor replaces dental film. A variety of manufacturers produce digital sensors. The clinician should seek professional advice from a digital-imaging manufacturer to evaluate a suitable sensor for the dental practice. For example, an endodontist requires immediate digital images during root canal therapy. The appropriate sensor for this procedure is a **charge-**

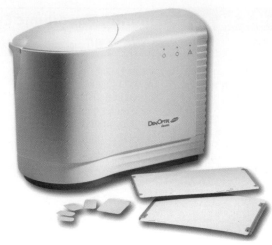

FIGURE 18-9
Laser scanning device and electronic processor used for indirect digital imaging. (Courtesy of KaVo Dental/Gendex Imaging, Lake Zurich, Ill.)

coupled device (CCD) in which the image is displayed on the monitor within an instant of exposure. Alternatively, a practice that uses dental hygienists and serves many recall patients might choose a **storage phosphor imaging system** (PSP). This system uses reusable imaging plates coated with phosphors that are placed into the oral cavity and exposed to radiation, much like traditional film. After exposure, a laser device in an electronic processor scans the plates and the image is transferred to the monitor (Figure 18-10). This processing procedure lasts up to 5 minutes because of the additional laser-scanning step.

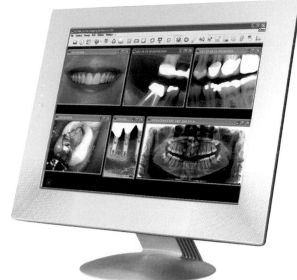

FIGURE 18-10
Computer monitor displays the digital image of a periapical radiograph. (Courtesy Eastman Kodak, Rochester, New York)

Computer

The third component of digital imaging is the computer. The computer digitizes, processes, and stores the incoming electronic signal from the sensor and converts each pixel on the sensor to a shade of gray for each corresponding pixel on the computer monitor.[6] Each pixel is given a value between 0 and 255. This creates the availability of 256 shades of gray, or the resolution of the image (Figure 18-10).

ADVANTAGES AND DISADVANTAGES

Adoption of digital imaging has increased because of the positive benefits it brings to dentistry. These benefits include the following:

- Reduction in patient exposure to radiation
- Increased diagnosis accuracy because of the superior gray-scale resolution
- Increased speed of viewing images
- Increased time efficiency for office personnel
- Elimination of environmental hazards associated with processing equipment, film, chemicals, and darkroom maintenance
- Improved patient education with increased patient trust and acceptance of treatment planning
- Improved patient documentation and case presentation

Digital imaging and traditional film are not significantly different when used for common diagnostic tasks. For example, dental caries identification using digital imaging is equal to or better than the diagnostic level achieved with conventional film, given the ability to manipulate contrast levels.[12] In addition, digital images can be stored in a compact manner without

deterioration in quality. Images can be shared between referring doctors because of the ease of transmitting electronically.

A disadvantage of digital-imaging systems is the initial purchase of equipment. Costs vary depending on the manufacturer and the type of equipment needed (e.g., whether existing equipment requires upgrading or the purchase of new computer equipment). Additional auxiliary equipment can be purchased such as an intraoral camera. Infection control should be considered, because digital receptors cannot be sterilized by conventional means. The clinician or hygienist may disinfect sensors by wiping them with mild agents such as isopropyl alcohol; they should never be immersed in disinfecting solutions. Heat will ruin electronic components in CCD and complementary metal oxide semiconductor (CMOS) sensors and will distort the polyester base of PSP plates.[13] In the past, sensors were bulky and uncomfortable for the patient. These thicker sensors have been replaced with thinner, more flexible sensors, created to mimic the size and shape of traditional intraoral film. Figure 18-11 illustrates a PSP sensor next to a size no. 2 intraoral film.

Cone-Beam Imaging

Periapical and panoramic imaging have served dentistry well for many years. However, these imaging modalities produce magnification, distortion, and overlap of anatomy. Imaging technology has become available to view the oral and maxillofacial complex in three dimensions. This technology is termed **cone-beam imaging.** Some of the uses of cone-beam imaging include the following:

- Visualization of the cross-sections of the maxilla and mandible for dental implant imaging
- Localization of erosion or hard tissue formation within the temporomandibular joint (TMJ) complex and trauma to the maxilla and mandible
- Formation of hard tissue within salivary glands (sialoliths)
- Visualization of the paranasal sinuses

Cone-beam imaging centers are becoming more commonplace throughout the country as this type of technology becomes important in dentistry.

Cone-beam technology uses ionizing radiation, just as in traditional radiography. Radiation rotates 360 degrees around the patient's head in the shape of a cone, and the information received is translated into 512 images called **DICOM** (digital imaging and communications in medicine) data. Computer software manipulates the DICOM data to produce two-dimensional images in any plane, as well as three-dimensional renderings without the pitfalls of magnification, distortion, or overlap of anatomy. Because no magnification exists, measurements are exact (i.e., to the millimeter). The DICOM data may also be used in computer-guided dental implant software to aid in secure placement of dental implants. Understanding and interpreting three-dimensional image information may be overwhelming at first, however, through education, the information offered through cone-beam technology allows unparalleled

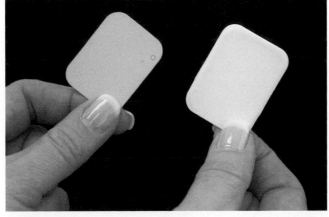

FIGURE 18-11
Example of a PSP (photostimulable phosphor plate) intraoral sensor used in digital imaging. Conventional no. 2 size film (*right*). The size, shape, and thickness of the sensor and film are very similar.

insight into the oral and maxillofacial complex (leading to better patient treatment). Disadvantages of cone-beam technology are the high cost of equipment and the knowledge required to produce appropriate images for a desired task.

✴ CASE APPLICATION 18-4.1

Cone-Beam Application for Delayed Eruption

Review Figure 18-4, *B;* it is a posterior coronal image of the area in question that reveals the reason for the delayed eruption: the crown of tooth #16 is located just beneath the buccal cusps of tooth #15. (This posterior coronal image is viewed as if standing behind the patient.) A three-dimensional volume rendering of the maxilla and mandible seen from an inferior position is seen in Figure 18-4, *C.* From this projection, the exact locations of teeth #15 and #16 can be viewed.

Intraoral Photographic Imaging

IPI allows patients an opportunity to see a magnified view of the oral cavity in an effort to aid in understanding their oral health. For years, dental clinicians have used intraoral photography for the purpose of case documentation. Better equipment in IPI has improved the ease of acquiring images. The standard of care in many dental communities is the comparison of pretreatment and posttreatment photographic images.

> *Note*
>
> Today, many patients are well-educated and respond favorably to viewing intraoral images and becoming involved with their care.

The dental hygienists' communication with patients can have a positive effect on treatment acceptance. Helping patients understand their current oral health needs is vital to patient acceptance of a comprehensive care plan, and IPI is a useful, modern adjunct to dental care. IPI can aid in diagnosis, allow patients to visualize oral health problems, illustrate options during treatment planning, and provide valuable documentation for dental insurance claims.[7,9] In addition, IPI gives a patient a sense of ownership of his or her mouth, the improved magnification helps the patient and clinician visualize detailed oral

---

✴ CASE APPLICATION 18-5.1

Education, Acceptance, and Motivation

For the first time, Ms. Winston can see the results of her disease process and is shocked. As you explain your observations and their meaning to the health of her teeth and gums, she becomes convinced that it is time to seek treatment. Ms. Winston agrees to the needed treatment and is motivated to comply with the necessary oral self-care to restore optimal health.

---

structures, and the clinical images may be saved and stored in the patient's file.

Some factors to consider when selecting an appropriate IPI system for dental practices include the following:
- System is user friendly
- Training of staff is straightforward
- Images produced are sharp and exhibit true colors
- Infection control procedures are easily accomplished
- System can be integrated into dental office software
- System provides durable equipment with service support readily available
- Cost is reasonable[2]

TYPES OF INTRAORAL PHOTOGRAPHIC IMAGING SYSTEMS

Camera systems used in dental practices today include the traditional 35-mm intraoral camera and various types of digital-imaging units. Three types of IPI systems are presented in the following sections, including advantages and disadvantages of each system.

35-mm Camera System

The gold standard in dentistry for many years of intraoral imaging has been the 35-mm camera (Figure 18-12). Earlier 35-mm intraoral cameras were cumbersome and difficult to use because of the tedious manipulation of exposure settings. However, current 35-mm cameras are all-in-one systems. Camera functions, such as focus and flash, are performed electronically, producing excellent intraoral images without changing camera settings. The recommended focal length for intraoral clinical photography is 105 mm. This is an advantage because the longer focal length permits a better working distance from the subject, thereby making intraoral posterior photography easier for the clinician and more comfortable for the patient. In addition, this length allows an appropriate distance between the camera and the sterile environment. Another advantage is the optional ringlight flash, which surrounds the lens of the camera and illuminates the area to be photographed, simulating true clinical light (Figure 18-13). Conventional 35-mm cameras use film that has to be developed, processed, and printed. The addi-

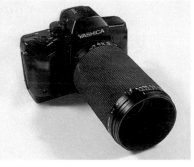

FIGURE 18-12
A 35-mm camera. (Courtesy Kyocera Optics Inc, Somerset, NJ.)

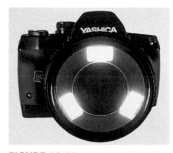

FIGURE 18-13
Ringlight flash. (Courtesy Kyocera Optics Inc, Somerset, NJ.)

tional time required for this step may be a disadvantage of this system, because the results cannot immediately be shared with the patient or used in treatment planning or evaluation.

Digital Cameras

A second option for IPI technology in dentistry is the digital camera (Figure 18-14). Digital cameras are physically smaller than their 35-mm equivalents.[11] During the photographic session, digital cameras are not attached to a computer and are able to be moved freely within the operatory. A removable memory card within the camera records the images. Modern computers are suitable for the retrieval of the images from the memory card and contain software to perform basic manipulations, such as cropping, magnification, brightness, and contrast. Digital cameras record images in different file sizes; higher-resolution images will produce larger file sizes. To maximize the hard drive space on the computer, the clinician should choose an appropriate resolution for the clinical task.

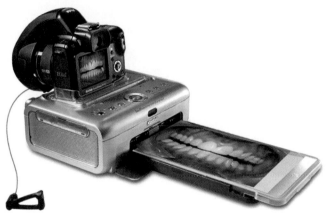

FIGURE 18-14
Example of an intraoral digital camera attached to a printer. (Courtesy Eastman Kodak Company, Rochester, NY.)

Advantages of digital cameras are easy and simple image storage and retrieval. Although digital photography is expensive, improvements in technologies and reduced costs are expected in the future. Another possible disadvantage is that digital cameras can be unreliable in the dental office because of interference from other dental equipment or fluorescent lighting.

Intraoral Video Systems

Intraoral video systems have been used in dentistry since the early 1990s. A video system consists of a microcamera, typically in the shape of a wand that can be held like a hand instrument and positioned in the mouth to create video clips of the oral cavity (Figure 18-15). Various hand piece adapters provide different angles of view for both extraoral and intraoral videos. The light that enters the intraoral video camera is automatically regulated, allowing a consistent amount of brightness for the images seen on the video.

The video captured by the microcamera is stored on the digital camera in analog form. Special software on a computer receives the analog video, converts it to digital video, and stores

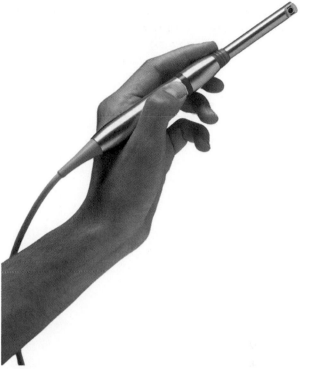

FIGURE 18-15
Example of an intraoral video camera. Reader should note the slender design, much like a dental hand piece. (Courtesy Eastman Kodak Company, Rochester, NY.)

it on the hard disk. (Note: Digital video files are large, so computers used to store them must have plenty of memory.) After the digital video is viewed on a monitor and edited, it can be saved onto a compact disk (CD) for later use. Additional software can be purchased that will compress the large digital file sizes to be used for online purposes.

Advantages of intraoral video systems include the ability to easily edit and transfer files across the Internet. Large file sizes, initial cost, and limited mobility of the microcamera (because of the wire connection to the computer) may make this system prohibitive.

Photographic Accessories

CHEEK, LIP, AND TONGUE RETRACTORS

To improve visibility and establish a clear field of view, the clinician often finds it necessary to use intraoral devices to retract tissues that may interfere with structures being photographed. Retractors are available in a variety of shapes and sizes to accommodate most patients and are produced in clear plastic or metal with single-ended or double-ended styles (Figure 18-16). All photographic accessories should be sterilized before intraoral use. Figure 18-17 demonstrates various techniques used to retract the lips and cheeks.

INTRAORAL MIRRORS

Intraoral mirrors are used to capture areas that are visually inaccessible, such as the palatal aspect of the maxillary molars. Intraoral mirrors come in a variety of shapes (Figure 18-18) and

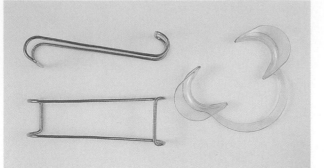

FIGURE 18-16
Plastic and metal cheek retractors.

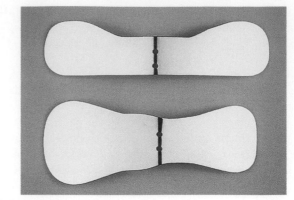

FIGURE 18-18
Intraoral mirrors.

must be sterilized before use. Metal mirrors with reflective surfaces are recommended. Figure 18-17 demonstrates techniques using an intraoral mirror. Compressed air may be sprayed onto the mirror surface if fogging occurs; in addition, patients should be instructed to breathe through the nose.

Photographic Exposures

The number of different intraoral images required is based on the needs of the clinical task. If the focus is a single tooth, then one intraoral photographic image may be sufficient (Figure 18-19). However, Figure 18-20 demonstrates 12 images taken when a comprehensive set of intraoral images is required.

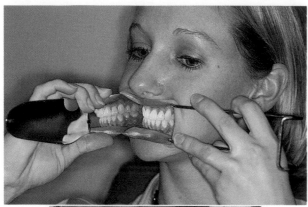

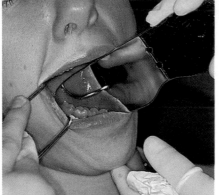

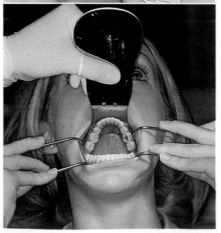

FIGURE 18-17
Cheek and lip retractors and intraoral mirror in use.

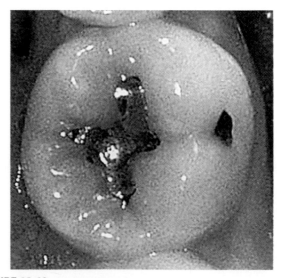

FIGURE 18-19
Single-tooth intraoral image, as would be used when the clinician is focused on only one tooth.

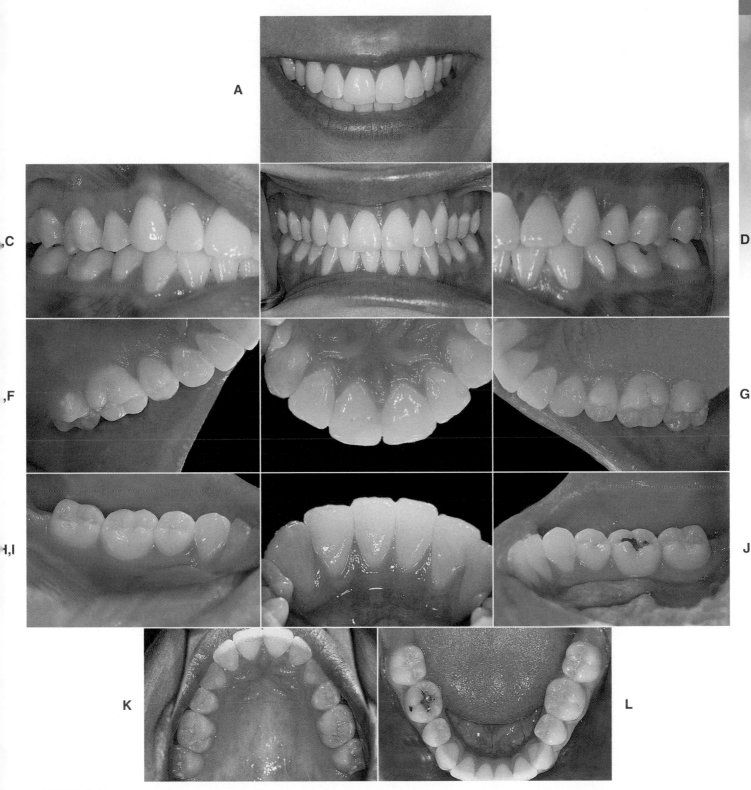

FIGURE 18-20
Examples of a comprehensive set of intraoral images (set of 12 images). **A** to **D,** Facial views: **A,** Close-up of smile. **B,** Maxillary and mandibular right posterior facials. **C,** Maxillary and mandibular anterior facials. **D,** Maxillary and mandibular left posterior facials. **E** to **G,** Palatal views: **E,** Maxillary left posterior palatal. **F,** Maxillary anterior palatal. **G,** Maxillary right posterior palatal. **H** to **J,** Lingual views: **H,** Mandibular left posterior lingual. **I,** Mandibular anterior lingual. **J,** Mandibular right posterior lingual. **K** to **L,** Occlusal views: **K,** Maxillary occlusal. **L,** Mandibular occlusal.

References

1. American Dental Association Council on Scientific Affairs: The use of dental radiographs: update and recommendations, *J Am Dent Assoc* 137(9):1304-1312, 2006.
2. Blaisdell L: One practice's intraoral camera success story, *Dent Econ* 85(1):48-54, 1995.
3. Delrose DC, Steinberg RW: The clinical significance of the digital patient record, *J Am Dent Assoc* 131:57S-60S, 2000.
4. Haring JI, Howerton LJ: *Dental radiography: principles and techniques,* ed 3, St Louis, 2006, Elsevier.
5. Hujoel PP et al: Antepartum dental radiography and infant low birth weight, *JAMA* 291(16):1987-1993, 2004.
6. Jameson C, Jameson JH: Incorporating high-tech equipment into your practice, *Dent Econ* 83(12):51-58, 1993.
7. Levin R: Increasing treatment acceptance with the intraoral camera, *Dent Econ* 84(11):84, 1994.
8. National Council on Radiation Protection and Measurement: *Radiation protection in dentistry,* Pub No 145, Bethesda, Md, 2003, The Council.
9. Reis-Schmidt T: Intraoral video cameras show increased visibility and usefulness in US general practices: survey report, *Dental Product Reports* 31(9):19-29, 1997.
10. Schleyer TKL et al: The technologically well-equipped dental office, *J Am Dent Assoc* 134:30-40, 2003.
11. Sharland MR: Digital imaging for the general dental practitioner: getting started, *Dent Update* 31:266-272, 2004.
12. Wenzel A: Digital radiography and caries diagnosis, *Dentomaxillofac Radiol* 27(1):3-11, 1998.
13. White SC, Pharoah MJ: *Oral radiology principles and interpretation,* St Louis, 2004, Mosby.

Nutritional Assessment

Cynthia A. Stegeman

INSIGHT

Nutrition has a tremendous affect on both oral and overall general health. Dental hygienists must recognize the relationship among dental health, disease prevention and wellness, and nutrition.

✸ CASE STUDY 19-1   Effects of Nutrition on Oral Health

John Chen, a 14-year-old boy, has been seen for routine supportive care appointments since age 4. His health history is unremarkable. Throughout the years, his dental history has included several discussions on the importance of adequate bacterial plaque biofilm removal caused by poor oral hygiene. His periodontal health has been acceptable, and he has not exhibited dental caries.

During the most recent supportive care appointment, the dental hygienist records six new areas of decay that were not noted in the previous 6 months, as well as several incipient carious lesions. On further investigation, John states that he does not floss but tries to remember to brush daily. His oral hygiene is fair.

John began high school this year. He thinks it is "so cool" to be able to drink sodas during class and notes that soda machines are present in almost every hall. John is an active teen and is involved in several sports throughout the year. He prefers to consume sports drinks to hydrate before, during, and after practice or events. "I just don't like water." In addition, he carries a roll of mints to keep his breath fresh. On further questioning, the hygienist determines that John consumes 8 to 10 mints during the day.

Table 19-1 outlines information obtained from John's 24-hour food recall.

Table 19-1	John's 24-Hour Food Recall	
MEAL	**FOOD AND QUANTITY**	**LOCATION**
Breakfast	Two large blueberry muffins 16-oz chocolate milk	Vehicle
Snack	20-oz soda	Classroom
Lunch	Two cheeseburgers 16 onion rings 20-oz soda	School cafeteria
Snack	Four large chocolate-chip cookies Mints (throughout day) 20-oz sports drink (before, during, and after game)	Classroom Bus (traveling to sports event)
Dinner	Six fried chicken wings One large baked potato with 3 tsp butter Four biscuits with 4 tsp honey 16-oz fruit punch	Kitchen
Snack	Four scoops chocolate-chip ice cream	Bedroom

NOTE: Did not brush or floss this day.

375

KEY TERMS

ameloblasts	disaccharides	fermentable carbohydrates	odontoblasts
anticariogenic	discretionary calorie allowance	monosaccharides	polypharmacy
cariogenic	dysgeusia	nonacidogenic	polysaccharides
catabolism	early childhood caries	nonnutritive sweeteners	remineralization
demineralization	enamel hypoplasia	nutritive sweeteners	

LEARNING OUTCOMES

After reading this chapter the student will be able to:

1. Discuss dental conditions associated with nutrient imbalances.
2. Outline conditions in the oral cavity that inhibit food intake.
3. Describe conditions under which fermentable carbohydrates are cariogenic or noncariogenic.
4. Assess the dental patient to determine whether nutritional care is needed and the type and amount of nutritional intervention that is required.
5. Develop strategies to provide the highest-quality health care that will correct the diet-related dental situation.
6. Evaluate the effectiveness of nutritional intervention in a dental patient.

Nutrition in Dental Hygiene Practice

Nutrition has a tremendous impact in both oral and overall general health. Dental hygienists must recognize the relationship among dental health, disease prevention and wellness, and nutrition.

The oral cavity exhibits many characteristic abnormalities of nutritional discrepancies (deficiencies and excesses) during growth, development, and maintenance of oral tissues. Signs and symptoms of nutritional challenges are often first observed in the oral cavity and are used as a foundation to determine a diagnosis or medical cause. This chapter discusses the assessment process involved in identifying nutrition-related dental disorders that are necessary to treat and refer patients to the appropriate health professionals.

The dental profession is in a unique patient-care situation. A patient may not visit his or her physician for routine physicals but may maintain intervals of regular dental supportive care.

> *Note*
>
> Dental hygienists are often the first to recognize medical abnormalities for which their patients should seek further medical treatment, making the dental hygienist an integral part of the healthcare team. Addressing this point specifically is the goal of any dental hygienist: to enhance health promotion and disease prevention and to provide comprehensive patient care.

tient. When the nutrition or dental issue involves a medical condition that affects diet, a reduced eating ability, or a compromised nutritional status, the dental patient will need to be referred to a physician or a registered dietitian.

> *Distinct Care Modifications*
>
> Disease states or conditions such as eating disorders, diabetes, human immunodeficiency virus and acquired immunodeficiency syndrome (HIV/AIDS), osteoporosis, cardiovascular disease, Sjögren's syndrome, end-stage renal disease, and the effects of cancer treatment create additional diet-related dental concerns.

Effects of Nutrition on the Oral Cavity

19-1
19-2

Nutritional challenges change from decade to decade. Nutritional deficiencies can occur in a variety of circumstances—in medically compromised individuals, during periods of rapid growth, in the older adult, in inner city or rural areas of the United States, and in developing countries. Today's nutrition-related complications in the United States are often the result of overconsumption of food or supplements.

The oral cavity reflects many indiscretions related to an individual's nutrient intake. Table 19-2 presents a list of oral complications and links to nutrition. Growth, development, maintenance, and repair of oral tissues are also compromised because of improper nutritional balance. Periodontal tissues are metabolically active throughout life, and nutrients are regularly needed for such tissue maintenance. In many instances, clinical signs and symptoms of deficiencies or excesses are not noted until the problem is in an advanced state.

> *Prevention*
>
> An observant and knowledgeable dental hygienist can recognize subtle changes in an oral examination related to nutrition and can work toward a solution before such changes become uncontrolled, cause irreparable damage, or both.

DENTAL CONSIDERATIONS

Examples of oral conditions related to nutrition include soft tissue lesions, cheilosis, stomatitis, glossitis, dental caries, erosion, alveolar bone loss, and salivary gland dysfunction.

Dental hygienists are valuable resources on general health for patients, including accurate, current, and evidence-based nutrition information and obtaining reliable data to dispel myths or fads. Basic nutrition counseling is a meaningful component of the comprehensive dental services offered to the pa-

Table 19-2	Nutrition-Related Complications of the Oral Cavity
NUTRIENT	**DEFICIENCY SYMPTOMS**
Thiamin (B$_1$)	Increased sensitivity and burning sensation of oral mucosa, burning tongue, loss of taste and appetite
Riboflavin (B$_2$)	Angular cheilosis, blue-to-purple mucosa, inflamed mucosa, glossitis, magenta tongue, enlarged fungiform papillae, atrophy and inflammation of filiform papillae, burning tongue
Niacin (B$_3$)	Glossitis, ulcerations of tongue, atrophy of papillae, cheilosis, thin epithelium, burning of oral mucosa, stomatitis, erythremic marginal and attached gingiva, loss of appetite
Pyridoxine (B$_6$)	Cheilosis, glossitis, atrophy and burning of tongue, stomatitis
Cobalamin (B$_{12}$)	Stomatitis, hemorrhaging, pale-to-yellow mucosa, glossitis, atrophy and burning of tongue, altered taste, loss of appetite
Folic Acid	Glossitis with enlargement of fungiform papillae, ulcerations along edge of tongue, gingivitis, erosion and ulcerations on buccal mucosa, pale mucosa
Biotin	Glossitis, patchy atrophy of papillae, gray mucosa
Vitamin C	Odontoblast atrophy, porotic dentin formation, gingival inflammation with easy bleeding, deep-red–to–purple gingiva, ulceration and necrosis, delayed wound healing, muscle/joint pain, defects in collagen formation, petechia
Vitamin A	Ameloblast atrophy, faulty bone and tooth formation, accelerated periodontal destruction, hypoplasia, xerostomia, cleft lip, keratinization of epithelium, drying and hardening of salivary glands, impaired taste *Toxicity symptoms:* hypertrophy of bone, cracking and bleeding lips, thinning of epithelium, erythremic gingiva, cheilosis
Vitamin D, Calcium, and Phosphorus	Failure of bones to heal, mild calcification to enamel hypoplasia, loss of alveolar/mandibular bone, delayed eruption, increased dental caries rate, loss of lamina dura around roots of teeth
Phosphorus	*Toxicity symptoms:* poor tooth formation and bone demineralization
Vitamin K	Gingival hemorrhaging
Iron	Painful oral cavity; stomatitis; thinned buccal mucosa with ulcerations; pale-to-gray mucosa, lips, and tongue; angular cheilosis; burning tongue; reddening at lips and margins of tongue; atrophy of filiform papilla
Zinc	Thickening of epithelium, thickening of tongue with underlying muscle atrophy, impaired taste, atrophy of filiform papilla
Protein	Smooth, edematous tongue; angular cheilosis; fissures on lower lip; smaller teeth; delayed eruption; delayed wound healing; dental caries
Selenium	*Toxicity symptoms:* dental caries
Fluoride	Dental caries *Toxicity symptoms:* enamel fluorosis
Magnesium	Retardation in dentin formation, enamel hypoplasia, atrophy of ameloblasts and odontoblasts, enamel hyperplasia

Modified from Mahan LK, Escott-Stump S: *Food, nutrition, and diet therapy,* ed 11, Philadelphia, 2004, WB Saunders; Swartz, MH: *Textbook of physical diagnosis,* ed 4, Philadelphia, 2002, WB Saunders; Stegeman CA, Davis, JR: *The dental hygienist's guide to nutritional care,* ed 2, St Louis, 2005, Elsevier.

In general, B vitamins (Box 19-1) are necessary daily, and a deficiency affects primarily the tongue and oral mucosa. Cheilosis, gingival hypertrophy, and stomatitis are other common occurrences from a vitamin B deficiency. Deficiencies seldom occur in isolation but instead in combination with other vitamin deficiencies within the B complex. Deficiencies can be a result of low dietary intake; inadequate absorption or use; or increased body requirements, excretion, or destruction. Smoking, consuming large quantities of alcohol or caffeine, taking certain medications, and reacting to stress can increase the need for vitamins. A thorough assessment of the patient's medical, dental, and social history can help identify an individual's risk factors for nutritional imbalance (Box 19-2), which will require thorough assessment by the dental

---

BOX 19-1

WATER- AND FAT-SOLUBLE VITAMINS

Water-Soluble Vitamins	Fat-Soluble Vitamins
B complex	Vitamin A
Thiamin (B_1)	Vitamin D
Riboflavin (B_2)	Vitamin E
Niacin (B_3)	Vitamin K
Pyridoxine (B_6)	
Cobalamin (B_{12})	
Biotin	
Pantothenic acid	
Folic acid (folate, folacin)	
Vitamin C (ascorbic acid)	

BOX 19-2

GROUPS AT NUTRITIONAL RISK

Older Adults
Dentate status
Systemic diseases/conditions
Polypharmacy
Psychosocial issues
Xerostomia
Osteoporosis
Low income
Dysgeusia
Dysphagia

Individuals Undergoing Periods of Rapid Growth
Pregnant and lactating women
Infants, children, adolescents

Individuals Receiving Inadequate Calories, Protein, or Nutrients
Eating disorders
Long-term dieting, very–low-calorie diets or fad diets
Vegans
Low income

Immunocompromised Individuals
Human immunodeficiency virus infection
Cancer
Diabetes
Organ transplants
End-stage renal disease

Other Individuals
Individuals taking certain medications or multiple medications
Alcoholics

---

hygienist and possible referral to the physician or registered dietitian.

HARD AND SOFT TISSUE FORMATION

The role of nutrition and diet begins with tooth bud formation, approximately 6 weeks in utero. Most structures of the craniofacial area are developed during the first trimester of pregnancy.[12] Even one incidence of mild to moderate malnutrition during the first 12 months of life is associated with an increased risk for dental caries in deciduous and permanent teeth.[1] The systemic properties of nutrition continue until calcification is complete. Thus the development of enamel, dentin, cementum, and pulp are connected to dietary intake.

Vitamins A, D, and C and fluoride are among the nutrients that are considered important to preeruptive tooth growth and development. **Enamel hypoplasia,** delayed tooth eruption, tooth spacing, improper formation or atrophy of **ameloblasts,** and **odontoblasts** that affect enamel, dentin, and pulp development, as well as resistance to decay, are common results of improper nutrition during craniofacial development.

Collagen is present throughout the periodontium as the principal connective tissue fiber in the gingiva, the periodontal ligament, and the major organic component of alveolar bone. Collagen requires protein, vitamin C, iron, zinc, and copper for growth, development, and maintenance. Defective collagen formation negatively affects the mineralization of enamel, creating structural defects of the teeth.

Mineralization occurs after collagen formation. This process involves the deposition of inorganic materials into an inorganic matrix and requires the nutritional elements of protein, carbohydrates, fat, calcium, phosphorus, magnesium, sodium, and potassium. Therefore the integrity of the entire tooth structure relies on adequate nutrition.

DENTAL CARIES

Although posteruptive nutrition has a reduced systemic impact on tooth formation, nutrients do continue to support tooth maintenance. Systemic and topical fluoride help prevent dental caries in all age groups. Throughout the life span, fluoride is implicated in reducing the growth of **cariogenic** bacteria, inhibiting **demineralization,** and enhancing the **remineralization** of enamel.[6,7] Fat, protein, phosphorus, calcium, calcium lactate in milk, and sugar alcohols have local **anticariogenic** properties. These nutrients do not cause dental caries and may actually help prevent dental caries because they do not lower plaque biofilm pH. Box 19-3 provides examples of these protective foods.

Consumption of sugar and other fermentable carbohydrates is a significant factor in the progression of dental decay, not only because of acid formation, but also because of the production of plaque biofilm. An increase in the consumption of soft drinks in the United States, particularly among adolescents, is responsible for a rise in the rate of dental caries for this population group, as well as an increased risk of malnutrition. According to the American Beverage Association, carbonated soft

---

BOX 19-3

FOODS THAT PROTECT AGAINST DENTAL CARIES

Cheese	Butter
Milk	Cream
Nuts	Cream cheese
Products made with xylitol	Margarine
Meat, fish, poultry, and eggs	Oils
Fat	Sour cream

✴ CASE APPLICATION 19-1.1

Soda Consumption and Effects on Nutrition

As presented in Case Study 19.1, John is a representative of the most avid consumer group for carbonated soft drinks and sports drinks (boys and men, ages 12 to 19).[8,16] From a health standpoint, John may be at risk for malnutrition. Sodas contain little to no nutrient value yet are high in calories (except diet drinks). The caffeine in some soft drinks actually interferes with the absorption of nutrients consumed in foods. Consuming a large number of sodas daily correlates with low consumption of milk, which provides vitamins and minerals such as calcium, protein, and riboflavin that may promote remineralization. John's incidence of dental caries may be related to the constant bathing of the tooth surface in cariogenic carbohydrates.

---

drinks account for approximately one of every four (28%) beverages that Americans consume.[2]

PERIODONTAL DISEASE

Although inadequate nutrition alone does not cause a periodontal problem, it can be a factor influencing the severity of disease and wound healing.[3,5] Systemically, optimal nutrition is associated with the host defense mechanism, whereby the body can react rapidly to healing and prevent or minimize infections. When a surgical procedure is required, an adequate nutrient reserve is essential for the individual to withstand the stresses incurred by the procedure. Nutrient needs actually can double in situations such as blood loss, increased **catabolism,** tissue repair, and host defense mechanisms. The dental hygienist will promote a variety and balance of food, adequate calories, and sufficient fluids.

Another factor influencing the relationship between nutrition and periodontal disease is food texture. Soft, sticky, retentive foods cling to teeth and provide an environment that is conducive to plaque biofilm formation. Such foods are often carbohydrate-rich foods, such as bread or raisins. Such fermentable carbohydrates provide a substrate for bacterial growth. Therefore one of the roles of the dental hygienist is to educate the patient on nutrient-rich food choices that do not promote plaque biofilm formation, as well as on proper oral self-care techniques and fluoride therapy.

SALIVA

Nutrients, particularly vitamin A and protein, affect the development and secretory function of salivary glands. However, nutrient intake does not significantly affect saliva composition, volume, or antibacterial properties unless the patient is malnourished. The action of chewing and the taste of sour stimulate saliva flow, which is beneficial for controlling the rate of dental caries and overall health of the oral cavity.

A patient experiencing xerostomia may be sipping on fermentable carbohydrate fluids throughout the day to relieve the dryness. Even choices of 100% fruit juice and milk can be cariogenic when less saliva is available to neutralize the acid that the carbohydrate produces. Sucking on hard candy is another common practice that may be destructive. Sugar-free hard candies are an alternative. Remind patients that products containing sugar alcohols are to be used in moderation.

Effects of Oral Complications on Nutrition

Inadequate nutritional intake or use can result from any inhibitive oral condition that causes pain or reduces the ability to chew or swallow food. Individuals often modify food selection and quantity to accommodate compromising oral conditions. Therefore maintaining optimal oral health is essential in promoting and maintaining overall health.

Poor eating habits, inadequate nutrient intake, **dysgeusia,** and gastrointestinal disorders are associated with reduced masticatory ability.[14] The number of teeth, existence of a prosthesis, function of the prosthesis, or any combination of these factors often dictate food choices, particularly in the texture of food and quantity consumed. Individuals with such concerns often choose softer foods that are frequently high in carbohydrates and can be low in nutrient value, simply for ease and safety. These foods adhere to teeth, encouraging plaque biofilm growth and creating an unhealthy oral environment.

When a full upper denture located on the palate covers the taste buds, which are responsible for sour and bitter sensations, a decrease in taste sensations occurs. As the number of sensations for food (taste, texture, and temperature) decreases, the level of interest in eating declines, resulting in an increased risk of malnutrition.

In addition, xerostomia creates an unpleasant and often difficult eating situation to the extent that enjoying food becomes difficult for an individual. Functions of saliva include lubricating and moistening food to ease swallowing. A reduced salivary flow makes chewing and swallowing difficult. Without the protective buffering components of saliva, the individual with diminished saliva flow is at risk for increased incidence of dental caries and periodontal disease, just as the individual with a dry mucosa has difficulty removing oral debris. Xerostomia is most common in the older adult and is a side effect of numerous prescription and over-the-counter (OTC) medications.[15] Box 19-4 provides possible causes for

BOX 19-4

RISK FACTORS FOR XEROSTOMIA

Medications
Cancer treatment
Systemic conditions (Sjögren's syndrome, diabetes)
Stress and depression
Significant vitamin deficiency
Liquid diets (caused by lack of mastication)
Dehydration

Modified from Stegeman CA, Davis, JR: *The dental hygienists' guide to nutritional care,* ed 2, St Louis, 2005, Elsevier.

xerostomia that the dental hygienist can use to evaluate the patient further.

A painful and sore tongue, oral lesions, inflamed gingiva, tooth sensitivity, and dental caries are examples of complications that result in a reduced ability and diminished desire to eat. Box 19-5 identifies common oral issues related to dietary intake. Poor oral health may be an important contributing factor of unintentional weight loss and compromised nutrient intake.[13]

BOX 19-5

COMMON ORAL HEALTH PROBLEMS ASSOCIATED WITH FOOD INTAKE

Alveolar ridge resorption
Bleeding while chewing or brushing
Dental caries
Dentinal sensitivity
Denture sores
Fractured teeth
Glossitis
Inability to chew or swallow
Inadequate fit or lack of retention of prosthesis
Inadequately occluding teeth
Infection or inflammation
Lesions or ulcerations
Pain or soreness
Prosthesis-related problems
Root tips
Temporomandibular joint (TMJ) difficulties
Tooth mobility
Xerostomia

Modified from Steinberg L: The impact of oral health on diet, *Nutrition and the MD* [newsletter] 23:1, 1997.

Diet and Dietary Habits Contributing to Dental Caries

The dental hygienist is the expert in preventing and treating dental disorders. He or she becomes the primary educator in many dental issues that involve diet and diet behaviors and is alert to circumstances that may require collaboration with other members of the healthcare team.

Nutrition and dietary practices are significant components for the development of dental caries. The presence of cariogenic bacteria in the dental plaque biofilm, the amount and quality of saliva, fluoride status, oral hygiene regimen, and genetics are other etiologic factors associated with the development of dental caries. When isolated, none of these factors significantly affects oral health. Only when all the factors interact can dental caries develop.

FERMENTABLE CARBOHYDRATES

Candy, cookies, soda, ice cream, and other food products containing sucrose can cause enamel demineralization; this fact is well established. However, all carbohydrates have the potential to be fermentable. Several factors or behaviors will determine whether the situation is cariogenic.

Nutritive Sweeteners
Creation of an acidic environment

All **nutritive sweeteners** and any carbohydrate that contains calories have the potential to drop plaque biofilm pH to an acidic range, causing dissolution of enamel. Therefore **monosaccharides, disaccharides,** and **polysaccharides** are all considered **fermentable carbohydrates.** With the exception of sugar alcohols, each carbohydrate provides 4 calories per gram. A fermentable carbohydrate is any carbohydrate that has the potential to reduce plaque biofilm pH from neutral (approximately 7.0) to a critical level (5.5 or lower). Once pH is lowered, it remains at an acidic level for 20 to 40 minutes until the buffering capabilities of saliva return the pH to the neutral level. The MyPyramid Food Guidance System[17] and 2005 Dietary Guidelines for Americans[18] encourage the amount of added sugars to be within the **discretionary calorie allowance.** For example, an individual consuming 1600 calories each day should restrict added sugars to 132 calories per day.

Monosaccharides

Monosaccharides are single-unit carbohydrates (Figure 19-1). Fructose, for example, is the primary carbohydrate in fruit. Unless eaten in excessive quantities, fruit is not cariogenic, with the exceptions of bananas and dried fruit. Because most fruits are fibrous, additional chewing is required, increasing saliva flow and decreasing the chance for developing dental caries. In addition, the high water content of most fruit can dilute its fructose. The exception to this statement, however, is illustrated in the individual with **early childhood caries** who sips fruit juice at will from a baby bottle, a practice that permits the fluid to pool around the teeth for hours, producing an acidic environment and increasing the risk of decay.

Sugar alcohols

Sugar alcohols (sorbitol, mannitol, xylitol, and erythritol) are nutritive sweeteners that typically do not promote decay. Each of these sugar alcohols provides a small level of calories (approximately 2 calories per gram). Sugar alcohols are most

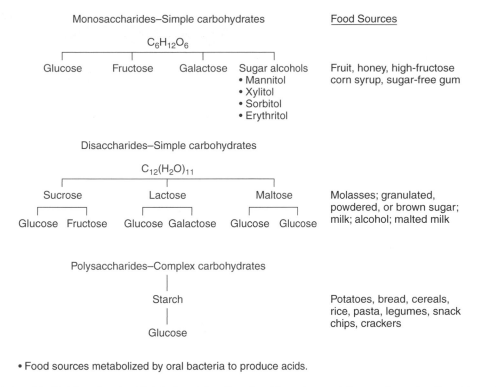

Monosaccharides–Simple carbohydrates   Food Sources

$C_6H_{12}O_6$

Glucose	Fructose	Galactose	Sugar alcohols	Fruit, honey, high-fructose

Sugar alcohols
• Mannitol
• Xylitol
• Sorbitol
• Erythritol

Fruit, honey, high-fructose corn syrup, sugar-free gum

Disaccharides–Simple carbohydrates

$C_{12}(H_2O)_{11}$

Sucrose   Lactose   Maltose

Glucose Fructose   Glucose Galactose   Glucose Glucose

Molasses; granulated, powdered, or brown sugar; milk; alcohol; malted milk

Polysaccharides–Complex carbohydrates

Starch

Potatoes, bread, cereals, rice, pasta, legumes, snack chips, crackers

Glucose

• Food sources metabolized by oral bacteria to produce acids.

FIGURE 19-1
Fermentable carbohydrates. (Modified from American Dietetic Association: Use of nutritive and non-nutritive sweeteners [position statement], J Am Diet Assoc 104:255-275, 2004.)

commonly found in sugar-free candy and chewing gum. The use of sugar-free gum, especially one containing xylitol, has actually been recognized as **nonacidogenic;** that is, such gums do not raise the plaque biofilm pH to an acidic range[10]; it may actually decrease the risk of dental caries and even remineralize some lesions.[9] The action of chewing, which stimulates saliva flow, in combination with the sugar alcohol promotes a healthy environment in the oral cavity.

However, because they contain calories, sugar alcohols can be cariogenic in some circumstances. One example of such an instance is the individual who experiences xerostomia and uses hard candy, sweetened with sugar alcohols, to relieve the dryness. The small amount of fermentable carbohydrate in the absence of the protective components of saliva can create an acidic environment. When recommending a product containing a sugar alcohol, the dental hygienist should inform the patient that such products may produce gastrointestinal distress and can have a laxative affect with as few as five to six pieces.

Disaccharides

Disaccharides are a combination of two carbohydrate units. Larger molecules of carbohydrates need to be hydrolyzed or broken down into the monosaccharide glucose before they can be digested and absorbed. Lactose, or milk sugar, is the least cariogenic of all disaccharides. The protective qualities of protein, phosphates, and calcium lend milk its low cariogenic potential. As with juice, however, when milk is permitted to sit on teeth for hours, a cariogenic environment is created.

Polysaccharides

Polysaccharides are actually many monosaccharides combined. A starch contains only glucose units. A starch molecule is large and cannot penetrate plaque biofilm. As salivary enzymes begin to hydrolyze starch to glucose, saliva can neutralize the acids easily. A cooked starch, such as instant oatmeal, is more readily hydrolyzed than a raw starch and lowers plaque biofilm pH but at a slower rate than sucrose.[11] The combination of a starch and sucrose, such as jelly on toast, creates an even greater cariogenic potential than toast alone.

★ CASE APPLICATION 19-1.2

Effect of Starch and Sucrose on Nutrition
John had eaten honey on biscuits for dinner, another example of a combination of sucrose and starch, which contributes to his increased rate of dental caries.

To label certain foods as cariogenic in all situations can be challenging because the multifactorial dental caries model acknowledges that an increase or decrease in any one factor can alter the cariogenic potential significantly. No food is cariogenic in all instances.

Nonnutritive Sweeteners

High-intensity, **nonnutritive sweeteners** provide negligible or no energy and do not promote dental caries.[4] Acesulfame-K, aspartame, neotame, saccharin, and sucralose are the five nonnutritive sweeteners approved by the U.S. Food and Drug Administration (FDA). Evidenced-based research does not support health claims associated with using nonnutritive sweeteners.

"Consumers can safely enjoy a range of nutritive and non-nutritive sweeteners when consumed in a diet that is guided by current federal nutrition recommendations" (position of the American Dietetic Association, 2004).[4]

PHYSICAL FORM OF FERMENTABLE CARBOHYDRATES

The demineralization potential of any fermentable carbohydrate is most related to the length of tooth exposure, the sticky and retentive nature of the carbohydrate, and the point at which it is consumed, not just the amount of fermentable carbohydrate present in food or in a meal. Therefore some foods are considered destructive to enamel because of their sucrose content (e.g., soft drinks) but may not be as cariogenic as a food lower in sugar (e.g., potato chips).

The physical form (solid or solution) of the fermentable carbohydrate affects its cariogenicity. Typically, a fermentable carbohydrate in solution form, such as a fruit drink, is less cariogenic than a solid because it is readily cleared from the oral cavity. A drop in pH can occur within 2 to 4 minutes and last up to 20 minutes for liquids until the buffers in saliva return the pH in plaque biofilm to a neutral level. A drink containing sucrose, such as soda, coffee or tea with sugar, or a sports drink, is even more damaging than fruit juice or milk.

Soft, sticky, or chewy fermentable carbohydrates are retained longer on the tooth surface than liquid forms and are therefore more cariogenic. The oral cavity can have a lowered pH for as long as 40 minutes with retentive food, such as bread, raisins, or bananas.

✦ CASE APPLICATION 19-1.3

Effect of Liquid Fermentable Carbohydrate on Nutrition

A solid food with a liquid fermentable carbohydrate can be as cariogenic as a solid alone. Vanilla ice cream, for example, is cleared readily from the oral cavity (within 20 minutes). However, the chips in chocolate-chip ice cream, as consumed by John, can adhere to the tooth surface, creating an even greater cariogenic potential. In addition, the sports drink with the cookies that John had as an afternoon snack is more cariogenic than the sports drink alone.

FREQUENCY OF FERMENTABLE CARBOHYDRATES

The point at which the fermentable carbohydrate is actually consumed is a second factor to consider in the potential of dental caries. A fermentable carbohydrate consumed as a snack alone, with no other protective food, is more harmful than the same food consumed with a meal.

The moment at which the fermentable carbohydrate is eaten during the meal affects the cariogenic potential significantly. When a fermentable carbohydrate is ingested over a period, the number of minutes of acid exposure increases.[15]

✦ CASE APPLICATION 19-1.4

Dietary Cariogenic Buffers

The soda that John drank as a morning snack has a greater cariogenic potential than the same amount of soda he drank during his lunch. The protein, lipids, calcium, and phosphorus in the cheeseburger he ate for lunch provided a buffer to help neutralize plaque biofilm pH. If the soda, however, were consumed at the very end of the meal, then John would have gained little to no benefit from the protective foods.

✦ CASE APPLICATION 19-1.5

Carbohydrate Exposure Time

If John drank his soda in the morning all at once, then he would have had only 20 minutes of acid exposure. If, however, he took the drink to class and sipped it all morning, the number of minutes of acid exposure would then equate to 20 minutes for each sip, easily adding up to many hours of acid exposure and leading to enamel demineralization. To determine the best intervention strategy for John's increased rate of dental caries, an observant dental hygienist would question him further regarding his diet and eating behaviors. One example would be as follows:

Do you typically drink soda during your classes?

Consulting John's food record in Table 19-1, do any other areas of concern related to the frequency of John's intake of fermentable carbohydrates exist?

Finally, fermentable carbohydrates consumed at bedtime are more cariogenic than those consumed at another time during the day. Salivary flow is reduced during sleep, resulting in less saliva to protect the teeth.

One of the goals of the dental hygienist should not be to eliminate all fermentable carbohydrates in any patient's dietary intake. A recommendation to reduce sugar or other fermentable carbohydrates is not effective and actually may lead the individual to select foods higher in protein or fat.

Acids in Drinks

Excessive consumption of diet sodas and canned or bottled flavored teas can also lower plaque biofilm pH and be a factor in dental erosion. Erosion will make the tooth susceptible to dental decay. In particular, malic, tartaric, citric, and phosphoric acids in these drinks create the environment for damage to the enamel.[19]

> *Prevention*
> Making the patient aware of the cariogenic potential of his or her existing diet, helping to modify the dietary intake, suggesting healthy snack alternatives, and recommending appropriate times to consume fermentable carbohydrates are considerations for patient education. Tailoring the information to the patient and changing the existing diet as little as possible results in a greater compliance rate and thus a greater success rate. Above all, proper oral hygiene techniques must be emphasized.

Nutritional Assessment

All dental patients can benefit from nutrition counseling. The goal of this section is to recognize individuals who are at the greatest risk for diet-related dental issues. To identify these patients and provide the highest quality and most appropriate care, the dental team must complete a thorough assessment. Analyzing the information provided ensures appropriate direction and helps prevent misinterpretation of the diet and dental situations. Figure 19-2 provides a summary of this process. A nutritional assessment involves four basic components:

1. Clinical evaluation (health, dental, and social history)
2. Anthropometric evaluation
3. Laboratory evaluation
4. Dietary intake evaluation

HEALTH, DENTAL, AND SOCIAL HISTORY

A thorough health, dental, and social history reveals risk factors that are suggestive of nutritional problems. A health history identifies individuals with conditions that can lead to malnutrition, such as **polypharmacy.** Extraoral and intraoral examinations can detect such problematic physical signs and symptoms as malnutrition, dentate status, poorly fitting dentures, and difficulty with chewing and swallowing. To gain further insight into dietary habits, the dental hygienist should ask open-ended questions to clarify or understand the patient's lifestyle. For example, the dental hygienist may have asked John from Case Study 19-1 how often he eats at home versus out and who prepares his meals.

ANTHROPOMETRIC EVALUATION

An anthropometric evaluation measures the physical characteristics of the body, such as height and weight. Most concerning

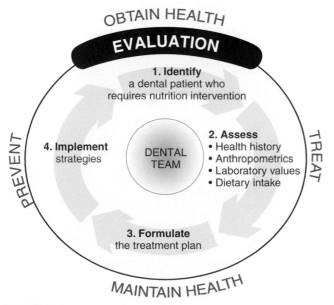

FIGURE 19-2
Each of the components of the inner ring is to be conducted by the dental team to promote and encourage the components on the outer ring. Both rings revolve around the dental team. Evaluation is ongoing and is performed at each step.

is the patient who has unintentionally lost or gained 10% or greater of his or her body weight in a 6-month period. Other measures are either impractical or irrelevant to dentistry.

LABORATORY EVALUATION

Findings from standard saliva tests, plaque biofilm–control indices, and dental caries risk-assessment activities are examples of laboratory evaluations that can target individuals who are at risk for diet-related dental problems. Biochemical tests, such as a complete blood count (CBC), although beneficial, are unrealistic in dental settings.

DIETARY INTAKE EVALUATION

The final element of the nutrition assessment process involves recording a patient's food intake. Obtaining a food diary for 3 to 7 days allows a dental hygienist and the patient to evaluate individual food habits, consumption of fermentable carbohydrates, food preferences, and nutrient adequacy.

> ### ★ CASE APPLICATION 19-1.6
>
> #### 24-Hour Food Diary
> Gathering data by patient interview and asking the patient to list the foods eaten the previous day is called a *24-hour recall.* John's case provides an example of this type of nutrition assessment (see Table 19-1).

Collecting data this way is easy, requires little time, and allows for an analysis of the foods. The greatest disadvantage is that a 24-hour recall represents only 1 day of food consumption and may not represent a person's true food intake pattern. A 3-day or 7-day food record, on the other hand, covers more days and is more representative of the individual's diet than a 24-hour record. The patient completes a food record through the stated period and returns it to the dental hygienist. Completing a 3- to 7-day food record allows patients to take responsibility for their personal health care by taking an active role. Dietary indiscretions are easier to identify when more days are recorded.

Analysis of Dietary Intake Data

Nutrient intakes from the diet history can be compared with a dietary standard, such as the U.S. Department of Agriculture (USDA) MyPyramid Food Guidance System[17] (Figure 19-3) and the 2005 Dietary Guidelines for Americans (Box 19-6).[18] The principles underlying these educational tools are appropriate for healthy Americans older than 2 years and coordinate with the information found in the nutrition facts label on food products. The patient's caloric level is to be determined to establish a tailored plan. John's caloric level is 2800 calories, based on his sex, age, and activity level. Table 19-3 provides a comparison John's food intake from Case Study 19-1 to the MyPyramid Food Guide System. The results identify nutrition elements in which John is doing well and areas he needs to modify. When fermentable carbohydrate intake increases the risk of dental caries, as in the case study, the dental hygienist or the patient should circle or highlight these items on the food record.

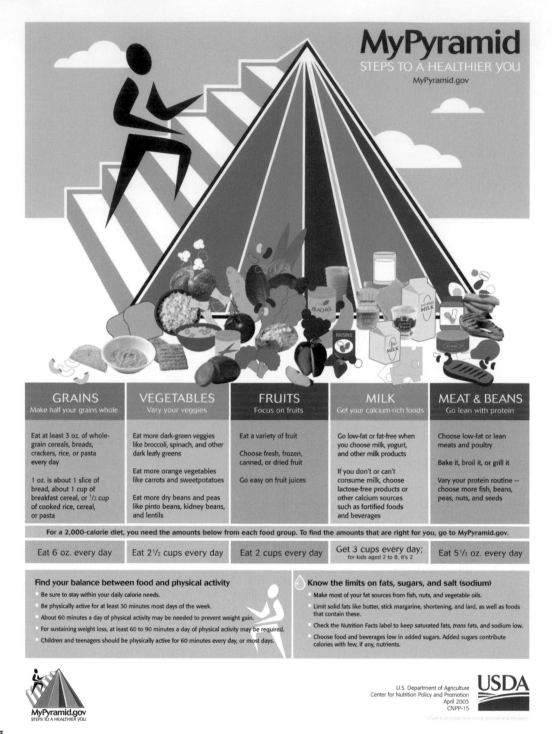

FIGURE 19-3
MyPyramid Food Guidance System. (USDA, Center for Nutrition Policy and Promotion 2005, [http://www.mypyramid.gov].)

TREATMENT PLAN

Once all the assessment information has been gathered, the dental team and patient can determine a realistic treatment plan that best suits the patient's needs. The counseling message therefore is tailored to the patient, and only information relevant to the individual needs to be discussed. This approach not only eliminates the standardized diet instruction, but also increases patient compliance. Therefore each diet instruction is different.

Concise documentation is essential and provides a means of communication among members of the dental team. Documentation may include the patient's goal or goals, expected compliance, and summary of the diet-related dental issue or issues.

BOX 19-6

DIETARY GUIDELINES FOR AMERICANS 2005

Summary of Key Recommendations for the General Population

Adequate nutrients within calorie needs
Choose a variety of nutrient-dense food and beverages
Choose a balanced eating pattern
Weight management
Balance calories from food and beverages with calories expended
Physical activity
Regular, moderate-intensity physical activity of 30-90 minutes on most days of the week

Food Groups to Encourage

Sufficient amount and variety of fruits and vegetables, whole-grain products, and milk products
Stay within a recommended calorie level

Fats

Limit saturated fats, cholesterol (300 mg/day), and trans fats
Choose polyunsaturated and monounsaturated fats

Choose and prepare low-fat or fat-free meat, poultry, beans, or milk products

Carbohydrates

Choose high-fiber foods
Limit added sugars

Sodium and Potassium

Consume less than 2300 mg sodium per day
Choose potassium-rich foods

Alcoholic Beverages

In moderation: one drink/day for women, two drinks/day for men
Sensibly

Food Safety

Clean hands, food-contact surfaces, and fruits and vegetables
Keep foods at safe temperatures
Separate raw, cooked, and ready-to-eat foods

Data from US Department of Agriculture, Department of Health and Human Services: *Dietary guidelines for Americans, 2005,* ed 6, Washington, DC, 2005, US Government Printing Office [www.healthierus.gov/dietaryguidelines].

Table 19-3 — Comparison of 24-Hour Recall to the MyPyramid Food Guidance System

FOOD AND QUANTITY	GRAINS	VEGETABLES	FRUITS	MILKS	MEATS AND BEANS	DISCRETIONARY CALORIES
Two Large *Blueberry Muffins*	6 oz	—	—	—	—	90
16-oz *Chocolate Milk*	—	—	—	2	—	150
Two 20-oz *Sodas*	—	—	—	—	—	520
Two Cheeseburgers	2 oz	—	—	2	4 oz	130
16 Onion Rings	—	½ cup	—	—	—	320
Four Large *Cookies*	2 oz	—	—	—	—	140
Mints	—	—	—	—	—	Approximately 100
20-oz *Sports Drink*	—	—	—	—	—	260
Six Fried Chicken Wings	—	—	—	—	6 oz	670
One Large Baked Potato	—	1½ cup	—	—	—	—
3 tsp Butter	—	—	—	—	—	105
Four *Biscuits*	4 oz	—	—	—	—	240
4 tsp *Honey*	—	—	—	—	—	65
16-oz *Fruit Punch*	—	—	—	—	—	230
Four Scoops *Ice Cream*	—	—	—	4	—	410
Total	14 oz	2 cups	0	8	10 oz	3430

Data from US Department of Agriculture and Center for Nutrition Policy and Promotion: *MyPyramid Food Guidance System,* Washington, DC, April 2005 [http://mypyramid.gov]. A comparison of John's 24-hour recall to the MyPyramid Food Guidance System was used to estimate his nutrient adequacy and eating patterns. His calorie level was determined to be 2800 calories. The fermentable carbohydrates are typically highlighted or circled. (They appear in *italics* within the table.)

Continued

Table 19-3	Comparison of 24-Hour Recall to the MyPyramid Food Guidance System—cont'd		
FOOD GROUP	**RECOMMENDED FOR 2800 CALORIES**	**ACTUAL**	**COMPARISON**
Grains	10 oz	14 oz	High
Vegetables	3½ cups	2 cups	Low
Fruits	2½ cups	0	Low
Milk	3 cups	8	High
Meat and Beans	7 oz	10 oz	High
Discretionary Calories	425	3690	High

EVALUATION

Distinct Care Modifications

Medically compromised patients require a referral to a dietitian or the primary care practitioner for nutrition intervention.

Note

One of the dental hygienist's roles is to be an oral health expert who is part of a healthcare team. The dental hygienist can report findings that are related to positive or negative changes observed in the oral cavity and can serve as an educational resource to others on the healthcare team.

During dental hygiene supportive care or other appointments, the dental team can monitor the patient's progress. The dental hygienist is there to support the positive changes made, review material as needed, and revise or add goals. As with all phases of patient care, the evaluation process is ongoing.

Clearly, every dental patient can benefit from nutrition counseling. The members of each dental environment must determine a philosophy as to which patients are appropriate candidates for more intense education.

References

1. Alvarez J: Nutrition, tooth development, and dental caries, *Am J Clin Nutr* 61(suppl):410-416, 1995.
2. American Beverage Association: *Product variety: what America's drinking* [Internet], Washington, DC, 2005 [http://www.ameribev.org].
3. American Dietetic Association: Oral health and nutrition [position statement], *J Am Diet Assoc* 103:615-625, 2003.
4. American Dietetic Association: Use of nutritive and nonnutritive sweeteners [position statement], *J Am Diet Assoc* 104:255-275, 2004.
5. Enwonwu C: Interface of malnutrition and periodontal disease, *Am J Clin Nutr* 61(suppl):430-436, 1995.
6. Featherstone J: The caries balance, *Dimens Dent Hyg* 2:14-18, 2004.
7. Featherstone J: Tipping the scales toward caries control, *Dimens Dent Hyg* 3:20-27, 2004.
8. Guthrie J, Morton J: Food sources of added sweeteners in the diets of Americans, *J Am Diet Assoc* 100:43-51, 2000.
9. Makinen K: Prevention of dental caries with xylitol—a potential dietary procedure for self-care and population-level use in young adults, *J Am College Health* 41:172-180, 1993.
10. Makinen K et al: Chewing gum and caries rate: a 40-month cohort study, *J Dent Res* 74:1904-1913, 1995.
11. Mormann J, Muhlemann H: Oral starch degradation and its influence on acid production in human dental plaque, *Caries Res* 15:166-175, 1981.
12. Pinkham J: *Pediatric dentistry: infancy through adolescence,* ed 4, St Louis, 2005, Mosby.
13. Ritchie C, et al: Nutrition as a mediator in the relation between oral and systemic disease: associations between specific measures of adult oral health and nutrition outcomes, *Crit Rev Oral Biol Med* 13:291-300, 2002.
14. Sheiham A, Steele J: Does the condition of the mouth and teeth affect the ability to eat certain foods, nutrient and dietary intake and nutritional status amongst older people? *Public Health Nutr* 4:797-803, 2001.
15. Stegeman C, Davis J: *The dental hygienist's guide to nutritional care,* ed 2, St Louis, 2005, Elsevier.
16. US Department of Agriculture: *Nationwide food consumption survey, 1977-78; continuing survey of food intakes by individual, 1987-88, 1994-96,* Washington, DC, 1998, US Government Printing Office.
17. US Department of Agriculture, Center for Nutrition Policy and Promotion: *MyPyramid Food Guidance System* [Internet], Washington DC, 2005, US Government Printing Office [http:www.mypyramid.gov].
18. US Department of Agriculture, Department of Health and Human Services: *Dietary guidelines for Americans,* ed 6, Washington, DC, 2005, US Government Printing Office.
19. VonFraunhofer J, Rogers M: Dissolution of dental enamel in soft drinks, *Gen Dent* 4:308-312, 2004.

Oral Risk Assessment and Intervention Planning

Sherry A. Harfst • Victoria C. Vick

INSIGHT

Dental hygienists often provide treatment, service, and care for individuals in a way these patients may have never before experienced. In Case Study 20-1, consider both the complexity and the opportunity to change a lifetime of dental neglect.

✦ CASE STUDY 20-1 Therapeutic Intervention with Risk Assessment

Robin Wallace, a 54-year-old woman who recently separated from her husband, arrives at your practice for a new patient examination. She reports inconsistent oral care during her lifetime and is currently experiencing pain caused by untreated dental caries. Ms. Wallace has no dental insurance at this time and needs significant restorative dentistry, as evidenced by her clinical oral examination and radiographic survey. Periodontally, she exhibits generalized gingivitis characterized by marginal inflammation of the gingiva and bleeding on gentle probing. Horizontal bone loss is evident radiographically; loss of attachment is noted in the premolar region.

When asked about her normal oral self-care habits, she confides that her toothbrush was "lost" in her recent move when she and her husband separated and that she just has not cared enough about her appearance to replace it. Ms. Wallace believes she has a promising job interview in a month, which she anticipates will offer dental insurance as a benefit. The job for which she is applying involves initial client contact for a major law firm in your community.

Think about the components involved in planning care for Ms. Wallace and the oral risk assessment steps that must occur before a plan is developed. How do you approach the pattern of dental neglect and lack of interest in self-care? What motivational factors can you isolate and use to help her gain optimal self-care? Where do you start? How do you individualize the treatment plan that is appropriate for this patient? This seemingly overwhelming function of dental hygiene diagnosis and patient care planning is manageable when broken down into a series of steps, particularly when the patient is involved as a participant.

KEY TERMS

intervention	prevention	risk assessment	therapeutic intervention strategy
patient-centered care	risk	risk factors	

LEARNING OUTCOMES

After reading this chapter the student will be able to:

1. Determine a working definition for the following terms: intervention, oral risk assessment, prevention, risk, and risk assessment.
2. Compare and contrast a patient-specific approach to care with a standardized routine.
3. Give examples of patient-centered oral care.
4. Cite examples of therapeutic intervention in dentistry.
5. Cite examples of prevention strategies in dentistry.

6. Cite examples of when therapeutic intervention and prevention overlap in dentistry.
7. Describe the benefits of oral risk assessment to individualizing preventive and therapeutic strategies.
8. Develop a clinical goal, therapeutic intervention, and evaluation measure based on a given oral risk concern.

Careful and appropriate planning of patient care affords dental hygienists the opportunity to touch a life and to influence the oral health—and potentially the systemic health—of individuals in their care. Dental hygienists often provide treatment, service, and care for individuals in a way they may have never before experienced (see Case Study 20-1).

Patient-Specific Approach to Oral Care

Initially, it might appear that a standard course of therapy can be applied to each patient who exhibits a specific set of clinical criteria; and to some extent, this statement is true. For example, a patient with marginal gingivitis will be clinically treated to remove the bacterial plaque biofilm and associated toxins and provided with appropriate self-care techniques to prevent and lessen plaque biofilm accumulation to a level that is biologically acceptable so that health is promoted and maintained. As a *standard of care,* this treatment rationale is sound by today's criteria. However, every patient exhibits not only clinical findings, but a biopsychosocial history as well. Each patient brings unique histories (medical and health, dental, biological, psychologic, sociologic, and cultural), including prescription and over-the-counter medications, beliefs, behaviors, unique clinical and radiographic findings, and expectations, all of which must be factored in providing appropriate clinical and oral self-care therapy. Patient-centered care—the method of care driven by a specific set of individualized needs—expresses the dictates of the

> *Note*
>
> The diagnosis and planning of dental hygiene therapy are two of the more complex and ultimately rewarding aspects of patient care. Numerous physical and cognitive steps must be carefully evaluated and weighed to arrive at an appropriate plan of therapy and education, leading to ongoing, supportive care.

surgeon general's *Report on Oral Health in America* (see Chapter 2); presents a holistic approach to care; and is the currently accepted method of patient care, planning, and delivery.[19]

ORAL RISK ASSESSMENT
Concept

Driving the concept of **patient-centered care** is oral **risk assessment.**[*] The basic premise of this concept states that each patient has a set of historical data—facts about genetic predisposition, previous oral and systemic disease experiences, medication regimens, fluoride history, habits, practices, behaviors, and beliefs. Each patient also has a specific set of current medical-dental data that reveal the patient's current oral status. Dental hygienists have the data that are necessary to complete an oral risk assessment when both the historical and the current information are evaluated for a given patient. Once the data are evaluated, a clear picture of potential and clinical oral risk concerns begins to emerge. Not only can a patient's current oral conditions be determined, but a listing of *potential* oral risk concerns (conditions, manifestations) can also be generated. This listing is based on current and past health histories, including dental history, for which therapeutic **intervention** strategies and personalized **prevention** strategies can then be developed (Box 20-1).

> *Note*
>
> Understanding the way in which intervention and prevention can and do occur simultaneously is critical in planning successful therapies.

Please refer to Case Study 20-1 for background information concerning the patient discussed throughout the chapter.
*References 1, 6, 17, 18, 20.

BOX 20-1

INTERVENTION AND PREVENTION

An explanation of the terms *intervention* and *prevention* is warranted as the discussion of patient-care planning begins. Although each term is clearly and distinctly defined, in dentistry, however, these terms overlap, making their application less clear. For example, *to intervene* implies a step or a measure designed to halt or significantly alter the current course of an event. In the case of removing demineralized tooth structure and replacing it with a restorative material, the process of dental caries development has been arrested by the intervention of a restorative dental procedure. To give a periodontal example, debriding a 4-mm pocket should result in eliminating gingival inflammation and in arresting bone loss and gingival attachment. Both procedures are clear examples of intervention.

Prevention is defined as the method that stops or prevents an expected or anticipated outcome from occurring. Removal of bacterial plaque biofilm to biologically acceptable levels can prevent both dental caries and gingival or periodontal diseases. The application of topical fluoride can prevent demineralization and enhance remineralization. This procedure is a clear example of prevention.

However, understanding the way in which intervention and prevention can and do occur simultaneously is critical in planning successful therapies. For example, when topical fluoride is applied to an incipient carious lesion, what happens?

First, the lesion remineralizes (intervention), and the process of dental caries development is arrested. At the same time, the tooth structure becomes less pervious to an acid challenge, thus preventing future demineralization from occurring (see Chapter 25). Removal of plaque biofilm and associated toxins, as in debridement, can be both an intervention to a disease process and a prevention of a disease process, as in daily oral self-care to prevent toxins from accumulating at the gingival margin (see Chapter 24).

This chapter uses these two terms in their simplest forms: *intervention strategies* are designed to stop the disease process, and *prevention strategies* are designed to ensure that a disease process will not occur. However, it should be noted that intervention and prevention often occur simultaneously.

Definition

The term **risk** is defined as the probability that an event will occur, such as a loss or injury. The term *risk* can be further defined as the probability of a person experiencing a change in health status over time.[12] In oral risk assessment, knowledge of risk factors—known associates to specific diseases or conditions—is used to partially determine a course of therapy and to design self-care interventions, as appropriate to a given patient (Box 20-2). **Risk factors**, then, are specific conditions or behaviors associated with risk occurrence.[3]

Application to Medicine and Dentistry

Medicine has provided dentistry a model for applying oral risk assessment. For decades, through the use of oral risk assessment, the medical community has targeted groups of individuals who are at risk for certain diseases (e.g., stroke, cancer, diabetes, heart disease), with intervention strategies specific to the particular disease.[4] This type of **therapeutic intervention strategy** is also appropriate for dentistry. Research has confirmed that certain subgroups are at an increased risk for certain oral disease populations. In planning appropriate dental hygiene care, clinicians need to be aware of these subgroups and realize that aggressive disease states are often defined by biological, psychologic, and sociologic components.[2,5,7,10]

> *Note*
>
> Use of a system-driven, clinical decision-making tool assists in collecting, assessing, and implementing this process.

Gathering, reviewing, and assessing patient data to perform an oral risk assessment can indeed be a time-consuming function for the oral health care provider, yet it is probably one of the most important functions that is integral to determining risk factors and potential oral conditions, designing appropriate supportive therapy, and planning patient self-care prevention strategies based on specific patient need.

Oral Risk Assessment System or Process

In dentistry, an organizational tool that helps gather and review data systematically, analyze and assess risk, and provide appropriate oral care recommendations provides a clinical framework for oral risk assessment. Following an oral risk assessment process helps provide a more holistic approach to patient data collection and subsequent course of therapy, which can result in early disease intervention.[6,11,14]

Oral risk assessment should then include a simple, clinical data-gathering and decision-making tool for chairside use. It incorporates a five-phase approach to the design of therapeutic intervention and prevention strategies based on numerous health-promotion stratagems and decision support systems.* Data are gathered via a standard health history form and by using a specialized patient questionnaire termed the *prevention survey* (Figure 20-1).

An oral risk assessment process follows the traditional dental hygiene model of assessment, diagnosis, planning, implementation, and evaluation[13] (Box 20-3).

ORAL RISK ASSESSMENT WORKSHEET

The five columns on the oral risk assessment worksheet (Figure 20-2) provide a template for the clinician to record the following:

- Summary findings from the review of pertinent histories and current clinical findings
- Listings of current and potential oral symptoms and conditions based on oral risk
- Established goals of therapy (therapeutic intervention strategies) and patient self-care prevention goals, including appointment planning
- Specific oral care recommendations
- Reevaluation

---

*References 6, 8, 11, 14-16.

BOX 20-2

KNOWLEDGE OF RISK FACTORS

Benefits to be gained from oral risk assessment, as presented by Douglas, include four basic tenets. Knowledge of risk factors can facilitate the following:

1. Increase the chances of correctly predicting an oral disease instance (e.g., dental caries, periodontal disease)
2. Help identify individuals and groups who would benefit from targeted interventions
3. Stimulate increased clinician awareness and level of suspicion, which prompts increased acuteness in the assessment process
4. Provide a foundation for early disease recognition, which identifies candidates for new and emerging disease-management technologies

From Douglas CW: Oral risk assessment in dentistry, *J Dent Ed* 62(10):756-761, 1998.

BOX 20-3

FIVE-STEP PROCESS IN ORAL RISK ASSESSMENT

1. *Gather and review assessment data.* Gather and review all patient data.
2. *Assess and analyze data for oral risk concerns.* Assess and analyze patient data for potential oral concerns (oral risk).
3. *Plan.* Outline goals of therapy for professional and patient self-care.
4. *Recommend.* Provide specific oral care products and an oral self-care regimen.
5. *Evaluate or reevaluate.* Evaluate outcomes of clinical dental hygiene therapy and recommend alternatives as appropriate.

DENTAL HISTORY

Name _____ Date _____

A — Prevention Survey

1. **In the past two years, have you experienced any of the following symptoms?**
   (If yes, please check all that apply.)
   - ☐ Sensitive teeth
   - ☐ Bleeding gums
   - ☐ Bad breath
   - ☐ Swelling inside mouth
   - ☐ Sore jaw
   - ☐ Difficulty chewing
   - ☐ Burning sensation
   - ☐ Tartar buildup
   - ☐ Toothache
   - ☐ Filling fell out
   - ☐ Abscess
   - ☐ Yellowing teeth
   - ☐ Sore gums
   - ☐ Dry mouth
   - ☐ Swollen face
   - ☐ Difficulty swallowing
   Comments _____

2. **When you look inside your mouth, do you know what to look for?**

	Yes	No
Tooth Decay	☐	☐
Oral Cancer	☐	☐
Gum Disease	☐	☐

3. **For the past two years, what is your best estimate of the number of times you have been to see a dental professional for each of the following:**
   - _____ Checkups and cleanings
   - _____ Other dental treatment such as fillings, gum treatment, crowns (caps), bridges, dentures
   - _____ Dental emergencies

4. **Do you clench or grind your teeth in the daytime or at night?**
   ☐ Yes ☐ No
   If yes, do you wear a bite guard? _____ For how long? _____

5. **In the past two years, have you been concerned about the appearance of your teeth?**
   (If yes, please check all that apply.)
   - ☐ Yellowing/graying teeth
   - ☐ Stains
   - ☐ Crowded, crooked
   - ☐ Spacing between teeth
   - ☐ Other _____

6. **Check any of the following you regularly use at home:**
   - ☐ Soft toothbrush
   - ☐ Hard toothbrush
   - ☐ Medium toothbrush
   - ☐ Oral irrigator
   - ☐ Denture adhesive
   - ☐ Dental floss
   - ☐ Special brush
   - ☐ Fluoride toothpaste
   - ☐ Rubber tip
   - ☐ Denture cleanser
   - ☐ Floss threader
   - ☐ Toothpick
   - ☐ Fluoride rinse or gel
   - ☐ Mouthrinse
   - ☐ Whitening product
   - ☐ Powered interdental cleaner
   - ☐ Powered brush
   - ☐ Other_____

7. **Check the type of toothpaste you use:**
   - ☐ Fluoride
   - ☐ Sensitivity protection
   - ☐ Tartar control
   - ☐ Baking soda
   - ☐ Gum benefit
   - ☐ Peroxide
   - ☐ Whitening
   - ☐ Multiple benefit

8. **Estimate how long it takes you to clean your teeth and gums each time:**
   Please indicate your best and most reliable estimate.
   Brushing_____ (time)   Flossing_____ (time)

9. **About how many times each day/week do you brush and floss?**
   I brush about _____ times per day OR _____ per week
   I floss about _____ times per day OR _____ per week

10. **Do you find it difficult to maintain an oral hygiene schedule due to your job/profession or other reasons?**
    ☐ No ☐ Yes

11. **Do any conditions make it difficult for you to adequately clean your teeth?**
    (If yes, please check all that apply.)
    - ☐ Hold a toothbrush
    - ☐ Use dental floss
    - ☐ Brush/floss for any length of time
    - ☐ Don't see well

12. **Generally, how have you felt about your previous dental appointments?**
    - ☐ Very anxious and afraid
    - ☐ Somewhat anxious and afraid
    - ☐ Don't care one way or the other
    - ☐ Look forward to it

FLUORIDE HISTORY

B

1. ☐ Yes ☐ No Are you on a fluoridated public water system?
   If yes, for how long? _____

2. ☐ Yes ☐ No Do you use any type of water filter or bottled water for your main water source?
   If yes, what type of filter? _____
   If yes, what brand of water? _____
   For how long? _____

3. ☐ Yes ☐ No If you are on a fluoridated public water system, does your job/profession keep you away from home more than 4 days per week?
   If yes, do you use any fluoride supplements during that time?
   (For example: a fluoridated mouthrinse) ☐ Yes ☐ No

4. ☐ Yes ☐ No Do you drink bottled fruit juices? _____
   If yes, how many per day? _____

5. ☐ Yes ☐ No Do you currently use a fluoridated toothpaste?
   If yes, how often? _____
   If yes, for how many years? _____
   If yes, what brand? _____
   If no, why not? _____

6. ☐ Yes ☐ No Do you use an oral rinse containing fluoride?
   If yes, how often? _____
   If yes, what brand? _____

7. ☐ Yes ☐ No Do you use any additional sources of fluoride (such as drops, tablets)?
   If yes, what sources? _____
   For how long? _____

For Child Patient

8. ☐ Yes ☐ No Are the children in your home in childcare, daycare, or school where they **do not receive** fluoridated public water? _____
   If yes, how many days per week? _____

9. ☐ Yes ☐ No Do you or anyone in your home use a fluoridated supplement (drops or tablets?)
   If yes, what dosage? _____
   If yes, for how long? _____

FIGURE 20-1

The prevention survey is a specialized, four-part patient questionnaire used to gather data on dental history **(A)**, fluoride history **(B)**, health behaviors **(C)**, and diet recall and health beliefs **(D)**.

BEHAVIORS

1. Do you have an annual physical examination?
   ❑ No ❑ Yes

2. When you are ill, do you:
   ❑ See your physician? ❑ Seek care in an emergency room?
   ❑ Wait to see if the condition goes away?

3. When your physician recommends a change in health behavior, do you follow his/her advice?
   ❑ No ❑ Yes ❑ Sometimes

4. When your dental professional recommends a change in health behavior, do you follow his/her advice?
   ❑ No ❑ Yes ❑ Sometimes

5. When your dental professional recommends a specific oral care product or self-care regimen do you follow his/her advice?
   ❑ No ❑ Yes ❑ Sometimes

6. Do you have regular hobbies/interests outside of work?
   ❑ No ❑ Yes

7. Do you strive to reach a balance between work and relaxation?
   ❑ No ❑ Yes

8. Are your eating habits out of control?
   ❑ No ❑ Yes

9. Do you feel your stress level has increased in the past 6 months?
   ❑ No ❑ Yes

10. Do you use tobacco in any form? If yes, what form and frequency?
    ❑ No ❑ Yes ❑ Sometimes Type _____ Frequency/Quantity _____
    For how long? _____

11. Do you consume alcohol?
    ❑ No ❑ Yes ❑ Sometimes Type _____ Frequency/Quantity _____

12. Do you consume caffeine?
    ❑ No ❑ Yes ❑ Sometimes Type _____ Frequency/Quantity _____

13. Do you exercise daily?
    ❑ No ❑ Yes ❑ Sometimes Type _____ Frequency/Quantity _____

14. Do you participate in sports/recreation activities?
    ❑ No ❑ Yes ❑ Sometimes Type _____ Frequency/Quantity _____

C

DIET SURVEY

Please indicate which sweets and cooked starches you eat between meals.

Food	Frequency	✓ if between meals
Breath mints		
Cough drops		
Chewing gum		
Dried fruits		
Canned/bottled beverages		
Sugared liquids		
Chips		
Crackers		
Cookies		

D

BELIEFS

1. In your opinion, compared with the average person, how likely do you think you are to have cavities or other problems with your teeth and/or gums?
   ❑ Much more likely ❑ About average ❑ Much less than average
   ❑ More than average ❑ Less than average

2. How important is it for you to prevent cavities, gum problems, or other diseases of the mouth?
   ❑ Very important ❑ Somewhat important ❑ Not at all important

3. Would you like your dental professional to make specific product recommendations to meet your oral care needs?
   ❑ Yes ❑ I am not sure ❑ No

4. There are times in our lives when it seems we have the energy and time to tackle new projects or to make changes.
   At this time, I ❑ can ❑ cannot imagine trying to change a habit

5. I believe that I have control over the condition of my mouth.
   ❑ Firmly believe ❑ Somewhat believe ❑ Do not believe

FIGURE 20-1, cont'd

Oral Risk Assessment Worksheet

Patient Name_____

I   II

REVIEW			ANALYZE — Oral Risk Concerns	
Health History	**Medications & Dose**	**Duration**	**At risk for**	**Clinically Evident**
❑ Cardiovascular (heart)	(prescription and OTC)		**Hard Tissues**	
❑ Central nervous system (nerves)			❑ Abrasion/Attrition/Erosion	❑
❑ Endocrine (endocrine glands)			❑ Bone Loss	❑
❑ Gastrointestinal (stomach, intestines)			❑ Bruxism/Occlusal Trauma	❑
❑ Genitourinary (sex organs, urinary tract)			❑ Calculus	❑
❑ Head, eyes, ears, nose, throat			❑ Caries: coronal/interproximal	❑
❑ Hematologic (blood)			❑ Caries: root surface	❑
❑ Integumentary (skin)			❑ Chipped broken teeth	❑
❑ Musculoskeletal (muscles, bones, joints)			❑ Extrinsic staining	❑
❑ Psychologic			❑ Fluorosis	❑
❑ Respiratory			❑ Intrinsic staining	❑
Vital Signs BP / Pulse			❑ Malaligned teeth	❑

PREVENTION SURVEY

Dental History				
❑ Sensitive teeth	❑ Sore jaw	❑ Toothache	❑ Sore gums	❑ Clenching
❑ Bleeding gums	❑ Difficulty chewing	❑ Filling fell out	❑ Dry mouth	❑ Grinding
❑ Bad breath	❑ Burning sensation		❑ Abscess	❑ Swollen face
❑ Swelling inside mouth	❑ Tartar buildup	❑ Yellowing teeth	❑ Difficulty swallowing	
❑ Adequate OH time	❑ Anxiety/Pain	❑ Oral self-care difficulty		

Right-column continued (At risk for / Clinically Evident):
❑ Mobile teeth ❑ · ❑ Sensitive teeth ❑ · ❑ Trauma ❑ · ❑ Other ❑

Oral Health Products:

Fluoride History

❑ Fluoridated water	❑ Away from home >4 days/week	❑ Oral rinse w/fluoride	
❑ Water filter	❑ Bottled juice	Child:	
❑ Bottled water	❑ Fluoridated dentifrice	❑ In daycare w/out fluoride	❑ Supplements

Soft Tissues
❑ Abscess: carious ❑
❑ Abscess: periodontal ❑
❑ Atrophic ulcer ❑
❑ Aphthous ulcer ❑
❑ Burning tongue/mouth ❑
❑ Candidiasis ❑

Behaviors

❑ Annual physical	❑ Balance work/relaxation	❑ Tobacco use	❑ Exercise
❑ Follows medical advice	❑ Eating habits controlled	❑ Alcohol use	
❑ Follows dental advice	❑ Increased stress	❑ Caffeine use	
Diet Survey	❑ Carbohydrate/Sucrose intake (excessive/moderate/minimal)		

❑ Ecchymosis ❑
❑ Gingival recession ❑
❑ Gingival hyperplasia ❑
❑ Gingivitis ❑
❑ Herpetic lesions ❑
❑ Increased plaque ❑

Beliefs

❑ Understands oral status	❑ Values prevention	
❑ Wants product recommendations	❑ Open to change	❑ Feels in control of oral condition

❑ Leukoplakia ❑
❑ Lichen planus ❑
❑ Oral cancer ❑
❑ Periodontal disease ❑
❑ Petechiae ❑
❑ Salivation – increased ❑
❑ Salivation – decreased ❑
❑ Trauma ❑
❑ Xerostomia ❑
❑ Other_____ ❑

Clinical and Radiographic Findings

Intraoral/Extraoral Examination	❑ Within normal limits		❑ See chart
Caries	❑ Coronal	❑ Interproximal	❑ Root surface
Restorations/Prosthetics			
Restorations	❑ Amalgam	❑ Composite	❑ Crowns/inlays/onlays ❑ Bridges
Dentures	❑ Complete	❑ Partial	
Periodontium			
❑ Recession	❑ Plaque ❑ Bleeding on probing	❑ Loss of attached gingiva	❑ Pockets <3mm
❑ Mucogingival defects			
Occlusion/TMJ	❑ Traumatic occlusion	❑ Crepitus	
Bone Loss	❑ <25%	❑ 25-50%	❑ Horizontal ❑ Vertical

Consult   **Referral**
❑ Consultation with physician ❑
❑ Consultation with dental specialist ❑

FIGURE 20-2
Five columns of the oral risk assessment worksheet, a form used to summarize, analyze, and plan patient treatment. **A,** Column I is used to summarize a review of patient data. **B,** Column II is used to analyze the assessment data reviewed in column I for oral risk concerns.

Date_____

III			IV			V
PLAN			**ORAL CARE RECOMMENDATIONS**			**EVALUATE**
Clinical Goals	Therapeutic Intervention	Patient Goals	Prevention Strategy		Product	Clinical Goals
				Toothbrush		
				❑ Mechanical		
				❑ Child ❑ Youth ❑ Compact ❑ Full		
				❑ Soft ❑ Extra Soft		
				❑ Powered		
				Brushing frequency		
				Brushing duration		
				Interdental Cleaning Products		
				❑ Floss Type Frequency		
				❑ Oral Irrigator Frequency		
				❑ Interdental Brush Frequency		
				❑ Other		
				Dentifrice		
				❑ Fluoride ❑ Whitening		
				❑ Sensitivity ❑ Multiple Benefit		
				❑ Tartar Control ❑ Gingival Benefit		
				❑ Children's		
				Oral Rinse		
				❑ Fluoride		
				❑ Cosmetic		Patient Goals
				❑ Alcohol-free		
				❑ Tartar Control		
				❑ Chlorhexidine		
				❑ Essential Oil/Phenol Compound		
				Prosthodontic Care		
				❑ Adhesive ❑ Denture Brush		
				❑ Denture Bath/Cleanser		
				Self Evaluation		
				❑ Disclosing tablets or solutions		
				❑ Evaluate bleeding points		
				Other		

FIGURE 20-2, cont'd
C, Column III is used to plan therapeutic intervention. **D,** Column IV is used for specific product and procedure recommendations for patient oral self-care. **E,** Column V is used for therapeutic and patient-goal reevaluation.

This chapter addresses the first three steps of an oral risk assessment process. Steps 4 and 5, which involve individualized prevention strategies, appointment planning and sequencing, and reevaluation, are discussed in Chapter 21.

Column I: Gather and Review Patient Data

In Step 1, the clinician gathers and records a summary of all documented histories and clinical and radiographic findings (see Figure 20-2, *column I*).

Column II: Assess and Analyze

In Step 2, the patient information gathered is assessed and analyzed relative to both current and potential oral disease and conditions (see Figure 20-2, *column II*).

Column III: Plan Strategies for Therapeutic Intervention, Individualized Prevention, and Appointment Planning

Step 3 formalizes the process of establishing therapeutic intervention and prevention strategies that are essential to appointment planning and the reevaluation process (see Figure 20-2, *column III*).

Column IV: Recommend

In Step 4, the clinician actively recommends specific products and procedures to the patient for implementing prevention strategies (see Figure 20-2, *column IV*).

Column V: Evaluate or Reevaluate

In Step 5, both clinical therapy and patient oral self-care must be evaluated or reevaluated after therapy and intervention recommendations. Oral care habits can be evaluated for successful outcomes; new suggestions can be made as appropriate. This reevaluation is sometimes done during the course of treatment, as in the case of multiple appointments, or it can occur at a subsequent supportive care appointment (see Figure 20-2, *column V*). Whatever the continuum of care may be, the reevaluation phase is a critical component of competent oral care; the design of appropriate, individualized oral self-care prevention strategies; and the patient's involvement in the process of care. This step is addressed in Chapter 21.

The oral risk assessment tool described in this chapter provides a linear format; that is, it is followed from the far left column to the far right column. The patient data in the Case

---

✸ CASE APPLICATION 20-1.1

Assessing Health Beliefs and Practice

Initial Clinic Impression
The patient, 54-year-old Ms. Wallace, has generalized, marginal gingivitis and dental caries.

Biopsychosocial Inventory and Dental History
The biopsychosocial data for this case were gathered using a personal inventory tool called a *prevention survey* (see Figure 20-1), which collects the patient's dental history, fluoride use, health behaviors, and health beliefs.

Clinical Data
The clinical data are provided via a standard health history form, along with a clinical narrative.
Ms. Wallace, who reported for a new patient examination, revealed the following information in her oral risk assessment survey:

Health History
- Her health history indicates that she is being treated for cardiovascular disease, for which she takes diltiazem (Cardizem), a calcium channel blocker.
- Her blood pressure is 179/80 mm Hg (right arm, sitting); her pulse is 82 beats per minute (strong and regular).

Prevention Survey
- Her self-reported prevention survey (Figure 20-3) reveals the following:

Dental History
- Bleeding gingiva
- Calculus accumulation
- Toothache
- Unaware of signs of oral disease
- Irregular dental visits
- Indicates that her teeth appear yellow and that she would like them to be whiter
- Cannot find her toothbrush
- Does not use dental floss (unable to coordinate her fingers)
- Spends an inadequate amount of time in oral self-care
- Unsure of type of toothpaste used
- Seeks dental care only when in pain

Fluoride History
- Is not currently benefiting from fluoridated public water source
- Unsure whether her dentifrice contains fluoride; uses any sale brand (when she brushes)

CASE APPLICATION 20-1.1–cont'd

Prevention Survey

DENTAL HISTORY

Name _Robin Wallace_   Date _MM/DD/YY_

1. In the past two years, have you experienced any of the following symptoms?
(If yes, please check all that apply)

- ☐ Sensitive teeth
- ☒ Bleeding gums
- ☐ Bad breath
- ☐ Swelling inside mouth
- ☐ Sore jaw
- ☐ Difficulty chewing
- ☐ Burning sensation
- ☒ Tartar buildup
- ☒ Toothache
- ☐ Filling fell out
- ☐ Abscess
- ☐ Yellowing teeth
- ☐ Sore gums
- ☐ Dry mouth
- ☐ Swollen face
- ☐ Difficulty swallowing

Comments _____

2. When you look inside your mouth, do you know what to look for?

	Yes	No
Tooth Decay	☐	☒
Oral Cancer	☐	☒
Gum Disease	☐	☒

3. For the past two years, what is your best estimate of the number of times you have been to see a dental professional for each of the following:

_____ Checkups and cleanings
_____ Other dental treatment such as fillings, gum treatment, crowns (caps), bridges, dentures
_3_ Dental emergencies

4. Do you clench or grind your teeth in the daytime or at night?
☐ Yes ☒ No
If yes, do you wear a bite guard?_____ For how long?_____

5. In the past two years, have you been concerned about the appearance of your teeth?
(If yes, please check all that apply)

- ☒ Yellowing/graying teeth
- ☐ Other_____
- ☐ Stains
- ☐ Crowded, crooked
- ☐ Spacing between teeth

6. Check any of the following you regularly use at home:

- ☐ Soft toothbrush
- ☐ Hard toothbrush
- ☐ Medium toothbrush
- ☐ Oral irrigator
- ☐ Denture adhesive
- ☐ Dental floss
- ☐ Special brush
- ☐ Fluoride toothpaste
- ☐ Rubber tip
- ☐ Denture cleanser
- ☐ Floss threader
- ☐ Toothpick
- ☐ Fluoride rinse or gel
- ☐ Mouthrinse
- ☐ Whitening product
- ☐ Powered interdental cleaner
- ☐ Powered brush
- ☐ Other_____

lost my toothbrush

7. Check the type of toothpaste you use:

- ☒ Fluoride ?
- ☐ Sensitivity protection
- ☐ Tartar control
- ☐ Baking soda
- ☐ Gum benefit
- ☐ Peroxide
- ☐ Whitening
- ☐ Multiple benefit

8. Estimate how long it takes you to clean your teeth and gums each time:
Please indicate your best and most reliable estimate.
Brushing _15 seconds_ Flossing _0_
(time)   (time)

9. About how many times each day/week do you brush and floss?
I brush about _____ times per day OR _7_ per week _-when I have a toothbrush_
I floss about _____ times per day OR _____ per week

10. Do you find it difficult to maintain an oral hygiene schedule due to your job/profession or other reasons?
☐ No ☒ Yes _I don't have a toothbrush_

11. Do any conditions make it difficult for you to adequately clean your teeth?
(If yes, please check all that apply) _-my fingers don't work that way_

- ☐ Hold a toothbrush
- ☒ Use dental floss
- ☐ Brush/floss for any length of time
- ☐ Don't see well

12. Generally, how have you felt about your previous dental appointments?

- ☐ Very anxious and afraid
- ☐ Somewhat anxious and afraid
- ☒ Don't care one way or the other _I go when I have a problem_
- ☐ Look forward to it

FLUORIDE HISTORY

1. ☐ Yes ☒ No Are you on a fluoridated public water system?
If yes, for how long? _____

2. ☐ Yes ☒ No Do you use any type of water filter or bottled water for your main water source?
If yes, what type of filter? _____
If yes, what brand of water? _____
For how long? _____

3. ☐ Yes ☐ No If you are on a fluoridated public water system, does your job/profession keep you away from home more than 4 days per week?
If yes, do you use any fluoride supplements during that time?
(For example: a fluoridated mouthrinse) ☐ Yes ☐ No

4. ☐ Yes ☒ No Do you drink bottled fruit juices?
If yes, how many per day?_____

5. ☐ Yes ? ☐ No Do you currently use a fluoridated toothpaste?
If yes, how often? _not sure_
If yes, for how many years? _____
If yes, what brand?_____
If no, why not?_____

6. ☐ Yes ☒ No Do you use an oral rinse containing fluoride?
If yes, how often? _____
If yes, what brand? _____

7. ☐ Yes ☒ No Do you use any additional sources of fluoride (such as drops, tablets)?
If yes, what sources? _____
For how long? _____

For Child Patient

8. ☐ Yes ☐ No Are the children in your home in childcare, daycare or school where they do not receive fluoridated public water?
If yes, how many days per week?_____

9. ☐ Yes ☐ No Do you or anyone in your home use a fluoridated supplement (drops or tablets)?
If yes, what dosage? _____
If yes, for how long?_____

BEHAVIORS

1. Do you have an annual physical examination?
☒ No ☐ Yes

2. When you are ill, do you?
☐ See your physician? ☒ Seek care in an emergency room?
☐ Wait to see if the condition goes away?

3. When your physician recommends a change in health behavior, do you follow his/her advice?
☐ No ☐ Yes ☒ Sometimes

4. When your dental professional recommends a change in health behavior, do you follow his/her advice?
☐ No ☐ Yes ☒ Sometimes

5. When your dental professional recommends a specific oral care product or self-care regimen do you follow his/her advice?
☐ No ☐ Yes ☒ Sometimes

6. Do you have regular hobbies/interests outside of work?
☒ No ☐ Yes

7. Do you strive to reach a balance between work and relaxation?
☒ No ☐ Yes

8. Are your eating habits out of control?
☒ No ☐ Yes

9. Do you feel your stress level has increased in the past 6 months?
☐ No ☒ Yes

10. Do you use tobacco in any form? If yes, what form and frequency?
☒ No ☐ Yes ☐ Sometimes Type _____ Frequency/Quantity _____
For how long? _____

11. Do you consume alcohol?
☐ No ☐ Yes ☒ Sometimes Type _beer_ Frequency/Quantity _weekends only_

12. Do you consume caffeine?
☐ No ☒ Yes ☐ Sometimes Type _coffee_ Frequency/Quantity _6-8 cups a day_

13. Do you exercise daily?
☒ No ☐ Yes ☐ Sometimes Frequency/Quantity _____

14. Do you participate in sports/recreation activities?
☒ No ☐ Yes ☐ Sometimes Type _____ Frequency/Quantity _____

FIGURE 20-3
Prevention survey filled out by Robin Wallace, the case study patient, showing the dental history (**A**), fluoride history (**B**), and health behavior (**C**) portions.

Continued

DIET SURVEY

Please indicate which sweets and cooked starches you eat between meals.

Food		Frequency	✓ if between meals
breath mints			
cough drops			
chewing gum			
dried fruits			
canned/bottled beverages			
sugared liquids			
chips			
crackers	either peanut butter or plain	after breakfast, lunch, dinner and snacks	✓
cookies			

D

BELIEFS

1. In your opinion, compared to the average person, how likely do you think you are to have cavities or other problems with your teeth and/or gums?
   ☒ Much more likely   ☐ About average   ☐ Much less than average
   ☐ More than average   ☐ Less than average

2. How important is it for you to prevent cavities, gum problems or other diseases of the mouth?
   ☒ Very important   ☐ Somewhat important   ☐ Not at all important

3. Would you like your dental professional to make specific product recommendations to meet your oral care needs?
   ☒ Yes   ☐ I am not sure   ☐ No

4. There are times in our lives when it seems we have the energy and time to tackle new projects or to make changes.
   At this time, I ☒ can   ☐ cannot imagine trying to change a habit

5. I believe that I have control over the condition of my mouth.
   ☐ Firmly believe   ☒ Somewhat believe   ☐ Do not believe

FIGURE 20-3, cont'd
Diet recall and health beliefs (**D**) portions of Robin Wallace's prevention survey.

Health Behavior
- Seeks medical attention only on an emergency basis
- Occasionally follows medical and dental care providers' recommendations
- Feels stressed
- Does not use tobacco products
- Occasionally consumes alcohol
- Drinks six to eight caffeinated beverages a day
- Does not exercise

Diet Survey
- Consumes crackers between meals

Health Beliefs
- Believes she is more likely than others to have dental problems
- Believes prevention of oral problems is important
- Likes to get recommendations from dental professionals
- Believes she can tackle a new project or make a change
- Somewhat believes she has control over her oral condition

Clinical and Radiographic Findings
- Extraoral and intraoral examination (Figure 20-4) reveals several breaks in the integrity of the buccal mucosa at the line of occlusion (consistent with cheek biting).
- Root surface caries are noted in the mandibular premolar area (Figure 20-5).
- Numerous restorations indicate previous carious experience; restorative materials present include amalgam, composite, and gold alloy (Figure 20-6; see also Figure 20-5).
- Periodontium exhibits recession, bacterial plaque biofilm, bleeding when probed, and loss of attached gingiva (Figure 20-7).
- Horizontal bone loss is noted (see Figure 20-6).
- No pathologic processes noted radiographically (see Figure 20-6).

CASE APPLICATION 20-1.1–cont'd

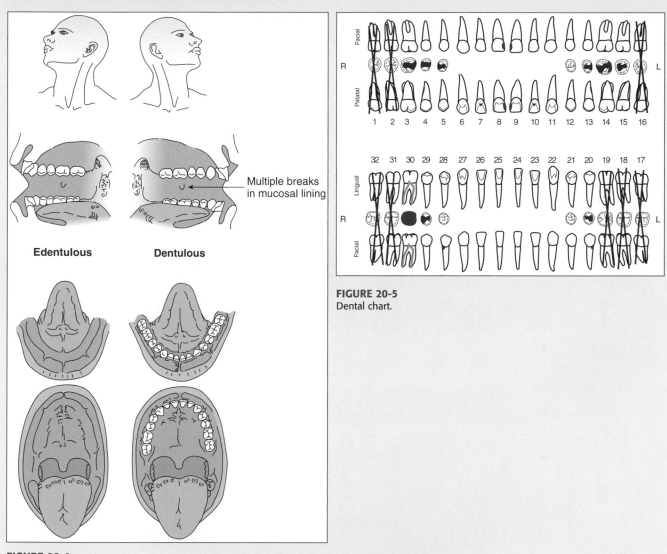

Multiple breaks
in mucosal lining

Edentulous   **Dentulous**

FIGURE 20-4
Intraoral-extraoral chart form.

FIGURE 20-5
Dental chart.

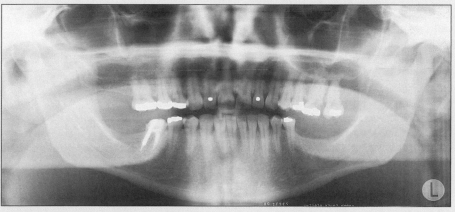

FIGURE 20-6
Dental panoramic radiograph.

Continued

☆ CASE APPLICATION 20-1.1–cont'd

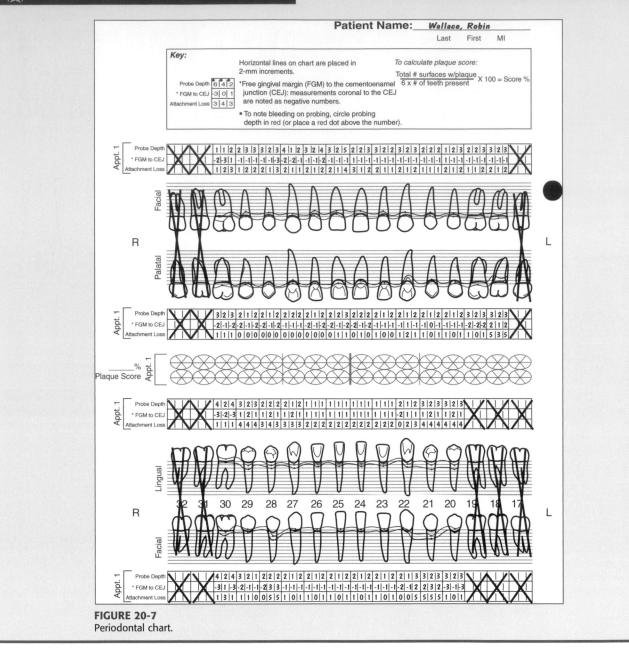

FIGURE 20-7
Periodontal chart.

Study 20-1 provides an example of the value of an oral risk assessment process to patient outcomes.

Although the clinical data presented in the case study concerning Ms. Wallace appears somewhat similar to many others, the fact that she also exhibits her own unique background and circumstances that provide clues that are necessary to the planning of appropriate and successful therapeutic strategies should be evident. The designs of both the clinical therapy and the patient intervention therapy are unique to this patient's circumstances and are based on the concepts of oral risk assessment.

Oral Risk Assessment Application to Case Study

STEP 1: GATHER AND REVIEW ASSESSMENT DATA

Health History

Figure 20-8

- Ms. Wallace's health history indicates that she is being treated for cardiovascular disease, for which she takes diltiazem (Cardizem), a calcium channel blocker.
- Her blood pressure is 179/80 mm Hg (right arm, sitting); her pulse is 82 beats per minute (strong and regular).

Dental History

Figure 20-9; see also Figure 20-3, *A*

- Bleeding gingiva
- Calculus accumulation
- Toothache
- Unaware of signs of oral disease

- Irregular dental visits
- Indicates that her teeth appear yellow and that she would like them to be whiter
- Cannot find her toothbrush
- Does not use dental floss (unable to coordinate her fingers)
- Spends an inadequate amount of time on oral self-care
- Seeks dental care only when something hurts

Fluoride History

Figure 20-10; see also Figure 20-3, *B*

- Is not currently benefiting from fluoridated public water source
- Unsure whether her dentifrice contains fluoride; uses any sale brand (when she brushes)

Health Behavior

Figure 20-11; see also Figure 20-3, *C*

- Seeks medical attention when only appropriate
- Occasionally follows medical and dental care providers' recommendations

Health History	Medications & Dose	Duration
☑ Cardiovascular (heart)	(prescription and OTC)	
❑ Central nervous system (nerves)	*Cardizem*	
❑ Endocrine (endocrine glands)		
❑ Gastrointestinal (stomach, intestines)		
❑ Genitourinary (sex organs, urinary tract)		
❑ Head, eyes, ears, nose, throat		
❑ Hematologic (blood)		
❑ Integumentary (skin)		
❑ Musculoskeletal (muscles, bones, joints)		
❑ Psychologic		
❑ Respiratory		
Vital Signs BP	*(RAS) 179/80*	Pulse *82 bpm (S+R)*

FIGURE 20-8
Summary of information from health history applied to column I of the oral risk assessment worksheet.

Dental History				
❑ Sensitive teeth	❑ Sore jaw	☑ Toothache	❑ Sore gums	❑ Clenching
☑ Bleeding gums	❑ Difficulty chewing	❑ Filling fell out	❑ Dry mouth	❑ Grinding
❑ Bad breath	❑ Burning sensation		❑ Abscess	❑ Swollen face
❑ Swelling inside mouth	☑ Tartar buildup	☑ Yellowing teeth	❑ Difficulty swallowing	
❑ Adequate OH time *NO*	❑ Anxiety/Pain	☑ Oral self-care diffuculty		
Oral Health Products: *No flossing, inconsistent brushing — can't find brush*				

FIGURE 20-9
Dental history portion of the prevention survey applied to column I of the oral risk assessment worksheet.

Fluoride History		
❑ Fluoridated water *NO*	❑ Away from home >4 days/week	❑ Oral rinse w/fluoride
❑ Water filter *NO*	❑ Bottled juice *NO*	Child:
❑ Bottled water *NO*	☑ Fluoridated dentifrice	❑ In daycare w/out fluoride ❑ Supplements

FIGURE 20-10
Fluoride history portion of the prevention survey applied to column I of the oral risk assessment worksheet.

Behaviors			
❑ Annual physical *NO*	❑ Balance work/relaxation	❑ Tobacco use	❑ Exercise *NO*
❑ Follows medical advice *some*	❑ Eating habits controlled	☑ Alcohol use	
❑ Follows dental advice *some*	❑ Increased stress	☑ Caffeine use *6-8 cups a day*	

FIGURE 20-11
Health behavior portion of the prevention survey applied to column I of the oral risk assessment worksheet.

- Feels stressed
- Does not use tobacco products
- Occasionally consumes alcohol
- Drinks six to eight caffeinated beverages a day
- Does not exercise

Diet Survey

Figure 20-12; see also Figure 20-3, *D*

- Consumes crackers between meals

Health Beliefs

Figure 20-13; see also Figure 20-3, *D*

- Believes she is more likely than others to have dental problems
- Believes prevention of oral problems is important
- Likes to get recommendations from dental professionals
- Believes she can tackle a new project or make a change at this time
- Somewhat believes she has control over her oral condition

Clinical and Radiographic Findings

Figure 20-14; see also Figures 20-4 through 20-7

- Extraoral and intraoral examination reveals several breaks in the integrity of the buccal mucosal at the line of occlusion (consistent with cheek biting).
- Root surface caries are noted in the mandibular premolar area.
- Numerous restorations indicate previous carious experience; restorative materials present include amalgam and composite.
- Periodontium exhibits recession, bacterial plaque biofilm, bleeding when probed, and loss of attached gingiva.

- Horizontal bone loss is noted.
- No pathologic processes are noted radiographically.

STEP 2: ASSESS AND ANALYZE ORAL RISK CONCERN

Based on the review of the patient findings recorded in column I of the oral risk assessment worksheet, some evidence-based assumptions of *potential* oral risk concerns can be made. The *first* analysis is for *potential risk concerns,* not actual or clinically evident risk concerns. This process is now applied to Ms. Wallace.

Potential Risk Concerns

The health history findings for Ms. Wallace indicate that she is taking a calcium channel blocker for cardiovascular disease. Based on pharmacologic studies, several oral sequelae to this drug include xerostomia, lichenoid reactions, altered taste, gland pain, and gingival hyperplasia.[9] These oral risk concerns would be indicated on the left side of column II of the worksheet (Figure 20-15).

Based on the patient's dental history, gingivitis may be expected (she does not use dental floss). She reports bleeding gingiva and calculus accumulation, both of which indicate an oral risk concern for gingivitis, increased plaque biofilm, and periodontal disease. As potential oral risk concerns, these findings would be noted on the left side of column II of the worksheet (see Figure 20-15).

Reading her self-reported fluoride history, dental caries would be checked as a *potential* oral finding because she does not have access to a public fluoridated water source, and she is unsure whether her toothpaste contains fluoride (when she brushes; see Figure 20-15).

Ms. Wallace's diet survey indicates a source of refined carbohydrates consumed between meals, which may potentially

Diet Survey	❑ Carbohydrate/Sucrose intake (excessive/moderate/minimal)

FIGURE 20-12
Diet survey portion of the prevention survey applied to column I of the oral risk assessment worksheet.

Beliefs		
❑ Understands oral status	☑ Values prevention	
☑ Wants product recommendations	❑ Open to change ☑ Feels in control of oral condition – *somewhat*	

FIGURE 20-13
Health beliefs portion of the prevention survey applied to column I of the oral risk assessment worksheet.

Clinical and Radiographic Findings			
Intraoral/Extraoral Examination	❑ Within normal limits	*Cheek biting* ☑ See chart	
Caries	❑ Coronal	❑ Interproximal	☑ Root surface
Restorations/Prosthetics			
Restorations	☑ Amalgam	☑ Composite	☑ Crowns/inlays/onlays ❑ Bridges
Dentures	❑ Complete	❑ Partial	
Periodontium			
☑ Recession	☑ Plaque ☑ Bleeding on probing	☑ Loss of attached gingiva	❑ Pockets <3mm
❑ Mucogingival defects	*Bone loss – horizontal*		
Occlusion/TMJ	❑ Traumatic occlusion	❑ Crepitus	
Bone Loss	❑ <25%	❑ 25-50%	❑ Horizontal ❑ Vertical

FIGURE 20-14
Clinical and radiographic findings portion of the prevention survey applied to column I of the oral risk assessment worksheet.

contribute to both coronal and root surface caries (see Figure 20-15).

Clinically Evident Concerns

Clinical and radiographic findings for this patient reveal the following:

- Loss of integrity of the oral mucosa (trauma)
- Root surface caries
- Gingivitis
- Periodontitis

The clinical findings are recorded on the right side of column II of the worksheet as *clinically evident* (Figure 20-16). Based on this review and assessment, a sense is developed of the types of therapeutic intervention strategies that need to be planned and of the self-care measures that should be recommended based on specific patient need.

Now that a summarized picture of this patient's therapeutic needs has been developed, the therapeutic intervention can be mapped through defining the goals of therapy.

STEP 3: PLAN THERAPEUTIC INTERVENTION

Strategies for therapeutic intervention follow the data review and assessment phase of oral risk assessment and begin by establishing goals of therapy (Box 20-4). Stated in other terms, the first portion of this phase sets expected *clinical* outcomes.

When a patient's oral conditions are within normal limits of health, goals for clinical therapy will include maintaining health and preventing disease. This goal will be achieved when no change in oral health status occurs within a stated evaluation period. Although this evaluation or reevaluation period should be established for every patient, it typically equates to a patient's next supportive care appointment at 3, 4, 6, or even 12 months. When active disease is present, goals become more complex and include broader categories such as identifying disease origin, eliminating the disease process, and establishing and maintaining health.

Corresponding goals to address patient self-care health behavior and beliefs also need to be established (phase two of Step 3) and are addressed in the Chapter 21.

ANALYZE
Oral Risk Concerns

At risk for		Clinically Evident
	Hard Tissues	
☐	Abrasion/Attrition/Erosion	☐
☒	Bone Loss	☐
☐	Bruxism/Occlusal Trauma	☐
☐	Calculus	☐
☒	Caries: coronal/interproximal	☐
☒	Caries: root surface	☐
☐	Chipped broken teeth	☐
☐	Extrinsic staining	☐
☐	Fluorosis	☐
☐	Intrinsic staining	☐
☐	Malaligned teeth	☐
☐	Mobile teeth	☐
☐	Sensitive teeth	☐
☐	Trauma	☐
☐	Other	☐
	Soft Tissues	
☐	Abscess: carious	☐
☐	Abscess: periodontal	☐
☐	Atrophic ulcer	☐
☐	Aphthous ulcer	☐
☐	Burning tongue/mouth	☐
☐	Candidiasis	☐
☐	Ecchymosis	☐
☐	Gingival recession	☐
☒	Gingival hyperplasia	☐
☒	Gingivitis	☐
☐	Herpetic lesions	☐
☒	Increased plaque	☐
☐	Leukoplakia	☐
☒	Lichen planus	☐
☐	Oral cancer	☐
☒	Periodontal disease	☐
☐	Petechiae	☐
☐	Salivation – increased	☐
☐	Salivation – decreased	☐
☐	Trauma	☐
☒	Xerostomia	☐
☒	Other *altered taste, gland pain*	☐
Consult		**Referral**
☐	Consultation with physician	☐
☐	Consultation with dental specialist	☐

FIGURE 20-15
Potential oral risk concerns recorded in column II of the oral risk assessment worksheet.

ANALYZE
Oral Risk Concerns

At risk for		Clinically Evident
	Hard Tissues	
☐	Abrasion/Attrition/Erosion	☐
☒	Bone Loss	☒
☐	Bruxism/Occlusal Trauma	☐
☐	Calculus	☐
☒	Caries: coronal/interproximal	☐
☒	Caries: root surface	☒
☐	Chipped broken teeth	☐
☐	Extrinsic staining	☐
☐	Fluorosis	☐
☐	Intrinsic staining	☐
☐	Malaligned teeth	☐
☐	Mobile teeth	☐
☐	Sensitive teeth	☐
☐	Trauma	☐
☐	Other	☐
	Soft Tissues	
☐	Abscess: carious	☐
☐	Abscess: periodontal	☐
☐	Atrophic ulcer	☐
☐	Aphthous ulcer	☐
☐	Burning tongue/mouth	☐
☐	Candidiasis	☐
☐	Ecchymosis	☐
☐	Gingival recession	☒
☒	Gingival hyperplasia	☐
☒	Gingivitis	☒
☐	Herpetic lesions	☐
☒	Increased plaque	☒
☐	Leukoplakia	☐
☒	Lichen planus	☐
☐	Oral cancer	☐
☒	Periodontal disease	☒
☐	Petechiae	☐
☐	Salivation – increased	☐
☐	Salivation – decreased	☐
☐	Trauma	☒
☒	Xerostomia	☐
☒	Other *altered taste, gland pain*	☐
Consult		**Referral**
☐	Consultation with physician	☐
☐	Consultation with dental specialist	☐

FIGURE 20-16
Completed oral risk concerns.

BOX 20-4

THERAPEUTIC INTERVENTION

- Identify patient needs.
- Establish goals.
- Plan executional tactics for the goals.
- Define treatment sequence.
- Reevaluate outcomes, and modify goals as necessary.

Measurable Goals

Every phase of treatment must be accompanied by a set of measurable clinical outcomes. Returning to the information in the case application (see Figures 20-15 and 20-16), the reader should refer to the second column of the oral risk assessment worksheet developed for Ms. Wallace. The following oral findings for which this patient is

> *Note*
>
> Every phase of treatment must be accompanied by a set of measurable clinical outcomes.

| Table 20-1 | Steps in Therapeutic Intervention Planning |

ORAL RISK CONCERN	CLINICAL GOAL	THERAPEUTIC INTERVENTION	EVALUATION MEASURE
Bone Loss (Clinical Finding)	• Arrest bone loss • Prevent future bone loss	• Periodontal therapy • Patient goals (see Chapter 21)	• No increase in attachment loss at supportive care intervals
Gingival Recession (Clinical Finding)	• Arrest gingival recession • Prevent future recession	• Patient goals (see Chapter 21) • Periodontal therapy	• No additional recession at supportive care intervals • No increase in current recession
Gingival Hyperplasia (Potential Finding)	• Prevent future gingival hyperplasia (because problem is potential, not diagnostic)	–	–
Gingivitis (Clinical Finding)	• Arrest gingival inflammation	• Periodontal debridement	• No bleeding on probing at reevaluation interval • Tissue color, contour, and consistency within normal limits
Increased Plaque Biofilm (Clinical Finding)	• Reduce plaque biofilm quantity to biologically acceptable level	• Patient goals (see Chapter 21)	• No bleeding on probing at reevaluation interval • Improved plaque biofilm index
Periodontal Disease (Clinical Finding)	• Arrest periodontal disease activity	• Periodontal therapy	• No bleeding on probing at reevaluation interval • No increased probing depths at reevaluation interval • No new evidence of radiographic bone loss at reevaluation interval
Coronal Caries (Potential Finding)	• Prevent future caries (because problem is potential, not diagnostic)	• Patient goals (see Chapter 21)	• No coronal caries at supportive care intervals
Root Caries (Clinical Finding)	• Arrest demineralization • Promote remineralization	• Plaque biofilm control • Diet survey and discussion • Fluoride application • Oral self-care evaluation	• No new dental caries at supportive care appointment • Arrested or reversed dental caries process
Trauma (Clinical Finding)	• Determine cause of trauma	• Patient goals (see Chapter 21)	• No evidence of trauma
Taste Alteration (Potential Finding)	• No treatment goal	• Patient goals (see Chapter 21)	• Patient interview
Xerostomia (Potential Finding)	• No treatment goal	• Patient goals (see Chapter 21)	• Patient interview
Gland Pain (Potential Finding)	• No treatment goal	• Patient goals (see Chapter 21)	• Patient interview

either *at risk* or for which she has *exhibited symptoms* should be noted: bone loss, coronal caries, root caries, gingival recession, gingival hyperplasia, gingivitis, increased bacterial plaque biofilm, periodontal disease, trauma, taste alteration, and gland pain. The clinical goal, therapeutic intervention, and evaluation goals for Ms. Wallace are charted in Table 20-1.

20-1 to 20-9

Case Summary

Designing therapeutic intervention is not an easy task, especially when therapy is based on individualized needs. By using an organized oral risk assessment system, this complex task becomes a series of manageable steps.

STEP 1: GATHER AND REVIEW ASSESSMENT DATA

In applying this step to the patient, the oral risk assessment worksheet has been completed for Ms. Wallace (Figure 20-17). Her health history, prevention survey, and clinical and radiographic findings were reviewed and then summarized in column I of the oral risk assessment worksheet (see Figure 20-17, *A*).

STEP 2: ASSESS AND ANALYZE ORAL RISK CONCERN

The data from column I (see Figure 20-17, *A*) was analyzed to make evidence-based assumptions about Ms. Wallace's *potential oral concerns* (*risk assessment,* which was placed in column II to the left of listing). Ms. Wallace's clinical and radiographic findings were reviewed to reveal her *current oral status,* which was also placed in column II to the right of the listing (see Figure 20-17, *B*).

STEP 3: PLAN THERAPEUTIC INTERVENTION

Based on the notations of oral risk, both potential and actual, the therapeutic intervention for the patient was planned (see Figure 20-17, *C,* and Table 20-1).

This step completes the portion of patient care planning that primarily involves the clinician. It is now time to explore how the patient is involved in the management and prevention of oral conditions and disease, an aspect that is critical to a successful outcome of therapy. To complete the oral risk assessment process, see Chapter 21 for Step 4 (recommend) and Step 5 (evaluate/reevaluate).

I

A — PREVENTION SURVEY

REVIEW				
Health History			**Medications & Dose**	**Duration**
☒ Cardiovascular (heart)			(prescription and OTC)	
☐ Central nervous system (nerves)			*Cardizem*	
☐ Endocrine (endocrine glands)				
☐ Gastrointestinal (stomach, intestines)				
☐ Genitourinary (sex organs, urinary tract)				
☐ Head, eyes, ears, nose, throat				
☐ Hematologic (blood)				
☐ Integumentary (skin)				
☐ Musculoskeletal (muscles, bones, joints)				
☐ Psychologic				
☐ Respiratory				
Vital Signs BP		*(RAS) 179/80*	Pulse *82 bpm (S+R)*	
Dental History				
☐ Sensitive teeth	☐ Sore jaw	☒ Toothache	☐ Sore gums	☐ Clenching
☒ Bleeding gums	☐ Difficulty chewing	☐ Filling fell out	☐ Dry mouth	☐ Grinding
☐ Bad breath	☐ Burning sensation		☐ Abscess	☐ Swollen face
☐ Swelling inside mouth	☒ Tartar buildup	☒ Yellowing teeth	☐ Difficulty swallowing	
☐ Adequate OH time *NO*	☐ Anxiety/Pain	☒ Oral self-care diffuculty		
Oral Health Products: *No flossing, inconsistent brushing — can't find brush*				
Fluoride History				
☐ Fluoridated water *NO*	☐ Away from home >4 days/week		☐ Oral rinse w/fluoride *NO*	
☐ Water filter *NO*	☐ Bottled juice *NO*	Child:		
☐ Bottled water	☒ Fluoridated dentifrice	☐ In daycare w/out fluoride		☐ Supplements
Behaviors				
☐ Annual physical *NO*	☐ Balance work/relaxation	☐ Tobacco use		☐ Exercise *NO*
☐ Follows medical advice *some*	☐ Eating habits controlled	☒ Alcohol use		
☐ Follows dental advice *some*	☐ Increased stress	☒ Caffeine use *6-8 cups a day*		
Diet Survey	☒ Carbohydrate/Sucrose intake (excessive/moderate/minimal)			
Beliefs				
☐ Understands oral status	☒ Values prevention			
☒ Wants product recommendations	☐ Open to change	☒ Feels in control of oral condition *somewhat*		
Clinical and Radiographic Findings				
Intraoral/Extraoral Examination	☐ Within normal limits		*Cheek biting*	☒ See chart
Caries	☐ Coronal	☐ Interproximal		☒ Root surface
Restorations/Prosthetics				
Restorations	☒ Amalgam	☒ Composite	☒ Crowns/inlays/onlays	☐ Bridges
Dentures	☐ Complete	☐ Partial		
Periodontium				
☒ Recession	☒ Plaque ☒ Bleeding on probing		☒ Loss of attached gingiva	☐ Pockets <3mm
☐ Mucogingival defects	*Bone loss – horizontal*			
Occlusion/TMJ	☐ Traumatic occlusion		☐ Crepitus	
Bone Loss	☐ <25%	☐ 25-50%	☒ Horizontal	☐ Vertical

II

B

At risk for	ANALYZE — Oral Risk Concerns	Clinically Evident
	Hard Tissues	
☐	Abrasion/Attrition/Erosion	☐
☒	Bone Loss	☒
☐	Bruxism/Occlusal Trauma	☐
☐	Calculus	☐
☒	Caries: coronal/interproximal	☐
☒	Caries: root surface	☒
☐	Chipped broken teeth	☐
☐	Extrinsic staining	☐
☐	Fluorosis	☐
☐	Intrinsic staining	☐
☐	Malaligned teeth	☐
☐	Mobile teeth	☐
☐	Sensitive teeth	☐
☐	Trauma	☐
☐	Other	☐
	Soft Tissues	
☐	Abscess: carious	☐
☐	Abscess: periodontal	☐
☐	Atrophic ulcer	☐
☐	Aphthous ulcer	☐
☐	Burning tongue/mouth	☐
☐	Candidiasis	☐
☐	Ecchymosis	☐
☐	Gingival recession	☒
☒	Gingival hyperplasia	☐
☒	Gingivitis	☒
☐	Herpetic lesions	☐
☒	Increased plaque	☒
☐	Leukoplakia	☐
☒	Lichen planus	☐
☐	Oral cancer	☐
☒	Periodontal disease	☒
☐	Petechiae	☐
☐	Salivation – increased	☐
☐	Salivation – decreased	☐
☐	Trauma	☒
☒	Xerostomia	☐
☒	Other *altered taste, gland pain*	☐
Consult		**Referral**
☐	Consultation with physician	☐
☐	Consultation with dental specialist	☐

FIGURE 20-17
The completed oral risk assessment worksheet showing column I **(A)** and column II **(B)**.

Continued

III

PLAN		
Clinical Goals	**Therapeutic Intervention**	**Patient Goals**
Bone Loss • Arrest bone loss. • Prevent future bone loss. Gingival Recession • Arrest gingival recession. • Prevent future recession. Gingival Hyperplasia • Prevention goal only. Gingivitis • Arrest gingival inflammation. Increased Plaque • Reduce plaque quantity to a biologically acceptable level. Periodontal Disease • Arrest periodontal disease activity.	• Periodontal therapy • Debridement	• Acknowledge the signs of gingival disease. • Understand the role of plaque in gingival disease. • Understand the role of the host response in gingival inflammation. • Understand/demonstrate patient role in treatment and prevention of gingival disease. • Purchase and use recommended products for the treatment and control of gingival disease. • Understand personal role in compliance. • Appreciate the benefits of supportive care appointments.
Coronal Caries • Prevention goal only. Root Caries • Arrest demineralization. • Promote remineralization. Trauma • Determine cause of trauma. Taste Alteration • No treatment goal. Xerostomia • No treatment goal. Gland Pain • No treatment goal.	• Plaque control • Diet survey and discussion • Fluoride application • Oral self-care evaluation	• Understand the role of plaque, diet, and saliva in the caries process. • Acknowledge the difference between coronal and root surface caries. • Understand/demonstrate patient role in treatment and prevention of dental caries. • Purchase and use recommended products for the prevention of dental caries. • Understand personal role in compliance.

FIGURE 20-17, cont'd
The completed oral risk assessment worksheet showing column III **(C)**.

References

1. Beck JD: Risk revisited, *Community Dent Oral Epidemiol* 26(4):220-225, 1998.
2. Beck JD: Issues in assessment of diagnostic tests and risks for periodontal disease, *Periodontol 2000* 7:100-108, 1995.
3. Beck JD: Methods of assessing risk or periodontitis and developing multifactorial models, *J Periodontol* 65:468-478, 1994.
4. Beck JD, Kahout F, Hunt RJ: Identification of high caries risk adults: attitudes, social factors and diseases, *Int Dent J* 38(4):231-238, 1988.
5. Disney JA et al: The University of North Carolina Caries Risk Assessment Study: further developments in caries risk prediction, *Community Dent Oral Epidemiol* 20:64-75, 1992.
6. Douglas CW: Risk assessment in dentistry, *J Dent Educ* 62(10):756-761, 1998.
7. Edelstein BL: Case planning and risk management according to caries risk assessment, *Dent Clin North Am* 39(4):721-758, 1995.
8. Frank MS: Embodying medical expertise in decision support systems for health care management: techniques and benefits, *Top Health Inf Manage* 19(2):44-54, 1998.
9. Gage TW, Pickett FA: *Mosby's dental drug reference*, ed 6, St Louis, (in press), Mosby.
10. Hildebrandt GH: Caries risk assessment and prevention for adults, *J Dent Educ* 59(10):972-980, 1993.
11. Karlsson D, Aspervall O, Forsum U: Concepts, contexts, and expert systems, *Stud Health Technol Inform* 68:713-715, 1999.
12. Kleinbaum D, Kupper L, Morgenstern H: *Epidemiologic research: principles and quantitative methods,* Belmont, Calif, 1982, Lifetime Learning Publications.
13. Mueller-Joseph L, Petersen M: *Dental hygiene process: diagnosis and care planning,* Albany, NY, 1995, Delmar.
14. Novak B: Intelligent systems in medical diagnosis, *Stud Health Technol Inform* 68:700-702, 1999.
15. Saunders RP: What is health promotion? *Health Educ* 19(5):14-18, 1998.
16. Slavkin HC: Placing health promotion into the context of our lives, *J Am Dent Assoc* 120(1):91-95, 1998.
17. Stamm JW et al: Risk assessment for oral diseases, *Adv Dent Res* 5:4-17, 1991.
18. Stoddard JW: Caries risk assessment used as a determinant for caries management and prediction, *J Dent Educ* 59(10):957-961, 1995.
19. US Department of Health and Human Services, National Institute of Dental and Craniofacial Research, National Institutes of Health: *Oral health in America: a report of the surgeon general,* US Department of Health and Human Services, Rockville, Md, 2000, US Government Printing Office.
20. Vick VC, Harfst SA: The Oral Risk Assessment and Early Intervention System: a clinician's tool for integrating the bio/psycho/social risk into oral disease interventions, *Compendium* 30(21 suppl):57-67, 2000.

Individualizing Preventive and Therapeutic Strategies

Sherry A. Harfst • Victoria C. Vick

INSIGHT

The ultimate success of any dental hygiene therapy is the restoration of oral health and prevention of future disease. Engaging the patient in developing his or her own prevention strategies is challenging but also arguably the most rewarding aspect of delivering oral care (and

an aspect of the profession that depends entirely on the philosophy of practice that includes the patient as a partner). This chapter details the final two steps of the oral risk assessment process, focusing on oral self-care recommendations.

✦ CASE STUDY 21-1   Individualizing Prevention Strategies

In Case Application 20-1.1, Assessing Health Beliefs and Practices, presented in Chapter 20, the following information from 54-year-old Robin Wallace's prevention survey was noted under the section titled Health Beliefs (see Figures 20-3, *D,* and 20-13). The patient's health beliefs were as follows:

- Feels she is more likely than others to have dental problems
- Believes prevention of oral problems is important
- Likes to get recommendations from dental professionals
- Feels she can tackle a new project or make a change at this time
- Somewhat believes she has control over her oral condition

Based on previous knowledge of patient and human behavior, will the outcome of prevention discussions with Ms. Wallace will be positive? What if Ms. Wallace did not believe prevention of oral problems was important? In this case should the hygienist address her needs differently? What if Ms. Wallace did not feel she could make any changes in personal habits at this time? Should the hygienist's course of action and/or patient goals change?

KEY TERMS

implementation	prevention strategy	therapeutic intervention

LEARNING OUTCOMES

After reading this chapter the student will be able to:

1. State rationale for the engagement of the patient as a partner in the oral care process.
2. Compare and contrast a therapeutic intervention and a prevention strategy.
3. Explain, by way of a patient example, four logical small steps in the process of recommending products and practices for oral self-care.
4. Differentiate between a goal and a strategy.
5. Cite several obstacles to seeking dental care.

6. Discuss components important to consider in planning oral care.
7. Defend the value of evaluation and reevaluation as a way of ensuring optimal oral health.
8. Map a patient's care plan in therapeutic intervention, prevention, and evaluation and reevaluation.
9. Apply Steps 4 and 5 of the oral risk assessment process to any patient.
10. Recognize the value of a systematized holistic approach to oral care.

This chapter is written in conjunction with Chapter 20, which the reader is advised to consult for prerequisite information.

Patient as a Clinical Partner

The more a patient is involved in his or her dental hygiene therapy, and ultimately oral self-care, the greater the chances are for successful outcomes. Involving patients in their care implies that intervention strategies are individualized. As stated previously, this is a complex but ultimately rewarding process that, to many clinicians, is the core of dental hygiene care. To design successful clinical therapy and to realize a short-term goal of a successful initial clinical outcome is satisfying. However, to witness the failure of therapy when the patient returns with the same (or perhaps worse) level of disease causes frustration for dental hygienists and, ultimately, can lead to career burnout. Although individualizing prevention strategies and involving patients in their oral self-care cannot ensure 100% success, these practices do go a long way toward promoting optimal oral health for each patient, adding to the personal satisfaction of the healthcare provider.

> *Note*
>
> The more a patient is involved in his or her dental hygiene therapy (and ultimately oral self-care), the greater the chances are for successful outcomes.

The determination of clinical treatment goals and corresponding **therapeutic intervention** is more or less empiric (i.e., based on supporting evidence), and it addresses oral conditions present at the time of therapy. The establishment of patient goals and course of action is based on dental science plus an understanding of each specific patient's needs, individual background, health beliefs, and health habits. It also addresses long-term patient intervention and prevention.

Step 4: Recommend

As Step 4 of the oral risk assessment system is explored, dental hygienists should realize the crucial need to treat each individual patient based on his or her unique needs and circumstances.

When broken into logical planning steps Step 4, *recommend*, does the following:

1. Reviews the oral risk concerns for the patient (column II of the oral risk assessment worksheet; see Figure 20-16)
2. Determines the specific patient goal in managing the prevention of the risk concerns and designs the **prevention strategy** necessary to reach the goal, based on specific patient needs
3. Recommends specific products and procedures to help each patient reach the stated goals and records the recommendations on the oral self-care recommendation form
4. Determines the measure of evaluation

ORAL RISK CONCERNS

By reviewing a patient's oral risk concerns, four main topic areas can be determined for which patient goals will be developed.

Periodontal Concerns

- Bone loss
- Gingivitis
- Increased plaque biofilm
- Periodontal disease
- Gingival recession

> *Note*
>
> Because patient goals and strategies for this oral risk concern are interrelated, presenting them as one category in planning prevention strategies is most efficient.

Dental Caries

- Coronal caries
- Root caries

Trauma or Medication-Induced Oral Risk Concerns

- Lichen planus
- Gingival hyperplasia
- Altered taste
- Gland pain
- Xerostomia

> *Note*
>
> Because patient medication-induced oral risk concerns are interrelated, presenting them as one category in planning prevention strategies is most efficient.

★ CASE APPLICATION 21-1.1

Examination of Oral Risk Concerns

Based on Ms. Wallace's history and clinical findings, her oral risk concerns are examined in Table 21-1.

PATIENT GOAL

Addressing each area of oral risk concern involves understanding not only the clinical aspects of the therapeutic intervention strategy but also the biological, psychologic, and sociologic components.

★ CASE APPLICATION 21-1.2

Review of the Prevention Survey

From Ms. Wallace's prevention survey, the hygienist can see that she lacks a basic understanding of the following primary topics:

- The role of plaque biofilm in both gingival and hard tissue disease
- Her role in the prevention process
- The benefits of regular dental care
- Knowledge of products and practices used to promote the prevention of oral disease
- Awareness of a cheek-biting habit
- Potential side effects of prescription medications

Table 21-1	Application of Step 4 to Robin Wallace*		
ORAL RISK CONCERN	**PATIENT GOAL**	**PREVENTION STRATEGY**	**EVALUATION**
Bone Loss Gingivitis Increased Plaque Biofilm Periodontal Disease Gingival Recession	• Acknowledge signs of gingival disease • Understand role of plaque biofilm in gingival disease • Understand role of host response in gingival inflammation • Understand and demonstrate patient role in treatment and prevention of gingival disease • Purchase and use recommended products for treatment and control of gingival disease • Understand personal role in compliance • Appreciate benefits of supportive therapy appointments	• Discussion and discovery (with patient) of intraoral conditions contributing to gingival disease • Discussion of host response and immune defenses • Discussion with patient of oral self-care strategies for treatment and prevention of gingival disease • Recommendation of products for oral self-care for prevention of gingival disease • Demonstration of oral self-care techniques for treatment and prevention of gingival disease • Discussion and plan of supportive therapy appointments	*At appropriate supportive care appointment, patient should do the following:* • Describe oral changes noticed in gingival inflammation, dental caries, and esthetics • Describe or demonstrate oral self-care regimen appropriate for disease prevention • Describe role plaque biofilm plays in process of oral disease • Arrive for appointment and schedule next one
Root Caries Coronal Caries	• Understand role of plaque biofilm, diet, and saliva in dental caries process • Acknowledge difference between coronal and root surface caries • Understand and demonstrate patient role in treatment and prevention of dental caries • Purchase and use recommended products for prevention of dental caries • Understand personal role in compliance • Appreciate benefits of supportive care appointments	• Discussion and discovery (with patient) of intraoral conditions that contribute to dental caries • Determination of habits that place patient at risk for dental caries • Discussion with patient of oral self-care strategies for treatment and prevention of dental caries • Recommendation of products for oral self-care for prevention of dental caries • Demonstration of oral self-care techniques for prevention of dental caries	*At appropriate supportive care appointment, patient should do the following:* • Describe or document changes in diet and oral self-care that have contributed to reduction or prevention in dental caries
Trauma	• Understand result of trauma-inducing oral habits	• Discussion and plan of supportive care appointments • Discussion and discovery (with patient) of intraoral conditions that contribute to breaks in oral mucosa	*At appropriate supportive care appointment, patient should do the following:* • Describe or demonstrate cessation of traumatic oral habit
Lichenoid Lesions	• Understand result of trauma-inducing oral habits	• Discussion of possible oral effects of current medication	*At appropriate supportive care appointment, patient should do the following:* • Evaluate occurrence or lack of occurrence of oral side effect
Taste Alteration	• Increase awareness of oral side effects of current medication (as explained by clinician)	• Discussion of possible oral effects of current medication	*At appropriate supportive care appointment, patient should do the following:* • Evaluate occurrence or lack of occurrence of oral side effect
Gingival Hyperplasia	• Increase awareness of oral side effects of current medication (as explained by clinician)	• Discussion of possible oral effects of current medication	*At appropriate supportive care appointment, patient should do the following:* • Evaluate occurrence of lack of occurrence of oral side effect
Xerostomia	• Increase awareness of oral side effects of current medication (as explained by clinician)	• Discussion of possible oral effects of current medication	*At appropriate supportive care appointment, patient should do the following:* • Evaluate occurrence or lack of occurrence of oral side effect
Gland Pain	• Increase awareness of oral side effects of current medication (as explained by clinician)	• Discussion of possible oral effects of current medication	*At appropriate supportive care appointment, patient should do the following:* • Evaluate occurrence or lack of occurrence of oral side effect

*Refer to Chapter 20, Case Studies 20-1 and 21-1, and the case applications for more information.

Periodontal Concerns

Patient goals that address these oral risk concerns in the periodontal concerns category would include the following:

- Acknowledge the signs of gingival disease
- Understand the role of plaque biofilm in gingival disease
- Understand the role of the host response in gingival inflammation
- Understand and demonstrate the patient role in the treatment and prevention of gingival disease
- Purchase and use recommended products for the treatment and control of gingival disease
- Understand the personal role in compliance
- Appreciate the benefits of supportive therapy appointments

Prevention Strategy for Periodontal Concerns

The prevention strategy statements outline how the patient goals can be reached for each of the concern areas. For example, the prevention strategy that would be used to reach the patient goals for the category of periodontal concerns would include the following:

- Discussion and discovery (with patient) of intraoral conditions contributing to gingival disease
- Discussion of host response and immune defenses

- Discussion with patient of oral self-care strategies for the treatment and prevention of gingival disease
- Recommendation of products for oral self-care for the prevention of gingival disease
- Demonstration of oral self-care techniques for the treatment and prevention of gingival disease
- Discussion and planning of supportive therapy appointments

★ CASE APPLICATION 21-1.3

Prevention Strategies

Review Table 21-1 to determine how such prevention strategies were applied to Ms. Wallace.

PRODUCT RECOMMENDATION

For a patient to fully comply with any given prevention strategy, he or she needs to know what tools (i.e., specific procedures and products) are recommended for use. Chapters 24, 25, 26, 27, and 30 outline personal self-care procedures and detailed product options. For Ms. Wallace, products and procedures are recommended in the following categories: toothbrush, interdental cleaning, dentifrice, oral rinse, and self-evaluation (Figure 21-1).

ORAL CARE RECOMMENDATIONS

Prevention Strategy	Toothbrush	Product
	❑ Mechanical	
• Discussion and discovery (with patient) of intraoral conditions	❑ Child ❑ Youth ❑ Compact ❑ Full	
	☑ Soft ❑ Extra Soft	
	☑ Powered	*Spinbrush*
	Brushing frequency *2X daily*	
• Discussion of host response and immune defenses	Brushing duration *2 minutes*	
	Interdental Cleaning Products	
	☑ Floss Type *waxed* Frequency *1X day*	*Oral B*
• Discussion with patient of oral self-care strategies	☑ Oral Irrigator *w/water* Frequency *1X day*	
	❑ Interdental Brush Frequency	
• Recommendation of products for oral self-care	❑ Other	
	Dentifrice	
• Demonstration of oral self-care techniques	❑ Fluoride ❑ Whitening	*Crest*
	❑ Sensitivity ☑ Multiple Benefit	*Multicare*
	❑ Tartar Control ❑ Gingival Benefit	*w/whitening*
• Discussion and planning of supportive care appointments	❑ Children's	
	Oral Rinse	
	❑ Fluoride	
• Discussion and discovery (with patient) of intraoral conditions	❑ Cosmetic	
	❑ Alcohol-free	
	❑ Tartar Control	
• Determination of habits that place her at risk for dental caries	❑ Chlorhexidine	
	❑ Essential Oil/Phenol Compound	
	Prosthodontic Care	
• Discussion with patient of oral self-care strategies	❑ Adhesive ❑ Denture Brush	
	❑ Denture Bath/Cleanser	
• Recommendation of products for oral self-care	**Self-Evaluation**	
	☑ Disclosing tablets or solutions	
	☑ Evaluate bleeding points	
• Demonstration of oral self-care techniques	**Other**	
• Discussion and planning of supportive care appointments		
• Discussion of possible oral effects of current medication		

FIGURE 21-1
Column V of an oral risk assessment worksheet: Evaluate.

Note

For a patient to fully comply with any given prevention strategy, he or she needs to know what tools (i.e., specific procedures and products) are recommended for use.

To complete the product recommendation process, the patient can be provided with personalized, written instructions, as shown in Figure 21-2.

The process for personalizing prevention strategies is the same for each area of oral risk concern identified, as presented in Table 21-1.

Prevention Strategy Implementation

To ensure the successful **implementation** of any prevention strategy, dental professionals must first apply a logical approach blended with an understanding of how adults learn. For example,

discussing all patient goals at the first appointment can be overwhelming to the patient. Just as dividing dental hygiene therapy between appointments is necessary, presenting patient goals in a series of small steps is also important. Depending on patient success in mastering a goal, more goals can be added at subsequent appointments. When a patient has difficulty mastering concepts of oral self-care, goals can be revised. Although frustrating and disappointing, clinicians must realize that not all patients will act on their recommendations. Constant evaluation and revision of goals is necessary to provide optimal oral health care.

At this point in the planning stage, several elements should be taken into

Note

To ensure the successful implementation of any prevention strategy, dental professionals must first apply a logical approach blended with an understanding of how adults learn.

Personalized Oral Care Recommendations

For _Robin Wallace_
Date _MM/DD/YY_

Services provided at today's visit:

☑ Oral hygiene instructions
☐ Prophylaxis (dental cleaning)
☐ Therapeutic debridement
☑ Fluoride treatment
☐ Sealant/Varnish
☐ Nutrition evaluation
☐ Other

Plaque was noted in the following areas

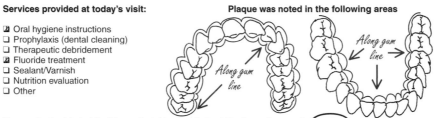

Along gum line / *Along gum line* / *Along gum line*

Your next scheduled visit with our dental hygienist should be in ___1___ months/(weeks)

Recommended oral care products

Toothbrush				Product
☐ Mechanical				
☐ Child	☐ Youth	☐ Compact	☐ Full	
☑ Soft	☐ Extra Soft			
☑ Powered				*Spinbrush*
Brushing frequency *2x day*				
Brushing duration *2 minutes*				

Interdental Cleaning Products			
☑ Floss Type *waxed* Frequency *1x day*			*Oral B*
☑ Oral Irrigator *w/water* Frequency *1x day*			
☐ Interdental Brush Frequency			
☐ Other Frequency			
☐ Other			

Dentifrice		
☐ Fluoride	☐ Whitening	
☐ Sensitivity	☑ Multiple benefit *w/whitening*	*Crest Multicare Whitening*
☐ Tartar control	☐ Gingival benefit	
☐ Children's		

Oral Rinse *none*	
☐ Fluoride	
☐ Cosmetic	
☐ Alcohol-free	
☐ Tartar Control	
☐ Chlorhexidine	
☐ Essential Oil/Phenol Compound	

Prosthodontic Care *none*		
☐ Adhesive	☐ Denture Brush	
☐ Denture Bath/Cleanser		

Self-Evaluation	
☑ Disclosing tablets or solutions	*Use 1X a week*
☑ Evaluate bleeding points	*Check floss daily*
Other	

FIGURE 21-2
Oral care recommendations for 54-year-old Robin Wallace, whose case is presented in Case Studies 20-1 and 21-1.

consideration that can significantly affect successful appointment planning: appointment flow, appointment times, and engagement of the patient in his or her oral care.

TREATMENT SEQUENCING

Determining appropriate clinical treatment planning involves the following:

- Identifying all necessary therapeutic interventions (see Chapter 20) and required armamentarium
- Understanding obstacles to care
- Planning appropriate appointment sequencing
- Gaining patient feedback in the reassessment process
- Reevaluating and retreating as appropriate

Identifying Armamentaria

Although this is not a crucial planning step, being certain that all necessary armamentaria are available for use is important. For example, being aware that only four air-polishing units are available for use among 16 clinicians can help prevent a potential problem in patient completion. If the patient appointment calls for special supplies, such as a sealant kit or a specific type of fluoride, then it may be necessary to check supplies well in advance of the patient's arrival.

Understanding Obstacles to Care

Appointment planning is influenced by many variables—some patient driven, some clinician determined. Patients may face several obstacles to obtaining the health care they need, for valid reasons (Box 21-1). Being sensitive to these issues can help the clinician establish successful appointment habits. Understanding the adult as a learner is also important (Box 21-2). Adults learn differently from children and prefer practical and problem-centered learning that does not put them at risk of exposing an inadequate skill (e.g., demonstrating flossing to a room of other adults). By keeping just a few adult learning principles in mind, the adult learning curve can be greatly enhanced.

Planning Appropriate Appointment Sequencing

Once appointment times have been established and possible obstacles have been examined and overcome, the dental hygienist must plan care for each patient visit. This process, once again, involves weighing variables to provide the necessary data on which to plan appropriate treatment sequencing.

Gauging patient comfort or pain

If a patient experiences oral pain and a diagnosis has been established in which dental hygiene therapy will help alleviate the discomfort, that section or area of the oral cavity might be treated first.

If, however, a patient is not experiencing oral discomfort, the therapy might be initiated in a specific, standardized sequence of either sextants (i.e., six oral divisions), quadrants (i.e., four oral divisions), or half-mouth (i.e., maxillary and mandibular quadrants on one side). The selection of the sequencing depends on the disease classification, intraoral access, clinician proficiency, and patient factors (Figures 21-3 to 21-5) and clinic policy (if any).

Using a consistent starting point

By initiating consistent and specific predetermined dental hygiene therapy, record keeping and subsequent appointments can be more efficient. For example, the right-handed clinician can begin treatment in the upper right quadrant or sextant, at the posterior surface of the most posterior tooth (e.g., distobuccal of tooth #1), or the clinician can begin on the lower right, at the posterior surface of the most posterior tooth (e.g., distobuccal of tooth #32). (Left-handed hygienists would begin on the opposite side.) Clinical faculty may have additional suggestions and recommendations on this topic.

BOX 21-1

OBSTACLES TO OBTAINING HEALTH CARE

Ethnic and cultural beliefs
Differences in terms used by professionals and nonprofessionals
Negative views of the medical setting
Personal and group values
Group memberships and attitudes
Ineffective form and content of message delivery
Illiteracy
Poverty
Lack of technical sophistication
Habit
Availability of services
Confidence in treatment outcomes

Denial of illness
Belief in personal invulnerability
Differing opinions
Risk of suggested procedure
Transportation difficulties
Convenience
Attitudes toward the body
Fear and anxiety level
Education level
Confusion regarding treatment options
Insincerity of educator or patient

From Debiase CB: *Dental health education: theory and practice*, Philadelphia, 1991, Lea & Febiger.

BOX 21-2

ADULTS IN THE LEARNING PROCESS

Adults prefer practical and problem-centered learning.

DO

- Give information specific to their oral condition.
- Clearly state the goals (expected outcomes).
- Direct conversation to solution-centered responses.
- Offer suggestions as to how they might integrate new information into what they already know.

DO NOT

- Let the discussion become too theoretical.
- State too many goals or give too many directions at one appointment.

Adults appreciate a boost to positive self-esteem.

DO

- Give praise for new tasks learned.
- Give anticipated results in concrete language (e.g., look better, feel better, smell better).
- Begin with easy changes and move to the more difficult ones.
- Respect the learner with eye-to-eye contact, organization, and engaging the learner in feedback.
- Avoid technical jargon (unless you thoroughly explain it and the use of jargon is somehow necessary to success).

- Validate and confirm their knowledge.
- Confront old beliefs gently: "we used to think . . ." "then we learned . . ." "and now we know . . ."

DO NOT

- Ignore the fact that the adult already knows some of what you are about to tell them.
- Overdirect or oversimplify instructions.
- Challenge their skills in a group setting.
- Expect total agreement or complete change just because you have given instructions.
- Mistake your enthusiasm for their motivation.

Four Critical Elements of Learning

1. Motivation (Knowing the *why* can be a powerful motivator.)
2. Reinforcement (Telling positive and negative aspects of changed behavior is helpful.)
3. Retention (Building knowledge session to session encourages retention.)
4. Transference (The taught behavior becomes internalized and is now a habit.)

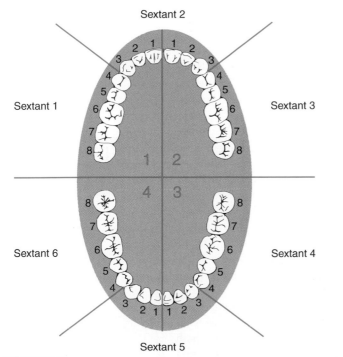

FIGURE 21-3
Sextant divisions of the dentition. (Modified from Liebgott B: *The anatomical basis of dentistry,* ed 2, St Louis, 2001, Mosby.)

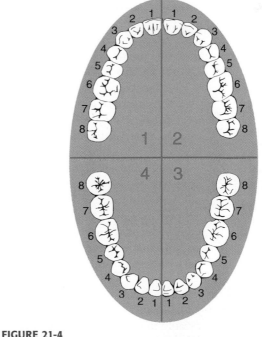

FIGURE 21-4
Quadrant divisions of the dentition. (From Liebgott B: *The anatomical basis of dentistry,* ed 2, St Louis, 2001, Mosby.)

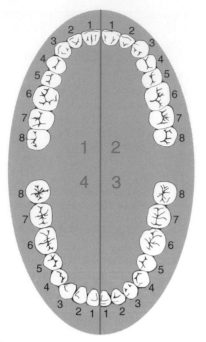

FIGURE 21-5
Half-mouth division. (Modified from Liebgott B: *The anatomical basis of dentistry,* ed 2, St Louis, 2001, Mosby.)

Determining the degree of difficulty

Occasionally it can be determined from radiographic interpretation and clinical charting that the disease status in a specific area of the mouth is more advanced. Initiating dental hygiene therapy in the more advanced disease sites gives the clinician more chances to reevaluate the success of therapy at sequential appointments.

Accommodating patient perceptions

A patient may direct where he or she wants the dental hygiene therapy started. Reasons a patient may provide these instructions could be esthetic (e.g., unsightly stains or calculus on the anterior facials) or driven by discomfort. Although total patient-directed care is not encouraged, accommodating such requests may provide an opportunity for fuller patient acceptance and participation in oral self-care.

Tips for Successful Treatment Sequencing
- Identify armamentaria
- Understand obstacles to care
- Plan appropriate appointment sequencing
- Gauge patient comfort or pain
- Use a consistent starting point
- Determine the degree of difficulty
- Accommodate patient perceptions

Realizing the Goal of Therapy

Whatever appointment sequencing is established and followed, the dental hygienist must realize the goal of any dental hygiene therapy—to complete whatever therapy is initiated.

The goal of any dental hygiene appointment is to complete any areas initiated for two reasons:

1. Wound healing is improved. Once an area is biologically stressed from a bioburden and inflammatory standpoint, all toxin and underlying gingival irritants must be removed so that the tissue can respond quickly and efficiently.
2. Assessing outcomes of dental hygiene therapy is accomplished only when the therapy is complete. In that way, any area requiring retreatment is easily identified. Patient self-care can likewise be addressed, and goals can be changed as appropriate.

Planning the Time Allotment

Appointment times have been carefully established by most dental hygiene programs and will be modified as clinical competence is gained. Typically, longer appointment schedules are established at the beginning of the student experience. As clinical competence is gained, each successive clinic session will provide more challenges in that appointment times will be shorter, allowing more patients to be seen in a single clinic session. The recommendations made in this chapter focus on *planning the allotted time*—not in suggesting the length of time a specific procedure should take.

Listening to Patient Feedback

As the name implies, patient-centered dental hygiene therapy *centers on the patient*. Although patients do not *direct* the therapy, they clearly need to be active participants.

Setting expectations of treatment involves clinical judgment and establishment of the patient as a fully active participant in his or her oral self-care. Although a complex process, establishing and evaluating patient goals is not only rewarding and satisfying but also essential to provide and promote optimal oral health.

Note
Although patients do not *direct* patient-centered therapy, they must be active participants in it.

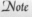

Step 5: Reevaluation

Evaluation and reevaluation of clinical outcomes (therapeutic intervention) and patient goals (prevention strategies) is the final step in dental hygiene care. Evaluation of the outcome is just as important as the first step and determines the type of supportive care each patent requires.

Each of the examples in the following case application requires a different form of supportive care. Taking the necessary time to evaluate outcomes is crucial to successful dental hygiene therapy, both in therapeutic intervention and in prevention strategies.

Note
Evaluation of the outcome is just as important as the first step and determines the type of supportive care each patent requires.

CASE APPLICATION 21-1.4

Supportive Care Recommendations

Ms. Wallace's sextant #1 was debrided (see Figure 20-6). At the end of 3 weeks, sextant #1 was evaluated for bleeding on probing and plaque biofilm accumulation. The recommendations for supportive care were different, based on the various outcomes (Figure 21-6). For each of the following clinical outcomes, what supportive care recommendations should the hygienist have made?

- Three sites that were initially charted as bleeding on probing were unchanged.
- Although no bleeding on probing was noted, a high plaque biofilm index was calculated, and the patient was unable to recall any signs of gingival inflammation.
- No bleeding on probing or discernible plaque biofilm was noted.
- The patient was unable to demonstrate interdental cleaning, and three sites exhibit bleeding on probing.

EVALUATE

Clinical Goals

- Attachment loss does not increase as measured at supportive care intervals
- No additional recession at supportive care intervals
- Current recession does not increase
- No bleeding on probing at reevaluation interval
- Tissue color, contour, consistency within normal limits
- Improved plaque index
- No bleeding on probing at reevaluation interval
- No increased probing depths at reevaluation interval
- No new evidence of radiographic bone loss at reevaluation interval
- No coronal caries evident at supportive care intervals
- No new dental caries at supportive care appointment
- Arrested/reversed dental caries process
- No evidence of trauma
- Patient interview

Patient Goals

At the appropriate supportive care appointment, the patient will:

- Describe the oral changes the patient has noticed in the area of gingival inflammation, dental caries, and esthetics
- Describe/demonstrate an oral self-care regimen appropriate for disease prevention
- Describe the role plaque plays in the process of oral disease
- Have been present for the appointment and scheduled the next one
- Describe/document changes in diet and oral self-care that have contributed to a reduction/prevention of dental caries
- Describe/demonstrate a cessation of the traumatic oral habit
- Evaluate the occurrence/lack of occurrence of the oral side effect

FIGURE 21-6
Personalized instructions for 54-year-old Robin Wallace (whose case is presented in Case Studies 20-1 and 21-1) to take home.

CASE APPLICATION 21-1.5

Treatment Sequencing

Initial treatment sequencing for Ms. Wallace now can be mapped. This appointment mapping uses a prevention survey, clinical and radiographic findings, and a specially designed worksheet.

For this case, care has been divided into sextants, requiring seven total appointments: six for therapeutic intervention and prevention strategy implementation and a final one for reevaluation (Tables 21-2 to 21-8).

Designing successful clinical therapy and appropriate personalized patient care requires the following careful steps:

- Gather and review all patient records.
- Assess and analyze oral risk concerns.
- Plan therapeutic intervention and prevention strategies.
- Recommend personalized oral self-care products and practices.
- Reevaluate all outcomes

The use of a system-based organization tool can help dental students and clinicians reach a holistic, patient-centered approach to oral care, providing optimal oral health and clinician satisfaction.

Table 21-2	Appointment One		
DENTAL HYGIENE THERAPY AND THERAPEUTIC INTERVENTION	**PATIENT DISCUSSION AND PREVENTION STRATEGY**	**EVALUATION**
• Review intraoral examination • Disclose patient • Engage patient in oral evaluation • Chart plaque biofilm index • Discuss patient education • Debride sextant #1 (assuming no variables need consideration in order of treatment of oral cavity) • Give postdebridement instructions	• Asking and answering of any new questions as needed • Discussion and discovery (with patient) of intraoral conditions contributing to gingival disease • Discussion of host response and immune defenses • Discussion with patient of oral self-care strategies for treatment and prevention of gingival disease • Recommendation of products for oral self-care for prevention of gingival disease • Demonstration of oral self-care techniques for treatment and prevention of gingival disease	• Verbal feedback to gain additional goals, ensuring that communication is clear

Table 21-3	Appointment Two		
DENTAL HYGIENE THERAPY AND THERAPEUTIC INTERVENTION	**PATIENT DISCUSSION AND PREVENTION STRATEGY**	**EVALUATION**
• Review intraoral examination • Disclose patient • Engage patient in oral evaluation • Chart plaque biofilm index • Debride sextant #2 • Give postdebridement instructions	• Discussion and discovery (with patient) of intraoral conditions contributing to dental caries • Determination of habits that place patient at risk for dental caries • Determination of why patient feels more likely than others to have dental problems • Discussion with patient of oral self-care strategies for treatment and prevention of dental caries • Asking and answering of any new questions as needed	• Plaque biofilm index should be lower • Patient should be able to articulate role of plaque biofilm in gingival disease • Patient should be able to demonstrate compliance with recommendations

Table 21-4	Appointment Three		
DENTAL HYGIENE THERAPY AND THERAPEUTIC INTERVENTION	**PATIENT DISCUSSION AND PREVENTION STRATEGY**	**EVALUATION**
• Review intraoral examination • Check BOP index on sextant #1 • Disclose patient • Engage patient in oral evaluation • Chart plaque biofilm index • Debride sextant #3 • Debride again any areas of BOP on sextant #1 • Give postdebridement instructions	• Determination of which oral changes patient may have noticed, such as improved gingival color and tone, no bleeding on brushing, no breath odor, and teeth "feeling" better • Discussion of importance in following healthcare provider recommendations • Raising of patient awareness to side effects of current medication • Asking and answering of any new questions as needed	• Plaque biofilm index should be lower • Patient should be able to articulate role of plaque biofilm in dental caries • Patient should be able to discuss changes made to diet to reduce acid challenge to hard tooth structures • Patient should be able to discuss why (in the past) oral disease has occurred and how (in the future) oral health can be controlled • Patient should be able to demonstrate compliance with recommendations

BOP, Bleeding on probing.

Table 21-5	Appointment Four	
DENTAL HYGIENE THERAPY AND THERAPEUTIC INTERVENTION	**PATIENT DISCUSSION AND PREVENTION STRATEGY**	**EVALUATION**
• Review intraoral examination • Check BOP index on sextant #2 • Disclose patient • Engage patient in oral evaluation • Chart plaque biofilm index • Debride sextant #4 • Debride again any areas of BOP on sextant #2 • Give postdebridement instructions	• Progress of therapy • Compliance with recommendations • Asking and answering of any new questions as needed	• Patient should be able to self-evaluate for oral change and comply with recommendations • Any BOP in sextant #2 needs careful notation and retreatment

BOP, Bleeding on probing.

Table 21-6	Appointment Five	
DENTAL HYGIENE THERAPY AND THERAPEUTIC INTERVENTION	**PATIENT DISCUSSION AND PREVENTION STRATEGY**	**EVALUATION**
• Review intraoral examination • Check BOP index on sextant #3 • Disclose patient • Engage patient in oral evaluation • Chart plaque biofilm index • Debride sextant #5 • Debride again any areas of BOP on sextant #3 • Give postdebridement instructions	• Progress of therapy • Compliance with recommendations • Asking and answering of any new questions as needed	• Patient should be able to self-evaluate for oral change and comply with recommendations • Any BOP in sextant #3 needs careful notation and re-treatment

BOP, Bleeding on probing.

Table 21-7	Appointment Six	
DENTAL HYGIENE THERAPY AND THERAPEUTIC INTERVENTION	**PATIENT DISCUSSION AND PREVENTION STRATEGY**	**EVALUATION**
• Review intraoral examination • Check BOP index on sextant #4 • Disclose patient • Engage patient in oral evaluation • Chart plaque biofilm index • Debride sextant #6 • Debride again any areas of BOP on sextant #4 • Give postdebridement instructions	• Progress of therapy • Compliance with recommendations • Asking and answering of any new questions as needed	• Patient should be able to self-evaluate for oral change and comply with recommendations • Any BOP in sextant #4 needs careful notation and re-treatment

BOP, Bleeding on probing.

Table 21-8	Appointment Seven (21 Days after Therapy)	
DENTAL HYGIENE THERAPY AND THERAPEUTIC INTERVENTION	**PATIENT DISCUSSION AND PREVENTION STRATEGY**	**EVALUATION**
• Review intraoral examination • Check BOP index on all sextants • Disclose patient • Engage patient in oral evaluation • Chart plaque biofilm index • Debride any areas of BOP • Polish as appropriate • Apply topical fluoride • Establish supportive care interval	• Summary of all previous discussions, time for questions, and clarification of responses • Summary of dental hygiene therapy outcomes, with notation of progress on charts such as plaque biofilm index • Reinforcement of progress • Suggestions for improvement, where appropriate • Establishment of interval of supportive care	• Any BOP in any sextant needs careful notation and retreatment • Changes in color, contour, or consistency in gingiva should be noted • Patient should be able to articulate own role in oral self-care for the prevention of gingivitis and dental caries • Patient should be able to discuss signs and symptoms of oral disease • Patient should be able to discuss recommended oral self-care regimens and products, specific to individual need • Patient should acknowledge appropriate supportive care interval

BOP, Bleeding on probing.

Posttreatment Assessment and Supportive Care

Jill Rethman

INSIGHT

The dental hygienist will treat a variety of patients who have periodontal conditions and other chronic oral ailments. Tailoring treatment to the specific needs of the patient is the first step toward improving and maintaining health. **Periodontal maintenance** (PM) and supportive care appointments designed with the patient's needs in mind are an essential part of dental hygiene practice.

CASE STUDY 22-1 Evaluating Periodontal Outcomes

Mrs. Lucy Lightfoot, age 62, who is one quarter Native American, completed active periodontal treatment 9 months ago. Mrs. Lightfoot is taking tolazamide (Tolinase) for non–insulin-dependent diabetes mellitus (NIDDM), as well as a diuretic and a calcium channel blocker to control her blood pressure. She is experiencing some osteoarthritis, for which she takes over-the-counter (OTC) naproxen as needed. Mrs. Lightfoot alternates her professional oral care every 3 months between the periodontal and the general dental office. This is her third 3-month supportive care visit but the first time the hygienist has seen her. She has been faithful in keeping her 3-month PM appointments but appears to be indifferent to the procedures performed during the appointment. (PM involves procedures performed at selected intervals to assist the periodontal patient in maintaining oral health. It was formerly referred to as **supportive periodontal therapy** (SPT), *preventive maintenance, or recall maintenance.*) During the periodontal assessment, the hygienist notices that the bleeding index has gradually increased; it now is 25%, and the hygienist thinks Mrs. Lightfoot's plaque biofilm control could be improved. Her recession has not increased, but she has five deeper probe measurements, 5 mm in two marginal and three interproximal sites.

As the hygienist prepares to ask the receptionist to make Mrs. Lightfoot's next appointment with the periodontist, Mrs. Lightfoot informs the hygienist that she will be traveling at that time and cannot keep the appointment.

KEY TERMS

adherence	full-mouth disinfection	supportive care	therapeutic alliance
compliance	interval	supportive periodontal care	transtheoretical model
concordance	periodontal maintenance	supportive periodontal therapy	

LEARNING OUTCOMES

After reading this chapter the student will be able to:
1. Identify patients whose oral health risks and problems require close intervals for supportive care or continuation of care for other oral problems.
2. Recognize symptoms or conditions that indicate referral or co-management with the periodontist and discuss them with the patient.
3. Plan a supportive care program based on the patient's disease control skills and the risk of disease recurrence.
4. Identify successful or reasonable outcomes, which may vary from patient to patient.
5. Document everything.
6. Evaluate current literature on the topic of supportive care intervals.

Implicit in the title of this chapter is the concept that patients with a persistent problem or chronic disease should receive professional care at regular intervals. An **interval** is the length of time between appointments. Reevaluation of a patient's periodontal status by the oral healthcare provider at regular intervals is an evidence-based practice. Dental research has shown that the combination of daily personal plaque biofilm control efforts and frequent professional care produces the most stable periodontal health.[10] Individuals who receive regular, professional periodontal **supportive care** have less gingivitis, loss of attachment, and tooth loss compared with individuals who do not receive periodic **supportive periodontal care** (SPC). The shortened intervals of care and specific periodontal procedures are based on patients who have demonstrated a risk of periodontitis.[2] Case Study 22-1 highlights the fact that even though Mrs. Lightfoot has been faithful in keeping her 3-month PM appointments, the amount of inflammation has increased (indicated by increased bleeding on probing).

✨ CASE APPLICATION 22-1.1

Appointment Intervals

One question the clinician should ask is whether 3-month PM appointments are frequent enough for Mrs. Lightfoot.

The most familiar example of regular professional supervision to control and mitigate a chronic disease in dentistry is the common 3-month appointment intervals of individuals who have had nonsurgical or surgical periodontal therapy. Supportive care focuses on individuals prone to periodontal diseases and is also important for patients with a high dental caries rate or other less common problems that require closer professional supervision.

The terminology for regular, periodic supervision of individuals with periodontitis has gone through several transitions. For procedures done after completion of active therapy, the terms *maintenance, therapy, care, recare, recall,* and *treatment* are all found in the literature. In 1989 the World Workshop in Periodontics adopted the name *Supportive Periodontal Therapy (SPT)* and defined it as the periodic care intervals for periodontal patients.[33] In January 2000 the Board of Trustees of the American Academy of Periodontology approved the name *Periodontal Maintenance (PM)* to replace SPT.[4]

In Europe the term *SPC* refers to three levels of care: (1) preventive, (2) posttreatment, and (3) palliative.[28] The three levels of assessment for periodontal patients are (1) the patient (or systemic level), (2) the tooth, and (3) the site at risk. In this chapter, *PM* refers to the SPC for an individual at risk for various periodontal problems. This could include as few as one site in an individual. In addition, supportive care for other chronic oral problems that benefit from regular professional intervention is discussed.

Risk Assessment

An individual who has had an infection or disease usually is considered at risk for recurrence unless the initial infection was one that could have resulted in immunity. When immunity is conferred, the disease is not chronic; the patient is then considered *protected* from future disease. However, the most common oral infections (e.g., periodontal diseases, dental caries, herpetic outbreaks, and certain oral mucosal lesions) are chronic conditions. Therefore a person who has lost clinical attachment, has had carious lesions in the past year, or has had a herpetic lesion ("cold sore") is at greater risk for future disease than a person who has never had an attachment loss, dental caries, or a herpetic lesion.

Four important factors can help identify patients at risk for a periodontal disease[42]:

1. Tobacco use
2. Age
3. Attachment loss
4. Abnormal tooth mobility

> *Patient Educational Opportunity*
>
> The clinician should explain to the patient that periodontitis is not cured; instead regular professional care is required to treat and manage it.

TOBACCO USE

The oral effects of tobacco use vary. Localized tissue changes are obvious when tobacco is held in direct contact with mucosal and gingival tissues. Smoking is a well-documented risk for periodontal problems.[25,46] The consequences of smoking include changes in the gingival crevicular fluid and oral microbiology and adverse effects on blood vessels, connective tissue, and the immune response.[8]

In the periodontium, tobacco smoking increases the prevalence and severity of periodontal diseases.[6] Studies in which plaque biofilm accumulation was adjusted for or kept to a minimum have shown that smoking groups had more sites with deeper probing depths and greater attachment loss.[11,29] From contemporary studies, a general pattern seems to be that smokers have greater attachment and bone loss, increased numbers of deep probing depths, and calculus formation.[11] Variable levels of plaque biofilm and inflammation seem to be present, although the signs of clinical inflammation are generally reduced.[18]

Although smoking appears to be one of the most significant risk factors for the development of periodontitis, smoking cessation is beneficial to periodontal health. Studies have shown that the periodontal status of former smokers is intermediate between the status of those who never smoked and those who are smoking currently.[13] In fact, research has shown that current smokers are about four times more likely than people who have never smoked to have an advanced periodontal disease. However,

> *Patient Educational Opportunity*
>
> The clinician should explain to the patient that once he or she stops smoking tobacco, periodontal health can be maintained just as well as if he or she had never smoked.

11 years after quitting, former smokers' likelihood of having a periodontal disease was not significantly different from those who had never smoked.[46] Based on current evidence, oral health professionals should incorporate tobacco cessation counseling for patients who smoke into their armamentarium (see Chapter 29).

AGE

Older adults (older than age 70) may require more intensive PM.[47] A decline in general health, increasing cognitive and physical impairments, and an increase in the number of medications taken may impair an older adult's ability for oral self-care.

Similarly, periodontitis diagnosed at an early age necessitates acute treatment and ongoing evaluations. An individual diagnosed with a periodontal condition at an early age may be prone to such conditions throughout his or her lifetime. In addition, periodontal diseases diagnosed at an early age are usually more aggressive and cause rampant destruction in a short period of time.[1]

ATTACHMENT LOSS

Patients at risk for a periodontal disease are those who have lost 2 mm or more of periodontal attachment. Although no test or index has been accepted as predictive of attachment loss, the correlation has been shown. Increasingly severe attachment loss has been associated with an increased risk for tooth loss[19] (see Chapter 16 for calculation of attachment loss).

ABNORMAL TOOTH MOBILITY

Physiologic mobility of 1 mm or less is normal. Teeth affected by a periodontal disease, however, are significantly more mobile. If the mobility is due to occlusal trauma, then it may or may not be pathologic (resulting in disease.) In other words, a tooth with an excessive occlusal load may adapt to that load by becoming mobile, but that mobility may stabilize. If the mobility becomes progressive over a period of time (days or weeks), then it could be considered pathologic. Therefore to adequately assess pathologic tooth mobility, two or more separate evaluations should be conducted.[36] Pathologically mobile teeth place stress on a weakened periodontium and may be treated with corrective restorative procedures, orthodontics, periodontal procedures, or a combination of these techniques.

OTHER FACTORS

Patients who cannot perform oral self-care or who have systemic medical conditions that influence oral health are at greater risk for recurrence of disease.

ADDITIONAL RISK ASSESSMENT TOOLS

Recently, a computer-based risk assessment tool was developed for periodontitis. The Oral Health Information Suite (PreViser Corporation, Mount Vernon, Wash.) analyzes clinical data collected during a periodontal examination and determines an individual's risk for developing a periodontal disease. Figure 22-1 is a sample from the PreViser software. The tool was designed to

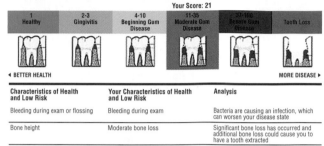

FIGURE 22-1
Sample from the PreViser Periodontal Risk and Disease Analysis. (Courtesy PreViser Corporation, Mount Vernon, Wash.)

overcome variations in risk assessment because of subjective analyses by clinicians. Clinical opinions are highly variable between practitioners and could result in the misapplication of treatment for some patients.[37] Computer analysis of the data eliminates subjective interpretation. Furthermore, use of the computerized risk assessment tool over time may result in more uniform and accurate periodontal clinical decision making.[35] In addition, reduction in the need for complex therapy and in healthcare costs could result.[34]

> ### Prevention
> When using new or technologically advanced techniques, explain to the patient that advances in dentistry and periodontics are ongoing and help improve diagnosis and treatment.

Rationale for Supportive Care

Periodic monitoring of a periodontal patient with a chronic condition is important for the following reasons:

- To help the patient achieve a stable dental condition and sometimes even attain a higher level of health
- To extend periods of disease remission

- To lessen the extent and severity of acute, episodic outbreaks (For patients susceptible to chronic infections, personal efforts at disease control alone are difficult and often inadequate for achieving continued remission.)

The goals of PM are to eliminate, prevent, or reduce these negative outcomes. The need for continuing professional care and monitoring to identify signs of the progression or recurrence of disease is part of the supportive care cycle (Figure 22-2).

Supportive care is recommended to periodontal patients for the following reasons:

- The outcome of periodontal therapy needs to be monitored at frequent intervals, because the patient has demonstrated a risk for periodontal breakdown.
- Tooth loss in some patients has been shown to be inversely proportional to the frequency of PM.[51]
- Surgery may not be possible for patients with general health problems (e.g., poorly controlled diabetes mellitus or immunosuppression) or for adult patients in active orthodontics because of the instability of the periodontal fibers.
- Teeth with a poor surgical prognosis may be improved by PM.
- Some patients may not be able to achieve sufficient plaque biofilm control unless they receive more frequent SPC. Data suggest that most patients with a history of periodontitis should receive PM at least four times per year.[21]
- A patient may simply refuse surgical correction or augmentation but may agree to SPC. Such situations require that the clinician explain the possible results of not obtaining needed surgical care, along with the patient signing an informed refusal form.
- Periodontal infections may significantly affect systemic health and may serve as risk indicators for certain systemic diseases or conditions.[4]

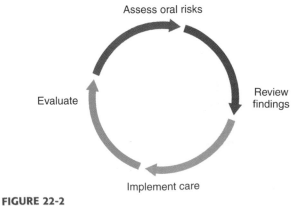

FIGURE 22-2
Cyclical nature of supportive care.

- PM should provide the following:[50]
  - Plaque biofilm control assistance and stability of the healthy periodontium
  - Protection from adverse effects on the periodontium related to systemic conditions
  - Lessening of suspected deleterious effects of periodontopathogenic microbes systemically, with particular attention to the possible relationships between periodontal diseases and stroke, heart attack, low–birth-weight infants, and diabetes mellitus.

✦ CASE APPLICATION 22-1.2

Periodontal Maintenance
Case Study 22-1 demonstrates the importance of frequent maintenance to disrupt pathogens in diabetics.

Patient Compliance

One critical factor in the control of chronic infections is patient **compliance.** Haynes defines compliance as "the extent to which a person's behavior coincides with medical or health advice."[23] Patient compliance in periodontal disease or dental caries control requires the following:

- Diligence with daily oral self-care
- Maintaining consistent appointments at the dental office for regular professional monitoring of oral health status

The terms **adherence** and **therapeutic alliance** are also used to describe the congruence between medical advice and individual behavior.[49] The medical literature also uses the term **concordance,** especially when describing patients' behaviors regarding prescription medications.[14]

✦ CASE APPLICATION 22-1.3

Patient Compliance and Adherence
Case Study 22-1 demonstrates the importance of a patient's commitment to compliance/adherence in performing oral hygiene self-care.

In recent years, renewed attention has focused on the **transtheoretical model** of behavioral change. This model suggests that individuals progress through a series of distinct stages when attempting to alter a behavior.[38,39] The transtheoretical model has four components[40]:

1. *The stages of change.* The stages of change include five different levels that individuals progress through when changing behavior.
2. *The processes of change.* The processes of change include techniques that are used to modify behavior and to help ensure successful adoption of the change.
3. *Decisional balance.* Decisional balance involves weighing the advantages and disadvantages of changing behavior.
4. *Self-efficacy.* Self-efficacy is an individual's ability to remain confident in making and maintaining change.

Although the transtheoretical model has been used for tobacco cessation, weight loss, psychologic concerns, alcohol abuse, and exercise programs, it has not been researched for changing oral hygiene behaviors. However, it has been suggested that the transtheoretical model could be used to develop individualized self-care strategies for patients and that it further could be applied to help with treatment acceptance.[9,45]

The clinician should impress on each patient his or her role in oral disease control and that attaining periodontal health requires a daily, lifetime commitment (Box 22-1). Stressing patient involvement in oral health maintenance is important from the first appointment through the ongoing phases of periodontal therapy, including each SPC appointment. Patients should demonstrate their involvement by the following:

- Learning and practicing oral care techniques
- Understanding the purpose and anticipated outcomes of periodontal care
- Learning how to evaluate the health of their own mouths

Many reasons have been suggested to explain why the average patient with a chronic disease is not particularly compliant (Box 22-2). (See Chapter 5 for a discussion of communication techniques.) For example, after nonsurgical therapy, surgery, or emergency treatment, patients often consider themselves healed, or at least improved, and often attribute the change to "seeing the doctor" or to the care the therapist provided. The healthcare professional, and in dentistry most often the dental hygienist, is responsible for helping patients recognize their daily role in maintaining oral health. This is probably the most challenging role in oral care—to teach patients with a chronic disease that they must take responsibility for daily self-care. Patients with periodontal or chronic oral diseases find it difficult to make the adjustments required to perform more frequent and often dexterity-challenging self-care procedures that require more time and special materials or equipment. Often family and friends fail to support the extra time, money, and commitment.

Another impediment to patients with a chronic disease is that they may not feel ill when they are symptom free. Periodontal diseases are typically painless. During periodontal therapy the dental hygienist must stress that healthy tissues do not bleed. The PM patient will come to understand that bleeding is a sign of disease. Absence of bleeding is one of the best clinical signs for the patient, whereas the dental hygienist looks for stability of the clinical attachment. Patients may become less diligent in following a demanding oral self-care program when the signs of gingival bleeding cease.

An attentive, caring, and competent dental hygienist is essential in helping the patient improve his or her chronic disease. Encouragement, support, external motivation, and advice are part of the dental hygienist's responsibility in patient relations and are essential components of each supportive care appointment.

BOX 22-1

SUGGESTIONS FOR IMPROVING PATIENT COMPLIANCE AND CONCORDANCE

- Set goals *with* the patient, not *for* the patient.
- Write down what you say and what the patient agrees to, possibly using the patient's signature to reinforce the importance of the goals and the patient's understanding of them.
- Simplify self-care as much as possible.
- Use positive reinforcement.
- Involve the entire office in encouraging the patient.
- Discuss lack of compliance/concordance with the patient and seek remedies.
- Use appointment reminders.

BOX 22-2

FACTORS CONTRIBUTING TO POOR PATIENT COMPLIANCE AND CONCORDANCE[50]

- The symptoms disappear.
- The patient feels better.
- The self-care regimen is inconvenient, demanding, or too difficult.
- The patient is not convinced of the value and efficacy of recommended self-care routines and treatment.
- The periodontal maintenance (PM) visits are too frequent, too expensive, or too uncomfortable.
- The patient is unsure whether a periodontist or a generalist will handle the PM visit.
- The patient exhibits general discouragement (common with chronic conditions).

Evaluation of Initial Therapy

Initial therapy usually consists of quadrant debridement with anesthesia. A more recent concept, **full-mouth disinfection,** has emerged. Full-mouth disinfection is a procedure combining complete debridement with the use of adjunctive antimicrobials; the procedure is completed within a 24-hour period to attempt to eradicate or diminish bacterial reservoirs in the mouth that could impede optimal healing. Full-mouth disinfection is an appealing concept, particularly because it could decrease the number of patient visits while allowing more efficient use of treatment times. Some research has shown that full-mouth disinfection can provide better clinical outcomes than quadrant therapy.[41] However, a recent review article suggests that larger study populations and corroborating data from different treatment centers are needed to determine whether full-mouth disinfection provides clinically relevant improvements beyond quadrant debridement.[20]

When disease has been reduced, whether through a series of quadrant debridements with anesthesia or through full-mouth disinfection, the results must be evaluated (Box 22-3). The interval for this evaluation usually is 4 to 6 weeks after initial therapy, which is differentiated from the less frequent (typically 3 months or less) maintenance interval. Tissue response and the patient's personal care effectiveness are the parameters of evaluation. The response to the initial debridement dictates the choice of further treatment options, which include the following:

- Site-specific debridement in areas of continued infection
- Consideration of adjunctive antimicrobial use
- Regular PM interval of every 3 months or less
- Surgical correction of periodontal defects

It has been recommended that surgery not be considered until at least several weeks or months after the initial debridement.[22]

When areas of infection persist (i.e., erythema, bleeding, exudate, or no decrease in probing depth), several causes can be considered. Minute areas of undisturbed dental plaque biofilm or calculus may be present, which the clinician can redebride where needed. The patient may not have mastered self-care procedures sufficiently to maintain gingival health; furthermore, conditions in the mouth, such as deep periodontal pockets, malaligned teeth, or poorly contoured margins, may thwart the patient's self-care efforts. Listening to the patient and watching him or her demonstrate self-care techniques are important keys to determining why the gingival tissue is not responding as anticipated. The clinician must continue to encourage and work with the patient to detect the problems in controlling plaque biofilm. It can be helpful to use plaque biofilm–staining products so that the patient can visualize areas routinely missed during self-care procedures. Problems with access may be improved only through surgery, or an underlying systemic problem may be retarding gingival healing. If systemic factors are suspected, then a physician should evaluate the patient.

Because of either anatomical factors associated with periodontitis or lack of patient compliance with self-care measures (or because of both), the dental hygienist will need to deplaque

> *Note*
>
> When inflammation and BOP are absent, the patient typically is placed on a supportive care interval appropriate for the level and type of disease.

BOX 22-3

PROCEDURE FOR EVALUATION OF INITIAL OR PRESURGICAL PERIODONTAL DEBRIDEMENT*

- Review the patient's record.
- Greet the patient.
- Update the patient's health history.
- Obtain the patient's evaluation of the success of the treatment and discuss any problems or complaints.
- Recheck any previously identified extraoral and intraoral irregularities that might affect the course of the appointment.
- Evaluate the gingival response.
- Check the patient's oral hygiene status (e.g., level of plaque biofilm control, reaccumulation of calculus, presence of stain from chlorhexidine or tobacco).
- If gingivitis remains with effective plaque biofilm control, evaluate for systemic factors (e.g., diabetes, pregnancy).
- Observe, adjust, and encourage the patient's plaque biofilm control skill if disease is still present.
- Debride and polish as necessary.
- Assist with determination of referral for surgical therapy or maintenance.

*This evaluation usually is performed 4 to 6 weeks after the debridement procedure.

tient learn effective methods to control dental plaque biofilm is an essential component to the patient's oral health.

24). Periodontal patients with chronic disease may benefit from the use of a local or systemic antimicrobial agent. At supportive-care appointments the clinician should consider the use of an antimicrobial agent if bleeding has not been controlled through mechanical means (see Chapter 27).

Persistent or unresolved periodontitis may be site specific or generalized and can be caused by several factors (Table 22-1). Incomplete debridement results in incomplete wound healing because sufficient bacteria to cause infection have remained in the periodontal pocket. The host immune response can become overwhelmed when the bacterial load or pathogenicity of the plaque biofilm is too great. In some patients, professional and self-care mechanical procedures cannot adequately reach and disrupt periodontal bacterial pathogens, such as in furcations, deep pockets, or around tooth defects. In these cases the dental hygienist and patient can discuss other options for attaining a healthy periodontium. Peri-

where the patient has not adequately disturbed bacterial activity. The dental hygienist also must determine whether the patient lacks motivation or skill, whether he or she needs a different self-care device (see Chapter 24), or whether adjunctive antimicrobial therapy should be considered. Helping the patient learn effective methods to control dental plaque biofilm is an essential component to the patient's oral health.

Refer to Chapters 20 and 21 for planning and executing individualized preventive and intervention strategies.

Periodontal patients typically have teeth that are more difficult to deplaque (because of tooth position and root exposure) and usually need to use more than a toothbrush and floss to effectively clean the dentition (see Chapter 24). Periodontal patients with chronic disease may benefit from the use of a local or systemic antimicrobial agent. At supportive-care appointments the clinician should consider the use of an antimicrobial agent if bleeding has not been controlled through mechanical means (see Chapter 27).

odontal surgery, among other procedures, is used to eliminate deep pockets that act as bacterial reservoirs. For chronic periodontitis patients, pharmacotherapy using local drug delivery systems may be helpful at nonresponding sites (see Chapter 27). Regenerative surgical therapies can help replace lost tissue and bone,

enabling patients to access sites more easily. Occlusal adjustments may aid in reducing tooth mobility and gaining some bone lost because of traumatic occlusal forces.[15]

Table 22-1	Treatments for Cases of Unresolved Healing
PROBLEM	**TREATMENT**
Incomplete Debridement	• Debride inflamed areas. • Consider obtaining a culture specimen to identify the bacteria causing the inflammation.
Poor Plaque Biofilm Control	• Reassess the patient's skills and attitude. • Change aids or modify the current procedure. • Consider irrigation or antimicrobial intervention.
Deep Bony Defect	• Refer for surgery.
Complicating Oral Conditions	• Refer for correction or improvement of oral conditions.
Complicating Systemic Conditions	• Consider medical and laboratory examinations for possible underlying systemic disease.

Supportive Care Intervals for Periodontal Patients

Regularly spaced intervals of professional care have proved beneficial for most individuals prone to a chronic disease.[10,30,51] The recommended average interval of supportive professional treatment for patients susceptible to a periodontal disease is 3 months.[4,50] This interval can be lengthened or shortened based on a number of individual factors (Box 22-4).

BOX 22-4

FACTORS AFFECTING THE INTERVAL OF SUPPORTIVE PROFESSIONAL CARE

• Patient's current oral condition and general health status
• Risk of reinfection
• Clinical evidence that more frequent professional monitoring and intervention result in improved patient health
• Patient's compliance or concordance regarding recommended personal oral health regimens
• Patient's willingness to return for regular supportive periodontal care (SPC) appointments

More frequent patient visits allow the oral healthcare professional to monitor for recurrence of infection, to encourage the patient to continue a daily regimen, and to provide preventive procedures if active infection is present. In fact, intervals of 2 weeks, 2 to 3 months, 3 months, 3 to 4 months, 3 to 6 months, 4 to 6 months, and up to 18 months have been evaluated.[2]

It should be noted that the typical 3-month PM interval is not the same as the 1- or 2-week appointment interval (for up to 6 weeks) that is scheduled after surgery. Generally 1- or 2-week reevaluation appointments after periodontal surgery improve oral health in the healing phase.[48]

Review of Patient Record

The American Academy of Periodontology recommends that all patients receive a thorough, systematic periodontal examination at regular intervals. The examination should include the patient's chief complaint, medical and dental histories, clinical examination, and analysis of appropriately updated radiographs.[7] However, just as the patient with blood pressure problems frequently has more difficulty regulating blood pressure, and the insulin-dependent person must take extra care to maintain a stable blood sugar, periodontal patients must work harder to maintain a healthy periodontium. Therefore the prevention and intervention plans must be realistic, and patients should feel that they can achieve the objectives.

To plan an individual prevention program, several questions must be answered:

- What is the patient's risk level for recurrence of the disease?
- What are the patient's attitude and psychomotor abilities in controlling the disease?
- Which kinds of supportive care procedures are best for different patients?
- Based on the patient's primary problem, what is the optimal interval length for supportive care?

These questions are challenging, and the answers differ from patient to patient. Patients' needs, problems, and general health status are not static; therefore a care plan including goals and evaluation measures is necessary for each supportive care appointment. Specific supportive care procedures require periodic reevaluation.

To focus the supportive care plan, one must identify the intended outcomes—the criteria by which patients and clinicians can judge success.

Note

Currently the desirable outcome in PM is stability; that is, attachment loss is halted. Complete absence of bleeding and exudate are end points of therapy that can be measured by the clinician and observed by the patient.

However, these are criteria for judging the *success* of preventive and therapeutic measures; the *prediction* of periodontal diseases or periodontal breakdown is considerably less well defined. Identifying the desired outcomes and reinforcing the patient's role in therapeutic outcomes is important. The following are the goals of periodontal therapy:

- To preserve the natural dentition
- To maintain and improve periodontal health, comfort, esthetics, and function
- To provide replacements (i.e., dental implants) where indicated[7]

The only successful interventions are those that help achieve those goals.

Elements of the Periodontal Maintenance Appointment

Sequencing of elements that make up the PM appointment is similar to that of the accepted annual examination for a person with no previous periodontal problems. The following are the primary differences between PM and annual examination appointments:

- Shortened interval between PM appointments versus annual examination appointments
- Particular time, care, and emphasis on the patient's periodontal status in PM appointments
- Types of interventions that may be necessary in PM appointments
- Such interventions used in PM appointments may include the following:
  - Use of antimicrobial agents
  - Reinstruction or changes in oral hygiene
  - Shorter interval of care for the next PM appointment
  - Consideration of a return to more aggressive therapy

Thorough attention to the site around each tooth is critical in PM appointments. All the components of the periodontal examination (see Chapter 16) generally are performed at each PM appointment, with particular attention given to any areas of change. A change of 2 mm or more of attachment loss, along with other clinical findings, is a suggested criterion for more aggressive intervention. Two millimeters accounts for the 1-mm accepted variation in probe depth measurements. However, for a patient with significant previous attachment loss, even a 1-mm increase in attachment loss may be an unfavorable clinical sign. BOP is an important clinical sign that must be recorded at each supportive care appointment.[26] The *absence of BOP* is considered more predictive of periodontal health than the *presence of BOP* is predictive of increased attachment loss. Although BOP has approximately a 30% predictive power for future attachment loss, its negative predictive power of 98% makes lack of bleeding after probing a very useful tool.[27]

DENTAL CONSIDERATIONS

The presence of bleeding does not necessarily mean that a site will progress to a more serious disease state; the absence of bleeding indicates health. An exception to this statement applies to individuals who smoke, because the use of tobacco products tends to decrease gingival inflammation and bleeding.

The following components may be part of a PM visit.[2] However, all treatment is dependant on individual patient circumstance. The clinician should use her or his best judgment when determining the proper protocol for a given patient.

REVIEW AND UPDATE OF MEDICAL AND DENTAL HISTORY

Updating the health history at every patient appointment is essential. General health and physiologic vigor, specific health problems and recent medical care, the patient's stress level, and medications must be reviewed, because positive responses to some of these questions have a significant effect on periodontal conditions (see Chapters 12). Research has shown evidence of connections between periodontitis and systemic risks or problems in addition to diabetes mellitus or bacterial endocarditis.[5] At each PM appointment the patient may present with similar plaque biofilm levels yet varying degrees of periodontal health. A thorough familiarity with each patient's systemic health allows the dental hygienist to modify the care plan and to help determine why the level of plaque biofilm evident at a previous PM appointment does not result in comparable periodontal health.

> **Prevention**
>
> Describe to the patient that research is showing a possible connection between poor periodontal health and certain systemic conditions (e.g., diabetes, poor pregnancy outcomes, cardiovascular diseases, respiratory diseases). Some of the research indicates a stronger link than others; although researchers cannot say that periodontitis *causes* these health problems, a connection seems to exist between oral health and good overall health.

Before the appointment a review of the patient's record, including chartings and radiographs, will familiarize the dental hygienist with the following:

- Patient's general health
- Extent of previous periodontal conditions
- Type of surgery performed, if any
- Level of stability currently attained
- Specific problem sites
- Patient's contribution to his or her own periodontal health

In addition, knowledge of the patient's need for anesthesia, antibiotic premedication, preference for a particular debridement and polishing technique, and other patient-specific concerns allows the clinician to prepare for a more beneficial and efficient appointment.

CLINICAL EXAMINATION

Extraoral and Intraoral Examinations

An extraoral and intraoral examination should be performed at every appointment. The examination is important for every patient; however, examination is particularly important for patients who have had a previous malignancy and those with high oral health risk behaviors (e.g., tobacco and alcohol use).

Dental Examination

The dental examination should include the recording of tooth mobility, fremitus and occlusal factors, coronal and root caries, restorative factors (e.g., defective restorations), and other tooth-related problems (e.g., open contacts or malpositioned teeth).

Periodontal Examination

The periodontal examination consists of recording probing depths, gingival recession, BOP, levels of plaque biofilm and calculus, furcations, and exudation. Recording of attachment levels, if indicated, may be performed. In addition, microbial testing could be done if indicated.

Examination of Dental Implants and Periimplant Tissues

If a patient has dental implants, probing depths, BOP, examination of the prosthesis and abutment, evaluation of stability, and occlusal examination should be performed. Other signs and symptoms of disease activity (e.g., pain, suppuration) should be noted.

Radiographic Examination

Radiographs of diagnostic quality are needed. They should be current and should permit high-quality evaluation and interpretation of the oral structures. Disease status or changes in status are determined by reviewing radiographs (compared with baseline) along with clinical findings.

Assessment of Personal Oral Hygiene

The best time to review psychomotor skills and have the patient practice in a problem area is after the mouth has been disclosed or before professional debridement. The patient should demonstrate the use of oral hygiene products so that the dental hygienist can provide guidance in proper use. Being attuned to the patient's mental and emotional status, attitude toward the mouth, sense of responsibility for the problems in the mouth, and ownership of successes is an important task for the dental hygienist. Through effective motivation and encouragement, the dental hygienist, the dentist, and the office staff serve as part of the patient's support group.

Treatment

Removal of subgingival and supragingival plaque biofilm and calculus is a key aspect of the PM appointment. The clinician must concentrate on sites that show *any* undesirable changes, from the most subtle rolled or shiny gingival margin or swollen interdental papilla to frank bleeding or pus-producing areas. These signs are evidence of the body's response to an infection. Deplaquing is particularly difficult for patients with periodontal problems. Exposed root surfaces, furcations, malpositioned teeth, and complex restorative correction frequently pose difficult challenges in oral self-care. The patient's self-care is not always sufficient to halt attachment loss.

Polishing is necessary to remove stains and other heavy plaque biofilm at and under the gingival margin. This process is particularly important when gingival disease is present.

New technologic advances in dentistry are making it possible to further investigate the actual site of inflammation. The periodontal endoscope provides visualization and magnification within the periodontal pocket, sulci, furcas, and crown margins and is indispensable for finding plaque biofilm missed, burnished calculus, or rough root surfaces responsible for plaque biofilm retention. Debridement disturbs the bacterial matrix, making plaque biofilm less pathogenic. Although calculus does not typically accumulate to become a large or tenacious deposit at a 3-month interval, all calculus deposits should be removed because they create a retentive area for bacterial plaque biofilm (see Chapter 31).

Additional treatment procedures that might be performed during the PM visit include occlusal adjustment, root desensitization, and the use of systemic antibiotics or local antimicrobials.

Communication

This aspect of the PM appointment involves informing the patient of current disease status and the need for additional treatment, if indicated. Consultations with other healthcare practitioners might also be warranted. No one is as familiar with a patient's oral condition as the patient; therefore it makes good sense to listen to the patient's evaluation of how the mouth "feels." Of particular interest to the dental hygienist are comments such as the following:

> **Note**
>
> In accepting the patient as a co-therapist in periodontal care, the value of listening to the patient cannot be overemphasized.

> **Prevention**
>
> Explain to the patient that a thorough periodontal evaluation takes time. In some cases more than one appointment may be needed to effectively perform an evaluation and the necessary debridement.

- Any kind of tooth sensitivity
- Mechanical problems
- Concerns with therapeutic drugs
- What does or does not "feel right" in the patient's mouth
- Any concerns about changes in oral condition

PLANNING SUBSEQUENT PERIODONTAL MAINTENANCE APPOINTMENTS

Because most PM intervals are established at 3-month intervals, a date for the next appointment often is made before the patient leaves the office. This is a common practice for any appointments that are not 6 months into the future so that the appropriate interval is maintained and not lengthened because of scheduling problems. Attention to maintaining the recommended interval of care is important whether the supportive care appointment is at the same office or alternates between the periodontist and the generalist.

One additional element that is vital to the success of PM is allowing for adequate appointment time. In 1981, Schallhorn and Snider[43] conducted a study of the average time required for different components of PM. One hour is the generally accepted minimum for a PM appointment, although some patients require more time. However, 26 years later, more activities are required during that hour. For example, the infection control protocol has become more involved, and intraoral preventive options (e.g., antimicrobial therapy and instruction) have increased. Patients who require full-mouth local anesthesia usually are scheduled for two appointments so that only the left or right half of the mouth is anesthetized at one visit.

Any treatment plan must include criteria for outcome assessment, which can be defined as results, completion, achievement, success, or simply progress (see Chapters 20 and 21). Outcomes goals can vary and may be established as short term or long range, but both the patient and the clinician must agree to them. Although the goals of therapeutic intervention and prevention strategies are not always the same for therapist and patient, the criteria for a successful outcome from PM appointments should be discussed and agreed upon with the patient.

Responsibility for Periodontal Supportive Care Appointments

The severity of the patient's periodontal condition and the extent of needed treatment are the most common determinants of the responsibility of care. Other factors might include the patient's preference, travel time for appointments, and insurance coverage. Patients with dental implants or extensive prostheses and those undergoing orthodontic therapy may require PM care to sustain health. Effective PM involves open and active communication between all parties, including the patient, referring (or general) dentist, and the periodontist.

After initial periodontal treatment, several courses of action are possible[2]:

- The patient may be seen in the periodontist's office for all supportive care appointments. This is recommended for patients with a history of severe periodontal attachment loss or aggressive forms of periodontitis.
- The patient may alternate 3-month visits between the general dental office and the periodontal office. This is

appropriate for patients with a history of chronic periodontitis with mild to moderate attachment loss.

- The general dental office may resume responsibility for all patient care. This option works best in recurrent gingivitis cases or slight, chronic periodontitis cases with minimal bone loss.
- The patient may decide not to seek SPC despite the clear advice given during the initial periodontal therapy.

The periodontist and generalist teams should determine which of the first three options is best, but the patient ultimately decides the course of action (see Appendix B).

Supportive Care for Dental Caries and Other Chronic Oral Conditions

DENTAL CARIES

Developmental pits and fissures at risk for dental decay should be protected with sealants. Patients with active dental caries or those who are at risk for smooth surface and root caries should be placed on a professionally supervised program of more frequent intervals for several reasons (see Chapters 25 and 28). The dental hygienist should advise the patient regarding the use of multiple forms of fluoride, which assist in remineralization, and other primary preventive agents for controlling and healing the incipient lesion. The dental hygienist may also consider the use of chlorhexidine as an anticarious agent. Frequent appointments for dental caries control include:

- intensive self-care instructions and motivation
- encouragement to reduce sugars and fermentable carbohydrates from the diet (see Chapters 19 and 25)

The dental hygienist must first update the individual's risk for dental caries (i.e., he or she reviews all the dental caries–producing influences pertinent to the individual patient to determine which risk factors must be reduced or modified). Risk factors may include dietary choices, frequency of eating, types of snacks, degree of exposure to topical fluoride, salivary influences, quality of tooth development, medications, and genetic and social factors. The *dental caries risk assessment form* is found in Chapter 25, along with the process for management by risk assessment.

Age is no longer as strong a risk factor for dental caries as other considerations. Occlusal caries are developing much later than the historical pattern of early dental caries formation. Changes in tooth position, root exposure, diet, medication, oral care, and lifestyle influence a person's susceptibility to dental caries, and these situations occur across the life span. Any patient who has had active dental caries in the past 12 months should be considered at high risk for the development of new dental caries and requires close professional supervision and modification of care for dental caries control.

The extent and effectiveness of patient concordance with the dental caries control program are assessed at each appointment. *Listening* to patients to determine their self-care regimens, their attitudes, and their feelings about oral self-care (its value, its success), as well as how the mouth feels physically, helps the clinician understand the level of patient concordance. The dental hygienist also should watch patients perform oral care in areas where they are having difficulty with plaque biofilm removal or fluoride application, as well as areas where a particular problem is noted. Plaque biofilm staining can be quite useful in this regard.

Use of fluoride considerably decreases dental decay. The patient's use of fluoride must be reviewed and reevaluated at each supportive care appointment, because exposure to frequent daily doses of fluoride is considered the best dental caries–preventive interval. The Centers for Disease Control and Prevention (CDC) have recommended frequent, daily exposure to topical fluoride via toothpastes, mouthrinses, and fluoridated water.[17] The need for professionally applied topical fluoride, as well as its frequency and type, also should be evaluated. For both personal and professional fluoride therapy, changes in application might be suggested based on the progress seen, the current severity of the disease, the patient's acceptance of products, or the availability of a new product. For example, the belief that fluoride enhances remineralization of enamel and has an effect on exposed dentin is widely accepted.[16,24,44] Clinicians also know that chlorhexidine has a deleterious effect on *Streptococcus mutans,* the putative organism in incipient caries.[31,52] Effective, efficient means of applying chlorhexidine, such as with varnish or spray, are being developed to help retard or prevent dental caries. In addition, fluoride varnish, although approved in the United States as a desensitizer only, has evidence to support its use as an anticaries agent.

> *Patient Educational Opportunity*
>
> The clinician should describe to the patient that new advances in dental caries prevention, both in-office and at-home, are available and highly effective if used as recommended.

Newer anticaries agents, such as xylitol and amorphous calcium phosphate (ACP), have emerged and proven useful in preventing decay (see Chapter 25).

OTHER CHRONIC ORAL CONDITIONS

Some patients may have other chronic oral problems, such as dentinal sensitivity, rapid deposit accumulation, herpetic lesions, aphthous ulcers, or the tissue conditions associated with Sjögren's syndrome. A more frequent interval of professional care is generally advisable for these patients. The dental hygienist can monitor the patient's condition and often reduce the severity of the tissue breakdown, with the expected result of improved oral comfort and health for the patient.

Changes in mental and emotional status affect health and chronic disease, even though their effects are less understood and documented. A patient suffering emotional or mental stress or trauma may precipitate a chronic condition or may cause a chronic condition to become acute. The interrelationship of the physiologic mechanisms, hormonal influences, patient psyche, and attention or skill with self-care is not completely clear. The oral mucosal tissue is a commonly affected area, and the multifactorial type of chronic problem includes the autoimmune classes of oral mucosal disease.

Chronic, infectious attacks of herpetic origin would not be a reason for more frequent supportive care. For some patients simple manipulation of the oral tissues during a dental appointment causes recurrence of a herpetic lesion. OTC products for alleviating the symptoms are the best therapy currently available for chronic herpetic lesions.

References

1. American Academy of Periodontology: Periodontal diseases of children and adolescents (position paper), *J Periodontol* 74(11): 1696-1704, 2003.
2. American Academy of Periodontology: Periodontal maintenance (position paper), *J Periodontol* 74:1395-1401, 2003.
3. American Academy of Periodontology: Academy report. Treatment of plaque-induced gingivitis, chronic periodontitis and other clinical conditions, *J Periodontal* 72:1790-1800, 2001.
4. American Academy of Periodontology: Parameter on periodontal maintenance, *J Periodontol* 71:849-850, 2000.
5. American Academy of Periodontology: Parameter on systemic conditions affected by periodontal diseases, *J Periodontol* 71: 880-883, 2000.
6. American Academy of Periodontology: Tobacco use and the periodontal patient (position paper), *J Periodontal* 70:1419-1427, 1999.
7. American Academy of Periodontology: Guidelines for periodontal therapy, *J Periodontol* 69:405-408, 1998.
8. American Academy of Periodontology: Consensus report. Periodontal diseases: pathogenesis and microbial factors, sec 11, *Ann Periodontol* 1:926-932, 1996.
9. Astroth D et al: The transtheoretical model: an approach to behavioral change, *J Dent Hyg* 76(4):286-295, 2002.
10. Axelsson P, Lindhe J, Nystrom B: On the prevention of caries and periodontal disease: results of a 15-year longitudinal study in adults, *J Clin Periodontol* 18:182-189, 1991.
11. Axelsson P, Paulander J, Lindhe J: Relationship between smoking and dental status in 35-, 50-, 65-, and 75-year-old individuals, *J Clin Periodontol* 25:297-305, 1998.
12. Baehni P: Supportive care of the periodontal patient, *Curr Opin Periodontol* 4:151-157, 1997.
13. Bolin A et al: The effect of changed smoking habits on marginal alveolar bone loss, *Swed Dent J* 17:211-216, 1993.
14. Britten N: Communication: the key to improved compliance, *Prescr J* 9(10):27-31, 1998.
15. Burgett F et al: A randomized trial of occlusal adjustment in the treatment of periodontitis patients, *J Clin Periodontol* 19:381-387, 1992.
16. Burt B, Ismail A, Eklund S: Root caries in an optimally fluoridated and a high-fluoride community, *J Dent Res* 65:1154-1158, 1986.
17. Centers for Disease Control and Prevention: *Oral health resources* [Internet], Atlanta, 2006 [www.cdc.gov/OralHealth/index.htm].
18. Dietrich T, Bernimoulin J, Glynn R: The effect of cigarette smoking on gingival bleeding, *J Periodontol* 75(1):16-22, 2004.
19. Gilbert G et al: Predicting tooth loss during a population-based study: role of attachment level in the presence of other dental conditions, *J Peridontol* 73(12):1427-1436, 2002.
20. Greenstein G: Efficacy of full-mouth disinfection vs quadrant root planing, *Compendium* 25:380-390, 2004.
21. Haffajee A et al: Relationship of baseline microbial parameters to future periodontal attachment loss, *J Clin Periodontol* 18:744-750, 1991.
22. Hall W: Sequence of treatment. In Hall W, ed: *Decision making in periodontology*, St Louis, 1988, Mosby.
23. Haynes R: A critical review of the "determinates" of patient compliance with therapeutic regimes. In Sackett D, Haynes R, eds: *Compliance with therapeutic regimens*, Baltimore, 1976, Johns Hopkins University Press.
24. Hunt RJ, Eldredge JB, Beck JD: Effect of residence in a fluoridated community on the incidence of coronal and root caries in an older adult population, *J Public Health Dent* 49:138-141, 1989.
25. Johnson G, Hill M: Cigarette smoking and the periodontal patient, *J Periodontol* 75(2):196-209, 2004.
26. Lang N, Joss A, Tonetti M: Monitoring disease during supportive periodontal treatment by bleeding on probing, *Periodontol 2000* 12:44-8, 1996.
27. Lang N et al: Bleeding on probing: a predictor for the progression of periodontal disease? *J Clin Periodontol* 13:590-596, 1986.
28. Lang NP, Karring T, eds: *Proceedings of the First European Workshop on Periodontology*, London, 1994, Quintessence.
29. Linden G, Mullally B: Cigarette smoking and periodontal destruction in young adults, *J Periodontol* 65:718-723, 1994.
30. Lindhe J, Nyman S: Long-term maintenance of patients treated for advanced periodontal disease, *J Clin Periodontol* 11:504-514, 1984.
31. Marsh P et al: Inhibition by the antimicrobial agent chlorhexidine of acid production and sugar transport in oral streptococcal bacteria, *Arch Oral Biol* 28(3):233-240, 1983.
32. Misselbrook D: Managing the change from compliance to concordance, *Prescriber* 9(8):23-33, 1998.
33. Nevins M, Becker W, Kornman K, eds: *Proceedings of the World Workshop*, Princeton, NJ, 1989, American Academy of Periodontology.
34. Page R et al: Longitudinal validation of a risk calculator for periodontal disease, *J Clin Periodontol* 30:819-827, 2003.
35. Page R et al: Validity and accuracy of a risk calculator in predicting periodontal disease, *J Am Dent Assoc* 133:569-576, 2002.
36. Palat M: Occlusal trauma. In Weinberg M et al, eds: *Comprehensive periodontics for the dental hygienist*, Upper Saddle River, NJ, 2001, Prentice Hall.
37. Persson R et al: Assessing periodontal disease risk—a comparison of clinicians' assessment versus a computerized tool, *J Am Dent Assoc* 134:575-582, 2003.
38. Prochaska J, DiClemente C: *The transtheoretical approach: crossing the traditional boundaries of therapy*, Chicago, 1984, Dow Jones/Irwin.
39. Prochaska J, DiClemente C: Transtheoretical therapy: toward a more integrative model of change, *Psychother: Theory, Res Pract* 20:161-173, 1982.
40. Prochaska J, Norcross J, DiClemente C: *Changing for good*, New York, 1994, Avon Books.
41. Quirynen M et al: Full- vs partial-mouth disinfection in the treatment of periodontal infections: short-term clinical and microbiological observations, *J Dent Res* 74:1459-1467, 1995.
42. Ramfjord S: Maintenance care and supportive periodontal therapy, *Quintessence Int* 24:465-471, 1993.
43. Schallhorn R, Snider L: Periodontal maintenance therapy, *J Am Dent Assoc* 103:227-232, 1981.

44. Stamm J, Banting D, Imrey P: Adult root caries survey of two similar communities with contrasting natural water fluoride levels, *J Am Dent Assoc* 120:143-149, 1990.

45. Tilliss T et al: The transtheoretical model applied to an oral self-care behavioral change: development and testing of instruments for stages of change and decisional balance, *J Dent Hyg* 77(I): 16-25, 2003.

46. Tomar S, Asma S: Smoking-attributable periodontitis in the United States: findings from NHANES III, *J Periodontol* 71(5):743-751, 2000.

47. Wennstrom J: Treatment of periodontal disease in older adults, *Periodontol 2000* 16:106-112, 1998.

48. Westfelt E: Significance of frequency of professional tooth cleaning for healing following periodontal surgery, *J Clin Periodontol* 10:148-156, 1983.

49. Wilson T: Compliance and its role in periodontal therapy, *Periodontol 2000* 12:16-23, 1996.

50. Wilson T: Supportive periodontal treatment introduction: definition, extent of need, therapeutic objectives, frequency, and efficiency, *Periodontol 2000* 12:11-15, 1996.

51. Wilson T et al: Tooth loss in maintenance patients in a private periodontal practice, *J Periodontol* 58:231-235, 1987.

52. Zickert I, Emilson C, Krasse B: Effect of caries preventive measures in children highly infected with the bacterium *Streptococcus mutans*, *Arch Oral Biol* 27(10):861-868, 1982.

Case Development, Documentation, and Presentation

Bonnie Francis

INSIGHT

The clinical dental hygienist works with various cases throughout the working day. Case development and documentation exercises provide the framework of information necessary for complex decision making and treatment recommendations for individual patient's needs and clinical situations. Developed cases can then be presented in various forms to promote learning and professional development.

✦ CASE STUDY 23-1   Use of Patient Case Documentation for Extended Learning

Jennifer Shaw, a senior dental hygiene student, has recently received an assignment to prepare a case for her periodontology course. She has thoroughly reviewed the criteria established for the assignment (see Case Application 23-1.1, Case Selection, later in this chapter) and is aware of the aspects required to complete the task. The patient scheduled for today's clinical session, 70-year-old Ann Cronin, appeared to have the necessary elements that would allow her to complete her case documentation assignment. Jennifer discussed the prospects with her faculty, informed Mrs. Cronin, and gathered the necessary clinical data for case development and documentation.

KEY TERMS

case development   case documentation   case presentations

LEARNING OUTCOMES

After reading this chapter the student will be able to:
1. Provide an example of how case development and documentation may be used.
2. Analyze the purpose, the intended audience, and the goal of case development in a given situation.
3. Identify the components that can be developed and documented on a given case.
4. Compile all material necessary to document the therapeutic interventions and strategies of patient care provided in the case being developed.
5. Demonstrate case presentation skills to peers and other professionals in either written or oral format.

Applications

Students and educators have favorably accepted case-based instructional methods.* When working with patients, the clinician should use the following case-based concepts†:

- Enhance learning.
- Promote self-directed learning.
- Expand critical thinking.
- Increase clinical reasoning skills and decision making.
- Allow students to solve real-world problems in the safe environment of the classroom.
- Promote life-long learning patterns.

The use of properly designed cases facilitates active learning and enhances higher levels of critical thinking, which requires the learner to integrate knowledge from basic science and dental science with clinical applications.[2,4,5]

Case representation of patient care can be used in several ways. The first and perhaps most obvious is patient education. "A picture is worth a thousand words" is true when motivating a person to change oral care behavior or to encourage a patient to continue the present course. Documenting the changes or progression of health may motivate the patient and the dental hygienist.

Cases may be used by the hygienist to review patient outcomes and to determine when goals are met and what adjustments may be needed either in the patient's self-care habits or in the clinician's strategies, skills, or both. Reviewing documentation of some patients who exhibit dramatic changes in tissue response and oral self-care is encouraging to the dental hygienist and the patient. Conversely, a patient may demonstrate subtle oral health changes, and the process of capturing this information visually may assist in the evaluation of the therapy provided. **Case documentation** may provide motivation and self-evaluation for both the patient and the dental hygienist.

LEGAL DOCUMENTATION AND INSURANCE SUBMISSION

Accurate and thorough records of patient care—an essential part of **case development**—serve as legal documents and may help form a valuable defense if needed. Additionally, case documentation is required when insurance claims are filed for some procedures. Submitting an organized, thorough, and accurate case documentation with accompanying visual images with an insurance claim form assists in claim reimbursement.

TEACHING TOOLS AND EDUCATION

Case documentation may be used for teaching in the academic setting and in professional presentations to peers. **Case presentations** are organized presentations of documented patient care. All components of a case are gathered and presented along with visual images to support objective clinical and radiographic findings. Chartings, radiographs, photographs, study models, and laboratory tests are combined with written documentation

*References 3, 8, 10, 11, 13, 14.
†References 1, 3, 6, 7, 9, 11, 13, 14.

to "tell the story" of the patient's care from the initiation of therapy through the post therapy evaluation.

CASE DEVELOPMENT

Case development and documentation require a visual and written representation of a patient's clinical case. Information to be considered in the development of a case may include specifics about the case, visual elements representing the case, and specific details of case management and proceedings.[15] Selection of a case to develop involves three considerations: (1) the purpose of developing the case, (2) the intended audience, and (3) the defined goals or expected outcomes.

Establishing Purpose

Various reasons for developing a case presentation may differ between clinicians. Case development and presentations may enhance any variety of learning processes. For example, a case may be developed to demonstrate clinical efficiency of a specific procedure or to showcase a unique clinical condition. Answering the following questions will help the clinician determine the purpose of a specific case development:

- Why document this case?
- Why is this case worth sharing?
- What makes this case different or unique?
- What should others learn or see from this case?

✦ CASE APPLICATION 23-1.1

Case Selection

When Jennifer realized that Mrs. Cronin had specific periodontal challenges, she recognized that the development of this case would satisfy her class assignment and provide an interesting learning experience for her and her classmates.

Considering the Intended Audience

Identifying the intended audience will help determine the quantity and quality of information to be collected and recorded. When routine, thorough documentation has been completed, information can be edited or targeted to accommodate the intended audience. Answering the following questions will help the clinician identify the audience of a specific case:

- Will this case be developed for personal viewing and professional development?
- Will this case be seen and evaluated by instructors, patients, or professional colleagues?

✦ CASE APPLICATION 23-1.2

Case Selection

Jennifer will be presenting her case to her classmates and faculty advisors. A clear understanding of the intended audience may help identify various components of the case that may need to be addressed more thoroughly, briefly, or not at all.

- Will this case be publication ready for use in professional journals or books?

Defining Goals or Expected Outcomes

The overall goal of developing each case should be thoroughly explored.

> **Note**
>
> Understanding why this case should be developed and the value of the finished product may stimulate the effort needed for appropriate case selection and review.

Developing and documenting a case can be time-consuming and demanding. Ideally, when these three issues are addressed, the resulting information can act as an outline for prompting content organization, thoroughness in the design, and precision and objectivity in the implementation and presentation of the case.

CASE DOCUMENTATION

Because the purpose, audience, and goals of each case are varied and unique, the actual components of each case also vary depending on the issues to be addressed. Each case presentation has a unique flow in response to the issues addressed previously. The following discussion of case development is

> **Note**
>
> For the purposes of this chapter, *documentation* refers to the process of recording events, words, or images to reflect aspects of preventive care, therapeutic care, or both.

intended to introduce ideas and options rather than to give specific guidelines. Essentially, proper case design and development centers on thorough and accurate documentation.

According to the *Merriam-Webster Online Language Center* (http://www.webster.com), the definition of *documentation* is the act or an instance of furnishing or authenticating with documents.

Documentation of procedures performed in the patient record is only one facet of case development. Cases may also include the following:

- Record of the patient's present health status
- Health history of patient and family
- Social history
- Beliefs and practices
- Extraoral and intraoral observations
- Charts
- Photographic or radiographic imaging (or both)
- Assessments of self-care
- Identification of oral risks

Notations of the therapeutic interventions and photographic images taken during the course of treatment also may be included to document the progress toward health. Any aspect of an interesting case, procedure performed, diagnostic aid used, or test result may become documented components of a case.

CASE CONTENT

Information about each case may include, but would not be limited to, obtaining information for the patient profile, supporting clinical evidence, and case management details.

Patient Profile

The objective of including a patient profile is to provide basic information about the individual, which introduces the patient to the audience. By sharing information such as age, gender, ethnicity, behavior and beliefs, and professional or familial roles, the case becomes "real" to the audience. Current and historical background information in health, dental, or personal categories often adds essential insight to the components of the case. These categories in case development provide an opportunity to inform the audience of significant and apparently insignificant information that has affected or may have a future influence on the events and strategies within the case. Any of the components of the patient assessment discussed in earlier chapters can provide information to be included in the patient profile.

Clinical Evidence

Clinical evidence representing the actual case may include data obtained from the initial clinical assessment including the following:

- Extraoral and intraoral examination (EIX)
- Periodontal examination
- Indices (gingival, plaque biofilm, and bleeding)
- Radiographic examination
- Oral hygiene assessment
- Caries Management by Risk Assessment (CAMBRA)
- Nutritional assessment

Clinical representation of the case may also include the following components:

- Intraoral photographs or images
- Radiographs
- Diagnostic study casts
- Supplementary diagnostic test results (e.g., genetic testing)
- Salivary testing
- Pulp testing

Because these items represent the patient and must accurately characterize the case when the patient is absent physically, they must be clinically accurate and of high diagnostic quality. Accurate, complete, and thorough documentation is essential to show the patient's current health, any disease progression, and changes that may have occurred because of therapy.

Case Management

Details of case management and proceedings are represented by the documentation of treatment goals and strategies introduced, implemented, and evaluated. Components may include strategies of treatment, instrumentation, oral self-care instruction, patient management, and follow-up evaluations. Organization and clinical accuracy of content must be observed.

Depending on the intended audience, this section could focus on specific strategies that were introduced and accepted by the patient, implemented, and then evaluated after therapy. The clinician may detail the discussion during the introduction of the strategy (or perhaps revisions to initial strategies implemented during the course of therapy) with explanations of when and why strategies needed to be revised. Any of these issues may affect the final outcome or course of the case. By reporting the strategies and variations in treatment, case documentation presents a more realistic case with explanations for and observations of the events or changes that occurred.

CASE PRESENTATION

Cases may be presented in a variety of formats. Oral presentations are the most widely used because of the variety of options in presenting and the interactivity between presenter and audience. Written format also may be developed for use in a document, such as for a journal article or electronic delivery. The purpose of the presentation, the intended audience, and the presentation goals must be addressed to determine the appropriate format. A case that has been thoroughly and accurately documented may be easily adapted to fit either presentation format.

Oral Case Presentation

Oral case presentations provide an opportunity for interaction between the presenter and the audience. The dialog may guide discussion topics and provide feedback toward specific items that may need clarification, further discussion, or both. The purpose of an oral presentation is to verbally address the important issues or elements of the case with the audience. The information may be presented in the following ways:

- In a one-to-one discussion (clinician to patient)
- In a small group such as a gathering of colleagues or patients
- In a large audience such as professional or public meetings

The composition and size of the audience and the amount of time permitted for discussion determines the content to be delivered and the discussion issues to be addressed. To effectively communicate with a given audience, terminology and professional jargon used needs to be appropriate to that audience, and correct pronunciation must be rehearsed.[12] The goal of an oral presentation is to provide an accurate representation of the case and to provide opportunities for discussion and learning at a level appropriate for the audience.

Written Case Presentation

Written case presentations demand a more organized and thorough presentation of the material to ensure all relevant data are covered. Discussion questions are generally included with the written presentation to provide guided-learning opportunities or objectives. The purpose of a written presentation is to distribute a case example that ensures learning opportunities to others. Because of the nature of publication distribution, the scope of the audience is not always known. Therefore when preparing a case presentation in written format, the clinician should avoid professional jargon or nomenclature that may be misinterpreted or misunderstood by the general population. Providing a thor-

> *Note*
> The goal of a written presentation therefore is to distribute a clinically accurate representation of a case that may be reviewed and discussed by anyone.

ough, accurate representation of the case, along with discussion issues that highlight or affect the learning points of the case, is important.

Summary of Case Development, Documentation, and Presentation
[23-1]

Case development requires attention to detail and organization; it forces the clinician to thoroughly seek and document all relevant information that may affect the case or the outcomes of various case specifics. Paying attention to the details of case development assists the clinician in recognizing the value of thorough, accurate record keeping and providing well-constructed strategies for quality patient care. The presentation of a case provides the clinician with an opportunity to design, implement, evaluate, and share the strategies used in the therapeutic management of a particular case. A case presentation may provide an opportunity to review, discuss, evaluate, and learn various aspects of patient care directly from the clinician. Case presentation may also assist the audience in recognizing the value of maintaining high standards of record keeping, therapeutic excellence, and comprehensive quality of oral care. Together, case development, case documentation, and case presentation provide an opportunity for dental professionals to share case examples and learn more about the strategies and challenges that arise during the daily clinical practice of their profession.

⭐ CASE APPLICATION 23-1.3

Example of Case Development and Documentation Guidelines

The following section is an example of case development and documentation guidelines for an upper-level periodontology course. The total assignment was given to Jennifer's class, with the instructions that the students were to complete sections 1 and 2 during the first semester and report their progress on those sections as a midterm assignment.

Case Development and Documentation Assignment
[23-2]

PURPOSE

The purpose of this periodontal case development and documentation exercise is to provide upper-level dental hygiene students the opportunity to select a periodontally involved patient and complete the case documentation, treatment, and posttherapy evaluation for discussion and learning purposes.

AUDIENCE

The audience for the case presentation will be the students' peers and faculty.

GOAL OR EXPECTED OUTCOME

This exercise will provide students with the opportunity to work through a difficult periodontal case, actually implementing treatment and evaluating the efforts of their treatment. The exercise provides students with the opportunity to share their case, strategies, and ideas with classmates. As a result of this exercise, the overall goal is to provide valuable learning experiences and increase understanding of the variety and complexity of treating periodontal cases. Ideally this exercise benefits the student developing the case and the students who view the case presentation.

PATIENT SELECTION GUIDELINES

The patient selected must have active periodontal disease and a plan for periodontal therapy. Ideally the patient should have some unique case feature or features, treatment, or outcome aspect that will provide learning opportunities. Students need to complete the assessment, planned treatment, and post-therapy evaluation on the patient to complete case documentation and presentation requirements for this course.

23-3 | CASE DOCUMENTATION GUIDELINES

Section I: Patient Information

This section is intended to introduce the patient to the audience. Thorough summaries of each of these components provide relevant background information that may affect oral health outcomes:

- *Patient profile.* Summary of basic patient information
- *Patient's chief concern.* Summary of primary purpose of dental visit or main dental concern as reported by patient
- *Health history.* Comprehensive summary of health-related findings
- *Dental history.* Comprehensive summary of dental-related findings
- *Diet history.* Comprehensive summary of diet-related issues
- *Health beliefs and behaviors.* Summary of behavioral characteristics noted during discussion and treatment

Section II: Clinical Evidence

Thorough summaries of each of these components provide descriptive information about the case:

- *Extraoral examination.* Summary of findings
- *Intraoral examination.* Summary of findings
- *Current dental conditions.* Summary of existing restorations, occlusal classification, dental caries risk assessment (CRA), or edentulous conditions
- *Radiographic examination.* Summary of periodontal, restorative, and pathologic findings
- *Periodontal examination.* General summary of periodontal status including probing depths, furcation involvement, mobility, levels of clinical attachment, a gingival

description, American Academy of Periodontology (AAP) classification, and bleeding index

Specific guidelines for clinical evidence

Clinical evidence is intended to provide visual or tangible representation of the patient's clinical findings. Clinical accuracy and thoroughness provide visual information and clinical data relating directly to the case (see Chapters 11 through 22).

- *Intraoral photographs.* Includes all photos necessary to adequately provide documentation and visualization of patient's existing gingival and periodontal condition (see Chapter 18)
- *Study models.* Trimmed and presented according to diagnostic study model guidelines
- *Intraoral radiographs.* Based on diagnostic need of patient; must be of diagnostic quality and mounted correctly (see Chapter 18)
  - *Current or previous complete radiographic series.* Includes all radiographs necessary to adequately assess the patient's oral health status
  - *Current bite-wing series (vertical or horizontal).* Includes radiographs that appropriately assess the proximal status of all teeth
- *Complete and accurate dental and periodontal chart.* (see Chapters 16 and 17)
  - *Existing restorations.*
  - *Existing pathologic condition.*
  - *Probe depths (PD).* Initial visit, posttherapy follow-up visit
  - *Clinical attachment levels.*
  - *Gingival recession.* Clinician should draw in gingival margin and identify mucogingival discrepancies when applicable
  - *Furcations.* Presence, location, and extent properly identified
  - *Mobility.* Classified as I, II, or III
  - *Bleeding.* Noted on chart and summarized as a percentage score
  - *Exudate.* Presence and types determined
  - *Presence and distribution of plaque biofilm and calculus.* Plaque index (PI) summarized as a percentage score
  - *Gingival description.* Color, contour, consistency, location, and extent of involvement (mild, moderate, or severe)
- *Oral health management by risk assessment.* Completed and assessed according to oral risk assessment guidelines; identifies systemic and oral-behavioral risk factors that may contribute to periodontal condition or may influence periodontal therapy (see Chapters 20 and 21)

Section III: Case Management
Planning phase

Thorough summaries of each of these components provide insight strategies in therapy and patient instruction:

- *Rationale for case selection.* Summary

- *Treatment goals and desired outcome.* Summary
- *Initial therapeutic strategy.* Must accurately reflect patient's chief complaint, treatment needs, psychosocial needs, and pain management
- *Preventive education strategy.* Oral heathcare aids to be introduced (when and why)
- *Instrumentation strategy.* Must accurately reflect patient's needs and operator skill level
- *Discussion points with patient.* Possible therapeutic alternatives, potential complications, expected results, patient's responsibility in treatment outcomes, and consequences of no treatment
- *Consent.* Informed or written consent (or both) of treatment strategies

Implementation phase

Thorough summaries of each of these components provide descriptive information about the actual therapeutic and preventive care of the patient during the implementation phase:

- *Date of appointment and number of appointments in series.* Necessary to provide information on spacing interval of treatment and timeline of therapy
- *Actual services completed or treatment performed.* What was actually accomplished on this date and appointment number
- *Treatment revisions with rationale.* Identifies changes in treatment plan and discusses reasons why changes to original therapeutic strategies were implemented
- *Patient care.* Identifies how the patient is responding to care and answers questions such as the following: Is the patient more or less motivated? Is the patient evaluating or noticing his or her own progress and healing? Is the patient having postoperative pain or sensitivity, and is that concern being addressed during the appointment?
- *Self-care.* Summarizes patient's progress with preventive education plan and discusses rationale for home care aids being introduced or changed to meet therapeutic and psychosocial goals

Posttreatment assessment (4 to 6 weeks)

The clinician should thoroughly describe the patient's post-therapy clinical evaluation findings. Summaries of each of these components provide descriptive information about the therapeutic and preventive outcomes and identify future needs of the patient, as follows:

- *Intraoral photographs.* As indicated
- *Review of chief complaint, health history, and EIX.* Whether completed care addressed goals, risks, and patient concerns; summary of health history update; and changes in EIX noted
- *Periodontal examination.* Summary of PDs, bleeding on probing (BOP), PI, and gingival description

- *Oral home care outcomes.* Summary of patient's understanding and effectiveness of oral hygiene, current recommendations based on CAMBRA, biological indicators (BIs), PI, PDs, and gingival description
- *Therapeutic outcomes.* Summary of effectiveness of previously performed periodontal therapy and assessment of patient's response
- *Discussion points with patient.* Based on results of examination, status of patient's disease, therapeutic alternatives, potential complications, expected results, and patient's responsibilities regarding treatment; explanation of consequences of no treatment
- *Future care recommendations.*
  - *Indications for referrals.* Clinician should specify referral protocol
  - *Active therapy continued.* Possible need for further active therapy, in which dental caries or periodontal management might include antimicrobial therapy (site-specific or systemic) or further debridement (localized or generalized); specific actions and therapeutic strategy for continued active therapy
  - *Dental caries management and periodontal maintenance therapy.* Interval recommended for the control of dental caries or maintenance of a healthy periodontium

Student evaluation of therapeutic and preventive outcomes

This section is intended to provide the student an opportunity to discuss planning, implementation, and evaluation of the therapeutic and preventive strategies as applied to the case. Supporting documentation from current scientific literature may be introduced at this time to validate the therapeutic strategies. Thorough summaries of each of these components provide self-evaluation opportunities and appraisal of lessons learned, as follows:

- What was learned from treating the case? (summary)
- Which modifications would enhance treatment outcomes? (summary)

Study questions and answers

A minimum of three study questions will need to be included in every section. This exercise is intended to identify discussion topics and items of clinical interest that may be addressed with the case. Evidence-based support for therapeutic strategies may be considered to encourage decision-making skills based on current scientific literature. (Three questions from each of the three sections are developed that can be drawn from the case as a learning or discussion point.)

Jennifer's Completed Case Assignment

The following information represents sections I and II of Jennifer's completed case documentation assignment.

Section I
Patient Profile
Ann Cronin, a 70-year-old retired seamstress, is a new patient to the dental practice. She recently has moved and now lives with her daughter, son-in-law, and three grandchildren. She is concerned that her small monthly pension will not cover her financial needs and has asked to delay any major dental treatment. (Mrs. Cronin's patient record can be located on this text's accompanying CD-ROM. All forms used to summarize the following information are included in the record.)

Chief Concern
Mrs. Cronin complains that her lower partial denture does not fit. She occasionally has not worn her partial denture for several days at a time.

Health History
Mrs. Cronin takes estrogen (Premarin) 1.25 mg once a day and celecoxib (Celebrex) 100 mg twice a day for arthritis. She began smoking when she was 16 years old but quit more than 5 years ago.

Dental History
Mrs. Cronin says that her teeth are sensitive to cold. She does not add ice to her beverages; she finds that her mouth is quite dry and believes that she needs to sip beverages or suck mints constantly to relieve her "dry throat." This visit is her first dental visit in 3 years. She uses a medium toothbrush with fluoridated toothpaste, brushes once a day, and uses an over-the-counter (OTC) mouthrinse. Mrs. Cronin reports that she has difficulty holding the toothbrush and does not think that she does an adequate job of cleaning her mouth.

Diet History
Mrs. Cronin sucks on mints throughout the day because of her dry mouth. Her sugar intake is also evident in the four cups of sweetened coffee she consumes during the day. Mrs. Cronin enjoys snacking on chips, cookies, and crackers.

Health Beliefs and Behaviors
Mrs. Cronin says that she believes that she is more likely than most people to have cavities. She feels that she has spent a good deal of her adult life in the dental chair. She also believes in the importance of oral self-care to prevent dental caries and periodontal disease and says she welcomes recommendations. She does not want to change any current habits and does not believe that she is in control of her oral health.

Mrs. Cronin receives a physical examination annually and adheres to her physician's advice but only sometimes changes her health behaviors on the recommendation of a dental professional. She reports that her eating habits are out of control and that she does not exercise or participate in sports or recreational activities.

Section I Questions
1. Of what relevance to the supportive care appointment is Mrs. Cronin's chief complaint?
2. Does her diet support oral disease?
3. What concerns do her current health beliefs and behaviors present to health promotion and disease prevention?

Section II
Extraoral Examination
Mrs. Cronin has bilateral 5-mm × 3- to 4-mm crusted areas at the commissures. No other extraoral findings were noted.

Intraoral Examination
Mrs. Cronin is partially edentulous (mandibular posterior regions with generalized multisurface amalgam restorations on remaining posterior teeth). She has buccal Class V composite restorations on most of her maxillary teeth, with evidence of 2- to 6-mm recession throughout. No active dental caries activity is apparent on hard tissue examination; her occlusal classification is a Class II incisor relationship. Mrs. Cronin's intraoral photographs are taken (Figure 23-1).

Radiographic Examination
Radiographic findings reveal vertical bone loss with apparent subgingival calculus present on the mesial of tooth #2. Vertical bone loss is apparent between teeth #3 and #4; however, on closer inspection the problem is determined to be horizontal bone loss (following the cementoenamel junction [CEJ] from tooth to tooth). Generalized minimal horizontal bone loss is evident through tooth #13, where once again vertical bone loss is seen around tooth #13. Mandibular posterior regions are edentulous with the exception of tooth #32 (with generalized 1- to 2-mm horizontal bone loss). Radiographs also reveal post buildup on tooth #20, several anterior composite restorations, and posterior amalgam restorations of varying condition. The pathologic condition observed is an apparent overhang (or overcontoured mesial #3) and possible dental caries under teeth #13 distal and #14 mesial; no other restorative areas of concern are noted.

Periodontal Examination
The patient has generalized 1- to 6-mm recession with PDs within normal range of 1 to 4 mm. She has Class I furcation involvement on the buccal furcation of teeth #1, #3, #14, and #15, with no mobility concerns. The clinician notes generalized healthy, pink, firm gingival tissue with an AAP periodontal classification of Class II chronic periodontitis; the patient's current condition is recorded as stable, with a 10% bleeding index.

Clinical Evidence
Intraoral images are taken—direct facial, right facial, left facial, maxillary occlusal, and mandibular occlusal views (see Figure 23-1). A complete series of radiographs is taken (Figure 23-2). Figure 23-3 shows the patient's dental chart, and Figure 23-4 shows her periodontal chart.

Section II Questions
1. Review Mrs. Cronin's intraoral photographs (see Figure 23-1) for the appearance of her soft and hard tissues. Given the narrative, were the findings what you expected?
2. Review findings of the CRA. Did the CRA findings correlate with radiographic and clinical assessment findings?

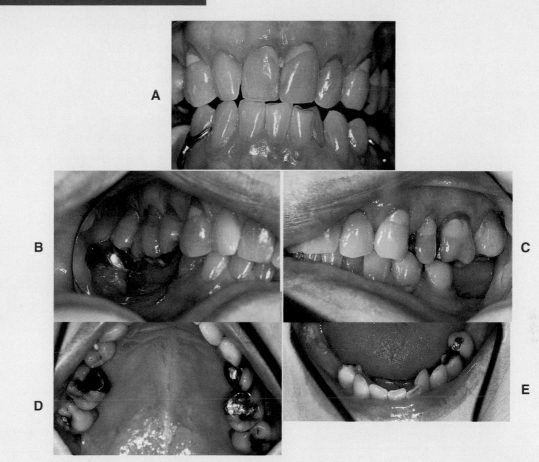

FIGURE 23-1
Intraoral images. **A,** Direct facial. **B,** Right facial. **C,** Left facial. **D,** Maxillary occlusal. **E,** Mandibular occlusal.

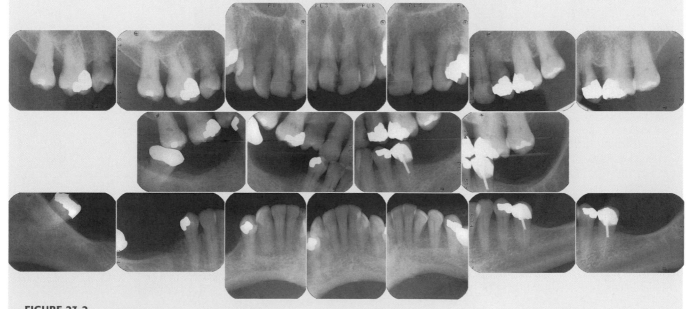

FIGURE 23-2
Complete series of radiographs of the patient's mouth.

Continued

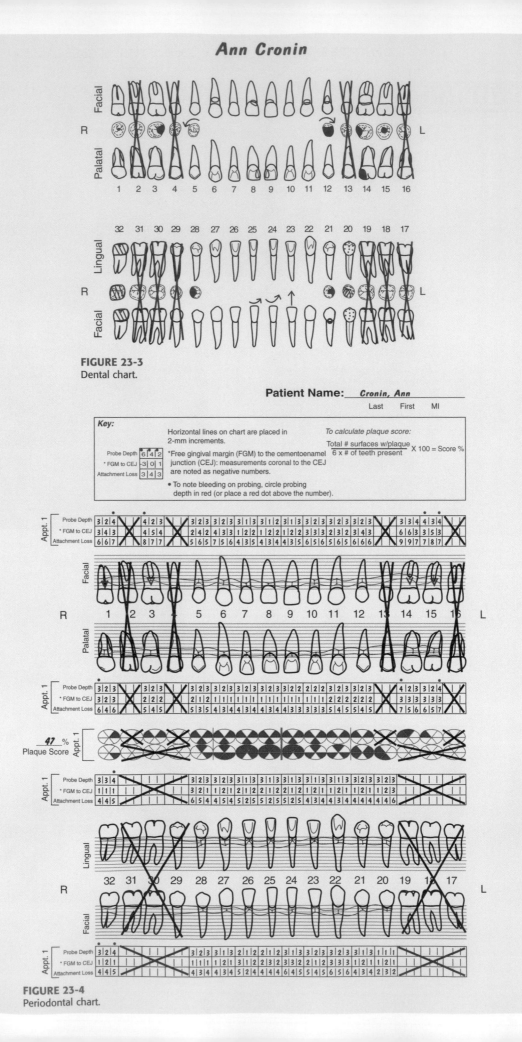

FIGURE 23-3
Dental chart.

FIGURE 23-4
Periodontal chart.

References

1. Belcher JV: Improving managers' critical thinking skills: student-generated case studies, *J Nurs Adm* 30(7-8):351-353, 2000.

2. Bowen DM: Integrating case-based instruction into dental hygiene curricula, *J Dent Educ* 62(3):253-256, 1998.

3. Clark GT, Koyano K, Nivichanov A: Case-based learning for orofacial pain and temporomandibular disorders, *J Dent Educ* 57:815 820, 1996.

4. Coleman PW: An overview of case-based test construction, *J Dent Educ* 62(3):242-247, 1998.

5. Daniel SJ: Case-based methods for dental hygiene faculty, *J Dent Educ* 62(3):230, 1998.

6. Dowd SB, Daviodhizer R: Using case studies to teach clinical problem-solving, *Nurse Educ* 24(5):42-46, 1999.

7. Engel FE, Hendricson WD: A case-based learning model in orthodontics, *J Dent Educ* 58:762-767, 1994.

8. Hendricson WD, Berlocher WC, Herbert RJ: A four year longitudinal study of dental students learning styles, *J Dent Educ* 41:175-181, 1987.

9. Jones DC, Sheridan ME: A case study approach: developing critical thinking skills in novice pediatric nurses, *J Contin Educ Nurs* 30(2):75-78, 1999.

10. Kassebaum KD, Averbach RE, Fryer GE: Student preference for a case-based vs lecture instructional format, *J Dent Educ* 44:781-784, 1991.

11. Lindesman HM, Bilan JP: Dental education and practice in the 21st century: opportunities for excellence, *J Prosthet Dent* 75:660-665, 1996.

12. Miller L: Presenting your case: solid verbal skills lay out the facts for periodontal treatment, *RDH* 17(5):26-28, 30, 58, 1997.

13. Norman GR, Schmidt HG: The psychological basis of problem-based learning: a review of the evidence, *Acad Med* 67:557-565, 1992.

14. Vaughan DA, DeBiase CB, Gibson-Howell JC: Use of case-based learning in dental hygiene curricula, *J Dent Educ* 62(3):257-259, 1998.

15. Woodall IR, Dafoe B: Case documentation. In Woodall IR, ed: *Comprehensive dental hygiene care,* ed 4, St Louis, 1993, Mosby.

CHAPTER

24

Devices for Oral Self-Care

Caren M. Barnes • Joan I. Gluch •

Deborah M. Lyle • Carol A. Jahn

INSIGHT

Dental plaque biofilm control is the most important factor in obtaining and sustaining optimal oral health. Plaque (i.e., dental biofilm) must be mechanically removed, and daily cleaning with a toothbrush and other interdental aids is the most dependable means by which to achieve and maintain this status. The role and professional responsibility of a dental hygienist is to provide oral health education and skill development for each patient as part of comprehensive dental hygiene patient care. Importantly, oral hygiene instruction for plaque biofilm control should be patient centered and individualized to meet the patient's oral conditions and biopsychosocial aspects and abilities to ensure optimal adherence to an oral self-care regimen.

✦ CASE STUDY 24-1   Specific Oral Self-Care Recommendations

Mrs. Ann Cronin (a patient included on the CD-ROM that accompanies this text) is a 70-year-old retired seamstress. She arrives at the clinic as a new patient who has recently moved to the area and is living in a multigenerational environment with her daughter and family. Mrs. Cronin is concerned that her small monthly pension will not cover her dental needs. She is arthritic, for which she takes extra-strength ibuprofen, and menopausal, for which she has visited a compounding pharmacy that has given her a "bioidentical hormone" supplement. On her prevention survey, Mrs. Cronin reports that she has sensitive teeth, a dry mouth, and a partial denture that does not fit. Her current oral hygiene measures include brushing once daily with a medium toothbrush, rinsing with a mouthrinse, and using whatever fluoridated dentifrice her daughter buys for the grandchildren. Her dental status reveals missing teeth; multiple restorations including crowns, amalgams, and composites; rotated teeth; a 47% plaque index (PI); and periodontal involvement of several teeth. The patient feels that prevention is important but that she is more likely than the average person to have oral problems. In addition, she does not see how she could change a habit at this time and does not believe she has control over the conditions in her mouth. Please access the patient schedule on the CD-ROM accompanying this textbook for Mrs. Ann Cronin's record.

KEY TERMS

anatomical considerations	evidence-based decision making	International Organization for Standardization	powered toothbrushes
Bass method	floss holder		rolling-stroke method
brush-head design	floss threader	manual toothbrush	rotating-oscillating
Charters method	Fones method	modified Stillman's method	rotating-oscillating-pulsating
dental floss	gingival architecture	multitufted	sonic
dental tape	handle design	oscillating-pulsating-pivoting	textured floss
disclosing solution	horizontal-scrub method	patient compliance	toothbrushing methods
end-rounded bristles	interdental brushes	plaque biofilm control	ultrasonic
end-tufted brush		power flossers	

LEARNING OUTCOMES

After reading this chapter the student will be able to:

1. Describe and explain the appropriate use of and oral health indications for the following categories of oral self-care devices: toothbrushes, interdental cleaners, dental floss, and dental water jet.
2. Identify the appropriate components of a randomized clinical trial.
3. Provide a rationale for oral self-care product selection based on evidence-based decision making, patient need, and anatomical considerations.
4. Explain the role of self-evaluation in plaque biofilm control. Explain how disclosing solutions or tablets can be used in a patient's individualized oral self-care plan.

5. Monitor and recommend modifications for patient use of oral self-care products based on therapeutic intervention planning.
6. Provide a rationale for recommending a manual or powered toothbrush to a patient.
7. Describe features that can be found on modern powered toothbrushes.
8. Identify differences in the mechanism of action among different types of powered toothbrushes.
9. Demonstrate the appropriate way to use the jet tip irrigator tip and the Pik Pocket tip to a patient.
10. Determine the appropriate irrigation tip to recommend to a patient.

Oral Self-Care Recommendations

CLINICAL CHALLENGE

Oral self-care instruction and self-care device and product recommendations are as important as the dental hygiene services provided for the long-term oral health of a patient. Failure to provide adequate oral self-care instruction is not only unethical but also can be viewed as supervised neglect. Conversely, patients have a responsibility to comply with oral self-care instructions; if a patient is noncompliant, then this must be documented in the patient's records. Oral hygiene instructions alone will not produce superior results, just as enthusiasm alone will not produce a plaque biofilm–free mouth. However, when patients have the appropriate knowledge, skill, and motivation to complete good home care procedures each day, optimal oral health can be achieved.

PATIENT EXPECTATIONS

Patients depend on dental hygienists for expert knowledge in oral health and gain confidence when they are provided with professional recommendations and counseling. The positive effect that oral care product recommendation and oral self-care instruction has on a patients' overall long-term oral health is significant.

When patients are confronted with hundreds of dental products to choose from, brand and formula-specific recommendations are important to eliminate confusion and frustration.[91]

Prevention

The role dental hygienists play in the recommendation of oral care products cannot be overemphasized. Consumers report that dental professionals are the most important source for oral self-care information. As consumers, patients are eager for specific information to help them make the right choices about their preventive oral care, especially given the multitude of products from which they can select.

MAKING DECISIONS BASED ON SCIENTIFIC EVIDENCE

The number of oral care products available for patients to choose from and for professionals to recommend is rapidly growing. Dental hygienists must keep up with oral care product development and have an ethical responsibility to maintain access to and stay current with the literature, the research, and the scientific knowledge regarding oral hygiene products.

Healthcare professionals should make decisions based on scientific literature and practice experiences, otherwise known as **evidence-based decision making**[68] (see Chapter 4). Dental hygienists need to continually keep abreast of new information by reading professional journals and accessing a number of the on-line literature databases and sources for systematic reviews. Evidence-based decision making requires the evaluation of the applicable and credible literature (Box 24-1) to determine whether the studies are well designed and appropriate for the patient's clinical conditions.

BOX 24-1

RESEARCH STUDY PARAMETERS TO BE USED IN EVIDENCE-BASED EVALUATIONS

- *Adequate size.* The study population is large enough to show a statistical difference ($p \geq .05$).
- *Study population.* The group of patients to be studied is appropriate for what is to be studied.
- *Blinded.* The study examiner does not know which patients are using which experimental product.
- *Experimental group.* This group receives the experimental product.
- *Control group.* This group receives the same product without the active ingredient (i.e., a placebo).
- *Duration.* The study is conducted long enough to show a difference in the parameter being studied.

Unfortunately, some randomized clinical trials that investigate the efficacy and safety of oral healthcare products and devices are inadequately reported or have poor design. The inadequate reporting of the results of clinical trials borders on unethical practice when biased results receive false credibility.[83] Examples of inadequate reporting or poor design include the following:

- Not truly randomizing subjects

- Failure to include adequate numbers of subjects to obtain credible results
- Unbalanced groups
- Not evaluating the success of "blinding" (masking) examiners
- Not including information regarding the calibration of examiners

For healthcare providers to evaluate the credibility of research, they must be able to understand the study design, how the study is conducted, as well as the analysis and interpretation of the results. For this understanding to be achieved, the authors must be forthcoming and transparent.[59] In the 1990s investigators and editors of scientific journals developed a document known as the *CONSORT* (Consolidated Standards of Reporting Trials) statement. The CONSORT statement is composed of a checklist and flowchart (Table 24-1) that has two important uses:

1. It serves as a guide for authors to improve reporting of clinical trials results.
2. It enables the reader to understand how clinical trials are conducted and how to assess the validity of reported results.

Patients will rely on the dental hygienist's knowledge and expertise as an oral care professional to provide them with the information and instruction they need to achieve and maintain a lifetime of optimal oral health. Dental hygienists recognize toothbrushing and interdental cleaning as an important element in the prevention of dental caries and periodontal disease;

Table 24-1	**CONSORT Checklist and Flowchart Guidelines for Improving the Reporting of Clinical Trials**	
PAPER SECTION AND TOPIC	**ITEM**	**DESCRIPTION**
Title and Abstract	1	How participants were allocated to interventions (e.g., random allocation, randomized, or randomly assigned).
Introduction and Background	2	Scientific background and explanation of rationale.
Methods and Participants	3	Eligibility criteria for participants and the settings and locations where the data were collected.
Interventions	4	Precise details of the interventions intended for each group and how and when they were actually administered.
Objectives	5	Specific objectives and hypotheses.
Outcomes	6	Clearly defined primary and secondary outcome measures and, when applicable, any methods used to enhance the quality of measurements (e.g., multiple observations, training of assessors).
Sample Size	7	How sample size was determined and, when applicable, explanation of any interim analyses and stopping rules.
Randomization—Sequence Generation	8	Method used to generate the random allocation sequence, including details of any restrictions (e.g., blocking, stratification).
Randomization—Allocation Concealment	9	Method used to implement the random allocation sequence (e.g., numbered containers or central telephone), clarifying whether the sequence was concealed until interventions were assigned.
Randomization—Implementation	10	Who generated the allocation sequence, who enrolled participants, and who assigned participants to their groups.
Blinding (Masking)	11	Whether or not participants, those administering the interventions, and those assessing the outcomes were blinded to group assignment. When relevant, how the success of blinding was evaluated.
Statistical Methods	12	Statistical methods used to compare groups for primary outcome(s); methods for additional analyses, such as subgroup analyses and adjusted analyses.

Adapted from CONSORT web site [http://www.consort-statement.org/]. Accessed June 5, 2006.

Table 24-1	CONSORT Checklist and Flowchart Guidelines for Improving the Reporting of Clinical Trials—cont'd

PAPER SECTION AND TOPIC	ITEM	DESCRIPTION
Results Participant Flow	13	Flow of participants through each stage (a diagram is strongly recommended). Specifically, for each group report the numbers of participants randomly assigned, receiving intended treatment, completing the study protocol, and analyzed for the primary outcome. Describe protocol deviations from study as planned, together with reasons.
Recruitment	14	Dates defining the periods of recruitment and follow-up.
Baseline Data	15	Baseline demographic and clinical characteristics of each group.
Numbers Analyzed	16	Number of participants (denominator) in each group included in each analysis and whether the analysis was by intention-to-treat. State the results in absolute numbers when feasible (e.g., 10/20, not 50%).
Outcomes and Estimation	17	For each primary and secondary outcome, a summary of results for each group, and the estimated effect size and its precision (e.g., 95% confidence interval).
Ancillary Analyses	18	Address multiplicity by reporting any other analyses performed, including subgroup analyses and adjusted analyses, indicating those prespecified and those exploratory.
Adverse Events	19	All important adverse events or side effects in each intervention group.
Discussion and Interpretation	20	Interpretation of the results, taking into account study hypotheses, sources of potential bias or imprecision and the dangers associated with multiplicity of analyses and outcomes.
Generalizability	21	Generalizability (external validity) of the trial findings.
Overall Evidence	22	General interpretation of the results in the context of current evidence.

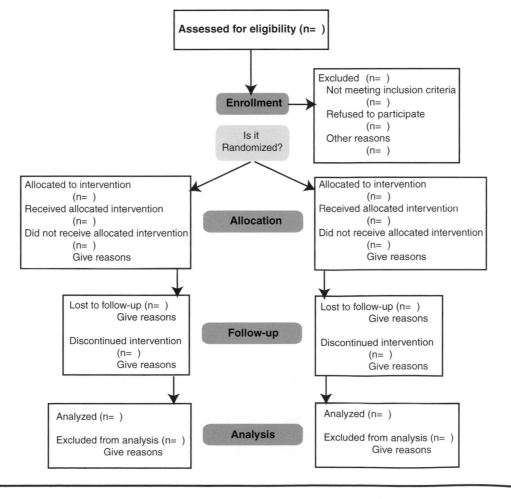

however, many patients view these efforts as merely a means to fresher breath and an esthetically pleasing smile.

Anatomical Considerations and Physical Challenges to Oral Self-Care

ANATOMICAL CONSIDERATIONS

Dental professionals need to identify and explain the topography of the oral structures to their patients and select self-care products that best help the patient in thorough biofilm removal. When patients have products that are easy to use and fit their oral conditions, they will perform self-care more skillfully and frequently. In addition, they will be more motivated and confident in their home care procedures.

> *Prevention*
>
> **Plaque biofilm control** is the consistent removal of dental plaque biofilm from teeth and gingival surfaces. However, complete and thorough removal of all dental plaque biofilm is not always readily accomplished because of the unique architectural features of the mouth, teeth, and tissues.

Just as an individual has a unique history and experiences, the physiologic condition of each person presents dental healthcare providers with challenges and distinct cues in selecting products and procedures to help achieve optimal oral self-care. Using the oral cavity architecture as a guide, the clinician can evaluate several specific elements to help formulate the appropriate recommendations:

- Lips
- Alveolar architecture and tooth position
- Tori and maxillary tuberosities
- Tongue mobility and dorsal surface
- **Gingival architecture**
- Interproximal embrasures

Lips

The width and elasticity of the opening to the oral cavity can have an effect on the size and shape of the toothbrush head and type of interproximal-cleaning procedures recommended. For example, if the lips are tight and nonelastic, then this makes the opening to the oral cavity small. A small oral cavity opening would make it frustrating for a patient to use a toothbrush with a large, square head or an interproximal cleansing method that requires the patient to see at least some posterior proximal surfaces.

> *Distinct Care Modifications*
>
> On opening the mouth, patients should be able to see at least the mesial of the first molars and place a toothbrush in the vestibular areas (both anterior and posterior). If this is not possible, then a toothbrush with a smaller head and thinner handle should be recommended for the patient.

To facilitate ease of oral self-care procedures, the elasticity of the lip and degree to which the mouth can be opened should be assessed.

In addition, patients should be able to manipulate an interproximal-cleaning device or product to the distal of the distal-most tooth present. If this is not possible, then recommendations should be amended to accommodate the specific abilities of the patient.

Alveolar Architecture and Tooth Position

The next step in selecting an appropriate oral self-care device is to evaluate the size and shape of the teeth, the overall alveolar architecture of the attached and unattached gingiva, and the teeth together (as a unit).

The brushing plane of a toothbrush, or the surface used to actually perform the cleaning, varies from a fairly flat plane to one gently curved to one that is completely uneven (Figure 24-1). Although little evidence supports that any one brushing plane is superior to another, the American Dental Association's (ADA's) Council on Scientific Affairs lends credibility to the point that a brush must conform to an individual's needs.[3,69]

DENTAL CONSIDERATIONS

The position of the facial, lingual, and palatal surfaces in relationship to the alveolar mucosa should be taken into consideration when selecting the most appropriate toothbrush and toothbrushing method.

Teeth that are tilted toward the palatal surface of the maxilla or the lingual surface of the mandible require close scrutiny when selecting a brush, as well as in selecting a brushing method and advising patients on brush placement. When teeth are tilted this way, the palatal areas at the gingival one third of the tooth surface hold much more plaque biofilm than teeth that are more vertically aligned. Typically a patient with this type of oral architecture is completely unaware of the difficulty this type of tooth alignment presents in oral self-care. Most patients are not able to see these surfaces and, at best, can feel them only with the tongue to determine whether they feel free of biofilm.

Reviewing the vertical dimension of the teeth and alveolar process as a unit from the facial perspective should be completed. Questions to ask during this evaluation include the following:

- Do the teeth appear to be constricted at the neck or gingival one third of the tooth to the extent that a plaque biofilm–retentive area is formed?
- Are teeth malpositioned, creating plaque biofilm traps?
- Will a typical brush stroke, if not appropriately placed, actually miss the critical area of plaque biofilm retention?
- What size brush head will be the easiest for this patient to manipulate?

Teeth with no adjacent tooth can result in an unusual interdental space and interdental papilla configuration; such teeth may require special brushing instructions and interdental cleaning recommendations. In addition, teeth with no opposing tooth, crowded teeth, and teeth with large diastemas pose challenges to oral care recommendations.

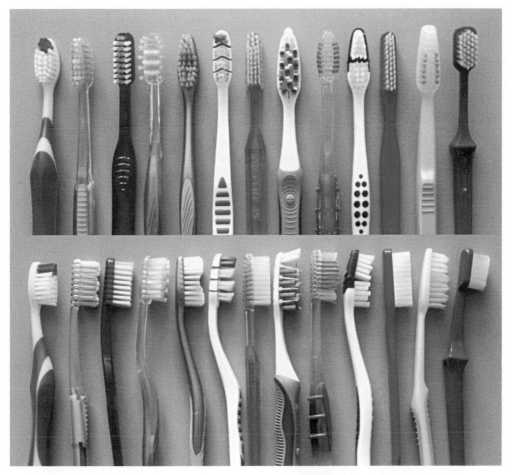

FIGURE 24-1
Example of brushing planes of various toothbrushes. (From Cappelli DP, Mobley CC: *Prevention in Clinical Oral Health Care,* St Louis, 2008, Mosby.)

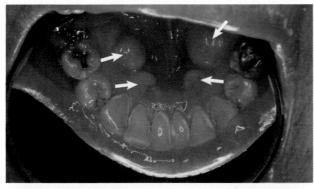

FIGURE 24-2
Manidbular tori. (From Ibsen OAC, Phelan JA: *Oral pathology for the dental hygienist,* ed 4, Philadelphia, Saunders, 2004.)

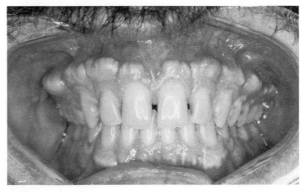

FIGURE 24-3
Maxillary exostoses. (From Ibsen OAC, Phelan JA: *Oral pathology for the dental hygienist,* ed 4, Philadelphia, Saunders, 2004.)

Tori and Maxillary Tuberosities

Tori (Figure 24-2) pose additional **anatomical considerations** to recommended oral self-care regimens. Large mandibular tori may require the use of a very small toothbrush head, such as a child's brush, used only in a vertical direction. Maxillary exostoses (Figure 24-3) on the facial aspects of the alveolus likewise should be evaluated in toothbrush and brushing method selection.

Tongue Mobility and Dorsal Surface

The mobility of the tongue is important to functions of speech, mastication, and self-evaluation of plaque biofilm removal. The inability of a patient to place his or her tongue at the distal-most surface of the distal-most tooth in either arch significantly alters the ability to determine successful plaque biofilm removal and will require the suggestion of alternative methods for oral self-care evaluation.

The dorsal surface of the tongue is replete with thousands of plaque biofilm–retentive spaces. Selecting the best plaque biofilm removal method will require close examination of this surface to determine whether the surface is fissured or fairly smooth. In addition, the hygienist should determine whether the tongue is coated and the reason for the coating so that he or she is able to recommend the best products to patients. When patients have highly fissured and coated tongues, the hygienist should recommend more frequent tongue cleaning, the use of a specific tongue scraper, or chemotherapeutic products (or a combination of these techniques) to aid in thorough plaque biofilm removal. (See Chapter 38, which includes images of tongue cleaners and cleaning.)

Gingival Architecture

Gingival recession, clefting, and rolled gingival margins (Figure 24-4) are not only the result of inappropriate plaque biofilm removal techniques but also create plaque biofilm–retentive areas difficult to reach without special and very specific instructions. Each area needs to be carefully evaluated and solutions discussed with the patient.

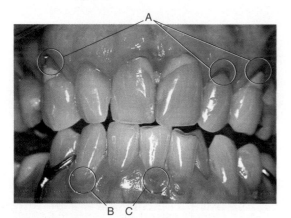

FIGURE 24-4
This patient has several areas of gingival recession as seen in *A*, examples of rolled margins at *B*, and gingival clefting at *C*.

✦ CASE APPLICATION 24-1.1

Oral Considerations in Oral Self-Care Device Recommendation

The intraoral examination of Mrs. Cronin reveals several significant findings that will affect the oral self-care device recommendations. Her crusted commisures, xerostomia, and sensitive teeth (in concert with the anatomical observations) should lead to numerous questions for the dental hygienist. What questions would the hygienist have?

The hygienist working with Ann had the following questions: Will her lips be elastic enough to get a cleaning device to the distal of the maxillary second molars with ease? How much room is there between the cheeks and the gingival one third of the tooth? How can Ann be guided to more effectively clean the gingival margins?

What questions would the hygienist have regarding tooth positions, recession, clefting, rolled margins, and interproximal embrasure spaces?

Interproximal Embrasures

The anatomical factors affecting the selection of interdental cleaning aids include the following:
- Size and shape of the embrasure
- Tooth position and alignment
- Contour and consistency of gingival tissues

The shape of the interdental space can vary from tooth to tooth and can range from no recession and a tight healthy papilla to no papilla present at all. Selecting the best interproximal-cleaning aid will be based on efficiency in removing plaque biofilm from the interproximal space and the consistency of the gingival tissues.

Embrasure spaces (Figure 24-5) have been classified in three basic classes:

Class I—No gingival recession with the interdental papilla filling the space
Class II —Moderate papillary recession
Class III—Complete loss of the interdental papilla

PHYSICAL CHALLENGES

After a careful evaluation of the oral architecture for the acceptance and selection of an oral cleaning device, the clinician should gain an appreciation of the patient's physical abilities in terms of dexterity and eyesight.

Dental professionals should work with patients to understand their capabilities and limitations and to recommend specific products to address their needs. For example, many patients prefer **powered toothbrushes** because they are easier to use and reduce the skill necessary to brush independently. As the patient ages, family members or caregivers may have to complete oral hygiene for the patient (especially when disabilities are more severe). However, promoting independence as long as possible is best, especially when adaptive oral hygiene aids are available.

> *Distinct Care Modifications*
> Conditions of the hands such as arthritis can make oral self-care difficult and painful. In addition, diminished eyesight or any vision problems can make it more difficult for patients to identify plaque biofilm and **disclosing solution** in their mouths, as well as to check that they are using proper technique.

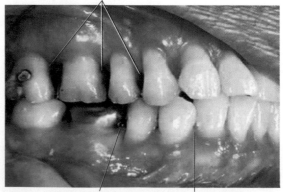

FIGURE 24-5
This patient's mouth exhibits Class I, II, and III embrasures.

Device Modifications

For example, the handle can be wrapped in foam or soft tubing to increase the width and comfort, or the handle can be placed

in a slit cut in a tennis ball so that patients have a wider and more stable grasp (Figure 24-6). The handles of most powered toothbrushes are longer and wider and can provide a more secure grip in addition to easier access. In addition, a toothbrush can be placed in a Velcro strap that many disabled individuals use to hold spoons or other adaptive aids to allow brushing with little finger or hand movement. Last, the clinician can angle a toothbrush handle by placing it under hot running water and bending it to provide additional adaptation to make oral hygiene easier for patients.

✳ CASE APPLICATION 24-1.2

Modifications of Oral Self-Care Devices

Mrs. Cronin, a retired seamstress, does have arthritis evident in both hands, predominantly in her fingers. The ultimate oral self-care devices selected will probably have to be modified to accommodate this physical challenge. The degree of difficulty she will experience will have to be assessed.

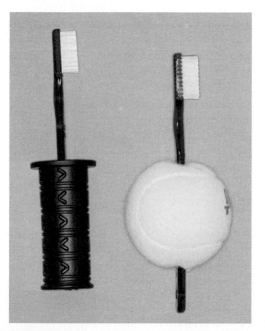

FIGURE 24-6
Toothbrush modifications.

Oral Self-Care Devices

DISCLOSING AGENTS

Both the dental professional and the patient use disclosing agents to determine the exact location of plaque biofilm.

Composition

Disclosing agents are usually composed of an erythrosine dye, are manufactured as a liquid or a tablet (Figure 24-7), and are designed to make plaque biofilm visible (Figure 24-8). Some agents stain plaque biofilm pink or red, whereas others are two-toned and show mature plaque biofilm in purple or violet and immature plaque biofilm in red or pink. The disclosing solutions containing fluorescein dye stain plaque biofilm yellow and are then viewed using a battery-operated blue light that causes the disclosed plaque biofilm to fluoresce. The fluorescein dye is available in small bottles or in prefilled applicators. A battery-operated light is available for use in the operatory, and a pen light version is designed for the patient's personal use.

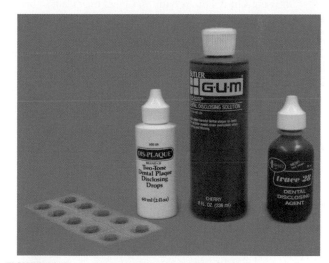

FIGURE 24-7
Disclosing solutions and tablets. (Courtesy Peggy Cain, College of Dentistry, University of Nebraska Medical Center, Lincoln, Neb.)

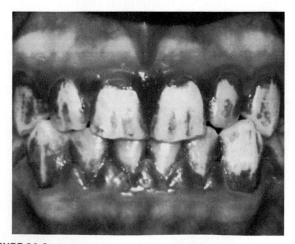

FIGURE 24-8
Disclosed plaque biofilm.

Uses

Disclosing agents can be used to do the following:

- Educate patients to the cause of disease
- Motivate patients for better self-cleaning
- Evaluate the effectiveness of oral self-care

> ### Patient Education Opportunity
>
> Educating the patient to the presence of disease, presence of plaque biofilm, and the removal or disturbance of the bacteria is essential. Disclosing agents provide patients with an image of the location of plaque biofilm and therefore can assist the patient with removal.

Patients cannot see plaque biofilm and are often unaware that red and bleeding gingiva are a result of the bacteria present within the plaque biofilm.

Disclosing agents can be used to measure the amount of plaque biofilm on the teeth and provide objective evidence of the success of plaque biofilm removal. The patient can be advised to use the disclosing agent before brushing and cleaning interdentally to disclose the plaque biofilm and then check for any stained areas that are missed. On the other hand, patients may elect to brush and clean interdentally first (then use a disclosing agent to check to see if they have missed any areas).

A number of PIs are available that dental professionals can use to quantitatively record and evaluate the effectiveness of patients' home care procedures (see Chapters 16 and 20). Disclosing agents allow assessment of these indices and can be used at maintenance appointments to evaluate a patient's progress and compliance with oral hygiene instruction.

DENTAL CONSIDERATIONS

The clinician should note that tissue assessment should be complete before the use of a disclosing agent, otherwise the tissues will also be stained from the solution and a misdiagnosis could occur.

TOOTHBRUSHES

Historical Perspective

Since ancient times people have made devices for cleaning their teeth. Chewing sticks were most likely the first toothbrushes made by Babylonians as early as 3500 BC. These chew sticks, also called *siwaks* (Figure 24-9), were small twigs that were frayed by chewing on the ends and rubbing the frayed ends against the teeth.[108,111] Bristle toothbrushes (made from coarse, stiff hog's hair attached to handles made of bone or bamboo) appeared in China around 1498. These toothbrushes were exported to Europe, where people found the boar bristles to be too stiff (causing their gums to bleed); they substituted horsehair for the boar's hair. By the seventeenth century, Europeans were using rags or sponges dipped in sulfur oil or salt to rub their teeth clean, so they were essentially mopping their teeth instead of brushing.

The first mass-produced toothbrushes appeared in England around 1780. William Addis of Clerkenwald, England, made these brushes. The first American to patent a toothbrush was H.N. Wadworth in 1857; mass production of toothbrushes in the United States began after the Civil War, around 1885.

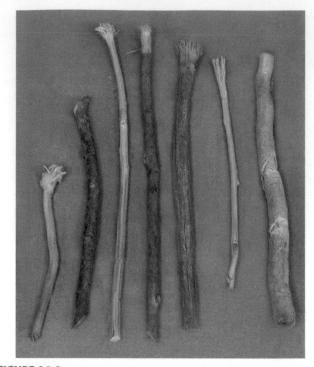

FIGURE 24-9
Ancient chew sticks, known as *siwaks* for tooth cleaning used by Babylonians as early as 3500 BC. (Courtesy the Dental Museum, College of Dentistry, University of Nebraska Medical Center, Lincoln, Neb.)

Wallace H. Carothere, who worked for the DuPont Laboratories, invented nylon in 1937; in 1938 nylon bristle toothbrushes were produced and marketed.[65] The first nylon-bristled American toothbrush was marketed as Dr. West's Miracle Toothbrush[79] (Figure 24-10). Another early mass-produced toothbrush was the Pro-phy-lac-tic Brush (Figure 24-11), made by the Florence Manufacturing Company of Massachusetts. It was not until after World War II that that regular toothbrushing became common in all parts of the United States (soldiers returning from the war brought this habit home from Europe).

The toothbrush remains the most effective and widely used device with which to remove dental plaque biofilm, with 80% to 90% of people in industrialized countries brushing their teeth at least once daily.[55,98,99] An international patent search for the years 1963 to 1998 revealed approximately 3000 toothbrush patents for both manual and power toothbrushes, reflecting the seemingly endless variations in design. In the United States alone, more than 50 million brushes are sold each year.[108]

MANUAL TOOTHBRUSH

24-1

For many patients, selecting a **manual toothbrush** is a matter of finding one that matches the bathroom decor. However, toothbrush selection is truly a serious issue, because toothbrushing is the sole method of oral hygiene practiced by many people.[30]

Efficacy

The effectiveness of a toothbrush is generally based on two factors:

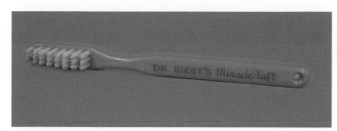

FIGURE 24-10
The first marketed nylon bristle toothbrush in the United States: Dr. West's Miracle Toothbrush. (Courtesy the Dental Museum, College of Dentistry, University of Nebraska Medical Center, Lincoln, Neb.)

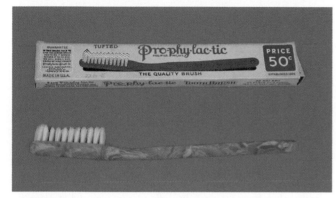

FIGURE 24-11
The Pro-phy-lac-tic Brush, another early mass-produced toothbrush in the United States. (Courtesy the Dental Museum, College of Dentistry, University of Nebraska Medical Center, Lincoln, Neb.)

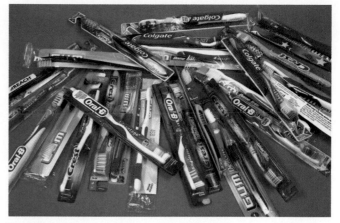

FIGURE 24-12
Assorted manual toothbrushes. (Courtesy Peggy Cain, College of Dentistry, University of Nebraska Medical Center, Lincoln, Neb.)

1. The product's design and materials
2. How well the patient uses the product to remove plaque biofilm, control gingivitis, and reduce bleeding.

Conflicting studies have been published in the literature regarding the comparative effectiveness of manual toothbrushes. More exact clinical and laboratory methods now provide standardization to objectively show differences between toothbrushes.[14,105] However, a study evaluating eight branded manual toothbrushes concluded that variations in toothbrush design are of little importance—the user is more important to successful plaque biofilm removal than the type of brush he or she is using.[39] Another study of four different commercially available manual toothbrushes compared plaque biofilm removal after a single brushing and found that all toothbrushes removed plaque biofilm equally well, with no single design being superior to the other.[38] Examples of the multitude of designs available for manual toothbrushes can be seen in Figure 24-12.

AMERICAN DENTAL ASSOCIATION ACCEPTANCE PROGRAM GUIDELINES

The ADA has Acceptance Program Guidelines that apply to both manual and powered toothbrushes, which can be seen in Box 24-2. Among the important requirements that the ADA has for toothbrushes are the following:

- Bristles must be soft.[4] Notably, the ADA requires that manufacturers make toothbrush bristles that meet standards of the **International Standardization Organization** (ISO).

BOX 24-2

AMERICAN DENTAL ASSOCIATION (ADA) SAFETY ACCEPTANCE GUIDELINES FOR MANUAL AND POWERED TOOTHBRUSHES*

- Evidence must be provided that the components of the toothbrush are safe for use in the oral cavity. Components and colorants should comply with applicable FDA standards.
- Toothbrush bristles shall be free of sharp or jagged edges and endpoints.
- In relation to bristle stiffness, reference should be made to the test methods in ISO 22254 (2005). Brushes having a stiffness index greater than 6 will usually not be considered for Acceptance. If the measured stiffness index is found to be greater than 6, clinical data demonstrating the safety of a toothbrush's bristles to oral hard and soft tissues will be required. In addition, abrasivity testing should be conducted using a toothbrush brushing machine (see ISO 11609: 1995, Annex A).
- Manual toothbrushes shall also comply with the requirements of ISO 20126 (2005).
- For powered toothbrushes, the product must have been submitted to an examination by and met the requirements of an appropriate technical safety laboratory such as Underwriters Laboratory, Inc. This requirement may be waived for products operating from nonrechargeable batteries of low voltage. The product shall also comply with the requirements of ISO 20127 (2005).
- For powered toothbrushes, adequate evidence must be provided from at least one clinical investigation of at least 25 subjects per group to show that the product is safe to oral hard and soft tissues and dental restorations.

---

*This is a portion of data required by the ADA when manufacturers of manual and powered toothbrushes submit a product for acceptance from the ADA Council on Scientific Affairs.

Adapted from American Dental Association Council on Scientific Affairs: *Acceptance guidelines—toothbrushes,* Chicago, 1998, The Association.

- Toothbrush bristles must be free of sharp or jagged edges.
- The brush must be made in a manner in which the bristles will be retained.

Obviously, toothbrush bristles with rounded ends allow for removal of bacterial plaque biofilm without producing traumatic lesions to the gingival and dental tissues.[32] Manual toothbrush handles are manufactured in a myriad of designs. The only acceptance requirement that the ADA has for manual toothbrush handles is that they be durable under normal use.

All patients should use a soft bristle toothbrush, but patients with sensitive teeth and esthetic restorations should be encouraged to use the softest bristle toothbrush available. How does a dental hygienist determine which toothbrush has the softest bristles? Toothbrush softness depends on many factors:

- Diameter of the bristles
- Length of the bristles
- Material used to make the bristles
- Number of bristles packed into each tuft

Simply reading on a package that a toothbrush is *sensitive* or *ultrasoft* may not accurately describe the bristle softness. Dental hygienists should try as many brands and types of brushes possible to determine which brushes are the softest and which ones are the best to meet the individual needs of their patients.

POWER TOOTHBRUSHES

Although the first generation of modern power toothbrushes was introduced in the early 1960s, Fredrik Wilhelm Tornberg, a Swedish watchmaker, patented the theory and design for the first "powered" (i.e., mechanical) toothbrush in 1885. He received patents for this invention in Sweden and Britian.[1,8,95,106] The wording accompanying the drawing of his invention (Figure 24-13) states, "This invention relates to an improved toothbrush by means of which the teeth may be cleaned as easily on the inner or backside as on the other side, the brushing being performed vertically instead of horizontally."[106] If Tornberg ever actually made one of these devices, then it has never been discovered or made commercially available.

The first electric toothbrush was marketed in the United States in 1880.[118] According to the manufacturer this toothbrush was "permanently charged with electro-magnetic current." Of course, these early toothbrushes were not powered by electricity. The first modern electrically powered toothbrush was reported in the literature in 1938,[104] and Bergmann and Woog developed a more-advanced version in Switzerland after

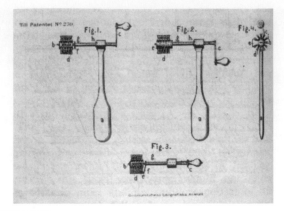

FIGURE 24-13
Patent of first powered toothbrush. (Reprinted by permission from Macmillan Publishers Ltd. Scutt JS, Swann CJ: The first mechanical toothbrush? *Br Dent J* 139(4):152, 1975.)

World War II,[17] which E.R. Squibb & Sons Company manufactured and introduced in 1960 under the name *Broxodent* (Figure 24-14). In 1961, General Electric introduced a rechargeable cordless model (Figure 24-15). These early powered toothbrushes were of the simplest design, modeled after the manual brush.[95,96] Early powered toothbrushes consisted of an electric motor with detachable and interchangeable toothbrushes.[18] The motor units were encased in watertight plastic and operated on an alternating current or rechargeable battery.

Some dental professionals did not embrace this device. Although the rationale behind the development of powered toothbrushes was to make it easier for people to clean their teeth, many clinicians feared that compulsive brushers in particular would use the excessively, causing damage to the supporting soft tissues.[57,82] However, this was not confirmed by clinical research. Most research in the 1960s on the reciprocating toothbrush (Broxodent) and the arcuate type of toothbrush (General Electric) was conducted to determine the effectiveness of the powered toothbrush compared with manual toothbrushing. The results on these second-generation powered toothbrushes varied from finding no significant difference between manual and electric toothbrushing[33,112] to reporting that the control of gingivitis was improved by use of a powered toothbrush.[10] Even though no evidence indicated that powered toothbrushes caused undue harm, dental professionals continued to limit their recommendations of powered toothbrushes well into the 1970s to individuals who were physically impaired, had orthodontic appliances, or otherwise had a special need.[22]

Efficacy and Safety

Since the early 1980s technologic advances in the design of powered toothbrushes have resulted in unique brushing instruments proven to be safe when applied to hard and soft dental tissues.[10,11,22] Furthermore, exhaustive laboratory and clinical testing has shown powered toothbrushes to be more effective

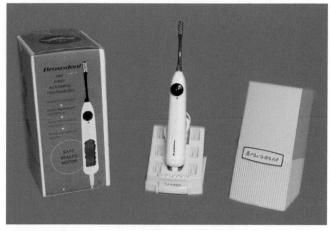

FIGURE 24-14
The Broxodent, the first modern electric toothbrush introduced by E.R. Squibb & Sons Company in 1960. (Courtesy the Dental Museum, College of Dentistry, University of Nebraska Medical Center, Lincoln, Neb.)

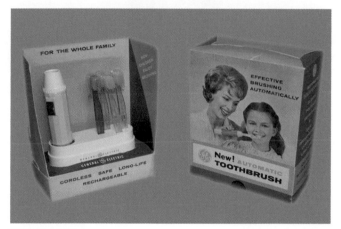

FIGURE 24-15
General Electric rechargeable cordless power toothbrush, introduced in 1961. (Courtesy the Dental Museum, College of Dentistry, University of Nebraska Medical Center, Lincoln, Neb.)

than manual toothbrushes in reducing dental plaque biofilm and gingivitis.*

Some powered toothbrushes enhance patient motivation by incorporating distinctive functions such as liquid crystal display (LCD) messages, 2- or 3-minute timers, and timers for quadrant brushing. The timers extend brushing time, which most patients fail to meet or exceed with manual toothbrushing.

A wide array of powered toothbrushes are available that vary by type of power source, mode of action, speed, and **brush-head design.**

Although numerous studies indicate that power brushing is superior, only one type of powered toothbrush has been demonstrated to be more effective than manual toothbrushing. In a systematic review conducted by the Cochrane Collaboration,[63] colleagues completed a systematic review that pooled the data for 29 clinical studies and found that only one type of powered

brush, the brush with a rotation oscillation action (Figure 24-16), removed more plaque biofilm and reduced gingivitis more effectively than manual brushes. The authors found that no other powered brush designs were consistently superior to manual toothbrushes. However, the authors acknowledged the limitations of the pooled research studies because of their variable nature and urge further study regarding comparative effectiveness of both manual and powered toothbrushes.[101] Does this mean that the only type of powered toothbrush that is effective is an oscillating-rotating brush? Quite simply, the answer is *no*. Other types of powered toothbrushes may be equally effective in plaque biofilm removal, as is the case with manual toothbrushes; much of the efficacy of a powered toothbrush depends on whether the patient knows how to use it properly for thorough plaque biofilm removal and then actually uses it accordingly.

Despite the wide variety of powered toothbrushes on the market with purchase prices that range from less than $10 to more than $100, 90% of toothbrushes sold are manual.[6]

> *Distinct Care Modifications*
> It has been demonstrated that plaque biofilm removal with powered toothbrushes is achieved more easily, faster, and more efficiently than with manual toothbrushes.*
>
> *References 4, 10, 11, 33, 34, 39, 43, 61, 84, 85, 119.

> *Note*
> A comparison of the efficacy and features of each of these powered toothbrushes reveals that although the various brands have different and widely varying mechanisms of action, they reliably remove plaque biofilm and reduce gingivitis, bleeding, stain, calculus, and probe depths (PDs).[22]

> *Note*
> Toothbrushing technique is much more critical than the type of brush used.

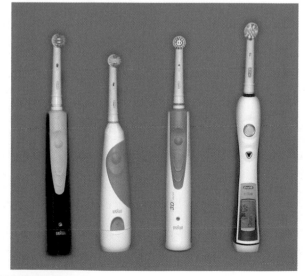

FIGURE 24-16
Rotating-oscillating powered toothbrushes, rotating-oscillating-pulsating powered toothbrushes, and oscillating-pulsating and pivot action powered toothbrushes. (Courtesy Peggy Cain, College of Dentistry, University of Nebraska Medical Center, Lincoln, Neb.)

---

*References 11, 13, 21-23, 84, 85, 89, 90, 94, 103, 113, 120, 125.

Recommendation of Powered Toothbrushes

The decision to recommend a powered toothbrush versus a manual toothbrush depends on a variety of circumstances. Certainly as has been documented many times in the literature, patients with compromised physical and mental conditions, as well as those with orthodontics and implants, can benefit from the use of a powered toothbrush.[126] However, other patients can also benefit from these devices.

> *Patient Education Opportunity*
>
> If a patient has used a manual toothbrush for a long period of time and his or her oral hygiene status requires improvement that is not occurring, recommending a powered toothbrush is a prudent intervention.

Power Toothbrush Instruction

Oral healthcare providers should request that patients bring in their powered toothbrushes for instructions on the most effective product use.[58,97,123] Because of the various actions of the powered brushes, becoming familiar with the suggested action of the brand recommended by the practice is helpful. Showing patients how to use the powered brush and having them demonstrate this new skill can be a useful tool in acceptance and effectiveness of the powered toothbrush. Professional instruction is extremely important to ensure a positive outcome with the use of powered toothbrushes.[105]

> *Distinct Care Modifications*
>
> Some individuals, regardless of health or physical status, cannot master dental plaque biofilm removal with a manual toothbrush. Switching to a powered toothbrush may be the perfect solution for these patients.

> *Patient Education Opportunity*
>
> Use of a videotape or instruction booklet does not take the place of professional one-on-one instruction to provide the patient with actual in-use instruction.

Types of Powered Toothbrushes

Dental hygienists should be familiar with the various types of powered toothbrushes available to better assist patients with making a selection, because powered toothbrushes have significant variations in action, design, brush-head design, filament patterns, speed, and type of motion. A simple way of describing the types of powered toothbrushes is to group them according to *type of power and action*. It should be noted that some variations of powered toothbrushes that use combined actions might not be covered in this chapter, because powered toothbrushes evolve and are introduced to the market frequently.

Three types of powered toothbrushes are **rotating-oscillating, rotating-oscillating-pulsating,** and **oscillating-pulsating-pivoting.** Rotating-oscillating-pulsating toothbrushes (see Figure 24-16) have a small round head with stationary tufts that move in a 60-degree counter-rotational motion with approximately 7600 strokes per minute. Models exist that have three-dimensional movement that adds a pulsating action of 20,000 to 40,000 movements per minute. Rotating-oscillating and rotating-oscillating-pulsating powered toothbrushes are distinctive in that the brush head is meant to

be moved from tooth to tooth instead of using it in a manner similar to a manual brushing technique. An exclusive feature of one of the rotating-oscillating-pulsating toothbrushes is the inclusion of bristles that are molded from elastomer. These elastomer bristles are designed to clean interproximal spaces, whereas the fixed bristles are designed to clean the other surfaces. Examples of rotating-oscillating and rotating-oscillating-pulsating powered toothbrushes can be seen in Figure 24-16. The rotating-oscillating powered toothbrushes have timers and are rechargeable.

Counter-rotational powered toothbrushes

The head of the counter-rotational toothbrush (Figure 24-17) is similar in shape to a manual toothbrush and can be purchased full-sized or compact, with 10 tufts of rotating bristles that are 0.0005 in diameter. Each tuft of bristles rotates 1.5

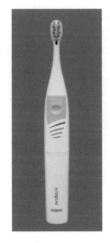

FIGURE 24-17
Powered toothbrush with counter-rotational bristles. Interplak (Conair, Shelton, Conn.). (Courtesy Peggy Cain, College of Dentistry, University of Nebraska Medical Center, Lincoln, Neb.)

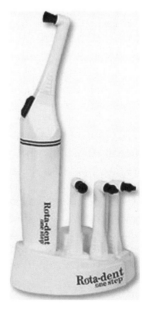
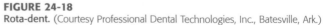

FIGURE 24-18
Rota-dent. (Courtesy Professional Dental Technologies, Inc., Batesville, Ark.)

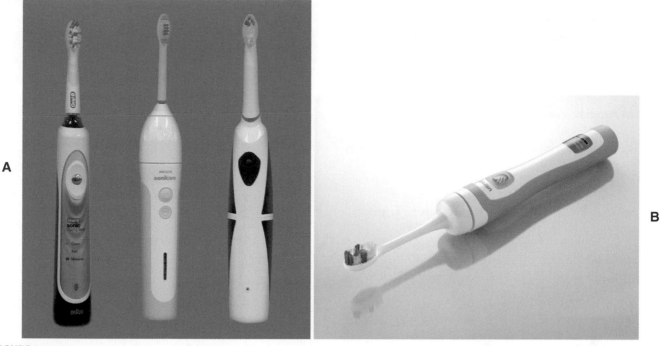

FIGURE 24-19
A, Sonic powered toothbrushes. *Left to right:* Sonic Complete (Oral-B, Boston, Mass.), Sonicare (Phillips Medical Systems, Andover, Mass.), SenSonic (Water Pik, Inc., Fort Collins, Colo.). **B,** Ultrasonic Ultreo. (A, Courtesy Peggy Cain, College of Dentistry, University of Nebraska Medical Center, Lincoln, Neb. B, Courtesy Ultreo, Inc., Redmond, Wash.)

turns in one direction and then reverses 1.5 turns in the opposite direction at a rate of 4200 rpm.

Rotary toothbrushes

A rotary-powered toothbrush (Figure 24-18) is available; it resembles a dental professional rotary instrument and is uniquely different from a traditional powered toothbrush. Consequently, additional instruction may be required for the patient to become adept at using this device effectively. This powered brush has three interchangeable tips that include a single tuft of bristles, a hollow cup brush, and an elongated brush tip that rotates.

Sonic and ultrasonic toothbrushes

Several manufacturers make **sonic** toothbrushes (Figure 24-19, A). Sonic toothbrushes vibrate at a rate of at least 30,000 brush strokes per minute (260 Hz), creating acoustic energy; these brushes have a side-to-side action and are available with 2-minute timers, with one brand offering a 2-minute timer incorporated with a 30-second indicator for quadrant brushing. An ultrasonic toothbrush is available that combines sonic bristle action with ultrasonic frequency. This **ultrasonic** brush combines high-frequency bristle motion (18,000 strokes per minute) with ultrasonic vibration that produces greater than 20,000 Hz. The head of this toothbrush has a traditional design and is equipped with a signal to indicate 30 second brushing intervals and an auto-shut off timer (Figure 24-19, B).[46]

Battery-Powered Toothbrushes

A variety of affordable battery-powered toothbrushes are on the market and commonly cost less than $10. Most of these

brushes have a circular motion and can be an inexpensive method of introducing powered toothbrushes for a patient who wants to try a powered toothbrush for the first time without a higher monetary investment. Most battery-powered toothbrushes operate on C-cell batteries or are disposable after the battery life is depleted. A hybrid battery-powered manual brush has recently been introduced in which the toothbrush vibrates but the bristles do not move. Examples of battery-powered toothbrushes can be seen in Figure 24-20.

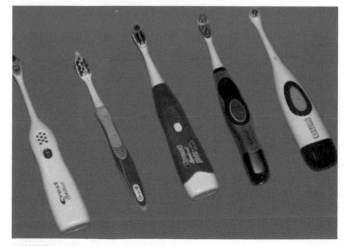

FIGURE 24-20
Composite of battery-powered toothbrushes. *Left to right:* CrestBrush Classic (Procter & Gamble, Cincinnati, Ohio), Oral B Pulsar (Oral-B, Boston, Mass.), Crest Spinbrush Multi-angle (Procter & Gamble, Cincinnati, Ohio), Crest ProClean (Procter & Gamble, Cincinnati, Ohio), Butler Gum Rotapower (Sunstar Butler, Chicago, Ill.). (Courtesy Peggy Cain, College of Dentistry, University of Nebraska Medical Center, Lincoln, Neb.)

In summary, powered toothbrushes have been shown to be effective, safe, and beneficial to patients as evidenced by long-term in vivo studies that offer compelling evidence of the benefits of powered toothbrushes along with the available **patient compliance** data.

Toothbrushing Techniques

The hygienist should do the following:

- Instill in individuals the importance and goals of toothbrushing.
- Teach a brushing method or combination of methods that will meet the needs of that specific patient.
- Assess thorough and effective toothbrushing as part of a total oral hygiene preventive program.[41]

Keeping in mind the need to evaluate specific design attributes of the oral care device being recommended (Box 24-3), as well as patient factors (Box 24-4), the hygienist should give each patient specific technique instructions.

BOX 24-3

BRUSH ATTRIBUTES TO CONSIDER WHEN MAKING ORAL SELF-CARE RECOMMENDATIONS

- Does the brush have tufted bristles that will increase interproximal cleaning?
- Are the bristles end rounded?
- Does the angulation of the brush head aid in accessing difficult-to-reach areas?
- Is the size of the brush head appropriate for the size and age of the patient?
- Does it have soft bristles to reduce the potential for tissue abrasion caused by overaggressive brushing?
- Does the design of the brush handle facilitate ease of use?

BRUSHING SEQUENCE

Patients often have areas that are particularly difficult for them to reach, in which case the hygienist might suggest that they start with those areas first. In general, a right-handed person will find it more difficult to brush the teeth on the right side; likewise, a left-handed individual will find it more difficult to brush the teeth on the left side.

Prevention

Recommend a specific brushing sequence to patients to encourage the development of a brushing pattern.

Patients should be instructed to begin on the distofacial surface of the distal-most tooth in the maxillary arch on their dominant side and to continue around the arch, including the occlusal and incisal surfaces, until they have reached the distal-most surface of the distal-most molar on the opposite side. They should then repeat the same sequence on the palatal surfaces. This process is then repeated on the mandibular arch.

BOX 24-4

PATIENT FACTORS TO CONSIDER WHEN MAKING ORAL SELF-CARE RECOMMENDATIONS

- Does the patient have any physical challenges that might require modifications to oral self-care devices or regimens?
- Is the brush the right size for the patient's mouth?
- What anatomical considerations need to be accommodated?
- Is the current brushing style safe and effective?
- Is the current brushing frequency sufficient?
- Does the patient's age affect brush selection?
- How motivated is the patient to comply with brushing instructions? If not motivated, what needs to be done to change level of motivation?
- Are the patient's expectations for plaque biofilm removal consistent with those of the dental professional?

OCCLUSAL SURFACES

The patient should be instructed to clean the occlusal surfaces using a short back-and-forth motion, forcing the bristles to gain access (as much as possible) to pits and fissures, followed by a sweeping motion to remove debris. A long sweeping stroke is not suggested because it does not allow the bristles' tips to penetrate sufficiently into the pits and fissures.

ANTERIOR, LINGUAL, AND PALATAL SURFACES

The best toothbrush placement to gain access to the anterior lingual and palatal areas is a vertically positioned brush. The heel of the brush should then be placed at the gingival margin and brought forward; this motion should be repeated several times.

FREQUENCY AND DURATION

A common question often asked by patients is, "How frequently and for how long should I brush?" The most commonly accepted recommendation among dental professionals is that patients should brush twice a day.[41,62,70] Research has documented that thorough plaque biofilm removal every 48 hours is the longest interval that will control gingivitis.[41] The ADA recommends that patients brush "regularly" and that oral hygiene routines be customized for patients based on their thoroughness of plaque biofilm removal and history of adherence to recommended protocols.[4]

For some patients, brush placement and toothbrushing procedures are easy. For others, malpositioned teeth and other anatomical and physical challenges may require a longer brushing session.

Note

The length of time a patient should brush needs to be determined by the length of time it takes to thoroughly remove plaque biofilm.

Prevention

Observe a patient during a toothbrushing procedure and assess the results rather than prescribing an arbitrary amount of toothbrushing time.

By observing the patient while he or she is brushing the teeth, more (or less) time may be recommended, depending on the thoroughness achieved. Research has demonstrated that unsupervised brushing by patients results in brushing times of 1 minute or less, even though they report their brushing times to be between 2 and 3 minutes.[55,64,128] Some dental hygienists recommend the use of an egg timer to time the brushing duration. Yankell suggested that patients brushing time should be customized based on their oral health status and history of adherence to oral hygiene programs.[128] Other factors that affect the amount of time needed by an individual to thoroughly brush the teeth include the tendency to accumulate plaque biofilm, psychomotor skill ability, and the clearance rate of foods and bacteria by saliva.

METHODS

Although patients have a wide variety of acceptable toothbrushes to choose from in the marketplace, they can remove plaque biofilm thoroughly only when the toothbrush is used routinely and in an effective manner that is safe to the oral tissues. Table 24-2 summarizes the following six **toothbrushing methods** that most commonly are taught to patients[15,54,116,128]:

1. **Bass method**
2. **Rolling-stroke method**
3. **Modified Stillman's method**
4. **Charters method**
5. **Fones method**
6. **Horizontal-scrub method**

Distinct Care Modifications

When a patient has healthy gingiva and few plaque biofilm deposits, arbitrarily recommending a change is counterproductive. This patient should be coached to continue his or her safe, effective pattern of brushing.[58]

The clinician should assess a patient's oral health status and observe the toothbrushing technique before recommending a particular brushing method.

Many patients may require only minor modifications to their brushing technique, which often results in their successful long-term adherence to oral self-care routines.

When teaching patients new oral hygiene protocols, the hygienist should provide both information and skills training in combination with motivational messages to ensure an appropriate level of understanding by the patient.[34] For example, use of a large mirror allows patients to observe the proper technique and retain tips for how to improve performance in specific areas. Whatever toothbrushing method is taught, the instructions given must be clear and specific. Directions and demonstrations, whenever possible, should be made using the patient's mouth.

Patients should be given written materials to reinforce the concepts presented in the oral health lesson.[64] Sample patient education pamphlets are available from a variety of dental organizations and product manufacturers.

Note

Note the exact instructions given to a patient in their chart so that they can be reviewed at the next visit (not all patients will remember the exact instructions that they were given).

⭐ **CASE APPLICATION 24-1.3**

Toothbrush Selection

Mrs. Cronin's hygienist initially selected an ultrasoft, small, oval-headed toothbrush with **multitufted, end-rounded bristles** in a flat-plane configuration. Using a large hand mirror, she showed Ann the areas of plaque biofilm retention in her mouth and how the ultrasoft brush and the modified Stillman's brushing method easily removed the disclosed plaque biofilm. When Ann was asked to demonstrate the technique, she did so quite slowly and with apparent difficulty. After five or six brushing repetitions, Ann dropped the toothbrush. After a flushed apology, Ann stated, "I guess these old hands just don't want to work today." Looking at Table 24-2, which consideration has the hygienist overlooked in selecting this brushing recommendation? What method should the hygienist have recommended? Would a powered toothbrush have been a better recommendation?

Toothbrush Replacement and Care

For a toothbrush to remain effective, it must be replaced periodically. The brushing method and force used by the patient determine toothbrush wear more than frequency of use. Wear can be exhibited in many ways—bristles can become splayed, bent, or even broken.

After each use the toothbrush should be cleaned by placing it under a stream of warm water to force any debris or remaining dentifrice from between the bristles. The brush handle should then be tapped against the sink top to remove the remaining water. Brushes should be kept with the head upright in the open air to enhance drying and minimize the development of bacterial growth.

Patient Education Opportunity

Although the average manual toothbrush can be expected to last approximately 3 months, this time span can vary widely because of differences in brushing habits. Other reasons to replace a toothbrush include illness, continuous exposure to water or other foreign substances, and damage to the handle.[86,122,128]

Prevention

Brushes should not be kept in contact with other toothbrushes, because proximity is a rich source of bacterial cross-contamination.

Tongue Brushing

Patients often complain of mouth odor, not realizing that it may be caused by bacterial accumulation on the tongue. Papillae on the tongue provide a perfect place to harbor bacteria and debris that can lead to the development of malodor. Unless instructed to do so, patients often do not know that they should clean the tongue much in the same way as they should clean their teeth. Tongue brushing can be accomplished by placing the side of the toothbrush near the middle of the tongue. The brush is then swept forward, and this step repeated

Table 24-2　Toothbrushing Methods

METHOD	DESCRIPTION	CONSIDERATIONS	INITIAL BRUSH PLACEMENT
Bass	• Bristles placed directly into sulcus at 45-degree angle to the tooth • Gentle short strokes in sulcus • Followed by rolling-stroke method because Bass method cleans only sulcus	• Good plaque biofilm removal from gingival margin and sulcus • Limited cleaning on remainder of tooth surface • Easy to learn	
Rolling Stroke	• Bristles placed against attached gingiva at a 45-degree angle to the tooth • Brush rolled slowly by flexing wrist to drag bristles against tooth with gentle, firm motion • Brush rolled at least five times for each area	• Used for removing plaque biofilm at gingival margin and clinical crown • Limited plaque biofilm removal at gingival margin	
Modified Stillman's	• Bristles placed onto the attached gingiva at a 45-degree angle to the tooth • Bristles pressed (enough to cause slight gingival blanching) and vibrated to promote circulation • Rolling stroke added to cleanse the tooth • Action repeated sequentially throughout mouth • In the anterior lingual area, heel or toe of brush placed on the gingiva, rotating and sweeping toward incisal edges	• Good gingival stimulation • Good (clinical crown) coronal and interproximal cleaning • Limited sulcular cleaning • Dexterity required	
Charters	• Side of brush placed against tooth with bristles facing occlusally • Brush slid to a 45-degree angle at the gingival margin • Bristles then pressed into the margin and proximal areas and vibrated for at least 10 strokes for each area of mouth • Rolling stroke is recommended before use of this technique to cleanse coronal surface	• Good interproxmial cleaning • Limited sulcular cleaning • Useful around orthodontic bands, fixed prostheses	
Fones	• With teeth closed, brush placed against the cheek with bristles directed to posterior teeth • Circular motions used in a quick, sweeping motion • Anterior teeth placed end-to-end and cleansed in same manner • In-and-out strokes used to cleanse the palatal and lingual areas	• Easy-to-learn first technique for children • Possibly detrimental for vigorous adult brusher	
Horizontal Scrub	• Bristles placed at a 90-degree angle to the tooth and brush moved back and forth or in a large circular motion	• Removes plaque biofilm successfully from facial and lingual surfaces (unless hard brush is used) • If hard brush is used, damage to tooth structure and soft tissues is possible • Inability to access interproximal areas	

several times. A dentifrice may be used to improve cleansing if it does not prove unpleasant to the patient. Plastic tongue scrapers are also available; patients with elongated papilla and deep grooves may find this type of device beneficial. (See Chapter 38 for more information on tongue brushing.)

Interdental Cleaning

Although some toothbrush bristles are contoured to reach around line angles and into the proximal area, they cannot adequately clean the entire proximal surface. The inaccessible proximal areas are those near the contact point and those located subgingivally. Recommendations for self-care interdental cleaning aids should be based on the following:

- Architecture of the oral anatomy
- Dexterity of the patient
- Patient preference
- Desired clinical outcomes

The primary reason to remove biofilm from the interdental space is to reduce gingival inflammation and prevent periodontal disease. It has been routinely demonstrated that periodontal disease is most frequent and severe in the interproximal areas. Periodontal disease commonly starts in the col area, which is difficult to clean and provides a haven for biofilm accumulation. Thus interproximal cleaning becomes essential to supporting a healthy periodontium. When periodontal structures are lost because of periodontal destruction, interproximal-cleaning aids become more important; in this case cleaning aids need to be chosen that reflect the needs and ability of the patient to access and effectively remove the plaque biofilm accumulations from interdental spaces.

DENTAL FLOSS

Historical Perspective

The development of **dental floss,** the most commonly recommended interdental device, is attributed to Levi Spear Parmly, a New Orleans dentist. He recommended that waxed silken thread be passed between the teeth "to dislodge that irritating matter which no brush can remove and which is the real source of distress."[50] The Johnson & Johnson Company obtained the first patent for dental floss in 1898. Later, Dr. Charles Bass, a physician, developed nylon floss as a replacement for silk.[53] Today, in addition to nylon, floss may be made out of a Gore-Tex type of material called *polytetrafluoroethylene* (PTFE). Floss may be waxed or unwaxed, and flavoring often is added to improve patient compliance. Floss may be enhanced with fluoride in addition to other therapeutic or cosmetic agents. However, the efficacy of additives has not been evaluated in clinical trials.

Efficacy

Research has shown that individuals who floss regularly have less biofilm, gingivitis, bleeding, and calculus.[60,77] The assumption that regular flossing correlates with a significant reduction in interproximal dental caries is not supported by research.[59,67,78] The reduction of dental caries or dental caries risk is most

strongly correlated with fluoride use. Interdental cleaning is an important component of a comprehensive self-care routine. (For more information on reduction of dental caries and dental caries risk, refer to Chapter 25.)

Adherence

Before World War II, most people did not use dental floss; however, with the advent of nylon floss, which did not shred as easily as silk, acceptance increased.[53] Despite improvements in materials and widespread advocacy by most dental professionals, the majority of people still do not perform regular interdental cleaning. Self-reporting has shown approximately two thirds of individuals do not floss regularly. Only 22% of the individuals observed while flossing demonstrated effective flossing technique.[77] When the patient is not complying with flossing recommendations or has more-advanced interproximal plaque biofilm–removal needs (e.g., open embrasure spaces because of periodontal destruction), restorative challenges (e.g., pontics, bridges, implants), or orthodontic appliances, other effective options for interdental cleaning may be considered:

- Floss holders
- Floss threader
- Powered flossers
- Interproximal (interdental) brushes
- End-tufted brushes
- Toothpicks and wood sticks
- Irrigating devices

Manual floss continues to be the primary focus of interdental cleaning recommendation among dental hygienists. However, clinicians should remember that when given a choice, many individuals will choose products other than dental floss.* This indicates a considerable gap in behavior between professionals and patients and is not reflective of patient-centered approach or evidence-based practice. By providing choices and including the patient in the decision-making process, the clinician can significantly increase compliance—resulting in improved oral health (Table 24-3).

Flossing Methods

Self-cleaning of the proximal tooth surfaces for Class I embrasures (Figure 24-21) can usually be accomplished with dental floss. Dental floss is a thin-diameter thread that slides easily into tight contacts and is available as a waxed or unwaxed product. The thin diameter of dental floss allows easy access through the contact point and subgingival cleaning between the interdental papilla and tooth.

Dental floss is manufactured in single-dose units and on spools of several yards (Figure 24-22). **Dental tape,** a flattened and wider form of dental floss, is recommended for cleaning Class I to Class II embrasures (Figure 24-23). Studies have shown no difference in clinical outcomes between waxed and unwaxed floss.[36,76,92,93] Either type can be recommended. In some instances, clinical findings such as tight contacts or defective restorations may make waxed floss a better choice.

---

*References 29, 35, 56, 72, 114

Table 24-3	Interdental Aids for Embrasure Types		
INTERDENTAL AID	**CLASS I EMBRASURE**	**CLASS II EMBRASURE**	**CLASS III EMBRASURE**
Dental Floss	X		
Dental Tape	X		
Power Flosser	X		
Textured Floss		X	X
Floss Holder	X		
Floss Threader	X		
Interdental Brush		X	X
End-Tufted Brush			X
Toothpicks		X	X
Wood or Plastic Sticks		X	X

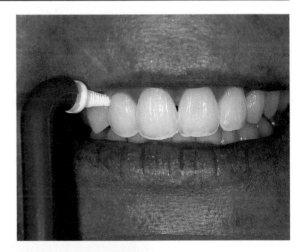

FIGURE 24-21
Self-cleaning of the proximal tooth surfaces for Class I embrasures. (From Bird DL, Robinson DS: *Modern dental assisting,* St Louis, 2006, Saunders.)

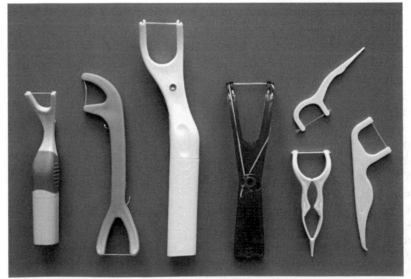

FIGURE 24-22
Assortment of single-unit floss devices and floss threaders. (From Cappelli DP, Mobley CC: *Prevention in Clinical Oral Health Care,* St Louis, 2008, Mosby.)

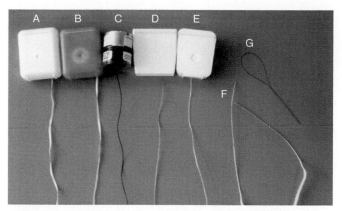

FIGURE 24-23
Examples of dental floss. **A,** Dental tape. **B,** Polytetrafluoroethylene (PTFE), a slippery substance that makes the floss slide easily between tight contacts and is also shred-resistant. **C,** Unwaxed nylon; the black contrasts with the tooth so that the user can see it. **D,** Waxed dental floss flavored with mint. **E,** Traditional waxed floss. **F,** Examples of textured dental floss. **G,** A floss threader. (From Cappelli DP, Mobley CC: Prevention in Clinical Oral Health Care, St Louis, 2008, Mosby.)

Two common methods of flossing exist: (1) the spool method and (2) the loop or circle method. The spool method is recommended for individuals with good manual dexterity. Children and individuals with poor manual dexterity may be more successful with the loop method (Box 24-5). Manual flossing is technique sensitive; if done incorrectly, then it may result in floss cuts and clefts (Figure 24-24).

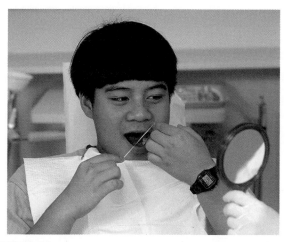

FIGURE 24-24
Manual flossing is technique sensitive; if done incorrectly, then it may result in floss cuts and clefts. (From Bird DL, Robinson DS: *Modern dental assisting,* 2006, St Louis, Saunders.)

Power Flossers

The introduction of **power flossers** has provided an alternative to manual floss (Figure 24-25). Evidence indicates that these devices can remove biofilm and reduce gingivitis and bleeding similar to manual floss.[5,76,110] Expectations of similar clinical outcomes between devices cannot be assumed. The clinical evidence specific to that brand must be reviewed before determining the product's effectiveness. Tip or filament shape, speed,

---

BOX 24-5

TRADITIONAL USE OF FLOSS

Flossing Technique
- When using both hands, a sufficient supply of floss (approximately 16 inches) is removed from the spool.
- Wrap one end of the floss loosely on the middle finger of one hand enough to secure the floss (4 to 5 inches).
- Wrap the remainder of the floss on the middle finger of the other hand (loosely so as not to cut off the circulation) leaving 2 to 3 inches between the fingers.
- The middle fingers act in a scroll-like fashion, holding the floss and wrapping and unwrapping to provide a clean area on the floss for each proximal area. (Using the same piece of floss from one proximal area to the next can introduce bacteria from one area to another.)
- Using the first finger and thumb, grasp the floss that has been left between the two middle fingers. The first finger and the thumb provide stability by keeping the floss tight for insertion between the teeth.
- Insert the floss between the teeth with a gentle back-and-forth (sawing) motion until the floss has moved apical to the contact.
- Slide the floss gently apically under the gingival tissue without cutting the gingival tissues, and encircle the proximal surface onto the line angles.
- Move the floss coronal to the contact and then apically along the proximal surface at least two times to remove soft deposits.
- Remove the floss from the proximal area, wind the used portion of the floss on the middle finger, unwind on the finger with the most floss, and move to the next proximal area.
- If the floss gets caught in the contact, do not force the floss coronally. Instead, release one end of the floss, pull the other end facially, and slide the floss out of the proximal area. If floss remains in the contact, then try to reinsert the floss or have waxed floss or polytetrafluoroethylene (PTFE)-coated floss to assist in removal of the floss threads.
- Discard floss when finished flossing.

Loop Method
- An alternative flossing method to wrapping or anchoring the floss on the fingers of each hand involves the use of dental floss tied in a circle. This is also called the *circle method.*
- Cut a piece of floss that is approximately 18 inches long, and tie it securely in a circle.
- Place all of the fingers, except the thumb, within the loop.
- Use the index fingers to guide the floss through the lower teeth, and use your thumbs to guide the floss through the upper teeth, making sure to go below the gum line, forming a "C" on the side of each tooth.
- A new section of the floss can be easily accessed for each proximal surface.

---

and mechanism of action vary between brands and can affect clinical outcomes.

Textured Floss

Tufted or **textured floss** is a type of floss that offers additional features (compared with traditional floss varieties) for cleaning

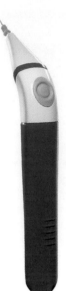

FIGURE 24-25
WaterPik Power Flosser. (Courtesy of Water Pik, Inc, Fort Collins, Colo.)

proximal surfaces and subgingival areas (see Figure 24-23). Some dental floss manufacturers have added a spongy or textured surface to floss to assist in proximal cleaning for Class II and III embrasures, around fixed orthodontic appliances, under pontics, and around abutments of crowns and implants. Textured dental floss is usually dispensed as a single strand and may have additional features such as a stiff-nylon end for threading and regular floss for Class I embrasures.

Floss Holder

A **floss holder** is designed to assist individuals whose dexterity or oral architecture cannot accommodate traditional manual flossing methods. A variety of floss holders are available. They range from small plastic disposable units with floss attached to handles that have spools of floss contained in the handle (see Figure 24-22). Figure 24-26 shows a sterling silver floss holder from the late 1800s. Units with preloaded floss are convenient for patients and allow for a clean piece of floss for each interproximal space. Other floss holders are sold as a handle without

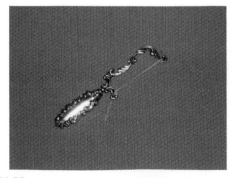

FIGURE 24-26
Sterling silver floss holder from the late 1800s.

floss; the floss is wound around a central button, guided between two "fingers," and secured around the button (Figure 24-27). Thus the taut floss in the holder can be substituted for the use of fingers. New floss can be pulled into place for the next proximal surface with the floss holder. Research studies have documented that the floss holders are as effective as manual flossing and suggest that patient compliance is increased with the disposable floss units.[29,73,114]

Floss Threader

A **floss threader** is a device that allows floss to be pulled through the interdental space (buccal to lingual) under the contact point for Class I embrasure. Floss threaders resemble a sewing needle with a loop for the floss and have sufficient flexibility and strength to be easily threaded under the contact point (Figure 24-28). The dental floss is then used to clean each proximal surface. Floss threaders support interdental cleaning for individuals with orthodontic appliances, and they provide access above a pontic and around abutment teeth of a fixed prosthetic bridge or other dental work that prevents passage of floss through the contact.

INTERDENTAL BRUSHES

Interdental brushes are appropriate for Class II and III embrasures and furcations, for tooth surfaces adjacent to missing teeth, and for orthodontic appliances. In conjunction with

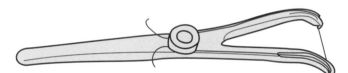

FIGURE 24-27
Rethreading of floss is necessary with some floss handles.

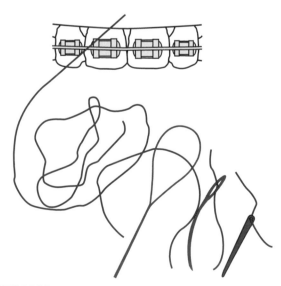

FIGURE 24-28
Floss threaders and precut floss units.

toothbrushing, interdental brushes have been found to be more effective in the removal of plaque biofilm from proximal tooth surfaces and considered preferable to floss for interdental plaque biofilm removal in patients with moderate to severe periodontitis or patients with loss of periodontium from a history of periodontitis[35,56,72] (Figure 24-29). Interdental brushes have also been found to be a very effective form of plaque biofilm control at the proximal area of abutment teeth.

The interdental brush handle is designed with contraangled ends that provide a place for insertion of a disposable brush. Cylindric or cone-shaped brushes in varying diameters are attached to a handle. The interproximal space size will determine the size and shape of brush to be used (selecting a larger-diameter brush for a larger embrasure space and vice versa). The reusable handle may be contraangled for better access posteriorly. Some handles are short, have a cover, and can be used while traveling (or away from home); these devices are disposed of after limited use.

Instructions for Use

Even though using the interdental brush is somewhat easier than dental floss for most patients,[35,72] a few simple instructions will make the overall process more effective and efficient. The patient should be instructed to do the following:

- After loading the appropriate-size brush in the reusable handle, insert the tip of the brush gently into the interproximal space similar to the placement of a toothpick.
- With a gentle motion, slightly wiggle or ease the brush into the interproximal embrasure space as far as the brush will allow (see Figure 24-29, *C*). If the brush is bending, then most likely too much pressure is being applied. Lighten up on the grasp, decrease the pushing force, and gently wiggle the brush into the interproximal space for maximal efficiency.
- Gently remove the brush from the embrasure space and move to the next contact area. The brush may not go all the way through the embrasure space, but it can still be very effective by the action of working the bristles interproximally.

For most effective interdental cleaning, the brush also needs to be reinserted from the opposing facial and palatal or lingual surface.

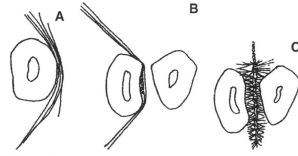

FIGURE 24-29
A, Floss conforms to proximal convex surface. **B,** Floss does not conform to proximal concave surface. **C,** Proxy brush cleans concavities.

DENTAL CONSIDERATIONS

Using the interdental brush between anterior teeth with intact interdental papillae is not recommended. Some reports describe the papillae being flattened by repeated use, causing some esthetic concerns in this area.[35]

Interdental brushes are also a vehicle for chemotherapeutic delivery interproximally. A small application of fluoride, chlorhexidine, desensitizing agent, or other antimicrobial on the brush will work the agent directly into the interdental space supporting desired therapeutic effects.

Even though the brushes are disposable, they can be reused several times before they need to be changed. The patient should be advised to treat the used interdental brush similarly to a toothbrush (rinsing it under running water and storing it until the next use). Powered interproximal brushes also may be used to clean proximal surfaces (Figure 24-30).

END-TUFTED BRUSHES

An **end-tufted brush** has tufts of bristles affixed to the end of a handle and is best used to clean proximal surfaces of teeth where an adjacent tooth is missing or in the posterior of the

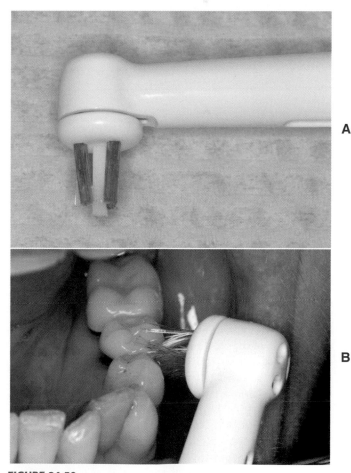

FIGURE 24-30
A, Powered proximal brush. **B,** Powered proximal brush in use.

mouth on the distal-most surface in the mouth. Unlike the interdental brush, the tip is not replaceable and is replaced much like a toothbrush.

TOOTHPICKS AND WOOD STICKS

Toothpicks have been used for centuries and were a part of early toiletry kits dating back to 3000 BC. Toothpicks were made out of gold, silver, and bronze and were carried on a chain or in fancy cases. It was also common to provide toothpicks at the dinner table for guests. For the less affluent, slivers from the mastic tree (the toothpick tree) provided a sufficient alternative. The early use of toothpicks was for the appearance of teeth and to remove food debris (not for prevention of oral disease).

Toothpicks are widely used because they are readily available and easy to use. Evidence indicates that they are effective in reducing biofilm and gingival bleeding. Toothpick holders are commercially available, provide better control and access to lingual and posterior regions, and reduce the potential for trauma.

Interdental wood sticks are made of soft balsa wood; their working ends are triangular in shape and tapered for access into the proximal space. Plastic versions of toothpicks and sticks with a tapered triangular shape are available from multiple manufacturers (Figure 24-31).

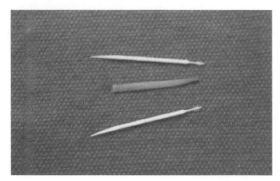

FIGURE 24-31
Wooden and plastic picks used for interdental cleaning.

OTHER PROXIMAL-CLEANING AIDS

The following aids can also be used for interdental cleaning and were often recommended because products available for Class II and Class III embrasures were limited. Today they are seldom used because of the plethora of effective and widely distributed products designed for multiple patient needs.[42] In instances in which cost or availability is an issue, knitting yarn, pipe cleaners, and gauze strips may be recommended.

24-10 Dental Water Jet

The first dental water jet was developed in 1962 in Fort Collins, Colorado, by a dentist, Dr. Gerald Moyer, and his patient, John Mattingly, a professor of engineering at Colorado State University. Numerous studies indicate that the dental water jet

is a safe and effective self-care tool for everyone (especially those who fail to comply with traditional self-care recommendations[12] and those with special needs such as periodontal maintenance,* crowns and bridges,[73] orthodontics appliances,[27,94] and diabetes[2]).

Mechanism of action

The mechanism of action of a dental water jet is through a process called *irrigation*. Irrigation works through the direct application of a pulsed or steady stream of water or other solution. Pulsation and pressure are critical to the efficacy of the dental water jet.[19,20,107]

Compared with a continuous-stream irrigating syringe, a pulsating device has been shown to be three times more effective.[107] Pulsation is critical because it creates hydrokinetic activity.[40] Two zones of activity occur: (1) the impact zone, where the solution initially contacts in the mouth, and (2) the flushing zone, where the solution reaches into the subgingival sulcus or pocket. The benefit of this of hydrokinetic activity is subgingival penetration. The majority of studies documenting this effect have been on dental water jets with a pulsation rate of 1200. A second critical component of the dental water jet is pressure control. A medium- to a high-pressure setting, generally in the range of 50 psi to 90 psi,[19,20,107] has been demonstrated for both safety and efficacy. When combined with pulsation, the pressure rate can be controlled.

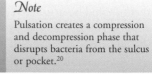

Note

Pulsation creates a compression and decompression phase that disrupts bacteria from the sulcus or pocket.[20]

Depth of delivery

A dental water jet delivers water or other agents subgingivally. The depth of delivery of that solution is dependent on the type of tip that is used on the dental water jet. Both a standard jet tip and a soft site-specific subgingival tip (Pik Pocket subgingival irrigation tip, Water Pik, Inc., Fort Collins, Colo.) have shown the ability to penetrate into a sulcus or pocket.[25,45] Figure 24-32 depicts placement of the jet tip, and Figure 24-33 depicts placement of the Pik Pocket. It has been found that average depth of penetration into a pocket with the standard jet tip was approximately 50%; however, in 60% of deep sites, penetration was 75% or greater[40] (Table 24-4).

Use of the jet tip is generally referred to as *supragingival irrigation,* whereas the use of the site-specific tip is called *subgingival irrigation*. The jet tip is used for full-mouth irrigation, whereas the site-specific tip is recommended for difficult-to-access areas such as a deep pocket, furcation, implant, or crown and bridge.

When compared with other self-care devices, the evidence seems to indicate that the dental water jet has the greatest potential for reaching deeper into a pocket than other traditional

---

*References 7, 40, 41, 43-45, 47-49, 51, 71, 88.

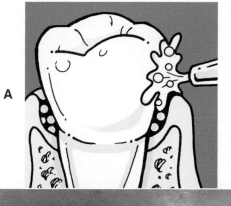

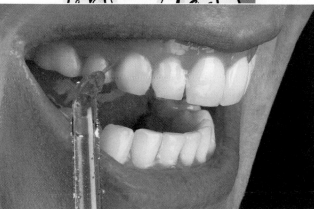

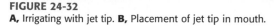

FIGURE 24-32
A, Irrigating with jet tip. **B,** Placement of jet tip in mouth.

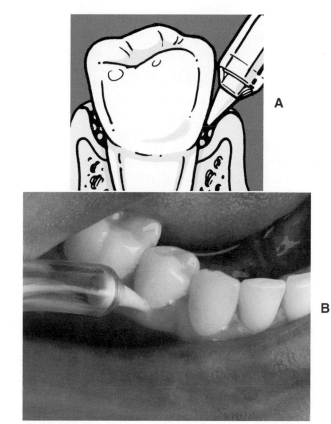

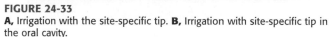

FIGURE 24-33
A, Irrigation with the site-specific tip. **B,** Irrigation with site-specific tip in the oral cavity.

self-care devices.[24,25,45] Studies documenting subgingival access for toothbrushing or flossing are limited or nonexistent. The ability of a sonic toothbrush to affect bacteria up to 3-mm thick has been tested only in the laboratory setting and has not been proven definitively on a live subject.[81,115,127] One study that looked at the subgingival disruption of plaque biofilm and bacteria by either a sonic toothbrush or manual toothbrush after 15 seconds of brushing time found both removed plaque biofilm and microbes up to only 1-mm thick.[124]

SAFETY

Because the dental water jet works differently from traditional self-care tools such as a toothbrush or floss, misconceptions about the device and its benefits have been cited, especially as it relates to tissue damage, penetration of bacteria, and deepening of pockets. Although several studies have included the reporting of adverse effects, no harm was found.*

The dental water jet has been tested to determine its effect on the soft tissue of a periodontal pocket and the penetration of bacteria into a pocket. Teeth diagnosed for extraction were used. Pockets in the treatment group were irrigated for 8 seconds via a pulsating dental water jet (Water Pik, Inc., Fort Col-

*References 7, 25, 31, 40, 45, 52, 66, 74, 80, 93.

Table 24-4	Depth of Delivery		
Attachment	**Depth of Delivery**		
	0-3 mm	**3-6 mm**	**7+ mm**
Jet Tip[17]	71%	44%	68%
Pik Pocket Tip[8]	90%	90%	64%

lins, Colo.) set at 60 psi (medium pressure). The control group received no irrigation. Extractions included the junctional epithelium. After examination with a scanning electron microscope, it was determined that no differences existed between test and control specimens in relationship to epithelial topography, cavitation, microulcerations, spacial relationships, and individual cell appearance.[40] Regarding bacteria, plaque samples showed that irrigated pockets had considerable reductions in microorganisms up to 6 mm in depth in irrigated pockets, compared with nonirrigated sites.[40] This concurs with early work by Drisko and colleagues, who also found that microorganisms were reduced up to 6 mm in irrigated pockets.[44]

The ability of a dental water jet to increase probing depth has been answered indirectly. Several clinical trials have investigated the effect a dental water jet has on probing depth. Rather than increasing depth, most have demonstrated statistically significant reductions generally ranging from 0.1 to 0.4 mm.* Although not clinically significant from a periodontal improvement standpoint, this evidence supports the safety of the dental water jet and refutes the notion that it causes a deepening of periodontal pockets.

Bacteremia

The advisability of recommending dental water jet for an individual at risk for infectious endocarditis (IE) has been debated, producing no clear answer.[16,47,102,117] The incidence of bacteremia from a dental water jet ranges from 7% in individuals with gingivitis[102] to up to 50% in those with periodontitis.[47] These percentages of bacteremia are similar to those found with other self-care devices.[28,100,121] Toothbrushing alone has been shown to cause bacteremia in 38.5% of cases.[37] No bacteremia was found in *daily* flossers but occurred 86% of the time in people who delayed flossing for 1 to 4 days.[28] Similar rates of bacteremia (10% to 14%) for brushing, flossing, and use of the Perio-Aid have been identified by others.[121]

> *Distinct Care Modifications*
>
> Before recommending a dental water jet, practitioners need to consider the patient's overall medical and oral health status. A consultation with the patient's physician may be necessary to assess the patient's risk and execute the best clinical judgment.

REDUCTION IN CLINICAL PARAMETERS

The dental water jet has been scientifically proven to reduce numerous clinical parameters including the following:

- Calculus[48,66,80]
- Biofilm (plaque)[†]
- Bacteria[‡]
- Gingivitis[§]
- Bleeding[‖]
- Inflammation and inflammatory mediators[2,43]

Calculus and Biofilm (Plaque) Removal

When the dental water jet was developed in the early 1960s, calculus was thought to be integral in the cause of periodontal disease. Therefore the fact that one of the earliest studies on the dental water jet investigated calculus reduction is not surprising. That study showed that adding a dental water jet to toothbrushing reduced calculus by 50%.[80] Others have found similar findings.[48,66]

In contrast, studies that have evaluated plaque biofilm removal have had inconsistent results, with some showing reduction and others not showing reduction.* Adding to the confusion, in most instances bleeding and gingivitis were generally significantly reduced regardless of changes in the PI.[26,31,51,52,80] Why this occurs is not completely known. Some of the answer may lie in the measurement of clinical indices. Traditional PIs measure supragingival plaque biofilm only. Additionally, the index is a measure of quantity not quality. Measurement of subgingival biofilm and its pathogens is more complex and less frequently done, yet it may provide better data on the true relationship between plaque biofilm and disease.

Reduction in Bacteria

As theories about the etiology of periodontal disease shifted from calculus and plaque biofilm to bacteria, scientific evidence seems to indicate that regardless of the effect on supragingival plaque biofilm, the dental water jet is capable of reducing subgingival microbiota[†]—some cases up to a depth of 6 mm.[40,44] When compared with other self-care routines such as toothbrushing or mouthrinsing, only a dental water jet with either water or 0.04% chlorhexidine reduced subgingival pathogens. Neither toothbrushing nor mouthrinsing with 0.12% chlorhexidine achieved the same results.[31] This is most likely because rinsing provides very little subgingival penetration compared with a dental water jet.[9] The Pik Pocket tip also has been shown to be effective at reducing subgingival pathogens.[49,71] Although an antimicrobial agent has been used in studies with the Pik Pocket tip, water may also be effective.[71]

Bleeding and Gingivitis

Evidence indicates that a dental water jet is a proven means for significantly reducing bleeding and gingivitis.[‡] In some cases these reductions are better than what can be achieved by routine oral hygiene.[12,43,51,87] A dental water jet has been shown to reduce bleeding by 50% over a 6-month time frame.[51] When a dental water jet and toothbrushing were compared with toothbrushing alone, adding the dental water jet was 73% more effective in reducing bleeding than brushing alone.[80]

DENTAL CONSIDERATIONS

When compared with dental floss, the addition of a dental water jet was up to 93% more effective at reducing bleeding and up to 52% more effective at reducing gingivitis than manual brushing and flossing.[1]

Periodontal maintenance patients who have added a dental water jet to their self-care routine have better reductions in bleeding and gingivitis versus those who do not.[51,87] Daily use of a dental water jet with water has been found to be more

---

*References 27, 37, 43, 51, 52, 71, 88.
†References 12, 31, 37, 43, 52, 66, 93, 121.
‡References 31, 37, 40, 44, 49, 71, 88.
§References 3, 4, 12, 26, 27, 37, 43, 49, 52, 66, 71, 80, 87.
‖References 3, 4, 12, 27, 31, 43, 51, 52, 66, 87, 93.

---

*References 12, 26, 31, 37, 43, 49, 51, 66, 77, 80, 87, 93, 121.
†References 31, 36, 40, 44, 49, 71, 88.
‡References 2, 7, 12, 26, 27, 31, 37, 40, 43, 48, 52, 71, 75, 80, 87, 93, 121.

effective than daily rinsing with 0.12% chlorhexidine for reducing bleeding.[52]

Inflammation and Inflammatory Mediators

The dental water jet reduces bleeding and gingivitis regardless of the amount of supragingival plaque biofilm removed.* What is only beginning to be known is how the dental water jet is able to do this. Some had hypothesized that the reductions were likely related to changes in the host inflammatory response.[11] Emerging information seems to confirm this.[3,24]

Two recent studies have included measures of inflammatory mediators, also called *cytokines,* as outcomes measures. Measures of both proinflammatory and antiinflammatory cytokines were chosen so that a true host modulation effect could be determined. The investigators also measured traditional clinical outcomes. The findings showed that the addition of a dental water jet to routine oral hygiene not only reduced the traditional measures of periodontal disease (i.e., bleeding, gingivitis, plaque biofilm) but also reduced the destructive cytokines, interleukin-1β (IL-1β), and prostaglandin E_2 (PGE$_2$), while increasing the antiinflammatory cytokine, interleukin-10 (IL-10), and maintaining interferon-γ (INF-γ)—a cytokine key in killing bacteria. Measures were taken 8 hours postirrigation. These results seem to indicate that the dental water jet produced a selective modulation of the host inflammatory response, thus potentially inhibiting periodontal disease activity.[43] In a study with similar measurements, twice-daily use of a dental water jet (with a Pik Pocket tip and plain tap water in a population with diabetes) reduced both traditional clinical outcomes and serum measures of the proinflammatory cytokines IL-1β and PGE$_2$ and reactive oxygen species.[2]

_____

*References 7, 40, 43, 51, 52, 87.

ROLE OF THE DENTAL WATER JET IN EVERYDAY SELF-CARE

Traditionally, dental hygienists have recommended that patients brush and floss. With the development of new and innovative devices in the past few years, alternative interdental aids are slowly being accepted as effective tools for interproximal cleaning. The role of the dental water jet in everyday self-care has remained less well defined.

The dental water jet is an appropriate self-care tool for almost any patient, including adolescents. A recent study conducted at the University of Nebraska found that a dental water jet paired with either a manual or a power toothbrush was as effective as a manual toothbrush and floss at reducing bleeding, gingivitis, and plaque biofilm; in some cases it was superior for reducing bleeding and gingivitis. Regardless of brush type, significant improvements in oral health occurred; therefore many patients currently using a power toothbrush may get further improvements in oral health by the addition of a dental water jet[12] (Table 24-5).

Based on these study results, the most obvious candidate for using a dental water jet is any individual who is noncomplaint with self-care or fails to improve or achieve optimal oral hygiene through traditional means.[12] Specifically, dental water jets have been tested and found safe and effective on individuals with the following:

- Orthodontic appliances,[27] including those in maxillary fixation[93]
- Crowns and bridges[74]
- Implants[48]
- Diabetes[2]

Table 24-5	Percent Reductions in Clinical Parameters at Day 28[13]		
CLINICAL REDUCTION	**MTB + OI GROUP 2**	**PTB + OI GROUP 3**	**MTB + FL GROUP 1**
Gingivitis (Facial)	15.1%*	11.4%	9.9%
Gingivitis (Lingual)	14.2%*	10.8%	9.4%
Bleeding (Facial)	59.2%*	50.6%*	30.6%
Bleeding (Lingual)	37.7%	36.2%	26.9%
Plaque Biofilm (Facial)	8.8%	17.3%*	9.0%
Plaque Biofilm (Lingual)	10.2%	9.4%	8.1%

*Statistically significant difference compared with MTB + FL at Day 28.
MTB + OI, Manual toothbrush plus oral instruction; *PTB + OI,* powered toothbrush plus oral instruction; *MTB + FL,* manual toothbrush plus fluoride.

ADHERENCE

> **Note**
>
> As with any self-care device, daily adherence to a regimen is key to obtaining good results.

It has been observed that individuals like and regularly use a dental water jet.* When subjects were followed up 1 year after the completion of participation in a dental water jet study, two thirds of the subjects were still using the pulsating dental water jet. Importantly, those using the water jet had significant reductions in gingivitis compared with those who stopped using the device.[75]

INSTRUCTING PATIENTS TO USE A DENTAL WATER JET

When giving instructions for the use of the dental water jet, some general suggestions can make learning an easy and quick process. Because many different types of units are available, the hygienist should be sure to review manufacturer's complete instructions before recommending or demonstrating a particular unit. Figure 24-34 shows a home water jet unit. Recommending and instructing is easier if the hygienist has read all instructions and tried the product (Box 24-6).

The subgingival irrigation tip has been designed for low-pressure delivery. Because this tip is site specific, individuals will need to know exactly where in the mouth it should be used. Extra tips should be available to demonstrate the placement to the individual; this will also help with compliance (Box 24-7).

---

*References 7, 51, 52, 66, 75.

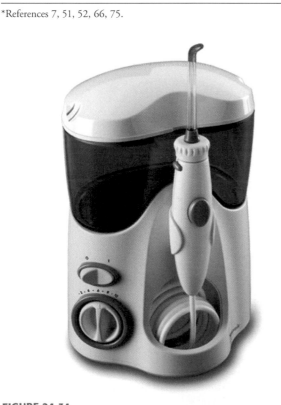

FIGURE 24-34
Waterpik Ultra Dental Jet for home use. (Courtesy Water Pik, Inc., Fort Collins, Colo.)

See Chapter 22 for more information on compliance and adherence.

USE OF ANTIMICROBIALS

Many solutions can be used in a dental water jet, but most beneficial is a solution that is acceptable to the individual (otherwise compliance may be compromised). The clinician should remind patients that when using a solution other than water, the unit must be flushed by filling the reservoir half full with water, removing the tip, and activating the system. If not, then the life of the unit could be shortened.

BOX 24-6

STEPS FOR USE OF THE DENTAL WATER JET

- For practical purposes, the unit should not be turned on until the tip is in the mouth.
- Bend from the waist over the sink and hold the arm up perpendicular to torso.
- The lips should be slightly closed to avoid splashing, but open enough to allow the water to flow freely from the mouth into the sink.
- Before removing the tip from the mouth, pause the flow of water or turn the unit off.
- Remember that for comfort, any solution used should be at room temperature.
- Begin at the lowest pressure setting when using the dental water jet for the first time.

The jet tip is recommended for general, full-mouth irrigation. When using the jet tip, the patient should do the following:

- Begin in the molar area and follow a pattern throughout the mouth. This helps avoid missing areas.
- Place the tip between the teeth at a right (90-degree) angle to the long axis of the tooth at the interproximal space. (The following figure shows the two zones of hydrokinetic activity and compares the impact zone and flushing zone.)

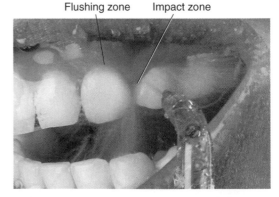

Flushing zone   Impact zone

- After the unit has been turned on and water has begun pulsating, briefly hold the tip in place at the interproximal area. This allows adequate penetration of the solution into the gingival crevice or pocket.
- Move the tip around the mouth in a linear fashion following the gingival margin. Make sure that all areas are irrigated from both the buccal and the lingual surfaces.

Three different types of agents have a body of evidence to support their use:

1. Water*
2. Chlorhexidine†
3. Essential oils[37,49]

Water is a very effective agent. Some of the benefits of using water are the following:

- True "natural" product
- No side effects
- Cost-effective
- Readily available
- Numerous studies to demonstrate efficacy‡

Chlorhexidine has frequently been evaluated in dental water jet studies.§ One of the benefits of using chlorhexidine is that because of better interproximal and subgingival penetration

✷ CASE APPLICATION 24-1.4

Oral Self-Care Evaluation and Modification

An evaluation of the proximal plaque biofilm retention and the embrasure configuration coupled with Mrs. Cronin's dexterity challenge leave the hygienist with several concerns. What should the hygienist's concerns be?

The hygienist helped Ann with the use of a disclosing agent and a small disposable mouth mirror, coaching her in seeing most of the posterior surfaces. Ann can reach the distal surfaces of her posterior teeth with her tongue and can tell the difference between a plaque biofilm–filled and plaque biofilm–free surface. Because of the difficulty Ann experienced in trying to thread a floss threader, the hygienist opted to recommend an ultrafine interdental brush. She wrapped the handle with foam, for which Ann was most grateful. With minimal coaching, Ann was able to clean all proximal surfaces with the interdental brush. In selected areas, the hygienist would like to encourage Ann to use a slightly larger brush but determined she would introduce that to Ann at the reevaluation appointment. If Ann experienced any difficulty with the recommended oral self-care devices, then she was instructed to call the office. Otherwise the hygienist felt that an assessment of these recommendations would best be made at the 6-week posttreatment appointment.

---

*References 2, 7, 27, 40, 43, 51, 75, 80, 87.
†References 26, 31, 48, 52, 71, 87, 121.
‡References 2, 12, 27, 40, 43, 51, 81, 87.
§References 26, 31, 48, 52, 71, 87, 121.

when compared with rinsing, diluting chlorhexidine is acceptable for use in a dental water jet.

The following dilutions (based on a 0.12% concentration) have been shown to be effective via randomized clinical trials:

- 0.02%—Five parts water to one part chlorhexidine[120]
- 0.04%—Two parts water to one part chlorhexidine[29,71]
- 0.06%—One part water to one part chlorhexidine[26,48,52,88]

Essential oils have also been studied as irrigants.[37,49] The most common brand of essential oils is Listerine antiseptic. However, several hundred generic brands exist. The reader should note that the effectiveness of Listerine antiseptic is based on studies using it at full strength only.

For a full review of chemotherapeutic agents, see Chapter 27.

References

1. Ainamo J et al: Assessment of the effect of an oscillating/rotating electric toothbrush on oral health. A twelve-month longitudinal study, *J Clin Periodontol* 24:28-33, 1997.
2. Al-Mubarek S et al: Comparative evaluation of adjunctive oral irrigation in diabetics, *J Clin Periodontol* 29:295, 2002.
3. American Dental Association Council on Scientific Affairs: *Acceptance guidelines—toothbrushes,* Chicago, 1998, The Association.
4. American Dental Association Seal-of-Acceptance Program: *The ADA seal of acceptance program* [Internet], Chicago, 1999, American Dental Association [http://www.ada.org].
5. Anderson NA et al: A clinical comparison of the efficacy of an electromechanical flossing device or manual flossing affecting interproximal gingival bleeding and plaque accumulation, *J Clin Dent* 6:105-107, 1995.
6. Anton P: *Oral health fast facts* [Internet], Chicago, 2004, American Dental Hygienists' Association [http://www.adha.org/media/facts/oral_health_fast_facts.htm].
7. Aziz-Gandour IA, Newman HN: The effects of simplified oral hygiene regime plus supragingival irrigation with chlorhexidine or metronidazole on chronic inflammatory periodontal disease, *J Clin Periodontol* 13:228, 1986.
8. Babb DA, Johnson RH: The effect of a new electric toothbrush on supragingival plaque and gingivitis, *J Periodontol* 60:336-341, 1989.
9. Bader HI: Review of currently available battery-operated toothbrushes, *Compend Cont Educ Dent* 13:1162, December 1992.
10. Barnes CM: Powered toothbrushes: a focus on the evidence, *Compend Oral Hyg* 7(2):3-10, 2002.
11. Barnes CM, Russell CM, Weatherford TW 3rd: A comparison of the efficacy of 2 powered toothbrushes in affecting plaque accumulation, gingivitis and gingival bleeding, *J Periodontol* 70(8):840-847, 1999.
12. Barnes CM et al: Comparison of irrigation to floss as an adjunct to toothbrushing: effect on bleeding, gingivitis and supragingival plaque, *J Clin Dent* 16(3):7, 2005.
13. Barnes CM et al: A comparison of a Waterpik dual-motor powered toothbrush and a manual toothbrush in affecting interproximal bleeding reduction and dental biofilm accumulation, *J Clin Dent* 14(3):49-52, 2003.
14. Bass CC: The optimum characteristics of toothbrushes for personal oral hygiene, *Dent Items Interest* 70:697-718, 1948.

15. Bass CC: An effective method of personal oral hygiene: II, *J La State Med Soc* 108:100-112, 1954.

16. Berger SA et al: Bacteremia after the use of an oral irrigation device, *Ann Intern Med* 80:510, 1974.

17. Bergmann M, Woog PGL: Presentation d'dune brose a'dents actionee electriqument, *Rev Fr Odontostomatol* 6:378-382, 1959.

18. Berman, CL et al: Observations of the effects of an electric toothbrush, *J Periodontol* 33:195-198, 1962.

19. Bhaskar SN, Cutright DE, Frisch J: Effect of high-pressure water jet on oral mucosa of varied density, *J Periodontol* 40:593, 1969.

20. Bhaskar SN et al: Water jet devices in dental practice, *J Periodontol* 42:593, 1971.

21. Biesbrock AR, Walters PA, Bartizek RD: The relative effectiveness of six powered toothbrushes for dental plaque removal, *J Clin Dent* 13(5):198-202, 2002.

22. Bowen D: An evidence-based review of power toothbrushes, *Compend Oral Hyg* 9(1):3-18, 2002.

23. Boyd RL: Clinical and laboratory evaluation of powered electric toothbrushes: review of the literature, *J Clin Dent* 8(3 spec no): 67-71,1997.

24. Boyd RL, Hollander BN, Eakle WS: Comparison of a subgingivally placed cannula oral irrigator tip with a supragingivally placed standard irrigator tip, *J Clin Periodontol* 19:340, 1992.

25. Braun RE, Ciancio SG: Subgingival delivery by an oral irrigation device, *J Periodontol* 63:469, 1992.

26. Brownstein CN et al: Irrigation with chlorhexidine to resolve naturally occurring gingivitis: a methodologic study, *J Clin Periodontol* 17:588, 1990.

27. Burch JG, Lanese R, Ngan P: A two-month study of the effects of oral irrigation and automatic toothbrush use in an adult orthodontic population with fixed appliances, *Am J Orthod Dentofacial Orthop* 106:121, 1994.

28. Carroll GC, Sebor RJ: Dental flossing and its relationship to transient bacteremia, *J Periodontol* 51:691, 1980.

29. Carter-Hanson, C, Gadbury-Amyot C, Killoy W: Comparison of the plaque removal efficacy of a new flossing aid (Quik Floss) to finger flossing, *J Clin Periodontol* 23:873-878, 1996.

30. Chava VK: An evaluation of the efficacy of a curved bristle and conventional toothbrush. A comparative clinical study, *J Periodontol* 71:785-789, 2000.

31. Chaves ES et al: Mechanism of irrigation effects on gingivitis, *J Periodontol* 65:1016, 1994.

32. Checchi L et al: Toothbrush filaments end-rounding: stereomicroscope analysis, *J Clin Periodontol* 28(4):360-367, 2001.

33. Chilton NW, DiDio A, Rothner JT: Comparison of the effectiveness of an electric toothbrush and a standard toothbrush in normal individuals, *J Am Dent Assoc* 64:777-782, 1962.

34. Choo A, Delac DM, Messer LB: Oral hygiene measures and promotion: review and considerations, *Aust Dent J* 46:166-173, 2001.

35. Christou V et al: Comparison of different approaches of interdental oral hygiene: interdental brushes versus dental floss, *J Periodontol* 69:759-764, 1998.

36. Ciancio SG, Shibly O, Farber GA: Clinical evaluation of the effect of two types of dental floss on plaque and gingival health, *Clin Prev Dent* 14:14, 1992.

37. Ciancio SG et al: Effect of a chemotherapeutic agent delivered by an oral irrigation device on plaque, gingivitis, and subgingival microflora, *J Periodontol* 60:310, 1989.

38. Claydon N, Addy M: Comparative single-use plaque removal by toothbrushes of different designs, *J Clin Periodontol* 23:1112, 1996.

39. Claydon N et al: Comparative professional plaque removal study using 8 branded toothbrushes, *J Clin Periodontol* 29:310-316, 2002.

40. Cobb CM, Rodgers RL, Killoy WJ: Ultrastructural examination of human periodontal pockets following the use of an oral irrigation device in vivo, *J Periodontol* 59:155,1988.

41. Corbet EF, Davies WR: The role of supragingival plaque in the control of progressive periodontal disease: a review, *J Clin Periodontol* 20:307-313, 1993.

42. Cronin MJ et al: A 30-day clinical comparison of a novel interdental cleaning device and dental floss in the reduction of plaque and gingivitis, *J Clin Dent* 16:33-37, 2005.

43. Cutler CW et al: Clinical benefits of oral irrigation for periodontitis are related to reduction of pro-inflammatory cytokine levels and plaque, *J Clin Periodontol* 27:134, 2000.

44. Drisko C et al: Comparison of dark-field microscopy and a flagella stain for monitoring the effect of a Water Pik on bacterial motility, *J Periodontol* 58:381, 1987.

45. Eakle WS, Ford C, Boyd RL: Depth of penetration in periodontal pockets with oral irrigation, *J Clin Periodontol* 13:39, 1986.

46. Emling RC, Yankell SL: The application of sonic technology to oral hygiene: the third generation of powered toothbrushes, *J Clin Dent* 8:1-3, 1997.

47. Felix JE, Rosen S, App GR: Detection of bacteremia after the use of an oral irrigation device in subjects with periodontitis, *J Periodontol* 42:785, 1971.

48. Felo A et al: Effects of subgingival chlorhexidine irrigation on perio-implant maintenance, *Am J Dent* 10:107, 1997.

49. Fine JB et al: Short-term microbiological and clinical effects of subgingival irrigation with an antimicrobial mouthrinse, *J Periodontol* 65:30, 1994.

50. Fischman SL: The history of oral hygiene products: How far have we come in 6000 years? *Periodontol 2000* 15:7-14, 1997.

51. Flemmig TF et al: Adjunctive supragingival irrigation with acetylsalicylic acid in periodontal supportive therapy, *J Clin Periodontol* 22:427, 1995.

52. Flemmig TF et al: Supragingival irrigation with 0.06% chlorhexidine in naturally occurring gingivitis: I—6 month clinical observations, *J Periodontol* 61:112, 1990.

53. Floss.com: *The world of dentistry online. Dental trivia and tips/ origins of toothpaste and floss* [Internet], Garden City, NY, 2006, Floss.com [http://www.floss.com].

54. Fones AC: Home care of the mouth. In Fones AC, editor: *Mouth hygiene*, ed 4, Philadelphia, 1934, Lea & Febiger.

55. Fransden A: Mechanical oral hygiene practices. State-of-the-science review. In Loe H, Kleinman DV, eds: *Dental plaque control measures and oral hygiene practices. Proceedings for a state of the science workshop*, Oxford, 1986, IRL Press Ltd, pp 93-116.

56. Gjeremo P, Flotra L: The effect of different methods of interdental cleaning, *J Periodontol Res* 5:230-236, 1970.

57. Glass RL: A clinical study of an electric toothbrush, *J Periodontol* 36:322-327, 1965.

58. Glutch-Scranton J: *Collaboration and empowerment in educational activities during dental hygiene care,* Ann Arbor, Mich, 1992, University Microfilms.

59. Granath LE et al: Intra-individual effect of daily supervised flossing on caries in school children, *Commun Dent Oral Epidemiol* 7:147-150, 1979.

60. Graves RC, Disney JA, Stamm JW: Comparative effectiveness of flossing and brushing in reducing interproximal bleeding, *J Periodontol* 60(5):243-247, 1989.

61. Grossman E et al: A comparative study of extrinsic stain removal with two electric toothbrushes and a manual brush, *Am J Dent* 9:25-29,1996.

62. Hancock EB: Prevention. In Genco RJ, Newman MG, eds: *Annals of periodontology,* Chicago, 1996, American Academy of Periodontology.

63. Heanue M, Deacaon SA: Manual versus powered toothbrushing for oral health, *Cochrane Database Syst Rev* (1):CD002281, 2003.

64. Heasman PA, Jacobs DJ, Chapple IL: An evaluation of the effectiveness and patient compliance with plaque control methods and prevention of periodontal disease, *Clin Prev Dent* 11:24-28, 1989.

65. Hine M: Toothbrush, *Int Dent J* 6:15, 1956.

66. Hoover DR, Robinson HBG: The comparative effectiveness of a pulsating oral irrigator as an adjunct in maintaining oral health, *J Periodontol* 42:37, 1971.

67. Horowitz AM et al: Effects of supervised daily dental plaque removal by children II: 24 months' results, *J Public Health Dent* 37:180-188, 1977.

68. Innes NP et al: Obtaining an evidence-base for clinical dentistry through clinical trials, *Prim Dent Care* 12(3):91-96, 2005.

69. International Organization for Standardization Dentistry: *Stiffness of the tufted area of toothbrushes,* Ref ISO 8627, Jersey City, NJ, 1987, The Organization.

70. Jepson S: The role of manual toothbrushes in effective plaque control. In Lang NP, Attstrom R, Loe H, eds: *Proceedings of European workshop on mechanical plaque removal,* Chicago, 1998, Quintessence Books.

71. Jolkovsky DL et al : Clinical and microbiological effects of subgingival and gingival marginal irrigation with chlorhexidine gluconate, *J Periodontol* 61:663, 1990.

72. Kiger RD, Nylund K, Feller RP: A comparison of proximal plaque removal using floss and interdental brushes, *J Clin Periodontol* 18(9):681-684, 1991.

73. Kleber CJ, Putt MS: Formation of flossing habit using a floss-holding device, *J Dent Hyg* 64:140-143, 1990.

74. Krajewski J, Giblin J, Gargiulo AW: Evaluation of a water pressure-cleansing device as an adjunct to periodontal treatment, *Periodontics* 2:76, 1964.

75. Lainson PA, Bergquist JJ, Fraleigh CM: A longitudinal study of pulsating water pressure cleansing devices, *J Periodontol* 43:444, 1972.

76. Lamberts DM, Wunderlich RC, Caffesse RG: The effect of waxed and unwaxed dental floss on gingival health: I—plaque removal and gingiva response, *J Periodontol* 53:393, 1982.

77. Lang WP, Ronis DL, Farghaly MM: Preventive behaviors as correlates of periodontal health status, *J Public Health Dent* 55(1): 10-17, 1995.

78. Lewis DW, Ismail AI: Periodic health examination, 1995 update: 2. Prevention of dental caries. The Canadian Task Force on the Periodic Health Examination, *CMAJ* 15:836-846, 1995.

79. Library of Congress: *Everyday mysteries. Fun science facts from the Library of Congress,* Washington DC, 2006, Library of Congress.

80. Lobene RR: The effect of a pulsed water pressure-cleansing device on oral health, *J Periodontol* 40:51, 1969.

81. McInnes C, Engel D, Martin RW: Fimbria damage and removal of adherent bacteria after exposure to acoustic energy, *Oral Microbiol Immunol* 8:277-282, 1993.

82. Menaker LM, Morhart RE, Navia JM: *Biological basis of dental caries: an oral biology textbook,* Hagerstown, Md, 1980, Harper & Row, pp 482-496.

83. Mills EJ et al: The quality of a randomized trial reporting in leading medical journals since the revised CONSORT statement, *Contemp Clin Trials* 26(4):480-487, 2005.

84. Moritis K, Delaurenti M: Comparison of the Sonicare Elite and a manual toothbrush in the evaluation of plaque reduction, *Am J Dent* 15(spec no):23B-25B, 2002.

85. Mueller LJ et al: Rotary electric toothbrushing: clinical effects on the presence of gingivitis and supragingival dental plaque, *Dent Hyg* 61:546-550, 1987.

86. Nelson D: *Review of dental hygiene,* Philadelphia, 2000, Saunders.

87. Newman MG et al: Effectiveness of adjunctive irrigation in early periodontitis: multi-center evaluation, *J Periodontol* 65:224, 1994.

88. Newman MG et al: Irrigation with 0.06% chlorhexidine in naturally occurring gingivitis: II—6 months microbiological observations, *J Periodontol* 61:427, 1990.

89. Niederman R, ADA Council on Scientific Affairs, ADA Division of Science: Manual versus powered toothbrushes: the Cochrane Review, *J Am Dent Assoc* 134(9):1240-1244, 2003.

90. Nunn ME et al: Plaque reduction over time of an integrated oral hygiene system, *Compendium* 25(10suppl 1):8-14, 2004.

91. O'Neil HW: Opinion study comparing attitudes about dental health, *J Am Dent Assoc* 109:910-915, 1984.

92. Ong G: The effectiveness of 3 types of dental floss for interdental plaque removal, *J Clin Periodontol* 17:463, 1990.

93. Phelps-Sandall BA, Oxford SJ: Effectiveness of oral hygiene techniques on plaque and gingivitis in patients placed in inter-maxillary fixation, *Oral Surg Oral Med Oral Pathol* 56:487, 1983.

94. Platt K et al: Clinical evaluation of the plaque removal efficacy and safety of the Sonicare Elite toothbrush, *Am J Dent* 15(spec issue):19B-22B, 2004.

95. Prader M: The toothbrush and other mechanical devices. In Prader M: *Oral hygiene products and practice,* New York, 1988, Marcel Dekker Inc, pp 141-194.

96. Rainey BL, Ash MM: A clinical evaluation of an electric toothbrush, *J Periodontol* 34:127-136, 1963.

97. Renton-Harper P, Addy M, Newcombe RG: Plaque removal with the uninstructed use of electric toothbrushes: comparison with a manual brush and toothpaste slurry, *J Clin Periodontol* 28:325-330, 2001.

98. Ring ME: *Dentistry—an illustrated history,* New York, 1985, Abradale Press, Harry N Abrams Inc Publishers, pp 34-141.

99. Ring ME: The "electric" toothbrush of one hundred years ago, *Periodontal Clin Invest* 21(1):23, 1999.

100. Roberts GJ et al: Dental bacteremia in children, *Pediatr Cardiol* 18:24, 1997.

101. Robinson PG et al: Manual versus powered toothbrushing for oral health, *Cochrane Database Syst Rev* Apr 18(2):CD002281, 2005.

102. Roman AR, App GR: Bacteremia, a result from oral irrigation in subjects with gingivitis, *J Periodontol* 42:757, 1971.

103. Rosema NA et al: An oscillating/pulsating electric toothbrush versus a high-frequency electric toothbrush in the treatment of gingivitis, *J Dent* 33(suppl 1):29-36, 2005.

104. Rosenthal PO: Toothbrushing, yesterday, today, tomorrow, *J South Calif Dent Assoc* 30:210-213, 1962.

105. Saxer U: Impact of improved toothbrushes on dental diseases. II, *Quintessence Int* 28(9):573-593, 1997.

106. Scutt JS, Swann CJ: The first mechanical toothbrush? *Br Dent J* 139:152, 1975.

107. Selting WJ, Bhaskar SN, Mueller RP: Water jet direction and periodontal pocket débridement, *J Periodontol* 43:569, 1972.

108. Sembera K: Evolution and analysis of the toothbrush, The American Society of Mechanical Engineering, *ASME Mechanical Advantage*, March 2001.

109. Sharma NC et al: Single-use plaque removal efficacy of three power toothbrushes, *J Dent* 33(suppl 1):11-15, 2005.

110. Shibly O et al: Clinical evaluation of an automatic flossing device vs manual flossing, *J Clin Dent* 12(3):63-66, 2001.

111. Smith C: Toothbrush technology—even the pharaohs brushed their teeth, *J Dent Technol* 17(4):26-27, 2000.

112. Smith WA, Ash MM: A clinical evaluation of an electric toothbrush, *J Periodontol* 34:127-136, 1963.

113. Sowinski JA et al: Comparative efficacy of Colgate battery-powered toothbrush and Colgate Plus (manual) toothbrush on established plaque and gingivitis: a 30-day clinical study in New Jersey, *Compend Contin Educ Dent Suppl* 31:S4-8, 2000.

114. Spolsky VW et al: Evaluating the efficacy of a new flossing aid, *J Clin Periodontol* 20:490-497, 1993.

115. Stanford CM, Srikantha R, Wu CD: Efficacy of the Sonicare toothbrush fluid dynamic action on removal of human supra-gingival plaque, *J Clin Dent* 8:10-14, 1997.

116. Stillman PR: A philosophy of the treatment of periodontal disease, *Dent Dig* 38:315-319, 1932.

117. Tamimi GA, Thomassen PR, Moser EH: Bacteremia study using a water irrigation device, *J Periodontol* 40:4, 1969.

118. Travers B, editor: *World of invention,* Detroit, 1994, Gale Research Inc, p 635.

119. Van der Weijden GA et al: The role electric toothbrushes: advantages and limitations. In Lang NP, Attstrom R, Loe H, eds: *Proceedings of European workshop on mechanical plaque removal,* Chicago, 1998, Quintessence Books.

120. Versteeg PA et al: Sonic-powered toothbrushes and reversal of experimental gingivitis, *J Clin Periodontol* 32(12):1236-1241, 2005.

121. Walsh TF, Glenwright HD, Hull PS: Clinical effects of pulsed oral irrigation with 0.0% chlorhexidine digluconate in patients with adult periodontitis, *J Clin Periodontol* 19:245, 1992.

122. Warren PR et al: A clinical investigation into the effect of toothbrush wear on efficacy, *J Clin Dent* 13:119-124, 2002.

123. Westfelt E: Rationale of mechanical plaque control, *J Clin Periodontol* 23:263-267, 1996.

124. Williams KB et al: Effect of sonic and mechanical toothbrushes on subgingival microbial flora: a comparative in vivo scanning electron microscopy study of 8 subjects, *Quintessence Int* 32:147-154, 2001.

125. Williams K et al: Plaque removal efficacy of a prototype power toothbrush compared to a positive control manual toothbrush, *Am J Dent* 16(4):223-227, 2003.

126. Wolf L, Kim A: Effectiveness of a sonic toothbrush in maintenance of dental implants, *J Clin Periodontol* 25:821-828, 1998.

127. Wu-Yuan CD, Anderson RD, McInnes C: Ability of the Sonicare electric toothbrush to generate dynamic fluid activity that removes bacteria, *J Clin Dent* 5:89-93, 1994.

128. Yankell SL, Saxer UP: Toothbrushes and toothbrushing methods. In Harris NO, Garcia-Godoy F, editors: *Primary preventive dentistry,* ed 6, Stamford, Conn, 2004, Appleton & Lange.

Dental Caries and Caries Management

Douglas A. Young • John D.B. Featherstone •

Alan W. Budenz

INSIGHT

Dental caries continues to be a principal reason for dental treatment and tooth loss. Although the widespread application of topical and systemic fluoride has helped reduce this dental challenge, it has not been able to eliminate the disease completely. One of the primary responsibilities of the dental hygienist is to understand the dental caries process and to educate patients about the cause and treatment and how to manage risk factors that affect this common infectious disease by recommending and using appropriate prevention strategies for each patient visiting the dental practice.

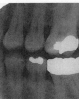

CASE STUDY 25-1 | Remineralization of the Early Carious Lesion

Frances Svensen, a 25-year-old sixth-grade teacher, reports to the dental office for a supportive care appointment. She and her husband have recently relocated to the area because of her husband's job transfer. She has brought her previous set of bitewing radiographs, which was taken 3 years before the current appointment, during which a current set is ordered. Her radiographs are reviewed for signs of hard tissue disease.

In comparing the radiograph taken 3 years ago **(A)** with that taken at the current appointment **(B),** what is evident about the following teeth?

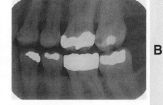

A   B

Tooth	3 Years Earlier	Now
#11 distal	Incipient lesion	Incipient lesion unchanged
#12 mesial	Incipient lesion	Lesion progressed through dentinoenamel junction (DEJ)
#13 distal	Incipient lesion	Lesion remineralized
#14 mesial	Carious lesion	Lesion restored
#15 mesial	No lesion noted	Carious lesion evident
#18 occlusal	Recurrent dental caries	Dental caries restored
#21 distoocclusal	Dental caries evident	Dental caries restored

KEY TERMS

acidogenic bacteria
body of the lesion
buffering
carbonated apatite
caries management by risk assessment
caries risk assessment
cavitation
cavity
demineralization
dental caries

diffusion channels
fluorapatite
fluoride
fluorosis
hydroxyapatite
lactobacilli
mutans streptococci
parts per million
remineralization
white spot lesion

LEARNING OUTCOMES

After reading this chapter the student will be able to:
1. Use CAMBRA to assess dental caries risk on a patient.
2. Develop dental caries prevention and disease intervention strategies for a patient, based on CAMBRA.
3. Recommend the appropriate fluoride products for an individual.
4. Select appropriate therapeutic strategies for implementation in the dental office.
5. Establish an appropriate interval for evaluation of the suggested strategies.
6. Work with other oral healthcare providers in the management of dental caries.

Chapter 17 emphasizes the detection of **dental caries** as part of the hard tissue evaluation. This chapter focuses on the molecular mechanisms of dental caries and the management of this infectious disease, including preventive and conservative treatment protocols and chemical treatment of early lesions. The chemical aspects of demineralization and remineralization and the role of **fluoride** are discussed to solidify the scientific basis for dental caries management by risk assessment. Fluoride products and their proper uses are also reviewed.

Dental Caries and Oral Hygiene

Studies in the 1950s implied that oral hygiene programs reduced the incidence of dental caries. Later, clinical studies compared fluoride-containing dentifrice to placebo dentifrice and reported dental caries reductions of approximately 30%, clearly showing that the addition of fluoride was important for beneficial anticaries effects related to toothbrushing.[88]

Dental caries remains a major problem in many developing countries. Although declining in most Western countries over the past 2 decades, dental caries continues to be the principal reason for dental treatment and tooth loss.[53,96]

> *Note*
>
> Approximately 80% of dental caries in U.S. children is found in 25% of the population.[53] Dental caries also remains a major problem in U.S. adults, with 94% reporting dental caries in one survey.[96]

The reasons for the reported reductions in tooth decay during the last 20 years have not been precisely determined, but evidence indicates that the use of fluoride products is the major reason.[49,52] Such products include fluoride toothpaste, fluoride mouthrinses, and topical fluorides in the dental office. In addition to fluoride products, many public water supplies are fluoridated, resulting in a reported 40% to 70% reduction in dental caries.[14,65,73,76]

Dental Caries Process

The basic process of dental decay is simple in concept. A biofilm called *pellicle,* derived from saliva, is strongly bound to the tooth surface. This coating has many beneficial effects, including protecting the surface from direct acid exposure and thus inhibiting demineralization. The pellicle, however, is in turn covered by the bacteria that form a biofilm called the *dental plaque.*[65,67] If the bacterial plaque contains significant numbers of the bacterial groups **mutans streptococci** (MS) or **lactobacilli** (LB), then the by-products of their metabolism will be small-chain organic acids, such as formic, lactic, acetic, and propionic. MS includes several species, classified into eight serotypes, two of which—*Streptococcus mutans* and *Streptococcus sobrinus*—cause dental caries in humans. These acid-producing bacteria are called **acidogenic bacteria.** They can also live in an acid environment and are called *aciduric* bacteria because of this. In other words, they not only can live in an acid environment but can also produce acids when they metabolize fermentable carbohydrates.[65,67,75] Any fermentable carbohydrate, such as glucose, sucrose, fructose, or cooked starch, can be metabolized by these bacteria to produce acid as a by-product of their metabolism,[45] dispelling the myth that only *sweets* containing sucrose cause dental caries.

DEMINERALIZATION

The organic acids produced by pathogenic bacteria can dissolve the calcium phosphate mineral of the tooth enamel or dentin through the process of **demineralization**.[25,32,35] When taken into the mouth, fermentable carbohydrates are metabolized by the bacteria, creating acid as a by-product. The acid then diffuses from the *plaque fluid* (the water-based fluid among the bacteria in dental plaque) through the pellicle covering the tooth and into the tooth itself. Surprisingly to many, the enamel is porous to small molecules and ions, such as calcium, phosphate, fluoride, and the small-chain organic acids. Movement of these small molecules and ions into the tooth is driven by passive diffusion from an area of high concentration to an area of low concentration. Thus the diffusion of molecules follows a simple concentration gradient and continues until the concentration reaches equilibrium. The small-chain organic acids readily diffuse, following the concentration gradient into the enamel or dentin, if exposed, and dissociate to produce hydrogen ions as they travel.[24,35] The dissociated hydrogen ions then dissolve the mineral, freeing calcium and phosphate into solution, which can then diffuse from the tooth through a similar concentration gradient.

When demineralization is not halted or reversed, the carious lesion progresses and can eventually lead to a **cavity** or **cavitation.** The spaces between the enamel crystals that allow these small molecules to diffuse are called **diffusion channels** (see Composition of Tooth Mineral later in this chapter). This process of demineralization continues until equilibrium is again reached.

REMINERALIZATION

Only if the acid is neutralized first and the concentration of calcium and phosphate ions becomes higher outside the tooth than inside will the calcium and phosphate ions reverse direction and diffuse back into the tooth, again through a concentration gradient. This replacement of mineral back into the tooth is called **remineralization**.[25,90,91] The saliva plays numerous roles, including neutralization of acid, which is called **buffering,** and providing the minerals (calcium and phosphate ions) that can replace those dissolved from the tooth during a demineralization challenge.

The earliest clinically detectable sign of dental caries is the **white spot lesion** of enamel. This lesion consists of a demineralized region called the **body of the lesion** just below what appears to be an intact surface layer.[86] This subsurface area may have lost up to 50% of its mineral and can be distinguished in the laboratory by specialized histologic techniques such as microradiography or polarized light microscopy. Clinically, the lesion appears white because the loss of mineral changes the refractive index compared with that of the surrounding translucent enamel.

DENTAL CONSIDERATIONS

The ability to recognize clinically a white spot lesion is a valuable asset for the clinician. A shiny white spot is usually a sign of arrested or remineralized lesions, and a dull appearance may indicate that the lesion is still actively demineralizing (see Chapter 17).

Why does the surface layer remain intact, or does it? In the early stages of dental caries, the surface crystals are partially dissolved by the plaque acids, and during subsequent repair they are partially remineralized as subsurface demineralization progresses. This process makes the surface appear *intact,* and the mineral is less soluble than it was originally. This remineralized surface accounts for the apparently intact surface layer observed with microradiography or polarized light microscopy in an early enamel lesion. This surface generally *feels* sound to gentle probing by the dental explorer.

COMPOSITION OF TOOTH MINERAL

Enamel is the hardest substance of the human body. The enamel and dentin of a tooth comprise millions of tiny mineral crystals embedded in a protein-lipid matrix. The individual crystals of enamel are only about 40 nm in diameter, approximately $\frac{1}{1000}$ of the thickness of a human hair. These small crystals lie approximately perpendicular to the tooth surface and are clustered into enamel rods approximately 4 to 5 mcm in diameter.[40] The tiny spaces or pores between the individual crystals and the larger spaces between the enamel rods are filled with protein, lipid, and water, which make up small passageways called *diffusion channels*. The diffusion channels between enamel rods form larger passageways than the channels between the individual crystals. The rod channels are large enough to allow the passage of small molecules and ions, such as hydrogen, calcium, phosphate, fluoride, and the organic acids produced by MS and LB, but they are too narrow to allow entry of bacteria.

The percent by volume is relevant to the diffusion processes that are the basis of dental caries progression. As the enamel is demineralized during dental caries progression, the mineral removed makes the carious enamel even more porous.[86]

For years the dental profession has referred to the tooth mineral as **hydroxyapatite,** although pure hydroxyapatite does not exist in real teeth. Rather than *pure,* the mineral of enamel, dentin, and bone may be viewed as *contaminated* by carbonate and other minerals, making the substance much more soluble in acid. Thus tooth mineral can be described best as a highly substituted **carbonated apatite.**[60,61] Although related to hydroxyapatite $[Ca_{10}(PO_4)_6(OH)_2]$, carbonated hydroxyapatite differs from pure hydroxyapatite in two ways. First, carbonated apatite is calcium deficient, with some calcium replaced by sodium, magnesium, zinc, and other substitutes. Second, some of the phosphate ions in the crystal lattice are replaced by carbonate, which can be as much as 3% to 6% by weight.* All these substitutions occur during tooth development, when the mineral is first laid down. The carbonate-rich areas represent major defects in the crystal structure. The three-dimensional size and shape of the carbonate ion differs from the phosphate ion, causing major crystal imperfections that are more susceptible to acid attack during demineralization.[30,33] The calcium substitutions (e.g., sodium, magnesium, zinc) also cause similar defects in the crystal lattice, although to a lesser extent than the carbonate defects. The combined effect of calcium deficiency and carbonate rich tooth mineral is that the carbonated hydroxyapatite is significantly more soluble in acid than pure hydroxyapatite.

As previously discussed, substitutions make the crystal less perfect and more soluble; the fluoride ion (F^-) can substitute for the hydroxyl ion (OH^+) of hydroxyapatite and make the crystal more perfect and less soluble. This improved crystal is called **fluorapatite** $[Ca_{10}(PO_4)_6F_2]$, which is very resistant to dissolution by acid. The solubility differential can be ranked as follows:

- Dental *mineral,* or *carbonated hydroxyapatite,* is the most soluble in acid.
- Hydroxyapatite is less soluble in acid.
- Fluorapatite is least soluble in acid.

*References 13, 16-17, 31, 34, 60-61.

> **Note**
> Mature enamel is approximately 85% by volume mineral and 15% lipid, protein, and water; thus 15% is the volume available for diffusion (Table 25-1).

> **Note**
> Dentin and cementum are roughly 47% by volume mineral and 53% lipid, protein, and water, illustrating their more porous nature.

Table 25-1	Approximate Composition of Enamel and Dentin			
	Enamel		**Dentin**	
TISSUE COMPONENT	**% BY WEIGHT**	**% BY VOLUME**	**% BY WEIGHT**	**% BY VOLUME**
Mineral: Carbonated Hydroxyapatite	96	85	70	47
Protein or Lipid	1	3	20	33
Water	3	12	10	20

The composition of crystal surfaces in remineralized enamel is a blend of hydroxyapatite and fluorapatite, and the remineralized crystals are therefore much less soluble than the original mineral.[91]

Fluoride

TOPICAL VERSUS SYSTEMIC UPTAKE

Another misconception in dentistry is that the major dental caries-inhibiting effect of fluoride is caused by its systemic uptake and incorporation into the enamel during tooth development before eruption. This misconception led to water fluoridation and the use of oral fluoride supplements prescribed for children without access to fluoridated water. As the mechanism of dental caries was elucidated in the 1970s and 1980s, the importance of fluoride in dental caries prevention became apparent. However, the effects were found to be *topical* via the surface of the tooth, not systemic.* *Topical uptake* means the fluoride diffuses into the surface of the enamel of an erupted tooth rather than being incorporated preeruptively during development (systemic incorporation). Surprisingly, this fact is still not widely known, and the standard of care still recommends *dietary fluoride supplements* for children in nonfluoridated communities.

Fluoridated water and prescription supplements systemically incorporate insufficient amounts of fluoride into the dental mineral to play a significant role in dental caries prevention.[44,91] Systemic delivery incorporates only about 1000 to 2000 **parts per million** (ppm) of fluoride in the outer enamel surface and 20 to 100 ppm of fluoride below the surface, depending on the fluoride ingestion during tooth development.[82] Other experiments show that systemic uptake of fluoride during tooth development results in no measurable benefit against acid-induced dissolution.[25,39,74,91] In contrast to systemic delivery, topical sources of fluoride can deliver as much as 30,000 ppm to the surfaces of the individual crystals of enamel, which significantly reduces mineral solubility in acid.[25] Thus the effect of systemically ingested fluoride on dental caries is negligible compared with topical uptake. Prescription supplements are still the standard

of care for children in nonfluoridated communities, but considering the risks of **fluorosis** (disturbance of enamel formation by fluoride during tooth development), the use of systemic fluoride supplements may soon be questioned. Currently, if prescribed, fluoride supplements should be used as a topical delivery system, with patients sucking or chewing tablets or lozenges before ingestion.

ROLE OF SALIVA

Saliva may represent the single most important group of components in the maintenance of oral health because it contains many protective proteins and minerals and keeps them available in solution (Box 25-1). Laboratory studies have shown that a significantly low level of fluoride in the saliva (0.04 ppm) is sufficient to produce beneficial anticaries effects through remineralization.[25,28,40] As the fluoride concentration increases above 0.04 ppm, the amount of remineralization also increases, with an optimal level at 0.08 ppm or greater. Clinically, these data indicate that small increases in the background level of fluoride in saliva and plaque fluid may provide important dental caries protection for erupted teeth of both children and adults.

When topical fluoride products are used in the mouth—whether a dentifrice (toothpaste), fluoride mouthrinse, or prescribed agent—the increased fluoride levels in the saliva diminish over time as the fluoride is cleared from the mouth. Beneficial levels of fluoride between 0.03 and 0.1 ppm can be sustained for as long as 2 to 6 hours, depending on the product and the individual.[12] For example, researchers have shown that a 0.05% sodium fluoride (NaF) mouthrinse (225 ppm fluoride) used for 1 minute not only provides increased salivary levels of fluoride for 2 to 4 hours but also remains in plaque biofilm for significantly longer.[99] Other researchers also demonstrate that daily use of both a fluoride-containing dentifrice and a 0.05% NaF topical rinse can completely prevent formation of white spot lesions (early demineralization) around orthodontic brackets *in vivo* (on human patients).[78]

BOX 25-1

GROUPS OF SALIVARY COMPONENTS

1. Proteins that form pellicle and protect the tooth surface (proline-rich proteins, statherins, histatins, cystatins)
2. Proteins that maintain the calcium and phosphate in solution in a supersaturated state (proline-rich proteins, statherins)
3. Proteins with antifungal and antibacterial properties (histatins, lysozyme, lactoferrin, lactoperoxidase)
4. Immunoglobulins (IgG, IgA)
5. Lipids that form part of the pellicle
6. Minerals, including calcium, phosphate, fluoride, and bicarbonate, that keep the teeth intact and buffer acids produced in the plaque biofilm
7. Proteins with other functions, such as inhibition of proteases (cystatins), lubrication (mucins), and neutralization of acids (peptides)

---

*References 5, 25, 29, 38, 41, 44, 90, 91.

early studies were approximately 0.005 to 0.01 ppm fluoride. As fluoride use became more common in the late 1980s, clinical studies involving 7- to 12-year-old children in the United States reported mean baseline fluoride concentrations in saliva of 0.02 to 0.04 ppm in both fluoridated and nonfluoridated drinking water areas.[62,63] Clearly, these higher salivary fluoride levels were achieved from topical fluoride sources other than the public water supplies; thus the salivary fluoride concentration (from all sources) rather than drinking water concentration is predictive of dental caries status.[62] In the 1990s, similar studies on 7- to 12-year-old children reported slightly higher mean salivary levels of approximately 0.05 ppm fluoride; but again, this mean was the same for both fluoridated and nonfluoridated communities.[84,85] Not surprisingly, these studies also showed that children with high individual salivary fluoride (0.075 ppm or greater) were more frequently dental caries free.

MECHANISMS OF ACTION

Topical fluoride prevents and inhibits dental caries progression in three ways:

1. Inhibition of demineralization
2. Enhancement of remineralization, including the deposition of a more dental caries–resistant surface (fluorapatite) on the remineralized individual crystals
3. Inhibition of bacterial activity*

These fluoride mechanisms rely on the fluoride being available in solution at the surface of the tooth.

Inhibition of Demineralization

When present in solution among the carbonated apatite (enamel mineral) crystals inside the tooth, fluoride inhibits demineralization by strongly *adsorbing* to the surfaces of these crystals, acting as a barrier against acid dissolution of surface sites.

Thus when cariogenic bacteria generate acid, the fluoride present in the plaque fluid (even at low levels) travels with the acid into the subsurface of the tooth, adsorbs to the crystal surface, and protects it from being dissolved.[25,91]

The beneficial effects of a 0.05% NaF mouthrinse on patients with xerostomia have been clearly demonstrated.[70]

Reviewing the success of topical fluoride both in access to the public and in reducing the incidence of dental caries is interesting. Before fluoride in toothpaste was commonplace, the salivary fluoride concentrations reported in

Enhancement of Remineralization

Fluoride enhances, or *speeds up*, remineralization by adsorbing to the crystal surfaces and attracting calcium ions, which attract phosphate ions, leading to rapid crystal growth.

The acid created by the plaque bacteria is slowly neutralized by the buffering components (bicarbonate, phosphate, and peptides) in healthy saliva as it flows over the plaque biofilm, causing the pH to increase toward neutral (Figure 25-1). This buffering action eventually halts the subsurface dissolution of the mineral.

Along with the buffering components, the saliva is supersaturated with calcium and phosphate, acting as a reservoir until the chemistry (pH and concentration) is conducive for these essential minerals to diffuse back into the tooth and *remineralize* or regrow a new crystal surface on the already partially demineralized surface of the crystal remnants inside the carious lesion. The partially dissolved crystals act as nucleators for new crystal formation, and fluoride adsorption to the crystal's surface greatly accelerates the entire process.

Incorporation of fluoride and phosphate instead of carbonate during remineralization creates a more perfect crystal with a highly acid-resistant new crystal surface similar to the mineral called *fluorapatite*. During remineralization the newly forming crystal surface preferentially takes up fluoride and phosphate from the surrounding solution and excludes carbonate.[91] Therefore this veneer has a composition between hydroxyapatite and fluorapatite, as previously described. Fluorapatite contains

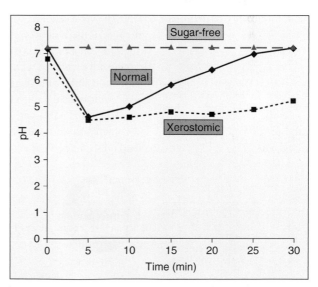

FIGURE 25-1
Typical pH curve in dental plaque (*normal*) after ingestion of fermentable carbohydrate is characterized by a fall in pH as a result of a generation of plaque acids and a return to neutral caused by buffering by salivary components. Typical pH–time curves for a patient with xerostomia and a normal patient with a sugar-free test are shown for comparison. (Modified from Featherstone JDB: Prevention and reversal of dental caries: role of low level fluoride, *Community Dent Oral Epidemiol* 27[1]:31-40, 1999.)

---

*References 5, 25, 37, 47, 90-91.

about 30,000 ppm fluoride through topical fluoride uptake, creating a new surface that is fluorapatite-like in its properties and less soluble in acid than the more highly soluble carbonated apatite of the original crystal surface.[25] Figure 25-2 outlines the demineralization-remineralization process.

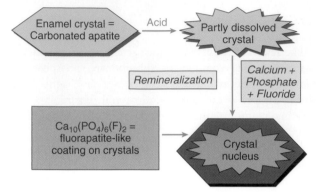

FIGURE 25-2
Demineralization and remineralization processes that lead to remineralized crystals with surfaces rich in fluoride and low in solubility. (Modified from Featherstone JDB: Prevention and reversal of dental caries: role of low level fluoride, *Community Dent Oral Epidemiol* 27[1]:31-40, 1999.)

Inhibition of Bactericidal Activity

After it enters the cell, fluoride is toxic to plaque bacteria because it both acidifies the cytoplasm and interferes with key enzyme pathways. Fluoride, in its ionized form (F^-), cannot cross the bacterial cell wall and membrane. Fluoride can rapidly travel through the cell wall and into the cariogenic bacteria only in the form of undissociated hydrofluoric (HF) acid.[47,93,95] The cariogenic bacteria produce acids during metabolism of fermentable carbohydrates, causing a fall in the pH (see Figure 25-1). A portion of the fluoride (F^-) present in the plaque fluid then combines with hydrogen ions (H^+) to form HF acid, which can then rapidly diffuse into the cell, effectively drawing more HF acid from the outside, and so on (Figure 25-3). Once inside the cell, the HF acid dissociates again, acidifying the cell and releasing F^-, which interfere with enzyme activity (e.g., enolase, adenosine triphosphatase [ATPase])

> *Note*
>
> The bacteria take up fluoride from topical sources when they produce acid, thereby inhibiting essential enzyme activity.

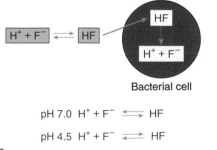

Bacterial cell

pH 7.0 $H^+ + F^- \rightleftharpoons HF$

pH 4.5 $H^+ + F^- \rightleftharpoons HF$

FIGURE 25-3
Fluoride enters a bacterial cell in the form of hydrofluoric (HF) acid at lower pH values, dissociates, and thereby provides H- and F ions inside the cell. At pH 7.0, almost no HF acid is present. (Modified from Featherstone JDB: Prevention and reversal of dental caries: role of low level fluoride, *Community Dent Oral Epidemiol* 27[1]:31-40, 1999.)

in the bacterium. F^- and H^+ become trapped in the cell, and the process is cumulative, eventually becoming toxic to the bacterium.

This process is the third topical mechanism of action of fluoride against the progression of dental caries.

Management of Dental Caries

Dental caries was once a life-threatening disease and even today remains a major problem in many developing countries. Although declining in the United States over the past 2 decades, dental caries continues to be the major reason for dental treatment and the primary cause of tooth loss.[53,96] Thus from a public health standpoint, identifying and targeting appropriate treatment to those individuals at greatest risk makes sense. Treatment of dental caries in the United States is beginning to change from the conventional *surgical* approach proposed by Black in the early 1900s to more contemporary methods. Research has clearly elucidated the mechanism of dental caries,[*] and the literature has suggested that dentists change the way they manage this infectious disease.[2,3,58] Newer concepts include the following:

- Treatment based on dental caries risk assessments
- Treatment of dental caries as a curable and preventable infectious disease
- Nonsurgical, chemical approaches to repair and reverse early lesions
- Minimally invasive tooth restoration if needed using new diagnostic methods[†]

Although their adoption has been slow in the United States, these new methods have been used in European countries with great promise. Lack of acceptance in the United States may be a result of inadequate compensation for preventive procedures by insurance companies and patients. However, *cosmetic* procedures initially had the same problem, which were helped by the increase in consumer demand and education of third-party payers. A similar approach in addition to more clinical trials that scientifically prove the benefits may help in the adoption of new caries management techniques.

> *Distinct Care Modifications*
>
> A recently completed clinical trial conducted in adults at high risk for dental caries showed that reducing the risk status by combined antibacterial treatment (chlorhexidine rinses) and fluoride treatment (fluoride rinses) resulted in reduced dental caries increment. This study was a longitudinal caries clinical trial in which each subject participated for 3 years, with bacteria and fluoride levels monitored every 6 months. The results of the study provide clinical proof of the concept of managing dental caries by reducing the bacterial challenge with antibacterial therapy and increasing the remineralization by additional fluoride therapy.[42]

*References 5, 25, 28, 36, 38, 90, 91.
†References 3, 6, 27, 50, 59, 61, 77, 80, 89.

TEAM APPROACH AND THE DENTAL HYGIENIST

The dental profession is advancing beyond the days when dentists were merely *drilling and filling,* assistants were simply passing instruments, and hygienists were exclusively cleaning teeth. The traditional view held that the hygienist was vital only to the periodontal management of patients and played little or no role in dental caries management. If this was intentional, why then is the dental hygienist routinely in charge of fluoride treatments in practice? Clearly, topical fluoride is an intervention used to treat dental caries, not periodontal disease. The modern dental office, however, emphasizes expanded duties for staff members, with the dental hygienist focusing on patient satisfaction, providing service, and promoting oral health. Modern dental caries management requires all dental team members, including the patient, to be actively involved in prevention and early intervention. Although surgical restorative repair will be needed in many patients, at least in the near future, the goal is to minimize this role through the elimination of the source of the disease through patient education and chemical therapies.

Before a diagnosis can be made, dental personnel must provide information and gather data through patient education, oral hygiene instruction, dietary counseling, salivary testing, dental caries risk assessment, dental charting, and bringing suggested lesions to the dentist's attention. Once the dentist has made the diagnosis and outlined the treatment plan, other staff members can perform much of the implementation. For example, dental hygienists can place sealants, perform fluoride therapies, and provide chlorhexidine antibacterial rinse instruction in many states; clinicians should check local regulations for their state.

> *Note*
>
> The dental hygienist is uniquely positioned to implement remineralization strategies and plays a major role in preventing damage to these early lesions through unnecessary root planing, coronal polishing, or improper hand instrumentation.

The dental hygienist is in the best position to educate patients and implement dental caries risk assessment, including the saliva test. The dental hygienist and dental assistant must participate in the team approach to modern dental caries management.

Implementing changes in the standard of care is no easy task, and it will require a team approach with strong leadership. Although it remains to be seen which team member—the dentist, hygienist, or dental assistant—will ultimately take this leadership responsibility, it is clear that all need to be involved. One problem in dentistry is that few organizations exist where all team members can be equally involved in learning and implementing this new standard of care. Recently, one such organization, the World Congress of Minimally Invasive Dentistry (WCMID), reached out to educators, researchers, and those responsible for the delivery of care—the dentist, hygienist, assistants, and other office staff—to join the fight to improve conservatively the oral health of their patients.

CARIES MANAGEMENT BY RISK ASSESSMENT

As previously described in detail, the cause of dental caries is multifactorial and involves plaque microorganisms, fermentable dietary carbohydrates (including frequency of ingestion), saliva, and the tooth surface itself.[71] The specific plaque hypothesis[64] states that only a limited number of organisms in plaque can cause disease. The primary organisms involved in human dental caries are MS and LB.[65] These organisms should be targeted, as with any bacterial infection in the human body. Filling teeth does not eliminate infection, and oral hygiene alone has not been proven to eliminate dental caries.[97]

> *Distinct Care Modifications*
>
> The medical model of dental care involves treatment of the disease, not the symptoms.[2,3] Treatment should be directed at reducing or eliminating MS and LB and enhancing repair by remineralization, not simply tooth restoration. Management of dental caries requires a multifaceted approach.

Dental caries is an infectious disease transmittable from mother to child[15] and even iatrogenically transferred from one carious site to a previously uninfected site.[19,66] Therefore the clinician must use *sterile* techniques during examination and restorative procedures.

The traditional surgical method used to treat dental caries often included only the restoration of carious teeth, the teaching of oral hygiene, and perhaps advice to avoid eating sweets. In the last decade, however, researchers and clinicians have demonstrated that these traditional methods alone do not guarantee oral health. Restorative dentistry and oral hygiene have not proven adequate to eliminate dental caries. Newer management techniques treat dental caries on the basis of risk assessment of the patient. This type of dental caries management has several names in the literature, suggesting the need for common nomenclature. In this text the term **caries management by risk assessment** (CAMBRA) is used.

Whereas traditional methods treat the consequences of infection (carious lesions), CAMBRA stipulates that the dentist treats those at risk first, identifying these individuals and then treating the infection (pathogenic bacteria). Dentists no longer need to wait until teeth are damaged to begin dental caries treatment. CAMBRA is a major step toward preventing and eliminating dental caries disease.

> *Distinct Care Modifications*
>
> CAMBRA accurately describes the process in which clinicians deal with dental caries as an infectious disease first by gathering information about the patient's dental caries risk status (risk assessment) and then by planning intervention or treatment (dental caries management) based on that risk.

DENTAL CARIES RISK ASSESSMENT

Caries risk assessment (CRA) begins with an understanding of the chemical nature of the demineralization-remineralization process and the way in which it is affected by the following:

- Fluoride
- Saliva

- Pellicle
- Diet
- Bacterial environment[36]

Xerostomia, a high-sucrose diet, frequent snacking, a lack of fluoride, and the presence of pathogenic organisms can affect the patient's dental caries risk status. In each individual the unique balance between these pathologic and protective components determines risk and ultimately disease progression or reversal (Figure 25-4). Under average conditions, with an individual whose protective components are not compromised, this delicate balance is tipped either way several times a day.

The demineralization-remineralization process is a simple, reversible chemical reaction that can be manipulated (through its pathologic and protective components) to benefit patient health.[28] To perform CRA, the clinician must qualitatively weigh the pathologic and protective factors of the patient and make a judgment call on which way the balance will tip. A CRA is accomplished via a thorough patient interview in the context of the medical and dental histories, which include the following:

- Dietary habits
- Frequency of eating
- Complaints of xerostomia
- Oral hygiene
- Fluoride use

The dentist will use all the information available, including the CRA and medical and dental history, when interviewing and examining the patient. Pathologic factors include the amount of pathogenic (cariogenic) bacteria and adequacy of salivary flow, both of which can be determined by saliva testing (see the following section, Salivary Analysis). The dietary

interview helps the clinician assess the amount and frequency of fermentable carbohydrate intake. In addition, lack of saliva (xerostomia) is a major pathologic factor that may be caused by damaged salivary glands secondary to radiation therapy or certain medications (e.g., antidepressants).[48] On the other side of the dental caries balance, adequate amounts of saliva (e.g., calcium, phosphate, fluoride), use of fluoride products, use of antimicrobial agents, and good dietary habits constitute the major protective components. Dental caries is an ever-changing balance between pathologic and protective factors.

Although many forms and formulas have been proposed to document the CRA quantitatively, most are time-consuming and intimidating and can deter clinicians from performing the CRA. Again, except for the quantitative saliva testing, each patient's CRA may be better thought of in qualitative terms; that is, as a scale that balances protective factors on one side and pathogenic factors on the other to determine whether the balance is favoring health or disease (see Figure 25-4).

SALIVARY ANALYSIS

For the salivary analysis the clinician measures the stimulated salivary flow rate and bacterial loading for both MS and LB. Stimulated saliva provides an easy means to sample the plaque from the whole mouth and reflects the cariogenic bacteria in the plaque on the teeth. Some commercially available kits also include a pH test to evaluate the buffering capacity of the saliva. Although the ability of salivary buffers to neutralize acid in the mouth is an important protective function of saliva, caution should be used in the interpretation of this test; the overriding influence is sufficient salivary flow to buffer and provide calcium, phosphate, and protective proteins. In other words, the patient could have a normal pH test but simply not enough saliva.

Bacterial testing is needed to determine whether cariogenic pathogens are present both before and after dental caries treatment and at what level these bacteria are present in the mouth. Although pathogenic organisms are present with an active carious lesion and it may seem that pretreatment bacterial testing is unnecessary, a baseline measurement is always needed for comparison at the post-

treatment recall visit. Furthermore, placement of a restoration after removal of the active lesion does not reduce the bacterial loading in the rest of the mouth.[97] Testing is beneficial even in patients without other signs of dental caries risk but where the lesion is probable because these individuals may have early enamel lesions that are identifiable only by a positive result for pathogens in a bacterial test for MS and LB. In these patients, chlorhexidine treatment may be instituted before any visible signs of demineralization. Bacterial testing for both MS and LB

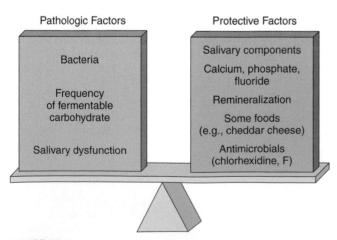

FIGURE 25-4
Balance between protective and pathologic factors in dental caries is illustrated. (Modified from Featherstone JDB: Prevention and reversal of dental caries: role of low level fluoride, *Community Dent Oral Epidemiol* 27[1]:31-40, 1999.)

Distinct Care Modifications

By definition, infection and dental caries can be diagnosed based on a high bacterial count of MS or LB, or some combination of both, and qualitative risk assessment alone. This approach indicates chemical and preventive treatment of early lesions that might otherwise be missed.

can be easily performed with one test with commercially available kits. The Ivoclar Vivacare system (Ivoclar North America, Amherst, NY, and Vivadent Co., Liechtenstein, Germany) uses selective media to provide counts of MS and LB and requires a 2-day incubation period to obtain the results. More rapid chairside methods that use monoclonal antibodies to surface antigens on the cariogenic bacteria are currently in development and will become available in the next few years.[83] Both groups of organisms should be tested because it is possible to have a low count of one organism and a significantly high count of the other and still have a high bacterial challenge.

PATIENT INVOLVEMENT

Once the patient is diagnosed with an active infection of dental caries, CAMBRA begins with patient education. Proper risk assessment permits early diagnosis even without visible evidence of a carious lesion.

Note

The patient's understanding of the disease process is pivotal because successful treatment depends on patient involvement in treatment recommendations and preventive strategies.

Without patient involvement, efforts to minimize pathologic factors and to maximize protective factors would be difficult because patients are ultimately responsible for dietary, fluoride, and chlorhexidine compliance.[4] Patients can begin active involvement by complying with dietary recommendations and topical fluoride use. Topical fluoride is an important step in the management of patients at risk for dental caries as described previously. Topical fluoride can come from multiple sources, such as fluoridated water, fluoridated toothpaste, fluoridated home rinses and gels, professional office gels, and varnishes. Recommendations on which fluoride product to use are based on an estimate of patient compliance; in other words, the product the patient is more likely to use is the best product for that patient. Low concentrations (0.04 ppm or greater) of fluoride in saliva are all that is required for the beneficial effects during remineralization.[26,36,37]

CAMBRA MADE EASY

Now that the science supporting CAMBRA has been reviewed and the concepts of CRA, salivary analysis, and patient involvement have been explained, it is time to put these concepts all together to implement on a real patient. All this information can make patients feel a little overwhelmed, but ways are available to make this process easier. In February and March of 2003 the *Journal of the California Dental Association* published two back-to-back issues completely devoted to CAMBRA. These issues include important review articles and a consensus statement of leading experts around the world. Within the

consensus statement a link to CRA forms (with permission to use them) is provided. In addition to a simple form to perform the CRA, the forms also include patient education and a checklist of patient interventions. All the review articles, the consensus statement, and forms are available to download for no charge at www.cdafoundation.org/journal/.

A modification of the published form that is in use at the University of the Pacific, School of Dentistry, is presented here for example purposes only (Figure 25-5). Readers should feel free to use the form and modify it for their own use.

The forms are designed as two double-sided pages but are presented here as four separate pages. The first page is the written CRA *(A)*, which is nothing more than an organized way to measure the dental caries balance of the patient at a particular point in time. This process takes approximately 2 minutes for the dental hygienist or assistant to fill out with the patient. Part of page one is a place to record the salivary flow rate test (to diagnose or rule out xerostomia) and a bacterial culture (to diagnose or rule out cariogenic bacterial infection). On the back of the first page *(B)* are directions for first-time users of the form. This page explains how to fill out the form and perform a saliva test. On the front of page two of the form is a checklist of possible interventions *(C)* that the dentist will recommend for the patient based on the risk determined by CRA data collected on page one. Based on risk level, the clinician has only three simple patient options: (1) healthy and low-risk patient, (2) moderate- to high-risk patient, and (3) patient with xerostomia.

Option 1: Healthy and Low-Risk Patient
Treatment options for this patient group include oral hygiene instruction, dietary counseling, regular (twice daily) fluoridated toothpaste (1000 ppm), the patient's choice to use xylitol gums or mints, and the choice to rinse with a 0.05% NaF over-the-counter (OTC) mouthrinse.

Option 2: Moderate- to High-Risk Patient
Treatment options for this patient group include everything listed in option 1 plus a higher concentration of topical fluoride and, if a bacterial culture was done, antimicrobial treatment using topical chlorhexidine or topical iodine or both. Xylitol gums or mints listed in option 1 become mandatory.

Option 3: Patient with Xerostomia (Highest Risk)
Treatment options for this patient group include everything checked in options 1 and 2 plus the choice of using baking soda

Patient Education Opportunity

Many offices copy key review articles for patients to take home to read. The job of the dental team is to act as the advocate for patients, by providing them with the best available evidence to help ensure they make the best possible decisions for their own health. The dentist no longer *dictates* to the patient needed treatment; thus rather than being viewed as *selling* dentistry, the dental team is viewed as a valued information-gathering resource.

CARIES RISK ASSESSMENT FORM FOR CHILDREN 6 YEARS AND OLDER/ADULTS

Instructions on reverse

Patient Name: _____ I.D. # _____ Age _____ Date _____

Initial/baseline exam date_____ Recall/POE date_____

A

Respond to *each* question in sections 1, 2, and 3 with a check mark in the yes or no column	Yes	No	Notes
1. High Risk Factors **			
(a) Visible cavitation (carious) or caries into dentin by radiograph			
(b) Caries restored in past three years			
(c) Readily visible heavy plaque on teeth			
(d) Frequent (greater than three times daily) between meal snacks of sugars/cooked starch			
(e) *Saliva-reducing factors:*			
1. Hyposalivatory medications			
2. Radiation to head and neck			
3. Systemic reasons, e.g. Sjögren's			
(f*) Visually inadequate saliva flow. (If yes, measure) less than 0.7 ml/min by test= low salivary flow or dry mouth			Amount: _____ ml/min
(g) Appliances present, fixed or removable, e.g. orthodontic brackets/bands/retainer or removable partial denture(s)			
2. Moderate Risk Factors			
(a) Exposed roots			
(b) Deep pits & fissures/developmental defects			
(c) Interproximal enamel lesions/radiolucencies			
(d) Other white spot lesions or occlusal discoloration			
(e) Uses recreational drugs			
3. Protective Factors			
(a) Lives /works/school in fluoridated community			
(b) Uses fluoride toothpaste daily			type _____
(c) Uses fluoride mouthwash/rinse/gel daily			type _____
(d*) Salivary flow visually adequate >1 ml/min by test			
(e) Uses xylitol gum or mints 4 x day			Type _____ and % xylitol_____
(f) Mother/caregiver has no caries activity			Brand _____ Frequency_____

**If yes to 1 (a) or any two of 1 (b)-(g), perform bacterial culture*	High Count Date: _____	Moderate Count Date: _____	Low Count Date: _____	
(a) Mutans streptococci				(Place a check in the box below the count)
(b) Lactobacillus				(Place a check in the box below the count)
Caries risk overall* (see over)	High	Moderate	Low	Circle High, Moderate or Low

Recommendations given: yes_____ no: _____ Date given:_____ or Date follow up:_____

*Indicates that test descriptions for these procedures are on the following pages

---

B

CARIES RISK ASSESSMENT FORM FOR CHILDREN AGE 6 YEARS AND OLDER/ADULTS

Instructions

1. Respond to questions 1, 2, and 3 with yes or no answers. You can make special notations such as the number of caries present, the severity of the lack of oral hygiene, the brand of fluorides used, the type of snacks eaten, or the names of medications/drugs that are causing dry mouth.

2. If the answer is yes to question 1(a) or any two of questions 1(b) through 1(g), then a bacterial culture should be taken using the **CRT bacteria test*** (Vivadent) — see below. Make an overall judgment as to whether the patient is at high, medium, or low risk depending on the balance between the pathological factors (sections 1 and 2) and the protective factors (section 3). **Note!** Determining the caries risk for an individual requires evaluating the number and severity of the risk factors. Certainly, an individual with caries presently or in the recent past is at high risk for future caries. A patient with low bacterial levels would need to have several other risk factors present to be considered at moderate risk. Some clinical judgment is needed while also considering the protective factors to determining the risk. **Note!** Children with developmental problems or low socioeconomic status are automatically at high risk. Place the completed form in the patient chart.

3. Provide the patient with recommendations based on your clinical observations and the responses to the questions and discuss strategies for caries control and management. Give the patient the sheet that explains how caries happens and the sheet with your recommendations. Copy the recommendations for the patient chart.

4. Inform the patient of the results of any test results. Showing the patient the bacteria grown from their mouth (CRT test result*) can be a good motivator, so have the culture tube handy at the next visit (or schedule one for this purpose — the culture keeps satisfactorily for some weeks), or give/send them a picture.

5. After the patient has been following your recommendations for three to six months, have the patient back to re-assess how well he or she is doing. Ask if he or she is following your instructions — how often. If the bacterial levels were moderate or high initially, repeat the bacterial culture to see if bacterial levels have been reduced. Make changes in your recommendations or reinforce protocol if results are not as good as desired or the patient is not compliant.

*Test procedures — Saliva Flow Rate and Caries Bacteria Testing

*1. **Saliva flow rate:** Have the patient chew a paraffin pellet (included with the CRT test — see below) for three to five minutes and spit all saliva generated into a cup. At the end of the three to five minutes, measure the amount of saliva (in milliliters) and divide that amount by time to determine the ml/minute of stimulated salivary flow. A flow rate of 1 ml/min and above is considered normal. A level of 0.7 ml/min is low, and anything at 0.5 ml/min or less is dry, indicating a high-risk situation. Investigation of the reason for the low flow rate is an important step in the patient treatment.

*2. **Bacterial testing: CRT bacteria test:** In the United States, the currently available chairside test for cariogenic bacterial challenge is the Caries Risk Test (CRT) marketed by Vivadent (Amherst, N.Y.). It is sufficiently sensitive to provide a level of low, medium, or high cariogenic bacterial challenge. It can also be used as a motivational tool for patient compliance with an antibacterial regimen. Other bacterial test kits will likely be available in the near future. The following is the procedure for administering the currently available CRT test. Results are available after 48 hours.

The kit comes with two-sided selective media sticks that assess mutans streptococci on the blue side and lactobacilli on the green side.

a) Remove the selective media stick from the culture tube. Peel off the plastic cover sheet from each side of the stick.

b) Pour the collected saliva over the media on each side until it is entirely wet.

c) Place one of the sodium bicarbonate tablets (included with the kit) in the bottom of the tube.

d) Replace the media stick in the culture tube, screw the lid on, and label the tube with the patient's name, registration number, and date. Place the tube in the incubator at 37 degrees Celsius for 48 hours. Incubators suitable for a dental office are also sold by the company.

e) Collect the tube after 48 hours and compare the densities of bacterial colonies with the pictures provided in the kit indicating relative bacterial levels. The dark blue agar is selective for mutans streptococci and the light green agar is selective for lactobacilli. Record the level of bacterial challenge in the patient's chart as low, medium, or high.

FIGURE 25-5

Caries Risk Assessment (CRA) forms. Forms can be downloaded from www.cdafoundation.org/journal and are also available for children ages 0 to 5 years. **A,** Caries Risk Assessment form for children 6 years old and older and adults. **B,** Reverse side of part **A** with instructions and test procedures. (©2002 California Dental Association.)

PATIENT RECOMMENDATIONS FOR CONTROL OF DENTAL DECAY (AGES 6 AND OLDER/ADULT)

Daily Oral Hygiene (Aimed at reducing the overall bacteria in the mouth, especially at sites likely to decay. Choose the recommendations based on the danger sites and the condition of the mouth)

___ brush twice daily (with fluoride toothpaste, all patients)   ___ floss daily

___ interproximal brush   ___ Stimudents   ___ toothpick   ___ Superfloss

___ other: _____

Diet (The most important thing is to reduce the number of between meal sweet snacks that contain carbohydrates, especially sugars. Substitution by snacks rich in protein, such as cheese will also help)

___ OK as is ___ limit snacking ___ limit sodas ___ other _____

Fluorides (All patients should use a fluoride toothpaste twice daily. Additional fluoride products should be added, depending on whether the risk level is medium or high. These fluoride products must be used daily to be effective)

___ fluoride-containing toothpaste 2X/day (all patients regardless of caries risk status)

___ fluoride rinse (0.05% NaF, **Act** or **Fluorigard**) 1X or 2X/day (use in addition to toothpaste. Patients at medium risk should rinse in the morning or last thing at night. For high risk patients use twice a day, once in the morning and once last thing at night. Continue long term with older patients or those who need or want extra protection)

___ **Prevident** "brush-on" nightly, **OR** ___ gel (**Prevident**) in custom tray 10 min./night (For high-risk patients, especially those with low saliva flow, or root caries, or active cavities. Continue until the risk status is lowered, then revert to fluoride as above)

___ fluoride lozenges (**Lozi-Flur or Fluor-a-day**) 1X/day (use for high-risk patients with low saliva flow, such as radiation xerostomia. By dissolving in the mouth, these lozenges provide a concentrated fluoride reservoir to protect against mineral loss and to enhance repair by remineralization. Dissolve slowly in mouth by holding the lozenge in a convenient place)

Sugar-free gum/mints (recommend for high risk patients, especially those with low saliva flow, and/or those who need to reduce in between meal snacking. The gums or mints that contain xylitol also have an antibacterial effect against the decay-causing bacteria. Preferably use a xylitol-containing gum.)

___ Chew after meals when you cannot brush (xylitol preferred). ___ Use Xylitol mints 3-4 times daily.

Antibacterial rinse

___ Chlorhexidine gluconate, 0.12% (**Periogard, Peridex, Oral Rx**, available on prescription). Rinse with 10 ml at bedtime for 1 minute, 1X/day for 2 weeks. Stop for two months. Repeat rinsing for 2 weeks. Use fluoride rinse (see above) every day during the weeks in between.

For dry mouth

___ baking soda tooth paste with fluoride ___ baking soda gum – **Dental Care Gum** (Arm & Hammer. It contains baking soda and xylitol) or similar product. Chew frequently throughout the day.

___ rinse frequently with baking soda suspension during the day (fill sports water bottle with water and add 2 teaspoons of baking soda for each 8 oz. of water.)

Practitioner signature _____ Date: _____

C

PATIENT INFORMATION ON TOOTH DECAY

How Tooth Decay Happens

Tooth decay is caused by certain types of bacteria (mutans streptococci and lactobacilli) that live in your mouth. When they attach themselves to the teeth and multiply in dental plaque, they can do damage. The bacteria feed on what you eat, especially sugars (including fruit sugars) and cooked starch (bread, potatoes, rice, pasta, etc.). Within about five minutes after you eat or drink, the bacteria begin producing acids as a byproduct of their digesting your food. Those acids can penetrate into the hard substance of the tooth and dissolve some of the minerals (calcium and phosphate). If the acid attacks are infrequent and of short duration, your saliva can help to repair the damage by neutralizing the acids and supplying minerals and fluoride that can replace those lost from the tooth. However if your mouth is dry, you have many of these bacteria, or you snack frequently; then the tooth mineral lost by attacks of acids is too great and cannot be repaired. This is the start of tooth decay and leads to cavities.

Methods of Controlling Tooth Decay

Diet: Reducing the number of sugary and starchy foods, snacks, drinks, or candies can help reduce the development of tooth decay. That does not mean you can never eat these types of foods, but you should limit their consumption particularly when eaten between main meals. A good rule is three meals per day and no more than three snacks per day.

Fluorides: Fluorides help make teeth more resistant to being dissolved by bacterial acids. Fluorides are available from a variety of sources such as drinking water, toothpaste, over-the-counter rinses, and products prescribed by your dentist such as brush-on gels used at home or gels and foams applied in the dental office. Daily use is very important to help protect against the acid attacks.

Plaque removal: Removing the plaque from your teeth on a daily basis is helpful in controlling tooth decay. Plaque can be difficult to remove from some parts of your mouth, especially between the teeth and in grooves on the biting surfaces of back teeth. If you have an appliance such as an orthodontic retainer or partial denture, remove it before brushing your teeth. Brush all surfaces of the appliance also.

Saliva: Saliva is critical for controlling tooth decay. It neutralizes acids and provides minerals and proteins that protect the teeth. If you cannot brush after a meal or snack, you can chew some sugar-free gum. This will stimulate the flow of saliva to help neutralize acids and bring lost minerals back to the teeth. Sugar-free candy or mints could also be used, but some of these contain acids themselves. These acids will not cause tooth decay, but they can slowly dissolve the enamel surface over time (a process called erosion). Some sugar-free gums are designed to help fight tooth decay and are particularly useful if you have a dry mouth (many medications can cause a dry mouth). Some gums contain baking soda, which neutralizes the acids produced by the bacteria in plaque. Gum that contains xylitol as its first listed ingredient is the gum of choice. If you have a dry mouth, you could also fill a drinking bottle with water and add a couple teaspoons of baking soda for each 8 ounces of water and swish with it frequently throughout the day. Toothpastes containing baking soda are also available from several companies.

Antibacterial mouthrinses: Rinses that your dentist can prescribe are able to reduce the number of bacteria that cause tooth decay and can be useful in patients at high risk for tooth decay.

Sealants: Sealants are plastic coatings bonded to the biting surfaces of back teeth to protect the deep grooves from decay. In some people, the grooves on the surfaces of the teeth are too narrow and deep to clean with a toothbrush, so they may decay in spite of your best efforts. Sealants are an excellent preventive measure for children and young adults at risk for this type of decay.

D

FIGURE 25-5

Caries Risk Assessment (CRA) forms. Forms can be downloaded from www.cdafoundation.org/journal and are also available for children ages 0 to 5 years. **C,** Patient recommendation form. **D,** Reverse side of part **C** with patient information. (©2002 California Dental Association.)

products (e.g., rinse, gum, toothpaste) to neutralize acid immediately after a snack, fluoride lozenges, and the use of a product that delivers calcium and phosphate, which are all listed in option 3 on the forms.

On the back of page two is a letter to the patient *(D)* describing a new way to think of dental decay. The second page is designed to be printed on NCR (no carbon required) paper so that the original copy goes to the patient and the NCR copy, along with page one (the CRA), goes into the patient record as medical-legal documentation.

Both pages of the CAMBRA form (the CRA and intervention sheet) should be completed at baseline and at each dental caries recall maintenance appointment. This approach will not only help determine the effectiveness of treatment, but it will hopefully serve as a source of encouragement for patients. Patient acceptance increases when they actually see the results of the saliva test. The saliva test can be photographed and sent to the patient or printed as a color print, or they can be shown the actual culture slides together with the scale of colony intensity.

> *Patient Education Opportunity*
> Patients should be informed that pathogen reduction might be gradual rather than instantaneous because of the lack of totally effective antimicrobial agents.

This increased patient involvement leads to better compliance when things are checked on the second page (the intervention checklist).

Some of the items listed in the intervention checklist are now examined in greater detail.

25-2 | CHEMICAL THERAPIES

Antimicrobial Treatments

Currently, the main chemotherapeutic agents shown to reduce the dental caries pathogenic bacterial load include chlorhexidine,[1] iodine,[18] and xylitol.[68] Of the three therapeutic agents, xylitol has demonstrated superior ability to interrupt the vertical transmission from caregiver (primarily the mother) to infants in some studies.[51]

A patient might require one or all of these chemical treatments on a regular basis before a significant reduction in bacteria is realized. More research is needed to study the combined effects of treatment interventions.

Chlorhexidine

Chlorhexidine is used in the treatment of dental caries in two ways:

1. As a *cavity cleanser,* it reduces the chance of bacteria remaining in the cavity preparation. No evidence indicates that this practice is clinically beneficial, but it seems logical because bacteria have been observed in dentinal tubules with microscopy.
2. It reduces the number of bacteria in dental caries patients with high bacterial challenge.[1]
   - The patient should be started on a prescription for 0.12% chlorhexidine gluconate oral rinse with instructions to rinse ½ ounce for 1 minute once a day for 7 days. The chlorhexidine should be started as soon as

possible and initially used while restorative work is in progress; a recent longitudinal clinical trial shows this timing to be most effective.[42] The daily chlorhexidine rinsing for 1 week should be repeated monthly until the bacterial load is reduced as measured by the salivary bacterial culture. The goal is to reduce the number of remaining pathogens, especially MS (chlorhexidine is not very effective against LB), to a safe level for the patient.[58] Once this goal is accomplished, the chlorhexidine rinse is discontinued, as in any other antibacterial treatment of infection. The week of the chlorhexidine treatment is usually followed by the addition of daily topical fluoride, such as mouthrinses (0.05% NaF), a high-concentration (5000 ppm F) fluoride-containing dentifrice, and xylitol gum or mints three times per day.

Iodine

Iodine has been studied in the operating room treatment of early childhood caries (ECC). Studies have demonstrated that a one-time exposure of 10% povidone-iodine (which is 1% free iodine) swabbed in the mouth in surgery significantly decreased the number of both MS and LS in children.[18] More studies are needed to validate this treatment on children and adults outside the hospital setting. DenBesten and co-workers showed that iodine treatment every 2 months reduces dental caries in young children. This office procedure is not recommended for patient home use. Of course, patients should be screened for any iodine allergies.

Xylitol

As previously stated, xylitol, when used by mothers of young children in the first 2 years, was more effective than chlorhexidine and fluoride varnish in interrupting the vertical transmission of bacteria from caregivers to infants.[51] This consumption of xylitol gum by the mothers during the first 2 years of the

> *Prevention*
> Xylitol is a noncariogenic sugar (not fermentable by dental caries–causing bacteria); it appears to also have powerful anticaries effects. The proposed mechanism is that it inhibits the attachment of MS to the tooth surface.[1]

children's lives resulted in significantly lower levels of dental caries 6 years later. Xylitol is a naturally occurring 5-carbon sugar polyol, which is not fermentable by MS or LB.

A recent study shows that chewing xylitol gum results in a significant decrease in bacterial levels in 5- to 6-year-old children.[68] The amount of xylitol used in these studies was 5 to 9 g per day, usually by chewing a xylitol-containing gum three to five times a day, depending on the amount of xylitol per piece of gum.

Topical Fluoride

Although topical fluoride has some antimicrobial effects, it is usually given to enhance remineralization and to produce a dental caries–resistant crystal surface called *fluorapatite.* A high-risk

Prevention

The strongly cationic (positively charged) chlorhexidine rinse should not be combined with the strongly anionic (negatively charged) fluoride rinse, especially in the same bottle, because of some negating effect based on charge.

patient should be actively involved immediately in his or her treatment and intervention strategies (decisions) and remineralizing techniques initiated. The patient is educated about the disease process and CRA. Using the first page of the CRA form, the patient is educated about his or her unique dental caries risk status. This tool is quite powerful in the review of dietary habits, oral hygiene, and pathogenic developments, as well as in remineralization strategies. The patient is then instructed in the recommended treatment interventions and given a copy (page 2 of the CRA form) to take home. Treatment may include the use of a topical fluoride product personally selected and based on compliance. In most patients the use of daily home fluoride products, such as an OTC 0.05% NaF mouthrinse, is preferred. A very effective home use fluoride regimen for high-risk patients is a prescription toothpaste with 5000 ppm fluoride (e.g., Prevident 5000 Plus from Colgate, Control Rx from OMNII Oral Pharmaceuticals). The high fluoride concentration toothpaste can simply be substituted for a regular toothpaste. The extra daily fluoride application for remineralization is discontinued only if the patient is to receive a 1-week chlorhexidine treatment, to prevent confusing the patient with two different rinse therapies.

Prevention

Young children under age 6 years should not use fluoride rinses or high fluoride concentration toothpastes to reduce the risk of excess fluoride ingestion.

Calcium and Phosphate Products

Recently, products designed to deliver additional calcium and phosphate for remineralization have arrived on the market. Although sufficient amounts are present in healthy saliva for remineralization, this approach could be beneficial to the patient with xerostomia. More studies are needed to see whether these products will have beneficial effects in patients with xerostomia and whether these products will have additional effects in individuals with normal saliva. Such products include MI Paste (GC America, Alsip, Ill.) and SootheRx (OMNII Oral Pharmaceuticals, West Palm Beach, Fla.).

Baking Soda Products

Healthy saliva contains all the buffers needed to neutralize an acid attack after a meal or snack. Similar to the concept of delivering more calcium and phosphate, studies are needed to answer the question whether additional buffering in the presence of healthy saliva will lead to beneficial dental caries preventive effects.

Prevention

Baking soda in a patient with xerostomia may be the first line of defense after the ingestion of food.

With inadequate saliva, the buffering capacity may be insufficient, and baking soda should be implemented as soon as possible after eating.

Baking soda can be used in the form of baking soda gum—*Dental Care Gum* (Church & Dwight, Princeton, NJ)—or by simply mixing 2 teaspoons of baking soda in an 8-ounce bottle of water and rinsing. The patient must be instructed to rinse and spit to minimize the ingestion of excessive sodium. Baking soda toothpastes are also available; however, most patients will not always brush after each snack, and many clinicians believe patients will become confused by the recommendation of two different toothpastes, especially if they are already using one containing fluoride.

Note

A neutral pH is necessary before fluoride can help remineralize a lesion.

MANAGEMENT OF A CARIOUS LESION

25-3
25-4

If CRA and salivary testing reveal that the patient is at high risk for dental caries, then CAMBRA requires the clinician to decide whether to treat lesions chemically or surgically.[3] Chemical treatment modalities consist of some combination of topical fluoride; xylitol; iodine; chlorhexidine; and, in the case of the patient with xerostomia, baking soda products, calcium, and phosphate.

Note

The location and extent of a lesion, whether it is cavitated, and whether it is active or inactive, all help the dentist determine whether a lesion should be restored or remineralized.

The absence of cavitation is significant because an intact enamel surface prevents bacteria from penetrating the tooth; the smaller enamel diffusion channels do not allow bacteria to enter. Thus noncavitated lesions can be remineralized. If the surface is substantially cavitated or presents a cosmetic problem, then the tooth should undergo restorative treatment.

Location is important because the three sites on a tooth—pits and fissures, proximal surfaces, and cervical surfaces—are each unique and should not be treated the same. For example, most pits and fissures cannot be cleaned and are associated with both poor dental caries–detection techniques and no reliable way to monitor remineralization procedures. Therefore relying on remineralization therapy on the occlusal surface is currently problematic. In contrast, remineralization on early, proximal, and smooth-surface enamel lesions and on root caries lesions offers better results because these lesions do not have deep occlusal anatomy and can be monitored more easily with bitewing radiographs or visually. Finally, cervical carious lesions often involve the root surface and are difficult to restore because the root has less mineral content and is, therefore, more porous than enamel. Cervical carious lesions do, however, respond well to fluoride and preventive treatments.

Management of the Occlusal Surface

Because of the large amount of surrounding sound tooth tissue, conventional radiography cannot detect lesions in occlusal surfaces until they are well advanced. Because pit and fissure lesions are now the most common type and currently cannot be monitored for remineralization, the first step in restorative procedures should be surgical dental caries control (temporary or permanent), with conservative preparations when possible, along with the use of pit and fissure sealants to eliminate potential niches for pathogenic bacteria to thrive. The clinician may inspect any areas of possible decay (e.g., deeply stained pits or fissures) using the DIAGNOdent (KaVo America Corp., Lake Zurich, Ill.) dental caries detector. This fluorescence device detects and measures bacterial by-products, providing a number to indicate whether to *open up* (fissure widening) the area. If this device is not available and the clinician suspects a hidden lesion, then a dental caries biopsy (fissure widening) is appropriate, a process that entails the removal of the smallest amount of enamel with a ¼- or ⅛-round or smaller bur (or perhaps a laser) to determine the presence or absence of hidden decay. Studies have shown that widening the fissures improves detection of the so-called hidden occlusal decay.[79]

If decay is found, then only the infected tooth structure is removed. Then the clinician selects an appropriate restorative material and the proper preparation, often a conservative preventive resin restoration or flowable composite.

⭐ CASE APPLICATION 25-1.1

Dental Caries Detection Devices

Of the new dental caries–detection devices, which one would be recommended for use on Mrs. Svensen?

This approach is the opposite of conventional methods, in which the material is chosen first and the tooth is prepared with the G. V. Black *extension for prevention* philosophy (i.e., to include all pits and fissures in the outline form to a depth of at least 1.5 mm) even before the presence or extent of dental caries is determined. If the dental caries biopsy identifies no active infection, then a sealant is placed with a filled, flowable composite resin. The benefits of dental sealants have been well described in the dental literature* but remain underused in clinical dentistry. The downside to resin sealants is that they need to be properly placed without compromise to moisture control. Some studies suggest that a better bond is achieved by conservative fissure preparation to remove debris and to get clean prismatic enamel to which to bond.[87]

> **Prevention**
>
> If the patient is at high risk for dental caries and aggressive preventive treatment is indicated, then sealants can be used in adults and children to seal all pits and fissures and marginal discrepancies.

Other studies show that resin sealants should be monitored annually and repaired when needed.[43]

The use of glass-ionomer products is one option to resin-based sealants. The advantage of using glass-ionomer products is the bonding mechanism itself. Glass ionomers chemically bond in a moist environment rather than micromechanically, requiring a dry environment as in the case of resin-based products. No polymerization shrinkage occurs, and the marginal seal is excellent. Although they will not bond to plaque biofilm and debris, glass ionomers will bond equally well to aprismatic and prismatic enamel. In the case where minimal or no tooth preparation is desired or where moisture control is possible, glass ionomers may prove to be the material of choice. In addition, the ability to deliver fluoride and have ion exchange with the mineral in the tooth and the mineral in the glass-ionomer material itself is unique, which is the basis of the *chemical bond*. Fluoride released from the surface of glass-ionomer restorations has been shown to inhibit decay on neighboring teeth.[46,92] Given that it delivers mineral and fluoride to the tooth, speculation suggests that an internal remineralization occurs underneath glass-ionomer restorations. More research is needed to validate this internal effect. The literature often reports studies on the *bond strength* and *retention rate* of restorative materials. Limiting the study parameters to these factors may bias studies to favor resin-based products over glass-ionomer products. Perhaps it would be just as important, if not more important, to study the ability of the restoration to create a long-term marginal seal and to inhibit the dental caries process around the restoration. In addition, bond-strength studies often measure bond strength immediately after placement and in a dry environment when resin-based products have the highest strengths and the glass ionomers are at their weakest strengths. Glass ionomers must be tested in a moist environment simulating the saliva; they have been shown to increase strength for months after placement by way of its incorporation of mineral from the saliva.

Management of the Proximal Surface

As previously stated, early enamel lesions without cavitations are the best candidates for successful remineralization techniques. The task is much easier if the lesion is on a smooth enamel surface that is easily visible, such as a white or brown spot lesion on the facial or lingual enamel surfaces. However, many smooth-surface lesions occur in the proximal area directly below the proximal contact and are not visible with direct visual inspection. Until better detection methods are available, dentists must rely on bite-wing radiographs and good clinical judgment. One recommended rule of thumb is to use remineralization therapies on radiographic E1 (enamel) lesions (see Chapter 17), and only those *touching* or penetrating the dentinoenamel junction (DEJ) should be restored. More accurate quantitative methods in the near future should improve these crude guidelines. Two such technologies, DIFOTI and QLF, are discussed in Chapter 17. Although both technologies are very sensitive at picking up early surface changes, studies have not demonstrated that DIFOTI or QLF can measure lesion depth, thus they may have limited ability to help in the decision on when to restore.

Once surgical repair is chosen, the priority shifts to the confirmation of the extent of both cavitation and active dental caries progression into dentin through a dental caries biopsy. One method for a proximal lesion is to start from an area close to the marginal ridge, such as a mesial or distal pit, then use a

---

*References 4, 10, 11, 22, 57, 81, 94.

small dental bur, laser, or micro–air abrasion to tunnel internally to the DEJ area of the lesion. This process often reveals only affected (stained but hard) dentin and no sign of cavitation. In this case the dentist can simply back-fill with an occlusal composite. If decay is found, then only the decayed tissue is removed; a restorative material is selected, and the cavity preparation is chosen for the selected material. Preferably a conservative approach can be implemented, such as a *slot preparation* or *tunnel preparation*. A slot preparation is simply the proximal box of a traditional Class II Black preparation (without the dovetail and isthmus) and is as retentive as the traditional Black preparation.[20] In a tunnel preparation the dental caries biopsy continues from the DEJ through the proximal enamel, following the cavitation from the inside to the outside. Although these contemporary restorative materials and conservative preparations, sometimes called *microdentistry,* are esthetically pleasing and minimize loss of tooth structure, they are not yet accepted as the standard of care.

Management of the Cervical Region

Although remineralization on a root surface is possible, this approach carries more inherent risk because of the high porosity of the root surface compared with enamel, the proximity of the root to the pulp, the vulnerability of exposed collagen in the tooth root to collagenase,[55] and the low mineral content of cementum and dentin. In addition, the porous structure of dentin or cementum makes placing restorations difficult and leakage of the restoration probable. For these reasons, treatment of cervical lesions requires special consideration.

> **Note**
>
> If pit and fissure lesions are the most difficult lesions to detect and smooth-surface lesions the most easily remineralized, then cervical lesions can be characterized as the most difficult to restore. All these differences result from the lesion's location.

As the number of older patients increases, more root caries will occur. Root caries is caused by the same bacteria that cause dental caries in enamel—MS and LB.[23,98] Ideally, cementum was designed to be covered by attached gingiva, and therefore an exposed root surface is at risk for dental caries.[54] Preventive strategies are essential in root caries because infections are usually severe and teeth are difficult to restore. Lesions may not be readily visible or may be advanced by the time they are visible. Bacterial enzymes such as collagenase can dissolve the collagen matrix of the root surface after partial loss of mineral by bacterially generated organic acids in the early stages of root caries. Despite the drawbacks, the demineralization-remineralization process in roots is similar to that of enamel, and fluoride still has beneficial effects on roots. However, the most effective concentration and frequency of fluoride use for root caries remain undetermined.

> **Prevention**
>
> Fluoride dentifrice is effective in the prevention of root caries, as are OTC fluoride rinses (0.05% NaF) and high-concentration fluoride gels.

Clinically, active dental caries on the root should be distinguished from inactive

or arrested dental caries. If no active dental caries is evident, then the lesion may be a result of abfraction or abrasion (see Chapter 17). In the absence of active dental caries, removal of tooth structure should be minimized, often restricted to a simple *roughening up* of the surface, especially if bonding techniques are being used with composite resins, glass ionomers, or compomers. Clearly, classic Black retention preparations should be rethought in light of current bonding studies and the porous nature of cementum and dentin, which makes leakage probable. Deep preparations in areas already close to the pulp and with a high chance of leakage are problematic. In the United States, controversy surrounds which material is best for the cervical area, although composite resin is popular now because of its superior esthetic results. However, composite shrinkage during the curing phase and subsequent gap formation have challenged the integrity of the cervical margin in these restorations.[56] Thus an esthetic result is negated if the cervical margin leaks. Glass ionomers are very popular in other countries[72] and may be the material of choice because of enhanced fluoride release and lack of shrinkage.[8]

Because no ideal restorative material has yet been found for the cervical area, dentists may better serve patients by educating them and offering a second treatment option involving the use of glass ionomer as a fluoride delivery device that does not leak, rather than the traditional *permanent* esthetic restoration.[7,8] Dentists should rethink the ways these cervical restorations are marketed to patients.

> **Note**
>
> Glass ionomers may be the material of choice for cervical restoration because of enhanced fluoride release and lack of shrinkage.[8]

REEVALUATION PERIOD

Treatment with chlorhexidine, iodine, or xylitol does not guarantee that the patient will have an immediate reduction in bacteria nor will these treatments ensure that the patient will remain disease free; the patient should be reevaluated for risk indefinitely, just as in the prevention of periodontal disease. CRA with saliva testing can be performed as often as once a month if indicated to evaluate the possibility of reinfection. Unlike the traditional approach, in which the next dental caries intervention would not be until another carious lesion is detected, the CAMBRA approach relies on immediate early intervention if pathogens are detected in significant numbers during the recall appointment. As previously described, this procedure permits chemical reversal of demineralization that is not yet visible, resulting in a surface that is resistant to dental caries. The patient is either placed on another appropriate dental caries recall if he or she is considered at low risk on CRA or given additional chlorhexidine and preventive treatments if bacterial test results are high.[2,4]

> **Distinct Care Modifications**
>
> Using CRA and salivary testing results to determine the next dental caries reevaluation period is an improvement over the use of unrelated periodontal maintenance schedules.

Clinical Implications: Fluoride-Delivery Systems

Fluoride is one of several protective factors and part of an overall plan to manage and prevent the occurrence and progression of dental caries.[29] Small adjustments can tip the dental caries balance one way or the other (see Figure 25-4), leading to dental caries arrestment, reversal, or progression. The delivery of fluoride to the surfaces of the teeth on a frequent (at least daily) basis is essential. The topical effects of fluoride are overriding, whereas the systemic incorporation of fluoride in the tooth mineral has no major benefit.[28,29,44] Dentists must use this information to manage dental caries more effectively in both adults and children. Fluoride in drinking water reduces dental caries but does not eradicate it. Fluoride in the drinking water provides fluoride at levels in the mouth that can inhibit demineralization and enhance remineralization, tipping the dental caries balance toward protection, provided the challenge is not too great.

> **Note**
>
> Concentration of fluoride in dental enamel and dentin provided systemically by fluoridation of drinking water or by natural fluoride water levels alone is insufficient to provide complete protection against dental caries.

The mechanism of action of fluoride in the drinking water is therefore an effective topical delivery system.

Fluoride-containing products such as dentifrice, mouthrinses, and topically applied gels provide dental caries–preventive benefits through the topical mechanisms previously described. The effects involve the mechanisms of inhibition of demineralization, enhancement of remineralization, and action on the bacteria. With high bacterial challenges and xerostomia or salivary dysfunction, even high levels of fluoride therapy may be insufficient to balance the effect of the pathologic factors and dental caries progression. Each individual has some level of challenge beyond which fluoride is insufficient to swing the balance. Fluoride products used frequently can maintain salivary fluoride levels in excess of 0.04 ppm, thereby providing significant dental caries protection. The major problem with the home-use products is the need for daily patient compliance.

✦ CASE APPLICATION 25-1.2

Nonfluoridated Water

Mrs. Svensen's prevention survey indicates that she has been exposed to a number of sources of fluoride. She was raised and lived in a community with fluoridated water until 12 months ago, when she moved to a rural area. Currently, her primary source of water is from a well, and her usual beverage of choice during the day is bottled water. She is using dentifrice with fluoride and brushes once a day. Mrs. Svensen does not use an oral rinse.

What recommendations would be suggested for Mrs. Svensen, based on the previous information and on her clinical and radiographic findings?

Professional Applications

PATIENT EDUCATION

The benefits of topical fluoride include the following:
- Prevention of demineralization
- Remineralization of early decay
- Decrease in enamel solubility
- Maximization of enamel resistance to decay

Professionally applied fluoride is effective in the reduction of coronal caries by 30%. Fluoride treatments, however, are not limited to use on children. Many adults with high dental caries rates or root exposure also can benefit from professional and self-care topical fluoride applications.

Fluoride solutions for professional application, available as gels, rinses, or foams, include 1.2% NaF, 8% stannous fluoride, and 1.23% acidulated phosphate fluoride (APF). APF gel or solution is used most often and has a concentration of 1.23% sodium fluoride plus 0.1 M orthophosphoric acid. The gel form also contains a thixotropic agent, which maintains the gelatinous state, becoming fluidlike under stress. This property allows the material to adhere to the teeth while flowing into interdental areas. Although the use of APF and stannous fluoride is safe on all tooth surfaces because of their acidic pH levels, a neutral NaF gel or solution should be used on patients with porcelain or composite restorations to prevent surface etching of these materials. Stannous fluoride is available in solution and gel form; the gel is recommended as an at-home, brush-on therapy, and the solution is available in combination with APF as a professional rinse. In addition, acidic fluoride (APF and stannous) can cause severe erosion of tooth structure if used routinely at home in devices that restrict salivary clearance, such as custom trays or night guards, and should not be used.

The gel and foam fluoride formulas are applied to the teeth through the use of a tray or can be painted on with cotton-tipped applicators. Fluoride varnish is painted on the teeth in the dental office and has an effect that is at least as good as the gels or foams (see the next section).

> **Note**
>
> Many practitioners now use varnish as the office topical application of choice rather than gels or foams in trays.

TRADITIONAL PAINT-ON TECHNIQUE

The paint-on technique to apply fluoride formulas requires isolation of the treatment areas with cotton rolls. With the patient in an upright position, one half of the mouth is isolated with cotton rolls, which are placed in holders for the mandibular arch and by hand for the maxillary arch. The teeth are dried with compressed air, and the fluoride gel or solution is painted on the teeth with a cotton-tipped applicator. A saliva ejector should be positioned near the cotton roll holder. A timer is set for 4 minutes, and the surfaces remain wet for this period. After 4 minutes the clinician removes the saliva ejector and cotton rolls, then wipes off the superficial gel or solution, allowing the patient to expectorate. The opposite side of the mouth then is isolated and fluoride is applied. After the fluoride paint-on procedure is complete, the patient is instructed not to rinse, eat, drink, or brush the teeth for at least 30 minutes.

FLUORIDE VARNISH

Fluoride varnish products have been approved by the U.S. Food and Drug Administration (FDA) for the reduction of dental caries. These contain 5% NaF and are very effective in the prevention of dental decay in all age groups. The simplest versions to use are those that come in unit-dose packaging, which require little preparation and are easy to apply. They are applied as discussed in the previous section but are not wiped off the teeth after application. Once painted on dry teeth, the varnish gels are removed after several hours with normal toothbrushing and expectoration. The amount of fluoride delivered is comparable with topical gels or foams. This delivery system provides a high concentration of fluoride with all of the benefits previously described.

> ### Prevention
> Fluoride varnish is an excellent treatment modality to use for individuals at high risk for dental caries with whom compliance of home-use products is uncertain.

Studies have shown that three to four treatments per year are effective in patients at high risk for dental caries.[73,99]

FLUORIDE TRAYS

A variety of fluoride tray designs are available for professional application. Most are constructed of disposable foam with a spongelike lining or molded interior. Trays are single-arch design or hinged for dual-arch applications, and sizes include child, small, medium, and large. The dentition is evaluated to ensure proper tray selection. The tray should cover the most distal tooth and provide enough depth and width for gel contact against the tooth surface.

Amount of Fluoride

A maximum 2 ml of fluoride per tray is recommended for an application. Most commercial fluorides are supplied in dispensing bottles. The use of a graduated medicine cup to dispense and place 2 ml of fluoride into the application tray can help the clinician determine the appropriate amount for future applications.

Insertion of Tray

After the tray is selected and loaded with fluoride gel, the patient should be prepared for the application, seated in an upright position. Using compressed air, the teeth should be dried thoroughly. The clinician should then insert the tray or trays, using light pressure to ensure gel contact with the teeth. The saliva ejector should be placed between the trays. Allowing the patient to close down gently against the saliva ejector helps maintain the adaptation of the gel to the tooth surfaces. A timer is then set for 4 minutes. On completion, the clinician should remove the trays and use the saliva ejector and gauze to remove excess fluoride, instructing the patient to expectorate thoroughly. Although a 4-minute application is recommended for optimal benefits, some manufacturers recommend 1-minute applications. Research is insufficient to support the claim that a 1-minute application is as effective as a 4-minute application.

> ### Patient Education Opportunity
> The patient should be instructed not to rinse, eat, drink, or brush for 30 minutes after the fluoride application.

PATIENT MONITORING

As with any dental procedure, the patient should be closely monitored while the fluoride application is in progress. The tray or paint-on application procedures may elicit a gag response. Leaning forward during the application allows the patient to feel that the gel is not flowing down the throat. Other gag-control techniques include deep nasal breathing and toe wiggling. The clinician also must ensure that the patient does not swallow the fluoride during or on completion of the application, possibly by allowing the patient to hold or move the saliva ejector during application.

If a stannous fluoride solution is used, then gingival sloughing may occur, particularly if the gingival tissues were inflamed before application.

Fluoride Toxicity

Fluoride is safe when used as directed but can prove to be damaging in chronic overexposure or in acute excess doses. Chronic overexposure to fluoride in children younger than age 6 years through excessive ingestion of fluoride dentifrice or OTC fluoride rinses can lead to fluorosis. *Fluorosis* is enamel hypomineralization and appears as a white stain that may later become discolored and brown. Excessive fluoride ingestion during tooth development can produce a pitted or mottled enamel surface.

Abuse of high-concentration gels or solutions and accidental ingestion of a concentrated fluoride preparation can lead to an acute toxic reaction. Acute fluoride poisoning is rare. The amount of fluoride likely to cause death is the *certainly lethal dose*. The safely tolerated dose is the amount that can be consumed without producing symptoms of serious acute toxicity; the safely tolerated dose is one fourth the certainly lethal dose (Box 25-2 and Table 25-2).

BOX 25-2

LETHAL AND SAFE DOSES OF FLUORIDE FOR ADULTS (70 KG)

Certainly Lethal Dose	Safely Tolerated Dose*
5 to 10 g of sodium fluoride	1.25 to 2.5 g of sodium fluoride
or	*or*
32 to 64 mg fluoride/kg	8 to 16 mg fluoride/kg

*One quarter of the certainly lethal dose.

Table 25-2	Lethal and Safe Doses of Fluoride for Children and Adolescents (18 Years)		
AGE (YEAR)	**WEIGHT (lb)**	**CERTAINLY LETHAL DOSE (mg)**	**SAFELY TOLERATED DOSE (mg)**
2	22	320	80
4	29	422	106
6	37	538	135
8	45	655	164
10	53	771	193
12	64	931	233
14	83	1206	301
16	92	1338	334
18	95	1382	346

From Heifetz SB, Horowitz HS: The amounts of fluoride in current fluoride therapies: safety considerations for children, *ASDC J Dent Child* 51(4):257, 1984.

Self-Applied Topical Fluoride Products

Self-applied topical fluoride products are available for patients with increased rates of dental caries, rampant enamel or root caries, xerostomia, exposure to radiation therapy, root surface sensitivity, or orthodontic bands or bonded appliances. Topical fluoride is available by prescription or OTC for lower concentrations.

Dental Considerations

Self-applied fluoride methods include the use of a custom tray, rinsing, or toothbrushing; the method should be selected based on the patient's ability to follow the prescribed method of application. A mouth tray requires dexterity to place and remove, adherence to the correct amount of gel to be dispensed, correct timing, and expectoration. Fluoride mouthrinses are easy to dispense and use but are contraindicated in children younger than 6 years of age. Fluoride brush-on gels are used after normal toothbrushing and flossing. The gel is applied with a toothbrush and brushed on for 1 minute. The APF and stannous formulas should not be used on porcelain or composite restorations or allowed to remain in contact with teeth for extended periods of time when salivary clearance is impeded (with custom trays and night guards).

Fluoride Supplements in Dental Caries Prevention

The so-called fluoride supplements (e.g., tablets, lozenges, drops) were initially used as a dietary supplement to make up for what was supposedly inadequate fluoride ingestion and thus protect against dental caries by incorporating fluoride into the tooth. For the reasons previously described, however, this is not the case.

Researchers gave fluoride tablets to children in Scotland either to swallow or to hold in the mouth (sucking or chewing).[69,87] The groups who dissolved the fluoride in the mouth and thereby *applied* fluoride topically had dramatic dental caries reductions (approximately 80%) compared with those who swallowed the tablets. Prescribed fluoride supplements should have instructions that the product be chewed or sucked to provide dental caries–protective benefits.

When fluoride tablets are swallowed, fluoride returned via the plasma to the saliva may be insufficient to provide a topical benefit. Research shows that after ingestion of a fluoride tablet, fluoride is elevated transiently in the plasma only.[21] Levels in saliva resulting from once-a-day fluoride tablet ingestion are not likely to have much, if any, topical benefit on their own, although these levels add to the topical fluoride from other sources. This point further illustrates the need to use fluoride supplements directly as a fluoride topical delivery mechanism if they are to be effective.

Note

To be effective against dental caries, fluoride supplements should be thought of as a means to supplement the topical mechanisms of fluoride action and not the minimal systemic action of fluoride.

Note

The anticaries effects of fluoride are primarily topical for children and for adults. The mechanisms of action of fluoride are (1) inhibition of demineralization at the crystal surfaces, (2) enhancement of remineralization at the crystal surfaces, and (3) inhibition of bacterial activity. The systemic effects of fluoride are minimal.

References

1. Anderson M: Chlorhexidine and xylitol gum in caries prevention, *Spec Care Dent* 23(5):173-176, 2003.

2. Anderson MH, Bales DJ, Omnell K-A: Modern management of dental caries: the cutting edge is not the dental bur, *J Am Dent Assoc* 124:37-44, 1993.

3. Anusavice KJ: Treatment regimens in preventive and restorative dentistry, *J Am Dent Assoc* 126(6):727-743, 1995.

4. Anusavice KJ: Chlorhexidine, fluoride varnish, and xylitol chewing gum: underutilized preventive therapies? *Gen Dent* 46(1):34-38, 40, 1998.

5. Arends J, ten Bosch JJ: In vivo de- and remineralization of dental enamel. In Leach SA, ed: *Factors relating to demineralization and remineralization of the teeth,* Oxford, 1995, IRL Press.

6. Benn DK et al: Standardizing data collection and decision making with an expert system, *J Dent Educ* 61:885-894, 1997.

7. Billings RJ: Restoration of carious lesions of the root, *Gerodontology* 5(1):43-49, 1986.

8. Billings RJ, Brown LR, Kaster AG: Contemporary treatment strategies for root surface dental caries, *Gerodontics* 1(1):20-27, 1985.

9. Billings RJ, Meyerowitz C, Featherstone JDB: Retention of topical fluoride in the mouths of xerostomic subjects, *Caries Res* 33:306-310, 1988.

10. Bohannan HM: Caries distribution and the case for sealants, *J Public Health Dent* 43:200-204, 1983.

11. Bohannan HM, Disney JA, Graves RC: Indications for sealant use in a community-based preventive dentistry program, *J Dent Educ* 48(2 suppl):45-55, 1984.

12. Bruun C, Givskov H, Thylstrup A: Whole saliva fluoride after toothbrushing with NaF and MFP dentifrices with different F concentrations, *Caries Res* 18:282-288, 1984.

13. Budz JA, LoRe M, Nancollas GH: Hydroxyapatite and carbonated-apatite as models for the dissolution behavior of human dental enamel, *Adv Dent Res* 1:314-321, 1987.

14. Burt BA, Fejerskov O: Water fluoridation. In Fejerskov O, Ekstrand J, Burt BA, eds: *Fluoride in dentistry,* ed 2, Copenhagen, 1996, Munksgaard.

15. Caufield PW, Cutter GR, Dasanayake AP: Initial acquisition of mutans streptococci by infants: evidence for a discrete window of infectivity, *J Dent Res* 72(1):37-45, 1993.

16. Curzon MEJ, Cutress TW, eds: *Trace elements and dental disease,* Littleton, NY, 1983, Wright-PSG.

17. Curzon MEJ, Featherstone JDB: Chemical composition of enamel. In Lazzari EP, ed: *Handbook of experimental aspects of oral biochemistry,* Boca Raton, Fla, 1983, CRC Press.

18. DenBesten P, Berkowitz R: Early childhood caries: an overview with reference to our experience in California, *J Calif Dent Assoc* 31(2):139-143, 2003.

19. D'Hondt DG, Pape H, Loesche WJ: Reduction of contamination on the dental explorer, *J Am Dent Assoc* 104:329-330, 1982.

20. Eakle WS et al: Mechanical retention versus bonding of amalgam and gallium alloy restorations, *J Prosthet Dent* 72(4):351-354, 1994.

21. Ekstrand J: Fluoride metabolism. In Fejerskov O, Ekstrand J, Burt BA, eds: *Fluoride in dentistry,* Copenhagen, 1996, Munksgaard.

22. Ekstrand KR et al: Detection, diagnosing, monitoring and logical treatment of occlusal caries in relation to lesion activity and severity: an in vivo examination with histological validation, *Caries Res* 32(4):247-254, 1998.

23. Ellen RP, Banting DW, Fillery ED: *Streptococcus mutans* and *Lactobacillus* detection in the assessment of dental root surface caries risk, *J Dent Res* 64(10):1245-1249, 1985.

24. Featherstone JDB: *Diffusion phenomena and enamel caries development.* Paper presented at the Cariology Today International Congress, Zurich, 1983, 1984.

25. Featherstone JDB: An updated understanding of the mechanism of dental decay and its prevention, *Nutr Q* 14:5-11, 1990.

26. Featherstone JDB: Fluoride, remineralization and root caries, *Am J Dent* 7:271-274, 1994.

27. Featherstone JDB: *Clinical implications of early caries detection: new strategies for caries prevention.* Paper presented at the 1st Annual Indiana Conference: Early Detection of Dental Caries, 1996.

28. Featherstone JDB: Prevention and reversal of dental caries: role of low level fluoride, *Community Dent Oral Epidemiol* 27(1):31-40, 1999.

29. Featherstone JDB: The science and practice of caries prevention, *J Am Dent Assoc* 131(7):887-899, 2000.

30. Featherstone JDB, Goodman P, MacLean JD: Electron microscope study of defect zones in dental enamel, *J Ultrastruct Res* 67:117-123, 1979.

31. Featherstone JDB, Mayer I, Driessens FCM: Synthetic apatites containing Na, Mg, and CO_3 and their comparison with tooth enamel mineral, *Calcif Tissue Int* 35:169-171, 1983.

32. Featherstone JDB, Mellberg JR: Relative rates of progress of artificial carious lesions in bovine, ovine and human enamel, *Caries Res* 15:109-114, 1981.

33. Featherstone JDB, Nelson DGA, McLean JD: An electron microscope study of modifications to defect regions in dental enamel and synthetic apatites, *Caries Res* 15:278-288, 1981.

34. Featherstone JDB, Pearson S, LeGeros RZ: An IR method for quantification of carbonate in carbonated-apatites, *Caries Res* 18:63-66, 1984.

35. Featherstone JDB, Rodgers BE: The effect of acetic, lactic and other organic acids on the formation of artificial carious lesions, *Caries Res* 15:377-385, 1981.

36. Featherstone JDB, Silverstone LM: The caries process: morphological and chemical events. In Nikiforuk G, ed: *Understanding dental caries,* Basel, Switzerland, 1985, Karger.

37. Featherstone JDB, ten Cate JM: Physicochemical aspects of fluoride-enamel interactions. In Ekstrand J, Fejerskov O, Silverstone LM, editors: *Fluoride in dentistry,* Copenhagen, 1988, Munksgaard.

38. Featherstone JDB, Zero DT: Laboratory and human studies to elucidate the mechanism of action of fluoride-containing dentifrices. In Emberry G, Rolla R, eds: *Clinical and biological aspects of dentifrices,* Oxford, 1992, Oxford University Press.

39. Featherstone JDB et al: Acid reactivity of carbonated-apatites with strontium and fluoride substitutions, *J Dent Res* 62:1049-1053, 1983.

40. Featherstone JDB et al: Enhancement of remineralization *in vitro* and *in vivo.* In Leach SA, ed: *Factors relating to demineralization and remineralization of the teeth,* Oxford, 1986, IRL Press.

41. Featherstone JDB et al: Dependence of in vitro demineralization and remineralization of dental enamel on fluoride concentration, *J Dent Res* 69:620-625, 1990.

42. Featherstone JDB et al: A randomized clinical trial of caries management by risk assessment, *Caries Res* 39:295 (abstract 25), 2005.

43. Feigal RJ: Sealants and preventive restorations: review of effectiveness and clinical changes for improvement, *Pediatr Dent* 20(2): 85-92, 1998.

44. Fejerskov O, Thylstrup A, Larsen MJ: Rational use of fluorides in caries prevention, *Acta Odontol Scand* 39:241-249, 1981.

45. Geddes DAM: Acids produced by human dental plaque metabolism in situ, *Caries Res* 9:98-109, 1975.

46. Gorton J, Featherstone JD: In vivo inhibition of demineralization around orthodontic brackets, *Am J Orthod Dentofacial Orthop* 123(1):10-14, 2003.

47. Hamilton IR, Bowden GHW: Fluoride effects on oral bacteria. In Fejerskov O, Ekstrand J, Burt BA, eds: *Fluoride in dentistry,* Copenhagen, 1996, Munksgaard.

48. Handelman SL et al: Hyposalivatory drug use, whole stimulated salivary flow, and mouth dryness in older, long-term care residents, *Spec Care Dent* 9:12-18, 1989.

49. Hargreaves JA, Thomson GW, Wagg BJ: Changes in caries prevalence in Isle of Lewis children between 1971 and 1981, *Caries Res* 17:554-559, 1983.

50. Hume WR: *Need for change in dental caries diagnosis.* Paper presented at the 1st Annual Indiana Conference: Early Detection of Dental Caries, 1996, Indianapolis.

51. Isokangas P et al: Occurrence of dental decay in children after maternal consumption of xylitol chewing gum, a follow-up from 0 to 5 years of age, *J Dent Res* 79(11):1885-1889, 2000.

52. Jenkins GN: Recent changes in dental caries, *Br Med J* 291:1297-1298, 1985.

53. Kaste LM, Selwitz RH, Oldakowski RJ: Coronal caries in the primary and permanent dentition of children and adolescents 1-17 years of age: United States, 1988-1991, *J Dent Res* 75:631-641, 1996.

54. Katz RV: Assessing root caries in populations: the evolution of the root caries index, *J Public Health Dent* 40(1):7-16, 1980.

55. Kawasaki K, Featherstone JDB: Effects of collagenase on root demineralization, *J Dent Res* 76:588-595, 1997.

56. Kemp-Scholte CM, Davidson CL: Marginal scaling of curing contraction gaps in class V composite resin restorations, *J Dent Res* 67:841-845, 1988.

57. Kidd EA, Joyston-Bechal S: Update on fissure sealants, *Dent Update* 21(8):323-326, 1994.

58. Krasse B: Biological factors as indicators of future caries, *Int Dent J* 38:219-225, 1988.

59. Lagerlof F, Oliveby A: *Clinical implications: new strategies for caries treatment.* Paper presented at the 1st Annual Indiana Conference: Early Detection of Dental Caries, 1996, Indianapolis.

60. LeGeros RZ: Calcium phosphates. Oral biology and medicine, *Monogr Oral Sci* 15:1-201, 1991.

61. LeGeros RZ et al: Carbonate substitution in the apatite structure, *Bull Soc Chim Fr* (Special issue):1712-1718, 1968.

62. Leverett DH et al: Caries risk assessment by a cross-sectional discrimination model, *J Dent Res* 72:529-537, 1993.

63. Leverett DH et al: Caries risk assessment in a longitudinal discrimination study, *J Dent Res* 72:538-543, 1993.

64. Loesche WJ: Chemotherapy of dental plaque infections, *Oral Sci Rev* 9(9):65-107, 1976.

65. Loesche WJ: Role of *Streptococcus mutans* in human dental decay, *FEMS Microbiol Rev* 50:353-380, 1986.

66. Loesche WJ: Antimicrobials in dentistry: with knowledge comes responsibility, *J Dent Res* 75:1432-1433, 1996.

67. Loesche WJ, Hockett RN, Syed SA: The predominant cultivable flora of tooth surface plaque removed from institutionalized subjects, *Arch Oral Biol* 17:1311-1325, 1973.

68. Makinen KK et al: Six-month polyol chewing-gum programme in kindergarten-age children: a feasibility study focusing on mutans streptococci and dental plaque, *Int Dent J* 55(2):81-88, 2005.

69. McCall D, Stephen KW, McNee SG: Fluoride tablets and salivary fluoride levels, *Caries Res* 15:98-102, 1981.

70. Meyerowitz C et al: Use of an intra-oral model to evaluate 0.05% sodium fluoride mouthrinse in radiation-induced hyposalivation, *J Dent Res* 70:894-898, 1991.

71. Moss ME, Zero DT: An overview of caries risk assessment, and its potential utility, *J Dent Educ* 59(10):932-940, 1995.

72. Mount GJ, Hume WR: *Preservation and restoration of tooth structure,* St Louis, 1998, Mosby.

73. Murray JJ, Rugg-Gunn AJ, Jenkins GN: *Fluorides in caries prevention,* ed 3, London, 1992, Wright.

74. Nelson DGA et al: Effect of carbonate and fluoride on the dissolution behaviour of synthetic apatites, *Caries Res* 17:200-211, 1983.

75. Newbrun E: *Cariology,* ed 3, Chicago, 1989, Quintessence.

76. Newbrun E: Effectiveness of water fluoridation, *J Public Health Dent* 49:279-289, 1989.

77. Nyvad B, Fejerskov O: Assessing the stage of caries lesion activity on the basis of clinical and microbiological examination, *Community Dent Oral Epidemiol* 25:69-75, 1997.

78. O'Reilly MM, Featherstone JDB: De- and remineralization around orthodontic appliances: an in vivo study, *Am J Orthod* 92:33-40, 1987.

79. Pereira AC, Verdonschot EH, Huysmans MC: Caries detection methods: can they aid decision making for invasive sealant treatment? *Caries Res* 35(2):83-89, 2001.

80. Pitts NB: Patient caries status in the context of practical, evidence-based management of the initial caries lesion, *J Dent Educ* 61: 895-905, 1997.

81. Ricketts D et al: Hidden caries: What is it? Does it exist? Does it matter? *Int Dent J* 47(5):259-265, 1997.

82. Robinson C, Kirkham J, Weatherell JA: Fluoride in teeth and bone. In Fejerskov O, Ekstrand J, Burt BA, eds: *Fluoride in dentistry,* ed 2, Copenhagen, 1996, Munksgaard.

83. Shi W, Jewett A, Hume WR: Rapid and quantitative detection of *S. mutans* with species specific monoclonal antibodies, *Hybridoma* 17:365-371, 1998.

84. Shields CP et al: A longitudinal chemical analysis of saliva, *J Dent Res* 76(Special issue, IADR meeting), 1997.

85. Shields CP et al: Chemical analysis of saliva: a longitudinal study, *J Dent Res* 74:15, 1995.

86. Silverstone LM: The structure of carious enamel, including the early lesion, *Oral Sci Rev* 3:100-160, 1973.

87. Stephen KW, Campbell D: Caries reduction and cost benefit after 3 years of sucking fluoride tablets daily at school: a double blind trial, *Br Dent J* 144:202-206, 1978.

88. Stookey GK: Are all fluoride dentifrices the same? In Wei SHY, ed: *Clinical uses of fluorides,* Philadelphia, 1985, Lea & Febiger.

89. Suddick RP, Dodds MW Jr: Caries activity estimates and implications: insights into risk versus activity, *J Dent Educ* 61:876-884, 1997.

90. ten Cate JM, Duijsters PPE: Influence of fluoride in solution on tooth demineralization: II—microradiographic data, *Caries Res* 17:513-519, 1983.

91. ten Cate JM, Featherstone JDB: Mechanistic aspects of the interactions between fluoride and dental enamel, *Crit Rev Oral Biol Med* 2:283-296, 1991.

92. ten Cate JM, van Duinen RN: Hypermineralization of dentinal lesions adjacent to glass-ionomer cement restorations, *J Dent Res* 74(6):1266-1271, 1995.

93. van Louveren C: The antimicrobial action of fluoride and its role in caries inhibition, *J Dent Res* 69:676-681, 1990.

94. Weintraub JA et al: A retrospective analysis of the cost-effectiveness of dental sealants in a children's health center, *Soc Sci Med* 36:1483-1493, 1993.

95. Whitford GM et al: Fluoride uptake by *Streptococcus mutans* 6715, *Infect Immun* 18(3):680-768, 1977.

96. Winn DM et al: Coronal and root caries in the dentition of adults in the United States, 1988-1991, *J Dent Res* 75:642-651, 1996.

97. Wright JT et al: Effect of conventional dental restorative treatment on bacteria in saliva, *Community Dent Oral Epidemiol* 20:138-143, 1992.

98. Zambon JJ, Kasprzak SA: The microbiology and histopathology of human root caries, *Am J Dent* 8(6):323-328, 1995.

99. Zero DT et al: Fluoride concentrations in plaque, whole saliva and ductal saliva after applications of home-use fluoride agents, *J Dent Res* 71:1768-1775, 1992.

Dentifrices

Caren M. Barnes

INSIGHT

One of the most frequently asked questions dental hygienists receive from their patients is, "What toothpaste should I be using?" It is imperative that dental hygienists have a clear understanding of the differences between the numerous dentifrices available for consumers and be able to make recommendations based on the needs of the individual patient.

✺ CASE STUDY 26-1 Selecting the Correct Dentifrice

A hygienist is the main resource for dental product information for patients in a busy, small-town practice. One of the most common questions is, "What is the best toothpaste?" The stock answer is, "It depends," and then the hygienist tries to assess the needs of the individual patient and makes an appropriate recommendation. With current patients, however, the answer is more complex.

Cynthia Courtland has been a patient in the practice for several years, along with her husband, Cal; daughter, Amber; and son, Brandon. Mrs. Courtland is 45 years old, and the hygienist enjoys her routine supportive care visits. She has some localized areas of mild gingivitis, mostly the result of infrequent flossing. Currently, she has some concerns she wants to discuss.

Mr. Courtland needed extensive oral self-care reinstruction at his last appointment. He is 52 years old and has a history of periodontitis that has been successfully controlled for approximately 10 years. He has some exposed root surfaces that are vulnerable to root caries and occasionally complains of cold sensitivity.

Amber's dental care team is concerned for her oral health. She recently had her orthodontic appliances removed because she had not been compliant with oral self-care or diet. Generalized enamel demineralization is present, as well as several carious lesions that need to be restored. Brandon, age 5, had no dental caries or plaque biofilm at his last visit, and he has his first loose tooth.

Mrs. Courtland wants to help her family maintain an optimal level of dental health, but she is confused by all the options when she shops for dental care products. She asks, "Which toothpaste should we use?" The dental hygienist pauses as the individual needs of the family members are considered. This situation may require more than a simple, single-product recommendation for the whole family.

KEY TERMS

active (therapeutic) agents	crossover study	halitosis	substantivity
basic ingredients	dentifrice	hydrodynamic theory	systematic reviews
blinding (masking)	efficacy	over-the-counter	superiority studies
calibration	erosion	parallel study	therapeutic approval
chemotherapeutic agents	fluorosis	relative dentin abrasivity index	washout
cosmetic approval			

LEARNING OUTCOMES

After reading this chapter the student will be able to:

1. Describe the difference between basic and active ingredients in a dentifrice.
2. List active and basic ingredients in dentifrices, and describe their functions.
3. Discuss compatibility of ingredients in a dentifrice and understand the reasons each is critical to the formulation.
4. Describe adverse effects that can be associated with the use of a dentifrice.
5. Explain the process necessary for a new product to receive U.S. Food and Drug Administration approval for marketing.
6. Discuss the process necessary for a product to receive the American Dental Association's Seal of Acceptance.
7. Differentiate between the roles of the U.S. Food and Drug Administration and the American Dental Association in product marketing.
8. Describe the differences between cosmetic approval and therapeutic approval.
9. Describe the different types of studies used to evaluate agents in dentifrices.
10. Explain the process by which a systematic review is conducted.
11. List the agents used in a dentifrice for the treatment of dental caries, sensitivity, gingivitis, calculus, stain removal, whitening, plaque biofilm removal, oral malodor, and inflammation.
12. Discuss the history of the evolution of dentifrices.
13. Distinguish between stain removal and whitening.
14. Recommend the appropriate dentifrice for each member of the family in this chapter's case study.
15. Discuss the ingredients and function of each used in natural dentifrices.

Patient Education Opportunity

The daily use of a dentifrice, usually a paste or gel, is one of the most beneficial recommendations that dental professionals can make to their patients in preventing and controlling dental diseases.

Certainly, one of the most frequently asked questions a dental hygienist receives is, "What kind of toothpaste should I use?"

The use of a fluoride dentifrice, beginning in the late 1950s, is widely acknowledged as a major reason for the decrease in dental caries in many parts of the world.[34] Over the years, dental professionals have helped patients realize the benefits of oral hygiene, specifically by recommending a toothbrush and toothpaste for the mechanical removal of plaque biofilm. Together with toothbrushes, dentifrices are the most widely recommended and used oral hygiene products, and they offer increased oral health benefits beyond simple mechanical removal of plaque biofilm.[16] In more recent years, various agents, such as fluoride, pyrophosphate, triclosan, hydrogen peroxide, and calcium carbonate, have been added to dentifrice formulations. The addition of these agents enhance the benefits of the dentifrice delivery system that can now address not only the prevention of dental caries and periodontal disease but also whitening, stain removal, oral malodor, calculus formation, and enamel remineralization.

When patients shop for toothpaste, they are faced with an overwhelming array of products with various claims. Distinguishing products with proven therapeutic effects from those with only cosmetic benefits is difficult for patients and oral healthcare providers. As part of individualizing prevention strategies, the dental professional must be prepared to help patients make informed choices about oral care purchases to maximize product benefits.

Composition of Dentifrice

Dentifrice is an inclusive term used to describe a powder, paste, or gel used with a toothbrush to aid in the removal of plaque biofilm, materia alba, and stain from teeth and soft tissues. The earliest commercial products were simple powder mixtures; modern dentifrices are generally toothpastes or gels that are complex formulations of many ingredients, some of which are active and some of which are basic and found in most formulations[94] (Table 26-1 and Figure 26-1).

Some early attempts to add **chemotherapeutic agents** to dentifrices were unsuccessful, largely because of reactions among ingredients.[92] As new agents are incorporated into dentifrices, such issues help explain the need for the extensive evaluations required by the U.S. Food and Drug Administration (FDA) before products can be released on the market.[87] Examination of the evolution of dentifrices and their active ingredients underscores the need for FDA evaluation.

Figure 26-2 illustrates the evolution of dentifrice formulations.[89] The first generation of dentifrice formulations was

---

Prevention

Compatibility of the components in dentifrices is critical to ensure that the chemotherapeutic and other types of agents are stable during storage and are biologically active when used in the mouth.[17]

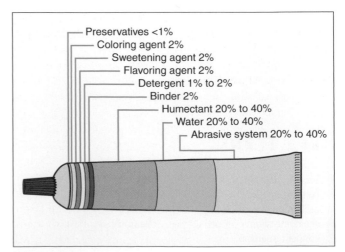

FIGURE 26-1
Dentifrice ingredients.

Preservatives <1%
Coloring agent 2%
Sweetening agent 2%
Flavoring agent 2%
Detergent 1% to 2%
Binder 2%
Humectant 20% to 40%
Water 20% to 40%
Abrasive system 20% to 40%

Table 26-1	**Basic Dentifrice Ingredients**			
COMPONENT	**PURPOSE**	**PERCENT**	**EXAMPLES**	**COMMENTS**
Abrasives	Varying particle sizes create an abrasive system that cleans and polishes	20 to 40	Calcium carbonate, calcium pyrophosphate, aluminum oxide, silicone oxides, bicarbonate, chalk	Must be compatible with other ingredients; must not damage teeth or soft tissues.
Detergents	Help loosen debris; have foaming action; act as surfactant moisture	1 to 2	Sodium lauryl sulfate (SLS), sodium lauryl sarcosinate	Some patients may have mucosal reaction to SLS.
Water and Humectants	Maintain moisture and consistency	20 to 40	Sorbitol, glycerin, propylene glycol, mannitol	Some humectants also add a sweet taste and require a preservative to prevent bacterial and mold growth.
Binders (Thickeners)	Prevent separation of ingredients	2	Alginate, gums, synthetic celluloses	High percentage of binders is found in gel formulations.
Preservatives	Prevent mold and bacterial growth	<1	Alcohols, sodium benzoate, dichlorinated phenols	Contact allergens occur in some patients.
Sweetening Agents	Imparts pleasant flavor	2	Saccharine, sorbitol, mannitol, xylitol, glycerin	Some also act as humectants.
Flavoring Agents	Give immediate pleasant taste sensation that lingers as an aftertaste	2	Essential oils (peppermint, spearmint, wintergreen, cinnamon), menthol	Contact allergens occur in some patients.
Coloring Agents	Give attractive and desirable appearance	2	Vegetable dyes	Must not stain teeth or soft tissues.

Data from Wilkins EM: *Clinical practice of the dental hygienist,* ed 8, Philadelphia, 1999, Lippincott Williams & Wilkins.

created in the twentieth century and targeted basic hygienic and cosmetic needs—the cleaning of teeth and the improvement of mouth odor. These formulations were very simple. The second generation of dentifrice formulations became more complex, containing calculus preventive or therapeutic ingredients that targeted the treatment of gingivitis or sensitivity. The third and fourth generations of dentifrice formulations combined two or more active ingredients but were aimed at treating or preventing a specific condition such as tobacco stains, gingivitis, or dental caries. Examples of these combined active ingredients are dentifrices containing sodium fluoride and sodium monofluorophosphate to strengthen the anticaries activity of the dentifrice. The fifth generation of dentifrice formulations is integrated with multiple active ingredients that target several conditions, such as anticaries and whitening or antigingivitis and antiplaque. Examples of these integrated ingredients include sodium monofluorophosphate (anticaries ingredient), calcium carbonate, perlite (whitening agents), hexametaphosphate (stain inhibition), or 0.3% triclosan plus 1000 parts per million (ppm) fluoride, 0.13% calcium glycerophosphate, calcium carbonate, Gantrez, and silica (antigingivitis and antiplaque ingredients).[69] The types of ingredients that will most likely be incorporated in future generations of dentifrices will be agents such as antioxidants that will boost host antioxidant defenses in combating periodontal diseases.[8]

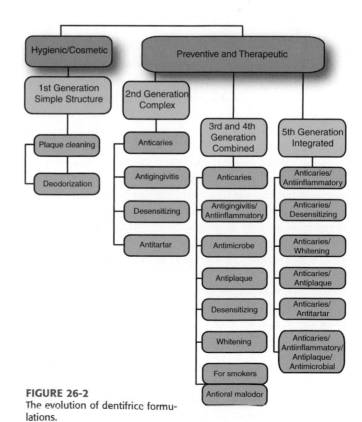

FIGURE 26-2
The evolution of dentifrice formulations.

Adverse Effects

Dental literature reports allergic reactions to many common ingredients in dentifrice formulations, most often contact-type reactions. The most common allergens are certain types of flavorings, detergents, and preservatives. Problems have been reported in 1.5% to 2.0% of users; immediate sensitivity reactions such as bronchospasm and asthma are rare.[75] Although implicated in allergic reactions,[80] acnelike eruptions,[76] and ulcerative stomatitis,[23] fluoride has been safely used for nearly 50 years. Reports detail oral mucosal desquamative effects and increased gingival blood flow associated with the use of the detergent ingredient sodium lauryl sulfate (SLS).[38] Recurrent aphthous ulcers may be related to SLS and cocoamidopropyl betaine detergents,[39] and perioral contact urticaria has been associated with sodium benzoate.[63]

> *Distinct Care Modifications*
>
> The most critical time to avoid excess fluoride is during the development of the anterior permanent teeth, which occurs up to 3 years of age.[66] The American Dental Association (ADA) and the American Academy of Pediatric Dentistry have recommended that children younger than the age of 3 years should use only a *pea-sized* smear of fluoride dentifrice for brushing. Intentional ingestion of fluoride dentifrice should also be discouraged in children.

Mucosal reactions to *tartar control* dentifrices that contain pyrophosphates include ulceration, sloughing of soft tissues, erythema, and migratory glossitis.[48]

Another concern is the increased risk of **fluorosis** in children, which may be partly caused by ingestion of fluoride dentifrices during tooth development.[83] Improper use of fluoride supplements also can be a major contributing factor in fluorosis.

Safety and Efficacy

The FDA is responsible for protecting the public from unsafe products. All **over-the-counter** (OTC) and prescription drugs require research studies that demonstrate proof of product safety. The FDA recognizes two categories of approval for products.[87] **Cosmetic approval** requires only proof of safety and does not allow claims of therapeutic value. **Therapeutic approval** requires extensive testing that shows efficacy before products can be marketed. For a product with a new active ingredient and therapeutic claims, the manufacturer must undergo a formal new drug application (NDA) process with the FDA. The stages of the FDA approval process begin with preclinical research and development to prove safety related to allergenicity and carcinogenicity. After product safety is established, investigatory new drug approval is required before clinical research and development can be performed. Three phases of testing are performed:

1. Pilot studies to determine safe doses for humans
2. Large human studies to prove **efficacy** and define the effective dosage range (phase 1 studies)
3. Large, long-term, double-blind controlled clinical trials (phase 2 studies)

The manufacturer then submits all these data to the FDA as part of the NDA and eventually receives approval from the FDA to market the product. The approval requires a period of postmarketing surveillance once the product is made available to the general public.[35]

The FDA also has established the monograph process to allow manufacturers to market dentifrices that meet specified compositional and technical requirements without going through the expensive and time-consuming NDA process. For example, one anticaries monograph permits dentifrices with sodium fluoride, stannous fluoride, or sodium monofluorophosphate to be marketed as long as the fluoride level is 1000 to 1100 ppm. The manufacturer also must generate data showing acceptable fluoride stability. Other ingredients (e.g., pyrophosphate) can be added to a fluoride dentifrice without the need for an NDA, as long as the ingredient is present for a cosmetic benefit and has an established safety pedigree for oral use. In addition, a desensitization monograph exists that allows the use of 5% potassium nitrate in conjunction with fluoride in a dentifrice.

The manufacturer can apply for the ADA Seal of Acceptance. This program is administered by the ADA's Council on Scientific Affairs (CSA) and is designed to help dental professionals advise patients and the public worldwide. The ADA Seal of Acceptance is a voluntary process and often requires an exhaustive review of the product, depending on the amount of preexisting information on products of similar formulation. The manufacturer must reapply for the Seal every 3 years, and the review committee can withdraw acceptance at any time. The Seal applies to products used in the practice of dentistry and to those sold commercially to the public. When used on labeling, the Seal is meaningful only for those specific therapies for which acceptance has been issued. Both dental professionals and patients can be assured that products receiving the Seal have been shown to be safe and effective when used as directed, based on the rigorous standards that the ADA has developed and continues to revise since the Council on Dental Therapeutics (predecessor to the CSA) was formed in 1930.[71]

> *Patient Education Opportunity*
>
> Dental professionals should talk to their patients about the meaning of the ADA Seal of Acceptance. When used on labeling, the Seal is meaningful only for those specific therapies for which acceptance has been issued. Both dental professionals and patients can be assured that products receiving the Seal have been shown to be safe and effective when used as directed, based on the rigorous standards that the ADA has developed and continues to revise since the Council on Dental Therapeutics (predecessor to the CSA) was formed in 1930.[71]

Evaluating Clinical Studies

Dental professionals and patients rely on the FDA to regulate availability of products based on safety and effectiveness and on the ADA for additional scrutiny of products. In addition to these extensive product evaluations, dental professionals also must be able to evaluate clinical studies performed on products.

Data from well-designed clinical trials are invaluable as the dental professional attempts to select appropriate products to meet each patient's unique needs. Studies involving agents for the control and prevention of oral diseases require appropriate analysis using specific criteria to assess credibility and prevent unfounded conclusions.

STUDY DESIGN

Accepted study designs use randomized, controlled clinical trials to evaluate chemotherapeutic agents in dentifrices, usually through efficacy studies or superiority studies. Efficacy studies compare a product with a placebo. **Superiority studies** compare products with one another, one of which has an accepted therapeutic value (positive control). The design is usually either a **parallel study,** with groups of patients assigned to one treatment for the duration of the study, or a **crossover study,** during which treatment groups are reversed midway through the study. Crossover studies require a period for the groups to return to baseline levels (a **washout** period) before starting the other treatment; crossover studies are difficult to interpret because of a possible carryover effect from one treatment to the other.[28] Patients are assigned to treatment groups in a randomized fashion, and the groups are stratified to balance groups for factors such as age and disease severity.[41] The end points of the study should address the variable of interest.[33]

Observed changes in plaque biofilm accumulation can occur hourly and gingival changes within days, but changes in periodontal attachment levels take months to years to be observed clinically. Chemotherapeutic dentifrice studies usually evaluate plaque biofilm and gingival changes but not attachment level changes. Some studies monitor the oral microflora to assess changes; others assess supragingival calculus accumulation. Evaluation of all the potential changes in the mouth resulting from the use of the chemotherapeutic agents is demanding and challenges researchers to select the appropriate indices.

Safety issues must also be addressed in the study design, with emphasis on standardized monitoring and reporting. Side effects in human studies can be difficult to assess; some effects are observed immediately, whereas others may take months or years to develop. Side effects are usually reported as adverse events, both serious and nonserious, and must be considered relative to the benefit of the agent.[64]

DURATION

Duration of the study depends on the agent being studied and the intended use. Well-designed studies of plaque biofilm and gingival changes usually last at least 3 months; the ADA guidelines for the Seal of Acceptance program require studies that last 6 months.[71]

STUDY POPULATION

The population chosen for the study is also a critical point of the study design. To demonstrate effectiveness of the chemotherapeutic agent, the study population must represent the consumer population; that is, patients must have the same level of the disease as the intended users of the product.[64]

EFFICACY CLAIMS

Efficacy or superiority claims can be extrapolated theoretically to the larger group only when the population studied in a clinical trial of an agent in a dentifrice formulation is similar to the population who will use the drug. Variations in populations studied are present in long-term controlled clinical trials for formulations containing chemotherapeutic agents. These variations make comparisons among studies difficult, and claims of efficacy may be difficult to apply to populations other than the specific study population.

> *Note*
>
> Conclusions about the effects of a chemotherapeutic agent are of significant value for the population studied, but extension of these effects to a general population is not always possible or appropriate.[40]

EXAMINER RELIABILITY

Controlled clinical trials on chemotherapeutic agents in dentifrices reported in the literature should contain statistical information or confirmation of examiner **calibration.** Calibration of examiners in the use of the indices is important to ensure consistency and validity of results.[29] Some studies use only one examiner for all clinical evaluations during the study, but intraexaminer reliability should be reported to allow for appropriate statistical analysis. In studies that use multiple examiners, interexaminer reliability is also needed.[70] Without confirmation of examiner calibration, the interpretation of the overall reliability of the studies is difficult.

Blinding (masking), or protecting the examiner from knowledge of information concerning the specific groups in the study, is also critical to protect the validity of the results. Ideally, neither the patient nor the examiner or clinician knows the treatment identity (double-blind design). In single-blind study designs, only the examiner is unaware of the treatment identity.

Evaluating all factors that may influence the outcome of a study is difficult. Ensuring that the results truly reflect the activity of the chemotherapeutic agent alone is challenging, especially in complex disease entities such as dental caries or gingivitis, which can be influenced by many factors. Studies analyzing chemotherapeutic agents in dentifrice formulations based on well-designed clinical trials are useful for the dental practitioner. Each study should be carefully evaluated, however, according to the inherent problems with applying information based on a specific population to an individual patient.

SYSTEMATIC REVIEWS

Another method for evaluating clinical trials is through **systematic reviews.** As the dental hygiene practice becomes evidence based, it is critical that dental hygienists locate sources for credible information that evaluates research on treatment interventions, in other words, systematic reviews. Systematic reviews are not literature reviews. Authors of systematic reviews identify a treatment intervention to evaluate how it works. The authors locate, evaluate, and appraise as many scientific studies as possible. Using specific criteria for inclusion, scientific studies that meet the criteria are summarized into a comprehensive report on the effectiveness of the treatment intervention. Sources for systematic reviews of clinical trials conducted on treatment interventions include the Cochrane Collaboration (International), the National Institute of Clinical Excellence (in the United Kingdom), and the Agency for Healthcare Research and Quality (in the United States). These agencies report on all aspects of health, and oral health is only one area for which systematic reviews are conducted. Under the heading of oral health, hundreds of reviews are available on a variety of types of oral healthcare interventions, including the effectiveness of fluoride, various restorative materials, power toothbrushes, and orthodontic treatments. Dental organizations, such as the American Academy of Periodontology, also conduct systematic reviews.

Dentifrice Formulations

> *Distinct Care Modifications*
>
> Patients with special needs such as contact allergies, high dental caries rates, sensitivity, calculus, staining, or periodontitis require the best efforts of the dental hygienist to advise them in the use of specialized products.

With the wide availability of effective agents in dentifrice products, all patients can benefit from appropriate use. Although these products will enhance mechanical hygiene, they clearly are not a substitute for constant vigilance in oral self-care efforts.

ANTICARIES

As early as 1942, fluoride added to drinking water has been found to reduce the incidence of dental caries. Early attempts to add fluoride to dentifrices were not successful, mostly because of the tendency of abrasives used at that time to inactivate the fluoride.[60] Continued testing found that stannous fluoride, when used with a compatible abrasive system, inhibited the formation of carious lesions. The ADA recognized the value of a stannous fluoride dentifrice as an anticaries agent by granting the Seal of Acceptance to Crest in 1960. Problems with shelf life and staining for products containing stannous fluoride led to further research on additional fluoride formulations. As a result, products containing sodium monofluorophosphate and sodium fluoride were recognized as equally effective or slightly more effective anticaries agents. Dentifrices containing these types of fluoride are desirable because of stability and compatibility with many abrasive systems.[65]

Topical fluoride acts as an effective dental caries–preventive agent in several ways. Fluoride acts in conjunction with the calcium and phosphate in saliva to remineralize the earliest stages of dental caries, the hypomineralized or white spot enamel. Fluoride also exhibits some **substantivity,** or the ability to be held in reservoirs within the oral cavity; it is released over time, creating continual exposure of hypomineralized enamel to fluoride. Several areas of the mouth can be considered fluoride reservoirs, including oral mucosa, plaque biofilm, and enamel. Rinsing with water after brushing is not recommended; the greater the concentration of fluoride left in the mouth to form a reservoir, the less the chance of decay.[61]

⁂ CASE APPLICATION 26-1.1

Selection of an Anticaries Dentifrice

Which member of the Courtland family could benefit from a dentifrice with anticaries properties? What oral conditions does this family member have that present the need for an anticaries dentifrice?

A systematic review of randomized clinical trials investigating the efficacy of fluoride toothpastes, mouthrinses, gels, and varnishes concluded that fluoride toothpastes have a similar degree of effectiveness for the prevention of dental caries in children.[55]

> *Prevention*
>
> Frequent exposure to a fluoride dentifrice is the most effective preventive method for dental caries in both children and adults.

The fluoride concentration of most dentifrices in U.S. OTC products is 1000 to 1100 ppm. High-potency dentifrices that contain fluoride at up to 5000 ppm are also available by prescription. Dental caries prevention is directly proportional to fluoride concentration, and compliance improves with the use of a paste rather than a fluoride gel because patients have to use only one product.[21] For populations at risk for severe dental caries, a high-potency fluoride dentifrice is an appropriate choice.

ANTIPLAQUE, ANTIGINGIVITIS, ANTIINFLAMMATORY

Most patients receiving treatment in a dental care setting have some level of gingival inflammation. Gingivitis is prevalent in the general population at a high rate, with as few as 15% of individuals free of signs of periodontal diseases.[12] Development of periodontitis is usually preceded by gingivitis, but not all sites with gingivitis progress to periodontitis. Currently, predicting the likelihood of developing attachment loss does not exist, and no evidence shows that control of gingivitis with topical agents decreases the progression of periodontitis or affects eventual tooth loss. Treatment of all gingivitis is generally recommended to prevent periodontitis. Dentifrices with chemotherapeutic agents that are successful in controlling or eliminating gingivitis, when combined with mechanical therapy, can improve oral health.

Evidence suggests strong relationships between periodontal disease and systemic health. This relationship is centered on the local inflammatory nature of periodontal disease and its link to systemic inflammatory diseases, cardiovascular disease, and atherosclerosis.[18,26] Certainly, no one would suggest that a dentifrice is a therapeutic treatment for periodontal inflammation. However, tight control of bacterial plaque is an essential arm of periodontal treatment, and the use of a dentifrice in an oral hygiene regimen can play a role in the control of periodontal inflammation and thus influence the systemic inflammatory status.

CALCULUS CONTROL

Dental professionals expend significant time and effort in the removal of calculus deposits. Similar to stains, patients often see supragingival calculus as an esthetic problem, and dental professionals are concerned about the role of calculus in the development of gingivitis. The rough surface of calculus can retain bacterial plaque close to the gingival tissues, and calculus is often located in areas that are difficult for patients to clean thoroughly.[1] Supragingival calculus can become easily discolored, and many extrinsic stains on teeth are actually stained calculus deposits.

For patients who form supragingival calculus, daily application of an anticalculus dentifrice to inhibit supragingival calculus deposition can be beneficial. Unfortunately, anticalculus dentifrices have little or no effect on subgingival calculus.

Occasionally, patients will question some commercially prepared dentifrices because they contain ingredients that are perceived to be controversial, such as fluoride and saccharin, although the FDA recognizes fluoride to be the only toothpaste ingredient to prevent dental caries. As consumers, patients have a choice among natural dentifrices that contain ingredients such as pure, natural-flavoring oils (e.g., peppermint, anise). Other ingredients in these natural toothpastes include tea tree oil, sodium bicarbonate, sea salt, boron, chlorophyll, potassium nitrate, aloe vera, grapefruit seed extract, vitamins C and E, and sanguinarine. Natural toothpastes can be found with other dental products in most retail stores or in health foods stores.

ORAL MALODOR CONTROL

Oral malodor, also called **halitosis** or bad breath, is universally experienced and has a variety of etiologic factors. Offensive mouth odors can be attributed to odoriferous foods, systemic illnesses, some medications, infections, and dry mouth, but oral malodor is most commonly attributed to bacteria. The oral cavity has a multitude of sites that harbor bacteria and contribute to oral malodor. Poor oral hygiene, bacterial coating of the tongue, food impaction, and microorganisms that are associated with gingivitis and periodontitis contribute to oral malodor.[52] Periodontal disease probably does not cause oral malodor, but strong evidence suggests that periodontal disease certainly increases the intensity and severity of oral malodor.[95] Numerous oral hygiene devices and chemical agents, including dentifrices, have been developed to control oral malodor. The first-generation dentifrices contained sweeteners and flavoring agents and could mask some oral malodors. Since that time, however, numerous active ingredients have been compounded with denti-

frices and have proven to eliminate some of the bacteria associated with oral malodor or, at the least, assist in the control of oral malodor. Many of these active oral malodor–fighting ingredients are quite effective; however, a comprehensive evaluation should be performed on patients with chronic malodor to ensure an effective diagnosis and appropriate treatment plan to eliminate the causes when possible.[45] For those who have oral malodor as a result of oral hygiene and in whom more serious etiologic factors have been eliminated, these new dentifrice compounds for fighting oral malodor are quite effective. (For more information on oral malodor, refer to Chapter 38.)

REMINERALIZATION

Recently, the remineralization of enamel has been the focus of dentifrices, with the intent to improve tooth surface smoothness and the luster of the teeth. Tooth structure destruction through dental caries and erosion occurs by acid attacks that affect the tooth in two different ways: (1) Through cariogenic bacteria, acid attacks initiate subsurface lesions and, if left untreated, progress through the enamel and dentin. (2) **Erosion** by acid attacks removes minerals from the enamel surface and can lead to the severe loss of enamel thickness and contour and surface luster. One approach to combat acid attacks is to use amorphous calcium phosphate compounds in dentifrices because calcium phosphates rapidly hydrolyze to form apatite.[13,88] These calcium phosphate compounds readily precipitate onto and into the tooth surface, thereby accomplishing the goal of improving the cosmetic appearance of the teeth, as well as providing anticaries efficacy.[52] One study found that the remineralization dentifrices containing calcium carbonates can be found, compounded with additional therapeutic ingredients such as sodium monofluorophosphate and sodium bicarbonate to improve remineralization and fluoride uptake.[78]

SENSITIVITY CONTROL

Localized, sharp, and instant pain, usually elicited when cold or other stimuli make contact with the cervical area of a tooth, characterize *dentin sensitivity*. Other oral conditions can mimic sensitivity, but the examiner can rely on the patient to point to the area. A short puff of air from the air/water syringe usually confirms the exact location, which is associated with an area of exposed root surface. The accepted theory of pain transmission in dentin sensitivity (i.e., **hydrodynamic theory** of dentinal hypersensitivity) involves delivery of stimuli through hydrodynamic movement of fluid in the dentinal tubule, activating pulpal tissues and inducing the sensation of pain.[56] Any procedures involving root surfaces can cause dentin sensitivity. Patients may complain of dentin sensitivity after periodontal debridement or restorative procedures. Others experience sensitivity after consuming acidic foods or after a period of poor oral hygiene. The concern that some ingredient in tartar-control dentifrice formulations may promote dentin sensitivity[5] has not been substantiated by clinical studies.

Because dentin sensitivity is associated with exposed dentinal tubules at the root surface, a course of treatment is sometimes directed at blocking or obfuscating the opening to the tubules. If left untreated, dentin sensitivity may subside. However, treatment usually begins with specific plaque biofilm–control instructions on the use of a sensitivity-control dentifrice formulation. The most common active ingredient in commercial sensitivity-control dentifrices is potassium nitrate. Other salts of potassium, such as potassium citrate, have also demonstrated effectiveness.[56] Additionally, strontium chloride and sodium citrate are used as active ingredients in sensitivity-control dentifrices.

✦ CASE APPLICATION 26-1.4

Desensitizing Dentifrice Needed

Which member of the Courtland family has sensitive teeth? What is the action of a desensitizing dentifrice?

> *Note*
>
> Sensitivity-control dentifrices require time to be effective; consequently, combining an in-office application of a dentin-blocking agent or fluoride varnish with the use of a sensitivity-control dentifrice at home is a common technique.

If these methods do not produce relief after 4 to 6 weeks, then more aggressive means include in-office applications of bonding agents, placement of permanent restorations, and gingival grafting for root coverage.

STAIN REMOVAL

Distinguishing between stain removal dentifrices and those dentifrices that claim to *whiten* teeth as a result of the fact that their ingredients produce a whitening effect via stain removal, is difficult in some cases. True whitening dentifrices produce the effect by changing tooth color.[79] The agents responsible for stain removal do so physically or chemically; however, some formulations do both—whiten by changing tooth color and chemically or physically remove stains using abrasives. Whitening dentifrices usually contain hydrogen peroxide, whereas abrasive dentifrices usually contain calcium carbonate, calcium phosphate dehydrate, alumina, aluminum silicate, sodium bicarbonate, and sodium metaphosphate.[36]

Dental hygienists have several issues to consider when recommending a dentifrice for a patient. Those considerations include whether the patient needs a dentifrice that will provide fluoride for dental caries prevention, antimicrobial medications for the prevention and control of gingival inflammation,

sensitivity ingredients to control dentinal hypersensitivity, or odor-controlling ingredients to manage oral malodor. Another important issue that must be considered is the type of restorative materials in the patient's mouth, especially the esthetic restorative materials that can be damaged by physical abrasives contained in dentifrices. The selection of an appropriate dentifrice to protect esthetic restorations is as important as selecting an appropriate polishing paste for esthetic restorative materials to prevent damaging surface integrity. Although not inclusive of all brands, Figure 26-3 provides a toothpaste abrasive index. Dentifrice abrasiveness is determined by the **relative dentin abrasivity** (RDA) **index.** The higher the score, the more abrasive the dentifrice.

> *Note*
>
> Dental hygienists have several issues to consider when recommending a dentifrice to patients. Those considerations include whether the patient needs a dentifrice that will provide fluoride for dental caries prevention, antimicrobials for the prevention and control of gingival inflammation, sensitivity ingredients to control dentinal hypersensitivity, or odor-controlling ingredients for managing oral malodor.

> *Patient Education Opportunity*
>
> A record of each patient and the type of dentifrice he or she needs, based on the patient assessment, interview, and treatment plan, should be maintained for 1 month. Findings should be discussed as a class.

WHITENING

Tooth discoloration is a patient concern that is addressed by various methods, both in-office treatments and at-home bleaching techniques. Intrinsic stains, such as fluorosis or tetracycline staining, can be treated using in-office vital bleaching techniques, with bleach containing hydrogen peroxide or carbamide peroxide. The patient can also use bleaching trays for a few hours daily at home.[37] Newer products, such as whitening strips, allow the patient convenient, comfortable options to whiten teeth. Scaling and polishing can remove extrinsic stains in the office, but controlling the staining at home has always been difficult for patients. Many dentifrices use "whitening" in labeling, but until recently, no consistent guidelines existed for claims of whitening dentifrices. The ADA's CSA criteria for whitening dentifrices call for the demonstration of change in tooth color of two or more shades on a value-ordered shade guide over 6 months. The ADA Seal of Acceptance has been awarded to few OTC tooth-whitening dentifrices. The first accepted product has a mild abrasive that removes extrinsic stains by a gentle polishing action and contains a tartar-control ingredient.[6]

Ingredients for Dentifrices

All dentifrices contain **basic ingredients** (see Table 26-1), which allow the dentifrice to include the **active (therapeutic) agents** and make the dentifrice palatable. In addition to basic ingredients, numerous active or therapeutic ingredients are included in dentifrices, which target the prevention of oral disease

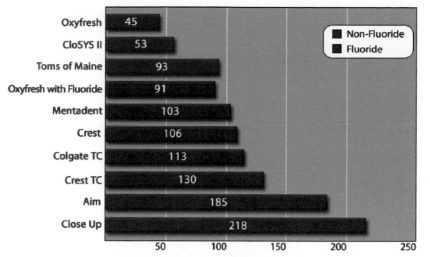

FIGURE 26-3
Comparison of toothpaste abrasiveness based on relative dentin abrasitivity (RDA).

or a specific condition such as stain removal or remineralization, sensitivity, or inflammation.

ACTIVE INGREDIENTS IN DENTIFRICES

Hydrogen Peroxide

Hydrogen peroxide is added to dentifrices for several purposes; it has some antigingivitis properties, it can serve as a chemical whitening agent, and it is used to assist in the control of oral malodor.

The safety of long-term use of hydrogen peroxide has been debated, especially regarding its effects on healing and potential co-carcinogenicity.[91] (It must be noted that hydrogen peroxide was identified as a potential co-carcinogen only at concentration levels of 30%.) It is generally accepted that the use of hydrogen peroxide in oral care products presents no long-term safety concerns, especially since most dentifrices contain a low level (<1%) of hydrogen peroxide.[58] Hydrogen peroxide is commonly found in dentifrices that contain other active ingredients, such as sodium bicarbonate and fluoride.

Sanguinarine

Sanguinarine, an alkaloid plant extract, is currently used in both dentifrice and mouthwash formulations. In many of the research studies of sanguinarine dentifrices, the dentifrice contains other active ingredients, such as zinc, or is combined with the use of sanguinarine-containing mouthrinses. Although conflicting reports of efficacy exist, some 6-month studies using the dentifrice and mouthwash in combination demonstrate a reduction in plaque biofilm and gingivitis. The formulations that contain zinc showed improved results.[46] Other agents evaluated in short-term studies include enzyme systems such as amyloglucosidase-glucose oxidase,[62] lactoperoxidase,[44] triclosan combined with silicon oil,[74] and cetylpyridinium chloride in a foam formulation.[2] An analysis of the use of sanguinarine in mouthwashes and toothpaste compared with other antimicrobial agents concluded that sanguinarine has some potential for decreasing supragingival plaque biofilm; it appears to be more

effective in a mouthrinse rather than in a dentifrice.[32] The more serious issue with sanguinarine is its association with oral leukoplakia. A case-controlled study found a significant association between the use of sanguinarine products and the development of oral leukoplakia.[3] A larger 58-participant, matched-case control study supported the findings that the use of sanguinarine products was a risk factor for oral leukoplakia.[59]

Sodium Bicarbonate

Sodium bicarbonate, or baking soda, has been used in dentifrices in the United States since the 1830s. Initially, sodium bicarbonate was mixed with water to form a paste. Even with no added active ingredients, sodium bicarbonate dentifrices have several benefits.[7] Because sodium bicarbonate is a buffering agent, it neutralizes bacterial acids that initiate demineralization and dental caries. Although sodium bicarbonate has a very low abrasivity, it effectively removes extrinsic stains and notably inhibits volatile sulfuric compounds to reduce oral malodors. Additionally, clinical and laboratory studies have established that sodium bicarbonate is effective in reducing cariogenic bacteria.[24,49,84-86] Modern-day sodium bicarbonate dentifrices are formulated into pastes and gels with other active ingredients such as hydrogen peroxide to promote whitening and fluorides to prevent dental caries and enhance remineralization. Sodium bicarbonate is a mild abrasive and may produce a mild antibacterial effect. As a dentifrice, bicarbonate is incorporated into both toothpastes and gels, sometimes in combination with hydrogen peroxide. Patient acceptance of baking soda products may be related to an increasing interest in natural products or in taste and texture.

Sodium Hexametaphosphate, Tetrapotassium Pyrophosphate, Gantrez, Zinc Chloride, and Zinc Citrate

Several active ingredients added to dentifrice formulations have anticalculus capabilities. The most effective ingredient appears to be sodium hexametaphosphate, which may inhibit calcification in the conversion of amorphous calcium phosphate to hydroxyapatite. The next most effective ingredient, pyrophosphate (3.3% to 5%), comes combined with sodium hexametaphosphate or tetrapotassium pyrophosphate.[79] In addition, 1% to 2% Gantrez, a copolymer of methoxyethylene and maleic acid, provides some very modest anticalculus properties. Zinc chloride (2%) and zinc citrate (0.5% to 2.0%) are used alone or in combination with other anticalculus chemicals to prevent or break down calculus formation.[77,96]

In addition, both pyrophosphates and zinc salts contribute some minor abrasiveness. The use of anticalculus dentifrices may be indicated in patients with supragingival calculus, which may result in a reduced need for calculus removal during dental treatment.[93]

Stannous Fluoride, Sodium Fluoride, and Sodium Monofluorophosphate

The most common forms of fluoride that are added to dentifrice formulations include stannous fluoride, sodium fluoride, and sodium monofluorophosphate.

Stannous fluoride was the first chemotherapeutic agent added to a dentifrice formulation, but the usefulness of stannous fluoride was limited because of difficulties in formulation and short shelf life. Stannous fluoride dentifrices have had the potential for staining and taste side effects. However, current formulations contain flavorings that mask the bitter taste, and now stains can be readily removed. Stannous fluoride has not only anticaries effects but also antiplaque and antigingivitis effects, probably because of the effects of the tin ion.[14] A more stable form of stannous fluoride dentifrice with bioavailability comparable with nonaqueous gel and mouthrinse formulations has shown significant reductions in gingivitis scores and gingival bleeding but no decrease in plaque biofilm scores.[9] One stannous fluoride dentifrice consisting of a stabilized 0.0454% stannous fluoride/sodium hexametaphosphate formulation has been approved by the ADA for anticaries, antigingivitis, antiplaque, sensitivity, and stain reduction.

The most widely used dentifrices contain sodium fluoride (24%) or sodium monofluorophosphate (76%). The efficacy of these two fluorides is not clinically or statistically significant; however, evidence suggests that dentifrices containing sodium fluoride are retained longer in the oral cavity than those containing sodium monofluorophosphate.[25,81]

Triclosan

The most important dentifrice additive since the addition of fluoride is triclosan, which has proven to provide numerous benefits previously not found in dentifrices. Triclosan is a broad-spectrum antimicrobial agent that has antiplaque and antiinflammatory properties. Several therapeutic ingredients are considered to be antiplaque, antigingivitis, and antiinflammatory with the most effective additive being triclosan. With approximately 77% of the population having some form of periodontal disease, having an effective dentifrice that is readily available and provides antimicrobial and antiinflammatory properties is important.

Triclosan is a bisphenol and has no associated major side effects. First used in soaps and antiperspirants, it is considered safe for use in oral healthcare products.[22] In dentifrice formulations, triclosan has been combined with several other active ingredients, including sodium fluoride for dental caries control, a poly-vinylmethylether–maleic acid (PVM-MA) copolymer to increase substantivity, and pyrophosphates to add anticalculus properties.[57] The addition of the PVM-MA copolymer acts as a retention aid for triclosan in the mouth, increasing the potential duration of the antimicrobial effects of the triclosan on plaque bacteria. The PVM-MA copolymer also has been shown to have some anticalculus properties,[30] but it is not as effective as formulations containing zinc citrate or pyrophosphates.[27] The results of multiple long-term studies typically show significant reductions in plaque biofilm, gingivitis, and calculus in participants using triclosan and PVM-MA copolymer dentifrice compared with control participants.* Some published articles do not support triclosan as more effective than other therapeutic agents.[10,27] A dentifrice formulation containing triclosan, PVM-MA copolymer, and sodium fluoride has been ADA-approved as a decay-preventive dentifrice that also helps prevent and reduce gingivitis, plaque biofilm, and calculus.[4]

Xylitol

Xylitol is a naturally occurring sugar substitute that has anticariogenic properties. Pure xylitol is a white crystalline substance that looks and tastes just as sweet as sucrose and is found in nature in fruits, berries, mushrooms, and birch bark. Importantly, xylitol has several pathways by which it prevents dental caries. From a chemical standpoint, xylitol is not a sugar; rather, it is a sugar alcohol. Other sweeteners such as fructose and glucose contain six carbon atoms; xylitol has only five. This difference is important because most bacteria, especially the cariogenic *Streptococcus mutans,* are unable to metabolize xylitol, thus preventing the acid that is normally produced when oral bacteria metabolize sugars and fermentable carbohydrates, thus producing the acids that dissolve calcium and phosphate salts from the enamel surface. Xylitol has antiplaque properties and has also been demonstrated to reduce levels of *Streptococcus mutan* in saliva and plaque biofilm,[42] loosen plaque biofilm binding to tooth surfaces, and reduce amounts of plaque biofilm.[51,90] Some evidence suggest that xylitol may have the potential to play a role in remineralization; however, most of this evidence is associated with xylitol-containing chewing gums.

---

*11, 15, 19, 20, 27, 31, 43, 50, 53, 54, 67, 68, 72, 82.

CASE APPLICATION 26-1.5

Dentifrice Recommendations

All four members of the Courtland family have different needs that may not be met by one dentifrice product. Familiarity with the family enables the dental professional to decide how receptive each of them will be to compliance issues. In addition, estimating their ideal frequency of supportive care intervals will be based on each of their patterns of disease history and their ability to stay motivated to practice optimal oral self-care.

Mrs. Courtland appears to maintain her oral health effectively between supportive care appointments except for localized areas of gingivitis. If she is performing optimal oral self-care but is still having problems managing specific areas, she might benefit from an antigingivitis toothpaste. Options would include a product that uses triclosan or stabilized stannous fluoride as the active ingredient.

Mr. Courtland has a history of periodontal disease and sensitive root surfaces. Because root caries is also a concern, a desensitizing dentifrice that contains fluoride would address both the root caries and the sensitivity issues.

Amber and Brandon may present the most challenging problems. Amber's needs are multifactorial. Counseling services will involve maximum efforts at improving oral self-care motivation, as well as dietary intervention to reduce the effects of fermentable carbohydrates. The dental professional should also be alert to the possibility of an eating disorder such as bulimia, which is common in this age group and can lead to decalcification of enamel surfaces. Before orthodontics can be reconsidered, Amber should receive in-office fluoride treatments and daily fluoride-concentrated applications at home in the form of a high-potency fluoride dentifrice. The dentist must prescribe this and probably needs to perform some restorative work in the meantime. Although some of Amber's problems are still reversible or at least reparable, she and Brandon both have future preventive needs. Both will benefit from oral hygiene counseling services. Brandon needs to establish the lifelong habit of regular daily plaque biofilm removal using a simple, pleasant-tasting, agreeably textured fluoride dentifrice. Amber's high-fluoride dentifrice is not appropriate for Brandon. Eventually, when Amber has improved her compliance with oral self-care and diet and her dental caries problem is controlled, she might benefit from a whitening dentifrice that contains fluoride, which would meet all her other needs and, at the same time, appeal to her need for increased self-esteem.

References

1. Addy M, Koltai R: Control of supragingival calculus—scaling and polishing and anti-calculus toothpastes: an opinion, *J Clin Periodontol* 21:342-346, 1994.
2. Addy M, Moran J: The effect of a cetylpyridinium chloride (CPC) detergent foam compared to conventional toothpaste on plaque and gingivitis, *J Clin Periodontol* 16:87-91, 1989.
3. Allen CM, Loudon J, Mascarenhas AK: Sanguinaria-related leukoplakia: epidemiologic and clinicopathologic features of a recently described entity, *Gen Dent* 49(6):608-614, 2001.
4. American Dental Association: First whitening dentifrice gets Seal, *ADA News* 30(20):14, 1999.
5. American Dental Association: FDA okays gingivitis-fighting toothpaste for US market, *ADA News* 28(15):3, 1997.
6. American Dental Association: Hypersensitivity reports requested, *ADA News* 27(16):1, 1996.
7. Barnes CM: An evidence-based review of sodium bicarbonate as a dentifrice agent, *Compend Cont Educ Oral Hyg* 6(3):3-10, 1999.
8. Battino M et al: In vitro antioxidant activities of antioxidant-enriched toothpastes, *Free Radic Res* 39(3):343-350, 2005.
9. Beiswanger BB et al: The clinical effect of dentifrices containing stabilized stannous fluoride on plaque formation and gingivitis: a six-month study with ad libitum brushing, *J Clin Dent* 6(special issue):46-53, 1995.
10. Binney A et al: A 3-month home use study comparing the oral hygiene and gingival health benefits of triclosan and conventional fluoride toothpastes, *J Clin Periodontol* 23(11):1020-1024, 1996.
11. Bolden TE et al: The clinical effect of a dentifrice containing triclosan and a copolymer in a sodium fluoride/silica base on plaque formation and gingivitis: a six-month clinical study, *J Clin Dent* 3:125-131, 1992.
12. Brown LJ, Oliver RC, Loe H: Periodontal diseases in the US in 1981: prevalence, severity, extent, and role in tooth mortality, *J Periodontol* 60(7):363-370, 1989.
13. Charig A, Winston A, Flickinger M: Enamel mineralization by calcium containing bicarbonate toothpastes: assessment by various techniques, *Compend Contin Educ Dent* 25(9 suppl 1):14-24, 2004.
14. Ciancio SG: Agents for the management of plaque and gingivitis, *J Dent Res* 71(7):1450-1454, 1992.
15. Cubells AB, Dalmau LB, Petrone ME: The effect of a triclosan/copolymer/fluoride dentifrice on plaque formation and gingivitis: a six-month clinical study, *J Clin Dent* 2:63-69, 1991.
16. Cummins D: Vehicles: how to deliver the goods, *Periodontol 2000* 15:84-85, 1997.
17. Cummins D, Creeth JE: Delivery of anti-plaque agents from dentifrices, gels, and mouthwashes, *J Dent Res* 71(7):1439-1449, 1992.
18. Dave S, Batista EL, van Dyke TE: Cardiovascular disease and periodontal diseases: commonality and causation, *Compend Cont Educ Dent* Jul 25(7 suppl 1):26-37, 2004.
19. Deasy MJ et al: Effect of a dentifrice containing triclosan and a copolymer on plaque formation and gingivitis, *Clin Prev Dent* 13(6):12-19, 1991.
20. Denepitiya JL et al: Effect upon plaque formation and gingivitis of a triclosan/copolymer/fluoride dentifrice: a 6-month clinical study, *Am J Dent* 5:307-311, 1992.
21. DePaola PF: The benefits of high-potency fluoride dentifrices, *Compend Cont Educ Dent* 18(2):44-50, 1997.
22. DeSalva SJ, Kong BM, Lin YJ: Triclosan: a safety profile, *Am J Dent* 2:185-196, 1989.
23. Douglas TE: Fluoride dentifrice and stomatitis, *Northwest Med* 56:1037-1039, 1957.
24. Drake D: Antibacterial activity of baking soda, *Compend Cont Educ Dent* 18(suppl 21):S17-S21, 1996.
25. Duckworth RM, Morgan SN: Oral fluoride retention after use of fluoride dentifrices, *Caries Res* 25:123-129, 1991.
26. Ebersole JL et al: Periodontitis in humans and non-human primates: oral systemic linkage inducing acute phase proteins, *Ann Periodontol* 7(1):102-111, 2002.
27. Fairbrother KJ et al: The comparative clinical efficacy of pyrophosphate/triclosan, copolymer/triclosan, and zinc citrate/triclo-

san dentifrices for the reduction of supragingival calculus formation, *J Clin Dent* 8:62-66, 1997.

28. Fleiss JL: General design issues in efficacy, equivalency, and superiority trials, *J Periodontal Res* 27(special issue):306-613, 1992.

29. Fleiss JL et al: A study of inter- and intra-examiner reliability of pocket depth and attachment level, *J Periodontal Res* 26:122-128, 1991.

30. Gaffar A, Esposito A, Afflitto J: In vitro and in vivo anti-calculus effects of a triclosan/copolymer system, *Am J Dent* 3:S37, 1990.

31. Garcia-Godoy F et al: Effect of a triclosan/copolymer/fluoride dentifrice on plaque formation and gingivitis: a 7-month clinical study, *Am J Dent* 3:S15-S26, 1990.

32. Grenby TH: The use of sanguinarine in mouthwashes and toothpaste compared with some other antimicrobial agents, *Br Dent J* 178(7):254-258, 1995.

33. Hancock B: Prevention, *Ann Periodontol* 1:223-255, 1996.

34. Hargreaves JA, Thompson GW, Wagg BJ: Changes in caries prevalence of isle of Lewis children between 1971 and 1981, *Caries Res* 17:554-559, 1983.

35. Harris NO, Christen AG: *Primary preventive dentistry*, ed 4, Stamford, Conn, 1995, Appleton & Lange.

36. Hattab FN: The state of fluorides in toothpastes, *J Dent* 17(2):47-54, 1989.

37. Haywood VB et al: Effectiveness, side effects and long-term status of Nightguard vital bleaching, *J Am Dent Assoc* 125:1219-1226, 1994.

38. Herlofson BB, Barkvoll P: The effect of two toothpaste detergents on the frequency of recurrent aphthous ulcers, *Acta Odontol Scand* 54:150-153, 1996.

39. Herlofson BB, Brodin P, Aars H: Increased human gingival blood flow induced by sodium lauryl sulfate, *J Clin Periodontol* 23:1004-1007, 1996.

40. Hujoel PP: Logical and analytical issues in dental/oral product comparison research, *J Periodontal Res* 27(special issue):362-363, 1992.

41. Hyman FN, Welch ME, Cheever JR: Regulatory issues for evaluation of therapies to prevent or arrest disease progression, *Ann Periodontol* 2:166-175, 1997.

42. Jannesson L et al: Effect of a triclosan-containing toothpaste supplemented with 10% xylitol on mutans streptococci in saliva and dental plaque, a six month study, *Caries Res* 36(1):36-39, 2002.

43. Kanchanakamol J et al: Reduction of plaque formation and gingivitis by a dentifrice containing triclosan and copolymer, *J Periodontol* 66:109-112, 1995.

44. Kirstila B, Lenander-Lumikari M, Tenovuo J: Effects of a lactoperoxidase-system-containing toothpaste on dental plaque and whole saliva in vivo, *Acta Odontol Scand* 52:346-353, 1994.

45. Klokkevold PR: Oral malodor: a periodontal perspective, *J Calif Dent Assoc* 25(2):153-159, 1997.

46. Kopczyk R, Abrams H, Brown AT: Clinical and microbiological effects of a sanguinaria-containing mouthrinse and dentifrice with and without fluoride during 6 months of use, *J Periodontol* 62:617-622, 1991.

47. Kostelc JG et al: Oral odors in early experimental gingivitis, *J Periodontol Res* 19(3):303-312, 1984.

48. Kowitz G et al: The effects of tartar-control toothpaste on the oral soft tissues, *Oral Surg Oral Med Oral Pathol* 70(4):529-536, 1990.

49. Legier-Vargas K et al: Effects of sodium bicarbonate dentifrices on the levels of cariogenic bacteria in human saliva, *Caries Res* 29:143-147, 1995.

50. Lindhe J, Rosling B, Socransky SS: The effect of a triclosan-containing dentifrice on established plaque and gingivitis, *J Clin Periodontol* 20:327-334, 1993.

51. Lynch H, Milgrom P: Xylitol and dental caries: an overview for clinicians, *J Calif Dent Assoc* 31(3):205-209, 2003.

52. Lynch RJ, ten Cate JM: The anti-caries efficacy of calcium carbonate-based fluoride toothpastes, *Int Dent J* 55(3 suppl 1): 175-178, 2005.

53. Mandel ID: *Chemical agents for control of plaque and gingivitis*, Committee on Research, Science, and Therapy, Chicago, 1994, American Academy of Periodontology.

54. Mankodi SM, Walker C, Conforti N: Clinical effect of a triclosan-containing dentifrice on plaque and gingivitis: a six-month study, *Clin Prev Dent* 14(6):4-10, 1992.

55. Marinho VC et al: One topical fluoride (toothpastes, or mouthrinses, or gels or varnishes) versus another for preventing dental caries in children and adolescents, *Cochrane Database Syst Rev* (1): CD002780, 2004.

56. Markowitz K: Tooth sensitivity: mechanisms and management, *Compend Cont Educ Dent* 14(8):1032-1045, 1997.

57. Marsh PD: Dentifrices containing new agents for the control of plaque and gingivitis: microbiological aspects, *J Clin Periodontol* 18:462-467, 1991.

58. Marshall MV, Cancro LPO, Fischman SF: Hydrogen peroxide: a review of its use in dentistry, *J Periodontol* 66:786-796, 1995.

59. Mascarenhas AK, Allen CM, Moeschberger ML: The association between Viadent use and oral leukoplakia: results of a matched case-control study, *J Public Health Dent* 62(3):158-162, 2002.

60. Mellburg JR: Fluoride dentifrices: current status and prospects, *Int Dent J* 41:9-16, 1991.

61. Mellburg JR: The mechanism of fluoride protection, *Compend Cont Educ Dent* 18(2):37-43, 1997.

62. Moran J, Addy M, Newcombe R: Comparison of the effect of toothpastes containing enzymes or antimicrobial compounds with a conventional fluoride toothpaste on the development of plaque and gingivitis, *J Clin Periodontol* 16:295-299, 1989.

63. Munoz FJ, Bellido J, Moyano JC: Perioral contact urticaria from sodium benzoate in a toothpaste, *Contact Dermatitis* 35:51, 1996.

64. Newman MG: Design and implementation of clinical trials of antimicrobial drugs and devices used in periodontal disease treatment, *Ann Periodontol* 2:180-198, 1997.

65. O'Mullane DM: Introduction and rationale for the use of fluoride for caries prevention, *Int Dent J* 44:257-261, 1994.

66. Osuju OO et al: Risk factors for dental fluorosis in a fluoridated community, *J Dent Res* 67:1488-1492, 1988.

67. Palomo F, Wantland L, Sanchez A: The effect of three commercially available dentifrices containing triclosan on supragingival plaque formation and gingivitis: a six-month clinical study, *Int Dent J* 44:75-81, 1994.

68. Peter S et al: Anti-plaque and anti-gingivitis efficacy of toothpastes containing triclosan and fluoride, *Int Dent J* 54(5 suppl 1): 299-303, 2004.

69. Pickles MJ et al: In vitro efficacy of whitening toothpaste containing calcium carbonate and perlite, *Int Dent J* 55(3 suppl 1): 197-202, 2005.

70. Polson AM: The research team, calibration, and quality assurance in clinical trials in periodontics, *Ann Periodontol* 2:75-82, 1997.

71. Products of excellence: ADA Seal Program, *J Am Dent Assoc* (suppl):1-2, 1997.

72. Renvert S, Birkhed D: Comparison between 3 triclosan dentifrices on plaque, gingivitis, and salivary microflora, *J Clin Periodontol* 22:63-70, 1995.

73. Ripa LW, Leske GS, Triol CW: Clinical study of the anticaries efficacy of three fluoride dentifrices containing anti-calculus ingredients: three-year (final) results, *J Clin Dent* 2:29-33, 1990.

74. Rolla G, Gaare D, Ellingsen JE: Experiments with a toothpaste containing polydimethylsiloxane/triclosan, *Scand J Dent Res* 101:130-132, 1993.

75. Sainio E, Kanerva L: Contact allergens in toothpastes and a review of their hypersensitivity, *Contact Dermatitis* 33:100-105, 1995.

76. Sanders MA: Fluoride toothpastes: a cause of acne-like eruptions, *Arch Dermatol* 111:793, 1975.

77. Santos SL et al: Anti-calculus effects of two zinc citrate/essential oil-containing dentifrices, *Am J Dent* 13(spec no):11C-13C, 2000.

78. Schemehorn BR et al: Remineralization by fluoride enhanced with calcium and phosphate ingredients, *J Clin Dent* 10(1 spec no):13-16, 1999.

79. Sharif N et al: The chemical stain removal properties of whitening toothpaste products: studies in vitro, *Br Dent J* 189(4):182-182, 2000.

80. Shea JJ, Gillispie SM, Waldbott GL: Allergy to fluoride, *Ann Allergy* 25:388-391, 1967.

81. Shellis RP, Duckworth RM: Studies on the cariostatic mechanisms of fluoride, *Int Dent J* 44(3 suppl 1):263-273, 1994.

82. Svatun B, Sadxton CA, Huntington E: The effects of three silica dentifrices containing triclosan on supragingival plaque and calculus formation and on gingivitis, *Int Dent J* 43:441-452, 1993.

83. Szpunar SM, Burt BA: Trends in the prevalence of dental fluorosis in the United States: a review, *J Public Health Dent* 47:71-79, 1987.

84. Tanzer J, Grant L, Ciardi J: Bicarbonate-based dental powder fluoride and saccharin effects on dental caries and on *Streptococcus sobrinus* recoveries in rats, *J Dent Res* 66:791-794, 1987.

85. Tanzer J, Grant L, McMahon T: Bicarbonate-based dental power, fluoride and saccharin inhibition of dental caries associated with *S. mutans* infection of rats, *J Dent Res* 67:969-972, 1988.

86. Tanzer, McMahan T, Grant L: Bicarbonate-based powder and paste dentifrice effects on caries, *Clin Prev Dent* 12:18-21, 1990.

87. Trummel CL: Regulation of oral chemotherapeutic in the United States, *J Dent Res* 73(3):704-708, 1994.

88. Tung MS, Eichmiller FC: Amorphous calcium phosphates for tooth mineralization, *Compend Cont Educ Dent* 25(9 suppl 1):9-13, 2004.

89. Utilivoskiy B, Sergey B: *Toothpastes,* Monography, SPb, p 272, 2001 *(Russian publication)*.

90. van Loveren C: Sugar alcohols: what is the evidence for caries-preventive and caries-therapeutic effects? *Caries Res* 38:286-293, 2004.

91. Weitzman SA et al: Chronic treatment with hydrogen peroxide: is it safe? *J Periodontol* 55(9):510-511, 1984.

92. White DJ: A "return" to stannous fluoride dentifrices, *J Clin Dent* 6(special issue):29-36, 1995.

93. White DJ et al: Quanticalc assessment of the clinical scaling benefits provided by pyrophosphate dentifrices with and without triclosan, *J Clin Dent* 7:46-49, 1996.

94. Wilkins EM: *Clinical practice of the dental hygienist,* ed 9, Philadelphia, 1989, Lippincott, Williams & Wilkins.

95. Yaegaki K, Sanada K: Biochemical and clinical factors influencing oral malodor in periodontal patients, *J Periodontol* 63(9):783-789, 1992.

96. Yiu CK, Wei SH: Clinical efficacy of dentifrices in the control of calculus, plaque, and gingivitis, *Quint Int* 24:181-188, 1993.

Chemotherapeutics

Maria Perno Goldie • Rebecca S. Wilder •

Sebastian G. Ciancio

INSIGHT

The dental hygienist is vital to assessing, diagnosing, and treating periodontal diseases. Many treatment options are available for controlling supragingival and subgingival plaque biofilm. The dental hygienist must stay current regarding evidence-based treatments for gingivitis and periodontitis so that appropriate decisions can be made for individual patients.

CASE STUDY 27-1 Selecting a Chemotherapeutic Agent Based on Patient Need

Ms. Chlöe Tevus, who is 39 years of age and an apparently healthy white woman, was diagnosed with localized chronic periodontitis. She denies any medical problems, takes no medication, and does not smoke. As an adolescent, she had active orthodontics and retains 24 teeth. The first premolars and the third molars were sound and were previously extracted for orthodontic reasons. She has occlusal amalgams on her molars, occlusal wear, and interproximal restorations between some of the posterior teeth.

Ms. Tevus's private law practice specializes in contract law. She is the sole caregiver for her elderly parent.

Ms. Tevus completed periodontal therapy 18 months ago and has alternately visited the hygienists at her periodontist and general dentist's offices every 3 months. She demonstrates capable technique with the toothbrush and the interdental brush. Her bleeding-on-probing percentage has varied between 23% and 32% at the 3-month intervals, generalized to interproximal sites. She has also developed a probe depth of 7 mm on the palatal of tooth #10. O'Leary's Plaque Control Record has resulted in average scores of 15% to 20%, particularly on the facial and palatal of the maxillary molars.

KEY TERMS

adjunctive therapy
antigingivitis
antimicrobial
antiplaque
bacteriocidal
bacteriostatic
biofilm
cationic

chemotherapeutic
controlled delivery
delivery system
essential oils
host modulation
host response
irrigation

locally administered antibiotics
    or antimicrobials
local delivery
minimum inhibitory
    concentration
plaque biofilm
plaque biofilm–inhibitory effect

rinsing
site-specific
substantivity
sustained-release
systemic antibiotics
triclosan

LEARNING OUTCOMES

After reading this chapter the student will be able to:

1. Discuss the rationale for chemotherapeutic treatments for reducing and controlling plaque biofilm, gingivitis, and other periodontal disease and maintaining periodontal health.
2. Differentiate among chemotherapeutic agents and delivery systems to select the optimal intervention and sequence for patient care.
3. Discuss the evidence base for selecting the various chemotherapeutic agents.

4. Discuss the available chemotherapies and the advantages and disadvantages of each.
5. Discuss the American Dental Association and the U.S. Food and Drug Administration guidelines for accepting chemotherapeutic agents for the control of plaque biofilm, gingivitis, and periodontitis.
6. Discuss the need for and methods of staying informed regarding developments and changes in the standards for using chemotherapeutic agents as adjuncts to nonsurgical periodontal therapy.

The dental hygiene process of care has five components: (1) assessment, (2) diagnosis, (3) treatment planning, (4) implementation of the treatment plan, and (5) evaluation. Although this section primarily supports the treatment phase, the other components are equally important. In defining treatment of periodontitis, mechanical therapy has been the foundation of periodontal care. Also important is daily personal plaque biofilm control and periodic professional supportive periodontal care with a dental hygienist, dentist, or periodontist. Careful, daily disruption of plaque biofilm, especially interproximally and at the gingival margins, is an essential oral health habit for health maintenance; however, this task is tedious and uninteresting for the average individual. As a result, most people do not deplaque their mouths as thoroughly as needed to maintain health. In fact, dental hygienists are probably one of the few groups excited about plaque biofilm control! However, even with good daily personal plaque biofilm control, and regular professional debridement, some periodontally involved patients are unable to attain and maintain periodontal stability.

When mechanical disruption of plaque biofilm is insufficient to control gingival inflammation, using chemotherapeutics should be considered. Chemotherapeutics and pharmacotherapeutics are broad terms encompassing agents that may affect microorganisms and hard and soft tissues in the oral cavity. **Chemotherapeutic** agents are used to eliminate, reduce, or alter the effect of microorganisms in the oral cavity, preferably the pathogenic microorganisms, or to effect a change in the host response. The term **antimicrobial** refers to agents that kill microbes or affect the growth and multiplication of microorganisms.[3]

Chemotherapeutic agents have been demonstrated to reduce gingivitis, plaque biofilm, and gingival bleeding when used daily. Evidence is still insufficient to state the magnitude of the effect that chemotherapeutics have in the deeper periodontal tissues, such as bone height and attachment level. Differences in periodontal pockets after the use of **irrigation** or chemotherapeutics have been reported, typically by attachment gain and change in the pocket microflora.[3,65,97] Currently, using pharmacotherapeutics is still considered **adjunctive therapy,** not monotherapy, or a substitute for professional debridement and daily personal plaque biofilm control. However, as these treatment modalities are studied, their use becomes a welcome and effective supplement to mechanical therapy.

A new arena for the use of chemotherapeutics in oral health care is to influence the host response to periodontal infections rather than to affect the microbial status. This task is accomplished by using a subantimicrobial concentration of certain chemotherapeutic agents (e.g., tetracycline derivatives). This concept is discussed more fully in the section on **systemic antibiotics** delivery.

When oral health clinicians speak of the benefits of chemotherapeutics, they are most often referring to the effect on the periodontal status of the mouth. Nonetheless, chemotherapeutics are useful for more than preventing and controlling periodontal diseases. For example, fluoride, chlorhexidine, essential oils, and other substances are used in controlling dental caries and their cariogenic microbes, as well as oral malodor. However, this chapter focuses on the use of chemotherapeutics in periodontal diseases—the delivery systems and the agents.

Plaque Biofilm, Host Response, and Need for Chemotherapeutics

Plaque biofilm and **host response** content are discussed in detail in Chapters 6 and 31. To understand the effectiveness of the various chemotherapeutic agents on the market, reviewing the nature of plaque biofilm, how the host response of the patient affects the disease process, and how available chemotherapeutic agents work will be helpful. Once the dental hygienist understands the science behind the use of chemotherapeutics, he or she is then able to recommend appropriate, *evidence-based products* for patients. (Read Chapter 4 to learn more about evidence-based practice.)

A **biofilm** is a complex community of bacteria adhering to an inert or living surface[26] (Figure 27-1). Biofilms are the predominant mode of bacterial growth in nature. Many microbial species not only exist as attached bacteria in the biofilms, but also discharge free-floating single-cell bacteria known as *planktonic cells. Plaque biofilm* is the new term for dental plaque. Plaque biofilms play an integral role in the cause and progression of dental caries and periodontal disease. The oral cavity is an ideal location for the formation of plaque biofilms because they require moist environments to provide the necessary nutrients for growth and proliferation. Plaque biofilms are difficult to eradicate. To date, scientific evidence supports physical disruption of biofilm by mechanical means (toothbrushing, flossing, hand and power instrumentation) to interrupt biofilm formation and growth. Using chemotherapeutic agents is considered adjunctive to physical disruption.

In addition to plaque biofilm, the patient's *host response* also plays a large role in the progression of the disease process (see Chapter 6). The patient's response to a microbial challenge helps determine the amount of disease the patient exhibits. The microbial challenge consists of antigens, lipopolysaccharide (LPS), and other virulence factors that stimulate the host response, resulting in the infections, gingivitis, or periodontitis.[5] If the patient is healthy and the immune defense system is competent, then the patient may be able to defend against the negative effects of the plaque biofilm's ability to produce an inflammatory response. However, if the patient has certain systemic conditions and is immunosuppressed (diabetes, respiratory illnesses, and autoimmune illness), then the host may not be able to combat the disease process.

Chemotherapeutic agents are intended to be used as adjunctive agents or in addition to evidence-based mechanical therapies such as nonsurgical periodontal therapy (scaling, root planing, and debridement) to assist in improving or maintaining a level of health. Considering that no clinician can remove all biofilm and calculus deposits from the tooth

> *Patient Education Opportunity*
>
> Explain to patients how the role of plaque biofilm and the patient's host response may determine their level of health or disease.

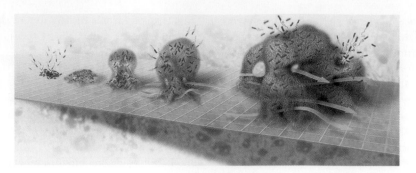

FIGURE 27-1
Different stages in a biofilm life cycle. (Images courtesy Joanna Heersink and Paul Stoodley, PhD, funded by Philips Oral Healthcare. Illustration by Keith Kasnot, Scientific American 2001, courtesy Philips Oral Healthcare.)

surface, chemotherapeutic agents are valuable home care or in-office adjuncts to treatment.[4,6] They are not intended to be used as the sole mechanism to control disease at this time, except in special circumstances in which the patient is unable to have mechanical therapy.

CONTROLLING PLAQUE BIOFILM WITH CHEMOTHERAPEUTICS

As mentioned previously, mechanical therapy is the first line of defense against dental biofilm. However, chemotherapeutic agents can be helpful adjuncts. The clinician must consider the types of bacteria being targeted, the chemotherapeutic agent being used, and the **minimum inhibitory concentration** (MIC), which represents the concentration of antibiotic required to inhibit growth of a planktonic bacterial population. The MIC has been used as a gold standard for determining antimicrobial sensitivities for animal and human pathogenic bacteria.[26] New techniques are now available to determine the types of bacteria present in the biofilm and for quantifying oral bacteria during biofilm formation.[87] New techniques using deoxyribonucleic acid–polymerase chain reaction (DNA-PCR) technology allow for DNA testing of live and dead bacteria, making timing a moot issue. Once mechanical debridement is accomplished, delivery of an adjunctive chemical agent may be accomplished in a variety of ways.

The delivery of therapeutic chemical agents to the site of infection is accomplished either systemically or locally and may be used during the presurgical, surgical, or supportive phases of periodontal care. The means by which the agent is applied or made available to the oral site is termed the **delivery system** and includes the drug carrier or vehicle, the route, and the target. Systemic or enteric delivery allows agents to flow through the body until reaching the diseased or intended site. Ingestion and intramuscular injection are common means of systemic delivery.

Topical drug-delivery systems deliver chemotherapeutic agents to the surface of mucosa or gingiva—for example with rinsing—or several millimeters below the gingival margin during supragingival irrigation. Site-specific delivery is accomplished with vehicles such as chips, powders, polymers, gels, and rinses. **Site-specific** delivery includes **sustained-release** and controlled delivery of a chemotherapeutic agent to a speci-

fied area of the mouth. Sustained release refers to systems and agents that are most active (provide drug delivery) for less than 24 hours, whereas **controlled delivery** means the agent is active longer than 1 day.[7] Controlled delivery is indicated for periodontal pockets deeper than 5 mm, and treatment is usually over a period of 7 to 28 days. In addition to rinsing, irrigation, and controlled delivery, vehicles such as lozenges, chewing gum, and sprays also have been employed to deliver chemotherapeutic agents. Irrigation with chemotherapeutic agents, as well as self-care devices, is covered in Chapter 24.

Antimicrobials: General Considerations and Specific Agents

QUALITIES OF THE IDEAL ANTIMICROBIAL AGENT

An ideal antimicrobial agent should possess certain qualities. The agent should be effective against specific microbes, they should inhibit the overgrowth of other organisms, and they should not cause an increase in bacterial resistance. The antimicrobial must be nontoxic to oral tissues and acceptable to the patient—for example, in taste, ease of use, and cost. A valuable quality for an antimicrobial is **substantivity,** or the persistence of antimicrobial activity[30] and the ability of an agent to remain in an area or site and resist becoming diluted or washed away by gingival crevicular fluid or salivary action. Substantivity is accomplished by adhering to the soft tissues in the oral cavity, which allows the agent to continue its antimicrobial action over a period of hours. Substantivity is assessed by measuring the changes in duration and numbers of bacteria.[30] Chlorhexidine[1] and tetracycline[71] have excellent substantivity. The usefulness of antimicrobials must be evaluated by site, concentration, and time.[20] In other words, the agent must be in a form that is capable of being delivered to the site in an effective concentration and work for a sufficient length of time.

SELECTION

Ideally, the clinician should determine the specific type of periodontal pathogens present and then select the optimal antimicrobial. In actual practice, clinicians have not readily used testing of periodontal pathogens before initiating antimicrobial therapy. One reason is that the antimicrobial recommendations are not yet specific enough for most oral periodontal pathogens. Another reason is that specific bacteria are implicated for only a few of the various types of periodontal infections, although periodontal research efforts continue to search for putative microbes. Although the in-office tests take only minutes of the clinician's time, the cost to the patient for these tests is significant. However, the ability to identify and target oral pathogens would permit clinicians to choose an antimicrobial agent with sufficiently narrow selectivity. Antimicrobial selectivity enhances microbial effectiveness and reduces antimicrobial resistance, thus improving patient care outcomes.

PATIENT CONSIDERATIONS

Using an antimicrobial involves several patient considerations:
1. Determination of any patient sensitivity
2. Determination of the area to be treated (the entire dentition or isolated areas)
3. Informed consent, advising the patient of the following:
   - Name of the agent
   - Method of use
   - Anticipated benefits
   - Possible side effects

4. Date for follow-up evaluation of the antimicrobial therapy
5. Evaluation of the results of chemotherapeutic use

CONCENTRATION, EFFECT, AND RESISTANCE

Chemotherapeutic agents should be used in the lowest concentration that achieves maximal benefit. Concentrations that are too low may be ineffective and increase the chance of microbial resistance, whereas excessive concentrations or length of use may have untoward tissue effects and be costly. For example, **local delivery** of chemotherapeutic agents allows high concentrations to be administered with relatively few side effects yet has a seemingly effective kill rate.

Evaluation of Chemotherapeutic Agents

AMERICAN DENTAL ASSOCIATION GUIDELINES FOR SEAL OF ACCEPTANCE PROGRAM

The American Dental Association (ADA) has established guidelines for accepting chemotherapeutic products for control of gingivitis (Box 27-1), as well as guidelines for chemotherapeutic agents to slow or arrest periodontitis (Box 27- 2). According to the ADA, "For more than 125 years, the ADA has sought to promote the safety and effectiveness of dental products."[19] The

---

BOX 27-1

GUIDELINES FOR CHEMOTHERAPEUTIC PRODUCTS FOR CONTROL OF GINGIVITIS

The ADA's Council on Scientific Affairs created *Acceptance Program Guidelines for Chemotherapeutic Products for Control of Gingivitis.* These guidelines maintain:

"The following guidelines are given for the design and conduct of clinical studies for the evaluation of chemotherapeutic agents to provide evidence of effectiveness and safety in the control of gingivitis and, if applicable, supragingival plaque. The clinical benefit of plaque biofilm control can best be demonstrated by a significant reduction in gingivitis.
- For products that accomplish their antigingivitis effectiveness through plaque biofilm reduction, it will be necessary to demonstrate statistically significant reductions in both plaque biofilm and gingivitis by the products.
- For products that do not exert their antigingivitis effect through plaque biofilm reduction, it will be necessary to demonstrate a statistically significant reduction in gingivitis and supporting data for the mechanism of action.

In each study, the active product should be compared with a placebo control. In addition, a positive control may be added. Designs employing either crossover or parallel groups are acceptable. Because of a possible retained effect of some agents, care must be taken in a crossover design to include an adequate latent period between study periods. Additionally, the crossover design may not be practical in the long-term studies required for adequate evaluation of product efficacy.

When the indices used allow accurate repeated measures, it is necessary to provide a measure of intra- and inter-evaluator variance. Examiners should be capable, at a minimum, of replicating their own

scores to a high degree on a site-by-site basis. A Kappa statistic of 0.6 would indicate satisfactory calibration for gingivitis. An attempt should be made to assess the level of compliance of the subjects in the study."*

For these guidelines the following information is required:
- Two 6-month studies conducted at two different centers
- Plaque biofilm and gingivitis assessments
- Safety to oral soft tissues, teeth, and restorations demonstrated
- Microbiological assessments
- Appropriate statistical analysis

Long-term studies with antimicrobial agents should demonstrate that, although a shift or change in the species of these bacteria may occur, a shift to predominately gram-negative, anaerobic, and motile forms should not occur. Evidence shall demonstrate that microorganisms that have been associated with periodontitis do not develop supragingivally during the course of a clinical study. Opportunistic organisms such as yeasts and gram-negative enteric bacteria shall also not develop during the study.

These guidelines are for products that are effective in controlling gingivitis. If a product significantly reduces plaque biofilm but does not significantly reduce gingivitis, then it cannot be ADA accepted.

Examples of chemotherapeutic products accepted under these guidelines include several versions of Colgate Total Toothpaste (triclosan), Crest Pro-Health Toothpaste (stannous fluoride), Peridex (0.12% chlorhexidine), several versions of Listerine Antiseptic Mouthrinses (Original, Cool Mint, Fresh Burst, Natural Citrus, and Tartar Control) (essential oils), and many generic (private label) copies of Listerine.

*From the ADA web site. Available at: http://www.ada.org/prof/resources/positions/standards/guide_chemo_ging.pdf.

BOX 27-2

GUIDELINES FOR CHEMOTHERAPEUTIC AGENTS TO SLOW OR ARREST PERIODONTITIS

The ADA has also provided guidelines for studies using chemotherapeutics to slow or arrest periodontitis. They may be accessed at: http://www.ada.org/prof/resources/positions/standards/guide_chemo_perio.pdf.

The benefit of periodontal therapy is best demonstrated by stabilization of clinical parameters of periodontal health. For products that accomplish their effectiveness by antiinfective or host modulation means, demonstrating significant reductions in clinical indices of periodontitis and including supporting data for the mechanism of action are necessary. In each study, the active product should be compared with:

- A positive control (scaling and root planing)
- A placebo nonactive product plus supragingival debridement and oral hygiene control

For approval of *test agent alone* products, a negative control (e.g., supragingival debridement and oral hygiene) is compared to the test agent.

Stand-alone therapies should show at least equivalent stability of periodontal health as thorough scaling and root planing. Evaluation of periodontal stability in nontreatment arms should be ongoing. Sites that exhibit attachment level loss of 2 mm or more occurring during the trials should be exited and treated by conventional methods, if appropriate. However, the 2-mm threshold may not be appropriate for all trials and may also depend on the measurement device used. The nature of the baseline disease diagnosis and the rate of expected change should be considered. In some cases, the threshold may be more or less than 2 mm.

For these guidelines, the following information is required:

- Two 6-month or longer studies shall be conducted at two different centers.
- Studies submitted shall present a clinical picture consistent with adult periodontitis.
- Frequency of use of the product should be representative of the actual use of the product in practice.
- Primary efficacy outcomes are beneficial attachment level changes, alveolar bone changes, or both.
- Secondary outcomes may include probing depth, bleeding on probing, microbial assessment (for antiinfective agents), and biochemical and metabolic by-products.
- Safety shall be demonstrated to oral soft tissues and restorations.
- Microbiological assessments shall be made.
- Information submitted for products containing active chemotherapeutic agents shall include assessments of possible side effects of the active agent or adverse effects of the product formulation.

For microbiological assessments, evidence should be provided that the development of resistant microorganisms or emergence of periodontal pathogens does not occur with the use of the product. Evidence that microbes associated with periodontitis, opportunistic organisms such as yeasts and gram-negative enteric bacteria, do not emerge subgingivally or supragingivally during the course of the study should be demonstrated.

Chemotherapeutic products accepted under these guidelines are doxycycline (Atridox and Periostat).

In general, these ADA Guidelines follow the principles of random controlled studies that represent an important pillar of evidence-based medicine and dentistry.

---

first Seal of Acceptance was awarded in 1931. In 1984, President Ronald Reagan gave the Association a certificate of commendation for the outstanding self-regulatory efforts of its Seal program.

Although compliance is strictly voluntary, more than 300 companies participate in the Seal program. Participating manufacturers commit significant resources to test and market products to obtain the Seal (Figure 27-2). More than 1100 dental products carry the Seal of Acceptance. Of these, approximately 40% are products sold to consumers, such as toothpaste, dental floss, manual and powered toothbrushes, and mouthrinses. The rest are products prescribed or used by dentists and dental hygienists, such as topical in-office fluorides, antibiotics, or dental restorative materials.

An important new development exists regarding how the ADA has decided to evaluate professional dental products. Starting in July 2006, the ADA launched a quarterly *ADA Professional Product Review* [PPR] *Newsletter* to replace the Seal Program for professional products, which will terminate at the end of 2007. The PPR has several enhancements as compared with the Seal Program for professional products.

Whereas the Seal Program is voluntary on the part of manufacturers, with the PPR, the ADA will choose which products to evaluate. The Seal means that a product has met ADA crite-

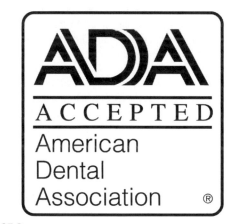

FIGURE 27-2
ADA Seal of Acceptance.

ria for safety and effectiveness, but no information is available about how products compare with others. Through focus groups and survey, ADA members have said that they want comparative product information. The PPR is designed to give the comparative information that dentists want. In each issue, many products in each of three different product categories will undergo ADA laboratory performance testing. In addition, clinical performance data will be included. Dentists can join the ADA Clinical Evaluator (ACE) Panel and receive periodic surveys to complete on their product use experience. The PPR also includes additional information such as expert panel discussions, buyer's checklists, new technology updates, and user tips to improve product performance. The PPR is provided free to ADA members as a member benefit and is available to anyone by subscription at pprclinical@ada.org.

One more important point is that the Seal Program for consumer (over-the counter [OTC]) products will continue. It is not being replaced and, in fact, will be made even better. Surveys continue to show that dentists and consumers highly value the Seal Program for consumer (OTC) products because of what the Seal means—that a product has met the ADA criteria for safety and effectiveness.

Products to be considered for acceptance are submitted to the ADA's Council on Scientific Affairs, which reviews data on product safety and effectiveness. Because a wide variety of dental products is available, the Council often calls on one or more of its approximately 200 expert dental consultants for assistance. By doing so, the Council is assured that knowledgeable individuals have examined all aspects of the submissions. The Council's *Guidelines for Participation in the ADA's Seal of Acceptance Program* provides overall guidance for companies that wish to submit products. In addition, specific product guidelines describe the clinical, biological, and laboratory studies that are necessary to evaluate safety and effectiveness for various product categories. These guidelines are subject to revision and may be updated at any time.

Once a product carries the ADA Seal of Acceptance, dental professionals and consumers can be assured that the product has met the ADA criteria for safety and effectiveness. For non–ADA-accepted products, dental professionals are encouraged to request from manufacturers the same information required for acceptance and base their recommendation on their own evaluation of the product.

> ### Patient Education Opportunity
> Talk to patients about the ADA Seal of Acceptance and what it means so that they will have a clearer understanding when purchasing dental products.

U.S. FOOD AND DRUG ADMINISTRATION REGULATIONS

The U.S. Food and Drug Administration (FDA) is in the process of developing guidelines for the dental industry entitled *Guidance for Industry—Gingivitis: Development and Evaluation of Drugs for Treatment or Prevention*. This document will assist sponsors of new drug applications (NDAs) with the development of drug products that treat or help prevent gingivitis in adults and children. This document will define gingivitis and clarify the distinction between gingivitis and periodontitis, as well as cover topics such as OTC versus prescription status and prevention versus treatment. The largest part of this guidance will focus on trial design issues and clinical assessments and will close with an examination of product safety determinations.[90]

Plaque Biofilm and Gingivitis Control with Chemotherapeutic Agents

Chemotherapeutic agents have been used over the years in an attempt to treat gingivitis and control plaque biofilm (Table 27-1). Dentifrices and mouthrinses are common agents used for this purpose. Typically, these agents are used for controlling supragingival plaque biofilm and gingivitis. They are usually not effective for periodontitis because they do not reach the bottom of the pocket unless they are delivered subgingivally (i.e., using irrigation). Even with subgingival application, the effectiveness for periodontitis varies. See Chapter 24 for more information on irrigation.

DENTIFRICES

Dentifrices are used to remove plaque biofilm and stains and may contain preventive or therapeutic agents that protect against oral malodor, dental caries, or periodontal diseases. Dentifrices are discussed in depth in Chapter 26, and oral malodor is discussed in Chapter 38. Two dentifrices with novel chemotherapeutic agents bear mention. The first chemotherapeutic is the antibacterial agent, **triclosan.** Triclosan can be considered to be a dual-action antiseptic because it has both antimicrobial and antiinflammatory properties. Although triclosan itself is not new, nor are dentifrices, the combination of the two products is a relatively new occurrence. Toothpastes with triclosan have been clinically proven to be effective against dental caries, gingivitis, plaque biofilm, and calculus. Triclosan has a wide spectrum of action against supragingival and subgingival bacteria found in biofilm, including many types of gram-positive and gram-negative nonsporulating bacteria, some fungi, *Plasmodium falciparum,* and *Toxoplasma gondii.* The combination of triclosan with a co-polymer in toothpaste allows the agent to remain on the tooth surface for a prolonged period, providing effective inhibition of biofilm formation and of gingivitis.[99] Triclosan with a co-polymer has been investigated in a dentifrice formulation and exhibited a 20% reduction in gingivitis and a 25% reduction in plaque biofilm formation.[27] In the United States, Canada, Europe, and other countries, Colgate Total toothpaste is available with triclosan and is ADA-accepted (Figure 27-3, A).

> ### Prevention
> Determine which of your patients might benefit from a therapeutic antimicrobial dentifrice with triclosan.

The most recent chemotherapeutic toothpaste on the market is a stabilized 0.454% stannous fluoride/sodium hexametaphosphate dentifrice. The toothpaste combines stannous fluoride for chemotherapeutic benefits while providing additional benefits of tartar protection and inhibition of extrinsic stain through the incorporation of hexametaphosphate. The dentifrice is stabilized in a low-water formulation to prevent hydrolysis and oxidation of the ionic stannous fluoride. One study found a 21.7% reduction in gingivitis, 57% reduction in bleeding, and 6.9% less plaque than the negative control.[59a] The

Table 27-1	Comparison of Topically Applied Antigingivitis Agents				
AGENT*	**NUMBER OF PATIENTS STUDIED**	**DECREASE IN GINGIVITIS (%)**	**DECREASE IN PLAQUE BIOFILM SCORES (%)**	**VEHICLE**	**MECHANISM OF ACTION**
Chlorhexidine[1-3]	612	18.2-43.5	21.6-60.9	Mouthrinse	Cell wall lysis, precipitation of cytoplasm
Essential oils[4-8]	866	14.0-35.9	13.8-56.3	Mouthrinse	Cell wall disruption, inhibition of enzyme production
Stannous fluoride[11-12]	450	19-22	0-6.9	Dentifrice	Alteration of cellular aggregation and metabolism
Triclosan and co-polymer[13-24]	1900	18.8-41.9	11.9-58.9	Dentifrice	Cell wall disruption, antiinflammatory
Cetylpyridinium[9-10]	230	15.4-24.0	15.8-28.2	Mouthrinse	Cell wall rupture

*A separate list of references for this table can be found under the Suggested References link for Chapter 27 on this text's Evolve site.

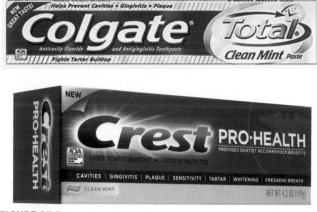

FIGURE 27-3
A, Triclosan-containing toothpaste. (Colgate Total, Colgate Palmolive, Inc.)
B, Stannous-fluoride–containing toothpaste. (Courtesy P&G Professional oral Health, Mason, Ohio.)

paste is approved by the ADA for anticaries, antigingivitis, antiplaque, and reduction of sensitivity and stain.

MOUTHRINSES

Rinsing is the action of swishing liquid forcefully around the mouth and between the teeth through the muscle action of the cheeks, lips, and tongue to dislodge particles and debris and to disperse agents. Antimicrobial agents reach mucosal and gingival surfaces effectively through a good rinsing pattern. However, rinsing is ineffective against the subgingival flora because the chemotherapeutic agent is not directed into the gingival margin. Additionally, some patients are able to rinse well, whereas other patients do not have adequate muscle action to move liquids around their mouth effectively.

Mouthrinses frequently contain alcohol as a common ingredient. Alcohol is used to dissolve the flavoring agents used to mask the taste of the active ingredient or to dissolve the active ingredient and stabilize the product. Some researchers believe that patients who have severely reduced salivary flow or xerostomia, alcohol-dependency problems, or tissues that are sensitive to alcohol should use an alcohol-free mouthrinse. In addition, comments have surfaced regarding an increase in oral cancer with the use of alcohol in excess of 20%. However, based on several studies reviewed by both the ADA and the FDA, conclusions were that the available data do not support a causal relationship between the use of alcohol-containing mouthrinses and oral cancer.[31] The same document states that "although some over the counter (OTC) mouthrinses contain alcohol, the potential for development of drug tolerance and addiction due to use of these products seems negligible."[31] Further, a recent review in the Journal of the American Dental Association and a meta analysis found no association between the use of alcohol in mouthrinses and oral cancer.[59a]

Mouthrinses can be cosmetic or therapeutic. Mouthrinses that are cosmetic *freshen breath* for a short period, but many have no long-lasting substantivity. Therapeutic mouthrinses are those that treat or prevent conditions or diseases, such as xerostomia, periodontal disease, and dental caries. Figure 27-4 shows various mouthrinses available for the consumer. The ADA and FDA have approved two mouthrinses, Listerine (essential oil) and Peridex (chlorhexidine), for controlling and treating plaque biofilm and gingivitis (Figures 27-5 and 27-6). Fluoride and other agents that fight dental caries are discussed in Chapter 25.

Mouthrinses fall into the following categories:
- Antimicrobial agents
- Plaque biofilm–reducing or plaque biofilm–inhibiting agents
- Anti–plaque biofilm agents; antigingivitis agents
- Antiperiodontitis agents

Mouthrinses are defined as follows:
- Antimicrobial agents: chemicals that have a bacteriostatic or bacteriocidal effect *in vitro* that alone cannot be ex-

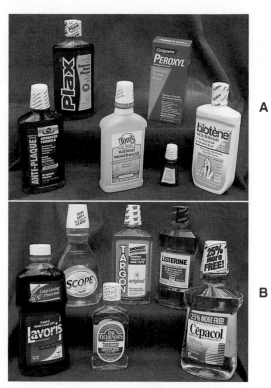

FIGURE 27-4
Mouthrinses. **A,** Two prerinses *(left)* and several non–alcohol-containing mouthrinses *(right).* **B,** Familiar brands of mouthrinses containing alcohol ranging from 8% to 27%. (Courtesy Dr. W. B. Stilley II, Brandon, Miss.)

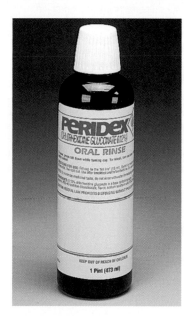

FIGURE 27-5
Peridex chlorhexidine rinse; by prescription only. (Courtesy OMNII Pharmaceuticals, West Palm Beach, Fla.)

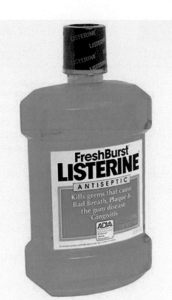

FIGURE 27-6
Listerine antiseptic mouthwash; available OTC. (Courtesy McNeil PPC, Morris Plains, N.J.)

or dental caries; also antigingivitis agents: chemicals that reduce gingival inflammation without necessarily influencing bacterial plaque biofilm (e.g., antiinflammatory agents)
- Antiperiodontitis agents: chemicals that are effective against subgingival biofilm[64]

Table 27-2 lists several common mouthrinse agents and their adverse effects, precautions, and contraindications. The following section will provide more detailed information about the specific agents.

Control of Plaque Biofilm and Gingivitis with Chemotherapeutic Agents

27-2

Killing bacteria alone is not sufficient to prove a product or agent useful. In addition to killing bacteria or modulating the immune system, the ultimate aim of a therapeutic agent is to improve tissue response and achieve a healthy state. That being stated, the plaque biofilm–inhibitory, antiplaque biofilm, and antigingivitis properties of these antimicrobial agents are considered along with their substantivity, safety, and possible clinical usefulness. The terms *plaque inhibitory, antiplaque,* and *antigingivitis* have been defined by the European Federation of Periodontology at its second workshop.[57] They define a **plaque biofilm–inhibitory effect** as one that reduces plaque biofilm to levels that are insufficient to prevent the development of gingivitis, an **antiplaque** effect as one that produces a prolonged and profound reduction in plaque biofilm sufficient to prevent the development of gingivitis, and an **antigingivitis** effect as one that has an antiinflammatory effect on the gingival health not necessarily mediated through an effect on plaque.[29] Plaque biofilm control can be accomplished using a variety of means. The next section explores other agents that may affect bacterial plaque biofilm.

trapolated to a proven efficacy *in vivo* against plaque biofilm
- Plaque biofilm–reducing or plaque biofilm–inhibiting agents: chemicals that have been shown to reduce only the quantity or effect, or both, of plaque biofilm but may or may not be sufficient to influence disease, such as gingivitis

Table 27-2   Mouthrinses: Adverse Effects, Precautions, and Contraindications

GENERIC NAME	ADVERSE EFFECTS	PRECAUTIONS AND CONTRAINDICATIONS
Chlorhexidine	Allergic reaction (skin rash, hives, swelling of face), alteration of taste, staining of teeth, staining of restorations, discoloration of tongue, increase in calculus formation, parotid duct obstruction, parotitis, desquamation of oral mucosa, irritation to lips or tongue, oral sensitivity	• Permanent staining of margins of restorations or composite restorations • Should not be used as sole treatment of gingivitis • Contraindicated in patients with sensitivity to chlorhexidine
Cosmetic Mouthrinses and Mouthrinses for Halitosis	Can have a drying effect on the oral mucosa because of alcohol content in these mouthrinses, particularly in people who have low salivary flow; however, may stimulate salivary flow because of the flowing agents in them	• Should be used cautiously in young children and in people who have low salivary flow caused by age or drugs • Contraindicated in patients with allergic reactions • Contraindicated in patients with oral ulcerations • Contraindicated in patients with oral desquamative diseases
Essential Oils	Burning sensation, bitter taste, drying out of mucous membranes	• Should not be used as sole treatment of gingivitis • Contraindicated in patients with oral ulcerations or desquamative diseases • Contraindicated in children (because of high alcohol content)
Fluorides	Ulcerations of oral mucosa, fluorosis, osteosclerosis, diarrhea, bloody vomit, nausea, black tarry stools, drowsiness, faintness, stomach cramps or pain, unusual excitement if swallowed	• Chronic systemic overdose may induce fluorosis and changes in bone • Contraindicated in patients with dental fluorosis • Contraindicated in patients who exhibit fluoride toxicity from systemic ingestion • Contraindicated in patients who have severe renal insufficiency
Oxygenating Agents	Chemical burns of oral mucosa, decalcification of teeth, black hairy tongue	• Should not be used for extended periods because of possible side effects mentioned at left • Contraindicated for treatment of periodontitis or gingivitis
Prebrushing Rinses	None reported	• Negligible effects on plaque biofilm make these agents of little use in the treatment of carious lesions or periodontal diseases, including gingivitis

From Mariotti AJ, Burrell KH: *Mouthrinses and dentifrices*. In Ciancio SG, ed: *ADA guide to dental therapeutics,* 3rd ed, Chicago, 2003, American Dental Association, p 213-231. Copyright © 2003 American Dental Association. All rights reserved. Adapted 2008 with permission.

WATER

For treating gingivitis, water has been the agent most used with irrigation. Using an intermittent (pulsed) stream of water is the least invasive procedure for supragingival and subgingival irrigation procedures. Although irrigation does not actually remove plaque biofilm, pulsed irrigation with ordinary water has been shown to alter plaque biofilm quality, rendering it less pathogenic by diluting or removing the bacterial toxins and therefore reducing bleeding and gingival inflammation.[21,23,35,65] The pulsating effect of water on bacteria in animal models has produced ruptured bacterial cell walls and production of bacterial ghosts, which are intact cell walls with no content, and imploded bacterial cell walls.[14] Research has demonstrated that a 14-day regimen of water irrigation produced therapeutic benefits in the gingiva and was accompanied by a reduction in the inflammatory cytokines in the gingival crevicular fluid.[13] Another study showed that when combined with toothbrushing, oral irrigation is an effective alternative to traditional dental floss for reducing bleeding, gingival inflammation, and plaque

biofilm in some areas of the mouth.[13] In some cases, daily pulsed irrigation with water is the extra help a patient needs to achieve healthy gingiva. See Chapter 24 for further information on irrigation.

CHLORHEXIDINE

Chlorhexidine digluconate (CHX) has been used in mouthrinses and dentifrices OTC in Canada and Europe for many years. In the United States, Peridex (OMNII Oral Pharmaceuticals, West Palm Beach, Fla.) was first available for oral use as a 0.12% prescription mouthrinse (see Figure 27-5). Later, PerioGard was introduced to the market (Colgate Oral Pharmaceuticals, Canton, Mass.). Peridex was the first CHX product to receive the ADA Seal of Acceptance in 1988 for reducing supragingival plaque biofilm and gingivitis.[10] Recently, an FDA-approved alcohol-free CHX mouthrinse was introduced to the U.S. market (Sunstar Americas, Chicago, Ill.). Currently, several brand and generic names of CHX are available with Peridex carrying the ADA acceptance seal. Reductions in plaque biofilm ranged from 22-61% and for gingivitis ranged from 18-44%.[15-17]

CHX is a **cationic** bisbiguanide and the most widely studied of the oral antimicrobials. Its mechanism of action is the rupture of the bacterial cell membrane and precipitation of the cytoplasmic contents. CHX can reduce the adherence properties of *Porphyromonas gingivalis,* a known periopathogen.[42] CHX binds well to oral tissues and continues to be released in its active form for 6 hours or more.[15] *In vitro* evidence shows that 0.12% chlorhexidine is cytotoxic to fibroblasts.[75] Specific protective factors may protect the fibroblasts in the oral tissues. Because its substantivity is superior to that of other known products, CHX is the recommended positive control in oral chemotherapeutic studies.[58]

Although disadvantages exist for CHX use, not every patient exhibits all the undesirable side effects. Table 27-2 lists the reported adverse effects of CHX as a rinse. The stain and calculus accumulation can be removed professionally; the other side effects disappear when use of the product is discontinued. Rinsing concomitantly with an oxidizing agent can also reduce stain from a CHX rinse.[43] The side effects are lessened when CHX is used in an irrigant rather than as a rinse.

Patients should be instructed to rinse with 15 ml for 30 seconds twice a day.[10] CHX interacts with and is inactivated by sodium lauryl sulfate and other positively charged detergents in dentifrices. Therefore patients should wait a minimum of 30 minutes between using a dentifrice and rinsing with CHX.[12] In addition, rinsing with water immediately after rinsing with CHX should be avoided because a bitter taste results.

For professional irrigation, 0.12% chlorhexidine is generally recommended, with 0.06% for at-home daily irrigation.[35] Data shows this is effective for gingivitis but not for periodontitis.

Dilutions (based on a 0.12% concentration) that have been shown to be effective via randomized clinical trials are as follows:

- 0.02% = 5 parts water + 1 part CHX
- 0.04% = 2 parts water + 1 part CHX
- 0.06% = 1 part water + 1 part CHX[39,45]

Use of chlorhexidine has also been incorporated in the concept of whole-mouth disinfection: debridement and antimicrobial therapy of the entire mouth within a 24-hour period.[78] Unlike the familiar quadrant scaling over a series of appointments at 1- or 2-week intervals, this 24-hour approach is designed to reduce the possibility of cross-infection and reinfection in areas that were treated.

To date, chlorhexidine is the only antimicrobial that has been used for full-mouth disinfection. In studies, scaling and root planing were accomplished within a 24-hour period, and the mouth was disinfected using CHX in professional subgingival irrigation 1%, brushing of tongue with 1% CHX gel, and rinsing with 0.2% CHX for 2 minutes daily for 2 weeks. A significant improvement was observed microbiologically and clinically after 2 months. Beneficial bacteria were found in periodontal pockets, with significantly fewer spirochetes and motile rods, and probing depths in deep pockets were reduced.[78] Further studies found beneficial clinical outcomes 8 months after a 1-day full-mouth scaling and root planing and disinfection[61] and a reduction in the microbial load.[77] One reported side effect was the temporary and slight increase in temperature experienced by some patients a day or two after the therapy. Although other studies either challenge the benefits of full-mouth disinfection or challenge the beneficial effects of the addition of chlorhexidine to the regimen, it is an area that warrants further investigation.

> **Patient Education Opportunity**
>
> Explain to patients about the benefits and disadvantages of using CHX mouthrinse. In addition, educate them about when and how to use the mouthrinse to obtain maximal results.

ESSENTIAL OILS

Essential oils of spices and herbs have antibacterial and antifungal properties, with thyme, oregano, mint, cinnamon, salvia, and clove found to possess the strongest antimicrobial properties.[52] Rinse formulations of phenol-related essential oils include thymol and eucalyptol with menthol and methylsalicylate. Essential oil rinses have a neutral electrical charge. The mechanism of action of the phenolics is to disrupt the bacterial cell wall and inhibit bacterial enzyme production. The most familiar essential oil mouthrinse is Listerine Antiseptic Mouthwash (McNeil PPC, Morris Plains, N.J.), which was awarded the ADA Seal of Acceptance in 1988 for the control of plaque biofilm and gingivitis[9] (see Figure 27-6). Recommended use is to rinse with 20 ml full strength for 30 seconds.[80] Studies have reported plaque biofilm reductions from 14% to 56% and gingivitis reductions from 14% to 39% with twice-daily use after toothbrushing.[30] Essential oils in mouthrinses have positive effects on plaque biofilm and salivary *Streptococcus mutans* levels. One study reported an essential oil mouthrinse produced respective reductions of 69.9% and 75.4% in total recoverable streptococci and in *S. mutans* in plaque biofilm and corresponding reductions of 50.8% and 39.2% in saliva.[32] Essential oils have also been studied as a preprocedural rinse before intraoral procedures. Fine and colleagues found a 94.1% reduction in bacteria collected from aerosols produced by ultrasonic scalers.[33] After more than a century of use of essential oils, no evidence exists of the emergence of opportunistic pathogens or resistant strains with the regular use of these rinses. Some individuals experience an initial burning sensation and an unpleasant taste with essential oil mouthrinses (see Table 27-2). For these individuals, Natural Citrus Listerine Antiseptic Mouthwash may be an alternative. Most of the Listerine antiseptics have alcohol contents in the 21.6% to 26.9% range, and Listermint is alcohol free. Other essential oil products are Advanced Listerine Antiseptic Mouthwash with Tartar Protection, Cool Mint Listerine Antiseptic Mouthwash, and FreshBurst Listerine Antiseptic Mouthwash, as well as several generic versions.

> **Note**
>
> After review from the National Cancer Institute, the ADA has stated that insufficient evidence exists to link oral cancer and mouthrinses containing alcohol in humans. The few studies available are not consistent in the findings on the relationship between smoking and using alcohol-containing mouthrinses.[20]

Concerns over the carcinogenic potential of preparations with a high alcohol content have been expressed. Studies reporting such carcinogenic potential have been fraught with problems— for example, inclusion of pharyngeal cancer, not controlling for other use of alcohol, and frequency and length of rinsing.[21] After review from the National Cancer Institute, ADA, and FDA, the ADA has stated that insufficient evidence exists to link oral cancer and mouthrinses containing alcohol in humans. The few studies available are not consistent in the finding on the relationship between smoking and the use of alcohol-containing mouthrinses.[20]

STANNOUS FLUORIDE

Stannous fluoride (SnF_2) is available in 0.63% (rinses), 0.4% (gels), and 0.454% (dentifrices) strengths. Studies with SnF_2 have shown an adverse bacterial effect[84] and a reduction in plaque biofilm and gingivitis for a short period. The antigingivitis action of SnF_2 is believed to be primarily through the stannous (tin) ion. However, a pilot study involving 70 sites in 10 patients found positive results using a 2.0% neutral gel as part of a supportive periodontal therapy program.[24]

One study demonstrated that the use of a SnF_2 rinse twice daily significantly reduced plaque biofilm index compared with placebo in both sites that received an oral prophylaxis and those that did not (29% overall).[22] No irritation was noted, although a trend toward lower gastrointestinal scores was observed at 3 weeks for the SnF_2 group. Therefore the study concluded that the product was effective in preventing new plaque biofilm accumulation, as well as reducing existing plaque biofilm. SnF_2 as a professionally applied subgingival irrigant was studied[56,60] and found to have little benefit.

The primary disadvantage of SnF_2 is the extrinsic black stain produced when used as a mouthrinse (see Table 27-2). The stain can be removed with a dental prophylaxis.

Stannous fluoride is also the active ingredient in Crest Pro-Health toothpaste, which contains stabilized 0.454% SnF_2 plus sodium hexametaphosphate as the abrasive system to reduce calculus and stain. It is accepted by the ADA for the reduction of plaque biofilm, gingivitis, dental caries, calculus, and tooth sensitivity. Reductions in plaque biofilm range from 0% to 7% and reductions in gingivitis range from 19% to 22%.

TRICLOSAN

Triclosan is a broad-spectrum antiseptic that has been used in many products, including soaps and antiperspirants.[48] It is a bisphenol with broad-spectrum antimicrobial activity. It has been incorporated into many oral products.[28] The dentifrice Colgate Total (Colgate Palmolive, Piscataway, NJ) contains triclosan and Gantrez, a co-polymer of poly-vinylmethyl-ether–maleic acid (PVM-MA) (see Figure 27-3). Triclosan with co-polymer has been studied as a dentifrice and found to reduce gingivitis by 19% to 42% and plaque biofilm by 12% to 59%.[27] It is the first dentifrice sold in the United States to receive the ADA's Seal of Acceptance for the reduction of plaque biofilm and gingivitis. In the United States, triclosan for oral benefit is currently available only in a dentifrice (see Chapter 26).

SANGUINARINE

Sanguinarine is an alkaloid extract obtained from the bloodroot plant *Sanguinaria canadensis* and is the active ingredient in both a rinse and a dentifrice for the treatment of gingivitis.[46] No benefits were obtained when only one of the products was used, but a decrease in plaque biofilm and gingivitis has been shown when both the dentifrice and mouthrinse were used together regularly. Reductions in plaque biofilm ranged from 17% to 42% and gingivitis reductions from 18% to 57%.[46] The only reported side effect has been a mild burning sensation when initially used.[7] It has been replaced in Viadent oral care products by zinc citrate in the dentifrice and by cetylpridinium chloride in the mouthrinse. It is found in some herbal products. Dentifrices with this herbal agent are not ADA accepted.

TETRACYCLINE AND ITS ANALOGS

The benefits of tetracycline (TCN) and its analogs, chemically modified TCN molecules (CMTs), are remarkable. TCNs can be used either as bacteriostatic agents to inhibit protein synthesis in the bacterial cells or, at subantimicrobial (lower) concentration, to modulate the host response.[93] Two useful properties of TCN are its ability to concentrate in gingival crevicular fluid and its long-established safety record in low systemic doses. The CMTs inhibit the destructive activity of mammalian collagenases and possess a powerful ability to inhibit osteoclastic activity, thus reducing bone loss.[94] TCN should not be administered to pregnant women or young children whose teeth are still calcifying because TCN's affinity for mineralizing tissue causes intrinsic staining in teeth.

As an irrigant, TCN (250-mg capsule in distilled water at 53° C) was reported to achieve clinical healing similar to scaling and root planing with an average attachment gain of 1.3 mm when the irrigant was delivered for 5 minutes per site.[18,85] If the entire mouth is periodontally involved, then using TCN as an antimicrobial irrigant is not practical because of the long application time. However, in an isolated site, the authors suggested this amount of time and concentration of TCN irrigant.

OXYGENATING AGENTS

Oxygenating agents such as urea peroxide, hydrogen peroxide, gaseous oxygen, and redox agents release oxygen for the resulting deleterious effect on anaerobic pathogens.[83] For periodontal problems, oxygenation is not retained sufficiently long in the pockets and produces untoward side effects. Oxygenating agents alter normal healing, have produced soft tissue lesions, and have been co-carcinogenic in an animal model.[20] The general belief is that overuse of oxygenating rinses, hydrogen peroxide in particular, causes the overgrowth of opportunistic organisms such as *Candida* species. In most studies, results of using oxygenating agents are similar to those of the placebo. However, using the redox agent methylene blue in a slow-release (controlled-delivery) device showed improvement in clinical and microbial pocket parameters beyond debridement alone[68] (see Table 27-2).

Rather than releasing oxygen, some oral antimicrobial agents such as Listerine, doxycycline, TCN hydrochloride (HCl), and sanguinarine have an antioxidant effect in the tissue, thus decreasing gingival inflammation.[34] This concept is not the same as that of oxygenation. Periopathogenic microbes produce oxygen free radicals (O^-) that are toxic to the gingival tissues. An antioxidant chemically reacts with these oxygen free radicals, thus reducing the inflammatory tissue response.

BAKING SODA, SALT, AND HYDROGEN PEROXIDE

Products that contain baking soda, salt, and hydrogen peroxide have been used together with hydrogen peroxide in a modality called *Keyes' technique*.[8] After mechanical instrumentation, a paste of baking soda, salt, and hydrogen peroxide were used as a dentifrice, and irrigation was performed with a saturated salt solution. Studies comparing this technique with other procedures showed no statistically different improvements in clinical efficacy.[41] Baking soda is also used in dentifrices as a cleaning agent.

QUATERNARY AMMONIUM COMPOUNDS

Agents that contain quaternary ammonium compounds are anionic and strongly positively charged and bind easily to oral tissues.[70] The most common quaternary ammonium compound is cetylpyridinium chloride (CPC) 0.05%. This cationic surface-active compound binds to oral tissues but less strongly than CHX. Its mechanism of action ruptures cell walls and alters cytoplasmic contents. Reported side effects are some staining, increased calculus formation, and an occasional burning sensation and epithelial desquamation.[24] Their activity is altered by anionic substances, such as flavoring agents, abrasives, and other charged particles sometimes found in dentifrices. Therefore, compliance could be problematic since a water rinse is recommended following use of traditional dentifrices to maximize their effect, which removes anionic substances. Cēpacol 0.05% CPC (Merrell Dow Pharmaceuticals, Inc., Kansas City, Mo.), Scope 0.045% CPC, Viadent 0.05% (Colgate Palmolive, Piscataway, NJ), and Crest Pro-Health Rinse 0.7% CPC (Procter & Gamble, Cincinnati, Ohio) are familiar brands. Six-month studies of CPC showed a 16% to 28% reduction in plaque biofilm and a 24% reduction in gingivitis.[59]

POVIDONE-IODINE

Povidone-iodine has been used for many years as a surgical hand-scrubbing agent. It is effective against many types of bacteria, viruses, and fungi.[76] A low concentration of povidone-iodine has been shown to be effective as a mouthrinse (in combination with hydrogen peroxide), a subgingival irrigant, and a preprocedural rinse.[38] Clinicians have generally avoided iodine preparations for their known caustic effect on tissue, staining, and the possibility of a sensitivity reaction to iodine. This agent should not be used in patients with known allergies to povidone-iodine or shellfish, with thyroid dysfunction, or who are pregnant or lactating.

PREBRUSHING RINSES

Plax (Johnson & Johnson, Morris Plains, NJ) is a detergent–sodium benzoate mixture sold as a prebrushing rinse. Generally, no benefit accrues because results from using the prebrushing rinse appear to be similar to placebo use [62] (see Table 27-2).

In summary, evidence suggests that some chemotherapeutic agents can control plaque biofilm and gingivitis or provide an effective adjunct to traditional therapies. Research efforts continue in the arena of antimicrobials in patient care, with the result that formulary changes, newer antimicrobials, new uses of familiar antimicrobials, and recommendations about how chemotherapeutics should be used are evolving and changing; thus the dental hygienist must stay up to date in this dynamic area of care.

Controlled Drug-Delivery Systems for Treating Chronic Periodontitis

Locally or controlled delivery products are a combination of antimicrobials or antibiotics and devices that deliver a drug directly to a periodontally diseased pocket. The term *controlled* is used to imply that the drug is released in the pocket at a controlled concentration over a period of time. The current products on the market deliver the drug from 7 to 14 days at a very low dose compared with a systemic antibiotic. In addition, the side effects are essentially nonexistent.

The effect of **locally administered antibiotics or antimicrobials** (LAAs) has been shown to produce better periodontal health effects than mechanical debridement alone. Although the effect of mechanical interventions may produce a positive change in the health of the periodontium, sites may attain a better response if an LAA is placed at the time of initial therapy or shortly thereafter. LAAs are designed to be used in periodontal pockets of 5 mm or greater that bleed on probing. They are not intended for patients with more aggressive forms of periodontal disease who might need more invasive procedures or systemic antibiotics to control the disease. They may be placed numerous times, if warranted.

What is the evidence supporting LAA? The Cochrane Oral Health Group (http://www.cochrane-oral.man.ac.uk/) conducts systematic reviews and develops protocols for treatment. *Protocols* are the introduction, objectives, materials, and methods for reviews currently being prepared and do not yet have abstracts. Local delivery of antimicrobials for chronic periodontitis is one such Cochrane protocol.[25] In addition, the Agency for Healthcare Research and Quality published a report in March 2004: *Effectiveness of Antimicrobial Adjuncts to Scaling and Root-Planing Therapy for Periodontitis*.[1] Conclusions reached were that "the difference in measurements between the treatment and control groups typically favored the treatment group, but was relatively modest. . . . Of the antimicrobials investigated, studies of locally applied tetracycline and minocycline—and locally delivered chlorhexidine—have fairly consistent results in moderately large studies that often reach statistical significance; improvements [in probing depths (PD)] observed in these studies typically average in the neighborhood of 0.3 mm to 0.6 mm. The other agents and delivery modes produced less consistent outcomes and fewer outcomes that reached statistical significance; the majority of studies showed small, statistically nonsignificant PD improvements. [Clinical attachment level (CAL)] outcomes were not as positive as those for PD. The question remains, the authors note, whether such improvements are clinically meaningful."[1]

The area of clinical significance has become a topic of interest to clinicians. Although knowing whether statistical significance has been achieved is important (to determine that a result did not happen by chance), it can provide little meaning when making clinical decisions. Killoy suggested that if a product or procedure achieved an improvement of 2 mm or more in probing depth or attachment gain, it might be deemed clinicially significant.[53] All of the LAA products in the U.S. market have published the clinically significant results of their clincal trials.

The first LAA on the U.S. market was a TCN fiber called Acticite. The fiber consisted of a woven tube made of the polymer ethylene vinyl acetate saturated with 25% TCN HCl. Even though the product was effective, placing it in a timely manner and retaining it in place for the duration needed was difficult. Currently, CHX (PerioChip), doxycycline hyclate (Atridox), and minocycline microspheres (Arestin) are the three controlled drug-delivery systems available in the United States. Products available in other countries include metronidazole gel, minocycline gel, and minocycline ointment.

ADVANTAGES

A controlled drug-delivery system has several advantages.

- Compliance with self-care is not an issue, and patients do not have to remember to take the medication because the dosing and timing are part of the delivery system.
- Dose concentration can be much greater, permitting a greater microbial kill rate and less opportunity for microbial resistance to develop.
- Side effects are often reduced because the agent is delivered to a particular site and not distributed throughout the mouth.
- The systemic effect on the body is also lessened because the agent is delivered locally rather than systemically.

CAUTIONS

Although an LAA is not typically used for generalized periodontitis, it is not contraindicated if a person has multiple pockets and will not or cannot undergo surgical therapy. The contraindication may be the result of medical or financial considerations or fear. Additionally, controlled drug-release delivery is not recommended for pockets less than 5 mm because retention may be an issue. Clinical trials have not included children younger than 18 years of age, pregnant women, and medically compromised individuals; therefore using controlled drug-delivery therapy in these population groups would be considered an *off label* use. Finally, individuals may respond differently to controlled drug-delivery systems, ranging from a worsened condition (infrequent) to a mild, moderate, or marked improvement. No single therapy is guaranteed, and all therapy should be monitored and evaluated.

CHLORHEXIDINE GLUCONATE

In 1998 the first subgingival sustained-release delivery system containing CHX became available to U.S. practitioners. PerioChip (manufactured by Dexcel Pharma and distributed by OMNII Oral Pharmaceuticals, West Palm Beach, Fla.) is a small orange chip, 4 mm × 5 mm × 350 mcm, weighing 7.4 mg (Figure 27-7, *A*). The prescription chip contains 2.5 mg of CHX, a broad-spectrum antimicrobial, in a biodegradable matrix of hydrolyzed gelatin cross-linked with glutaraldehyde, glycerin, and water. Gingival crevicular fluid concentration appears to be biphasic and varies among patients, peaking at 4 hours (more than 1000 mcg/ml) after insertion of the chip into the pocket, and then again at 72 hours (more than 480 mcg/ml) (Figure 27-7, *B*). Release of CHX lasts from 7 to 10 days. In patients with 5- to 8-mm pockets, depth reductions of 2 mm or more over scaling and root planing alone were reported in a 9-month period.[50]

Inserting the chip with forceps is simple, quick, and comfortable. Bacterial resistance to CHX in studies up to 2 years has not been observed.[15] Additionally, the customary side effects of CHX are not evident, most likely because CHX is released below the gingival margin.[11] This product is active in the pocket for 7 to 10 days. The patient is instructed to avoid brushing or flossing the area for 7 days.

DOXYCYCLINE HYCLATE

Doxycycline gel (Atridox) is a 10.0% concentration of doxycycline hyclate for controlled delivery subgingivally in treating chronic adult periodontitis. It is a liquid biodegradable polymer that hardens shortly following exposure to the fluid in the periodontal pocket. Marketed in the United States since 1998, Atridox is available by prescription and carries the ADA Seal of

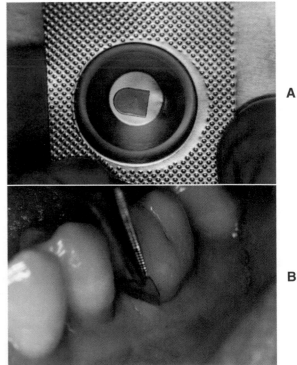

FIGURE 27-7
A, The PerioChip is a biodegradable film of hydrolyzed gelatin 0.35 mm in thickness and 4 × 5 mm, containing 2.5 mg chlorhexidine gluconate. **B,** The PerioChip is inserted into a 6-mm pocket on the mesial surface of tooth #19. (From Rose LF et al: *Periodontics: medicine, surgery and implants*, St Louis, 2004, Mosby.)

Acceptance. The polylactic acid gel and drug are mixed at chairside and delivered to the bottom of the pocket via a small cannula (Figure 27-8). The gel then solidifies, releasing doxycycline for a period of 7 days. Clinical trials have resulted in an increase in clinical attachment averaging 0.8 mm and a reduction of probe depths averaging 1.3 mm in a 9-month study.[37] Headache, common cold symptoms, and some toothache and gingival discomfort were the most common side effects. Interestingly, the difference in improvement between two groups, smokers and nonsmokers, was not evident when Atridox was used.[81] This product is active in the pocket for 7 to 10 days and usually dissolves in 28 to 30 days. The patient should be instructed to avoid brushing, flossing, or eating in the area of placement for 7 days.

MINOCYCLINE MICROSPHERES

Minocycline HCl is available in a controlled drug-delivery system with the brand name of Arestin (OraPharma, Inc.,

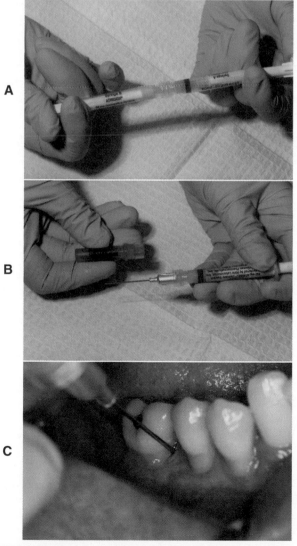

FIGURE 27-8
A, Atridox in two syringes that are coupled together for mixing. Atridox also comes in a single-syringe, premixed formulation. **B,** After mixing, the delivery syringe is attached to a blunt cannula. **C,** Atridox is placed into a 7-mm pocket on the mesial surface of tooth #30. (From Rose LF et al: *Periodontics: medicine, surgery and implants,* St Louis, 2004, Mosby.)

Warminster, Pa.). This TCN derivative is incorporated in a bioresorbable polymer in the form of a powder of bioadhesive microspheres and marketed in 1-mg unit-dose cartridges with accompanying delivery syringes. Minocycline is a member of the TCN class of antibiotics and has a broad spectrum of activity.[86] Minocycline inhibits protein synthesis in the bacterial cell wall that causes leakage and destroys the cell. At higher concentrations, minocycline is bacteriocidal, killing the bacteria. Laboratory testing has shown minocycline to be effective in eradicating the organisms that are associated with chronic periodontitis. *Porphyromonas gingivalis, Prevotella intermedia, Fusobacterium nucleatum, Eikenella corrodens,* and *Actinobacillus actinomycetemcomitans* are susceptible to minocycline at concentrations of up to and including 8 mcg/ml. A 2001 study reported the results of a 9-month multicenter trial on Arestin. The study compared scaling and root planing (SRP) alone, SRP plus minocycline microspheres, and SRP plus the placebo microspheres (not containing minocycline). The results showed a greater therapeutic effect of the SRP plus minocycline microspheres compared with the other treatment groups.[98]

Arestin has also been shown to maintain effective MIC of the drug for up to 14 days and, in some cases, 28 days.[17] The levels found were well above the MIC levels for common periodontal pathogens. Although the product maintains high local levels of drug, the systemic levels are minimal. In a pharmacokinetic study, results found mean dose saliva levels to be approximately 1000 times higher than serum levels (blood), indicating minimal absorption of the drug through the periodontal pocket into blood.[69]

BOX 27-3

TIPS FOR ARESTIN TIP PLACEMENT

- Ease of insertion may be facilitated by aligning the cartridge tip parallel to the long axis of the tooth, similar to a periodontal probe.
- In a pocket with *tight* tissue (smokers or maintenance patients), a probe may be inserted to retract the tissue before inserting the tip of the cartridge.
- For tight tissue, the orifice of the tip may be altered from a circle to an elliptical or flatter shape. Start at the end of the tip and run the end of the mirror handle up to the ring on the cartridge. Do this a few times.
- In a difficult-to-access pocket (i.e., distal of molars), the cartridge may be slightly bent to increase the angle at the existing angle of the cartridge, approximately 12 mm from the end of the tip. Do not bend the tip in the first 6 mm from the end of the tip because the plunger may rupture the cartridge and puncture the barrel wall.
- When inserting the cartridge tip, use a light grasp and an exploratory motion. When the pocket morphology or best access is identified, align the cartridge tip as parallel as possible to the long axis of the tooth; express the cartridge contents into the pocket.

Modified from Wilder RS: A new option for local delivery, *Dimens Dent Hyg* 1(2):24-27, April/May 2003.

The microspheres are dispensed subgingivally using a disposable premeasured plastic cartridge in a stainless steel handle. The tip is inserted to the base of the pocket and the material is activated into the pocket (Figure 27-9). Posttreatment instructions include avoiding eating hard, crunchy, or sticky foods for 1 week and postponing brushing for a 12-hour period and interdental cleaning for 10 days. Box 27-3 lists suggestions on Arestin placement.

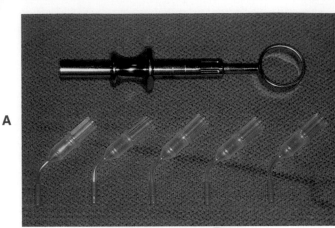

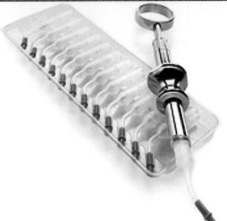

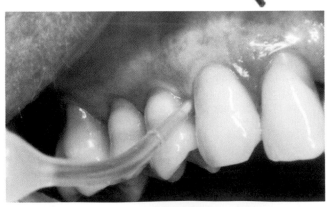

FIGURE 27-9
Minocycline microspheres (Arestin). **A,** Handle and premeasured cartridges. **B,** Handle with attached cartridge. **C,** Arestin is placed into a 6-mm pocket on the mesial surface of tooth #5. (**A** and **B** courtesy OraPharma, Inc.; **C** from Rose LF et al: *Periodontics: medicine, surgery and implants,* St Louis, 2004, Mosby.)

METRONIDAZOLE GEL*

Metronidazole gel contains 25% metronidazole in a glycerin mono-oleate and sesame oil base and is applied to the pocket using a syringe with a blunt cannula. This agent is not currently available in the United States. It is easy to place but may require multiple applications to achieve desirable results. Studies using metronidazole gel as a monotherapy show similar results compared with scaling and root planing.[2,39,73] When metronidazole gel was used in studies with two other adjunctive treatments to SRP and compared with SRP alone, all treatments improved over 6 months with no significant differences among treatment groups.[54,79]

MINOCYCLINE OINTMENT AND GEL

Minocycline ointment contains 2% minocycline HCl and is applied using a syringe with a blunt cannula. This agent is not currently available in the United States. A 2% minocycline gel has also been used in several studies. In a multicenter study of patients with moderate to severe periodontitis, results of treatment with minocycline ointment combined with SRP were found to be statistically significant when compared with treatment with a vehicle control with SRP.[91,92] When subgingivally applied minocycline gel was used as one of three adjunctive treatments to SRP compared with SRP alone, all treatments showed improvements with no significant differences among groups.[54,79]

Systemic Antibiotics

Antibiotics are organic substances that have the ability to destroy or inhibit the growth of bacteria and other microorganisms. Most antibiotics have been isolated and purified from their natural source and are prepared synthetically or semisynthetically. In contrast to antiseptics, they are administered orally, parenterally, and rarely topically. The topical route is not widely used because this route of administration may sensitize the patient to these agents, particularly when penicillin is concerned.

An ideal antibiotic should:
- Be selective and effective against microorganisms without injuring the host
- Destroy microorganisms (bactericidal action) rather than retard their growth (bacteriostatic)
- Not become ineffective as a result of bacterial resistance
- Not be inactivated by enzymes, plasma proteins, or body fluids
- Quickly reach bactericidal levels throughout the body and be maintained for long periods
- Have minimal adverse effects

Currently an ideal antibiotic for the treatment of periodontal disease does not exist. Depending on the antibiotic, several mechanisms of action are inherent. These mechanisms include the following:

---

*Text on metronidazole gel and minocycline ointment and gel borrowed with permission from Hill M and Moore R. In Rose LF et al: *Periodontics: medicine, surgery, and implants,* St Louis, 2004, Elsevier.

- Inhibition of bacterial cell wall synthesis
- Alteration of bacterial cell membrane permeability
- Alteration of bacterial synthesis of cellular components
- Inhibition of bacterial cell metabolism

Antibiotics are either bacteriostatic or bactericidal. **Bacteriostatic** antibiotics inhibit the growth and multiplication of microorganisms, whereas **bactericidal** antibiotics kill or destroy microorganisms. In general, bacteriostatic antibiotics alter the metabolic pathways or synthesis of cellular components. In contrast, bactericidal drugs interfere with the synthesis or function of the cell wall, the cell membrane, or both.

When two bactericidal antibiotics are given together, they may exert a greater effect than when each is given separately. This effect is called *antibiotic synergism*. Sometimes, however, when a bacteriostatic and a bactericidal antibiotic are given together, their effectiveness is negated or reduced. This effect is called *antibiotic antagonism.*

Their antimicrobial activity varies according to the agent selected, dose level, and route of administration. Some antimicrobials are effective against selected gram-positive and gram-negative bacteria, some are most effective against aerobic bacteria (although others act better on anaerobes), a few are effective against fungi, and most have no effect on viruses.

Susceptibility of various microorganisms to antibiotics is initially determined by laboratory tests. However, as with antiseptics, although an agent may be found to be active in laboratory tests, it may prove clinically ineffective if the dose is inadequate, a patient's resistance to infection is poor, or the wrong pathogen has been determined as the etiologic agent.

The advantage of a systemic antibiotic, assuming patient compliance in taking the oral medication, is that the drug reaches bacteria in deep periodontal pockets, gingival tissue, and other oral sites and leaves no reservoir or niche of microbes. The disadvantages of systemic delivery are the adverse side effects, such as gastrointestinal imbalance, nausea, diarrhea, and rash; the risk of producing antimicrobially resistant microbes; and patients not taking the pills as prescribed.[93] Another concern is that systemic antibiotics used to treat periodontal infections are not sufficiently narrow. Ideally, the putative organism should be identified so that the appropriate antibiotic can be selected. Because the causative organism or organisms and the destructive processes in periodontal diseases are not yet fully understood, selecting an antibiotic with a sufficiently narrow spectrum is difficult. Because antibiotics can produce adverse effects, knowledge of these side effects is essential for dental professionals because they may observe these side effects in their patients.[20] A major concern with antibiotics is the development of resistant strains of bacteria with the emergence of resistant strains considered to be one of the major therapeutic challenges facing practitioners in the next decade[63,89] (Box 27-4).

Antibiotics most often prescribed for dental therapy are shown in Box 27-5 and

> *Note*
>
> Antibiotics are either bacteriostatic or bactericidal. Bacteriostatic antibiotics inhibit the growth and multiplication of microorganisms, whereas bactericidal antibiotics alter the metabolic pathways or synthesis of cellular components.

BOX 27-4

POTENTIAL CONCERNS WITH SYSTEMIC ANTIMICROBIALS

- Interference with the body's normal microbial flora
- Side effects
- Drug pharmacokinetics (absorption, distribution, metabolism, and excretion)
- Drug pharmacodynamics (how the drug affects the body)
- Potential for development of microbial resistance
- Drug interactions
- Concerns with special populations (pregnant women, children, elderly, ethnicity, gender, general health status)
- Likelihood of increasing drug sensitivity
- Adherence and compliance to daily medication regimen

BOX 27-5

MOST COMMONLY PRESCRIBED ANTIBIOTICS IN DENTISTRY

- Amoxicillin
- Amoxicillin plus clavulanic acid
- Tetracyclines
- Tetracycline HCl
- Minocycline HCl
- Doxycycline HCl
- Metronidazole
- Clindamycin
- Combination of metronidazole and penicillins

HCl, Hydrochloride.

include penicillins, TCNs, metronidazole, and clindamycin. Other less often prescribed antibiotics that have been reported in the dental literature are ciprofloxin (alone or in combination with metronidazole) and azithromycin. Selecting an antibiotic for a patient may be based on microbiological evaluations of periodontal pathogens present in the patient, the clinical diagnosis, or both.

Antibiotic therapy should be an adjunctive treatment in managing periodontal diseases and not used as a monotherapy. This therapy should include SRP, optimal oral hygiene, and, as needed, surgical therapy.[51]

Systemic antibiotics have shown to be of minimal value in treating chronic periodontitis. However, they have been shown to be of value in treating localized aggressive periodontitis, generalized aggressive periodontitis, and unresponsive forms of periodontitis.[47,55,72,96]

ADVERSE EFFECTS OF ANTIBIOTICS

The adverse effects of the various antibiotic groups most commonly used as adjuncts to periodontal therapy are summarized in the following sections.

Amoxicillin

Amoxicillin toxicity is extremely low and, except for allergic reactions, it is one of the safest drugs known. Patients who are hypersensitive to one penicillin are most likely hypersensitive to all other penicillins. In addition, patients with a history of hypersensitivity to cephalosporins, griseofulvin, or penicillamine may show a similar response to penicillins. Moreover, the combination of amoxicillin and clavulanic acid (Augmentin) may produce diarrhea.

Tetracyclines

The side effects associated with TCN therapy are varied. These side effects and toxicities include photosensitivity, gastrointestinal upset, lymphoepithelioma, fetal tooth staining, and simulated lupus erythematosus. In addition, reports indicate that long-term TCN therapy with minocycline (as used for patients with acne) may discolor adult teeth and gingival tissue.[74,82]

Metronidazole

The main adverse effects of metronidazole are an interaction with alcoholic beverages, which can result in severe nausea and vomiting, metallic taste, gastric discomfort, and diarrhea.

Clindamycin

The main adverse effects of clindamycin are diarrhea and gastric upset. Therefore clindamycin should be taken with food. Pseudomembranous colitis has occurred during therapy with clindamycin, but its frequency of occurrence is less than that seen with ampicillin or the cephalosporins.

PREGNANCY CLASSIFICATION OF ANTIBIOTICS

All prescription medications are categorized according to their potential to produce adverse effects on the fetus.[19] These medications are listed in Table 27-3.

Host Modulation

Dentistry has had a long history of research into clarifying the role of the host in the pathogenesis of periodontal disease. Although the profession has long understood the importance of bacteria in disease causation, the understanding of how the host contributes to the periodontal disease process has emerged only since the 1970s. Although investigators have identified specific pathways and mediators of tissue destruction, logically, research effort has been undertaken into **host modulation** treatments that block or modulate these destructive pathways and mediators as a potential adjunctive way to treat periodontal disease. The following discussion is a summary of host modulation treatments for patient use.

PROTEASE INHIBITORS

Subantimicrobial dose doxycycline (SDD), 20 mg doxycycline twice daily over 6 to 9 months, has been proposed as an adjunctive treatment for periodontitis.[40] A recognized feature of doxycycline is its ability to downregulate the activity of matrix metalloproteinases (MMPs), which are active in tissue breakdown during periodontitis. The current understanding of periodontal pathogenesis suggests that MMPs play a major role in inflammation, tissue remodeling, and the destruction of collagen and bone within the periodontium, leading to clinical signs of periodontitis such as attachment loss, bone loss, and tooth mobility. Currently, multicenter clinical studies support the hypothesis that downregulation of MMPs by SDD confers measurable benefits to patients with periodontitis.

Caton and colleagues[16] reported on a 190-patient, placebo-controlled trial in which all patients received SRP; one half of these patients also received adjunctive SDD (20 mg doxycycline twice daily). Patients were examined every 3 months over a 9-month period, and for those receiving SDD, an improvement in attachment gain of 18% was noted (in patients with 4- to 6-mm pockets at baseline). The differences for SDD over SRP alone were greater in pockets of 7 mm or more, for attachment gain (33%), and for pocket depth reduction (40%). Thus the literature suggests that SDD, when prescribed as an adjunct to SRP, results in statistically significant gains in attachment levels and reduction in probing depth when compared with SRP alone. Although the adjunctive use of SDD in addition to mechanical therapy may provide statistically significant improvement in attachment gain when compared with mechanical therapy alone, many researchers have questioned the clinical significance of the differences, which average less than 0.5 mm.[40] One concern that arises with any antimicrobial usage is the emergence of resistant microbial strains, but research implies that SDD is not antibacterial at this dosage (20 mg), and it does not lead to the development of resistant strains or the acquisition of multi-antibiotic resistance.[88] The drug is well

Table 27-3	U.S. Food and Drug Administration Pregnancy Classifications
CLASSIFICATION	**DEFINITION**
A	No risk demonstrated to the fetus in any trimester
B	No adverse effects in animals; no human studies available—amoxicillin, amoxicillin plus clavulanic acid, clindamycin, metronidazole, azithromycin, erythromycin, cephalosporin
C	Only given after risks to the fetus are considered; animal studies have shown adverse reactions; no human studies available—clarithromycin
D	Definite fetal risks; may be given in spite of risks if needed in life-threatening situations—all tetracyclines
X	Absolute fetal abnormalities; not to be used at any time during pregnancy

tolerated by the body, and clinical trials have established that the incidence of unwanted effects is similar to that of the placebo. Walker and colleagues[95] concluded that SDD and placebo did not produce effects on vaginal or intestinal flora over 9 months of use. SDD is designed to be given over many months and may therefore suffer from compliance problems similar to other long-term medications used to treat chronic systemic conditions.[95]

SDD was evaluated as part of a systematic review and consensus report from the American Academy of Periodontology. SDD received the highest level of rating possible from a panel of periodontal thought leaders. The rating supported the efficacy and safety of SDD as an adjunct to conventional therapy in managing chronic periodontitis.[49]

NONSTEROIDAL ANTIINFLAMMATORY DRUGS*

Nonsteroidal antiinflammatory drugs (NSAIDs) are generally used in dentistry for treating pain. However, because these drugs inhibit antiinflammatory processes related to the cyclooxygenase pathway, such as prostaglandin, thromboxane, and prostacyclin production, they also have the potential to be beneficial as adjuncts in periodontal therapy. Researchers have recognized that prostaglandin E_2 and other arachidonic acid metabolites are important proinflammatory mediators in bone resorption and the various manifestations of periodontal disease.

NSAIDs are certainly of use after surgical periodontal procedures in reducing postoperative pain and inflammation. Ibuprofen, for example, has been shown to successfully inhibit prostaglandin E_2 production in the periodontal tissues after surgery, contributing to the healing process.[67] Ibuprofen as an adjunct for SRP, however, has not been demonstrated to be effective. Ng and Bissada,[66] for example, showed that ibuprofen (800 mg/day) administered as an adjunctive treatment to SRP did not improve the results on probing depth and clinical attachment levels when compared with SRP alone. Other drugs such as meclofenamate sodium (Meclomen) have been shown to produce positive results in patients with aggressive periodontitis. The use of systemically administered acetylsalicylic acid (aspirin; 500 mg daily for 6 weeks after mechanical debridement) has also been reported to be an effective adjunct in periodontal therapy.[36]

An important factor that must influence the decision on whether to use NSAIDs on a long-term basis is the gastrointestinal complications that may arise. Some cases may result in considerable ulceration of the gastric mucosa. Newer NSAIDs that selectively inhibit cyclooxygenase 2 (COX-2) inhibitors are much better tolerated by the gastric mucosa and may one day prove beneficial in modulating the host response in periodontitis.

Evaluation of Success

Evaluating the efficacy and the effects of chemotherapeutics is ultimately the responsibility of the clinician. Patients should be placed on a chemotherapeutic agent for a finite period and then return to the office for an evaluation. Currently accepted clinical signs of a healthy periodontium include the absence of inflammatory signs of disease such as redness, swelling, suppuration, and bleeding on probing; maintaining a functional periodontal attachment level; minimal or no recession in the absence of interproximal bone loss; and functional dental implants.[4] If these effects are not demonstrated when the use of irrigation and antimicrobials has been added to the patient's regimen, then the clinician should consider a sizeable number of possibilities, including the following:

- Was the agent used as directed?
- Did exudates, blood, calculus, or debris inactivate or block the action of the antimicrobial?
- Would a different chemotherapeutic agent be more effective?
- Is referral indicated?

If these questions do not provide the needed information, then the clinician must reinvestigate the oral condition, as well as the patient's general health and well-being. Adverse personal circumstances such as an increase in patient stress, a change in health status not reported by the patient, or an undiagnosed medical condition may contribute to the regression of the oral status. Although people are able to maintain their teeth longer—even seriously involved periodontal teeth—not every case always results in complete absence of bleeding and absence of attachment loss. The clinician must keep abreast of the patient's clinical signs and symptoms of health and treat the patient according to the best options available.

✦ CASE APPLICATION 27-1.1

Treatment Planning

What areas of concern do you have for Ms. Tevus's oral health? What treatment options might you offer her? Use a decision-tree diagram to illustrate your choices. (A decision tree is a pathway or diagram of lines indicating, at each problem point, the available choices or paths.) Some considerations to guide your thoughts may include the following:

- Does an adequate level of plaque biofilm control exist?
- What type of therapy you would recommend?
- Which chemotherapeutic agent would you recommend for the treatment of tooth #10?
- If SRP of tooth #10 does not improve the probing depth, what options will you suggest for that site?

Conclusion*

Using locally acting chemotherapeutic agents can be a valuable adjunct to conventional mechanical therapeutic treatments. Topically applied agents such as dentifrices and mouthrinses are useful in controlling gingivitis in patients who cannot perform traditional methods to control plaque biofilm or in patients who

---

*Adapted from Kinane DF: Systemic chemotherapeutic agents. In Rose LF et al: *Periodontics medicine, surgery, and implants,* St Louis, 2004, Elsevier.

*This section was adapted from Hill M, Moore R: Locally acting oral chemotherapeutic agents. In Rose LF et al: *Periodontics medicine, surgery, and implants,* St Louis, 2004, Elsevier.

need an adjunctive method to brushing and flossing. Although mouthrinses and dentifrices have been successful with gingivitis treatment, they have limitations for periodontitis cases because of issues with substantivity. In patients with chronic periodontitis, mechanical treatments with hand or powered instrumentation can provide an excellent clinical response in the majority of patients. However, locally delivered drugs placed subgingivally also represent a valuable adjunctive therapy for patients with chronic moderate periodontitis (5 to 8 mm) who have bleeding on probing. Locally delivered drugs can be used at the time of SRP or when the posttreatment evaluation indicates that the patient has not responded to mechanical therapy. A recent comprehensive meta-analysis demonstrated a statistically significant improvement in probing depth reduction and clinical attachment gain when these products were used as adjuncts to SRP.[45]

In some patients, adjunctive systemic agents will be indicated. In patients with aggressive forms of periodontitis and those who do not respond to mechanical therapy alone, adjunctive systemic agents may be indicated and should be considered as a viable therapeutic intervention.[44] Host response modulation using protease and inflammatory inhibitors may become widely accepted in the future as an adjunct to periodontal therapy. Furthermore, periodontal risk factor modification such as smoking cessation and simpler measures such as oral hygiene advice and motivation will continue to be crucial in the comprehensive treatment of periodontitis.

References

1. Agency for Healthcare Research and Quality: *Effectiveness of antimicrobial adjuncts to scaling and root-planing therapy for periodontitis,* March 2004. Available at http://www.ahrq.gov.

2. Ainamo J et al: Clinical responses to subgingival application of a metronidazole 25% gel compared to the effects of subgingival scaling in adult periodontitis, *J Clin Periodontol* 19:723-729, 1992.

3. American Academy of Periodontology: AAP position paper. The role of supra- and subgingival irrigation in the treatment of periodontal diseases, *J Periodontol* 76:2015-2027, 2005.

4. American Academy of Periodontology: AAP guidelines for periodontal therapy, *J Periodontal* 72:1624-1628, 2001.

5. American Academy of Periodontology: AAP position paper. Modulation of the host response in periodontal therapy, *J Periodontol* 73:460-470, 2001.

6. American Academy of Periodontology: AAP treatment of plaque-induced gingivitis, chronic periodontitis, and other clinical conditions, *J Periodontol* 72:1790-1800, 2001.

7. American Academy of Periodontology: The role of controlled drug delivery for periodontitis, *J Periodontol* 71:125-140, 2000.

8. American Academy of Periodontology: Current understanding of the role of microscopic monitoring, baking soda and hydrogen peroxide in the treatment of periodontal disease, *J Periodontol* 69:951-954, 1998.

9. American Dental Association, Council on Dental Therapeutics: Council on Dental Therapeutics accepts Listerine, *J Am Dent Assoc* 117:515-516, 1988.

10. American Dental Association, Council on Dental Therapeutics: Council on Dental Therapeutics accepts Peridex, *J Am Dent Assoc* 117:516-517, 1988.

11. AstraZeneca: *Monograph and full prescribing information* [brochure], Wilmington, Del, 1998, AstraZeneca Pharmaceuticals.

12. Barkvoll P, Rølla G, Svendsen AK: Chlorhexidine interactions with sodium lauryl sulfate in vivo, *J Clin Periodontal* 16(9):593-595, 1989.

13. Barnes CM et al: Comparison of irrigation to floss as an adjunct to toothbrushing: effect on bleeding, gingivitis, and supragingival plaque, *J Clin Dent* 16(3):71-77, 2005.

14. Brady JR, Gray WA, Bhaskar SN: Electron microscopic study of the effect of water jet lavage device on dental plaque, *J Dent Res* 52:1310-1315, 1973.

15. Briner WW, Kayrouz GA, Chanak MX: Comparative antimicrobial effectiveness of a substantive (0.12% chlorhexidine) and a nonsubstantive (phenolic) mouthrinse in vivo and in vitro, *Compend Contin Educ Dent* 15:1158-1168, 1994.

16. Caton JG et al: Treatment with subantimicrobial dose doxycycline improves the efficacy of scaling and root planing in patients with adult periodontitis, *J Periodontol* 71:521-532, 2000.

17. Christersson LA: *Tissue response and release of minocycline after subgingival deposition by use of a resorbable polymer* [unpublished data on file], Warminster, Pa, 1988, OraPharma, Inc.

18. Christersson LA, Morderyd OM, Puchalsky CS: Topical application of TCN-HCl in human periodontitis, *J Clin Periodontol* 20:88-95, 1993.

19. Ciancio SG ed: *ADA guide to dental therapeutics,* ed 3, Chicago, 2003, American Dental Association.

20. Ciancio SG: Antiseptics and antibiotics as chemotherapeutic agents for periodontitis management, *Compend Contin Educ Dent* 21(1):59-76, 2000.

21. Ciancio SG: Chemical agents: plaque control, calculus reduction and treatment of dentinal hypersensitivity, *Periodontol 2000* 8:75-86, 1995.

22. Ciancio SG: Clinical effects of a stannous fluoride mouthrinse on plaque, *Clin Prev Dent* 14(5):2730, 1992.

23. Ciancio SG et al: Effect of a chemotherapeutic agent delivered by an oral irrigating device on plaque, gingivitis, and subgingival microflora, *J Periodontol* 60:310-315, 1989.

24. Cleveland S, McLey L, Jones J: Irrigation of nonresponding periodontal pockets with neutral fluoride gel: a pilot study, *J Prac Hyg* 6(2):21-25, 1997.

25. Cochrane Protocol. Available at: http://www.update-software.com/Abstracts/ORALAbstractIndex.htm.

25a. Cole P, Rodu B, Mathisen A: Alcohol-containing mouthwash and oropharyngeal cancer: a review of the epidemiology. *J Am Dent Assoc* 134:1079-1087, 2003.

26. Costerton JW et al: Microbial biofilms, *Ann Rev Microbiol* 49:711-745, 1995.

27. Cubells AB et al: The effect of a triclosan/copolymer/fluoride dentifrice on plaque formation and gingivitis: a six month study, *J Clin Dent* 2:63-69, 1991.

28. DeSalva SJ, Kong BM, Lin YJ: Triclosan: a safety profile, *Am J Dent* 2:185-196, 1989.

29. Eley BM: Antibacterial agents in the control of supragingival plaque—a review, *Br Dent J* 186(6):286-296, 1999.

30. Elworthy A et al: The substantivity of a number of oral hygiene products determined by the duration of effects on salivary bacteria, *J Periodontol* 76:572-576, 1996.

31. Federal Register [Notices], vol 70, no 163, Wednesday, August 24, 2005.

32. Fine DH et al: Effect of an essential oil–containing antiseptic mouthrinse on plaque and salivary *Streptococcus mutans* levels, *J Clin Periodontol* 27(3):157-161, 2000.

33. Fine DH et al: Efficacy of preprocedural rinsing with an antiseptic in reducing viable bacteria in dental aerosols, *J Periodontol* 63: 821-824, 1992.

34. Firatli E et al: Antioxidative activities of some chemotherapeutics. A possible mechanism in reducing gingival inflammation, *J Clin Periodontol* 21:680-683, 1994.

35. Flemmig TF et al: Supragingival irrigation with 0.06% chlorhexidine in naturally occurring gingivitis: I—month clinical observations, *J Periodontol* 61:112-117, 1990.

36. Flemmig TF, Rumetsch M, Klaiber B: Efficacy of systemically administered acetylsalicylic acid plus scaling on periodontal health and elastase-alpha 1-proteinase inhibitor in gingival crevicular fluid, *J Clin Periodontol* 23:153-159, 1996.

37. Garrett S et al: Two multi-center studies evaluating locally delivered doxycycline hyclate, placebo control, oral hygiene, and scaling and root planing in the treatment of periodontitis, *J Periodontol* 70:490-503, 1999.

38. Greenstein G: Povidone-iodine's effects and role in the management of periodontal diseases: a review, *J Periodontol* 70: 1397-1405, 1999.

39. Greenstein G: The role of metronidazole in the treatment of periodontal diseases, *J Periodontol* 64:1-15, 1993.

40. Greenstein G, Lamster I: Efficacy of subantimicrobial dosing with doxycycline. Point/Counterpoint, *J Am Dent Assoc* 132:457-466, 2001.

41. Greenwall H, Bissada NF: A dispassionate scientific analysis of Keyes' technique, *Int J Periodontics Restorative Dent* 5:64-75, 1985.

42. Grenier D: Effect of chlorhexidine on the adherence properties of *Porphyromonas gingivalis*, *J Clin Periodontol* 23:140-142, 1996.

43. Gründemann LJ et al: Stain, plaque and gingivitis reduction by combining chlorhexidine and peroxyborate, *J Clin Periodontol* 27:9-15, 2000.

44. Haffajee AD, Socransky SS, Gunsolley JC: Systemic anti-infective periodontal therapy. A systematic review, *Ann Periodontol* 8: 115-181, 2003.

45. Hanes PJ, Purvis JP: Local anti-infective therapy: pharmacological agents. A systematic review, *Ann Periodontol* 8:79-98, 2003.

46. Harper DS et al: Clinical efficacy of a dentifrice and oral rinse containing sanguinaria-containing extract and zinc chloride during six months of use, *J Periodontol* 61:352, 1990.

47. Hayes C, Antczak-Bouckoms A, Burdick E: Quality assessment and meta-analysis of systemic tetracycline use in chronic adult periodontitis, *J Clin Periodontol* 19(3):164-168, 1992.

48. Hill M, Moore R: Locally acting oral chemotherapeutic agents. In Rose LF et al: *Periodontics medicine, surgery, and implants,* St Louis, 2004, Elsevier.

49. Host modulation, anti-infective agents, and tissue engineering. Proceedings of the 2003 Workshop on Contemporary Science in Clinical Periodontics. Oak Brook, Ill., July 26-29, 2003, *Ann Periodontol* 8(1):i, 1-352, 2003.

50. Jeffcoat MK et al: Adjunctive use of a subgingival controlled-release chlorhexidine chip reduces probing depth and improves attachment level compared with scaling and root planing alone, *J Periodontol* 69:989-997, 1998.

51. Jolkovsky DL, Ciancio SG: Chemotherapeutic agents in the treatment of periodontal diseases. In Newman MG, Takei HH, Carranza FA, eds: *Clinical periodontology,* ed 9, Philadelphia, 2002, WB Saunders.

52. Kalemba D, Kunicka A: Antibacterial and antifungal properties of essential oils, *Curr Med Chem* 10(17):813-829, 2003.

53. Killoy WJ: The clinical significance of local chemotherapeutics, *J Clin Periodontol* 29(Suppl 2):22-29, 2002.

54. Kinane DF, Radvar M: A six-month comparison of three periodontal local antimicrobial therapies in persistent periodontal pockets, *J Periodontol* 70:1-7, 1999.

55. Kornman KS, Robertson PB: Clinical and microbiological evaluation of therapy for juvenile periodontitis, *J Periodontol* 56(8): 443-446, 1985.

56. Krust KS et al: The effects of subgingival irrigation with chlorhexidine and stannous fluoride. A preliminary investigation, *J Dent Hyg* 65:289-295, 1991.

57. Lang NK, Karring T, Lindhe J, eds: *Proceedings of the 2nd European Workshop on Periodontology: chemicals in periodontics. Charter House at Ittingen Thurgau, Switzerland, February 3-6, 1996, under the auspices of the European Federation of Periodontology,* Quintessenz, 1997, Berlin, Chicago.

58. Lang NP, Brecx MC: Chlorhexidine digluconate, an agent for chemical plaque control and prevention of gingival inflammation, *J Periodontal Res* 21:74-89, 1986.

59. Lobene RR, Lovene S, Soparker PM: The effect of cetylpyridinium chloride mouthrinse on plaque and gingivitis, *J Dent Res* 56:595, 1977

59a. Mankodi S, et al: Anti-gingivitis efficacy of a stabilized 0.454% stannous fluoride/sodium hexametaphosphate dentifrice: a controlled 6-month clinical trial, *J Clin Periodontal* 32:75-80, 2005.

59b. Mascarenhas AK: Inconclusive evidence to suggest that alcohol-containing mouthwash increases the risk of oropharyngeal cancer, *J Evid Base Dent Pract* 4:249-250, 2004.

60. Mazza J, Newman M, Sims T: Clinical and antimicrobial effect of stannous fluoride on periodontitis, *J Clin Periodontol* 8:203-212, 1981.

61. Mongardini C et al: One stage full- versus partial-mouth disinfection in the treatment of chronic adult or generalized early-onset periodontitis: I—long-term clinical observations, *J Periodontol* 70:632-645, 1999.

62. Moran J, Addy M: The effects of a cetylpyridinium chloride prebrushing rinse as an adjunct to oral hygiene and gingival health, *J Periodontol* 62:562-564, 1991.

63. Murray BE: Problems and dilemmas of antimicrobial resistance, *Pharmacotherapy* 12:86S-93S, 1992.

64. Netuschil L, Hoffmann T, Brecx M: How to select the right mouthrinses in periodontal prevention and therapy: part I—test systems and clinical investigations, *Int J Dent Hyg* 1(3):143, 2003.

65. Newman MG et al: Effectiveness of adjunctive irrigation in early periodontitis: multi-center evaluation, *J Periodontol* 65:224-229, 1994.

66. Ng VW, Bissada NF: Clinical evaluation of systemic doxycycline and ibuprofen administration as an adjunctive treatment for adult periodontitis, *J Periodontol* 69:772-776, 1998.

67. O'Brien TP et al: Effect of a non-steroidal anti-inflammatory drug on tissue levels of immunoreactive prostaglandin E_2, immunoreactive leukotriene, and pain after periodontal surgery, *J Periodontol* 67:1307-1316, 1996.

68. Ower PC et al: The effects on chronic periodontitis of a subgingivally-placed redox agent in a slow release device, *J Clin Periodontol* 22:494-500, 1995.

69. Paquette D, Minsk L: A pharmacokinetic study of a locally delivered minocycline therapeutic system (MPTS), *J Clin Periodontol* 27(Suppl 1):27, 2000.

70. Paraskevas S: Agents for chemical plaque control, *Int J Dent Hyg* 3(4):162-178, 2005.

71. Pataro AL et al: Surface effects and desorption of tetracycline supramolecular complex on bovine dentine, *Biomaterials* 24(6): 1075-1080, 2003.

72. Pavicic M, van Winkelhoff A, de Graaff J: Synergistic effects between amoxicillin, metronidazole, and the hydroxymetabolite of metronidazole against *Actinobacillus actinomycetemcomitans*, *Antimicrob Agents Chemother* 35(5):961-966, 1991.

73. Pedrazzoli B, Williams M, Karring T: Comparative clinical and microbiological effects of topical subgingival application of metronidazole 25% dental gel and scaling in the treatment of adult periodontitis, *J Clin Periodontol* 19:715, 1992.

74. Polak SG et al: Minocycline-associated tooth discoloration in young adults, *JAMA* 254(20):2930-2932, 1985.

75. Pucher JJ, Daniel JC: The effects of chlorhexidine digluconate on human fibroblasts in vitro, *J Periodontol* 62:526-532, 1993.

76. Quirynen M et al: Topical antiseptic and antibiotics in the initial therapy of chronic periodontitis: microbiological aspects, *Periodontol 2000* 28:72-90, 2002.

77. Quirynen M et al: One stage full- versus partial-mouth disinfection in the treatment of chronic adult or generalized early-onset periodontitis: II—long-term impact on microbial load, *J Periodontol* 70:646-656, 1999.

78. Quirynen M et al: Full- versus partial-mouth disinfection in the treatment of periodontal infections: short-term clinical and microbiological observations, *J Dent Res* 74:1459-1467, 1995.

79. Radvar M, Pourtaghe N, Kinane DF: Comparison of 3 periodontal local antibiotic therapies in persistent periodontal pockets, *J Periodontol* 67:860-865, 1996.

80. Ross NM et al: Effect of rinsing time on antiplaque-antigingivitis efficacy of Listerine, *J Clin Periodontol* 20:279-81, 1993.

81. Ryder MI et al: Effects of smoking on local delivery of controlled-release doxycycline as compared to scaling and root planing, *J Clin Periodontol* 26:683-691, 1999.

82. Salman RA et al: Minocycline induced pigmentation of the oral cavity, *J Oral Med* 40(3):154-157, 1985.

83. Schlagenhauf U et al: Repeated subgingival oxygen irrigations in untreated periodontal patients, *J Clin Periodontol* 21:48-50, 1994.

84. Schmid E, Kornman KS, Tinanoff N: Changes of subgingival total colony-forming units and black pigmented bacteroides after a single irrigation of periodontal pockets with 1.64% SnF$_2$, *J Periodontol* 56:330-333, 1985.

85. Stabholz A et al: Clinical and antimicrobial effects of a single episode of subgingival irrigation with tetracycline HCl or chlorhexidine in deep periodontal pockets, *J Clin Periodontol* 25:794-800, 1998.

86. Stratton CW, Lorian V: Mechanisms of action of antimicrobial agents: general principles and mechanisms for selected classes of antibiotics. In *Antibiotics in laboratory medicine*, ed 5, Baltimore, 2005, Williams & Wilkins. 532-564.

87. Suzuki N et al: Real-time TaqMan PCR for quantifying oral bacteria during biofilm formation, *J Clin Microbiol* 42(8):3827-3830, 2004.

88. Thomas J, Walker C, Bradshaw M: Long-term use of subantimicrobial dose doxycycline does not lead to changes in antimicrobial susceptibility, *J Periodontol* 71:1472-1483, 2000.

89. Tomasz A: Multiple antibiotic resistant pathogenic bacteria, *N Engl J Med* 330(17):1247-1251, 1994.

90. US Food and Drug Administration, Center for Drug Evaluation and Research: *Guidance for industry—gingivitis: development and evaluation of drugs for treatment or prevention*, June 2005. Available at: http://www.fda.gov/cder/guidance/5146dft.htm.

91. van Steenberghe D et al: A 15-month evaluation of the effects of repeated subgingival minocycline in chronic adult periodontitis, *J Periodontol* 70:657-667, 1999.

92. van Steenberghe D et al: Subgingival minocycline hydrochloride ointment in moderate to severe chronic adult periodontitis: a randomized, double-blind, vehicle controlled, multicenter study, *J Periodotol* 64:637-644, 1993.

93. Van Winkelhoff AJ, Rams TE, Slots J: Systemic antibiotic therapy in periodontics, *Periodontol 2000* 10:45-78, 1996.

94. Vernillo AT et al: The nonantimicrobial properties of tetracycline for the treatment of periodontal disease, *Curr Opin Periodontol* 2:111-118, 1994.

95. Walker C et al: Effect of subantimicrobial dose doxycycline (SDD) on intestinal and vaginal flora, *J Dent Res* 79:608, 2000.

96. Walker CB et al: A role for antibiotics in the treatment of refractory periodontitis, *J Periodontol* 64(8 suppl):772-781, 1993.

97. Walker CB, Karpinia K, Baehni P: Chemotherapeutics: antibiotics and other antimicrobials, *Periodontol 2000* 36:146, 2004.

98. Williams RC et al: Treatment of periodontitis by local administration of minocycline microspheres: a controlled trial, *J Periodontol* 72:1535-1544, 2001.

99. Williams RC, Paquette DW: Periodontal disease diagnosis and treatment: an exciting future, *J Dent Educ* 62(10):871-881, 1998.

Sealants

Colleen Schmidt

INSIGHT

Dental caries is considered an infectious, transmissible disease. The Centers for Disease Control and Prevention report that dental caries is possibly the most prevalent infectious disease in American children. Dental caries is five times more common than asthma and seven times more common than hay fever in children.[136] The need to assess and recognize dental caries at its earliest stage is critical in preventing future restorative treatment. The dental hygienist is a specialist in preventing oral diseases and is in a primary role to assess a patient's risk for dental caries. The dental hygienist can recommend specific strategies, including the placement of dental sealants, to promote dental health.

CASE STUDY 28-1 · Pediatric Considerations for Sealant Application

Meghan Kopel, 6 years of age, comes into the office for routine cleaning and examination. The clinical evaluation reveals that all four first molars are partially erupted. Brown stain is evident in the mandibular molar fissures, but no explorer resistance or enamel opacity is evident in any of the four permanent molars. The radiographic examination reveals no incipient interproximal decay and sound tooth surfaces. The patient has not had restorative treatment in any of her primary teeth. Her snacking habits consist of moderate amounts of sweets, including chocolate, licorice, and bubble gum. Her oral hygiene habits include brushing in the morning before school and at night, "when my mom reminds me." Meghan is very active, is easily distracted, cannot keep her hands still, and likes to talk a lot about her new puppy.

KEY TERMS

acid etching	curing	microleakage	polymerization
air abrasion	estrogenicity	monomers	retention
bis-GMA	filled resin	polymers	viscosity

LEARNING OUTCOMES

After reading this chapter the student will be able to:

1. Recognize that sealants are a primary preventive means of reducing the need for future restorative treatment.
2. Discuss the types and general properties of dental sealant materials, including potential estrogenicity.
3. Discuss the indications for using pit and fissure sealants.
4. List the criteria for selecting teeth for the placement of sealant materials.
5. Using and applying the dental caries risk assessment principles, assess a patient's dental caries risk, and determine the need for sealant placement.
6. Describe how sealant materials are retained in the pits and fissures of enamel surfaces.
7. Describe the appropriate application technique of sealant materials.
8. Describe the efficacy and cost-effectiveness of dental sealants.
9. Apply the principles of sealant placement to clinical dental hygiene experiences.
10. Cite three reasons for dental practitioners' underuse of sealants.

Dental sealants were introduced more than 35 years ago and have demonstrated success as a primary dental caries–preventive procedure.* A pit and fissure sealant is a resin material that is placed into the occlusal pits and fissures of dental caries–susceptible teeth.[118] Sealant materials are micromechanically bonded to the enamel surface, providing a protective barrier between the enamel pits and fissures (areas inaccessible to toothbrush bristles) and dental caries–producing bacteria.[118] Dental pit and fissure sealants have three primary preventive effects:

1. Provide a mechanical barrier in the pit and fissure of the tooth
2. Eliminate the environment that is conducive to *Streptococcus mutans*
3. Make the occlusal pit and fissure easier to clean by toothbrushing and mastication [13,105,112]

With appropriate and conscientious placement and maintenance, sealants have been highly effective in preventing new pit and fissure decay since their introduction in the late 1960s.† Sealants effectively eliminate sites of bacterial growth by modifying the environment by blocking the exposed areas of the occlusal surface. Research indicates that clinicians can approach 100% dental caries prevention in pits and fissures with repeated sealant application.‡

Other preventive measures (e.g., oral hygiene instructions, dietary analysis and modification, fluoride application) are still advocated in oral health promotion, and other treatment modalities are still necessary for tooth surfaces that are not protected by dental sealants. Dental sealants provide a simple and effective means to reduce the incidence of occlusal dental caries and increase the prevalence of healthful habits, which ultimately leads to improved quality of life.[6,144] Dental hygienists must be familiar with the scientific evidence regarding dental sealants to use them properly and to identify patients for whom the preventive procedure is appropriate.

> ### Prevention
>
> As part of a comprehensive preventive dental caries program, sealants may reduce the incidence of new pit and fissure decay, as well as the need for future restorative treatment, provided the sealant material is retained.

Dental Caries and Risk Assessment

The decline in the rate of dental caries assessed in the general population can be directly related to the availability and efficacy of fluoride. However, fluoride is most efficacious on smooth tooth surfaces, leaving occlusal pits and fissures at high risk for dental disease.

"Changes in the distribution of caries in economically developed nations over the last 15-20 years include:

• An overall decline in prevalence and severity in child populations

• An increasingly skewed distribution, with most disease now found in a small number of children

• Concentration of caries in pit and fissure lesions"[20]

Some of the reasons for the decrease in the rate of dental decay in the American population is due, in part, to the increased availability of fluoride, improved dental materials, greater emphasis on oral health, and the rising expectations of patients in maintaining a healthy and functional dentition. Unfortunately, access to preventive dental services and early disease detection is still not accessible to all Americans.[32,36,78]

Numerous epidemiologic studies have evaluated the role of dental sealants in the declining rate of dental decay.[103-104,119-120,122] Before placing sealants, the dental clinician must assess the patient's risk for dental caries and complete a thorough dental caries–detection examination.

Effective management of dental caries includes developing specific risk assessment strategies. Recently, the American Academy of Pediatric Dentistry (AAPD) developed a dental caries–risk assessment tool that provides a framework for classifying dental caries risk (high, moderate, low) by patient age, as well as by environmental, physical, and general health factors.[2] Anyone who uses a risk assessment tool must recognize the balance that exists between the pathologic factors (cariogenic bacteria, fermentable carbohydrates, salivary dysfunction) and protective factors (saliva, fluoride, antibacterial agents) in the oral cavity. Additionally, using a dental–caries risk assessment tool is not equivalent to, nor is it a substitute for, a comprehensive dental caries diagnosis. Published literature supports that all individuals possess specific characteristics that either place them at higher risk for disease or decrease their potential for disease activity. Once a patient's specific disease risks are assessed, the clinician and patient can make informed decisions regarding the preventive and treatment measures that should be used in preventing or managing carious lesions.

> ### Prevention
>
> A dental–caries risk assessment tool assists clinicians in identifying patients who may benefit the most from preventive measures before the onset of dental caries.[2,11]

Action and Effectiveness of Sealants

Fluorides, both systemic and topical, increase enamel resistance to dental decay. However, pits and fissures do not benefit from the effects of fluoride to the degree that smooth enamel surfaces do. Dental pit and fissure sealants are an effective preventive measure for these surfaces because they provide a physical barrier from the oral environment by sealing the dental caries–susceptible pits and fissures. This barrier prevents oral bacteria and their nutrients from creating an environment that is conducive to the initiation of carious lesions. Because of the occlusal anatomy of posterior teeth and resultant topographic concavities, acid-producing microorganisms accumulate with the potential to demineralize untreated enamel (Figure 28-1). Application of a liquid resin to these dental caries–susceptible zones fills the areas not cleansed by toothbrushing. Clinical

---

*References 3, 4, 29, 85, 105, 120, 122.
†References 51, 56-57, 108-109, 130.
‡References 8, 47, 63, 120, 122, 140.

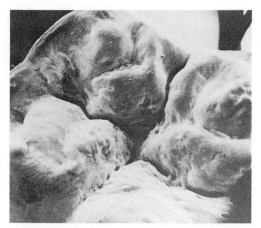

FIGURE 28-1
Scanning electron micrograph of occlusal pits and fissures.

research studies provide sufficient evidence of sealant efficacy when the pits and fissures of posterior teeth remain completely sealed.* In fact, dental caries protection approaches 100% by using pit and fissure resin sealants.[140]

The success of resin sealants depends on retaining the material in the enamel surface. For resin sealants to be mechanically retained within the pit and fissure, the enamel surface requires pretreatment with a 37% phosphoric acid etchant (Figure 28-2). Dr. Michael Buonocore developed the system of **acid etching** in the 1950s.[118] Focusing on the *bonding* of materials to enamel, Buonocore discovered that the enamel surface could be sufficiently roughened by the application of a phosphoric acid solution, which enhanced the **retention** of the applied dental material.[56] Acid etching chemically removes the contaminants found on the surface of enamel by creating an irregular enamel surface of microporosities. In addition, acid etching prepares the enamel surface by decalcifying portions of the rods in the enamel.[13] These porosities provide a surface for the resin material to adhere through the formation of resin tags. When the enamel surface is prepared in this manner, a low-

viscosity resin sealant material can flow more easily into the pit and fissures of the tooth because the enamel pores have been enlarged or opened by the acidic conditioning agent.

The resin sealant must have contact with or be bonded within the pit and fissures of the tooth during placement. *Mechanical bonding* results when the material becomes physically entrapped within the widened enamel pores. Provided the area conditioned with the acid is subsequently covered with the resin sealant, the tooth surface will remineralize. Once the tooth is re-exposed to the minerals naturally found in saliva, the tooth surface structure is replenished.

Two factors must be taken into consideration regarding sealant placement. First, if the resin cannot contact the base of the fissure, no bonding occurs to that specific area. Second, because of the inability to access the base of the fissure completely during the cleansing procedure, theories suggest that dental caries may develop apical to the sealant in the depths of the occlusal fissure (Figures 28-3 and 28-4). However, many clinical investigations have shown that resin pit and fissure sealants can be safely placed over early carious lesions and have demonstrated no progression

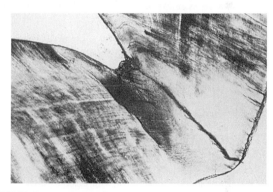

FIGURE 28-3
Scanning electron micrograph of wide V-shaped fissure.

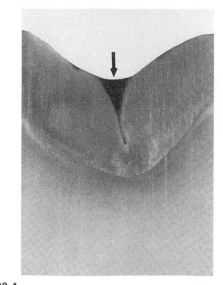

FIGURE 28-4
Scanning electron micrograph of penetration of resin sealant into occlusal fissure.

---

*References 39, 60, 86, 100, 120, 121, 140.

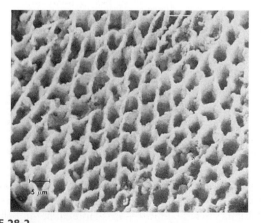

FIGURE 28-2
Scanning electron micrograph of etched enamel surface following acid conditioning.

of the early lesion.* Last, the **viscosity** of the resin sealant and the width of the enamel fissure affect the ability of the resin to penetrate to the depth of the fissure itself.

Routine clinical evaluations are necessary to determine whether resealing of teeth is necessary in cases of sealant loss caused by poor retention. Sealant retention reflects the sensitive nature of the application technique; the primary reason for inadequate sealant retention is often the result of salivary contamination during the application technique. Any form or amount of moisture contamination can influence the overall effectiveness and resultant use of a sealant intraorally, which diminishes its overall benefit to the patient. Rubber dam isolation is the most thorough means of isolating tooth surfaces to be sealed. Dental sealants placed by using cotton roll isolation and adequate evacuation has also been successful. Research has demonstrated that saliva reduces the strength of the bond between the etched enamel surface and the resin sealant.†

Additional factors that contribute to retaining dental sealants included the eruption status of teeth, the pit and fissure shape, the type of tooth and surface anatomy, the clinical setting, the clinician's level of experience, the age of the patient, and the type of sealant material.[44,70,117,132] The effectiveness of dental sealants has been scientifically proved, provided that the fissure remains sealed. In reviewing the data regarding sealant placement and retention, annual sealant loss was between 5% and 10%.[101] Dental manufacturers are continually improving the materials used for sealant placement and continue to simplify the application techniques to reduce the potential for sealant failure. Today, various materials from which to choose are available based on their composition, viscosity, type of **curing,** and color.

★ CASE APPLICATION 28-1.1

Identification of Dental Sealant Need

Refer to Case Study 28-1 while reading this section. Identify the indications for sealant placement that correspond with Meghan's case.

28-1 **INDICATIONS FOR DENTAL SEALANT PLACEMENT**

Three major factors must be considered before placing dental sealants (Box 28-1). First, the clinician must assess the anatomy of the tooth (Figure 28-5); deep occlusal fissures, fossa, cingula,

*References 64, 66, 86-90.
†References 15, 40-41, 131, 135.

BOX 28-1

FACTORS IN SEALANT PLACEMENT

Tooth anatomy
Location
Contours, depth, and irregularity of pits and fissures
Age of tooth
Tooth's proximity to other restorations
Future dental caries risk
Eruption patterns

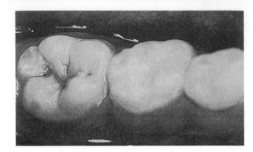

FIGURE 28-5
Fully erupted permanent first molar. (From Ryan JP: The clinical benefits of dental sealants, *J Pract Hyg* 6:13-17, 1997.)

and pits are ideal surfaces on which to place sealant materials. Second, with regard to tooth selection, the clinician must evaluate the following:

- Location
- Contours of the pits and fissures
- Depth and irregularity of the pits and fissures
- Age of the tooth
- Presence of interproximal decay
- Proximity to a restoration

Each patient's conditions should be evaluated for risk of future dental caries. These risk factors may predispose an identified tooth for future dental caries or for sealant placement challenges. If a restoration exists on an adjacent tooth, the tooth assessed for sealant placement may then already be at even greater

dental caries risk and may not benefit from the sealant. Third, in evaluating a mixed dentition, the clinician should be aware of the progression of dental eruption and should note the position of teeth for ease of access during sealant placement.

Patient population groups that benefit from the placement of dental sealants because of their intraoral status include the following:

- Children with newly erupted teeth with pits, fissures, or lingual pits
- Children whose lifestyle, developmental, or behavioral patterns or lack of fluoride exposure make them susceptible to occlusal or lingual caries

- Individuals with reduced salivary flow
- Other persons who desire sealant application and for whom sealant therapy is indicated and technically feasible*

The clinician must also assess the anatomy of the pit and fissures, the patients' future dental caries risk, dietary patterns, current and past exposure to fluoride, and ability to cooperate during the proposed treatment.

Sealants are most frequently indicated for children as a primary preventive measure to protect susceptible enamel surfaces before they have the opportunity to decay. Dental sealants are most frequently applied to molars and premolars of the permanent dentition; however, lingual pits located on the lingual surfaces of maxillary central and lateral incisors may be appropriate sites for sealant placement. Additionally, the margins of both amalgam and composite restorations require reassessment at each supportive care appointment. Because these areas are susceptible sites for recurrent dental caries, sealing of these restorative margins may improve marginal integrity.†

CONTRAINDICATIONS TO PLACEMENT

Contraindications to sealant placement include the following:
- Patients with clinically evident dental caries
- Proximal decay
- Insufficiently erupted teeth
- Enamel that is coalesced (fused), resulting in shallow or nonexistent fissures
- Primary teeth that are soon to be exfoliated
- Possibly patients with challenging behavioral characteristics that may make sealant placement difficult, decreasing the chances of long-term sealant retention

The patient's cooperation during the sealant placement procedure is critical because proper placement and maintenance of sealants requires a well-isolated, dry field.

With radiographic evidence of interproximal dental caries or in cases of self-cleaning pits and fissures, seal-ant placement provides no additional patient benefit. Dental professionals and the public should not view dental pit and fissure sealants as a substitute for other dental caries–control measures such as proper oral hygiene and diet. Pit and fissure sealants are an additional component to the patient's overall preventive oral self-care habits.

Sealant Composition and Types

Dental sealants are comparable in constitution with composite resins that are composed of dimethacrylate monomers, either bisphenol A-glycidyl methacrylate (**bis-GMA**) or urethane dimethacrylate (UDMA). Dental sealants are composed of polyurethane, cyanoacrylates, resin (filled or unfilled), and bis-GMA.[43,98,105,126] Sealant materials may also contain glass ionomer, resin-modified glass ionomer, fluoride, and color.*

Most commercial sealants are bis-GMA, in which **polymerization** is accelerated by light or another chemical compound.[25,27] Through the process of polymerization, **monomers** found in sealant resin become cross-linked **polymers,** adding strength to the material.

Sealant materials are polymerized by one of two mechanisms: (1) chemical activation (self-cure) or (2) light activation (light-cure). Chemical polymerization involves the mixing of an initiator and an accelerator (also known as a base and a catalyst, respectively), often referred to as a *two-component system*. The final setting of the material occurs within approximately 2 minutes following mixture of the initiator and the accelerator. One disadvantage of chemical polymerization is a result of mixing the chemicals; the potential exists for incorporating air bubbles into the mixture that may limit the retention of the sealant on the tooth surface. The light-cured system is referred to as a *one-component system* in which the chemical is polymerized by a 20-second application of visible light to each area under the coverage of the light source on each tooth.

Most sealant materials contain up to 50% inorganic filler to improve the material's durability[25,27] (Box 28-2). Fillers are often added to sealant materials to make them more resistant to occlusal wear.[123] "Unfilled sealant will abrade rapidly, probably within 24 to 48 hours, if it is left in occlusion with an opposing cusp tip. Filled sealant, however, will require occlusal adjustment included as a routine part of the application procedure, which not only increases the time and cost of the procedure,

---

*References 8, 9, 26, 35, 42, 45, 62, 68, 71, 74, 82-84, 93, 97, 106, 119, 145.

BOX 28-2

CLASSIFICATION OF SEALANTS

Filled
Unfilled
Fluoride-releasing
Autopolymerized
Photopolymerized (light polymerized)

---

*References 16, 18, 19, 29, 51, 109, 114, 125, 146.
†References 16, 30-31, 69, 86-91, 102.

but also may not allow all [allied dental professionals] who can apply sealant, to carry out the occlusal adjustment."[133]

Because most sealant materials contain a small amount of filler, the material has reduced viscosity, which allows the material to flow into the pits and fissures of the occlusal surface with greater ease. This reduced viscosity also increases sealant retention as a result of greater penetration into the enamel porosities by creating resin tags within the enamel surface. Today, flowable composites that contain an increased concentration of filler are often used as dental sealants because they demonstrate improved resistance to occlusal wear while also demonstrating sufficient viscosity for the application into the pits and fissures of teeth.[10,33,38]

When handling resin sealant materials, clinicians must follow specific guidelines. The resin materials must not be exposed to air or light to prevent evaporation and maintain the proper fluidity of the material and its ability to penetrate into the enamel pores. For optimal pit and fissure sealant placement, the clinician must use fresh materials and a well-maintained armamentarium.

> ### *Note*
> The resin materials must not be exposed to air or light to prevent evaporation and maintain the proper fluidity of the material and its ability to penetrate into the enamel pores.

A variety of delivery systems are available to clinicians. With a *chemically cured system,* the clinician physically mixes the base and catalyst and then applies the mixture to the tooth surface. The resin cures, or hardens, as a result of the chemical reaction between the base and the catalyst. The *photopolymerized system* requires exposure to visible light to cure the material. Currently, a one-step delivery system is available in which a light-protected syringe tip has been preloaded with resin material, ready for direct application to the prepared tooth surface, followed by light activation (3M Dental Products, St. Paul, Minn.).

Dental manufacturers have developed sealant materials in a variety of colors (white, clear, pink, tooth colored). The application of color to the sealant makes identifying the placement, location, and retention of the sealant material on the tooth surface easier for the dental professional, and most patients prefer clear sealants for their esthetic value.

Armamentarium and Application

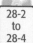

28-2 to 28-4

In preparation for placing a sealant on a tooth, a clinician must have the proper materials for the procedure (Box 28-3 and Figures 28-6 through 28-8).

The most important aspect of sealant placement procedures is appropriate and adequate isolation equipment and techniques. Adequate preparation before the patient appointment ensures efficiency and effectiveness during the procedure. Although many different sealant materials are available through various manufacturers, the steps involved in sealant application are similar (Box 28-4).

APPLICATION TECHNIQUE

1. Cleanse the *tooth surfaces* of hard and soft debris with a pumice and water paste with a prophylactic brush on a

---

BOX 28-3

ARMAMENTARIUM FOR SEALANT APPLICATION

Acid etchant	Gauze
Air/water syringe tip	High-volume suction
Articulating paper	Light-curing unit
Brush applicator	Light shield
Cotton pliers	Liquid resin
Cotton rolls	Rubber dam, including armamentarium (optional)
Explorer (Shepherd's hook)	

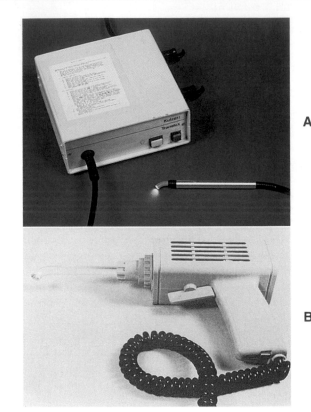

A

B

FIGURE 28-6
A, Visible white light wand. **B,** Visible white light.

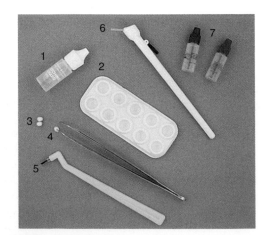

FIGURE 28-7
Armamentarium for sealant application: acid etchant *(1)*, dappen dish *(2)*, cotton pellets *(3)*, cotton pliers *(4)*, brush *(5)*, sealant applicator *(6)*, and sealant materials *(7;* base and catalyst).

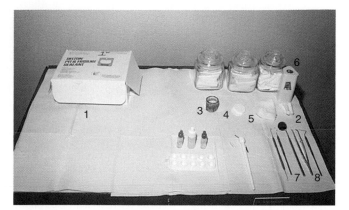

FIGURE 28-8
Armamentarium for sealant application and evaluation: pit and fissure sealant kit *(1)*, cotton rolls *(2)*, pumice *(3)*, dry angles *(4)*, cotton gauze *(5)*, floss *(6)*, mirror *(7)*, explorer *(8)*.

BOX 28-4

APPLICATION TECHNIQUE FOR DENTAL SEALANT

1. Tooth surfaces cleansed
2. Tooth isolated
3. Surfaces dried and etched
4. Acid washed away and surfaces dried
5. Sealant applied according to manufacturer's instructions
6. Sealant properly cured for polymerization
7. Sealant examined for appropriate placement
8. Patient evaluated for finishing and sealant bonding
9. Topical fluoride applied

Distinct Care Modifications

When working with children, organize and prepare all materials before bringing the patient back to the operatory.

Distinct Care Modifications

Tell, show, do. Patients, including children, are put at ease if they have an idea of what they are about to experience. Show them the items that will be used to place the sealant. Eliminate surprises that may startle them or make them nervous.

slow-speed hand piece or with an air polisher.* When the tooth is cleansed with an air polisher, the mechanical interlocking of the resin to the enamel surface improves with increased retention of the sealant material.[16,17] The cleansing agent should be rinsed from the tooth surface with water and high-speed evacuation. Previous thinking held that fluoride application before sealant placement would inhibit sealant retention.[43] However, recent research illustrates that exposure to fluoride before sealant placement has no effect on the effective bond strength between the enamel and the filled or unfilled sealant material.[72,73,139] Knowing this concept is beneficial in that sealant placement might occur within the same appointment as prophylactic dental hygiene procedures.

*References 17, 28, 77, 113, 118, 138.

2. Properly *isolate the tooth* to prevent any moisture contamination. The clinician may use triangular cotton isolation over the parotid papilla, known as *Driangles* (Dental Health Products, Youngstown, N.Y.), cotton rolls held with a metal clamp, or cotton roll holders and suction. Isolation may require placement of a rubber dam for application to multiple teeth in a quadrant or in situations in which other isolation techniques may not be useful (Figure 28-9).

3. Apply the *phosphoric acid* (30% to 50%, typically 37%) *enamel conditioner*, covering all areas of the enamel surface to be sealed (Figure 28-10). Apply the etchant for 20 to 60 seconds with a brush-tipped applicator or a cotton pellet, and then thoroughly rinse with water using high-speed evacuation (Figure 28-11). In a 3-year follow-up study of sealants that were placed following a 20-second etch, the retention rates were comparable with those placed following a 60-second etch.[37] This conclusion is supported by additional research stating that "the different etching times do not appear to affect the retention of fissure sealants."[34] Avoiding contact between the acid and oral mucosal tissues is important because contact may cause tissue discomfort and sloughing. The conditioning process may need to be repeated if an area of the tooth becomes contaminated with water or saliva on drying. In this case, repeat the

Distinct Care Modifications

If a dental assistant is available, ask him or her to help facilitate procedures and to ensure proper isolation techniques.

Prevention

Rubber dam isolation is often advised in applying dental sealants to prevent accidental swallowing of any dental material and to prevent salivary contamination.

Distinct Care Modifications

When placing dental sealants on children, using a rubber dam may not be practical. In these cases, using Driangles, cotton rolls, and cotton roll holders aids in properly isolating the tooth for sealant placement.

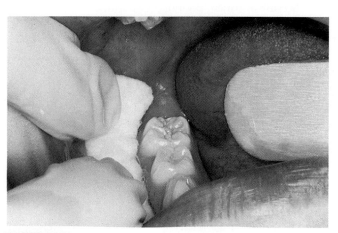

FIGURE 28-9
Isolate cleansed tooth with cotton roll and tongue depressor. (From Ryan JP: The clinical benefits of dental sealants, *J Pract Hyg* 6:13-17, 1997.)

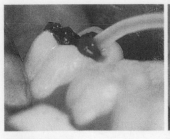

FIGURE 28-10
Apply acid etchant to enamel surface. (From Ryan JP: The clinical benefits of dental sealants, *J Pract Hyg* 6:13-17, 1997.)

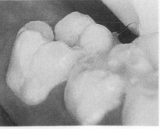

FIGURE 28-11
Rinse and dry etched surfaces. (From Ryan JP: The clinical benefits of dental sealants, *J Pract Hyg* 6:13-17, 1997.)

★ CASE APPLICATION 28-1.2

Patient's Movement Results in Etchant Burn

During the chairside application of the dental sealant, Meghan accidentally waves her arm upward just as the acid etchant is being moved to the mouth to the prepared and isolated tooth surfaces. This arm motion results in spilling a small amount of etchant on Meghan's right arm, causing a slight burn on her skin. How should this situation be handled?

---

conditioning process for 10 seconds, and completely dry the reconditioned surface or surfaces.

4. Evaluate the *tooth surfaces* for a frosty, white appearance of the areas to be sealed. This appearance ensures that the enamel fissures have been opened and made available to the sealant material (Figure 28-12). Again, take precautions to avoid salivary contamination of the conditioned surface.

5. Apply the *sealant material* according to the manufacturer's directions (Figure 28-13). Concentrate the sealant material in the central pit and fissure, and trace the resin material with an explorer to encourage flow into the prepared fissures. Even coverage on the maxillary molars is difficult because of patient positioning and the resultant mesial to

> ### Note
> Keep the patient interested and calm during the procedure by introducing each step and describing what you will be doing. Continue talking with the patient during the procedure.

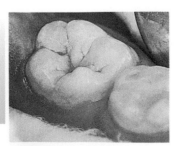

FIGURE 28-12
Thoroughly dry surface until frosty white. (From Ryan JP: The clinical benefits of dental sealants, *J Pract Hyg* 6:13-17, 1997.)

distal flow of the material. Care should be taken to avoid flowing the material into the contact area.

6. Ensure *proper sealant curing.* Polymerization of the sealant occurs through either light or chemical curing (Figure 28-14). If a light-cured material is being used, then the visible light must be correctly placed over the material and exposed for the required time (refer to manufacturer's instructions). The placement and timing of the light source must be properly maintained for successful material curing. The effectiveness of the light source diminishes once materials begin to accumulate on the light wand (see Figure 28-6). Both the patient and the clinician require protection from the intensity of the curing light. The sealant must not be disturbed until polymerization is complete. If a material requiring chemical polymerization is used, following the manufacturer's directions is imperative for proper and complete manipulation of the materials. The sealant must remain undisturbed until the polymerization process is complete, whether this is a result of chemical or light polymerization. Once the sealant has been light or chemically cured, wipe the surface with a wet cotton roll to remove the oxygen-inhibited layer of unpolymerized resin; this process also prevents an unpleasant taste.

7. Examine the *sealant* with an explorer for voids, undercuring, and proper extension into pits and fissures. With the explorer, attempt gentle removal of the sealant to determine whether an adequate bond exists be-

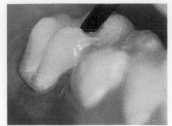

FIGURE 28-13
Apply sealant to conditioned surface. Overmanipulation of the resin material can lead to entrapment of air bubbles, leading to decreased material retention and voids on the sealant surface. (From Ryan JP: The clinical benefits of dental sealants, *J Pract Hyg* 6:13-17, 1997.)

> ### Prevention
> Be advised to avoid placing too much resin material into the central groove of a posterior tooth. Placing excessive material may result in significant postapplication adjustments but may also lead to overfill into the adjacent interproximal space. Place a small amount of resin into the central groove, and use an explorer to guide the resin into the adjacent pits and fissures. Interproximal areas should be flossed after sealant placement to confirm absence of sealant material.

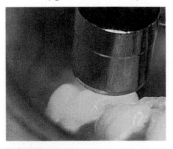

FIGURE 28-14
Polymerize with visible white light for the manufacturer's recommended exposure time. (From Ryan JP: The clinical benefits of dental sealants, *J Pract Hyg* 6:13-17, 1997.)

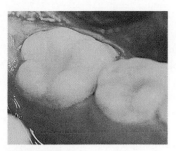

FIGURE 28-15
Occlusal sealant in place. Rinse thoroughly, evaluate occlusion, and assess interproximal areas with floss. (From Ryan JP: The clinical benefits of dental sealants, *J Pract Hyg* 6:13-17, 1997.)

tween the sealant and the tooth.

8. Evaluate the *patient's occlusion* with articulating paper, and smooth out any high areas with a finishing bur or a fine stone. Areas of high sealant material are often removed during masticatory action.[133] Evaluate the interproximal space to ensure the resin has not closed it. Any unnecessary resin material may require removal with a scaler (Figure 28-15).

9. Administer a *neutral sodium fluoride treatment* to ensure remineralization of the previously etched tooth surfaces before patient dismissal.

FISSURE PREPARATION AND ENAMELOPLASTY

Because reaching the base of a pit or fissure is impossible for the resin sealant material as a result of the presence of debris and trapped air owing to the anatomy of the pit or fissure, opening the fissure with a small-diameter bur is often helpful and necessary. This step removes any areas of potential decay with minimal removal of enamel and improves the penetration of the sealant material into the enamel porosities. This procedure is often referred to as an *enameloplasty* because removal of enamel surface is minimal and is a fissure-preparation procedure.[49,79,147,148]

Retention, Wear, and Replacement

Adequate retention in conjunction with the application technique is the principal predictor of dental sealant success.[22] Retention rates 1 year after application are 85% or greater and after 5 years are at least 50%.[61,120,122] Short-term sealant loss is often a result of technical application error rather than inadequate mechanical bonding.[14,24,122,140] The inability to maintain a dry field is the most frequent cause of sealant failure; therefore sealants often cannot be placed on the surfaces where they would be of most benefit.[48] Poor isolation and improper acid etching contribute to short-term sealant loss.[24] The majority of sealant materials used today are composed of the monomer bis-GMA, with titanium dioxide added to improve clinical identification and assessment.[122]

The two major factors affecting sealant durability are filler content and glass-ionomer content. A significant number of studies have confirmed that unfilled resin sealant materials are as effective as **filled resin** sealants.[45,68,93]

Two advantages of glass ionomer materials include:

- The ability to adhere chemically to the tooth surface
- The ability to release fluoride[50,105]

Theoretically, fluoride is incorporated into the surrounding tooth structure to prevent and arrest dental caries. Studies have shown the greatest fluoride release occurs 24 hours after application and steadily decreases with time.[105,106,115,127] Fluoride release from glass-ionomer materials inhibits both dentinal and recurrent marginal caries,[62] although it may not be the primary factor in dental caries prevention within enamel pits and fissures.[9] Other investigators state the dental caries–preventive effect of glass-ionomer sealant depends on both sealant retention and fluoride release.[74]

Again, retention is the prime determinant of dental sealant success.[104] The bond between the sealant and the enamel surface prevents significant marginal leakage.[104] Application of acid etchant before sealant placement enhances mechanical retention of sealants. Proper acid-etch bonding produces a mechanical bond strong enough to retain restorations, orthodontic brackets, bridges, and sealants.[98] This mechanical bond is unlikely to fail if the materials have been properly applied. Poor retention and excessive wear are frequently cited reasons for the current limited use of pit and fissure sealants.[99]

Fissure penetration is a result of both capillary action and the viscosity of the sealant material. If the site is well cleansed, etched, rinsed, and dried, then the acrylic monomers such as bis-GMA tend to wet, or spread, across the enamel surface. Sealant penetration only into the neck region (top opening) of the fissure has also shown clinically acceptable results; therefore complete fissure penetration is not critical.[25,27]

Evaluating the retention and effectiveness of sealants, researchers reported clinical success after one application.[122] Of all sealants placed, 27% were completely retained after 15 years and 35% partially retained. Of unsealed teeth surfaces, 82% became carious and 31% exhibited signs of decay. The author concluded that if sealants were reapplied when appropriate, 100% cavity protection might be realized.[92,140] Another researcher developed a similar conclusion provided teeth remain completely sealed. Typical sealant retention rates have been reported to be 60% at 2 years and 42% at 5 years.[103] After sealant placement, the rate of dental decay can be reduced by 80% after 1 year and 70% after 2 years. The decreased rate is a result of progressive loss of material over time.[103] Researchers have proposed that, if a sealant could endure 30 months of use, then progressive change was unlikely while the sealant continued to provide sufficient fissure protection from bacterial invasion.[99]

Other investigators report that most sealant losses occur shortly after placement, with the greatest loss and wear during the first 6 months after application.[9,56,69] Controversy has ensued regarding the clinical relevance of the observed volume of sealant loss. If anatomically critical areas remain safely obturated, then the amount of material loss may not be critical.[99]

The effectiveness of sealants improves when lost or partially lost sealants are repaired or replaced at subsequent visits. Therefore, with regularly scheduled maintenance appointments, clinicians should use explorers to examine the margins of sealants to determine whether the bond strength is still adequate or whether the sealant should be partially or completely replaced.[108,141-143]

Wear is a natural process resulting from movement between surfaces, which creates a damaged layer and subsequent loss of material.[12,80] Information is limited on the wear resistance of sealant materials.[8,24,76,133] Air polishing used during regular prophylaxis has been shown to increase the amount of wear of resin sealants.[65] Air polishing can also create resin surface roughness, leading to future material breakdown. The amount of wear increases with the longer time and exposure to **air abrasion.**[65] If replacement of sealant materials becomes necessary because of inadequate bond strength or wear, then any residual sealant material should be removed if possible, the tooth cleansed and re-etched, and a new resin placed and cured. Sealants have minimal to no filler particle; therefore these materials will wear faster and are subject to wear from occlusion. Wear is typically not a concern, provided that the sealant remains intact. If only part of the fissure is evident, then the sealant should be replaced.

Cost-Effectiveness

The cost savings and benefits of dental sealants has been questioned.[67,118] Given the overall decline in the dental caries rate in the United States, the cost of providing sealants to all teeth in all children exceeds the cost of providing restorative treatment.[67] As a result, a dental sealant is recommended to prevent overtreatment by targeting preventive resources to individuals at high risk for decay.[21,67,121,129] Sealant retention is the issue that is critical in determining the cost-effectiveness of the preventive procedure. Although carefully placed sealants are effective in preventing decay in occlusal pits and fissures, the cost-effectiveness of sealants is still questioned.

Potential Estrogenicity

Pit and fissure sealants and traditional composite materials have been based on bis-GMA or bis-GMA–like monomers. Sealants and composites may contain unpolymerized or only partially polymerized monomers. Under laboratory research conditions, leachable components such as bisphenol A (BPA) from the unpolymerized monomers of resin sealant materials have mimicked the naturally occurring female hormone estrogen.[94-96] Small amounts of unreacted monomer may remain within cured materials because light curing of plastic materials is inhibited by

oxygen. Therefore the oxygen-inhibited layer often present on the sealant surface may contain unreacted monomers. Unreacted monomer may be able to diffuse out of the restoration into either dentin or saliva. The biological acceptability of these unpolymerized materials has been studied.[54,94-96] Data suggest that BPA may be released from the resin matrix of sealants and composites.[95] This data might lead the clinician to question the safety of resin materials because of possible systemic absorption and carcinogenic properties (**estrogenicity**).[111]

Given this data in the 1990s, it is currently unclear what type of relationship exists between the elution of unpolymerized monomers from dental materials and their potential absorption into the bloodstream and whether this might result in any physiologic concerns. Evidence to suggest that the low concentration of inactivated monomers found in resin sealants poses a direct risk to dental patients is currently insufficient.[13] With negligible clinical evidence on the estrogenicity of these materials, the current standards for sealant placement seem appropriate. The indications for the continued clinical application of these materials should be encouraged. Recent research indicates that the chemical components of resin materials may not be absorbed or that they are present in nondetectable levels in the blood.[1,75,137] Investigators have suggested that dental professionals take precautions to prevent a patient's exposure to uncured resin following sealant placement, including removing the oxygen-inhibited layer of sealants following sealant polymerization.[1,12,46,110,126]

Preventing Restorative Microleakage

In addition to preventing dental caries in the pits and fissures of posterior teeth, sealants also protect the margins of dental restorations.[5,81,88,89] Marginal **microleakage** of dental composites is a potential concern because of material contraction during visible-light polymerization or debonding during tooth flexure or *in situ* occlusal loading. These gaps not only contribute to potential microleakage, but they also may result in marginal staining, recurrent decay, tooth sensitivity, and pulpal disease.[134] Clinical researchers have investigated the potential use of unfilled resins in reducing marginal microleakage.* Researchers observed that sealed composite restorations were clinically superior to unsealed restorations in their ability to maintain marginal integrity.[30]

Conclusion

The sealing of pits and fissures is an evidence-based preventive procedure that reduces the prevalence of dental caries.[101] Sealants serve to block biofilm accumulation by filling the occlusal anatomy. The presence of the sealant material also results in more effective toothbrushing. The reported numbers of children receiving sealants has increased over two decades. In 1995,

---

*References 5, 30, 81, 88-89.

10% to 15% of children ages 6 to 17 had received dental sealants[23,53]; whereas 32% of children ages 6 to 19 had received dental sealants by 2002.[136] Although reports indicate an increase in sealant placement, many underserved individuals have still not received this effective treatment to prevent dental caries in pits and fissures. Some of the reasons for irregularity of use include the following:

- Lack of insurance coverage for placement and maintenance
- Difficulty of the placement technique
- Concern that undetected dental caries would be sealed
- Maintenance and repair required for continued effectiveness
- Concern that sealants are not cost-effective[59,101,107,116]

Preventive dental procedures before the manifestation or spread of disease can conserve tooth structure.[7,85,89,127] Studies on using sealants in alternative preventive and therapeutic applications have shown that restorations sealed with unfilled resin:

- Have less microleakage
- Arrest the progression of dental caries
- Preserve existing restorations
- Increase marginal integrity
- Preserve tooth structure[5,81,88,89]

Sealants are effective preventive materials when used simultaneously with amalgam and composite resin as surface sealants.[5,30,88,128] Clinical research has found that early carious lesions have been arrested up to 6 years after placement of sealants over composite resin and amalgam restorations.* Research regarding pit and fissure sealants has demonstrated that dental sealants are an effective measure in preventing dental decay, particularly with ongoing evaluation and appropriate reapplication.

References

1. Adair SM: The role of sealants in caries prevention programs, *J Calif Dent Assoc* 31(3):221-227, 2003.
2. American Academy of Pediatric Dentistry: *Policy on use of a caries-risk assessment tool (CAT) for infants, children, and adolescents, 2002.* Reference Manual 2004-2005, pp 25-27.
3. ADA Council on Access, Prevention, and Interprofessional Relations, Council on Scientific Affairs: Dental sealants, *J Am Dent Assoc* 128(4):485-488, 1997.
4. ADA Council on Access, Prevention, and Interprofessional Relations: Intervention: pit and fissure sealants, *J Am Dent Assoc* 126:17-S, 1995.
5. Anderson KN, Anderson LE: *Mosby's pocket dictionary of medicine,* ed 3, St Louis, 1998, Mosby.
6. Anderson MH: Modern management of dental caries: the cutting edge is not the dental bur, *J Am Dent Assoc* 124(6):36-44, 1993.
7. Anusavice KJ: Treatment regimens in preventive and restorative dentistry, *J Am Dent Assoc* 126:727-743, 1995.
8. Aranda M, Garcia-Godoy F: Clinical evaluation of the retention and wear of a light-cured pit and fissure glass ionomer sealant, *J Clin Pediatr Dent* 19(4):273-277, 1995.
9. Arrow P, Riordan PJ: Retention and caries preventive effects of a GIC and a resin-based fissure sealant, *Community Dent Oral Epidemiol* 23:282-285, 1995.
10. Autio-Gold JT: Clinical evaluation of medium-filled flowable restorative material as a pit and fissure sealant, *Oper Dent* 27:325-329, 2002.
11. Barber LR, Wilkins EM: Evidence-based prevention, management, and monitoring of dental caries, *J Dent Hyg* 76(4):270-275, 2002.
12. Bayne SC: Dental biomaterials: where are we and where are we going? *J Dent Educ* 69(5):571-585, 2005.
13. Bayne SC, Thompson JY: Dental materials. In Roberson TM, Heymann HO, Swift EJ, eds: *Sturdevant's art and science of operative dentistry,* ed 4, St Louis, 2001, Mosby.
14. Boksman L et al: A 2-year clinical evaluation of two pit-and-fissure sealants placed with and without the use of a bonding agent, *Quintessence Int* 24:131-133, 1993.
15. Borem LM, Feigal RJ: Reducing microleakage of sealants under salivary contamination: digital-image analysis evaluation, *Quintessence Int* 25:283-289, 1994.
16. Brocklehurst PR, Joshi RI, Northeast SE: The effect of air-polishing occlusal surfaces on the penetration of fissures by a sealant, *Int J Paediatr Dent* 56:97-102, 1992.
17. Brockmann SL, Scott RL, Eick JD: A scanning electron microscopic study of the effect of air polishing on the enamel-sealant surface, *Quintessence Int* 21(3):201-206, 1990.
18. Brown LJ et al: Dental caries and sealant usage in US children, 1988-1991: selected findings from the Third National Health and Nutrition Examination Survey, *J Am Dent Assoc* 127(3):335-343, 1996.
19. Brown LJ, Selwitz RH: The impact of recent changes in the epidemiology of dental caries on guidelines for the use of dental sealants, *J Public Health Dent* 55(5 spec):274-291, 1995.
20. Burt BA: Prevention policies in the light of the changed distribution of dental caries, *Acta Odontol Scand* 56:179-186, 1998.
21. Burt BA: Fissure sealants: clinical and economic factors, *J Dent Educ* 48:96-102, 1984.
22. Charbeneau GT, Dennison JB, Ryge G: A filled pit-and-fissure sealant: 18-month results, *J Am Dent Assoc* 95:299-306, 1977.
23. Cherry-Peppers G et al: Sealant use and dental utilization in US children, *ASDC J Dent Child* 62:250-255, 1995.
24. Conry JP, Pintado MR, Douglas WH: Quantitative changes in fissure sealant six months after placement, *Pediatr Dent* 12(3):162-167, 1990.
25. Craig RG, Powers JM: *Dental materials: properties and manipulation,* ed 6, St Louis, 1996, Mosby.
26. Craig RG, Powers JM, Wataha JC: *Dental materials: properties and manipulation,* ed 8, St Louis, 2004. Mosby.
27. Craig RG, Powers JM, Wataha JC: *Dental materials: properties and manipulation,* ed 7, St Louis, 2000, Mosby.
28. De Craene GP et al: A clinical evaluation of a light-cured fissure sealant (Helioseal), *ASDC J Dent Child* 56:97-102, 1989.
29. Dental sealants in the prevention of tooth decay, *NIH Consensus Statement* 4(11):1-18, 1983.
30. Dickinson GL et al: Effect of surface-penetrating sealant on wear rate of posterior composite resins, *J Am Dent Assoc* 121:251-255, 1990.
31. Dickinson GL, Leinfelder KF: Assessing the long-term effect of a surface-penetrating sealant, *J Am Dent Assoc* 124:68-72, 1993.
32. Donly KJ, Brown DJ: Identify, protect, restore: emerging issues in approaching children's oral health, *Gen Dent* 53(2):106-110, 2005.

*References 30, 31, 52, 55, 66, 87, 89.

33. Duangthip D, Lussi A: Variables contributing to the quality of fissure sealants used by general dental practitioners, *Oper Dent* 28(6):756-764, 2000.

34. Duggal MS et al: The effect of different etching times on the retention of fissure sealants in second primary and first permanent molars, *Int J Paediatr Dent* 7:81-86, 1997.

35. Duke ES: Pit-and-fissure sealant materials, *Compendium* 22(7):594-596, 2001.

36. Eccles MF: The problem of occlusal caries and its current management, *NZ Dent J* 85:50-55, 1989.

37. Eidelman E, Shapira J, Houpt MJ: The retention of fissure sealants using 20-second etching time: 3-year follow-up, *ASDC J Dent Child* 55:119-120, 1988.

38. Eronat N, Bardakci Y, Sipahi M: Effects of different preparation techniques on the microleakage of compomer and resin fissure sealants, *J Dent Child* 70(3):250-253, 2003.

39. Feigal RJ: The use of pit and fissure sealants, *Pediatr Dent* 24(5):415-422, 2002.

40. Feigal RJ et al: Improved sealant retention with bonding agents: a clinical study of two-bottle and single-bottle systems, *J Dent Res* 79:1850-1856, 2000.

41. Feigal RJ, Hitt J, Splieth C: Retaining sealant on salivary contaminated enamel, *J Am Dent Assoc* 124:88-97, 1993.

42. Ferracane JL: *Materials in dentistry, principles and applications,* ed 2, Philadelphia, 2001, Lippincott Williams & Wilkins.

43. Ferracane JL: *Materials in dentistry: principles and applications,* Philadelphia, 1995, Lippincott Williams & Wilkins.

44. Folke BD, Walton JL, Feigal RJ: Occlusal sealant success over ten years in a private practice: comparing longevity of sealants placed by dentists, hygienists, and assistants, *Pediatr Dent* 26(5):426-432, 2004.

45. Forss H, Saarni UM, Seppa L: Comparison of glass-ionomer and resin-based fissure sealants: a 2-year clinical trial, *Community Dent Oral Epidemiol* 22:21-24, 1994.

46. Fung EY et al: Pharmacokinetics of bisphenol A released from a dental sealant, *J Am Dent Assoc* 131:51-58, 2000.

47. Futatsuki M et al: Early loss of pit and fissure sealant: a clinical and SEM study, *J Clin Pediatr Dent* 19(2):99-104, 1995.

48. Ganss C, Klimek J, Gleim A: One-year clinical evaluation of the retention and quality of two fluoride releasing sealants, *Clin Oral Investig* 3:188-193, 1999.

49. Garcia-Godoy F, de Araujo FB: Enhancement of fissure sealant penetration and adaptation: the enameloplasty technique, *J Clin Pediatr Dent* 19:13-18, 1994.

50. Garcia-Godoy F et al: Fluoride release from fissure sealants, *J Clin Pediatr Dent* 22:45-49, 1997.

51. Gilpin JL: Pit and fissure sealants: a review of the literature, *J Dent Hyg* 71(4):150-158, 1997.

52. Going RE et al: The viability of microorganisms in carious lesions five years after covering with a fissure sealant, *J Am Dent Assoc* 97:455-462, 1978.

53. Gonzalez CD et al: Sealant status and factors associated with sealant presence among children in Milwaukee, WI, *ASDC J Dent Child* 62:335-341, 1995.

54. Hamid A, Hume WR: A study of component release from resin pit and fissure sealants in vitro, *Dent Mater* 13:98-102, 1997.

55. Handelman SL, Buonocore MG, Heseck DJ: A preliminary report on the effect of fissure sealant on bacteria in dental caries, *J Prosthet Dent* 27:390-392, 1972.

56. Handelman SL, Shey Z: Michael Buonocore and the Eastman Dental Center: a historic perspective on sealants, *J Dent Res* 75(1):529-534, 1996.

57. Handelman SL, Washburn F, Wopperer P: Two-year report of sealant effect on bacteria in dental caries, *J Am Dent Assoc* 93(11):967-970, 1976.

58. Hassall DC, Mellor AC: The sealant restoration: indications, success and clinical technique, *Br Dent J* 191(7):358-362, 2001.

59. Hicks MJ, Call RL, Flaitz CM: Colorado pit and fissure sealant survey: attitudes toward and use of pit and fissure sealants by Colorado general dentists, *J Colo Dent Assoc* 68:8, 10-15, 1989.

60. Hicks MJ, Silverstone LM: Fissure sealants and dental enamel: a histological study of microleakage in vitro, *Caries Res* 16:353-60, 1982.

61. Horowitz HS, Heiferz SB, Poulsen S: Retention and effectiveness of a single application of an adhesive sealant in preventing occlusal caries: final report after five years of study in Kalispell, Montana, *J Am Dent Assoc* 85:1133-1139, 1977.

62. Houpt M, Fuks A, Eidelman E: The preventive resin (composite resin/sealant) restoration: nine-year results, *Quintessence Int* 25(3):155-159, 1994.

63. Houpt M, Shey Z: The effectiveness of a fissure sealant after six years, *Pediatr Dent* 5(2):104-106, 1983.

64. Houpt MI et al: Compressive strength of fissure sealant applied over cavities, *Pediatr Dent* 6(3):125-127, 1984.

65. Huennekens SC, Daniel SJ, Bayne SC: Effects of air polishing on the abrasion of occlusal sealants, *Quintessence Int* 22(7):581-585, 1991.

66. Jeronimus DJ, Till MJ, Sveen OB: Reduced viability of microorganisms under dental sealants, *J Dent Child* 42(4):275-280, 1975.

67. Kanellis MJ, Warren JJ, Levy SM: A comparison of sealant placement techniques and 12-month retention rates, *J Public Health Dent* 60(1):53-56, 2000.

68. Karlzen-Reuterving G, van Dijken JWV: A three-year follow-up of glass ionomer cement and resin fissure sealants, *J Dent Child* 62:108-110, 1995.

69. Kawai K, Leinfelder KF: Effect of surface-penetrating sealant on composite wear, *Dent Mater* 9(3):108-113, 1993.

70. Kersten S, Lutz F, Schupbach P: Fissure sealing: optimization of sealant penetration and sealing properties, *Am J Dent* 14(3):127-131, 2001.

71. Kilpatrick NM, Murray JJ, McCabe JF: A clinical comparison of a light-cured glass ionomer sealant restoration with a composite sealant restoration, *J Dent* 24(6):399-405, 1996.

72. Koh SH, Chan JT, You C: Effects of topical fluoride treatment on tensile bond strength of pit and fissure sealants, *Gen Dent* 46:278-280, 1998.

73. Koh SH et al: Topical fluoride treatment has no clinical effect on retention of pit and fissure sealants, *J Gt Houst Dent Soc* 67:16-18, 1995.

74. Komatsu H et al: Caries-preventive effect of glass ionomer sealant reapplication: study presents three-year results, *J Am Dent Assoc* 125(5):543-549, 1994.

75. Kostoryz EL et al: Biocompatibility of hydroxylated metabolites of BISGMA and BFDGE, *J Dent Res* 82(5):367-371, 2003.

76. Lekka M, Papagiannoulis L, Eliades G: Porosity of pit and fissure sealants, *J Oral Rehabil* 18:213-220, 1991.

77. Lupi-Pegurier L et al: Microleakage of a pit-and-fissure sealant: effect of air-abrasion compared with classical enamel preparations, *J Adhes Dent* 6:43-48, 2004.

78. Lussi AIS et al: Performance and reproducibility of a laser fluorescence system for detection of occlusal caries in vitro, *Caries Res* 33(4):261-266, 1999.

79. Lygidakis NA, Oulis KI, Christodoulidis A: Evaluation of fissure sealants retention following four different isolation and surface preparation techniques: four years clinical trial, *J Clin Pediatr Dent* 19:23-25, 1994.

80. Mair LH: Wear in dentistry: current terminology, *J Dent* 20(3):140-144, 1992.

81. May KN Jr et al: Effect of a surface sealant on microleakage of class V restorations, *Am J Dent* 9:133-136, 1996.

82. McCarthy MF, Hondrum SO: Mechanical and bond strength properties of light-cured and chemically cured glass ionomer cements, *Am J Orthod Dentofac Orthop* 105:135-141, 1994.

83. McLean JW, Wilson AD: Fissure sealing and filling with an adhesive glass-ionomer cement, *Br Dent J* 136(4):269-276, 1974.

84. Mejare I, Mjor IA: Glass ionomer and resin-based fissure sealants: a clinical study, *Scand J Dent Res* 98:345-350, 1990.

85. Mertz-Fairhurst EJ: Current status of sealant retention and caries prevention, *J Dent Educ* 48(2 suppl):18-26, 1984.

86. Mertz-Fairhurst EJ, Schuster GS, Fairhurst CW: Arresting caries by sealants: results of a clinical study, *J Am Dent Assoc* 112:194-197, 1986.

87. Mertz-Fairhurst EJ et al: Ultraconservative and cariostatic sealed restorations: results at year 10, *J Am Dent Assoc* 129(1):55-66, 1998.

88. Mertz-Fairhurst EJ et al: Cariostatic and ultraconservative sealed restorations: nine-year results among children and adults, *J Dent Child* 62:97-107, 1995.

89. Mertz-Fairhurst EJ et al: Cariostatic and ultraconservative sealed restorations: six-year results, *Quintessence Int* 23:827-38, 1992.

90. Mertz-Fairhurst EJ et al: Sealed restorations: 4-year results, *Am J Dent* 4:43-49, 1991.

91. Mertz-Fairhurst EJ et al: A comparative clinical study of two pit and fissure sealants: 7 year results in Augusta, GA, *J Am Dent Assoc* 109:252-255, 1984.

92. Mertz-Fairhurst EJ et al: A comparative study of two pit and fissure sealants: results after 4½ years in Augusta, GA, *J Am Dent Assoc* 103:235-238, 1981.

93. Moore BK, Winkler MM, Ewoldsen N: Laboratory testing of light-cured glass ionomers as pit-and-fissure sealants, *Gen Dent* 43:176-180, 1995.

94. Nathanson D et al: In vitro elution of leachable components from dental sealants, *J Am Dent Assoc* 128:1517-1523, 1997.

95. Olea N et al: Estrogenicity of resin-based composites and sealants used in dentistry, *Environ Health Perspect* 104:298-305, 1996.

96. Olio F: Biodegradation of dental composites/glass-ionomer cements, *Adv Dent Res* 6:50-54, 1992.

97. Ovrebo RC, Raadal M: Microleakage in fissures sealed with resin or glass ionomer cement, *Scand J Dent Res* 98:66-69, 1990.

98. Phillips RW, Moore BK: *Elements of dental materials for dental hygienists and dental assistants*, ed 5, Philadelphia, 1994, WB Saunders.

99. Pintado MR, Conry JP, Douglas WH: Fissure sealant wear at 30 months: new evaluation criteria, *J Dent* 19:33-38, 1991.

100. Pope BD et al: Effectiveness of occlusal fissure cleansing methods and sealant micromorphology, *J Dent Child* 63:175-180, 1996.

101. Primosch RE, Barr ES: Sealant use and placement techniques among pediatric dentists, *J Am Dent Assoc* 132:1442-1451, 2001.

102. Reid JS, Saunders WP, Chen YY: The effect of bonding agent and fissure sealant on microleakage of composite resin restorations, *Quintessence Int* 22(4):295-298, 1991.

103. Ripa LW: Sealants revisited: an update of the effectiveness of pit-and-fissure sealants, *Caries Res* 27(Suppl 1):77-82, 1993.

104. Ripa LW: The current status of pit-and-fissure sealants: a review, *J Can Dent Assoc* 51:367-380, 1985.

105. Roberson TM, Heymann HO, Swift EJ: *Sturdevant's art and science of operative dentistry*, ed 4, St Louis, 2002, Mosby.

106. Rock WP et al: A comparative study of fluoride-releasing composite resin and glass ionomer materials used as fissure sealants, *J Dent* 24(4):275-280, 1996.

107. Romberg E, Cohen LA, LaBelle AD: A national survey of sealant use by pediatric dentists, *ASDC J Dent Child* 55:257-264, 1988.

108. Romcke RG et al: Retention and maintenance of fissure sealants over 10 years, *J Can Dent Assoc* 56(3):235-237, 1990.

109. Rozier RG: The impact of recent changes in the epidemiology of dental caries on guidelines for the use of dental sealants, *J Public Health Dent* 55(5 Spec):292-301, 1995.

110. Rueggeberg FA, Dlugokinski M. Ergle JW: Minimizing patients' exposure to uncured components in a dental sealant, *J Am Dent Assoc* 130:1751-1757, 1999.

111. Ruse ND: Xenoestrogenicity and dental materials, *J Can Dent Assoc* 63(11):833-836, 1997.

112. Ryan JP: The clinical benefits of dental sealants, *J Pract Hyg* 6:13-17, 1997.

113. Scott L et al: Retention of dental sealants following the use of air polishing and traditional cleaning, *Dent Hyg* 62:402-406, 1988.

114. Selwitz RH et al: The prevalence of dental sealants in the US population: findings from NHANES III, 1988-1991, *J Dent Res* 75:652-660, 1996.

115. Sidhu SK, Watson TF: Resin-modified glass ionomer materials: a status report, *Am J Dent* 8(1):59-67, 1995.

116. Siegal MD et al: The use of dental sealants by Ohio dentists, *J Public Health Dent* 56:12-21, 1996.

117. Simecek JW et al: Dental sealant longevity in a cohort of young US naval personnel, *J Am Dent Assoc* 136:171-178, 2005.

118. Simonsen RJ: Pit and fissure sealant: review of the literature, *Pediatr Dent* 34(5):393-414, 2002.

119. Simonsen RJ: Glass ionomer as fissure sealant: a critical review, *J Public Health Dent* 56(3 spec):146-149, 1996.

120. Simonsen RJ: Retention and effectiveness of dental sealant after 15 years, *J Am Dent Assoc* 122:34-42, 1991.

121. Simonsen RJ: Cost effectiveness of pit and fissure sealant at 10 years, *Quintessence Int* 20:75-82, 1989.

122. Simonsen RJ: Retention and effectiveness of a single application of white sealant after 10 years, *J Am Dent Assoc* 115(7):31-36, 1987.

123. Simonsen RJ: Pit and fissure sealants. In *Clinical application of the acid etch technique*, ed 1, Chicago, 1978, Quintessence Publishing, pp 19-42.

124. Simonscn RJ, Geraldeli S, Perdigao J: Use of laser fluorescence for diagnosis of caries in pit and fissure surfaces, *J Dent Res* Abstract #1351, 2001.

125. Soderholm KM: The impact of recent changes in the epidemiology of dental caries on guidelines for the use of dental sealants: clinical perspectives, *J Public Health Dent* 55(5 Spec):302-311, 1995.

126. Soderholm K, Mariotti AL: BIS-GMA–based resins in dentistry: are they safe? *J Am Dent Assoc* 130(2):201-209, 1999.

127. Souto M, Donly KJ: Caries inhibition of glass ionomers, *Am J Dent* 7(2):122-124, 1994.

128. Stadtler P: A 3-year clinical study of a hybrid composite resin as fissure sealant and as restorative material for class I restorations, *Quintessence Int* 23:759-762, 1992.

129. Stahl JW, Katz RV: Occlusal dental caries incidence and implications for sealant programs in a US college student population, *J Public Health Dent* 53:212-218, 1993.

130. Swift EJ Jr: The effect of sealants on dental caries: a review, *J Am Dent Assoc* 116(6):700-704, 1988.

131. Thompson JL et al: The effect of salivary contamination on fissure sealant–enamel bond strength, *J Oral Rehabil* 8:11-18, 1981.

132. Thylstrup A, Poulsen S: Retention and effectiveness of a chemically polymerized pit and fissure sealant after 2 years, *Scand J Dent Res* 86:21-24, 1978.

133. Tilliss TS et al: Occlusal discrepancies after sealant therapy, *J Prosthet Dent* 68:223-228, 1992.

134. Tjan AHL, Tan DE: Microleakage at gingival margins of class V composite resin restorations rebonded with various low-viscosity resin systems, *Quintessence Int* 22(7):65-73, 1991.

135. Tulunoglu O et al: The effect of bonding agents on the microleakage and bond strength of sealant in primary teeth, *J Oral Rehabil* 26:436-441, 1999.

136. US Department of Health and Human Services: *Oral Health in America: A Report of the Surgeon General,* Rockville, Md, 2000, US Department of Health and Human Services, National Institute of Dental and Craniofacial Research, National Institutes of Health.

137. Wada J et al: In vitro estrogenicity of resin composites, *J Dent Res* 83(3):222-226, 2004.

138. Waggoner WF, Siegal M: Pit-and-fissure sealant application: updating the technique, *J Am Dent Assoc* 127:351-361, 1996.

139. Warren DP et al: Effect of topical fluoride on retention of pit-and-fissure sealants, *J Dent Hyg* 75:21-24, 2001.

140. Weintraub JA: The effectiveness of pit-and-fissure sealants, *J Public Health Dent* 49(5):317-330, 1989.

141. Wendt LK, Koch G: Fissure sealant in permanent first molars after 10 years, *Swed Dent J* 12:181-185, 1988.

142. Wendt LK, Koch G, Birkhed D: Long-term evaluation of a fissure sealing programme in Public Dental Service clinics in Sweden, *Swed Dent J* 25:61-65, 2001.

143. Wendt LK, Koch G, Birkhed D: On the retention and effectiveness of fissure sealant permanent molars after 15-20 years: a cohort study, *Community Dent Oral Epidemiol* 29:302-307, 2001.

144. Williams KB et al: Oral health–related quality of life: a model for dental hygiene, *J Dent Hyg* 72(2):19-26, 1998.

145. Winkler MM et al: Using a resin-modified glass ionomer as an occlusal sealant: a one-year clinical study, *J Am Dent Assoc* 127(10):1508-1514, 1996.

146. Workshop on Guidelines for Sealant Use: Recommendations, *J Public Health Dent* 55(5 Spec):263-273, 1995.

147. Xalabarde A et al: Fissure micromorphology and sealant adaptation after occlusal enameloplasty, *J Clin Pediatr Dent* 20:299-304, 1996.

148. Zervou C et al: Enameloplasty effects on microleakage of pit and fissure sealants under load: an in vitro study, *J Clin Pediatr Dent* 24(4):279-285, 2000.

Tobacco Dependence and Addictive Behaviors

Robert Ellis Mecklenburg • Cathy L. Backinger

INSIGHT

Addictive behaviors and the products that cause them significantly affect the practice of dental hygiene in numerous ways. Learning to connect the risks and associated substance-specific chronic, progressive, and relapsing challenges associated with addictions can help dental hygienists educate and support their patients through the challenges of cessation and improving overall health.

✲✲ CASE STUDY 29-1   Helping a Patient Quit Tobacco Use

Paula Evans is a 22-year-old woman who plans to begin a new job in 2 weeks. She wants to start with a good impression, so she is requesting dental hygiene services and a dental checkup before she enters her new position. She says, "I need this job to begin to pay off my school debts and become more independent."

When you inquire about her general health, Ms. Evans states that she tries to take care of herself. She says, "I exercise twice a week." On reviewing her health history forms, you verify that she is not aware of any illnesses, is not taking any drugs, and is not pregnant. She volunteers, "One day I want to settle down and have a family, but for now I enjoy being single." Her health history form discloses that she smokes, on average, approximately a pack of cigarettes a day and has for approximately 5 years. She has her first cigarette within a half hour of waking and smokes approximately 15 cigarettes a day. Inquiring about this habit, you learn that she smokes the most during social occasions, which are frequent. You learn that Ms. Evans began smoking when she was 13 years old and never intended to be smoking after she graduated from high school. She tried to quit twice. Approximately 4 years ago, she quit for a couple of weeks but then relapsed when drinking "maybe a little too much at a party." She tried to quit again 2 years ago but began again after a week because she was feeling irritable and "blue" and noticed that she had gained 4 pounds.

Diagnosis and Treatment Plan

Ms. Evans's vital signs are normal. An oral examination shows that she is free of dental caries and that the few restorations present are sound. Although her oral hygiene has been good, the upper anterior gingival area is fibrous, and the mesiopalatal probe depths of three molars measure 4 to 5 mm.

Ms. Evans is not aware that she has become nicotine dependent, nor that, as young as she is, her smoking is beginning to compromise her desire to be healthy and attractive. The peripheral vasoconstriction properties of nicotine inhibit gingival bleeding and are masking her early-stage periodontal disease.

KEY TERMS

acetylcholine	dopamine	nicotine dependence	serotonin
addiction	kretek	norepinephrine	tobacco
bidis	neurotransmitters	quid	tobacco-cessation

LEARNING OUTCOMES

After reading this chapter the student will be able to:

1. Recognize various ways that tobacco use undermines oral health and dental practice.
2. Recognize that nicotine and other chemical dependencies are chronic, progressive, and relapsing conditions of the brain, which alter vital neural functions.
3. Recognize common symptoms of nicotine and other drug dependencies and withdrawal.
4. Recognize that nicotine dependency can be effectively treated with modest, scientifically established methods and periodic reinforcement.

5. Use basic behavioral and pharmacotherapeutic intervention services in clinical practice.
6. Establish clinic policies and practices that ensure routine identification of patient tobacco use status and appropriate methods for care and follow-up.
7. Refer selected patients for specialized treatment of their nicotine and other drug dependencies.

Living in the thin moment of the present, animals do not share the human abilities of assigning meaning to observations, nor do they possess foresight, abstract thought, or self-consciousness. Beneath these human attributes, people do share with animals many basic drives that are essential to individual well-being and species continuity—drives such as drinking, eating, reproducing, socializing, and avoiding harm.

These basic survival attributes are finely developed in the central nervous system (CNS), especially the brain, as a result of eons of complex, continuing interaction between genetic architecture and environmental stimuli.[2] Early in a person's life, billions of dendritic connections form between neurons, as many as 10,000 per neuron. Many such pathways atrophy if they are not used during growth or if they fall into disuse later. Other pathways assume key roles in human interactions with the environment.

> ### Note
> Constant interplay between nature and nurture (between genetic makeup and experience) makes people who they are—unique but within limits.

At the chemical level, neurons communicate using **neurotransmitters.** These substances are monoamines such as **acetylcholine, norepinephrine, serotonin,** and **dopamine.** The release of neurotransmitters at neural clefts stimulates, inhibits, and modulates neural function, hormone production, and other processes through an unimaginably complex system. This system regulates automatic functions and willed behaviors that are needed to maintain life and a person's sense of well-being. Millions of monoamines are carefully metered out by neurons and then, within microseconds of transmitting their signals though synaptic clefts, are cleared away by reuptake into the producing neurons or destroyed by catalysts such as monoamine oxidase. In this symphony of interactions between neurons in the core structures of the brain and neocortex, the brain and mind merge. Other systems throughout the body exist primarily to provide the oxygen, food, and sensory stimuli that nurture the dynamic processes of being, which are expressed in the brain.

Seduction

The human brain is *vulnerable to devastation* by psychoactive chemicals. These substances subvert an individual's perceptions, feelings, personality, and judgment such that the mind gradually changes forever in both subtle and gross ways. Trauma, toxins, and infectious agents only threaten cell viability, but nicotine, alcohol, heroin, opium, cocaine, marijuana, hallucinogens, and other stimulants, depressants, and perception-altering chemicals transform neural cells themselves by altering neurotransmitter functions.

These substances create *liking* feelings that promote repetitive use. Neural pathways, neural receptors, and other cell and chemical structures change to compensate for the artificially produced stimuli. As neurons adjust to repeated exposure, the individual gradually increases exposure to achieve *once more* the desired mood-altering effect. The disease is progressive; it erodes basic animal drives and higher human satisfactions so that life gradually becomes centered on drug seeking, using, and recovery.

> ### Note
> Nicotine, alcohol, heroin, opium, cocaine, marijuana, hallucinogens, and other stimulants, depressants, and perception-altering chemicals transform neural cells themselves by altering neurotransmitter functions.

Addiction

Once neurons adjust such that their functions are *normal* only in the presence of a psychoactive substance, the sudden absence of the substance creates a neurotransmitter signal deficiency and hormone imbalances that clinically produce impaired emotions, motor skills, and thought processes. Without the artificial

> ### Note
> Feelings of acute anxiety and stress and an inability to concentrate and perform replace the sense of well-being that existed in the presence of the substance.

stimulus, brain and body react to a sudden plunge in mono-amine levels.

Other conditions commonly occur, such as the following:

- Insomnia
- Irritability
- Decreased heart rate
- Increased appetite
- Weight gain

> **Note**
>
> By definition, individuals who use **tobacco**, alcohol, or other psychoactive substances are at risk of developing a substance-specific chronic, progressive, relapsing disease.[19]

> **Note**
>
> Social and psychologic stimuli become part of the *dependence in addition to the drug* **addiction.**

Long-term psychoactive drug users receive little *pleasure* from their drugs. Rather, use is driven by a compelling need to prevent withdrawal symptoms. What users interpret as *pleasure* is merely relief from the symptoms of withdrawal. Users are trapped when the brain's delicate signal system has been altered, sometimes long before use has even become a daily preoccupation.

Environmental conditions are often as important as the substance's action. Environments associated with use trigger craving and anticipation. Certain times, places, or events act as cues that stimulate craving for the substance.

Ritual preparations for use heighten anticipation and concentrate perceptions. Motor pathways that develop with repetitive use become deeply imbedded in patterns of daily living.

Drug seeking, using, and recovery behaviors may overtake important basic motives and behaviors that are necessary for survival and fundamental to a sense of well-being. The subtle joys people experience from non–drug-related activities become dulled. They often experience the following:

- Diminished intellectual curiosity
- Lack of interest in accomplishment
- Inability to organize effectively
- Altered appetites and sexual desire
- Impaired social interaction
- Increased risk-taking behaviors
- Limited concern for personal integrity

Indeed, drug-dependent individuals often engage in risky and illegal behaviors to sustain their drug use. Dependency on nicotine, the most prevalent of the drugs that alter brain function, seldom leads to the ethical and legal compromises that are typically encountered when other drugs are used because tobacco is relatively inexpensive, easily obtained, and still socially acceptable in some environments.[21]

Table 29-1 provides a list of addictive chemicals, oral effects, and dental treatment concerns. Nicotine has not been included in this table but will receive the major focus of the chapter since dental hygienists can provide intervention for tobacco dependency.

Table 29-1	Addictive Substances, Oral Side Effects, and Treatment Concerns		
SUBSTANCE	**COMMON NAMES/ FORMS**	**ORAL SIDE EFFECTS**	**DENTAL TREATMENT CONCERNS**
Cannabinoids	Pot, weed, hash, hash oil, hashish, marijuana, mary jane, broccoli, cripple, and prescription	Leukoplakia; increased incidence of oral infections, dental caries, and periodontitis; "Cannabis stomatitis"; leukoedema; superficial anesthesia of the epithelium[c]	Avoid using local anesthetics with epinephrine[h]
Cocaine (Inhaled, Smoked, or Injected)	Blow, coke, everclear, crack, yeya, kryptonite, lady, kibbles n' bits, charlie, and biscuits	Gingival and alveolar bone necrosis in the maxillary premolar region; spontaneous gingival bleeding; palatal ulcerations/ischemic necrosis; bruxism; cracked lips[d,i,j]	Avoid using local anesthetics with epinephrine; surgical dental procedures should be preceded by a platelet count; concurrent use of the sedative, propofol, can induce grand mal seizures[h]

[a]Avon S: Oral mucosal lesions associated with use of quid, *J Can Dent Assoc* 70(4):244-248, 2004.

[b]Brazier WJ et al: Ecstasy related periodontitis and mucosal ulceration—a case report, *Br Dent J* 194(4):197-199, 2003.

[c]Cho CM et al: General and oral health implications of cannabis use, *Aust Dent J* 50(2):70-74, 2005.

[d]Faruque S et al: Crack cocaine smoking and oral sores in three inner-city neighborhoods, *J Acquir Immune Defici Syndr Human Retrovirol* 13(1):87-92, 1996.

[e]El-Hakim IE, Uthman MA: Squamous cell carcinoma and keratoacanthoma of the lower lip associated with "goza" and "shisha" smoking, *Int J Dermatol* 38:108-110, 1999.

[f]Klasser G, Epstein J: Methamphetamine and its impact on dental care, *J Can Dent Assoc* 71(10):759-762, 2005.

[g]Kuspis, DA, Krenzelok, EP: Oral frostbite injury from intentional abuse of fluorinated hydrocarbon, *Clin Toxicology* 37(7):873-875, 1999.

[h]Meechan, JG: Drug abuse and dentistry, *Dent Update* 26:182-190.

[i]Mitchell-Lewis DA et al: Identifying oral lesions associated with crack cocaine use. *J Am Dent Assoc* 125(8):1104-1108, 1110, 1994.

[j]Porter J, Bonilla L: Crack user's cracked lips: an additional HIV risk factor, *Am J Public Health* 83:1490-1491, 1993.

Continued

Table 29-1	Addictive Chemicals, Oral Side Effects, and Treatment Concerns—cont'd		
SUBSTANCE	**COMMON NAMES/ FORMS**	**ORAL SIDE EFFECTS**	**DENTAL TREATMENT CONCERNS**
Opioids	Heroin, smack, big H, china white, caballo, and horse	Rampant dental caries result from administration of methadone; thrombocytopenic purpura	Infective endocarditis in intravenous users; drug interactions with paracetemol and diazepam[h]
Methamphetamines	Meth, chalk, ice, crystal, glass, tina, speed, crank, and fire	Xerostomia; rampant dental caries; periodontal diseases[f]	
Benzodiazepine and Barbiturates	Barbs, reds, red birds, phennies, tooies, yellows, and yellow jackets	Xerostomia; fixed drug eruptions	Trouble with effective dental sedation[h]
Solvents	Paint thinner, glue, aerosols, and huff	Circumoral erythema; oral "frost bite"[g]	Avoid using local anesthetics with epinephrine; increased risk of seizures[h]
Anabolic Steroids	Roids, rocket fuel, and juice	Increased dental caries	Increased effect of epinephrine in local anesthetic; increased bleeding; aggressive behavior[h]
Hallucinogens/LSD	Acid, cid, and strawberry fields	Bruxism; trismus	
Amphetamines	Amp, ecstacy, X, black beauties, footballs, and bumblebees	Xerostomia; increased dental caries; bruxism; trismus; periodontitis; mucosal ulcerations; oral manifestations of malnutrition[b]	Increased bleeding[h]
Alcohol	Hooch, juice, wahoo juice, forty, and sauce	Prevalence of enamel erosion and pathologic tooth wear	Increased bleeding; sedative tolerance; adverse reactions with some antimicrobials (e.g., metronidazole, tinidazole, cephalosporins, ketoconazole)[h]
Quid	Tobacco mixed with areca nut	Squamous cell carcinoma of the lower lip[e]	
Goza and Shisha	Water pipe		
Betel Leaf		Desquamation and peeling of the mucosa; lesions similar to cheek biting	
Paan	Betel leaf and slaked lime	Lichenoid lesions; oral submucous fibrosis	

Intended Consequences

Most adverse mental and physical conditions are inadvertent, perhaps a result of injury, infection, aging, or a genetic glitch.

During the twentieth century, the tobacco industry has produced persuasive campaigns directed at girls and women.[7,29,30] In addition, this industry has secured many exemptions from government oversight, such as the Consumer Products Safety Act, and insulated itself from liability for tobacco-related injuries, such as by the 1998 settlement with state attorneys general.[22] Huge profits have helped tobacco companies secure a position of power and influence.

Results

- Approximately 23% of U.S. adults are current smokers, 23% are former smokers, and more than one half (54%) have never smoked cigarettes. Approximately 19% of adults smoke daily, and approximately 4% smoke less than daily.[10] More than 80% of daily users become dependent before they are legally old enough to buy tobacco; that is, before they are ready to make a rational choice.[39]

- Of the individuals who experiment with cigarette smoking, alcohol, cocaine, heroin, and other drugs, a higher proportion become dependent on using cigarettes.[3]
- Individuals who are dependent on multiple substances report that quitting tobacco use is more difficult than quitting use of other substances.[3]
- In addition to cigarette use, tobacco use involves smokeless tobacco (also called *spit tobacco,* including both oral snuff and chewing tobacco), cigars, pipe tobacco, and newer forms of tobacco such as **bidis** and **kretek.**
- In 2004, approximately 12% of middle school students and 28% of high school students used tobacco. The most common products used by high school students were cigarettes (22%), cigars (13%), smokeless tobacco (6%), pipes (3%), bidis (3%), and kretek (2%).[9]
- All forms of tobacco are harmful, accounting for 30% of all cancers. According to the Centers for Disease Control and Prevention, "About 4 in 10 current smokers (43%) attempted to quit smoking in the past year."[10]

Costs of Tobacco Habit

Each drug has its own constellation of adverse health consequences.

Individual differences in susceptibility lead to vulnerability for varying chronic diseases, different losses in quality of life, and different causes of death. Some tobacco users survive a long time. However, one half of smokers die of a tobacco-related disease. Who would fly if one half of all individuals who do so would die in an aircraft accident; perhaps not this flight, but one day?

In addition to the toll on tobacco users and their families, the social cost of tobacco use is high. Tobacco industry gross sales of $46 billion annually are not even a third of the estimated direct and indirect annual social costs of $157.7 billion.[15,38] Such costs include direct medical care, lost productivity, and neonatal care, but these costs do not include the following:

- Intangible costs such as impaired sexual function
- Pain and disfigurement
- Lost opportunities
- Costs to families and close associates when users are disabled or die prematurely as a consequence of tobacco use

Stated simply, tobacco use costs society nearly $3 for every $1 of tobacco sold.

Many oral diseases are caused or aggravated by tobacco use (Box 29-1).

- The prevalence and severity of adult periodontal diseases are directly related to the intensity and duration of smoking.[16,17,24]

> **Note**
> Tobacco dependence is responsible for more than one in every six deaths in the United States.[39]

> **Note**
> On average, cigarette smokers lose approximately 12 to 15 years of life, compared with similar groups of nonsmokers.[33]

BOX 29-1

TOBACCO-INDUCED AND TOBACCO-ASSOCIATED ORAL CONDITIONS

Oral Cancer
Leukoplakia
- Homogenous leukoplakia
- Nonhomogenous leukoplakia (precancer)
- Verrucous leukoplakia
- Nodular leukoplakia
- Erythroleukoplakia

Other Tobacco-Induced Oral Mucosal Conditions
- Snuff dipper's lesion
- Smoker's palate (nicotine stomatitis)
- Smoker's melanosis

Tobacco-Associated Effects on the Teeth and Supporting Tissues
- Tooth loss (premature mortality)
- Staining
- Abrasion
- Periodontal disease
  - Destructive periodontitis

- Focal recession
- Acute necrotizing ulcerative gingivitis

Other Tobacco-Associated Oral Conditions
- Gingival bleeding
- Calculus
- Halitosis
- Leukoedema
- Chronic hyperplastic candidiasis
- Median rhomboid glossitis
- Hairy tongue

Possible Association with Tobacco Use
- Oral clefts
- Dental caries
- Dental plaque biofilm
- Lichen planus
- Salivary changes
- Taste and smell

From Mecklenburg RE et al: *Tobacco effects in the mouth,* Bethesda, Md, 2000, US Department of Health and Human Services, Public Health Service, National Institutes of Health, NIH Publication No 00-3330. Reprinted September 2000, p. 548.

lowing:

- Carcinogenic effects
- Cardiovascular effects
- Reproductive and sensory effects
- Other adverse effects

Risks of developing these effects are generally a function of duration and intensity (often expressed in pack years).

DENTAL CONSIDERATIONS

Most non–diabetes-related adult periodontal disease may be attributed to smoking.[8,37] Withholding of or noncompliance with cessation services as a component of periodontal therapy dramatically lowers a favorable long-term outcome because a major contributor continues. Helping a patient quit is an essential component of his or her dental care.

BOX 29-2

TOBACCO EFFECTS ON CLINICAL CARE

Effects on Oral Health Care

- More difficult and less enduring oral hygiene services
- Twice the risk of experiencing dry socket
- Delayed wound healing
- Poorer prognoses after periodontal therapy, implant insertion, and other dental services that depend on healing and resistance to infection[15]
- Sinusitis
- Cosmetic dentistry

Effects of Fitness for Care

- Effects on immune system
- Increased medical emergencies
- Some treatment options, treatment, and prognoses precluded because tobacco use adversely affects oral health[27]
- More clinic time required for patients who are ill with tobacco-related diseases for medical consultation and provision of pretreatment medication
- Medications
- Disabilities

Effects on Family Health and Well-Being

- Premature death
- Involuntary tobacco smoke

Modified from Mecklenburg RE et al: *Tobacco effects in the mouth*, Bethesda, Md, 1994, US Department of Health and Human Services, Public Health Service, National Institutes of Health, NIH Publication No 96-3330.

- Patient tobacco use adds a preventable burden on practice (Box 29-2).

Nicotine is the psychoactive drug in tobacco but is not the substance that is most harmful.[5] Combinations of hundreds of tars, particulates, and gases produce the following:

Smokeless and Spit Tobacco

Boys and men are nearly eight times more likely to use spit tobacco than girls and women.[7] Oral cancer risks are even greater, especially when smokeless tobacco is combined with alcohol. One report demonstrates that spit tobacco users double their risk of cardiovascular death.[6] Nicotine from spit tobacco is absorbed through the oral mucosa in a basic environment. Youths begin the smokeless tobacco habit with nearly neutral pH forms that release little nicotine and are highly flavored to mask the bitter tobacco taste. As tolerance grows, users switch to products with higher pH levels to help transfer larger quantities of nicotine into the blood. Highly dependent users choose forms that are higher than pH 8 and have few, if any, masking flavors. Some spit tobacco users are so dependent that they sleep with a **quid** in their mouths for continuous nicotine absorption.

DENTAL CONSIDERATIONS

Approximately one half of users show tobacco-induced white lesions where they hold the quid. The juices are rich in tobacco nitrosamines that are powerful carcinogens.

Other Tobacco Products

Similar to spit tobacco juices, smoke from cigars, pipes, and bidis has a basic pH (above pH 7.0) and is harsh. Thus most nicotine is absorbed through the oral mucosa and upper brachial tree. Little nicotine reaches the lung alveoli. Cigarette smoke is acidic, having on average a 6.1 pH, and it must be inhaled deeply into the lung for nicotine absorption. Some cigarettes are treated with ammonia and other chemicals to increase absorption throughout the brachial tree and with still other chemicals to open and anesthetize the airway, permitting a deeper draw and greater nicotine absorption. The addition of sugars in cigarettes also increases the psychoactive *hit*.[4]

Essential Elements of Patient History

RISKS

The average age of smoking onset is 14.5 years.[39] The younger people begin smoking, the more likely they are to become long-term users, that is, to become nicotine dependent. Early tobacco use is often associated with early alcohol use. Children and youths who are users are at greatest risk of experimenting and becoming regular users of other psychoactive substances.

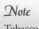

Note

Tobacco use, especially smoking, is considered a *gateway drug*.[39]

INITIATION

The onset of tobacco use usually begins for social or psychologic reasons. Other youths offer the product, and it is taken because of curiosity, a desire to fit in, as an act of rebelliousness against authority, to mimic an admired celebrity, or for no obvious reason. Intermittent use extends, on average, for approximately 4 years before regular (almost daily) use begins.[39]

CASE APPLICATION 29-1.1

Tobacco and Alcohol Use

Ms. Evans's history is typical. She began smoking during her early teens. Youths who have smoked as few as 100 cigarettes are likely to become daily smokers. She is past this point. She also drinks and may occasionally drink more than she intended. Alcohol use is both a common risk factor for relapse and a strong cofactor for oral cancer and other serious chronic health problems. Her routine use of two psychoactive drugs and her remark that she "likes socializing" may suggest that she is in a cluster of individuals who engage in multiple high-risk activities.

PROGRESSION

Nicotine mimics acetylcholine by binding to acetylcholine receptors at the autonomic ganglia, in the adrenal medulla at neuromuscular junctions, and in the brain. At low doses, nicotine stimulates the brain, primarily the cortex via the locus ceruleus. This stimulation produces increased alertness and cognition. At higher doses, nicotine tends to stimulate the production of dopamine, providing a *pleasure* effect and sense

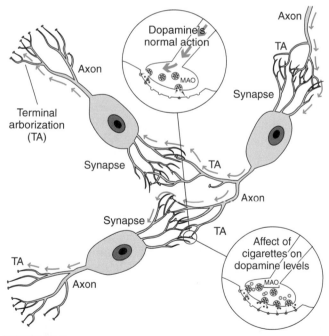

FIGURE 29-1
The addictive process. Nicotine is shown replacing the neurotransmitter acetylcholine at the receptor site, which results in increased alertness and cognition. With increased doses of nicotine at the receptor site, dopamine is produced, resulting in a feeling of pleasure and well-being. Because nicotine produced a large discharge of dopamine and this neurotransmitter does not clear from the receptor site as quickly as it would during normal functioning, the signal has an intense, lingering effect. Over time, more receptor sites are produced, returning signals to *normal* intensity and duration but only in the presence of nicotine. *MAO*, Monoamine oxidase.

of well-being (Figure 29-1). The nicotine promotes a more intense signal and, because the signal is not cleared normally, a lingering effect. In time, the CNS adjusts to these repeated stimuli by increasing the number of neuron receptor sites, returning signals to *normal* function but now only in the presence of nicotine. Thus to achieve the altered mood desired, higher doses are required over time (Box 29-3).

> *Distinct Care Modifications*
> Withdrawal from nicotine use creates a rebound effect that may extend for several weeks or longer, depressing cognitive ability, brain metabolism, emotional stability, and sense of well-being.

DEPENDENCE

The conversion from voluntary to involuntary use is gradual and is seldom recognized by the user. The search for reward through nicotine use and the avoidance of the penalties of stopping are embedded in the social and environmental context of use. *Tobacco dependence includes nicotine addiction,* but the social and environmental components make it more than a chemically induced behavior. Many compulsive behaviors are mischaracterized as addictive, such as compulsive eating, gam-

---

BOX 29-3

AMERICAN PSYCHIATRIC ASSOCIATION: DIAGNOSTIC CRITERIA FOR SUBSTANCE DEPENDENCY

The American Psychiatric Association (APA) diagnostic criteria applicable to nicotine dependency outline a maladaptive pattern of substance use, leading to clinically significant impairment of stress as exhibited by three or more of the following criteria, occurring at the same time in the same 12-month period.

A. Tolerance, as defined by one of the following:
   1. A need for markedly increased amounts of the substance to achieve intoxication or desired effects
   2. Markedly diminished effects with continued use of the same amount of the substance
B. Withdrawal, as exhibited by one of the following:
   1. The characteristic withdrawal syndrome for the substance
   2. Using the substance to relieve or prevent withdrawal symptoms
   3. Taking the substance in larger amounts and over a longer period than intended
   4. Persistent desire or unsuccessful effort to cut down substance use
   5. Spending a great deal of time in activities that are necessary to obtain the substance, use it, or recover from its effects
   6. Reducing or discontinuing important social, occupational, or recreational activities because of substance use
   7. Continued substance use despite knowledge of having a persistent or recurrent physical or psychologic problem that is likely to have been caused or exacerbated by the substance

From Hughes JR et al: Practice guideline for the treatment of patients with nicotine dependence, *Am J Psychiatry* 153(Suppl):1-31, 1996.

bling, sexual activity, and acquisition of money and goods, but these need not be driven by drug use. Both addictions and compulsions risk or compromise inherently advantageous fundamental behaviors.

Drug use is often differentiated as a *dependency,* connoting that chemicals directly alter the neurotransmitting functions of the brain. As is the case with purely behavioral compulsions, drug-taking behaviors are conditioned by the environment in which a drug is used and the reinforcement of learned, repetitive motor skills. Motor neuron pathways develop memory such that motions used to prepare and use tobacco products become refined and so ingrained within the individual that the user perceives them as efficient, *normal* motions.

RELAPSE

Women more than men state that they smoke to relieve anxiety, overcome depression, and manage weight gain. Unfortunately, the interruption of nicotine's action on neurotransmitters triggers much of such feelings a woman experiences and the decreased metabolism associated with her weight gain.

★ CASE APPLICATION 29-1.2

Tobacco Dependency

In Ms. Evans's case, social situations may be strongly reinforcing, as suggested by her remark that she smokes most heavily during such occasions. Whereas her first relapse was the result of a social situation, Ms. Evans's second relapse was caused by her nicotine dependency. She described typical withdrawal symptoms (Box 29-4).

BOX 29-4

AMERICAN PSYCHIATRIC ASSOCIATION: DIAGNOSTIC CRITERIA FOR NICOTINE WITHDRAWAL

A. The individual uses nicotine daily for at least several weeks.

B. The individual abruptly ceases nicotine use or the amount of nicotine used, followed within 24 hours by four or more of the following signs:
1. Dysphoric or depressed mood
2. Insomnia
3. Irritability, frustration, or anger
4. Anxiety
5. Difficulty concentrating
6. Restlessness
7. Decreased heart rate
8. Increased appetite or weight gain

C. The symptoms in criterion B cause clinically significant degrees of impairment in social, occupational, or other important areas of functioning.

D. The symptoms are not caused by a general medical condition and are not better accounted for by another mental disorder.

From Hughes JR et al: Practice guideline for the treatment of patients with nicotine dependence, *Am J Psychiatry* 153(Suppl):1-31, 1996.

DIAGNOSIS OF TOBACCO DEPENDENCY AND NICOTINE ADDICTION

Nicotine is rapidly metabolized so that the positive effects achieved through the use of a single cigarette may deteriorate within a half hour. Nicotine depletes when sleeping; therefore withdrawal symptoms are often most intense on waking. Smokers commonly report that the most *satisfying* or *enjoyable* cigarette is the one taken on waking. Without realizing it, they are reporting on their relief from withdrawal. Highly dependent smokeless or spit tobacco users may sleep with a chew so that some nicotine absorption occurs during sleep. Other indicators[10] that an individual is nicotine dependent are presented in Figure 29-2.[11]

RITUALS

Individuals who use tobacco or other substances develop rituals around use. For example, a pattern exists involving opening of the pack, tapping and removal of the cigarette, placing the cigarette into position, lighting, extinguishing the flame, and storing the pack and lighter, followed by a set means of holding and drawing on the cigarette and using the smoke in accord with the dose needed. Fine and often unconscious regulation of each dose occurs to adjust the amount of nicotine absorbed to maximize the effect without its reaching an unpleasant state of nicotine intoxication or overdose. On average, a cigarette smoker repeats puffing approximately 10 times per cigarette, receiving a dose that sustains comfort and avoids the onset of withdrawal symptoms for 20 to 40 minutes. A pack-a-day smoker might repeat the puffing act 73,000 times per year. The ritual provides an illusion of control and becomes a source of comfort.

ENVIRONMENTAL STIMULI

Nicotine dependency occurs in a social environment. Anticipation of use can trigger craving, and a social context in which the substance is used heightens desire for it. Cigarette smoking has been socially acceptable in a wide variety of environments, easily triggering a desire to use tobacco. This norm, coupled with the low cost, easy access, and seemingly ubiquitous encouragement by the tobacco industry has made cigarette smoking easy to develop and continue. An increasing number of policies to make public places smoke free are incentives for nicotine-dependent individuals to reduce use or quit, in spite of the physical withdrawal symptoms that occur while their brain readjusts to functioning without the presence of nicotine.

QUITTING

Most individuals who want to quit think about it for years before making their first quit attempt. Most people who attempt to quit require several attempts. Fewer than 10% of individuals who make a self-help quit attempt are capable of achieving long-

> *Patient Education Opportunity*
> Nearly one half of high school seniors and 60% to 70% of adults who smoke want to quit.[39]

Questions	Answers	Points
1. How soon after you wake up do you smoke your first cigarette?	Within 5 minutes	3
	6 to 30 minutes	2
	31 to 60 minutes	1
	After 60 minutes	0
2. Do you find it difficult to refrain from smoking in places where it is forbidden?	Yes	1
	No	0
3. Which cigarette would you hate most to give up?	The first one in the morning	1
	All others	0
4. How many cigarettes per day do you smoke?	10 or less	0
	11 to 20	1
	21 to 30	2
	31 or more	3
5. Do you smoke more frequently during the first hours of being awake than during the rest of the day?	Yes	1
	No	2
6. Do you smoke if you are so ill that you are in bed most of the day?	Yes	1
	No	0

Dependence score:

0 to 2	Very low
3 to 4	Low
5	Moderate
6 to 7	High
8 to 10	Very high

FIGURE 29-2
Items and scoring for the Fagerstrom Test for Nicotine Dependence. (Modified from Fagerstrom K, Schneider NG: Measuring nicotine dependence: a review of the Fagerstrom tolerance questionnaire, *J Behav Med* 12:59-182, 1989.)

term abstinence, that is, being free of tobacco for 6 months or longer. Thus only approximately 2% to 3% of smokers become abstinent each year.[12] Clinical and extra-treatment social support can double to triple long-term abstinence, and, with the use of a U.S. Food and Drug Administration (FDA)–approved pharmacologic agent, success rates can rise to 20% or more for a single quit attempt. Such rates are not as common among individuals who have low self-efficacy, multiple drug dependencies, or a psychiatric comorbidity, such as clinical depression.

Depressed neuronal function during the quitting process should be expected. Reduction in electroencephalographic (EEG)

waves, brain metabolism, and other functions become progressively more intense after quitting and peak within a few days. Most relapses occur within the first week.[20] Impaired neuronal function may extend more than a month, with recovery of neuronal function taking much longer. Learned, conditioned patterns of behavior exist indefinitely, requiring continued reinforcement of each former user coping strategies to counter them.

Techniques, Procedures, and Supportive Evidence

29-1

Who should help Ms. Evans, whose story was outlined in the case study at the beginning of the chapter? All healthcare providers can be effective in helping patients quit. Treatment delivered by a variety of clinician types increases cessation rates. Assistance by dentists and dental hygienists reinforces each other. Help in dental offices complements help provided in medical environments; therefore individuals who quit with the help of one discipline may have been prepared to do so earlier by someone of another discipline. The consistency and skill involved is more important than discipline. Of course, any patient who quits gains both dental and medical benefits simultaneously, which is not surprising because oral health is completely integrated with general health and well-being.

CASE APPLICATION 29-1.3

Tobacco Cessation

Ms. Evans is beginning to exhibit oral symptoms from her smoking. Stained teeth and restorations, fibrous gingiva, and the initial formation of pockets spell trouble ahead if she continues to smoke. Fortunately, scientifically sound **tobacco-cessation** services are a natural component of twenty-first century oral hygiene and periodontal dental services. Ms. Evans needs help and wants help, as signaled by her history of attempting to quit.

Dental hygienists are especially appropriate to provide tobacco-cessation services and to reinforce abstinence. Hygienist time is often long enough to integrate the discussion into the service. Hygiene services are quickly reversed by continued tobacco use. Tobacco-related conditions and the results of care are readily visible. Patients are willing to learn in a nonthreatening clinic environment. Evidence exists that dental hygienists can be effective.[23,32]

HELPFUL METHODS

Treatment of disease follows understanding the disease. Unfortunately, threatening or castigating patients or recommending actions or prescribing or recommending smoking-cessation drugs without knowing how they work is ineffective. Uncertain results and frustration in the attempt are likely outcomes. Dental staff members should choose methods that are proven to be effective and should know how each method helps each patient manage dependency. To keep the service effective and brief, clinic teams should follow a simple routine to identify tobacco use and respond appropriately.

The most widely used system for such identification and treatment uses the five *As*: *a*sk, *a*dvise, *a*ssess, *a*ssist, and *a*rrange. The steps involving the clinician were first advanced by the National Cancer Institute[28] and then organized into a clinical practice guideline by the Agency for Healthcare Research and Quality[1]; these steps were refined further to become the 2000 Public Health Service guideline entitled *Treating Tobacco Use and Dependence*.[13] The current guideline is the global standard inasmuch as it is based on more than 6000 clinical tobacco use–intervention studies.

✳ CASE APPLICATION 29-1.4

Identifying a Tobacco User

Ms. Evans was identified as a tobacco user before she spoke to anyone in the clinic. The patient history form given to her on her visit included routine questions such as, "Do you use tobacco?" and "How interested are you in quitting?" If Ms. Evans had not been a user, she might have been commended for being tobacco free. This commendation is especially important to reinforce abstinence among former users.

However, Ms. Evans is a user; therefore you should learn the extent of her problem and her interest in solving it. Clues that Ms. Evans is dependent on nicotine include the following:
- She has been smoking for several years and started when she was young.
- She is smoking daily, averaging three fourths of a pack to more than a pack of cigarettes a day.
- She begins smoking within the first hour of awakening.
- She tried to quit twice. Her second relapse was the result of withdrawal symptoms, anxiety, and depressed mood, as well as her concern for weight gain.

In addition, Ms. Evans may have a tendency toward multiple dependencies. Her first relapse followed drinking more than she intended. She likes socializing, thus she may be frequently in an environment in which alcohol is used.

FIRST VISIT

Ask

All patients are asked to fill out a health history that specifically asks questions to discern which patients are tobacco users, as well as the type and frequency of use. The receptionist routinely notes each patient's tobacco use status on the chart so that all team members are aware of it, often along with other vital signs.

Advise

The clinician should advise the patient to stop. A powerful motivator for an individual to stop smoking is a tobacco-related symptom or condition. The clinician should listen to the patient's reasons and reinforce them. This step is motivational. The clinician is reinforcing the tobacco user's determination to quit. Approximately a third of smokers are content with their use or at least have more reasons to continue use than to quit.

✳ CASE APPLICATION 29-1.5

Reinforce the Decision to Quit

If Ms. Evans had been in this group, then possible caring, positive advice is as follows:

"I think you would be doing yourself a huge favor by quitting. Even though you are only 22, I can see where smoking is damaging your gums. Most adult gum disease occurs among tobacco users, and it is hard to treat successfully when a person keeps using it. What are your reasons for wanting to stop?"

Whatever reasons she might have, you should reinforce to help quicken her decision to quit.

Assess

The assess step highlights the critical point when tobacco-using patients decide to make a quit attempt or not; it is a triage step in which a subset of patients who were routinely *asked* and *advised* agree to make a quit attempt. Some patients might have special problems, addressed later, which suggest that referral would be an option. However, the healthcare team can help most patients.

The majority of tobacco users are not ready to make a quit attempt. The clinician should offer motivational remarks. Of assistance are the five *Rs*: *r*elevance, *r*isks, *r*ewards, *r*oadblocks, and *r*epetition.

Relevance

The importance of quitting should be made real to each patient. The clinician should observe how patients' personal relations, career, hobbies, sports activities, or anything else might be better without tobacco.

Risks

Patients must understand the risks against quality-of-life issues such as threats to their oral health and life-threatening diseases, as well as threats to others about whom they care.

Rewards

The clinician should remind patients about the benefits of quitting in terms of health, money, protection of family, and positive feelings of being tobacco free.

Roadblocks

The clinician should help patients identify obstacles to quitting and suggest means to overcome each of these obstacles.

Repetition

Few individuals react positively to a new idea. People need time to think about advantages and disadvantages of doing something different. Periodic reminders are taken more seriously than constant reminders.

Assist

The assist step moves beyond the first three steps (ask, advise, and assess), which are routinely used with all patients. The clinician should offer to help the patient. Successful quitting, defined as 6 months or longer for this chronic disease, is much more likely with help than when attempted alone. The assist

step focuses on a subset of tobacco users who decide to quit and may address the following topics:

- *Setting a quit date.* The patient should select the date and take ownership of the attempt.
- *Coping with stress.* Because quitting smoking is a stressful time for the patient, the individual should try to avoid adding unnecessary stress to the situation, which may jeopardize success efforts.
- *Coping with physical withdrawal, including possible depression.* Both nicotine-replacement agents (patch, gum, lozenges, nasal spray, and oral inhaler) and bupropion (Zyban) reduce the duration and intensity of withdrawal from smoking. Both types of agents counter the depression that may occur during the quitting process. Both nicotine gum and bupropion temporarily postpone weight gain. Using at least one of these products is recommended during withdrawal, and sometimes a combination of nicotine replacement with bupropion is recommended for individuals who have difficulty maintaining abstinence using only one product. The patient may purchase some over-the-counter (OTC) nicotine-replacement agents, whereas others are available only by prescription

---

✳ CASE APPLICATION 29-1.6

Providing Motivation to Quit

At the very least you should say to Ms. Evans, "I'll be ready to help you *when* you are ready," implying that she will want to quit sometime. To underscore the message, you can provide her with a pamphlet tailored to her interests and situation.

Ms. Evans is already highly motivated. She has tried to quit twice, and she is on her way to a new job in which smoking might not be permitted. She wants to make a good impression. The same three parts to *advise* are important: First, you should tell Ms. Evans clearly, but with compassion, that she should quit. Second, you should relate her smoking to a tobacco-related health condition, for example, her halitosis, stained teeth, and most poignantly, the early signs of periodontal disease. A mirror is a helpful visual argument. You should tell Ms. Evans about the cost and problem of these teeth becoming loose and perhaps being lost and the difficulty of successful treatment in smokers. Third, you should solicit Ms. Evans's reasons for wanting to quit so that, as she speaks, they become stronger in her mind by having expressed them. Reinforcement of Ms. Evans's reasons, which may have little to do with health, is persuasive; you should expand on them when possible.

Because this patient is interested in her appearance, a powerful argument is how most people do not think smoking is attractive and that it leaves odors in hair, clothes, and breath. Users are not aware of this odor because the tobacco suppresses senses of taste and smell. In addition, attractiveness is defined primarily by a healthy appearance, and smoking promotes premature aging, pallor, and leads to conditions that damage the body long before they become clinically evident. The tobacco companies have promoted being thin as an attribute, but it is not the same as attractiveness. Indeed, tobacco company advertising promotes appearance, wealth, popularity, cleanliness, and other

features, which the use of their products destroys or with which it has no relationship. If Ms. Evans develops intractable periodontal disease, then loss of teeth is going to make her appear older, whereas a healthy dentition would help preserve her attractiveness indefinitely.

Another potential motivation for Ms. Evans to quit smoking includes wanting to protect her body for motherhood. Women who smoke have a harder time conceiving and carrying their babies to term than do women who do not.[35] The unborn baby is exposed to toxins in tobacco, and tobacco smoke produces a tobacco-induced restricted oxygen flow. Therefore women who smoke during pregnancy are at increased risk of having babies with physical problems and greater learning and behavioral problems as they grow.[34]

Ms. Evans may not be aware of special health risks for women. For the same amount of smoking, women are at a much higher risk than men for developing lung cancer. In addition to chronic, fatal diseases, smoking leads to more days of illness throughout life, especially respiratory illnesses. You may say to Ms. Evans:

"Better you should enjoy life tobacco free and accumulate earned sick leave; or, if you need sick leave for colds and influenza, then their symptoms will not be intensified by the burden that smoking places on the respiratory system."

Another useful argument in this patient's case is that by becoming tobacco free before beginning her new job, Ms. Evans may find that developing new friends among employees is easier if she is not a smoker among a majority of nonsmoking colleagues. You might remind Ms. Evans that nearly four of every five adults are now tobacco free and that the trend is toward being tobacco free because many are quitting every day.

⚜ CASE APPLICATION 29-1.7

Suggestions for Successful Tobacco Cessation

Ideally, Ms. Evans should first select a quit date in the next few days so that she can be smoke free for a week or more when she begins her new job. You might phrase this information in the following way:

"You are much more likely to succeed if you have only one stress to manage at a time. Beginning a new job is stressful, no matter how much people might welcome you, so the quit date should not be at the same time."

Second, Ms. Evans is concerned about her weight, but she should not try to diet at the same time. She should recognize that her metabolism may likely fall during the first few weeks after quitting; therefore she will not require as many calories as she usually consumes. She should eat well but avoid sweets and fats. This information is important because her periodic craving for nicotine may be interpreted as hunger. She should know that women usually find that quitting during their follicular, rather than luteal, phase is less stressful than at other times. A nicotine-replacement agent or bupropion may also dampen the stress of withdrawal.

Last, you might suggest that Ms. Evans increase her exercise program because exercise is a healthy way to manage both stress and weight. The moment she stops smoking, her blood oxygen will improve because she will no longer have the peripheral vasoconstriction from the nicotine and the oxygen binding from carbon monoxide and cyanide from the smoke. Nicotine artificially increases heart rate but restricts blood flow to heart muscles, a dangerous condition.

(Box 29-5). The *American Dental Association Guide to Dental Therapeutics* describes individual attributes, indications, and precautions for each drug.[26]

- Two other drugs may be helpful in special circumstances: (1) nortriptyline, a tricyclic antidepressant, and (2) clonidine, an antihypertensive agent. However, the FDA has approved neither of these agents for smoking cessation. Thus they should not be used in dental practice because the treatment of clinical depression and hypertension is commonly considered beyond the scope of dental practice. Herbal products such as mint leaf preparations that are commercially promoted for spit tobacco users, although harmless, have not been shown to be effective and are not recommended. Popular behavioral smoking–cessation methods such as hypnosis, acupuncture, and laser therapy have not been shown to be effective and are not recommended.[39]
- *Coping with environmental cues to smoke.* Because social events prompt urges to smoke, the dental hygienist should ask the patient whether he or she would stop going to events where smoking is likely or at least suspend going during the first weeks when resisting will be most difficult. If the patient is involved in a significant relationship with a smoker or is sure to be in situations in which smoking occurs, he or she should prepare and repeatedly

practice in advance how to refuse offers to smoke. Indeed, individuals whose friendship the patient regards highly should be specifically solicited to help by not smoking in the patient's presence and to help encourage others not to do so. Such social support should be sought in all family, community, work, and pastime environments.

- *Coping with deeply ingrained habits.* The clinician should remind the patient that all the rituals of smoking that he or she has repeated thousands of times over the years are well developed and cannot be expected to simply disappear. New rituals need to be established to override old ones. The clinician should ask about habits that involve smoking (e.g., driving, eating). In addition, the patient must consider alternative actions to carrying, taking out, lighting, and puffing on a cigarette. The patient may practice fun or distracting alternative behaviors to break the mold.
- *Coping with other common relapse risks.* The clinician may try to identify specific behaviors that have led that patient to break the resolve to quit and begin smoking again and suggest ways the patient can avoid such situations or substitute more healthful alternatives.

⚜ CASE APPLICATION 29-1.8

Avoid Alcohol

Ms. Evans may not be alcohol dependent, but she must be aware that her resolve may be easily undermined when she drinks, as experience has taught her. She should avoid alcohol during the quitting process, especially because drinking is one of the most common reasons people relapse. You should suggest substituting alcohol-like drinks, such as straight tonic water, that have low sugar. If she uses nicotine gum, she should know that acidic beverages (carbonated drinks, fruit juices, coffee, and tea) prevent absorption of the nicotine that suppresses her withdrawal symptoms. She should avoid drinking acidic beverages 15 minutes before and during nicotine gum or lozenge use.

- Provide the patient with (1) a reminder about the chosen quit date and (2) a booklet the patient can use to prepare for that date, such as the Public Health Service booklet, *You Can Quit Smoking Consumer Guide*[1] (or in Spanish, *Usted Puede Dejar de Fumar Guia del Consumidor*) and the National Cancer Institute booklet, *Clearing the Air: Quit Smoking Today.*[28] These sources are written in simple language and contain many tips to prepare individuals to quit and *then* to manage the quitting process.

Arrange

Quitting tobacco use is a process. Typically, developing nicotine dependence takes several months to a few years. Once nicotine dependence is firmly established, quitting may require months before the brain has readjusted to normal function in the absence of nicotine. Even so, learned patterns of behavior and

BOX 29-5

U.S. Food and Drug Administration: Approved Tobacco-Cessation Pharmaceutical Agents

General Information

All smokers who try to quit should receive pharmacotherapy as part of the quitting process, except in the presence of contraindications (e.g., pregnancy). Choices are among three drug types: varenicline, which eases withdrawal symptoms and partially blocks the effects of nicotine; buproprion, which partially blocks the "liking" effect of nicotine; and a variety of nicotine-replacement drugs that continue to provide patients with nicotine but are free of the dangerous chemicals and substances in and on tobacco leaves, added to tobacco products, and/or in tobacco smoke. None of the FDA-approved products for smoking cessation is known to create a cardiovascular risk. Both buproprion and nicotine gum have been shown to delay, but not prevent, weight gain. Bupropion may be the drug of choice if the patient exhibits symptoms of depression. However, varenicline has been shown to be significantly better in achieving long-term abstinence.[†] All FDA-approved drugs may be used longer than recommended treatment by patients who desire long-term therapy. Varenicline should not be used in combination with either buproprion or nicotine replacement drugs.[‡] Combining the nicotine patch with nicotine gum or nicotine nasal spray is more efficacious than a single form of nicotine replacement, and selected patients should be encouraged to use such combined treatment if they are unable to quit using a single type of nicotine replacement. In addition, combining bupropion with an FDA-approved nicotine replacement may be more effective than using either drug alone. Higher doses than recommended of nicotine-replacement products have not been shown to significantly increase long-term quit rates.

Nonnicotine Tobacco-Cessation Drugs
Varenicline (Chantix)

Precautions: No cardiovascular risks are known. The most common side effects are nausea and abnormal dreams.

Contraindications: Varenicline is contraindicated in individuals who use bupropion (Wellbutrin or Zyban), a nicotine replacement drug, youths, women who are pregnant, women who are breast feeding, or individuals who have used a monoamine oxidase inhibitor in the past 14 days.

Dosage: Patients should begin with one 0.5 mg tablet every day for 3 days, then one 0.5 mg tablet twice daily, and then 1.0 mg tablet daily for 12 weeks, that is, the 3 months after the quit date. Unlike with nicotine replacement products, patients should begin using varenicline 1 to 2 weeks before their quit date.

Instructions:

Spontaneous quitting: Some patients lose their desire to smoke before their quit date or spontaneously reduce the amount they smoke.

Scheduling of dose: If nausea and vomiting is severe, a nicotine replacement product should be used first.

Alcohol: The patient should use alcohol only in moderation.

Bupropion SR (Zyban)

Precautions: No cardiovascular risks are known. The most common side effects are dry mouth and insomnia.

Contraindications: Bupropion SR is contraindicated in individuals with a history of seizure disorder, with a history of eating disorder, who use another form of bupropion (Wellbutrin or Wellbutrin SR), or who have used a monoamine oxydase inhibitor in the past 14 days.

Dosage: Patients should begin with a dose of 150 mg every morning for 3 days, then increase to 150 mg twice a day. This dose should continue for 3 months after the quit date. Unlike with nicotine-replacement products, patients should begin bupropion SR treatment 1 to 2 weeks before their quit date.

Instructions:

Spontaneous quitting: Some patients lose their desire to smoke before their quit date or spontaneously reduce the amount they smoke.

Scheduling of dose: If insomnia is marked, taking the evening dose earlier (in the afternoon, at least 8 hours after the first dose) may provide the individual some relief.

Alcohol: The patient should use alcohol only in moderation.

Nicotine-Replacement Tobacco-Cessation Drugs
General Precautions for Nicotine-Replacement Therapy

This therapy is not an independent risk factor for acute myocardial events. Nicotine-replacement therapy (NRT) should be used with caution among particular cardiovascular patient groups, as well as persons in the immediate (within 2 weeks) postmyocardial infarction period, those with serious arrhythmias, and those with serious or worsening angina pectoris.

Nicotine Patch

Precautions: Up to 50% of patients using the nicotine patch have a local skin reaction. Skin reactions are usually mild and self-limiting but may worsen over the course of therapy. Local treatment with hydrocortisone cream (1% or 0.5%) and rotating patch sites may ameliorate such local reactions. In less than 5% of patients, such reactions require the discontinuation of nicotine patch treatment.

Dosage: Treatment of 8 weeks or less has been shown to be as efficacious as longer treatment periods. Based on this finding, the following treatment schedules are suggested as reasonable for most patients. Clinicians should consider individualizing treatment based on specific patient characteristics, such as previous experience with the patch, amount smoked, and degree of nicotine dependence. Finally, clinicians should consider starting treatment on a lower patch dose in patients who smoke 10 or fewer cigarettes per day or who weigh 100 pounds or less.

---

*Over-the-counter (OTC) drugs.

Modified from Fiore MC et al: *Treating tobacco use and dependence: clinical practice guideline,* Rockville, Md, 2000, US Department of Health and Human Services, Public Health Service.

[†]Gonzales D et al: Varenicline, an α4β2 nicotinic acetylcoline receptor partial agonist, vs stained-release buproprion and placebo for smoking cessation: a randomized controlled trial, *JAMA* 296:47-55, 2006.

[‡]Tonstad S et al: Effect of maintenance therapy with Varenicline on smoking cessation: a randomized controlled trial, *JAMA* 296:64-71, 2006.

Continued

BOX 29-5

U.S. FOOD AND DRUG ADMINISTRATION: APPROVED TOBACCO-CESSATION PHARMACEUTICAL AGENTS—CONT'D

Drug Name	Duration	Dosage
Nicoderm CQ*	4 weeks	21 mg/24 hours
Habitrol	Then 2 weeks	14 mg/24 hours
	Then 2 weeks	7 mg/24 hours
Prostep	4 weeks	2 mg/24 hours
	Then 4 weeks	11 mg/24 hours
Nicotrol*	8 weeks	15 mg/16 hours

Instructions:

Location: At the start of each day, the patient should place a new patch on a relatively hairless location between the neck and waist.

Activities: No restriction exists while using the patch.

Time: A patch should be applied as soon as the patient wakes on quit day. With Nicotrol patches, or in patients experiencing sleep disruption, consider removing the patch before bedtime.

Nicotine Gum

Side effects: Common side effects include mouth soreness, hiccups, dyspepsia, and jaw ache. These effects are generally mild and transient and often may be alleviated by correcting the patient's chewing technique.

Dosage: Nicotine gum is available in 2-mg and 4-mg (per piece) doses. Generally the gum should be used for up to 12 weeks, with no more than 24 pieces per day. The gum is most commonly used for the first few months of a quit attempt. Clinicians should tailor the duration of therapy to fit the needs of each patient. Patients using the 2-mg strength should not use more than 30 pieces per day, whereas patients using the 4-mg strength should not exceed 20 pieces per day.

Nicorette, Nicorette Mint (over the counter only)

Instructions:

Chewing technique: Gum should be chewed slowly until a *peppery* or *minty* taste emerges, then *parked* between the cheek and gum to facilitate nicotine absorption through the oral mucosa. Gum should be slowly and intermittently *chewed and parked* for approximately 30 minutes or until the taste dissipates.

Absorption: Acidic beverages (e.g., coffee, juices, soft drinks) interfere with the buccal absorption of nicotine; thus eating and drinking anything except water should be avoided for 15 minutes before and during chewing.

Scheduling of dose: Patients often do not use enough gum to get the maximum benefit; that is, they chew too few pieces per day, and they do not use the gum for a sufficient number of weeks. Instructions to chew the gum on a fixed schedule (at least one piece every 1 to 2 hours) for at least 1 to 3 months may be more beneficial than ad lib use.

Nicotine Lozenge

Precautions: Not indicated for children or patients who are in immediate postmyocardial infarction recovery, who have a history of gastrointestinal disorders, who are pregnant, or who continue using tobacco.

Side effects: Common side effects include mouth soreness, hiccups, and dyspepsia.

Dosage: Use 2-mg lozenges for patients who smoke their first cigarette more than 1 hour after waking. Use 4-mg lozenge for patients who smoke their first cigarette within one-half hour after waking. One lozenge every 1 to 2 hours during weeks 1 through 6, every 2 to 4 hours during week 7 through 9, and every 4 to 8 hours during weeks 10 through 12. The patient should not use more than one lozenge at a time, or more than 5 in 6 hours, or more than 20 per day.

Instructions: Lozenge should be held and sucked, not chewed or swallowed. Do not eat or drink 15 minutes before using lozenge or when it is in the mouth.

Nicotine Inhaler

Local irritation reactions: Local irritation in the mouth and throat was observed in 40% of patients using nicotine inhalers. Coughing (32%) and rhinitis (23%) were also common. Severity generally was rated as mild, and the frequency of such symptoms declined with continued use.

Dosage: A dose from the nicotine inhaler consists of a puff or inhalation. Each cartridge delivers 4 mg of nicotine over 80 inhalations, of which approximately 2 mg is absorbed. Recommended treatment is at least 6 cartridges every day, with a maximum limit of 16 cartridges per day.

Nicotine Inhaler (prescription only)

Instructions:

Ambient temperature: Delivery of nicotine from the inhaler declines significantly at temperatures below 40° F. In cold weather, the inhaler and cartridges should be kept in an inside pocket or warm area.

Dose reduction: Use is recommended for up to 6 months, with gradual reduction in frequency or use over the last 6 to 12 weeks of treatment.

Nicotine Nasal Spray

Nasal or airway reactions: 94% of users report moderate to severe nasal irritation in the first 2 days of use; 81% still reported nasal irritation after 3 weeks, although rated severity was mild to moderate. Nasal congestion and transient changes in sense of smell and taste were also reported. Nicotine nasal spray should not be used in persons with severe reactive airway disease.

Nicotrol NS (prescription only)

Instructions:

Dose delivery: Patients should not sniff, swallow, or inhale through the nose while administering doses. The spray is best delivered with the head tilted slightly back.

environmental cues continue in memory so that even a single use of tobacco years later may quickly precipitate a return to the previous pattern of use. As for other chronic diseases and conditions, nicotine dependence has a long recovery period and requires a lifetime of patient monitoring and reinforcement.

✸ CASE APPLICATION 29-1.9

Follow-Up Contacts

Ms. Evans's first visit should conclude with arrangements for follow-up contacts, ideally face-to-face meetings but at least by telephone. Timing, duration, and frequency of these contacts are important.

FOLLOW-UP VISITS

Timing

The first follow-up contact with a patient is usually conducted by telephone. This brief contact should occur a day or two before the scheduled quit date to accomplish the following:

- Determine whether the patient still plans to quit on that date
- Remind the patient to stop using and discard all tobacco products the evening before
- Ask the patient whether he or she has questions or wants to discuss anything after reading the booklet
- Ask the patient whether he or she is prepared

Interventions as brief as 3 minutes may help, but longer visits are more effective. Most contact lasts from 3 to 10 minutes.

Any follow-up visit increases the likelihood of long-term success, but four or more person-to-person sessions appear especially effective in increasing long-term abstinence.[14] Visits should occur at least once a month while a pharmacotherapeutic agent is being used and during the month after it is discontinued. After that, follow-up visits at regular intervals for routine hygiene services should be adequate. Because nicotine dependency is chronic and relapsing, reinforcement of the patient's abstinence should be provided at every dental visit as enthusiastically as possible. Simply being delighted with her being tobacco free is a lifesaving service.

✸ CASE APPLICATION 29-1.10

Scheduling the First Follow-Up Visit

Ms. Evans should be seen within the first week after she quits, perhaps in the third or fourth day, because physical withdrawal appears to be a major problem. During this visit, you should continue to provide encouragement, determine what problems she is experiencing, suggest means to overcome each problem, and ensure that the pharmacologic agent selected is being used properly. Are persons around her being helpful? You should reinforce the importance of her avoiding taking even a single puff from a cigarette and reassure her that physical symptoms of withdrawal are a normal part of the healing process and will start to subside in frequency and intensity as time passes.

Relapse

If the patient has relapsed, as most patients who quit will, the clinician should then congratulate the patient on making the attempt. The following techniques are helpful:

- Recognize any period of abstinence as a personal accomplishment—a victory.
- Make the session a learning experience.
- Determine what led to the relapse: a social situation, physical withdrawal symptoms, or an emotional state.
- Ascertain from where the tobacco came.
- Review the reasons why the patient wanted to quit and ask whether he or she is willing to try again.
- Encourage the patient to set a new quit date.
- Repeat the key steps: building the patient's determination to quit, helping manage the quitting process, using pharmacotherapy, and encouraging the patient that other individuals who are important to him or her also help in important ways.

Repeated quit attempts are important, with an aim to extend the duration of time the patient is tobacco free each time. Some patients want to continue using a nicotine replacement for an extended time to dampen their craving.

Common causes for relapse are drinking alcohol, having a significant other who smokes, or failing to use the pharmacologic agent properly. As stated, common causes for women include anxiety, depression, and weight gain. The clinician should help the patient develop a coping strategy for each factor. Repeated quit attempts are the norm; on average, approximately one in five individuals who quit with the help of clinical assistance and guideline-recommended methods achieve abstinence of 6 months or longer. Success rates increase as the duration and intensity of the help provided increases. Such continued care is similar to the strategy used to treat other chronic conditions.

Referral

The clinician should consider referring the patient if he or she is not willing to try again, not receptive to the suggestion to reconsider quitting in a few weeks, or needs more intensive help than the clinician can provide. Perhaps 10% to 30% of patients are good candidates for referral, which can take several forms:

- Patients who require more intensive help than the clinician can provide should be referred to a specialist in nicotine dependence or to a group program.
- Patients who have low self-efficacy or self-esteem, have overwhelming personal problems, or are mentally or emotionally disadvantaged should be referred to an appropriate counselor.
- Patients who have multiple drug dependencies should be referred to a drug treatment program.
- Patients who have psychiatric comorbidities, such as acute depression, should be referred for assessment for psychiatric assistance.

Avoiding the provision of additional assistance to the patient through referral is unethical. Tobacco use presents a clear threat to oral health and life. Abandoning the service is also not good business practice because tobacco use is a long-term liability to the practice. It might present a risk-management problem if a tobacco-related oral condition progressed in the absence of continued advice and encouragement to quit.

Team Approach

A few simple management steps permit tobacco-intervention services to be integrated into any clinic routine. First, the clinic should have a tobacco-intervention coordinator. This individual, usually not the primary care provider, ensures that all new employees are oriented to the system, that a mechanism is in place to identify and follow through with patients, and that appropriate motivational and quit method literature is available. Second, the clinic should have a tobacco-free policy such that signs are posted, tobacco-using staff members are offered help to quit, reception magazines and other materials are free of tobacco advertising, and other methods to convey that tobacco use is not encouraged. Third, patient records and the record-keeping system should facilitate clinical tobacco intervention services. Each chart should have a simple chart reminder, obvious to all staff, that identifies each patient's tobacco use status. The patient history form should determine whether tobacco is used. For example, the American Dental Association history form presents this question. Tobacco-intervention services should be coded. Records should provide for progress notes from follow-up visits.

> **Note**
>
> Since the second revision in 1994, the ADA's Current Dental Terminology lists under Other Preventive Services, code number 01320: *Tobacco Counseling For the Control and Prevention of Oral Diseases.* The statement accompanying this code is "Tobacco prevention and cessation services reduce patient risks of developing tobacco related oral diseases and conditions and improves prognosis for certain dental therapies."

Patients expect and respond to tobacco-intervention advice from respected clinicians. Dental teams enjoy providing this service for its ability to draw from an understanding of each patient's physical and mental status and social environment. Helping an individual become tobacco free, thereby reducing his or her risks to health and well-being, is extremely rewarding.

Nicotine dependence is a chronic, progressive, relapsing brain condition reinforced by certain social conditions, environmental cues, ingrained repetitive behavior, and tobacco industry strategies that attempt to give reasons to continue or start again. The action of nicotine in the CNS is similar to that of other psychoactive drugs, all of which deprive users of a degree of control over their capacity to think, do, and feel. Tobacco use adversely affects patients' oral health and the dental team's practice.

Although adult cigarette use declined during the 1970s and 1980s, it remained fairly stable in the 1990s and then continued to decline to the level that approximately 22% of adults are now smoking cigarettes.[31] Tobacco use by youth increased during the 1990s and then declined to 22%.[9]

In recent years, much has been learned about how the brain and mind work and how psychoactive substances alter func-

tion. In the future, a richer understanding of the underlying molecular and cellular neurologic processes should aid patient management in many ways. Although each psychoactive chemical has its own specific actions and effects, all of these substances act on the same system and in related ways. Clinicians who become competent in managing nicotine dependence improve their ability to diagnose and manage patients who have other drug-related and other neurologic conditions.

During the 1990s, remarkable progress was made in understanding how the tobacco industry conducts business and the social costs of tobacco use. Public awareness may convert this understanding to public outrage as more information is learned. Indeed, smoking is prohibited in an ever-increasing number of public environments. The global mortality for tobacco-caused disease is projected to rise from the current annual toll of 4 million deaths per year to 8.4 million per year by 2020.[41] However, the tobacco industry continues to market lethal products and to resist public health measures. A bright future depends on a well-informed, concerned public demanding better accountability from the tobacco industry.[18]

Clinically, brief, practical, and scientifically sound tobacco-intervention methods exist that should be routinely used in dental practice. Dental hygiene services are easily defeated by tobacco use. Dental hygienists have excellent opportunities to encourage their tobacco-using patients to quit and help them do so. Long-term abstinence is much easier to achieve when a caring person is encouraging and educates patients on how to manage the quitting process. Such help is ethically and morally sound and is satisfying with every success.

References

1. Agency for Healthcare Research and Quality: *You can quit smoking consumer guide,* Rockville, Md, 2000, US Department of Health and Human Services [Publications Clearinghouse: (800) 358-9295].
2. Allman JM: *Evolving brains,* New York, 1999, Scientific American Library.
3. Anthony JC, Warner LA, Kessler RC: Comparative epidemiology of dependence on tobacco, alcohol, controlled substances and inhalants: basic findings from the National Comorbidity Survey, *Exp Clin Psychopharm* 2:244-268, 1994.
4. Bates C, Jarvis M, Connolly G: *Tobacco additives: cigarette engineering and nicotine addiction,* Atlanta, Centers for Disease Control and Prevention Tobacco Industry Document web site at: http://www.cdc.gov/tobacco/industrydocuments/index.htm. Accessed July 14, 1999.
5. Benowitz NL, ed: *Nicotine safety and toxicity,* New York, 1998, Oxford University Press.
6. Bolinder G et al: Smokeless tobacco use and increased cardiovascular mortality among Swedish construction workers, *Am J Public Health* 84:399-404, 1994.
7. Brandt AM: Recruiting women smokers: the engineering of consent, *J Am Med Womens Assoc* 51:63-66, 1996.
8. Burgan SW: The role of tobacco use in periodontal diseases: a literature review, *Gen Dent* 45:449-460, 1997.
9. Centers for Disease Control and Prevention: Tobacco use, access, and exposure to tobacco in media among middle and high school

students in the United States, April 1, 2004, *MMWR Morbid Mortal Wkly Rep* 54(12):297-301, 2005.

10. Centers for Disease Control and Prevention: Health behaviors of adults: United States, 1999-2001, National Center for Health Statistics 2004, *Vital Health Stat* 10:219, 2004.

11. Fagerstrom K, Schneider NG: Measuring nicotine dependence: a review of the Fagerstrom tolerance questionnaire, *J Behav Med* 12:159-182, 1989.

12. Fiore MC: Trends in cigarette smoking in the United States: the epidemiology of tobacco use, *Med Clin North Am* 76:289-303, 1992.

13. Fiore et al: *Treating tobacco use and dependence: clinical practice guideline,* Rockville, Md, 2000, US Department of Health and Human Services, Public Health Service.

14. Fiore MC et al: *Clinical practice guideline number 18: smoking cessation,* Rockville, Md, 1996, US Department of Health and Human Services, Public Health Service, Agency for Health Care Policy and Research, AHCPR Publication No 96-0692.

15. Grossi SG et al: Response to periodontal therapy in diabetics and smokers, *J Periodontol* 67:1094-1102, 1996.

16. Grossi SG et al: Assessment of risk for periodontal disease: II—risk indicators for alveolar bone loss, *J Periodontol* 66:23-29, 1995.

17. Grossi SG et al: Assessment of risk for periodontal disease: I—risk indicators for attachment loss, *J Periodontol* 65:260-267, 1994.

18. Harris JE: American cigarette manufacturers' ability to pay damages: overview and a rough calculation, *Tobacco Control* 5: 292-294, 1996.

19. Henningfield JE, Cohen C, Pickworth WB: Psychopharmacology of nicotine. In Orleans CT, Slade J, eds: *Nicotine addiction: principles and management,* New York, 1993, Oxford University Press.

20. Hughes JR et al: Smoking cessation among self-quitters, *Health Psychol* 11:331-334, 1992.

21. Kaufman NJ, Nichter M: The marketing of tobacco to women: global perspectives. In *Women and the tobacco epidemic: challenges for the 21st century,* Geneva, Switzerland, 2001, World Health Organization.

22. Kelder G, Davidson P, eds: *The multistate master settlement agreement and the future of state and local tobacco control: an analysis of selected topics and provisions of the multistate master settlement agreement of November 23, 1998,* Boston, 1999, Northeastern University School of Law, Tobacco Control Resource Center.

23. Krall EA, Garvey AJ, Garcia RI: Alveolar bone loss and tooth loss in male cigar and pipe smokers, *J Am Dent Assoc* 130:57-64, 1999.

24. Little SJ, Stevens VJ: Dental hygiene's role in reducing tobacco use, *J Dent Hyg* 65(7):346-350, 1991.

25. Manley M et al: Clinical interventions in tobacco control, *JAMA* 266:3172-3173, 1991.

26. Mecklenburg RE: Cessation of tobacco use. In *ADA guide to dental therapeutics,* ed 3, Chicago, 2003, American Dental Association.

27. Mecklenburg RE et al: *Tobacco effects in the mouth,* Bethesda, Md, 1994, US Department of Health and Human Services, Public Health Service, National Institutes of Health, NIH Publication No. 96-3330.

28. National Cancer Institute: *Clearing the air: quit smoking today,* Bethesda, Md, 2003, The Institute, NIH Publication No 03-1647.

29. O'Keefe MA, Pollay RW: Deadly targeting of women in promoting cigarettes, *J Am Med Womens Assoc* 51:67-69, 1996.

30. Pierce JP, Lee L, Gilpin EA: Smoking initiation by adolescent girls, 1944 through 1988: an association with targeted advertising, *JAMA* 271:608-611, 1994.

31. Schoenborn CA et al: Health behaviors of adults: United States, 1999-2001, National Center for Health Statistics 2004, *Vital Health Stat* 10:219, 2004.

32. Severson HH et al: Using the hygienist visit to deliver a tobacco cessation program, *J Am Dent Assoc* 129:993-999, 1998.

33. Shopland DR, Burns DM: Medical and public health implications of tobacco addiction. In Orleans CT, Slade J, eds: *Nicotine addiction: principles and management,* New York, 1993, Oxford University Press.

34. Slotkin TA: The impact of fetal nicotine exposure on nervous system development and its role in sudden infant death syndrome. In Benowitz NL, ed: *Nicotine safety and toxicity,* New York, 1998, Oxford University Press.

35. Stein Z: Smoking and reproductive health, *J Am Med Wom Assoc* 51:29-30, 1996.

36. Teague C: *Survey of cancer research with emphasis upon possible carcinogens from tobacco,* RJ Reynolds internal report, February 2, 1953, Bates No 501932947-2968.

37. Tomar SL, Asma S: Smoking-attributed periodontitis in the United States: findings from NHANES III, *J Periodontol* 71: 743-751, 2000.

38. US Department of Health and Human Services: *The health consequences of smoking: a report of the Surgeon General,* Atlanta, 2004, Department of Health and Human Services, Centers for Disease Control and Prevention, Office on Smoking and Health.

39. US Department of Health and Human Services: *Preventing tobacco use among young people: a report of the Surgeon General,* Atlanta, 1994, US Department of Health and Human Services, Centers for Disease Control and Prevention, National Center for Chronic Disease Prevention and Health Promotion, Office on Smoking and Health.

40. US Department of Health and Human Services: *Reducing the health consequences of smoking: 25 years of progress,* Rockville, Md, 1989, US Department of Health and Human Services, Public Health Service, Centers for Disease Control, Office on Smoking and Health. DHHS Publication No (CDC) 89-8411.i.

41. World Health Organization: *Women and the tobacco epidemic: challenges for the 21st century,* Geneva, Switzerland, 2001, The Organization.

Care of Appliances and Dental Prostheses

Kenneth Shay

INSIGHT

Dental practices vary with respect to the role the dental hygienist is expected to play in educating patients about the care of intraoral appliances. Although the majority of a dental hygienist's training and professional practice is generally devoted to removing deposits from the teeth, patient education in oral health is an important and indispensable duty. The large number of patients with oral prosthetic appliances—dentures, bridges, splints, and orthodontic devices—must be taught and periodically reminded of the techniques for and importance of proper care of their appliances. In addition, the dental hygienist plays an essential role in the assessment of the integrity of such devices and the tissues they contact and in the referral of developing and extant problems before they worsen.

✺ CASE STUDY 30-1 | Caring for the Prosthodontic Patient

You have just begun employment in a thriving prosthodontics group practice headed by three young, full-time dentists. You are the first hygienist to be employed by the practice because, until lately, most of the patients had general dentists who oversaw the cases and provided preventive services, as needed. However, with the growth of the practice, the expanding number of patients with sophisticated oral reconstructions needing attentive preventive strategies has caused the partner dentists to realize that a dental hygienist dedicated to their patients would be an excellent patient service.

Your first patient illustrates the wisdom of their plan. Dr. Raj Basha, a 72-year-old retired professor of engineering at the nearby state university, has an edentulous maxilla that features a severely resorbed anterior ridge segment and a partially edentulous mandibular dentition. The maxillary arch is restored with a complete overdenture retained by a pair of implant-borne attachments that are connected with a gold bar that is in contact with the residual tissue. His mandibular dentition features a **porcelain fused-to-metal bridge** from canine to canine, full-coverage surveyed crowns with supragingival margins on all four premolars, and a removable **partial denture** that bilaterally replaces the molars. Dr. Basha is attuned to the *engineering* of his prostheses and takes good care of them, although he has noticed that the shiny silver metal of the lower partial is darkening and becoming dull.

Dr. Basha's mouth is rather dry, and the appearance of the periodontium around his remaining teeth is strongly suggestive of a history of resective periodontal surgery. The abundant exposed root surfaces are only moderately clean but appear free of dental caries. Despite the plaque biofilm, the gingiva appears healthy and features minimal bleeding on probing, and probe depths do not exceed 3 mm. Dr. Basha informs you that he uses a fluoride carrier each evening when he remembers to do so but admits that he dislikes the flavor of the topical fluoride he currently uses. He inquires as to whether you have a preferred type of fluoride gel and voices his hope that it might be a better-tasting product. Dr. Basha is familiar with floss, floss threaders, and interproximal brushes but prefers to use the last of these items in the mandible because of arthritic changes in his hands and right shoulder. The tissue around the splint bar in the anterior maxilla is inflamed, although the patient reports no discomfort in that area and seems confused when you inquire about his regimen for keeping the bar's tissue surface clean.

Dr. Basha is an overweight man who is a mouth breather. He requests to have his prophylaxis completed with the chair only partly reclined because he has even greater difficulty breathing when flat on his back. Further questioning reveals that this same problem has plagued him and his wife at night and that episodes of labored or even interrupted nocturnal breathing recently led to one of the prosthodontists fabricating a device for him to help manage his sleep apnea.

LEARNING OUTCOMES

After reading this chapter the student will be able to:

1. Correctly identify the following dental appliances: fixed partial denture, removable partial denture, complete removable denture, overdenture, splint, fluoride tray, bleaching tray, and maxillofacial prosthesis.
2. Practice role-playing a dental hygienist in assessing a patient with fixed and removable prosthetic replacements.
3. Detail the instruments, products, and procedures that are used to clean removable dental prostheses.
4. Explain the need for daily self-care of implant abutments, and specify how and why particular care must be taken.
5. Correctly identify and explain the cause of soft tissue pathoses associated with improperly maintained dental prostheses.
6. Explain to a patient the reason and method for cleaning a dental appliance and the abutment teeth, regardless of whether the appliance is fixed, removable, implant-borne, therapeutic, or prosthetic.

Intraoral appliances make up a varied, large, and important aspect of the practice of dentistry. Intraoral appliances may comprise the dental treatment itself, as with a denture or a **facial prosthesis.** They may also be the instrument by which care is affected, as with orthodontic appliances or bleaching trays. The appliance may play a key role in preventing disease, as with a fluoride carrier or a night guard. Finally, appliances may be used as a temporary measure, as with a **surgical stent,** or a long-lived measure, as with a **fixed bridge.**

Care of dental appliances is as varied as the devices themselves. Some prostheses are cleaned intraorally (e.g., fixed bridges, **implant abutments**), whereas others must be cared for extraorally (e.g., dentures, orthodontic appliances). Some appliances require the regular application of a material to accomplish their tasks (e.g., fluoride carriers, bleaching trays), whereas other devices may benefit from the addition of a material, but not all patients believe that this is necessary (e.g., using **denture adhesive** for dentures and certain maxillofacial prostheses). The cleaning of dental prostheses can involve brushing, soaking, immersing in ultrasonic baths, using microwave radiation, or combining these procedures. A variety of mechanical and chemical products is available, generally as over-the-counter products, for the care of dental appliances.

Some dental practices delegate all discussion of appliance care to the dental assistant, reserving the dental hygienist's time exclusively for intraoral care. Other dentists prefer to retain sole responsibility for instructing patients about the care and use of all dental devices. Most dental practices fall somewhere in the middle of these two preferences and have policies or practices that clarify the roles that team members are expected to play with respect to instructing patients on the care of dental appliances.

Role of the Dental Hygienist

The dental hygienist must:

- Be fully familiar with the range of dental appliances encountered in practice
- Know how to keep all dental appliances clean
- Be able to detect current or impending problems
- Be able to distinguish between clinical situations in which he or she is able to handle the patient's needs and those in which a dentist should be consulted

As a key member of the dental team, the dental hygienist is considered most focused on issues of prevention and patient education. For this reason, patients commonly direct many questions about self-care issues to the hygienist. Even if the dental practice's custom is to have the dentist provide information on the care of prostheses, deferring the answers to a patient's question may not be practical for a hygienist (Figure 30-1).

> *Patient Education Opportunity*
>
> Patients need to be educated as to which methods and compounds are or are not suitable for their own needs.

> *Note*
>
> The dental hygienist also must be familiar with dental appliances because no one in the dental office—except the dentist—devotes as much attention to detailed scrutiny of the oral cavity as does the hygienist. As such, the hygienist needs to be comfortable in recognizing intraoral conditions that represent heightened need for oral self-care and in situations that require a dentist's attention.

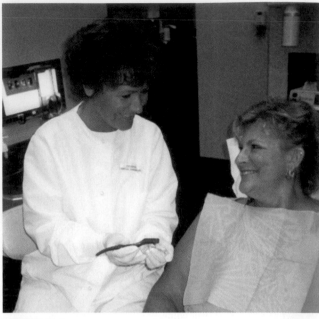

FIGURE 30-1
The role of the dental hygienist often includes the education of patients about the care of intraoral appliances.

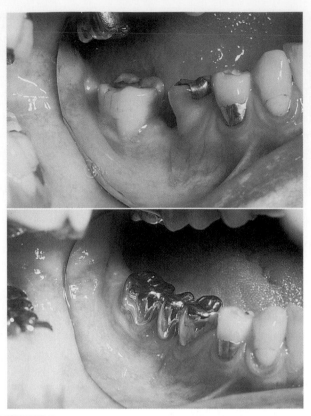

FIGURE 30-2
A, A common prosthetic dental solution for a missing single tooth is the fixed bridge. **B,** A three-unit bridge made of cast gold has been cemented into place, which provides the patient with additional occlusal function—and also with some new hygiene challenges.

Overview of Dental Appliances

FIXED PARTIAL DENTURES

Fixed partial dentures, also commonly called *bridges,* are multi-tooth devices that replace one or more missing teeth (Figure 30-2). Natural teeth, termed *retainers* or **abutments,** are located on either side of the artificial tooth (termed the **pontic**) or teeth and support one or more pontics, which the patient is not able to remove. Clinicians should be alert to the following four common problems to which bridges are prone:

- The connection between an abutment and a pontic may break, which results in excessive and adverse forces on the other abutment. A break between a pontic and an abutment is readily visualized as an irregular linear separation, usually in the area that mimics the interproximal region. The fracture usually permits independent, visible movement of the parts on either side of the break, and therefore it must be brought to a dentist's attention without delay. Although some bridges are designed in such a way as to permit independent movement of the pontic and one abutment, the connection in such a case is a *machined keyway* or *rest,* and the independent movements of the abutments are generally not visible.
- Because bridges use natural teeth to withstand the forces on the pontic, the abutment teeth experience increased occlusal forces and are prone to trauma from occlusion. Mobility of a bridge abutment that is more exaggerated than mobility of teeth elsewhere in the mouth should be brought to a dentist's attention without delay.
- Bridges are impediments to plaque biofilm control because they hinder the removal of plaque biofilm from the proximal surfaces of abutments and provide new surfaces on which plaque biofilm may collect, such as the side of the pontic facing the alveolar ridge tissue. In many cases, this side of the pontic has been designed for esthetic reasons with concavities that make hygiene impossible; in other cases, the pontic is fully convex, but the patient does not keep its undersurface clean. In either of these situations, the alveolar ridge tissue may be inflamed and can bleed spontaneously.
- The pontic of a fixed bridge undergoes a limited but still finite amount of bending under function. Porcelain is more inflexible than metal; thus, if deformation exceeds a certain level, then the porcelain of a porcelain-to-metal fixed bridge may exhibit fracture, particularly in the pontic and embrasure areas.

COMPLETE DENTURES

Complete dentures replace all of the teeth of either the mandible, the maxilla, or both. The hygienist may see complete dentures (also called **full dentures**) if the patient is edentulous in only one arch, which therefore requires care of the natural teeth of the opposing arch. If some of the teeth have been endodontically treated and contoured flush or nearly flush with the alveolar ridge, the denture resting over these structures is termed an *overdenture.* In this case, the remaining teeth (the *overdenture abutments*) still require periodic scaling (Figure 30-3).

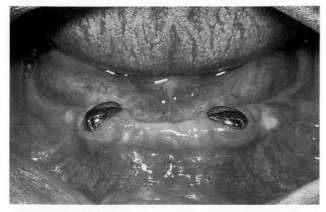

FIGURE 30-3
Overdenture abutments may be unrestored, restored only at the endodontic access, or restored to a contour that is most favorable for the retention of the prosthesis.

DENTAL CONSIDERATIONS

An **overdenture** is fabricated much as a denture, but the resulting prosthesis is far more stable and retentive than a denture, which allows the patient to exert more bite force. An overdenture may be preferable to a removable partial denture when the abutments are mobile or badly broken down or when the abutments disrupt the plane of occlusion.

✦ CASE APPLICATION 30-1.1

Patient with an Overdenture

Dr. Basha has an overdenture. As you continue to read, determine the steps you would take when caring for him.

Abutments are generally endodontically treated, but this procedure is not necessary if the pulp is not exposed when the abutment is reduced occlusally. Abutments may be unrestored, restored only at the endodontic access, or restored to a contour that is most favorable for retaining the overdenture.

Complete dentures are usually made of pink or clear acrylic resin, although some dentures may have metallic inserts for strength and rigidity. The teeth of dentures may be made from a material that bonds with the pink denture base (acrylic or composite) or from porcelain, which necessitates some means for mechanically connecting the teeth to the denture. The tissue surface of some complete dentures may have a lining of a material that is more resilient than acrylic. These *soft liners* can be temporary (placed by a dentist as a *tissue conditioner* to reduce trauma to the soft tissues) or permanent (placed by a dentist or a dental laboratory).

Patient Education Opportunity

Equivalent products to soft liners can be purchased over the counter by patients in pharmacies, but in most cases, these products cause oral trauma and irreparable damage to the denture itself.

As mentioned previously, some complete dentures are designed to sit over teeth that have been reduced (and sometimes crowned) to extend only slightly beyond the contour of the alveolar ridge. These overdentures may sit passively on the recontoured teeth or may actively engage some retentive device attached to the root face. In other cases, complete dentures, usually only mandibular ones, may have most of the portion of the base that contacts the tissues made from chrome-cobalt alloy, which affords increased accuracy and improved tissue reaction.

The clinician needs to be alert to the following dental considerations when caring for a patient with one or more removable complete dentures.

- Fractures in the acrylic base may readily reduce retention of the prosthesis, pinch the soft tissues, or cut the tongue. The flanges of dentures may have broken off if the appliance was dropped on a hard surface; the resulting sharp edges may traumatize adjacent tissues or the tongue. Fractures and dentures that are missing parts of their flanges need to be brought to the dentist's attention.

- Fractures in prosthetic teeth are common. Patients may be unaware of them, but they may be the source of vague complaints of poor chewing ability or impaired hygiene. Missing or damaged teeth need to be brought to the dentist's attention.

- Extreme wear of acrylic teeth, to the extent that mastication takes place against one or more areas of pink acrylic base material, which is much less resistant to wear, requires repair before perforation of the denture base occurs (Figure 30-4). Perforation through the denture base may be responsible for claims of looseness (as the *seal* of an upper denture is lost) or soreness (as the source of the perforation now traumatizes the underlying tissue). Perforation generally necessitates remake or at least major modification of the prosthesis and definitely needs to be called to a dentist's attention.

- Stained prosthetic teeth are common if the denture was made with porcelain teeth because no chemical bond exists—only an intimate fit that is prone to leakage—between porcelain teeth and the denture base, and thus stain accumulates along that interface (Figure 30-5).

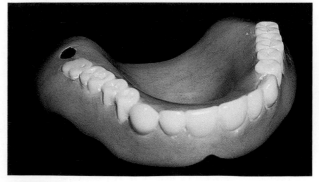

FIGURE 30-4
If extreme wear is apparent in an area of the denture base, then repair is required before perforation of the denture base and loss of retention occur.

- Overdentures with retentive elements generally require that parts of these elements be replaced once or more each year. Overdentures that fail to engage their retainers or engage some retainers more strongly and others less tightly need to be called to a dentist's attention.

- Soft liners of dentures often peel away from the base, which leads to odor, stains, and irritation. Soft bases may also be less resilient than when originally placed. Problems with soft liners should be brought to the dentist's attention.

REMOVABLE PARTIAL DENTURES

Removable partial dentures (RPDs), often termed *partials* or *removable bridges,* replace some, but not all, teeth in an arch. They generally attach to two or more remaining natural teeth with metallic clasps or wires or with soft plastic rings in the body of the denture that slip over the natural teeth. Partials are usually fabricated with a combination of metallic and acrylic elements. Some partials are wholly metal, with the prosthetic teeth made of porcelain, acrylic, or composite that is mechanically attached to the metal. Other partial dentures are wholly acrylic except for small wires that clip onto two or more natural teeth (termed *abutments* or *retainers,* as with fixed bridges). The simplest version of this form of partial denture is fabricated without any clasps and replaces one or a few anterior teeth. Called *flippers,* these devices stay in place with the engagement of small undercut areas on the palatal side of maxillary teeth between lingual palatal gingival papillae and interproximal contact areas. The most common partial has a cast metal framework that is largely encased in pink acrylic to which the prosthetic teeth are attached. In this partial, highly polished metal pieces of the framework extend beyond the acrylic to attach the appliance to the abutment teeth (Figure 30-6).

For a patient with RPDs, the clinician needs to be alert to the following dental considerations:

- Fractures within acrylic elements that pose a risk of laceration to the oral soft tissues

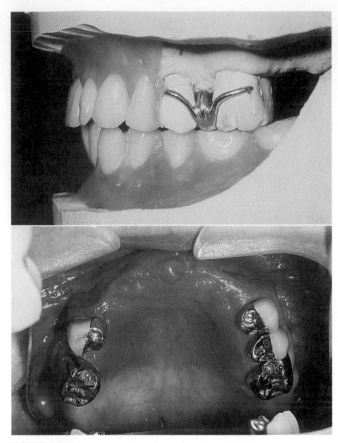

FIGURE 30-6
A, Esthetic results can be excellent, and the prosthesis allows natural teeth and soft tissues to distribute and share the added occlusal function. **B,** Removable partial dentures pose oral hygiene challenges by impeding the cleansing action of saliva and by placing large areas of soft and hard tissues in contact with materials that retain plaque biofilm and food debris.

- Metal portions, particularly smaller ones, that have broken off and thus pose a laceration hazard to the soft tissues of the oral cavity and indicate that the prosthesis is exerting forces onto teeth and tissues that vary from those intended by the original design
- Fractured teeth, worn teeth, stained areas around teeth, and signs of wear through the base acrylic, as described for complete dentures in the preceding section

IMPLANT AND IMPLANT-BORNE PROSTHESES

Implants and **implant-borne prostheses** have become widely used in dentistry. Many of the care issues associated with this form of treatment are identical to ones already discussed. Specifically, if the case has been restored with fixed bridgework, then the clinician needs to be alert for broken connectors, loss of porcelain, and the need for hygiene techniques to clean the surface of the prosthesis adjacent to alveolar ridge tissue. An additional consideration not present in tooth-borne fixed partial dentures is for the clinician to assess the integrity of the screws that attach the fixed bridgework to the implants scrupulously and to call to a dentist's attention any suspicious loosening or separation. If the case has been restored with a complete

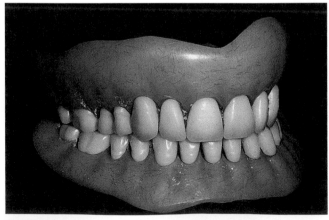

FIGURE 30-5
Because porcelain denture teeth do not bond to the denture base, many years of use may result in unaesthetic staining that cannot be removed between the porcelain prosthetic teeth and the denture base.

denture (specifically, an overdenture retained by attachments connected to the implants), then most of the issues raised previously in connection with complete dentures apply (e.g., damage to the base; need to assess retention of retainers; wear; fracture, or stain of prosthetic teeth).

The additional challenge that implants present to clinicians concerns the assessment and care of the **gingiva-implant interface.** As with the gingiva-tooth interface, an epithelialized sulcus exists along the subgingival surface of the implant. However, with implants, no junctional epithelium and no epithelial attachment exist. Failure on the part of the patient to remove plaque biofilm fastidiously from the supragingival and subgingival tissues around implants results in gingival inflammation (Figure 30-7) that may, in some cases, develop into the implant equivalent of periodontitis, termed **periimplantitis.** Periimplantitis involves inflammatory cell infiltration of the bone, purulent exudate around the implant, loss of bony support, and if not treated, eventual exfoliation of the implant. The clinician needs to devote the same level of meticulous assessment and removal of supragingival and subgingival deposits to implants as is expended on teeth. Instrumentation is slightly different, however.

> *Distinct Care Modifications*
> Special nonmetal scalers and curets are recommended for professional care of implants. Stainless steel instruments are contraindicated for instrumentation to eliminate the possibility of scratching or otherwise damaging the smooth, machined surface of the implants, which would lead to more rapid and tenacious plaque biofilm accumulation and greater hygiene difficulties.

ORTHODONTIC APPLIANCES

Orthodontic appliances may be fixed or removable and active or passive. The most common variety encountered outside of the orthodontic practice is the passive, removable variety, often called a **retainer** because its function is to retain the teeth in the position to which they were moved during the active phase of orthodontic therapy. Retainers are generally made from a tinted or colorless clear acrylic with one or more bent wire elements. Clinicians should examine retainers for sharp wires (usually an indication that an element has broken off as a result of metal fatigue) or cracks in the acrylic base. Either of these findings requires a dentist's attention.

SPLINTS

Splints are designed to take stresses off the temporomandibular joint by providing a healthful interocclusal resting position for the mandible. Splints are generally made to lock onto the maxillary arch, covering the occlusal surfaces and incisal edges. They may be retained by extensions of the acrylic base that lock into interproximal areas or with small ball clasps that extend beyond the acrylic. Splints are customarily made from clear acrylic and require periodic adjustment to continue to contact the mandibular teeth uniformly. As was specified for orthodontic appliances, a dentist needs to be informed when the hygienist finds sharp or broken wires and cracks or holes caused by excess wear in the acrylic base.

MOUTHGUARDS, NIGHT GUARDS, FLUORIDE CARRIERS, AND BLEACHING TRAYS

Mouthguards, night guards, fluoride carriers, and bleaching trays are made for patients by dentists but are rarely seen again in the dental office. They are made by drawing a heated sheet of plastic over a plaster or stone model of a patient's arch by using a vacuum apparatus. When cooled, the plastic is then trimmed just short of the gingival margin (sometimes more, sometimes less) and removed from the model so that the trimmed areas can be smoothed. These devices are usually made from 0.050-inch flexible clear acrylic that deforms elastically to a degree that undercut areas may be engaged, providing retention. Mouthguards are generally made for patients who are at risk, usually in sports, for blows or shocks to the jaws and dentition. Night guards are often recommended for bruxism.

> *Distinct Care Modifications*
> Patients with high rates of dental caries or with a risk for rampant dental caries should be considered candidates for fluoride carriers. Fluoride carriers and bleaching trays provide an intimate fit of appliance against teeth.

Current thinking suggests that the introduction of the additional occlusal material interrupts uncontrollable clenching and grinding or at least switches the trauma on irreplaceable tissues (teeth) to trauma on a material (the mouthguard) that is easier to replace.

In this way, when a small amount of remineralizing fluoride solution or an enamel-bleaching agent is placed into the tray before insertion, the desired chemical is brought into intimate contact with the teeth until the tray is removed (Figure 30-8). After the carrier is removed, excess gel in the mouth is expectorated. The carrier should then be rinsed thoroughly (brushing with a denture brush is also acceptable) and stored in a safe place. The patient spits out the excess medicament (either fluoride gel or bleaching solution) and must not rinse, eat, or drink for at least 30 minutes.

MAXILLOFACIAL PROSTHESES

Maxillofacial prostheses encompass a wide variety of removable appliances used to replace missing anatomical structures

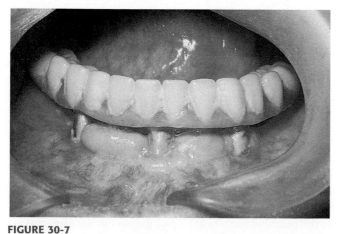

FIGURE 30-7
Failure to remove plaque biofilm from implant abutments may result in a disease process termed *periimplantitis,* which is similar to periodontitis.

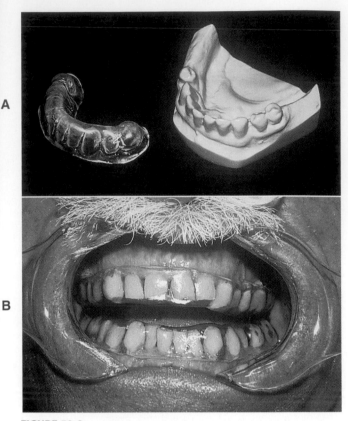

FIGURE 30-8
A, A model of the patient's dentition serves as the template for a vacuum-formed appliance that covers all buccal, lingual, and occlusal surfaces along with the gingiva immediately adjacent to the teeth. **B,** At the recommended frequency (usually daily), the patient places a drop or less of fluoride gel into each tooth hollow in the carrier and then inserts the carrier for the recommended period.

(loss caused by trauma, surgical resection for malignancy, or congenital defect) other than teeth or, less commonly, to supplement insufficient neuromuscular control. Maxillofacial prostheses may be entirely intraoral, such as when a complete or partial denture has an attached **obturator** that replaces all or part of the palate or maxilla (Figure 30-9) or has a posterior extension called a **palatal lift** that positions a flaccid soft palate superiorly and thereby aids speech and swallowing. The prosthesis may have both intraoral and extraoral components, such as when a maxillary prosthesis is connected to an extraoral piece that prosthetically replaces the nose, an eye, or another missing facial structure. Maxillofacial prostheses may be exclusively extraoral, replacing an ear, a nose, part of an orbit, or a cheek.

Not being under the care of a specialist would be unusual for a patient with a maxillofacial prosthesis; therefore the role the hygienist plays in the care of such prostheses is limited. Nevertheless, a hygienist should be alert to certain findings that are analogous to those of potential concern in the removable prostheses previously discussed (complete dentures, removable dentures). Thus perforations missing acrylic or metal elements, sharp edges of any material, peeling or flaking of a resilient material away from the more rigid base, and stains or cracks need to be brought to the dentist's immediate attention.

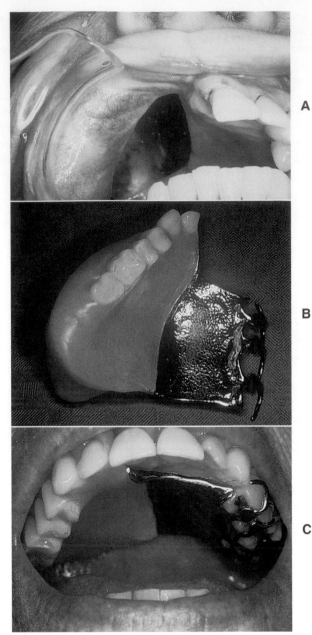

FIGURE 30-9
A, Resection of a maxillary tumor has left a large defect that affects the palate and sinus and impedes speech, swallowing, and chewing. **B,** A unilateral removable partial denture has been combined with an obturator *(the acrylic portion on the lower left)* that replaces contours of the missing palatal and antral structures. **C,** This treatment allows the patient to function in a more normal manner.

POSTSURGICAL STENTS AND SLEEP APNEA DEVICES

Two other varieties of prosthetic devices the hygienist encounters include postsurgical stents that protect graft sites or graft donor sites and sleep apnea devices that reposition the mandible anteriorly to ensure an open airway. Postsurgical stents may be removable, as when they cover a conservative graft site, such as the palatal donor site for a free gingival graft. They may be held in place with **circummandibular ligatures,** as is often the case following reconstructive oral surgery. Sleep apnea devices generally engage the coronal portions of both mandibular and maxillary teeth while flexibly directing the two jaws to relate in a slightly open, prognathic position.

Postsurgical stents, whether removable or affixed by ligatures, are generally used for a few days or weeks and then discarded. Patients do not usually bring sleep apnea devices to dental offices unless the patient requires an adjustment. As with all acrylic devices, the dental hygienist needs to be alert for cracked or missing pieces and sharp edges in both the acrylic and the metal components of the device.

✦ CASE APPLICATION 30-1.2

Sleep Apnea Device

Dr. Basha had been given a sleep apnea device. How would this effect his treatment?

Evaluating Oral Tissues Associated with Appliances

Dental appliances should not cause discernible changes in the adjacent oral soft tissues when the devices have been fabricated properly and maintained appropriately, unless, as with an orthodontic appliance or a bleaching tray, such is the stated purpose. Oral tissues in contact with, or near, dental appliances often display signals that call for dental attention, patient education, or both. Dental appliances may directly affect oral tissues, such as when a sharp edge lacerates or an acrylic component exerts undue pressure. Effects may also be indirect, such as the greater plaque biofilm accumulation on abutment teeth of fixed or removable partial dentures (Figure 30-10) or the reaction of gingival tissues to home-bleaching solutions. In the course of a thorough examination of the head and neck tissues, findings attributable to dental appliances are identifiable and may include the following:

> ### Note
> The astute hygienist needs to be open to the diagnosis of such findings until all data are collected; a poor-fitting denture that overlies a lesion may have caused the lesion or may be poor fitting because the lesion has altered the intraoral anatomy. In either case, both the lesion and the suspicion regarding the appliance need to be called to the dentist's attention.

- Erythema with or without edema
- Ulceration
- Hyperplastic tissue
- Microbial colonies
- Desquamative lesions

CONDITIONS ASSOCIATED WITH APPLIANCE WEAR

The most common condition associated with appliance wear is erythema, or redness of the tissues. Under close examination, erythematous tissue is seen to possess dilated vessels that account for its heightened color. Erythema may be associated with edema or, caused by the passage of fluid out of the dilated blood vessels

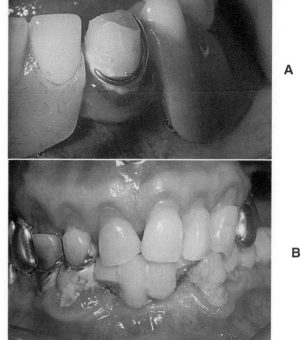

FIGURE 30-10
A, The clasp arm of a removable partial denture readily retains plaque biofilm in the gingival third of abutment teeth. **B,** A damaged lower anterior bridge traps food debris and calculus.

into the surrounding connective tissues, or edema may be absent. If erythema associated with an appliance is acute and localized, then it is likely accompanied by the patient's complaint of discomfort and is probably a result of trauma from the appliance in the area of the redness. Less common possibilities include lesions that are coincidentally located in the area of the appliance or perhaps worsened by its presence, such as erosive lichen planus, early herpes simplex lesions, and bullous mucous membrane pemphigoid. Erythema, neither asymptomatic nor associated with pain, is probably chronic and caused by a candidal infection attributable to inadequate hygiene of the prosthesis. Other possible diagnoses, coincidentally in the area of the appliance, are squamous cell carcinoma or its predecessor, carcinoma *in situ*.

Candida Infection

Many removable dental appliances, such as complete dentures, partial dentures, splints, and maxillofacial prostheses, are composed in large part of methyl methacrylate resin, a strong and stain-resistant material that is adjustable, polishable, and characterized to resemble oral mucosa. The curing process for methyl methacrylate resin results in a material that appears pockmarked on microscopic examination. These surface irregularities and chemical properties of the material lead readily to its colonization by species of the common oral yeast *Candida*, particularly *Candida albicans* and *Candida glabrata*. Adherent yeast organisms excrete metabolic by-products that irritate the mucosa. If various factors permit the uncontrolled colonization of the denture surface with *Candida*, then the result is a condition of tissue erythema and edema called *candidiasis,* or more correctly—though less commonly used—*candidosis.* The most common form of candidosis specifically associated with using removable dentures is termed *acute atrophic candidiasis* and is characterized by striking erythema of the part of the tissue in contact with the prosthesis (Figure 30-11). The following are two less common forms of candidosis:

- *Acute hyperplastic candidiasis.* Acute hyperplastic candidiasis, also termed *thrush,* is raised, loosely adherent, irregular white patches (composed of dead mucosal cells and colonies of the yeast organisms) that are disseminated across the surface of the tissue (Figure 30-12).

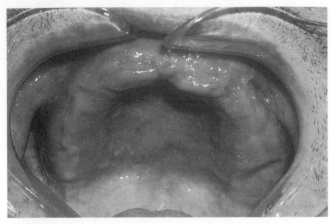

FIGURE 30-11
Acute atrophic candidiasis, also called *denture stomatitis,* features edematous, red tissue (usually palatal) that is in direct contact with a denture.

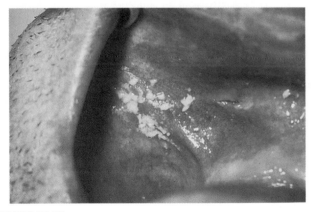

FIGURE 30-12
Acute hyperplastic candidiasis (thrush) comprises raised white plaques that, when removed, reveal a raw, bleeding surface underneath.

- *Chronic hyperplastic candidiasis.* Chronic hyperplastic candidiasis, also termed *palatal hyperplasia,* occurs when the surface mucosa (usually of the palate, but the alveolar ridges may also be affected) is covered by a continuous mat of small, spherical projections of tissue that readily bleed under moderate pressure (Figure 30-13).

In a healthy person, natural antifungal proteins in the saliva and the presence of other organisms stabilize the population of intraoral *Candida* species. However, the *Candida* organisms thrive under the following conditions:

- An acrylic substrate is present, especially one that is worn continuously.

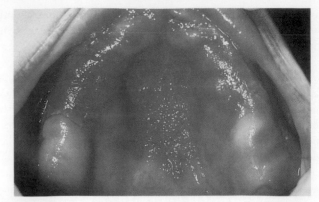

FIGURE 30-13
This patient has chronic hyperplastic candidiasis (palatal hyperplasia), a condition in which small rounded projections of epithelialized tissue grow into the space between the palate and an ill-fitting maxillary denture.

- Saliva is reduced as a result of medications or disease.
- Oxygen is sparse (a condition more easily attained between a prosthesis and the bearing mucosa).
- A glucose source is plentiful (caused by poor oral hygiene or poorly controlled diabetes).
- Antibiotics have disturbed the natural balance of intraoral microorganisms.
- The host's immunologic defenses are compromised (caused by chemotherapy, certain diseases, and certain medications).

DENTAL CONSIDERATIONS

The dental hygienist then needs to be observant for lesions of *Candida* associated with dental appliance use not only to ensure optimal oral health, but also because the presence of candidal lesions may indicate a more serious underlying health condition.[7]

Erythema and Edema

Erythema and edema caused by bacterial plaque biofilm may be present beneath the pontic area of a fixed bridge, where their presence is essentially invisible unless floss is passed between the pontic and the underlying tissue (in which case slight bleeding occurs). Bacterially mediated erythema and edema at the gingival margin are also, of course, hallmark signs of gingivitis and are commonly seen on abutment teeth because the appliance disrupts the hygienic contour of the tooth surface itself. Similar changes are observed in the tissues surrounding implants if plaque biofilm deposits are not scrupulously removed.

Ulcerations and Lacerations

Ulcerations and lacerations are also conditions often associated with dental appliance use. Ulceration may occur as a result of repeated abrasion of soft tissue by a dental appliance or excess pressure against tissue, which results in a localized pressure necrosis. Laceration, or cutting of the tissue, results from a rough edge or other sharp element that causes a break in the mucosa. In all of these cases, lesions are distinctly localized, with a reddish outline and a yellowish center that exposes the submucosal layer (Figure 30-14). The tissue immediately adjacent to the lesion or laceration may be erythematous and slightly edematous, or it may be normal in color and contour. Some ulcerations and lacerations are painful, although others are not. When the causative agent of this sort of lesion is not addressed (because the lesions are asymptomatic or beneath the patient's threshold to seek help), the mucosa may heal but often does so accompanied by a proliferation of soft tissue, which is, itself, subsequently traumatized. Patients with removable dental appliances should always be carefully examined for signs of redundant tissue at the border areas where the appliance terminates against mucosal tissue.

Desquamation

Areas in which a thin mucosal layer has been sloughed away from the underlying tissue are described as *desquamative*. Desquamative lesions in association with a dental appliance may be caused by direct trauma from the appliance before proper adjustment. Desquamative lesions associated with dental appliances are likely caused by chemical burns (Figure 30-15), such as a reaction to the surface of the appliance (e.g., when a denture has not been thoroughly rinsed after soaking in a disinfectant solution) or to its contents.

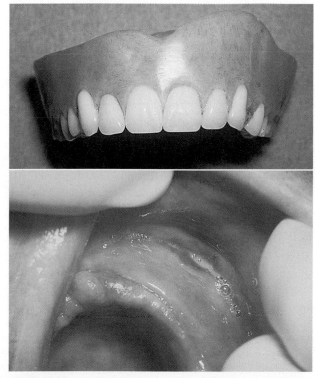

FIGURE 30-14
If denture flanges are made too long **(A)** or become too long as the denture *settles* as a result of gradual loss of the supporting bone, a painful denture ulceration results **(B)**.

Care and Cleaning of Dental Appliances

Removable dental appliances should not be continuously worn in the mouth. Oral tissues—whether teeth, gingiva, or mucosa—need to have some extended period, each day, during

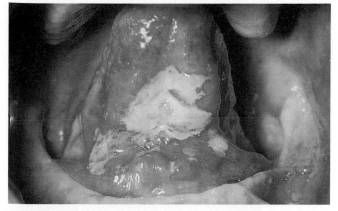

FIGURE 30-15
This patient has a desquamative lesion on the ventral surface of the tongue. The patient failed to rinse the mandibular denture after it had been soaked in a bleach solution. The resulting chemical burn caused sloughing of the mucosa of the underside of the tongue. The lesion is painful but will resolve in 7 to 10 days without treatment.

which they are in unrestricted contact with salivary components.

Regular cleaning of dental appliances is necessary to minimize unpleasant odors, sensations, and in particular, unwanted tissue reactions. Fixed bridges and fixed bridgework over implants should be cleaned several times a day with a toothbrush; toothpaste; and one or more supplemental hygiene aids, such as a floss threader, interproximal brush, or superfloss (Figure 30-16). The supplemental aids are necessary to clean the areas of the prostheses that are in contact with or facing the alveolar ridges. The hygienist needs to work closely with each patient to identify the self-care devices that are most appropriate for the patient's dental needs, manual dexterity, and visual acuity and to train the patient in the correct technique.

> ### Patient Education Opportunity
> Saliva provides an environment of essential lubricating, antimicrobial, remineralizing, hydrating, oxygenating, and buffering properties that ensure optimal tissue health.

Removable prostheses are cleaned outside the mouth. Patients should remove such appliances after every meal to rinse off adherent food and thereby minimize the substrate for development of bacterial plaque biofilm. Complete dentures, overdentures, and partial dentures should be gently but thoroughly scrubbed daily on all surfaces under running water, using a brush specifically designed for dentures. Patients should be instructed to always clean their oral prostheses over a sink in which several inches of water are present or in which a washcloth has been placed (Figure 30-17) so that the appliance will not break if it is accidentally dropped while being cleaned. Toothpaste should not be used with the denture brush because the abrasive properties of normal dentifrice actually wear away acrylic over time. Patients who desire a *fresh* or *minty* flavor or sensation once they have cleaned their dental appliance should be directed to one or more commercial products, either foaming denture cleansing pastes or soaking agents, that feature such a flavor.

Brushing, even with a denture dentifrice, does not adequately remove organisms that tightly adhere to the appliance surface

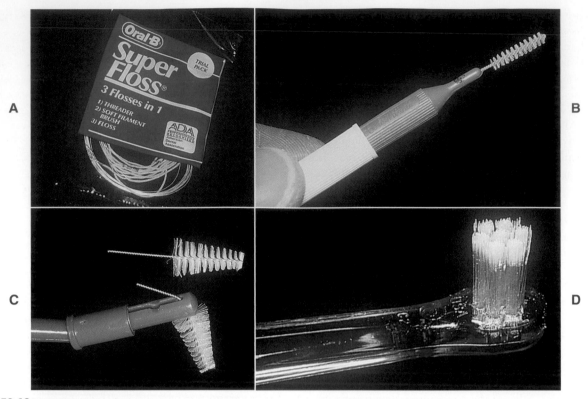

FIGURE 30-16
Floss can be introduced under a bridge pontic with a floss threader or a floss product with a stiffer end **(A)**. Interproximal brushes are also effective for cleaning between the pontic and the ridge tissue, whether held straight **(B)** or contraangled **(C)**. End-tuft or uni-tuft brushes are also useful **(D)**.

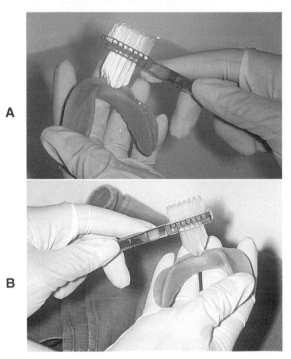

FIGURE 30-17
Brushing a denture should always be done over water **(A)** or a towel **(B)** so that the denture is not damaged if it is dropped.

and are sheltered within the acrylic pores.[1] Placing an acrylic appliance in a small ultrasonic cleaning bath effectively removes all microorganisms in a few minutes.[5] Small cleansing units that cost less than $100 can be obtained for patient use, but they are not widely available and are used by only a small minority of patients. Soaking overnight in a cup of 10% home-bleaching solution, with or without a teaspoon of dishwasher detergent, is also effective in the eradication of microbes on removable appliances.[2] More than 75% of patients with complete and removable dentures, however, use a commercial denture-soaking solution two or more times a week. In the United States, denture-cleaning products come as tablets that effervesce in water and release an effective bleach, chelation (for removing calcium), and detergent solution, which effectively eradicates more than 99% of adherent microbes in less than 15 minutes[8] (Figure 30-18). When an appliance is left overnight in such a solution, virtual sterilization of the device occurs. Appliances with metal elements, such as partial dentures and orthodontic retainers, should not be left for more than 20 minutes in such solutions (or in home-bleaching solutions, for that matter) because the metallic parts darken and become dull as a result of the powerful oxidization effects of the bleach. A recent development in commercially available appliance-soaking solutions is the introduction of a product that both cleans the dental device and coats it with a thin, insoluble layer of silicone polymer. This silicone polymer inhibits subsequent candidal colonization of the surface but wears off during the course of a day. This *preventive* approach to hygiene of dental devices is novel and logical.

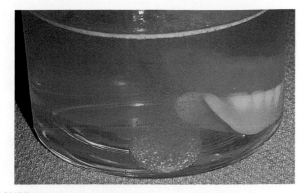

FIGURE 30-18
Commercial soaking agents effectively clean dentures in 10 to 20 minutes.

Several dental appliances either benefit from or actually require using materials that need periodic (usually daily or more frequent) reapplication or replenishment. Fluoride carriers are the best example; their proper use depends on the daily introduction of fluoride gel that is then held in proximity to the teeth by the appliance. The two most common formulations for topical fluoride gel are acidulated stannous fluoride (1100 ppm or 0.4%) and neutral sodium-fluoride gel (5000 ppm or 1.1%). Much clinical and experimental data support the use of one or the other of these for a given clinical situation. The most compelling criterion concerns the acidity of the compounds—stannous fluoride gel is distinctly acidic (with a pH of approximately 4.5) and should not be left in contact with the teeth for more than 3 minutes daily. After fluoride trays have been in the mouth for the desired interval, they are to be removed, cleaned under running water with a denture brush, and stored in clean water.

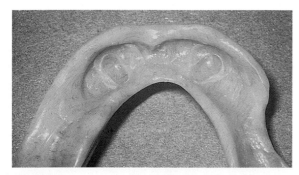

FIGURE 30-19
The undersurface of an overdenture clearly shows where the abutment teeth sit. Daily application of a single drop of topical fluoride gel into each of these sites will suppress plaque biofilm growth and metabolism and therefore help preserve abutment health and longevity.

Distinct Care Modifications

An empiric regimen used is the introduction of a drop of fluoride gel into the areas of an overdenture that correspond to the retentive abutment (Figure 30-19). Limited clinical data support this regimen, noting enhanced periodontal health and limited root caries in abutment teeth.[3]

As with fluoride trays, bleaching trays are specifically designed and used to place a therapeutic agent into contact with the dentition. Home-bleaching solutions are used under a dentist's supervision, and thus the material, its

amount, and all other patient instructions have been specified in advance. One of the dental hygienist's responsibilities is to assess the surrounding soft tissues and, as necessary, counsel the patient on providing or enhancing the necessary daily hygiene of the appliance.

Certain removable dental appliances benefit from using products applied to keep the device in place. Some maxillofacial prosthetic devices, particularly those with extraoral components such as eyes, ears, noses, and cheekbones, may require or benefit from using solvent-dissoluble adhesives that ensure esthetic, prolonged adaptation to the natural tissues. Increasingly, such appliances rely on osseointegrated implants for retention but still may benefit from the ability of adhesive material to ensure a less apparent transition from prosthetic to genuine skin. The adhesive material and its solvent are generally available only by prescription.

Denture adhesive is an over-the-counter product that is used by approximately 25% of patients with complete dentures. Sparingly soluble in water or saliva, powder and cream denture adhesives work by flowing into spaces between the denture and the bearing tissues. This action optimizes the *seal* that results from an intimate fit between the denture and the soft tissues. In addition, denture adhesive is sticky, thick, and effectively adheres to the tissues and the denture while also resisting disaggregation.[6] Use of denture adhesive improves the retention (resistance to displacement of the denture away from the bearing tissues) and stability (resistance to movement relative to the underlying bone, while being retained by the soft tissue) of all dentures, even well-fitting, new ones.[4] However, expense is involved in its use, and the product makes daily hygiene more complex because, by design, the material is not easily removed from either the denture or the oral tissues. Use of warm or hot water and a brush or washcloth assists in removing adhesive. Some dentists have strong feelings in opposition to patients' use of denture adhesive because of the providers' lack of familiarity with the high quality and efficacy of modern denture adhesives. For this reason, the dental hygienist needs to understand the practice's preference with respect to the use of denture adhesive before offering such a product to a patient.

References

1. Dills SS et al: Comparison of the antimicrobial capability of an abrasive paste and chemical-soak denture cleaners, *J Prosthet Dent* 60:467, 1988.
2. Ettinger RL, Bergman W, Wefel J: Effect of fluoride on overdenture abutments, *Am J Dent* 7(1):17, 1994.
3. Glass RT, Belobraydic KA: The dilemma of denture contamination, *Okla Dent Assoc J* 81(2):30, 1990.
4. Grasso JE, Rendell J, Gay T: Effect of denture adhesive on the retention and stability of maxillary dentures, *J Prosthet Dent* 72:399, 1994.
5. Gwinnett AJ, Caputo L: The effectiveness of ultrasonic denture cleaning: a scanning electron microscope study, *J Prosthet Dent* 50:20, 1983.
6. Shay K: Denture adhesives: choosing the right powders and pastes, *J Am Dent Assoc* 122:70, 1991.
7. Shay K, Renner RP, Truhlar MR: Oropharyngeal candidosis in the older patient, *J Am Geriatr Soc* 45:863, 1997.
8. Warner-Lambert Company: Discussion with product manager [oral communication], 1999.

CHAPTER

31

Powered Instrumentation and Periodontal Debridement

Bonnie Francis • Deborah E. Fleming

INSIGHT

Periodontal debridement is the foundation of treatment offered by the dental hygienist. The goals of periodontal debridement are to arrest infection and maintain a healthy periodontium by eliminating the pathogenic microorganisms on the tooth and root surface and removing hardened calculus deposits and dental plaque biofilm from the sulcus or pocket.

✦ CASE STUDY 31-1   Therapeutic Selections for the Periodontal Patient

Mrs. Melba Ray is a 55-year-old white woman seeking periodontal care for the first time in your office. She has recently moved to the area and indicates that she had previous periodontal problems that were treated with "deep cleanings several years ago, but it hurt so I didn't want to go back." She said that she has recently noticed bleeding in some areas of her mouth when she brushes, as well as a bad taste, so she thought it was time to come get her "teeth cleaned."

Mrs. Ray's health history reveals type II non–insulin-dependent diabetes mellitus and mild hypertension. She takes 10 mg of glipizide daily for her diabetes and is not taking medications for hypertension. Instead, she closely monitors her blood pressure, exercises, and modifies her diet to control both the hypertension and the diabetes.

The extraoral examination is within normal limits (WNL), or noncontributory, whereas the intraoral examination reveals a cheek bite on the right buccal mucosa. Also noted was that she has a partially erupted tooth, palatal to an existing fixed bridge. When questioned about the finding, she said that the tooth did not come in correctly, that a bridge was made a long time ago to fill in the space, and that she has not had any problems in the area. Clinical and radiographic findings are presented in the images of the mouth and the periodontal charting.

As you review the images and chart, you should use the process presented in Chapters 20 and 21 to identify risks and establish therapeutic and self-care strategies for patient care. This chapter will help you apply a therapeutic strategy that is consistent with Mrs. Ray's needs.

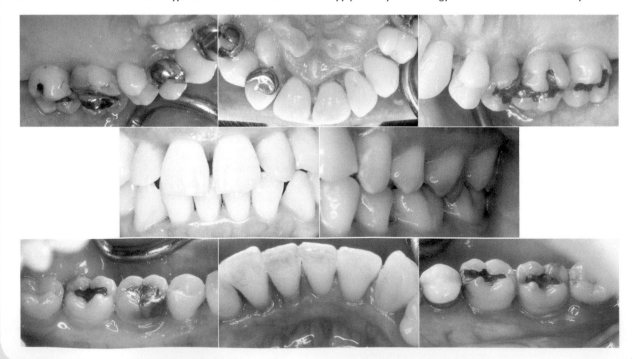

CASE STUDY 31-1 **Therapeutic Selections for the Periodontal Patient—cont'd**

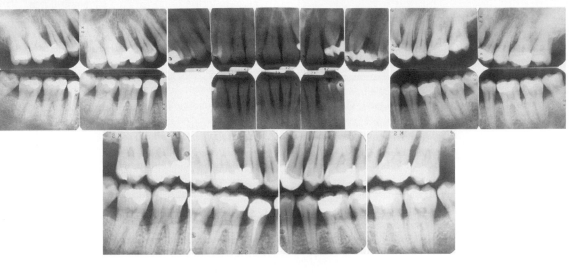

Periodontal Charting

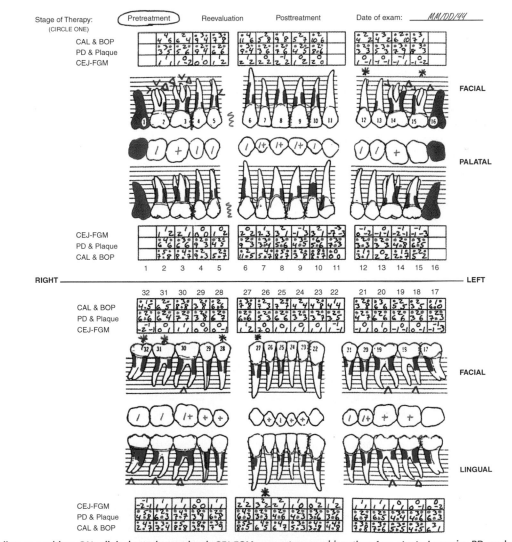

Stage of Therapy: (Pretreatment)   Reevaluation   Posttreatment   Date of exam: _MM/DD/YY_

(CIRCLE ONE)

BOP, Bleeding on probing; *CAL,* clinical attachment level; *CEJ-FGM,* cementoenamel junction–free gingival margin; *PD,* probe depth.

KEY TERMS

air turbine	dental plaque biofilm	lipooligosaccharide	piezoelectric
antigens	hertz (Hz)	magnetostrictive	power-driven
cavitation	host immune response	mechanical debridement	prostaglandins
cycles per second (cps)	interleukins	pathogenesis	sonic scalers
cytokines	lipopolysaccharide	periodontal debridement	ultrasonic
dental endoscope (endoscopy)			

LEARNING OUTCOMES

After reading this chapter the student will be able to:

1. Make appropriate instrument selections—manual or powered—for periodontal debridement.
2. Discuss the process of pathogenesis and wound healing relative to the need for periodontal debridement.
3. Select the appropriate tips for the debridement process based on patient need and access.
4. Set up a powered instrument for periodontal debridement.
5. Using information gathered during the assessment phase, select an appropriate debridement treatment plan for a patient.
6. Determine appropriate treatment codes for a patient who is undergoing periodontal therapy.
7. Assess treatment outcomes based on healing of periodontal structures following treatment.

Periodontal Debridement

Periodontal debridement is the foundation of dental hygiene care and is provided to patients daily by dental hygienists throughout the world. Debridement is the process by which hard and soft deposits are removed from the supragingival and subgingival surfaces of the teeth, including the disruption of bacterial cell walls of nonadherent plaque biofilm.[55] In patients who are having periodontal maintenance, **mechanical debridement** reduces inflammation and disturbs the bacterial biofilm, which is thought to be critical to disease control, including prevention of progression.[38] The goals of periodontal debridement are to arrest infection and maintain a healthy periodontium by eliminating pathogenic microorganisms on the tooth and root surface and removing hardened calculus deposits and dental plaque biofilm from the sulcus or pocket.* Because **dental plaque biofilm** is a dynamic, living organism and has been shown to repopulate the pockets within weeks following therapy,† the clinician must understand the ongoing role and commitment of both the patient and the dental hygienist in the thorough mechanical removal regularly of supragingival and subgingival microbial biofilms. The treatment that the dental hygienist offers is part of three critical elements toward achieving and maintaining a healthy periodontium. These elements are as follows:

- Thorough and definitive debridement as part of professional periodontal treatment by the dental hygienist
- The patient's compliance with the recommended self-care regimen
- The body's ability to fight infection and heal (host response)

All three factors play a key role in arresting disease and maintaining a healthy periodontium throughout the lifetime of each patient.*

The hygienist's role of providing a thorough periodontal debridement starts with the following:

- A clear understanding of the pathogenesis of the periodontal pocket
- Periodontal microbiology
- Wound healing
- Specific instrumentation techniques for achieving optimal therapeutic outcomes

Periodontal debridement as part of professional periodontal treatment starts with a thorough evaluation to determine the existing periodontal status and extent of treatment needed to achieve the goal of health. The dental hygienist then must select the appropriate manual or powered instruments or a combination of the two that will offer the best treatment and clinical outcome for the individual's needs. Knowledge of powered and

---

*References 8-10, 14, 25, 38.
†References 6, 23, 28, 29, 41, 44, 50.

---

*References 5, 8-10, 14-15, 24-26, 38.

manual instruments, tip design, and fundamentals for use is essential to achieving established goals. Routine and ongoing evaluation of tissue response and healing are critical elements in determining whether further intervention (professional or self-care) is required short or long term. Continuous and frequent monitoring of periodontally involved patients is necessary to prevent further tissue destruction; therefore placement on frequent intervals of supportive care that include instructions and monitoring of dental plaque biofilm–control procedures are necessary when providing optimal oral care.*

Previous chapters have provided a background of procedures and techniques used to assess a patient's health thoroughly, to develop therapeutic and preventive strategies, and to educate patients on appropriate preventive home-care strategies. Design and technique for using manual instruments is presented in Chapter 9. This chapter provides the foundation for periodontal debridement and procedures used by the dental hygienist for therapeutic delivery through powered instrumentation. The authors recognize that powered instrumentation is one part of the spectrum of instruments that can be used for periodontal debridement and in no way undervalue manual instrumentation or the synergy that occurs when powered instrumentation and manual instrumentation are used together for thorough and definitive periodontal treatment.

DEFINITION OF TERMS

Debridement ultimately reduces dental plaque biofilm, bacterial by-products (endotoxins), and plaque biofilm–retentive features (i.e., dental calculus) resulting in improvement and healing of the soft tissues. Depending on the clinical situation, as well as the clinical needs of the patient, debridement—as a general term—is a fundamental component, with varying degrees of technique and difficulty, applied to several different procedure codes as recognized by the American Dental Association Current Dental Terminology (CDT),[3] which will be discussed in detail later in this chapter (Table 31-1). The CDT codes for debridement procedures are listed below with clinical applications.

Debridement includes instrumentation of the supragingival and subgingival aspects of the tooth and reduction of viable bacteria within the periodontal pocket. Chemotherapeutic agents, both local (CDT code 4381)[3] and systemic, may be used in conjunction with instrumentation and have been noted to improve treatment outcomes in patients with periodontitis.[17,33,39] In addition, patients can be instructed to use adjunctive chemotherapeutic agents as part of their home-care routine to help reduce the recolonization and negative effects of virulent organisms.[†] (See Chapter 27, Chemotherapeutics.)

Reducing dental plaque biofilm can be accomplished through various methods involving physical or mechanical removal, such as brushing and interproximal cleaning, polishing, or using an exploratory stroke within the healthy sulcus. These methods, however, do not always affect the well-organized complex of dental biofilm in areas affected by periodontal disease, which generally include more complex root morphology and ideal environmental conditions for biofilm proliferation. Dental plaque biofilm has been described as a sophisticated network of well-organized microbes, complete with ventilation, plumbing, nourishment, communication, and modes of travel, held together within an extracellular matrix.[11] In cases of periodontal disease, debridement within the pocket by scaling and root planing is required to definitively remove the adherent calculus and soft deposits filled with plaque biofilm. The end result of periodontal debridement is not necessarily a glassy-smooth root surface, as was once the goal of root planing. However, thorough calculus and dental plaque biofilm removal is essential for the health of the periodontium.*

PERIODONTAL ASSESSMENT

Periodontal assessment is critical to determining the need for treatment, as well as evaluating treatment outcomes and determining supportive care intervals. Current status of self-care and deposit accumulation should be evaluated during each patient visit, before periodontal debridement, to determine specific therapeutic needs and treatment strategies for the patient's current clinical situation. Refer to Chapter 16 for thorough details of an initial periodontal assessment and Chapter 22 for details on posttreatment assessment and supportive care.

Evaluating risk factors has also been found to be of vital importance in the assessment phase of periodontal disease diagnosis and treatment. A myriad of etiologic risk factors has been found to be associated with inflammatory periodontal disease and, if not identified, may influence the success or failure of any debridement procedure.[10,15,31,49] Risk factors mentioned in Table 31-2 are environmental, behavioral, or biological factors that, if present, increase the probability of the disease occurring and, if absent or removed, reduce the probability of developing the disease.

Each of these risk factors in their own specific way inhibits plaque biofilm control and indirectly contributes to the development of gingivitis and periodontitis. Contributory factors that do not initiate gingivitis but foster increased or longstanding challenges to the periodontium are also mentioned in Table 31-2.

ATTAINING THERAPEUTIC GOALS

Arresting infection, resulting in the healing of inflamed tissue, and preventing further disease activity by maintaining a healthy periodontium are the primary goals of periodontal therapy.

> **Prevention**
> An environment that encourages the tissue to heal and prohibits microorganisms from collecting and colonizing on the surface through the process of thorough professional debridement and daily self-care will, in most patients, result in reduced inflammation and a return to periodontal health when the body is able to support the healing process.

---

*References 5, 8-10, 14-15, 24-26, 38.
†References 8, 14, 17, 26, 33, 39.

*References 6, 9, 26, 29, 38, 43, 44.

Table 31-1	CDT Codes that Correlate with Debridement	
CODE	**DESCRIPTION***	**CLINICAL APPLICATION**
1110—Prophylaxis (Adult)	Removal of plaque biofilm, calculus, and stains from the tooth structures in the permanent and transitional dentition. It is intended to control local irritation factors.	Supragingival debridement for the treatment of gingivitis, which is a basic debridement procedure focused on supragingival plaque biofilm and calculus removal on patients with no history of periodontal breakdown.
4910—Periodontal Maintenance	This procedure is instituted following periodontal therapy and continues at varying intervals, determined by the clinical evaluation of the dentist, for the life of the dentition or any implant replacements. It includes removal of the bacterial plaque biofilm and calculus from supragingival and subgingival regions, site-specific scaling and root planing where indicated, and teeth polishing. If new or recurring periodontal disease appears, then additional diagnostic and treatment procedures must be considered.	Procedures including the removal of supragingival plaque biofilm and calculus, as well as debridement of pocket areas, to maintain periodontal health in patients with a history of periodontal breakdown. This procedure is performed on patients who have completed initial periodontal treatment (surgical or nonsurgical periodontal therapies), at a frequent maintenance interval, and is mostly geared toward removing the soft deposits and light calculus that may have accumulated in a periodontal pocket since the previous debridement or periodontal maintenance procedure.
4341—Periodontal Scaling and Root Planing (Four or More Teeth per Quadrant)	This procedure involves instrumentation of the crown and root surfaces of the teeth to remove plaque biofilm and calculus from these surfaces. It is indicated for patients with periodontal disease and is therapeutic, not prophylactic, in nature. Root planing is the definitive procedure designed for the removal of cementum and dentin that is rough and/or permeated by calculus or contaminated with toxins or microorganisms. Some soft tissue removal occurs. This procedure may be used as a definitive treatment in some stages of periodontal disease or as part of presurgical procedures in others.	Definitive therapeutic action of scaling and root planing for patients with periodontal disease. This procedure is the most involved debridement procedure, usually associated with removing tenacious buildup of subgingival deposits that have accumulated over an extended period. Scaling and root planing is considered the gold standard periodontal treatment modality.[11] Scaling and root planing are generally completed in multiple appointments, completing a quadrant or sextant during each visit depending on the amount of deposit to be removed, the severity of the disease, and the patient's ability to respond and heal. Single-session, full-mouth treatment has also been found to be effective in the healing process for patients with chronic periodontitis.[63] Because of the complex nature of this treatment, the patient and operator often prefer local anesthesia when the scaling and root planing procedures are performed.
4342—Periodontal Scaling and Root Planing (One to Three Teeth per Quadrant)	See 4341 description.	See 4341 description.
4355—Full-Mouth Debridement to Enable Comprehensive Evaluation and Diagnosis	The gross removal of plaque biofilm and calculus that interfere with the ability of the dentist to perform a comprehensive oral evaluation. This preliminary procedure does not preclude the need for additional procedures.	Used to enable comprehensive periodontal evaluation and diagnosis before scaling and root planing when some type of initial cleaning is required to accurately assess the clinical needs of the patient. This procedure is generally completed in conjunction with thorough home-care education and instructions, then the patient is appointed to return for comprehensive examination and treatment planning.
4381—Localized Delivery of Chemotherapeutic Agents via a Controlled Drug-Release Vehicle into Diseased Crevicular Tissue, per Tooth, by Report	FDA approved subgingival delivery devices containing antimicrobial medication(s) are inserted into periodontal pockets to suppress the pathogenic microbiota. These devices slowly release the pharmacological agents so they can remain at the intended site of action in a therapeutic concentration for a sufficient length of time.	Used as an adjunct to periodontal treatment in conjunction with thorough scaling and root planing to support healing in diseased sites. Short-term use of the time-released therapeutic agent as supplemental or adjunctive therapy provides for reduction of subgingival flora. This procedure does not replace conventional or surgical therapy required for debridement, resective procedure, or regenerative therapy.

*Data from *American Dental Association Current Dental Terminology* 2007-2008.

Table 31-2	Risk Factors for Periodontal Disease
RISK FACTOR	**DESCRIPTION**
Periodontal Disease	Risk factors that have been associated with periodontal disease include, but are not limited to, the following: • Plaque biofilm or microbiota and poor oral hygiene • Tobacco use • Poor nutrition or diet • Stress Risk factors that have been associated with periodontal disease that cannot be modified include, but are not limited to, the following: • Genetics • Age • Gender • Race
Natural Risk Factors for Plaque Biofilm Retention	• Calculus • Crowding • Previous periodontal destruction leaving defects and complex root anatomy
Iatrogenic Risk Factors	• Restorations impinging on biological width • Open margins and overhangs that accumulate bacterial buildup • Poorly designed clasps or prostheses
Traumatic Risk Factors	• Occlusal trauma • Toothbrush abrasion to soft tissue • Piercings that cause trauma to adjacent soft tissue
Systemic Risk Factors	• HIV and other immunocompromised or immunosuppressed conditions • Endocrine and hematologic disorders • Hormones

HIV, Human immunodeficiency virus.

This process includes preventing, arresting, and stabilizing periodontal disease by removing supragingival and subgingival bacterial plaque biofilm and its by-products. Although calculus removal seems to be a secondary goal of the debridement process, it is important because of its plaque biofilm–harboring qualities. The healing of the periodontium can occur after the following:

- The root accretions and subgingival endotoxin are professionally removed
- The patient has adopted a thorough daily home-care routine to disturb the plaque biofilm
- The body's **host immune response** is able to support the challenge*

The following are other major factors that may determine the success or failure of treatment are:

---

*References 8, 14, 25, 38, 44.

- Patient compliance
- Disease severity
- Previous history of disease
- Corresponding loss of periodontal structures
- Host immune response*

Additional factors that affect the degree to which these goals can be attained are the dental professional's technique, skill, and expertise and using various instrumentation devices.[7,32,47,54]

Review of Pathogenesis and the Bacterial Challenge

Appreciating **pathogenesis** and the bacterial challenge is a critical link to understanding the importance of debridement and periodontal health. For detailed information on pathogenesis, refer to Chapter 6. Inflammatory periodontal diseases are caused, in part, by the result of the presence of plaque biofilm. Plaque biofilm is an organized cohesive mixture of cellular and acellular components, which is usually preceded by a bacterial pellicle and is difficult to remove.†

At birth, the oral cavity is sterile. Soon after birth, pioneer species bacteria start to appear. The first bacteria to alter the surface environment bring along attachment factors and nutrients for other species, such as the streptococci species (*Streptococcus salivarius, Streptococcus oralis,* and *Streptococcus mitis*). The early bacteria make the environment hospitable for other species and develop conditions that are ideal for bacterial growth and the proliferation of a multitude of species.

With the eruption of teeth, the environment begins to see the appearance of other bacteria, including *Streptococcus sanguis* and *Streptococcus mutans.* Without mechanical plaque biofilm removal, the development of plaque biofilm and microbial adherence occurs when the bacteria come into contact with the surface pellicle. The pellicle is derived from primarily saliva and is made up of glycoproteins, albumin, carbohydrates, and immunoglobulins. Initial adhesion occurs when the bacteria interact with the pellicle by means of weak bonds of Van der Waal's forces and hydrogen bonds. Later *Staphylococcus, Veillonella, Neisseria, Actinomyces, Lactobacillus,* and *Fusobacterium* species can attach and become part of the stable bacterial community. By this time, a complex community is present that represents a dynamic balance between the resident flora as a result of bacteria-bacteria and bacteria-host interactions.

Normal microbial flora of the oral cavity contains up to 500 species or more.[41] Approximately 200 species are found in dental plaque biofilm alone, but only between 12 and 15 species are considered to be pathogenic or accountable for tissue destruction found in individuals with periodontal disease.

Note

Estimates suggest that 75% of the adult population has some form of periodontal disease and 15% to 25% of it is tissue destructive. One significant correlation with the severity of disease is the amount and type of bacteria present in the biofilm.[28]

---

*References 8, 14, 31, 47, 49.
†References 9, 11, 24, 29, 38.

As indicated in Chapter 16, the periodontal diseases known as *gingivitis* and *periodontitis* originate from the presence of bacterial biofilm, which produces an immune response within the host. Initially, bacteria are deposited on the clinical crowns of teeth, primarily at the cementoenamel junction. When plaque biofilm remains undisturbed, it begins to migrate subgingivally. The two main forms of subgingival plaque biofilm are adherent and nonadherent (outlined in Table 31-3).

- Adherent subgingival plaque biofilm and the supragingival plaque biofilm are composed primarily of gram-positive rods and anaerobic forms of streptococci.
- Nonadherent or tissue-associated plaque biofilm is composed of both gram-positive and gram-negative species. Among the most common secretions of gram-negative bacteria is the potent endotoxin, **lipopolysaccharide** (LPS)[41] or **lipooligosaccharide** (LOS).

Some bacterial species invade the periodontal tissues and secrete a large number of by-products that can damage host tissues, invoking an immune response that can cause further damage. Bacterial **antigens** trigger the body's immune response by releasing neutrophils, monocytes, and macrophages to attack the by-products of the bacterial plaque that have both defensive and destructive properties. As these cells attempt to contain or reduce the bacterial biofilm, they release or stimulate the release of inflammatory mediators such as the following:

> **Note**
> Adherent plaque biofilm is dense, whereas the portion of plaque biofilm adjacent to the tissues (nonadherent) is more loosely organized than the adherent form and has been found to be much more virulent.

- Prostaglandins
- **Cytokines**
- Interleukins
- Enzymes collagenase and proteinase (Figure 31-1)

Prostaglandins and **interleukins** are released to assist in the battle, producing the inflammatory response seen clinically as erythema and edema accompanied by bleeding, increased temperature, and pain.[25] Table 31-4 shows Page and Schroeder's model of the development of the periodontal lesion in stages.

Table 31-3	Bacteria Associated with Periodontal Pathology
TYPE	**NAME**
Nonadherent Bacteria	• *Porphyromonas gingivalis* • *Prevotella intermedia* • *Fusobacterium* species • *Veillonella* species
Adherent Bacteria	• *Streptococcus mitis* • *Streptococcus salivarius* • *Streptococcus mutans* • *Actinomyces viscosus* • *Actinomyces naeslundii* • *Eubacterium* species

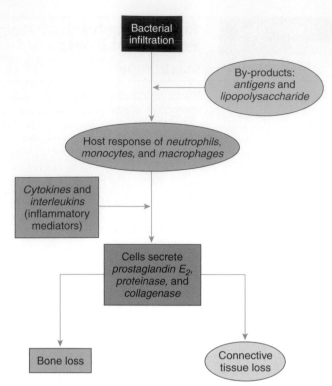

FIGURE 31-1
The immune response to the presence of periodontal pathogens.

This cascade of events of the bacterial complex and the immune system causes tissue breakdown and destruction, which results in destruction of the periodontal ligament and subsequent pocket formation when the bacterial biofilm is not reduced or removed.[25] Initial stages of this immune response are seen endoscopically (Figure 31-2) as a progression from healthy-pink firm sulcular epithelium (Figure 31-2, *A*), to initial stages of inflammation (Figure 31-2, *B*), and advancing stages of inflammation (Figure 31-2, *C*).

Although dental plaque biofilm and calculus are not the only factors in the pathogenesis of periodontal disease, they are the etiologic factors managed during debridement procedures.

> **Note**
> Endoscopic evaluation of periodontal pockets has shown the presence of residual calculus on the root surface adjacent to inflammatory redness in the epithelial lining of the pocket[43,63] (Figure 31-2, *D*).

Practically speaking, these images imply the importance of thorough deposit removal in the role of periodontal pathogenesis and wound healing.

Wound Healing

31-1
31-2

Understanding the process of wound healing helps the dental hygienist visualize the activity occurring within the tissues and sets expectations during the evaluation of a patient's tissues. A thorough review of wound healing is presented in Chapter 6. Any debridement procedure produces a wound. This wound goes through a large number of specific steps during the healing process. In *The Periodontic Syllabus,* Rapley writes the following: "Healing is the phase of the inflammatory response that

Table 31-4	Page and Schroeder's Model for Development of the Periodontal Lesion		
LESION	**CONSECUTIVE DAYS OF PLAQUE BIOFILM EXPOSURE**	**HISTOLOGICAL**	**CLINICAL**
Initial	2-4 days with plaque biofilm	PMNs, mononuclear cells subjacent to JE; decrease of some collagen fibers	Gingival fluid detectable in sulcus; vasculitis subjacent to JE
Early	4-7 days with plaque biofilm	Dense lymphoid cell infiltrate in CT; reduction in collagen by 70% in areas of inflammation	More gingival fluid detectable and increase in vasculitis subjacent to JE; possible BOP
Established	2-3 weeks with plaque biofilm	Plasma cells predominate within CT, producing IgG	JE and sulcular epithelium; continuation of signs of proliferation, with thickening of epithelium; inflammation present; BOP
Advanced	Variable	Extensive destruction of collagen fibers; predominance of plasma cell; regeneration of transseptal fibers as lesion moves apically	Continued progression of gingivitis with attachment loss; crestal alveolar bone resorbing

BOP, Bleeding on probing; *CT,* connective tissue; *IgG,* immunoglobulin G; *JE,* junctional epithelium; *PMNs,* polymorphonuclear neutrophils.

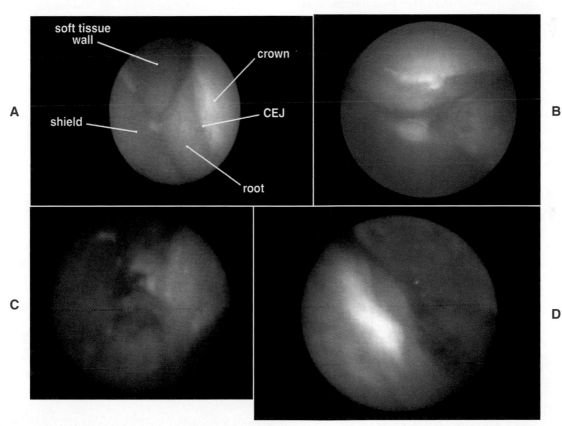

FIGURE 31-2
Endoscopic view of the subgingival space at 48× magnification. **A,** Healthy tissue. **B,** Initial stages of inflammation. **C,** Advancing stages of inflammation. **D,** 30-day posttreatment. Inflammation appears adjacent to the residual calculus deposit covered with biofilm. (Images courtesy Perioscopy Inc., Oakland, Calif. and Bonnie Francis, Dallas, Tex.)

leads to a new physiological and anatomical relationship among the disrupted body elements."[46]

Histologically, periodontal wound healing is initiated after instrumentation when a thin clot becomes interposed between the collagen fibers in the cementum and the collagen of the wound surface in the soft tissues. The healing wound surface consists of a base of moderately inflamed connective tissue covered with granulation tissue, a layered zone of neutrophils, and a clot. The epithelium begins to proliferate from the margins of the wound and migrates at approximately 0.5 mm per day. During this time, fibroblasts in the granulation tissue begin to produce collagen. Granulation tissue penetrates the thin clot and permits the fibers extending from the cementum to unite with the new collagen formed by gingival fibroblasts. The epithelial attachment usually remains at its original position on the tooth, or it may migrate a few cells coronally, producing a long junctional epithelial attachment.[46]

Thus periodontal debridement actually results in soft tissue reattachment, not regeneration as defined by new cementum, periodontal ligament, and bone attached to a previously diseased root surface. Awareness of the healing rate of the tissues involved in periodontal diseases is important in the monitoring of treatment outcomes. Epithelial tissue heals at a faster rate than connective tissue. Of all the periodontal tissues, bone takes the longest time to heal. This knowledge is essential to the development of appropriate intervention strategies and realistic expectations for clinical outcomes. Current research indicates that regeneration of periodontal structures occurs only routinely following surgical intervention.[22,61,62] Table 31-5 lists the tissues of the periodontium and associated healing rates.

Shifts in the composition of the subgingival microflora are found after periodontal debridement procedures.[6,50] Organisms associated with periodontal health are more prominent with an increase in gram-positive rods and cocci species. Gram-negative organisms, spirochetes, and motile forms are consistently reduced but not always eliminated from the pocket. *Actinobacillus actinomycetemcomitans*, one of the most virulent and pathogenic oral microorganisms, is more resistant to mechanical debridement than it is to periodontal debridement procedures. Additional systemic antimicrobial therapy is often needed to manage completely the aggressive diseases associated with this particular bacteria.[2,27,59]

Probing depth reduction results from tissue shrinkage and healing of the gingival structures, as evidenced by gingival recession and a gain of clinical attachment. Recession may be assessed 1 week after debridement procedures, and the amount of recession is gener-

> **Note**
> Reduced probing depth, decreased gingival inflammation, and decreased bleeding on probing are measurable clinical indicators of healing.

ally related to the initial probing depths and the amount of inflammation in the tissues before treatment. In studies,* deeper pocket depths exhibiting moderate to severe inflammation have exhibited greater healing and gain of clinical attachment, with the most gingival shrinkage occurring interproximally. Conversely, after instrumentation, a small amount of attachment loss has been noted in sites that are shallow, with little or no inflammation. Some loss of attachment does occur as a result of trauma inflicted during aggressive subgingival instrumentation. During the subsequent healing phase, however, this loss generally rebounds, with attachment levels returning to the positions they held before instrumentation.[9,14,24,38]

Selecting the best method, technique, or procedure to reduce dental plaque biofilm is constantly under review through additional scientific inquiry, generating knowledge and new questions. Continued advancements in dental technology and resulting therapies will add to the existing armamentarium in providing optimal periodontal health to all patients.

> **Prevention**
> Reducing the biofilm and creating an environment for tissue healing through therapeutic intervention is part of the dental hygienist's role in periodontal debridement. Another important role is to motivate and educate the patient on the significance of thorough, daily self-care and other positive behavioral changes that will affect disease progression or healing. Also critical to discuss are disease, treatment options, treatment outcomes, and maintenance, as well as emphasizing home care and routine biofilm control with the patient before treatment begins and during every subsequent visit, including maintenance visits, to reinforce the commitment of maintaining a healthy periodontium throughout the life time of the patient.[8-9,14,24,38]

★ CASE APPLICATION 31-1.1

Review Chart and Identify Factors

Review Mrs. Ray's periodontal charting and clinical photographs. Identify factors that may influence the success of periodontal debridement in the case of Mrs. Ray.

Powered Scaling Instruments

Periodontal debridement (scaling and root planing) was traditionally performed by manual instrumentation, with ultrasonic and sonic instrumentation, and was used primarily for supragingival gross deposit and stain removal. Today, scientific evidence supports using sonic and ultrasonic instruments as an integral and important part of periodontal debridement.

With advances in tip design offering longer shanks and smaller-diameter tips, powered scaling has become an increasingly efficient and effective option for subgingival instrumentation. Multiple studies have investigated the effectiveness of

Table 31-5	Healing Rates of Periodontal Tissues
TISSUE TYPE AND LOCATION	**HEALING RATE**
Junctional Epithelium	5 days
Sulcular Epithelium	7-10 days
Gingival Surface Epithelium	10-14 days
Connective Tissue	21-28 days
Bone	4-6 weeks

---

*References 5, 13, 37, 45, 57.

power-driven scalers. Studies comparing manual instrumentation with sonic, piezoelectric, and magnetostrictive scalers show similar clinical results in probing depth reductions and bleeding on probing.* In addition, studies have shown that powered scalers decrease subgingival microflora and root associated toxin and remove plaque biofilm similar to manual instrumentation when used correctly.†

When choosing an instrument for treatment of more involved periodontal pockets, an important point to remember is that adequate access for debridement is more difficult as probing depths increase. When treating pockets deeper than 3 mm, sonic and ultrasonic scalers provide better access to the base of pockets for the removal of plaque biofilm and calculus than manual instruments, although complete extension to the base of moderate to deep pockets (5.7 to 8.3 mm) is generally not achieved by any instrument.[13,25,47,54] Anatomical root features found in areas with loss of periodontal structure require a close look at appropriate instrument choices and techniques to be most effective at instrumenting or debriding these challenging areas. **Power-driven** scalers have demonstrated a more effective and efficient choice for scaling and root planing furcations than manual instruments when smaller tip sizes (less than 0.55 mm) are used,[20,56] but specially designed manual instruments such as Curettes, files, and hoes will often remove the accumulation of deposit in these hard-to-reach areas as well.

> **Note**
>
> Any type of powered instrumentation can be effective in improving clinical parameters as long as proper technique is used and sufficient time is spent to debride the entire root surface thoroughly.

Choosing the appropriate instrument for the degree of difficulty and using this instrument correctly becomes paramount in achieving the goal of periodontal debridement.

ULTRASONIC SCALERS

The term **ultrasonic** is described as inaudible acoustic vibrations that are reported in units by frequency referred to as **cycles per second (cps)** or **hertz (Hz).** The principles of ultrasonic physics and the mechanism of action for these powered scaling instruments are the passage of high-frequency current and the passage of compressed air into a vibrating tip of up to 18,000 to 50,000 cps while a cooling water spray is present. The two categories of ultrasonic scalers—magnetostrictive and piezoelectric—are based on this mechanism of conversion of the electrical power to the movement of the tip. Table 31-6 provides specifics on powered instrument characteristics.

Ultrasonic scalers require a power source and water supply. However, some ultrasonics are integrated into the dental unit, tapping into the dental unit water supply and power source, requiring only a hand piece connection to the tubing of the dental unit. Other ultrasonic systems are available with optional water reservoirs that are attached directly to the machine that can be interchanged with either water or various chemotherapeutic agents such as chlorhexidine, hydrogen peroxide, or phenolic compounds. Reviewing design specifics of each available unit is beyond the scope of this chapter. Reading the manufacturer's instructions or becoming familiar with the specific features of each powered instrument is important for safety, effectiveness, and efficiency.

Magnetostrictive

The first category of ultrasonic instruments is the **magnetostrictive** (Figure 31-3). With this mechanism of action, the working tip is part of an insert that fits into a hand piece located on the ultrasonic unit. The insert is composed of either a

*References 5, 16, 35-37, 45, 57, 63.
†References 16, 21, 24, 36, 37, 50.

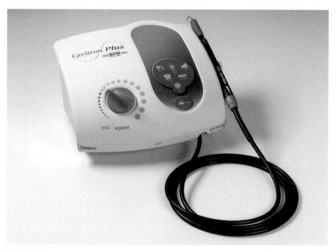

FIGURE 31-3
Components of magnetostrictive unit. (Courtesy DENTSPLY, York, Pa.)

Table 31-6	Comparison of Characteristics of Powered Instruments			
TYPE OF INSTRUMENT	**CYCLES PER SECOND (HERTZ)**	**MOTION OF TIP**	**TIP POWER DISPERSION**	**POWER TRANSDUCER**
Sonic	3500 to 8000	Elliptical or orbital	All surfaces active	Compressed air from dental unit
Magnetostrictive	18,000 to 45,000+	Elliptical	All surfaces active	Metal rod or stack of metal sheets
Piezoelectric	25,000 to 50,000+	Linear	Lateral surfaces active	Ceramic disks

stack of nickel alloy strips or a ferrous rod. The stack end inserts into the hand piece, and the other is a shaft where the working tip is connected (Figure 31-4). Water flows around the stack to cool as the stack transfers a magnetic vibratory motion of 18,000 to 45,000 cps or Hz.

Magnetostrictive ultrasonic units are available in the 25-kilohertz (kHz) or 30-kHz options. Differences between the two systems cannot always be easily detected, but the 30-kHz scaler is somewhat quieter during use than the 25-kHz unit. One obvious difference is the length of the *stack:* 30-kHz stacks are shorter in length than the 25-kHz options (Figure 31-5). Operating frequency is generally hard wired into the system equipment; thus 25-kHz and 30-kHz tips are not interchangeable. Dental hygienists should check with the manufacturer for specific guidelines on frequency and tip requirements.

Magnetostrictive action produces an elliptical motion by the tip, allowing for activation of all surfaces of the tip simultaneously with varying amounts of power dispersion. This feature provides the option to use the side, back, or front of the tip for adaptation to the root surface.[16,42]

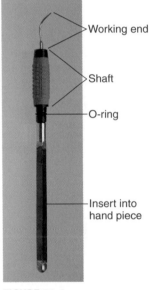

FIGURE 31-4
Parts of a magnetostrictive insert and tip. (Courtesy DENTSPLY, York, Pa.)

Working end

Shaft

O-ring

Insert into hand piece

Increasing the power of magnetostrictive systems increases the tip displacement (amplitude) for more robust scaling, but it may also decrease patient comfort. Power, tuning, tip selection, and technique all become critical to patient comfort and instrument effectiveness in varying clinical situations. Features in magnetostrictive technology improvements have come mostly in tip design features, which include fiberoptic lighting (Figure 31-6), color-coded hand pieces, swivel functions that improve ease of use and ergonomics, and smaller, longer, thinner tips designed for deeper penetration into periodontal pockets.

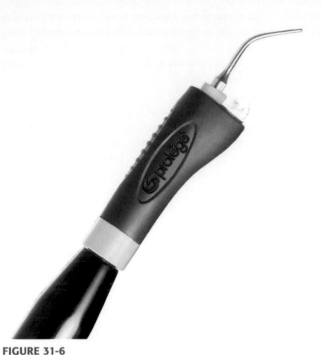

FIGURE 31-6
Protégé insert with fiberoptic lighting. (Courtesy Discus Dental, Culver City, Calif.)

Piezoelectric

The second category of ultrasonic instruments is **piezoelectric** (Figure 31-7). The mechanism for conversion of electrical power to tip movement uses a pulsing voltage applied to ceramic disks or quartz plates that flex to move the tip without producing heat. The vibratory motion is transformed to the tip to produce a linear movement at 25,000 to 50,000 cps. Unlike the magnetostrictive unit inserts, no magnetic field is present, and little heat is generated in the hand piece, but the high-speed movement of the active tip will generate heat, requiring water to cool the tissues in the working area.[42] The piezoelectric working tips screw onto the end of the hand piece and require a custom wrench to place and remove. Tips are available in an

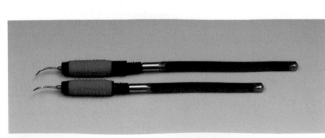

FIGURE 31-5
Comparison of the 25-kHz and 30-kHz magnetostrictive insert.

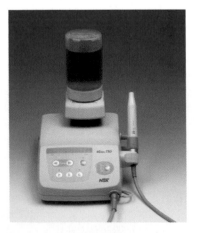

FIGURE 31-7
Piezoelectric system. (Courtesy NSK-Nakanishi, Inc., Japan)

assortment of styles for the varying clinical applications (Figure 31-8). Because of the linear movement of the tip, only the lateral surfaces are active, similar to a bladed hand instrument. When adapted incorrectly, the different sound from the tip alerts the clinician to adjust the adaptation to allow the proper working end to be effective.[16]

The wide assortment of tips on piezoelectric systems is probably the key benefit of this technology. Tip selections not only cover the range of periodontal debridement functions, they can be used in endodontics, surgery, and restorative dentistry as well. One of the disadvantages of piezoelectric technology is that their tips are generally not interchangeable among brands; however, future product developments may eliminate this issue. Some of the newer features on piezoelectric systems include fiberoptic lines into the hand piece that assist the clinician by improving visibility during scaling, as well as color-coding designs that make it easier to distinguish the tip applications and the appropriate power setting for the tips being used.

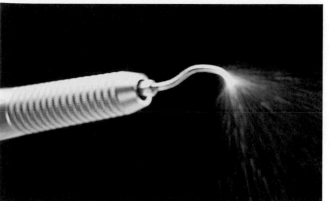

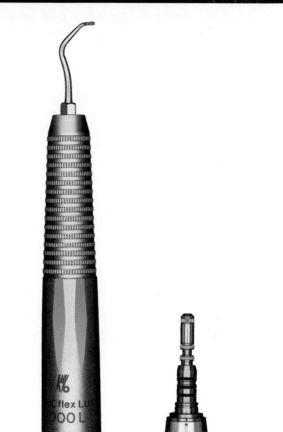

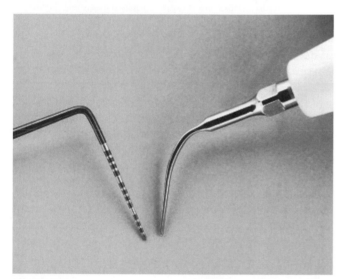

FIGURE 31-8
Piezoelectric tip in comparison to an UNC 15 probe. (Courtesy EMS America, Dallas, Tex.)

SONIC SCALERS

Sonic scalers operate under the same principles as ultrasonic with the exception of using an **air turbine** as the energy source. Sonic scalers are the size of a hand piece and attach to a conventional air/water hand piece connector on the dental unit (Figure 31-9). Some sonic scalers are equipped with fiber optics, with ergonomic handles, or both. The sonic scaler operates at a frequency of 3000 to 8000 cps, eliciting a variation of vibratory type of tip movements that are primarily linear or elliptical in direction using all surfaces of the tip.[52] Sonic scalers do not generate heat in the hand piece, but they need water to cool the working area. The water comes from the hand piece hose connection, and the dental unit foot pedal is used to control activation.

Sonic instruments have changeable tips. The tip design is based on the task to be performed and specific tooth anatomy. Most manufacturers' tips are designed to simulate curet and sickle scalers with recent design changes to improve effectiveness

FIGURE 31-9
A, Sonic instrument with fiber optics. **B,** Sonic tip connected to a fiber-optic coupler that connects to the dental unit air/water connection. (Courtesy KaVo America, Lake Zurich, Ill.)

and efficiency. Directions for use may vary slightly, depending on the manufacturer. When cross-sectioned, some tips are round, whereas others may have angles, producing flat sides and requiring a slightly different tip-to-tooth adaptation.

Tip Designs and Applications

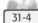

A wide variety of powered scaling instruments is on the market, with numerous tip designs. Primary features of common tip designs will be discussed in this chapter. Dental hygienists should thoroughly review and explore specific features and functions of the various instrumentation options, as well as manufacturer recommendations, before using any powered scaling system. Powered instrument tip options generally vary in length, shape, diameter, and function. Having an understanding of function, power recommendations, and applications is important when choosing an appropriate tip for the varying clinical situations. Figure 31-10 comparatively illustrates the sonic, magnetostrictive, and piezoelectric tips.

Tip designs have evolved over time to adapt to the various clinical applications that powered instrumentation offers. Magnetostrictive inserts were initially designed similarly to the manual instruments, including shapes such as the chisel; sickle; curet; probe; and a wide, flat instrument used for heavy stain removal and supragingival scaling. Recently, tips have been developed that are smaller, thinner, and curved to allow access to deeper pocket areas, difficult interproximal surfaces, and posterior areas. Water-delivery options also had to adapt to the changing tip dimensions with external water tube delivery—known as a *trombone*—or internal water-delivery source within the tip to control the water source and provide increased ease of use. Piezoelectric tips have gone through similar transformations and now offer numerous tip selections for a range of procedures. Powered instrumentation units offer a wide variety of system features, as well as specific tip designs, for various clinical applications.

Decision making for powered scaling requires consideration of numerous factors. The clinician needs to address the following:

- Access to the area requiring debridement
- Location and amount of deposit present
- Condition of the periodontal tissues
- Probing pocket depths
- Root morphology

UNIVERSAL TIPS—SUPRAGINGIVAL

All powered instruments have universal—supragingival—tip designs. The term *universal* refers to an instrument that can be used anywhere in the mouth and adapted to all surfaces of the teeth. These tips are generally designated by size for supragingival or subgingival scaling. Supragingival universal tip designs are generally thicker and wider, designed for removal of heavy supragingival plaque biofilm, calculus, and stain (Table 31-7). Examples of conic universal inserts include KaVo's Soniflex #5 and Titan's universal tip. Magnetostrictive universal design is the original standard diameter P-style, from Dentsply (York, Pa.), or Hu-Friedy #10

> *Note*
>
> Supragingival universal tips are ideal for the removal of moderate to heavy supragingival deposits and some subgingival deposit removal if the tissue permits tip entry into the pocket. These inserts may be operated on a medium to high power setting, depending on the amount of power needed for the debridement procedure.

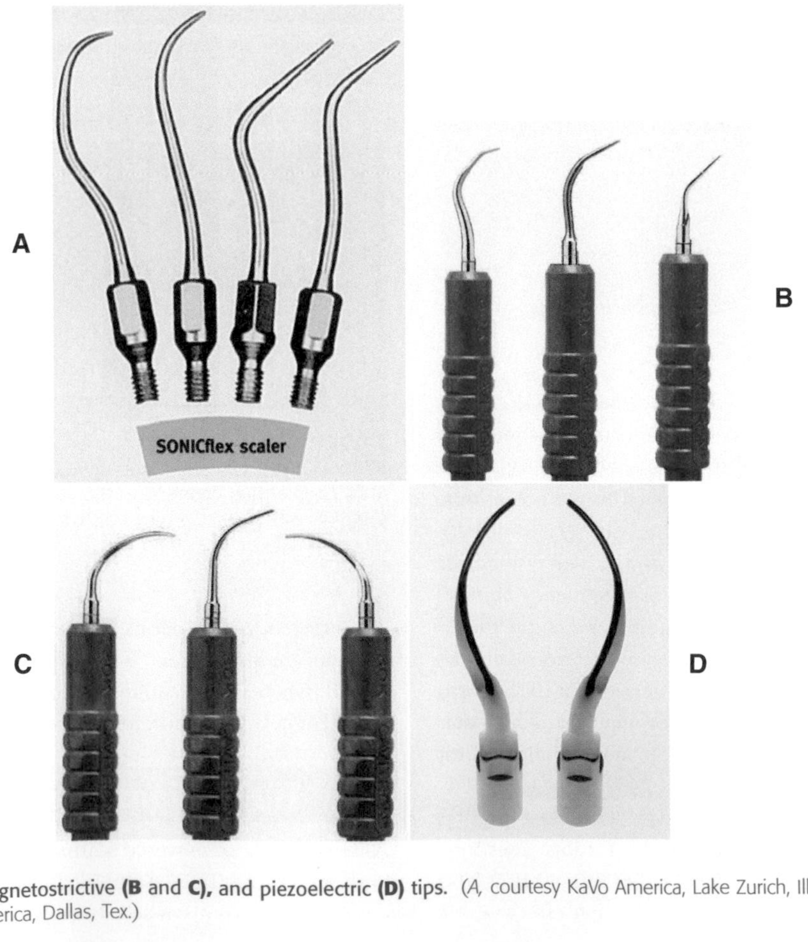

FIGURE 31-10
Comparison of sonic **(A)**, magnetostrictive **(B and C)**, and piezoelectric **(D)** tips. (*A*, courtesy KaVo America, Lake Zurich, Ill.; *B* and *C*, courtesy DENTSPLY, York, Pa.; *D*, courtesy EMS America, Dallas, Tex.)

Table 31-7	Tip Characteristics	
TYPE	**CHARACTERISTICS AND USES**	**SUGGESTED POWER SETTING**
Supragingival Universal Tip	• Larger in diameter • Used to remove gross supragingival and subgingival deposits.	• Can be used on medium to high power setting.
Modified Thin Periodontal Tips	• Smaller in diameter and longer in length. • Used for subgingival plaque biofilm and calculus removal.	• Use medium to low power settings. • Low power setting for biofilm removal.
SLIM UNIVERSAL STRAIGHT TIPS	• Designed for periodontal pockets and fine debridement procedures. They have the best overall performance because of the improved tactile sensitivity and better access but are not sturdy enough for heavy deposit removal.	• Medium power for removing hard calculus. • Higher power may be necessary to remove hard calculus in deeper periodontal pockets.[42]
RIGHT AND LEFT TIPS	• Designed as a complementary pair. Each is curved to access one half of the tooth surface, and together they provide superior adaptation to complete root anatomy. Right and left tips provide the best access to tight interproximal spaces and furcations but do not adapt to all surfaces; thus they need to be changed as indicated and used in conjunction with each other.	
Specialty Tips *FURCATION TIPS*	• Straight, right, or left with ball on the tip are designed to instrument contours of furcal walls and concavities. • Use slow, consistent movement to minimize iatrogenic damage to root surface.	• Use on low to medium power.
DIAMOND TIPS	• Large diamond tips are designed for gross deposit removal. • Fine diamond tips are designed for fine-tuning and removing imbedded and burnished calculus under direct visualization.	• Can be used on medium to high power. • Use only on low power settings.
IMPLANT TIPS	• Made of carbon composite or plastic tip that covers inserts. • Used for periodontal maintenance around implant and cosmetically restored surfaces.	• Use low to medium power setting.

universal insert. Examples of universal piezoelectric inserts include the P & PS (EMS) or 10Z (Acteon/Satelec).

MODIFIED TIPS—PERIODONTAL OR SUBGINGIVAL

In the 1980s, clinicians began to envision how tips might be altered to increase access and improve the overall effectiveness of ultrasonics for periodontal debridement. Tips were thinned and reshaped, enabling them to be placed subgingivally. Modifications were made to the original design resulting in a 40% thinner and longer probelike periodontal insert. The modified *periodontal inserts* feature straight and area-specific right or left design, which are longer and thinner than the standard-designed tips. These tips enhance access and adaptation in deeper periodontal pockets, particularly in posterior areas with complex anatomical features that may include concavities, convexities, and furcations. Modified periodontal designs feature thinner tips, approximately 0.5 mm at the tip, and longer shank than the standard-designed tips, which is ideal for debriding deep pocket areas (see Table 31-7). Figure 31-10, *B* and *C*, shows a comparison of the standard and slimline magnetostrictive inserts. Adjusting the power is necessary when using these

tips. Low to medium power is indicated when using the thinner type of insert.

Furcation tip inserts feature a 0.8-mm or a 0.5-mm ball end on the tip that reduces the likelihood of gouging the root surface and are available in a straight, right, and left option. These tips allow access into the variety and complexity of furcation anatomical sites (Figure 31-11).

Many companies now offer *diamond tips* that come in a variety of sizes and shapes and have very specific applications. DENTSPLY offers the Diamondcoat magnetostrictive insert that is intended for use in removing tenacious calculus, providing soft tissue debridement, and removing amalgam overhangs. This insert is essentially a universal tip with a coarse diamond coating covering the last 4 mm on the active tip end. It is a heavy-style tip for heavy applications.

Conversely, manufacturers of piezoelectric technology have produced tip designs that are very thin with options of a fine diamond coating on tips the size of explorers. The piezoelectric diamond-coated tips are designed for very fine, finishing-type procedures and are offered on most of the piezoelectric systems. As would be expected, to prevent breakage or damage to the

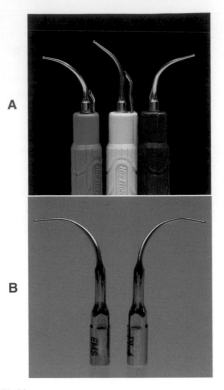

FIGURE 31-11
Furcation tips. **A,** Magnetostrictive inserts. **B,** Piezo furcation right and left tips. (*A,* courtesy Hu-Friedy, Chicago, Ill.; *B,* courtesy EMS America, Dallas, Tex.)

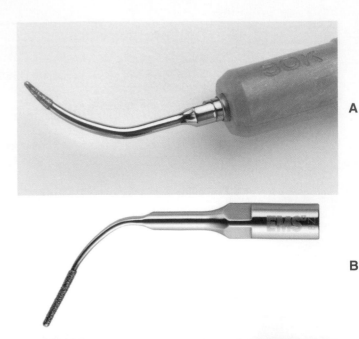

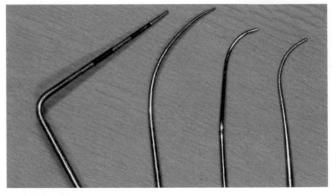

FIGURE 31-12
Diamond tips. **A,** DENTSPLY Cavitron diamond tip. **B,** Piezo diamond tip. **C,** Piezo diamond tip compared with other instruments. Left to right: Marquis periodontal probe, Piezo diamond tip, ODU 11/12 explorer, and Satelec H2-R diamond tip. (*A,* courtesy DENTSPLY, York, Pa.; *B,* courtesy EMS America, Dallas, Tex.; *C,* courtesy Mikelle Watson, Newport, Calif.)

root surfaces, the power level used with these tips needs to be on a low setting, and the touch and movement should be light, for proper use. Recommendations are that diamond tips be used only when the clinician has direct vision of the surfaces or is using very light touch with minimal stokes and a low power setting[42] (Figure 31-12; see also Table 31-7). Diamond-coated tips have been shown to be more efficient in removing calculus in moderate to deep pockets than regular ultrasonic tips,[65] and diamond-coated furcation inserts are also efficient and effective for removing debris within the furca.[51]

With the increased use of dental implants and cosmetic restorations, manufacturers of powered instruments have produced tips that permit the dental hygienist to debride these areas effectively without the concern of damaging restored surfaces. Plastic tip covers that can be placed on specific tips, as well as carbon composite inserts in various tip designs, can all be used effectively without scratching or damaging the restorative or implant surfaces (Figure 31-13). Refer to Tables 31-7 and 31-8 for general guidelines for tip selection.

Today, with the newly designed powered scaling systems and tip selections, the antiquated theories of periodontal therapy need to be eliminated from practice. Current tip design allows for access to root surfaces and reduction or elimination of dental plaque biofilm and hard deposits. Because of the ever-changing world of instrument design, checking with the product manufacturer for current tip design and recommendations is always valuable.

✳ CASE APPLICATION 31-1.2

Select Tip(s) for Debridement

Note the size, shape, and length of the tips in Figure 31-14 and determine which tip is used in which area of the mouth and for which type of debridement. Now select the tip or tips you would choose for Mrs. Ray's debridement.

Considerations for Use of Powered Instrumentation for Periodontal Debridement

31-5

Before any therapeutic or preventive measure is performed in the dental office, thorough assessment, diagnosis, and planning must occur. Identifying oral and systemic risks, current conditions, and a plan for preventive and therapeutic interventions is

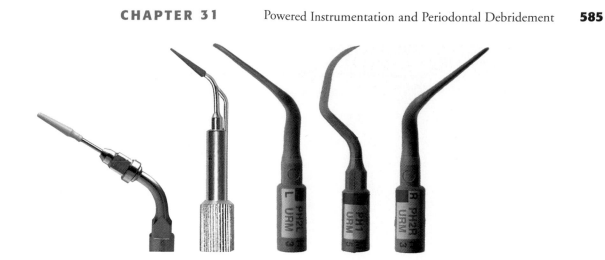

FIGURE 31-13
Various implant tip options. (Courtesy (1) EMS America, Dallas, Tex.; (2) Tony Riso Company, New York, NY; (3-5) Acteon/Satelec, Mt. Laurel, NJ.)

Table 31-8	Tip-Selection Guidelines
STEPS TO TAKE	**DESCRIPTION**
1. Look at the Patient Conditions Before Choosing the Tip	
STATE OF HEALTH OR DISEASE OF THE PERIODONTIUM	• Healthy tissue: Select smaller tip size on low power for biofilm debridement. One universal tip, followed up with manual instrumentation as indicated, may be adequate for biofilm and calculus removal in healthier patients. • Diseased tissue: Usually accompanied by heavier deposits. Start with heavier, universal tips for gross deposit removal, then move on to smaller tips for fine-tuning and deeper pocket penetration. • May require multiple visits for complete calculus removal and disease management.
TOOTH AND ROOT MORPHOLOGY	• Areas with furcation involvement may require using a furcation tip for more complete deposit removal. • Anatomically challenging areas such as deep interproximal pocketing may require modified right and left tips to access and instrument thoroughly.
TYPES AND LOCATION OF DEPOSITS	• Light, scattered deposit can usually be managed with smaller tip selection on lower power. • Heavier deposit removal will generally require multiple modes of instrumentation techniques. Consider using heavy, sturdier tips for gross deposit removal followed by hand instrumentation for most effective and thorough instrumentation.
2. Choose the Most Appropriate Tip for the Initial Treatment	• Change tips as necessary throughout the procedure to provide the most effective and efficient treatment for the case.
3. Start with the Heavier, Universal Supragingival Deposit Removal	
4. Move into the Pocket with a Tip that Allows Access to the Pocket	
5. Finish with Finer Tips at a Lower Power	• Allows complete instrumentation of root surface and affected periodontal site. • Use finishing diamond tips and furcation tips for specific treatment applications only. • Use caution on cosmetic and restorative work to avoid permanent damage to porcelain surfaces.

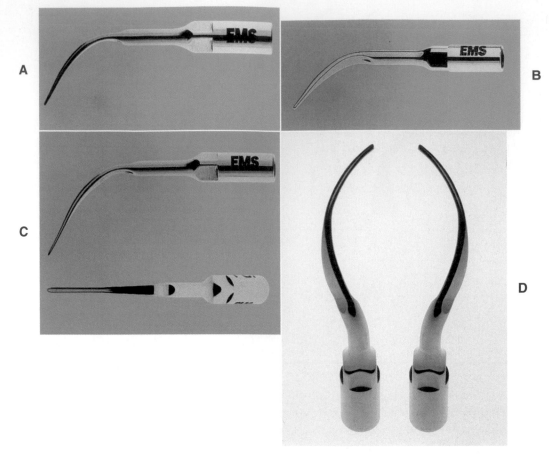

FIGURE 31-14
Various tip options for periodontal debridement. **A,** Perio regular tip P. **B,** Universal tip A. **C,** Perio slim tip PS. **D,** Curved tips. (Courtesy EMS America, Dallas, Tex.)

performed. During this process, the clinician identifies whether the patient has any medical or dental considerations that might prohibit the use of powered instruments.

HEALTH CONSIDERATIONS

Some concern surrounds the use of magnetostrictive ultrasonics on patients with pacemakers. In general, modern pacemakers are shielded against electromagnetic interference, with the exception of various sources in the medical field and in dentistry, which include magnetostrictive ultrasonic scalers and ultrasonic bath cleaners.[1,4,16] No reports of interference by piezoelectric scalers have surfaced.[1,4,16]

Other considerations for using powered instruments are patients with communicable diseases such as hepatitis, tuberculosis, or human immunodeficiency virus (HIV), primarily because of the amount of aerosols produced during the procedure and the immunocompromised status of these patients. Patients who are at an increased risk for infection because of medical conditions such as immunosuppression, diabetes, or organ transplants may exhibit complications from aerosols or contaminated dental-unit waterlines. Additional considerations include patients who are at risk for respiratory or breathing problems such as asthma, emphysema, cystic fibrosis, or pulmonary diseases. Because of the amount of aerosols and water produced during powered instrumentation, patients who are prone to gagging or dysphagia may not be good candidates.[16,58]

Prevention

For patients with a pacemaker, always have a medical consultation directed to the cardiologist before using magnetostrictive ultrasonic scalers. Manual instrumentation or piezoelectric scalers are acceptable debridement instruments for these patients.[1,4,16]

Distinct Care Modifications

Medical considerations with using powered instruments include patients who have communicable diseases such as hepatitis, tuberculosis, HIV, or acquired immunodeficiency syndrome (AIDS). Patients with increased risk of infection from aerosols and waterline contamination may include immunosuppressed patients or patients with diabetes; organ transplant recipients; or persons with respiratory problems such as asthma, emphysema, cystic fibrosis, or pulmonary diseases.

Standard precautions will protect the clinician, and therefore the decision to use powered instruments is based on the patient's health.[16]
- Consider the risk versus the benefits when selecting instruments to treat patients in these health categories.
- Manual instrumentation can always be considered for any debridement procedure when health considerations are present.

DENTAL CONSIDERATIONS

Caution also should be exercised when using powered instruments with certain dental conditions. Powered instrumentation is contraindicated on the following circumstances:

- Titanium implants can be easily damaged. Instruments made from carbon composite, plastic or other resin-type materials that are specifically designed for scaling implants are recommended.
- Certain restorative materials, including composite, porcelain, gold, and amalgam, can be damaged or scratched during instrumentation of the restored surface.
- Appropriate tip selection, which may include carbon composite or resin tips, proper technique, and proper power setting are essential to minimize permanent damage to the restorative material and restoration interface.
- Heat, water, and vibration associated with powered instrumentation may aggravate sensitive areas such as exposed dentin or demineralization and is generally contraindicated in such areas to minimize sensitivity and further breakdown.[16]

Tip selection: Use plastic or carbon composite tips when working around implants or cosmetic restorations.

Technique: Keep tip adapted to root surface below restorative margin, and keep tip from coming in contact with restoration surface.

- Once powered instrumentation has been established as an appropriate treatment modality, the preparation for treatment can begin.

Note

Attention and detail is needed when instrumenting around dental implants and restorative margins to reduce scratching or damaging the restorative material.

⊛ CASE APPLICATION 31-1.3

Contraindications

Review Mrs. Ray's medical and dental history. Does Mrs. Ray have any contraindications that would prevent you from using a powered instrument to complete her dental hygiene treatment plan? If so, explain the contraindication and steps that might be taken to minimize or manage the effects.

Preparation of Powered Instruments

OPERATOR AND WORKING AREA

Preparation of the operator and working area is the same as when the clinician is providing any form of patient care. Universal precautions are followed, as outlined in Chapter 7. The additional personal protective equipment (PPE) of a face shield is ideal during the use of power-driven instruments, and clinicians may also choose to wear a disposable head covering. Using high-volume suction with an aerosol-reduction device is recommended. Aerosol-reduction devices have been shown to reduce aerosols when attached to various types of powered instruments, including ultrasonics.[30,48] Preparation of the unit with appropriate coverings to prevent contamination is also necessary. Chapter 7 discusses work practice controls and PPE required for instruments that create aerosols.

SYSTEM SETUP

All powered scalers require an electrical power supply and a water supply for function. The clinician should check specific system instructions for information on connections and supplies. After connecting to the water line and before using the unit, the water line or water reservoir should be flushed to remove or reduce waterborne bacteria and biofilm in the unit.

Prevention

A general rule with all dental equipment is to flush the water lines before use on a patient. This process simply means turning on the power and water to the powered scaler and activating the foot control to run water through the system for a specified amount of time. This flushing of the water lines will reduce the patient's exposure to possible biofilms that have broken loose in the water tubing and are released in the water that comes out of the working end of the system.

ADJUSTING WATER VOLUME

Water is essential for all powered scaling applications, regardless of power setting or tip used. The amount of water should be adjusted on the system after the tip has been placed according to system-specific needs and clinical conditions. For example, piezoelectric systems do not require water to cool the machine or internal components of the hand piece but still need water to cool the working end of the tip. In contrast, in magnetostrictive systems, the water control adjusts the volume and temperature of the fluid flowing from the hand piece to cool the stack and insert tip and lubricates the tip for easy insertion. The volume of water also indicates the phase or tuning of the system. Water on all powered instruments acts as an irrigator to lavage and flush debris from the treatment site and cools the working end of the tip to prevent damage to the root surface and soft tissue during instrumentation.

Cavitation is another unique feature of water in powered instrumentation. **Cavitation** is a physiologic property associated with the operation of the ultrasonic generator that causes water to atomize as it passes over the vibrations of the moving tip creating air cavities that collapse and explode. This cavitational action has been shown to cause cell disruption within the periodontal pocket,[58] supporting the goals of periodontal debridement. All of these factors should be considered when instrumentation is initiated.

ADJUSTING POWER–TUNING

The power setting affects the length of stroke or amplitude of the vibrations. The higher power setting delivers a longer, more powerful stroke, and conversely, a lower power setting delivers a shorter, less powerful stroke. Because of the variation in tip size and clinical application, power settings need to be adjusted appropriately for each tip application on every powered scaling instrument. The dental hygienist should become familiar with the specific manufacturer power adjustments and recommendations before use on a patient.

Magnetostrictive scaling devices have power-control and water-control functions and can be either manually or automatically tuned. The frequency control on manually tuned units can be adjusted to fine-tune the tip vibration or adjust the number of tip cycles per second. When the appropriate water and power is selected, a fine water spray is observed from the tip when the unit is activated. The spray should deflect off the working tip in a fine spray, forming a halo appearance (Figure 31-15).

If, during activation of the magnetostrictive instrument, the hand piece begins to feel warm, then some adjustment is required. Increasing the water flow may reduce the heat; however, disadvantages are that this produces too much water for the clinician and patient, and the spray will no longer be directed onto the tip. Reducing the power setting may also decrease the generation of heat to the hand piece but may result in inefficient deposit removal. Minor adjustments to water or power

> ### Note
> Sturdier, supragingival tips can accommodate a higher power setting while finer precision thin tips require less power. Medium to high power settings are recommended for heavy debris removal, and a low to medium power setting is recommended for removing light debris and plaque biofilm. See specific tip guidelines for appropriate power setting range for each tip being used.

> ### Distinct Care Modifications
> Power selection can affect patient comfort and should be adjusted to accommodate certain procedures, particularly with areas of root sensitivity or patient apprehension with the procedure. Reducing the power setting will reduce the length of stroke and vibrations, minimizing patient discomfort levels. Appropriate water flow will reduce temperature sensitivity caused by heat from the tip movement.

settings, or both, can often manage the problem. If these adjustments do not change the temperature, then air bubbles may be trapped in the water line. The insert should be removed, and holding the hand piece upright while activating the rheostat should bleed the line. Water should be allowed to flow out of the hand piece while observing for bubbles. When the bubbles have subsided, the insert should be placed into the hand piece, and the procedure can then be resumed.

PATIENT PREPARATION

Patient preparation is also necessary when using powered instruments. Before using the powered instrument and at the time of informed consent, the dental hygienist should explain the procedure to the patient, reason for use, action of the powered instrument, necessity of suction and draping, and any anticipated response.

Before starting instrumentation, a signal can be agreed on that the patient can use if he or she feels the need to stop or communicate during the procedure. The clinician should be perceptive to body language indicating patient discomfort. Providing protection and a drape for the patient or providing some form of barrier protection from the water spray is also recommended. A cotton towel or a commercially available face shield may be provided to the patient to be placed over the nose and upper face to prevent the area from being covered with spatter from the procedure and reduce the inhalation of aerosols. Figure 31-16 illustrates patient, operator, and equipment readiness for use. Draping of the face and nose is optional; eyewear is essential.

> ### Patient Education Opportunity
> Explain the procedure to the patient in simple terms such as, "this instrument will create a lot of noise and vibration and has a water spray that may get things a little wet." This explanation will prepare the patient for the upcoming procedure and reduce anxiety when the actual procedure begins.

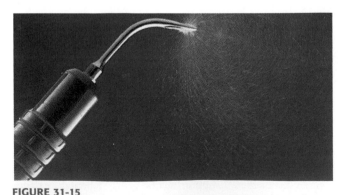

FIGURE 31-15
The spray should reflect off the working tip in a fine spray, forming a halo appearance. (Courtesy DENTSPLY, York, Pa.)

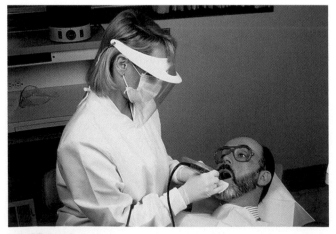

FIGURE 31-16
Patient preparation for ultrasonic treatment: patient, operator, and equipment readiness for use. Note protective gear on operator and patient.

PREPROCEDURAL RINSE

The clinician should recommend that the patient rinse before dental hygiene procedures are initiated to reduce the level of bacteria in the aerosols. This precaution is of great importance during powered instrumentation.[30,48,58] Studies have shown that using a preprocedural rinse can also decrease the number of microorganisms introduced in the bloodstream during ultrasonic therapy.[40] The recommendation for preprocedural rinse is to rinse for 1 minute with 0.12% chlorhexidine[19,58] or with an essential oil–containing antiseptic mouthrinse (Listerine Antiseptic) for 30 seconds before treatment is initiated.[18]

Fundamentals of Powered Instrumentation

PATIENT AND OPERATOR POSITIONING

The performance logic positioning as presented in Chapter 8 is recommended for powered instrumentation. Modifications can be made to the supine position if needed for patient comfort. The mouth mirror is used for illumination to enhance visibility.

PATIENT COMFORT

During powered debridement procedures, managing patient comfort is important. Power scaling can produce high-pitched sounds, increase tooth sensitivity, and generate excessive water that many patients may find uncomfortable. Communicating before starting the procedure is an important aspect of patient management. High power settings often cause excess heat and vibration, which can lead to patient discomfort. Selecting the proper power setting and using a thorough, gentle technique are of upmost importance in patient comfort.

> *Note*
>
> Adjust the power setting to as low a setting as possible to debride the surface effectively and efficiently. Power settings can and should be changed throughout the procedure to reflect the clinical situation, the tip that is being used, and patient comfort levels. Effective evacuation control of the aerosols and water produced also increase patient comfort and acceptance of the procedure.

> *Patient Education Opportunity*
>
> Removing biofilm and calculus in a periodontal pocket can be difficult to perform effectively when the tissue is inflamed and sensitive. If the clinician cannot access the pockets and debride effectively, then the infectious process of the disease will continue, and healing cannot take place. The analogy of removing a splinter is easy for the patient to understand and is applicable to the procedure being performed. A splinter of any size can cause discomfort and pain because the body is trying to deal with or expel the *foreign body or irritant*. Once the splinter is removed, then the area starts to feel better, and healing can occur.
>
> Topical or local anesthetics can be used to help reduce the discomfort from the scaling procedure, as well as allow the clinician the opportunity to debride these areas thoroughly without fear of *hurting the patient*.

✷ **CASE APPLICATION 31-1.4**

Pain Management Options

Referring to Mrs. Ray's initial evaluation and treatment needs, identify appropriate steps to support pain management options for this case.

For involved procedures such initial debridement in the presence of inflammation (CDT code 4355) or scaling and root planing (CDT code 4341),[3] preemptive pain management such as topical[12] or local anesthetics may be indicated to increase patient comfort and ensure a thorough, more complete debridement procedure. Pain management guidelines to follow are reviewed in Chapters 40-42.

GRASP

Similar to manual instrumentation, powered instruments require using a light, modified pen grasp at the junction of the handle and the shank (Figure 31-17, Table 31-9). A light grasp increases tactile sensitivity, increases patient comfort, and reduces clinician fatigue. A light grasp also allows the clinician flexibility in movement to roll the instrument between the fingers to access line angles and other subgingival anatomical features.

Both sonic and ultrasonic hand pieces are heavier than manual instruments. Additionally, weight from the cord causes drag and may require adjustments in cord placement. To reduce tension from the cord, many clinicians find it helpful to rest the cord in the palm of the hand around the thumb, wrap it around their forearms, and lay it across their laps or grasp it between their fingers in the grasp (Figure 31-18). Several companies that design and manufacture powered instruments have introduced hand pieces that have a moveable mechanism in the handle, or in the ultrasonic insert itself, that can help eliminate drag so that the clinician can spend less time managing the cord and can focus on the procedure.

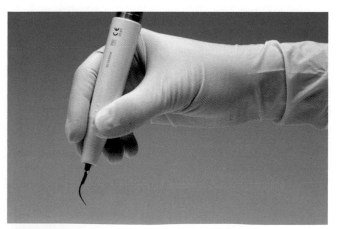

FIGURE 31-17
Light modified pen grasp.

Table 31-9	Similarities and Differences between Magnetostrictive and Piezoelectric Instrumentation		
Use	**Similarities**	**Differences**	
		Instrumentation Type	
		MAGNETOSTRICTIVE OR SONIC	**PIEZOELECTRIC**
Patient-Operator Positioning	Appropriate proprioceptive position for working in the selected area. Patient may be raised slightly to help with water control issues.		
Patient Comfort	Communication, appropriate power settings, adequate water evacuation, anesthesia (topical or local) as indicated for discomfort.		
Grasp	Light, modified pen grasp.	Position the grasp on the hand piece, and not the insert, when using an extraoral fulcrum.	
Fulcrum	Soft tissue external fulcrums are used more frequently during powered instrumentation than with mechanical instrumentation. Internal fulcrums may also be used for stability and control.		Internal fulcrums are used more with piezoelectric instrumentation than with other instrumentation because instruments are generally smaller and easier to manipulate.
Insertion	Similar to a bladed hand instrument or a periodontal probe. Start at the coronal edge of the calculus. Maintain angulation near 0 degrees.		
Adaptation	The instrument anterior 2-3 mm of the tip is placed on the tooth surface at nearly a 0-degree angulation and can be opened slightly. Tip-to-tooth adaptation should never exceed 15 degrees.	All surface areas of magnetostrictive tips are active during instrumentation with power dispersion ranging from the most powerful terminal 4 mm of the point of the tip, decreasing progressively from the concave side to the convex backside then the lateral surfaces generating with least amount of energy.	The lateral surfaces of piezoelectric tips must be adapted to the tooth or root surface, similar to a bladed hand instrument, for the most effective and efficient instrumentation to occur.
Activation		Tap at the calculus in an apical direction. Lead with the tip of the insert.	A light back-and-forth sweeping motion should be used keeping the side of the tip against the tooth.
Stroke		Use slow overlapping strokes and light pressure to tap, or push with the tip in an apical or oblique direction.	Use a variety of strokes, including horizontal, oblique, or vertical with very light pressure.

FULCRUM

Establishing a fulcrum when using powered instruments is as important as when using manual instruments (see Table 31-9). Soft tissue external fulcrums are used frequently in performance logic positioning and also when using powered instruments (Figure 31-19; refer to Chapter 8 for positioning content). The bulk of the powered instrument hand piece and attached cord may require using an extraoral fulcrum to maintain control of the instrument. An external fulcrum provides balance rather than strength. When using an external fulcrum with a powered instrument, having a stable extraoral hand rest by using a broad surface area of contact between the hand and the patient's face is necessary. Also critical is to position the grasp on the hand piece, not the insert, when using an extraoral fulcrum. Intraoral fulcrums may also be

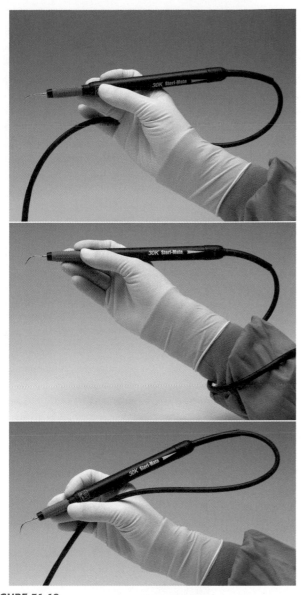

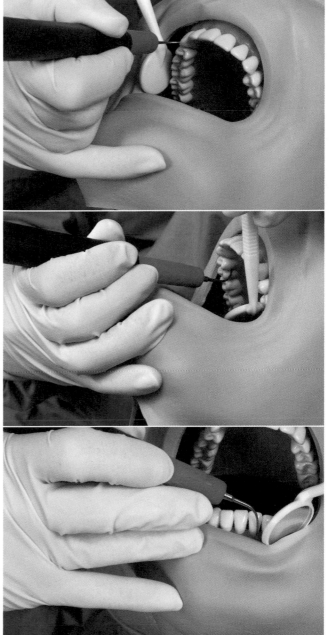

FIGURE 31-18
Cord management options. **A,** Grasped between the fingers.
B, Wrapped around the forearm. **C,** Resting in the palm of the hand
around the thumb.

FIGURE 31-19
A to **C,** External fulcrums that may be used during powered instrumentation.

beneficial and used in certain areas for additional support and
stabilization.

ADAPTATION

Powered instruments, similar to manual instruments, must always be adapted properly. Regardless of the type of powered
instrument used, the tip of the instrument should be kept parallel to the surface being treated and should always be adapted
as close to 0 degrees as possible. Keep in mind the anatomical
changes of the root surface as the instrument is moved in the
sulcus. The anterior 2 to 3 mm of the instrument tip is placed
on the tooth surface at nearly a 0-degree angulation and can be
opened slightly, but tip-to-tooth adaptation should never exceed 15 degrees.

DENTAL CONSIDERATIONS

Improper adaptation of the tip (more than 15 degrees)
causes gouging on the root surface and injury to surrounding soft tissues.

Tips that are similarly shaped to manual instruments should
be adapted to the tooth in the same way that manual instruments are adapted. The precision thin tips shaped as a periodontal probe can be inserted into the pocket similar to a probe
and adapted to the root surface as described previously. The
specific function and the motion of the tip of the various

powered scaling devices determine the appropriate adaptation of the working end of the instrument to the tooth surface.

ACTIVATION AND INSTRUMENTATION

Tip movements differ between the types of powered instruments, creating a difference in actual activation and instrumentation technique between the systems. Because of this difference, the details of activation and instrumentation will be described separately to accommodate the variation of action between the orbital or the elliptical movement of the sonic scalers and magnetostrictive inserts and the linear movement of the piezoelectric scalers.

With all powered instrumentation, the strokes should be close, making sure they are overlapping to cover all surfaces of the root. Powered scaling is most effective using a variety of strokes including horizontal, oblique, or vertical (Figure 31-20). Powered scaling strokes differ from manual instrumentation when positioning the tip under the gingiva and beneath the calculus is necessary. The concept for powered instrumentation is to position the tip on the coronal edge of the deposit and tap at the calculus in an apical direction.[42]

Periodically, the clinician may stop activation of the unit, pause, and use a cursory exploratory stroke to feel the tooth surface. If roughness or deposit is noted, immediate activation of the tip can occur, thus increasing time utilization. Tactile sensitivity develops with continued use of the powered instruments, as it does with the use of manual instruments. With an increased tactile sense, evaluation of the tooth surface can occur while the tip is activated. Finite evaluation of the tooth surface may be accomplished with an instrument designed for this purpose such as an ODU 11/12 explorer (see Chapter 9) or periodontal probe or dental endoscope that is described later in this chapter.

Sonic and Magnetostrictive

With sonic and magnetostrictive instruments, an important point to remember is that *all* surface areas of the tips are active during instrumentation. This circumstance means that the back, front, and sides of the tips can be adapted to access surface irregularities or difficult proximal surface root anatomy.

Power dispersion of the tips goes from the terminal 4 mm of the point of the tip being the most powerful, with power dispersion decreasing progressively from the concave side to the convex backside with the least amount of energy generated on the lateral surfaces (Figure 31-21). These levels of power dispersion need to be considered when adapting magnetostrictive instruments for effective and efficient powered instrumentation. Power to the system can be changed on the system power function control, but retuning may be necessary unless an auto-tune system is being used. The elliptical pattern of the tip movement removes calculus by going over the surface and smoothing off the calculus in layers (Table 31-10).

To begin instrumentation follow these steps:

- Adapt and maintain the terminal end of the ultrasonic tip to the tooth or root at an angle of 0 to 15 degrees to ensure that the direction of motion is working tangentially to the tooth rather than pulsing at it.
- Insert the tip like a scaling instrument or a probe and lead the stroke with the tip, moving in a coronal to apical direction.
- Keep the tip moving at all times to minimize unnecessary trauma to the root surface.
- Use slower strokes and light pressure to tap or push with the tip in an apical or oblique direction.[42]
- Use a combination of stroke patterns as mentioned previously to cover the root surface completely and debride the hard and soft deposits within the pocket thoroughly.

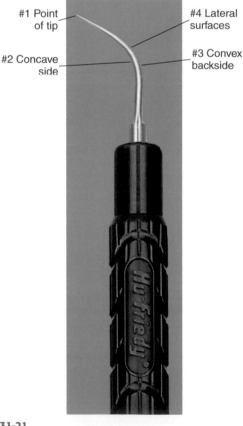

FIGURE 31-21
Power dispersion of a magnetostrictive scaler.

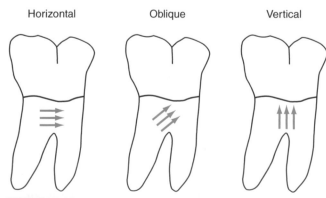

FIGURE 31-20
Strokes with powered instruments may be made in various directions: overlapping, horizontal, oblique, and vertical.

Table 31-10	**Debridement for Varying Clinical Conditions**	
USE	MAGNETOSTRICTIVE	PIEZOELECTRIC
Plaque Biofilm Removal	• Use the lateral surfaces for light deposit removal.	• Use the lateral surfaces on a low power setting.
Light Calculus Removal	• Maintain light pressure. Use the lateral surfaces of tip for light calculus removal.	• Maintain a light pressure. Use the lateral surfaces and adjust power on system for increased power needs.
Heavy Calculus Removal	• Rotate instrument to convex (back) surface for more powerful stroke on heavier deposits. • Use a probing or tapping motion to break up a ledge of large deposit.	• Heavy, sturdy tips on high power settings may be used to remove larger deposits. • Both downstrokes and upstrokes are active.

- Use the lateral surfaces of the tip for removing light deposits and rotate the instrument to the back (convex) surface for a more powerful stroke to remove heavier deposits.
- Maintain a light pressure and overlap strokes for thorough debridement. Severe root damage has been shown to occur with increased lateral force, improper angulation adaptation, or increased power settings.

These factors need to be properly adjusted to the various clinical needs for effective and safe magnetostrictive instrumentation to occur.[21]

Piezoelectric

The *piezoelectric* tips operate in a linear motion, with the lateral surfaces being the most active part of the tip. This feature makes adaptation of a piezoelectric instrument tip slightly different from the magnetostrictive tips but similar to the cutting edge of a manual instrument with primarily the lateral surfaces used for instrumentation. Calculus is removed by shearing off the calculus when the tip is adapted correctly (see Table 31-10).

- The *lateral surfaces* must be adapted to the tooth or root surface, similar to a bladed hand instrument, for the most effective and efficient instrumentation to occur.
- Insertion and activation of the piezoelectric tips is similar to the magnetostrictive and sonic tips. The instrument tip can be inserted similar to insertion of a manual scaling instrument or similar to a probe, but with piezoelectric technology, the lateral surfaces need to be adapted to the surface being instrumented for effective debridement to occur.
- For increased power needs when removing heavier deposits, power can be adjusted manually. Rotating the tip so that the back is adapted to the surface, as in magnetostrictive instrumentation, is not effective with piezoelectric scalers because the linear tip movement turns into a pounding motion rather than a scaling action.
- During instrumentation, a light back-and-forth sweeping motion should be used, keeping the terminal 2-3 mm of the lateral surface adapted to the root surface.
- Position tip apically with the entire tip placed parallel to the root surface.

- Move tip with a methodical stroke that is both overlapping and delivered with a featherlike touch.
- With the lateral surfaces of the tip, the curvatures of the root morphology are followed keeping the side adapted to convex and concave anatomical surfaces.
- The tip is maintained in continuous motion; the clinician uses little or no lateral pressure while moving around the tooth to cover all surfaces.

Piezoelectric tip design can be round, as found in a universal-type insert, or flat edged for dense supragingival calculus removal. Round and flat piezo tips can be used for removing stains, plaque biofilm, and calculus by adapting the round or flat edge of the top of the tip and the lateral sides of the tip on the tooth surface then using an up-and-down motion or sweeping motion to produce a smooth, stain-free surface. The most effective way to use the flat edge tip is to adapt the flat edge and the sides of the tip to the tooth, then use an up-and-down motion to sheer off heavy calculus. (Note: The tip is active in both the upstroke and downstroke and will remove calculus in both directions.) The paddle-shaped tips are effective for supragingival scaling and stain removal and particularly effective for removing amalgam or other restorative material overhangs.

★ CASE APPLICATION 31-1.5

Alleviate Discomfort

As you are instrumenting the lower anterior sextant, Mrs. Ray tells you that the water is starting to feel warm and that the tip is hot on her teeth. How would you modify the procedure to improve the situation and alleviate the discomfort that Mrs. Ray is feeling?

SYSTEMATIC APPROACH

After preparing the unit, using proper patient and clinician positioning, selecting an appropriate suction and water-evacuation device, and determining the ideal fulcrum, the clinician will begin powered instrumentation with the universal tip. The clinician should perform powered instrumentation in an orderly, methodical sequence that does not deviate from the treatment plan. Standard or universal tips should be used initially to reduce the supragingival calculus and begin deplaquing the teeth concurrently. Following the use of the standard tip, the clinician can proceed with the precision thin inserts for subgingival plaque biofilm and calculus removal. The intentional sequence should minimize the number of times the inserts or tips need to be changed, the unit retuned, or the power changed and should maximize the time spent on debridement.

Selecting a Tooth to Start Instrumentation

- Initially, ensure that the universal tip is parallel to the surface that requires scaling.
- Insert the tip at the distal line angle (facial, lingual), and position the tip to adapt to the distal line angle.
- Start activation and slowly move the tip, using small overlapping strokes into the interproximal space.
- Start most coronally and move the terminal third of the instrument tip to the base of the pocket, covering all accessible surfaces in the process.
- Use various stroke sequences and patterns to complete instrumentation on the distal surface of the tooth from the base of the pocket to the contact point of the interproximal space. If access is limited, then continue the sequence to the next accessible area and return to instrument incomplete areas when instrument tips are changed. Right and left inserts may be needed to complete instrumentation in these areas, particularly posterior.
- Reposition the insert at the distal line angle to proceed mesially, across the facial or lingual surface to the opposite line angle.
- Rotate the tip to adapt to the mesial line angle and interproximal space similar to distal adaptation; ensure that the tip is parallel to the deposit and beneath the contact.
- Proceed to the next tooth, starting again at the distal line angle, covering the distal aspect first, repositioning and moving mesially.
- Continue in a systematic approach using short overlapping strokes to completely instrument all surfaces requiring instrumentation.

The same concept will be applied when debriding anterior or posterior teeth with a universal tip. The clinician should begin the sequence at the line angle and use a sweeping or pushing stroke to reach the opposite line angle. If adequate instrumentation cannot be achieved on the proximal surfaces with the universal tip, the appropriate right or left tip should then be selected to gain better access to the surface and complete a thorough debridement of the entire tooth.

Right and Left Tip Designs

Right- and left-bend tips are ergonomically designed, area-specific tips with working end curvature to improve access to deeper pockets and proximal surfaces while keeping the handle parallel and manageable (Figure 31-22). To identify the correct working end, the clinician should direct the point of the tip toward the occlusal surface of the tooth and roll the tip toward the facial or the lingual and observe the direction that the curve is going. The surface that has the point or tip facing up is the surface that should be instrumented with this tip.

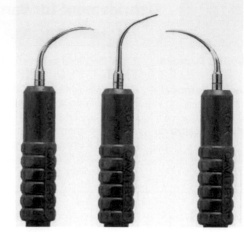

FIGURE 31-22
Right, straight, and left inserts. (Courtesy DENTSPLY, York, Pa.)

- Use a sweeping or pushing motion to remove the calculus from one line angle to the opposite line angle, again using strokes that will first remove the top of the deposit down to the bottom of the deposit.
- For the proximal surfaces on the lingual, roll the instrument to the line angle for overlapping coverage. When working in the posterior, perform the strokes from the anterior to the posterior using a pushing motion and then from the posterior to the anterior using a pulling motion (see Table 31-9).

✴ CASE APPLICATION 31-1.6

Powered Scaling Treatment Sequence Plan

Determine a powered scaling treatment sequence plan that would be the most appropriate for the debridement needs of Mrs. Ray, starting in the maxillary right quadrant:
- Which type of powered instrument would be used?
- Which tip would be used first, and at which power setting? Provide rationale for your decision.
- Which tip would be used next, and at what power setting? Provide rationale for your sequencing choices.
- How many tip changes would need to be made to complete the debridement sequence on the maxillary right quadrant?

MAINTENANCE

Following use, powered instrument tips should be removed from the hand piece and sterilized according to the manufacturer's recommendation. Dry heat and sterilization should be avoided as a means of sterilizing ultrasonic inserts because it has been shown to damage insert O-rings. Chemical vapor methods should also be avoided because they have been shown to prematurely damage the insert O-rings. Steam under pressure autoclaving achieves the best results while maintaining the integrity of the inserts and tips.

Ultrasonic inserts should not have anything placed on top of them when they are loaded in the sterilization unit. The magnetostrictive transducer or stack of the insert needs to be handled carefully so that it is not bent, remains closely approximated, and does not show signs of splaying. In addition, the precision thin insert or the piezoelectric tips can become bent if heavy instruments are placed on top of them, resulting in decreased performance following sterilization and potentially the need for premature replacement.

The O-rings of the magnetostrictive inserts are made of a rubber material and, over time, will weaken, lose elasticity, and need to be replaced. If the insert begins to leak or drips water from the connection between the hand piece and the insert, then the O-ring may be failing and will need to be replaced.

For resin handles, phenols and iodophors should be avoided. The plastic resin handles and metal components can be altered by immersion into chemical solutions. Corrosion or rust can occur and result in the need for replacement.

Maintaining the tips is critical to achieving adequate results of periodontal debridement, deplaquing, and all acceptable uses of ultrasonic inserts. Tips can become worn and no longer capable or efficient at removing deposits. Inserts should be examined before use to ensure that the tips or stacks are not bent or damaged. Use causes wear of tip and development of facets and pits, which alter tip performance. As with manual instruments, all powered instrument tips will show some wear over time. The length of the tip is critical to the effectiveness of the instrument. Over time, the length will shorten and need to be replaced. When an ineffective tip is used, several negative results can occur, including extended instrumentation time, increasing the power setting, burnishing the calculus, and the increased likelihood of damaging the root surfaces or causing root gouging. An insert tip worn down by 1 mm has lost 25% of its efficiency, and a tip worn down by 2 mm has lost 50% of its efficiency. Using a worn tip will also increase the chance of the tip fracturing.

Many powered instrument manufacturers have designed maintenance tip templates to compare when an insert is of ideal length and when it no longer has an effective tip (Figure 31-23). The wear indicator guides are an integral part of maintaining efficient powered instruments in dental hygiene practice.

Evaluation of Debridement during the Procedure

During the process of periodontal debridement, tactile and visual evaluation should be used. As previously mentioned, the nonactivated tip may be used during the procedure to perform a cursory evaluation of the tooth surface. However, feeling the tooth surface for deposits or roughness should be performed more definitively with an explorer. All tissue tags should be removed and bleeding stopped before dismissing the patient.

When multiple appointments are necessary to complete the periodontal debridement procedure, evaluating tissue response and self-care in previously treated areas is important. If an area previously treated still exhibits signs of bleeding and inflammation, then the area may need further instrumentation and/or closer self-care attention. As the treatment progresses, a common side effect of healing tissue is exposed dentin, which produces dentinal sensitivity. Refer to Chapter 22 for specifics on evaluation of care at the posttherapy evaluation.

Using the Dental Endoscope Technology in Periodontal Debridement

Even though the endoscope is still a relatively new instrument, it can affect periodontal debridement in several ways by adding direct, real-time visualization of the periodontal pocket before, during, and after periodontal therapy. The **dental endoscope (endoscopy)** was introduced to the dental community in the late 1990s and has slowly infiltrated into periodontal specialty offices, general dental offices, and educational settings (Figure 31-24, A).

The core of the dental endoscope starts with a 0.99-mm-diameter flexible bundle of imaging and illumination fibers. These fibers communicate the oral environment to a flat-screen monitor that essentially becomes the operator's mirror into the periodontal pocket. The fiberoptic bundle is protected from oral contaminants by a specially designed sterile, disposable

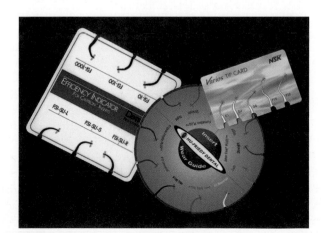

FIGURE 31-23
Maintenance tip templates from various companies.

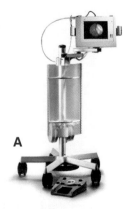
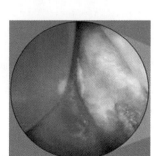

FIGURE 31-24
A, DentalView DV2 Dental Endoscope. **B,** Magnified view of subgingival environment on endoscope monitor. (Courtesy Perioscopy Inc., Oakland, Calif.)

sheath system, which also delivers water directly to the working site. The endoscope fits into specially designed manual instruments that carry the fiber bundle and reflect the soft tissue away from the small lens at the distal aspect of the sheath-covered fiber.

Once the instrument is inserted into the periodontal pocket, water is used to clear sulcular debris, bleeding, and plaque biofilm away from the lens. The operator controls the water flow with a foot pedal and watches the monitor rather than looking into the mouth. The image on the monitor reflects exactly what is in front of the lens, magnified up to 48× (Fiure 31-24, B). The operator can see not only tooth and root structure, but also changes in the soft tissue lining of the pocket, accretions that may be remaining on the root surface, and other etiologic factors that may be contributing to the destruction of the supporting periodontal structures.

USING THE ENDOSCOPE AS AN AID TO PERIODONTAL DEBRIDEMENT

The dental endoscope can be used to support visualization of subgingival conditions and during the actual debridement procedure.[34,43,53] As with the use of endoscopes in medicine, a two-handed technique is used to accomplish treatment under direct visualization.

- The endoscope is inserted into the pocket to identify areas needing further instrumentation.
- Once the area is identified, the operator will select a debridement instrument that is appropriate for the clinical situation. Many operators using the two-handed technique prefer to use the fine, thin periodontal tips designed for most ultrasonic scalers, which allow ease of access and instrumentation within the viewing area of the endoscope (Figure 31-25, Box 31-1).
- The instrument will then be inserted between the endoscope and the tooth surface until the instrument is seen visually on the monitor.
- To increase effectiveness and precision in the procedure, a few practice strokes are recommended to enable the

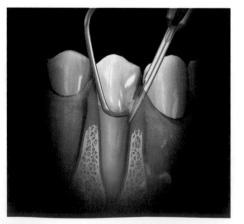

FIGURE 31-25
Two-handed instrumentation technique with dental endoscope.

BOX 31-1

TWO-HANDED ENDOSCOPIC INSTRUMENTATION TECHNIQUE

1. Identify a site to be treated.
2. Use endoscope explorer as *mirror* to reflect sulcular tissue and view root surface.
   a. Accomplished by holding endoscope explorer in dominant or non-dominant hand.
   b. If dominant hand is used initially, then transfer of hands will be necessary to instrument with dominant hand.
   c. If nondominant hand is used, then transfer is not necessary.
3. Select endoscope explorer that will provide the best access to the site without interfering with instrumentation (instrument selection may be different depending on the hand used, access, and adaptation).
4. Identify accretion to be removed on root surface.
5. Insert hand or powered instrument between root surface and endoscope explorer; follow the light of the endoscope for proper instrument placement.
6. View instrument placement on monitor adjacent to selected accretion before activating instrument.
7. Make a few practice strokes to ensure proper positioning and adaptation of instrument on tooth surface.
8. Activate hand or powered instrument and visualize removal of selected accretion on monitor.
9. Remove selected accretion from root surface to completion.
10. Progress to another area on the tooth surface until all areas are cleaned to completion.

---

clinician to determine the stroke direction and activation accuracy.

- Stroke activation can then occur and proceed until all visual signs of the accretion have been thoroughly removed.
- Activation of powered instruments is very specific and selective, with shorter phases of activation rather than the constant activation as is customary under nonvisual treatment.
- Once the area has been thoroughly debrided, the endoscope is repositioned to evaluate the other surface areas of the periodontal pocket.
- The endoscope is systematically moved around the circumference of the tooth to cover all anatomical surfaces of the root that have been affected by periodontal disease.

The endoscope is an aid in periodontal debridement that allows the clinician a highly specific treatment option that is based on visual feedback, as well as assurance that all bacterial accretions have been sufficiently removed from the root surface and that the body can now begin to recover from the effects of the biofilm accumulation.

Posttherapy Evaluation

Mrs. Ray's posttherapy evaluation revealed generalized healing of 2 to 3 mm, with reduction of inflammation and bleeding on probing. Most areas had healed to a stage at which oral self-care and routine supportive care might effectively maintain periodontal health, with the exception of teeth #10 and #14. Mrs. Ray had noticed less bleeding when brushing and seemed satisfied with the effort she was putting into her dental care.

Teeth #10 and #14 still exhibited probe depths of 7 to 8 mm, with bleeding on probing and interproximal inflammation. The areas were evaluated with the dental endoscope. Tooth #14 exhibited remaining deposits at the cementoenamel junction, in the buccal furcation, at the distobuccal line angle, and in the distal furcation. These areas were then thoroughly debrided again using manual and powered periodontal instruments under direct endoscopic visualization. Tooth #10 had deposit remaining in the mesial palatal line angle, which was also visualized and removed.

After 2 weeks, the site was evaluated for subsequent healing and desensitization of the treated areas. Healing was evident in all sites. Sensitive areas were treated with a desensitizer, and a desensitizing dentifrice was recommended for self-care.

Coding for Periodontal Debridement

In health care, the professional associations establish fees and codes for diagnoses and treatment and are linked with specific descriptions. The codes in dentistry are established by the American Dental Association and are accepted and used universally to achieve uniformity, consistency, and specificity in accurately reporting dental treatments. The codes are continually reviewed and periodically updated to reflect changes in procedures and nomenclature.

The existence of a code does not mean that the procedure is a covered or reimbursed benefit in a dental benefits plan; it is merely a way to describe the diagnosis and treatment that is often used for insurance submittals and reimbursement.

Fees within the office are established to reflect the level of disease and the treatment being offered to manage the level of disease. The fees should reflect the level of disease, the time involved in managing and treating the disease, and the degree of difficulty of the procedures involved. The dental hygienist provides different treatments for patients who have different periodontal conditions. Each treatment reflects the level of disease that is present at the time of examination and subsequent visits. Patients with advanced levels of periodontal disease will require a higher level of skill and intervention or prevention strategy than patients with minimal disease. Given the differences among patients and the disease each practice should establish a reasonable fee structure to reflect the disease level of the patient and the type of treatment provided for care.

Practicing dental hygienists should have a complete understanding of procedure codes to ensure that what is recorded in the patient's record, and subsequently filed with insurance

companies, accurately reflects the procedures performed. Application of these codes as a dental hygiene student will provide an understanding of the differences in levels of care required among patients with varying types and degrees of disease. Table 31-1 lists and describes each periodontal treatment code for the adult patient as described in the CDT 2005 users manual.[8]

Treatment Strategy

Outline a treatment strategy that would be appropriate for this patient's needs, and include appropriate procedure codes.

References

1. Adams D et al: The cardiac pacemaker and ultrasonic scalers, *Dent Health London* 22:6-8, 1983.
2. American Academy of Periodontology: Position paper: parameter on aggressive periodontitis, *J Periodontol* 71:867-869, 2000.
3. American Dental Association: *CDT 2007 2008 current dental terminology,* Chicago, 2007, ADA.
4. Anonymous: Recommended clinical guidelines for infection control in dental education institutions, *J Dent Educ* 55:621-627, 1991.
5. Badersten A, Nilveus R, Egelberg J: Effect of nonsurgical periodontal therapy: III—single versus repeated instrumentation, *J Clin Periodontol* 11:114-124, 1994.
6. Beikeler T et al: Microbial shifts in intra- and extraoral habitats following mechanical periodontal therapy, *J Clin Periodontol* 31(9):777-783, 2004.
7. Brayer WK et al: Scaling and root planing effectiveness: the effect of root surface access and operator experience, *J Periodontol* 60(1):67-72, 1989.
8. Cobb CM: Clinical significance of non-surgical periodontal therapy: an evidence-based perspective of scaling and root planing, *J Clin Periodontol* 29(2):6-16, 2002.
9. Cobb CM: Non-surgical pocket therapy: mechanical, *Ann Periodontol* 1:443-490, 1996.
10. Cohen RE et al: Position paper: periodontal maintenance, *J Periodontol* 74:1395-1401, 2003.
11. Costerton JW, Stewart PS: Battling biofilms, *Sci Am* 285(1): 74-81, 2001.
12. Donaldson D et al: A placebo-controlled multi-centered evaluation of an anesthetic gel (Oraqix) for periodontal therapy, *J Clin Periodontol* 30(3):171-175, 2003.
13. Dragoo MR: A clinical evaluation of hand and ultrasonic instruments on subgingival debridement, *Int J Periodontol Res Dent* 12:311-323, 1992.
14. Drisko CH: Nonsurgical periodontal therapy, *Periodontol 2000* 25:77-81, 2001.
15. Drisko CH: Trends in surgical and nonsurgical periodontal treatment, *J Am Dent Assoc* 131(6):31S-38S, 2000.
16. Drisko CL et al: Position paper: sonic and ultrasonic scalers in periodontics—research, science and therapy committee of the American Academy of Periodontology, *J Periodontol* 71(11): 1792-1801, 2000.
17. Ehmke B et al: Adjunctive antimicrobial therapy of periodontitis: long-term effects on disease progression and oral colonization, *J Periodontol* 76(5):749-759, 2005.

18. Fine DH et al: Reduction of viable bacteria in dental aerosols by preprocedural rinsing with an antiseptic mouthrinse, *Am J Dent* 6(5):219-221, 1993.

19. Fine DH et al: Efficacy of pre-procedural rinsing with an antiseptic in reducing viable bacteria in dental aerosols, *J Periodontol* 63(10):821-824, 1992.

20. Fleischer HC et al: Scaling and root planing efficacy in multirooted teeth, *J Periodontol* 60(7):402-409, 1989.

21. Flemmig TR et al: Working parameters of a magnetostrictive ultrasonic scaler influencing root substance removal, in vitro, *J Periodontol* 69:547-553, 1998.

22. Froum SJ, Gomez C, Breault MR: Current concepts of periodontal regeneration: a review of the literature, *NY State Dent J* 68(9):14-22, 2002.

23. Fux CA et al: Survival strategies of infectious biofilms, *Trends Microbiol* 13(1):34-40, 2005.

24. Greenstein G: Changing periodontal concepts: treatment considerations, *Compend Cont Educ Dent* 26(2):81-88, 2005.

25. Greenstein G: Nonsurgical periodontal therapy in 2000: a literature review, *J Am Dent Assoc* 131(11):1580-1592, 2000.

26. Greenstein G: Periodontal response to mechanical non-surgical therapy: a review, *J Periodontol* 63(2):118-130, 1992.

27. Guerrero A et al: Adjunctive benefits of systemic amoxicillin and metronidazole in non-surgical treatment of generalized aggressive periodontitis: a randomized placebo-controlled clinical trial, *J Clin Periodontol* 312(10):1094-1095, 2005.

28. Haffajee AD, Socransky SS: Microbial etiological agents of destructive periodontal diseases, *Periodontol 2000* 5:78-111, 1994.

29. Haffajee AD et al: Controlling the plaque biofilm, *Int Dent J* 53(Suppl)3:191-199, 2003.

30. Harrel SK, Barnes JB, Rivera-Hidalgo F: Aerosol and splatter contamination from the operative site during ultrasonic scaling, *J Am Dent Assoc* 129(9):1241-1249, 1998.

31. Hart TC, Korman KS: Genetic factors in the pathogenesis of periodontal disease, *Periodontal 2000* 14:202-215, 1997.

32. Keptic TJ, O'Leary TJ, Kafrawy AH: Total calculus removal: an attainable objective? *J Periodontol* 61(1):16-20, 1990.

33. Killoy WJ: The clinical significance of local chemotherapies, *J Clin Periodontol* 29(Suppl 2):22-29, 2002.

34. Kwan JY: Enhanced periodontal debridement with the use of micro ultrasonic, periodontal endoscopy, *J Calif Dent Assoc* 33(3):241-248, 2005.

35. Laurell L: Periodontal healing after scaling and root planing with the KaVo Sonicflex and Titan-S sonic scalers, *Swed Dent J* 14(4):171-177, 1990.

36. Loos B, Kiger R, Egelbert J: An evaluation of basic periodontal therapy using sonic and ultrasonic scalers, *J Clin Periodontol* 14(1):29-33, 1987.

37. Loos B et al: Clinical effects of root debridement in molar and non molar teeth: a 2 year follow up, *J Clin Periodontal* 16(8):498-504, 1989.

38. Matthews D: Conclusive support for mechanical nonsurgical pocket therapy in the treatment of periodontal disease, *Evid Based Dent* 6(3):68-69, 2005.

39. Mombelli A, Samaranayake LP: Topical and systemic antibiotics in the management of periodontal diseases, *Int Dent J* 54(1):3-14, 2004.

40. Muir KF et al: Reduction of microbial contamination from ultrasonic scalers, *Br Dent J* 145(3):76-78, 1978.

41. Paster BJ et al: Bacterial diversity in human subgingival plaque, *J Bacteriol* 183(12):3770-3783, 2001.

42. Pattison AM: A closer look at ultrasonic scalers, *Dimens Dent Hyg* 3:28-31, 2005.

43. Pattison, AM: Periodontal instrumentation transformed, *Dimens Dent Hyg* 2:18-22, 2003.

44. Petersilka GJ, Ehmke B, Flemmig TF: Antimicrobial effects of mechanical debridement, *Periodontol 2000* 28:56-71, 2002.

45. Proye M, Caton J, Polson A: Initial healing of periodontal pockets after a single episode of root planing monitored by controlling probing force, *J Periodontol* 53:206-301, 1982.

46. Rapley J: Wound healing. In Fedi PF, Vernino AR, Gray JL, eds: *The periodontic syllabus,* ed 4, Philadelphia, 2000, Lippincott Williams & Wilkins.

47. Rateitschak-Pluss EM et al: Non surgical periodontal treatment: Where are the limits? An SEM study, *J Clin Periodontol* 19(4):240-244, 1992.

48. Rivera-Hidalgo F, Barnes JB, Harrel SK: Aerosol and splatter production by focused spray and standard ultrasonic inserts, *J Periodontol* 70(5):473-477, 1999.

49. Salvi GE et al: Influence of risk factors on the pathogenesis of periodontitis, *Periodontol 2000* 14:173-201, 1997.

50. Sbordone L et al: Recolonization of the subgingival microflora after scaling and root planing in human periodontitis, *J Periodontol* 61(9):579-584, 1990.

51. Scott JB, Steed-Vellandis AM, Yukna RA: Improved efficacy of calculus removal in furcations using ultrasonic diamond-coated inserts, *Int J Periodontol Res Dent* 19:355-361, 1999.

52. Shaw S et al: Variability of sonic scaling tip movement, *J Clin Periodontol* 21(10):705-709, 1994.

53. Stambaugh RV: A clinician's 3-year experience with perioscopy, *Compend Cont Educ Dent* 23(11A):1061-1070, 2002.

54. Stambaugh RV et al: The limits of subgingival scaling, *Int J Periodontol Res Dent* 1(5):30-41, 1981.

55. Stutsman-Young NS, O'Heir TE, Woodall I: Periodontal debridement. In Woodall I, ed: *Comprehensive dental hygiene care,* ed 4, St Louis, 1993, Mosby.

56. Sugaya T, Kawanami M, Kato H: Effects of debridement with an ultrasonic furcation tip in degree II furcation involvement of mandibular molars, *J Int Acad Periodontol* 4(4):138-142, 2002.

57. Torfason T et al: Clinical improvement of gingival conditions following ultrasonic versus hand instrumentation of periodontal pockets, *J Clin Periodontol* 6(3):165-176, 1979.

58. Trenter SC, Walmsley AD: Ultrasonic dental scaler: associated hazards, *J Clin Periodontol* 30(2):95-101, 2003.

59. Walker C, Karpinia K: Rationale for use of antibiotics in periodontics, *J Periodontol* 74(4):566, author reply 566, 2003.

60. Walmsley AD et al: Effects of cavitational activity on the root surface of teeth during ultrasonic scaling, *J Clin Periodontol* 17:306-312, 1990.

61. Wang HL, Cooke J: Periodontal regeneration techniques for treatment of periodontal disease, *Dent Clin North Am* 49(3):637-659, vii, 2005.

62. Wang HL et al: Periodontal regeneration, *J Periodontol* 76(9):1601-1622, 2005.

63. Wennstrom JL et al: Full-mouth ultrasonic debridement versus quadrant scaling and root planing as an initial approach in the treatment of chronic periodontitis, *J Clin Periodontol* 32(8):851-859, 2005.

64. Wilson TG, Francis B: An endoscopic look at bleeding on probing and subgingival accretions, Paper in progress to submit to *J Periodontol.*

65. Yukna RA et al: Clinical evaluation of the speed and effectiveness of subgingival calculus removal on single-rooted teeth with diamond-coated ultrasonic tips, *J Periodontol* 68: 436-442, 1997.

Cosmetic and Therapeutic Polishing

Bonnie Francis • Caren M. Barnes

INSIGHT

This chapter assists the dental hygiene student in the understanding of dental stains, the professional treatment options available to remove those stains, and the attentiveness necessary to maintain tooth structure and esthetic restorations in the polishing process.

✦ CASE STUDY 32-1 Selecting the Appropriate Polishing Method

Bill Smith, a 28-year-old healthy white man, reports that he is concerned with health, works out daily, and has a diet filled with fruits and vegetables. On his visit to the clinic, Mr. Smith's chief complaint is to get his teeth cleaned. He knows that his smoking habit is ruining his health and the way his teeth look, and he has noticed some staining. Mr. Smith reported that he thought that getting his teeth cleaned would be a "good motivator to help me quit smoking."

The intraoral examination revealed stable periodontal status with generalized 2- to 3-mm pocketing and localized areas of slight recession. Gingival structures appear pink, firm, stippled, and healthy. Porcelain veneer restorations had been placed on the facial surfaces of teeth #6 through #11 to cover the tetracycline (TCN)-stained anterior teeth. No other apparent TCN stain is noted. Moderate tobacco stain is present, primarily on the lingual and palatal surfaces. Mr. Smith reports that he has smoked one pack of cigarettes a day for the past 10 years but is aware of its effect on his health and is "ready to quit."

KEY TERMS

abrasion	coronal polishing	grit	Porte polisher
abrasive	endogenous	hypoplasia	pounds per square inch
air-powder polisher	engine-driven polishing	intrinsic	pumice
calcium carbonate	esthetics	polishing	revolutions per minute
cleaning	exogenous	polishing agent	therapeutic polishing
cleaning agents	extrinsic		

LEARNING OUTCOMES

After reading this chapter the student will be able to:

1. Explain to a colleague, patient, or employer the relationship of polishing to the therapeutic and cosmetic goals for oral care.
2. Use cleaning agents rather than polishing agents when clinically appropriate. Select appropriate agents for cleaning and polishing esthetic restorative materials.
3. Classify the various dental stains as either *endogenous* or *exogenous* and be able to determine whether the stain can be removed and, if so, which polishing procedure can remove the stain.
4. Select Porte, engine, or air-powder polishing and the appropriate polishing agent, based on the requirements of the patient's oral condition, his or her response to care, and the equipment and time available.
5. Apply appropriate procedures for each of the polishing methods to remove stains without causing trauma to the oral structures and restorations or discomfort to the patient.
6. Summarize the research findings that suggest the limited therapeutic benefit for coronal polishing and the more relevant therapeutic value of root polishing.
7. Adopt and implement a successful policy of polishing for clinical practice.

A visit to the dental hygienist is often associated with the **polishing** procedure performed at the conclusion of the supportive care appointment.

Polishing traditionally has been associated with the prophylaxis procedure in most dental practices, which patients know and expect. Patients prefer this procedure over debridement with instruments for many reasons. An important factor is that patients respond positively to the smooth, clean feeling that polishing produces. Polishing is also less traumatic than scaling and less stressful and easier for a patient to understand and tolerate. Polishing often produces a benefit patients can see when they look in the mirror. Patients also know that polishing generally comes at the conclusion of the oral prophylaxis procedure. All of these factors play a role in the patient-operator interactions that take place daily in the dental office.

As with changing perspectives regarding scaling and root instrumentation, polishing principles have been reviewed and revised over time. Superficial polishing of the crown is now considered mainly cosmetic, with *minimal* therapeutic benefit. **Therapeutic polishing,** in contrast, refers to polishing of the root surfaces that are exposed during surgery to reduce endotoxin and the microflora on the cementum. Whether polishing for cosmetic or therapeutic benefit, an understanding of the polishing process and the resulting effects on the tooth surface and restorations is critical to dental hygiene professional development.

Polishing involves smoothing a surface to make it glossy or lustrous; **cleaning** is the act of removing of debris, impurities, or extraneous matter. **Cleaning agents,** unlike polishing agents, are nonabrasive, round, flat particles and do not scratch surface material. Although the term *polishing* has been used to describe the professional removal of soft deposits and stain from tooth surfaces, in reality this includes both cleaning and polishing. Removal of deposits has usually been achieved by friction created with the use of an **abrasive** agent and some form of mechanical device. Plaque biofilm, stain, and acquired pellicle (which is the acellular bonding apparatus for plaque biofilm and stain) are all removed during polishing. Although polishing does remove plaque biofilm and therefore may inhibit the occurrence of gingivitis,[71] the same benefit can be accomplished with thorough plaque biofilm–removal procedures at home. Therefore **coronal polishing** has questionable positive effects beyond creating a stain-free smile.[70] In fact, polishing is contraindicated in certain conditions (Box 32-1).

Historically, teeth were polished to remove all soft deposits and stains before the application of topical fluorides, because clinicians believed that it would allow for greater fluoride uptake in the enamel. However, studies have repeatedly demonstrated that polishing does not improve the uptake of professionally applied fluoride; therefore polishing is no longer a prerequisite to topical fluoride application.[61,66] At one time, polishing plaque biofilm off the patient's teeth and removing stains was considered the responsibility of the dental hygienist as opposed to a patient responsibility. As scientific knowledge has evolved, it has been demonstrated that professional polishing removes part of the fluoride-rich outer layer of enamel.[42,55]

BOX 32-1

CONTRAINDICATIONS FOR USE OF ORAL PROPHYLAXIS POLISHING PASTE[1,2]

Absence of extrinsic stain
Acute gingival or periodontal inflammation
Esthetic restorations
Allergy to paste ingredients
Dental caries
Decalcification
Enamel hypoplasia
Exposed dentin or cementum
Hypomineralization
Newly erupted teeth
Patients with respiratory problems
Recession
Tooth sensitivity
Xerostomia

Even though remineralization of tooth structure does occur under normal oral conditions[73] and exposure to fluoride,[16,40] continuous professional polishing over years of routine care may cause morphologic changes in the teeth. Essentially, routine polishing may abrade the tooth structure, especially at the cervix of cementum and dentin.[17] Therefore every dental hygienist must understand the delicate balance between cosmetic and therapeutic polishing.

Assessment of Need

As part of a clinical assessment, an identification of the types and amount of soft deposits present on patients' teeth should be made to aid in establishing an effective treatment plan. Obviously, a stain that cannot be removed by the patient is the primary factor that determines the need for cosmetic polishing. Once the type, amount, and distribution of stains have been assessed, the type of abrasive and mechanical device best suited for stain removal can be planned. With this information, a more appropriate treatment choice can be made to consider patients' expectations, effectiveness, and long-term effects of clinical decisions.

Theory

DENTAL STAINS

Classification of Dental Stains and Tooth Discoloration

Tooth discoloration and dental stains are often associated with the **exogenous, extrinsic** staining effects from food, drink, tobacco, and drugs. Although this type of staining is common, staining or discoloration actually may be attributed to three main sources: (1) direct adherence to tooth surfaces by bonding to the acquired pellicle, (2) containment within calculus and soft deposits, and (3) staining integral to the actual tooth structure.

Tooth staining and discoloration are categorized as either **endogenous** or *exogenous* in nature.[58,69] Endogenous stains originate within the tooth from developmental and systemic disturbances, whereas exogenous stains originate outside the tooth from exposure to environmental agents. Exogenous staining can be subcategorized even further as *extrinsic* and **intrinsic** stains, based on their ability to be removed mechanically by either the individual or the dental professional. Extrinsic stains are those stains that are on the exterior of the tooth and can be removed. Intrinsic stains are of exogenous origin but become incorporated into the tooth structure and cannot be removed by mechanical means.

Because many patients are more concerned with **esthetics** than with disease, the presence of these dental stains may be used to the patient's advantage as a motivating factor to improve oral hygiene.

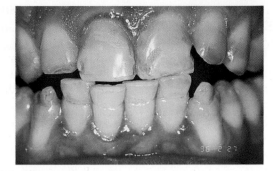

FIGURE 32-1
Endogenous developmental stain. Febrile illness. (Courtesy Dr. George Taybos, Jackson, Miss.)

★ CASE APPLICATION 32-1.1

Esthetic Concerns

A good example of motivation is the case of Mr. Smith, who wants to get his teeth cleaned because of esthetic concerns. Patients such as Mr. Smith may practice more thorough plaque removal and may be motivated to change some stain-promoting behaviors in an attempt to achieve a whiter and healthier appearance of the teeth.

DENTAL CONSIDERATIONS

As coronal surfaces are polished to remove the stain, soft debris, and acquired pellicle, the fluoride-rich outer layer of the enamel is also affected and potentially removed.

Because of this, clinicians should possess an understanding of the origins and manifestations of the various stains to help them determine whether stains can or cannot be removed by mechanical means.

Endogenous stains

Examples of stains that cannot be removed by mechanical means of scaling and polishing begin with endogenous developmental stains.

Endogenous stains are the result of the following:

- Heredity
- Developmental disturbances
- Genetic factors
- Drugs
- Trauma

Endogenous stains imbedded within the actual tooth structure often reflect the period of tooth development affected by the exposure. These stains manifest in newly erupted teeth and can be seen in both deciduous and permanent dentitions (Figure 32-1). Examples of endogenous developmental stains are found in Tables 32-1 to 32-4.

Endogenous stains that are developmental in origin include stains from medications that the mother or child takes during tooth development (see Table 32-2). Such medications may cause staining that occurs as a result of the deposition of substances circulating systemically at that time. TCN is one example of a medication that is known to cause developmental stains (Figure 32-2).

> ***Prevention***
>
> Exposure to TCN between the fifth month of fetal life and age 8 years often results in discoloration and sometimes **hypoplasia** of permanent and deciduous teeth.

TCN discoloration results because the drugs have an affinity for calcifying tissue, which is active during tooth formation. TCNs are incorporated chiefly into dentin but also may interfere with enamel formation. The tooth discolorations range from yellow through brown to gray and produce stains that are particularly visible on anterior teeth because of the thin enamel coating overlying the damaged TCN-stained dentin.[45]

Endogenous staining exhibiting enamel hypoplasia can be found when factors such as local infections or trauma and congenital illness have altered tooth form or color. Enamel hypoplasia results from a disturbance of or damage to ameloblasts during enamel matrix formation and exhibits defective enamel of normal hardness (Figure 32-3). Examples are summarized in Table 32-3. Excessive repeated intake of fluoride during tooth development is a classic example of enamel hypoplasia that is often referred to as *dental fluorosis* (Figure 32-4). This type of hypoplasia may cause tooth discoloration ranging from localized white flecks to irregular patterns of brown pitting of the enamel, often referred to as *mottled enamel*. The more fluoride that is ingested at the time of enamel formation, the more severe the staining and mottling.

Another endogenous stain category includes stains that are environmentally induced. Environmentally induced stains are the result of pathologic incursions into the tooth, such as the following:

- Dental caries
- Pulpal necrosis
- Metallic stains from dental restorations
- Prolonged exposure to metals in the air or water (see Table 32-4)

Stains associated with primary (i.e., initial lesions on unrestored tooth surfaces) and secondary (i.e., recurrent) caries

Table 32-1   Endogenous Stains: Developmental

TYPE	APPEARANCE	ETIOLOGY
Amelogenesis Imperfecta	Hypoplastic: Insufficient enamel ranging from pits and grooves to complete absence of enamel Hypocalcification: Normal quantity of enamel but soft and friable; color variable, from white opaque to yellow to brown and darkening with age	Genetic disorder of enamel formation affecting both dentitions
Dentinogenesis Imperfecta	Overall bluish translucence or opalescence; teeth variable in color from yellow-brown to gray; entire crown appearing stained because of underlying dentin malformation	Genetic disturbance in odontoblastic layer during dentin formation; may occur with osteogenesis imperfecta or as isolated trait
Dentin Dysplasia	Type I: Both dentitions normal color but have short roots or periapical inflammatory lesions Type II: Opalescent primary dentition, normal permanent dentition	Genetic autosomal-dominant trait affecting dentin
Congenital Porphyria	Teeth appearing red to brown and fluorescing red with ultraviolet light; enamel, dentin, and cementum all affected	Genetic disorder of hemoglobin formation
Rh Incompatibility	Primary teeth appearing green to brown	Maternal antibody destruction of fetal red blood cells
Liver Disease Biliary Atresia Neonatal Hepatitis	Primary dentition affected; green discoloration; yellowish-brown color	Secondary to the deposition of bilirubin in developing enamel and dentin

Table 32-2   Endogenous Stains: Drug Induced

ETIOLOGY	APPEARANCE	TOOTH STRUCTURE INVOLVED
Exposure to Tetracycline (TCN) between the Fifth Month of Fetal Life and Age 8	Discolorations ranging from yellow through brown to gray; stains particularly visible on anterior teeth because of thin enamel coating overlying damaged TCN-stained dentin	TCN's affinity for calcifying tissue incorporated chiefly into dentin but also may interfere with enamel formation; may affect permanent and deciduous teeth
Fluoride Ingestion (Dental Fluorosis)	Mottled discoloration of enamel ranging from white flecks and chalky opaque areas of enamel to brown or black staining and pitted or overall corroded enamel appearance; more fluoride ingested at time of enamel formation; more severe staining and mottling	Can affect any permanent or primary teeth exposed to fluoride during development; affected teeth generally resistant to decay

Table 32-3   Endogenous Stains: Enamel Hypoplasia

ETIOLOGY	APPEARANCE	TOOTH STRUCTURE INVOLVED
Dental Fluorosis: Excessive Repeated Intake of Fluoride during Tooth Development	See Table 32-2	See Table 32-2
Febrile Illness (Measles, Chicken Pox, Scarlet Fever) Vitamin Deficiency (A, C, or D)	Pitting of enamel of teeth developing at time of illness or deficiency	Teeth that form during first year of life (permanent central incisors, laterals, cuspids, and first molars)
Local Infections or Trauma of Primary Teeth	Color of enamel possibly ranging from yellow to brown or severe pitting and deformity; severity dependent on degree of infection or stage of underlying tooth development	Usually single tooth; permanent maxillary incisors and permanent mandibular premolars
Trauma during Tooth Maturation, Endocrine, Metabolic, or Unknown Causes	Enamel hypocalcification; localized chalky white flecks or spots in enamel, focally or linearly; normal amounts of enamel produced but hypomineralized; underlying enamel possibly soft and susceptible to dental caries	Possibly single tooth or all teeth being formed at time of disturbance

Table 32-4	**Endogenous Stains: Environmental**	
TYPE	**APPEARANCE**	**ETIOLOGY**
Incipient Caries	White, chalky	Acid-producing bacteria
Active Caries	Brown to black	Acid-producing bacteria
Secondary Caries	White, gray to brownish-black around existing restorations	Marginal leakage of restorations and acid-producing bacteria
Pulpless Teeth	Light yellow-brown, bluish-black, or black; possibly also tinted orange, pink, and green	Decomposed pulp tissue and hemoglobin penetrating dentin tubules
Pulpal Necrosis	Yellowish-black	Trauma
Iatrogenic Teeth	Variable from gray-brown to pinkish hues	Usually result of restorative materials, exposure of dentin to bleeding, and other problems of unknown cause

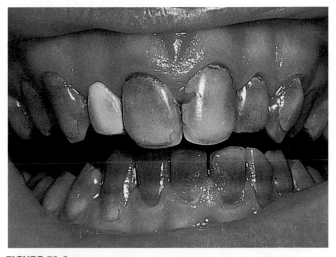

FIGURE 32-2
Endogenous developmental stain. Tetracycline (TCN). (Courtesy Dr. George Taybos, Jackson, Miss.)

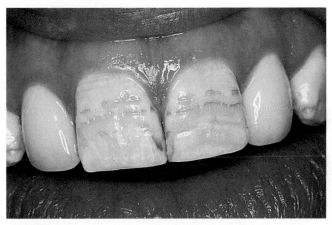

FIGURE 32-4
Endogenous developmental stain. Dental fluorosis. (Courtesy Dr. George Taybos, Jackson, Miss.)

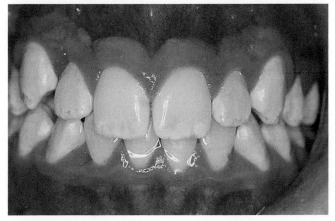

FIGURE 32-3
Endogenous developmental stain. Enamel hypoplasia. (Courtesy Dr. George Taybos, Jackson, Miss.)

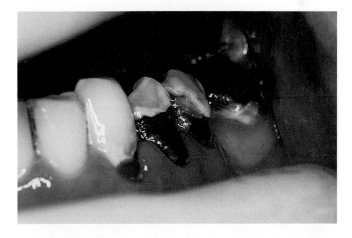

FIGURE 32-5
Endogenous stain. Cervical caries. (Courtesy Dr. George Taybos, Jackson, Miss.)

transform over time with exposure to the harsh oral environment. Initial (incipient) carious lesions appear slightly whiter, chalky, and dull in comparison with unaffected enamel. With increased dental caries development, the decalcified areas become stained with food and bacterial debris, and the degree of discoloration is proportionate to the duration of active decay (Figure 32-5). The second type of discoloration includes those stains adjacent to both intact and defective restorations. These stains may indicate the presence of secondary or recurrent caries and should be closely monitored (Figure 32-6). Stains resulting

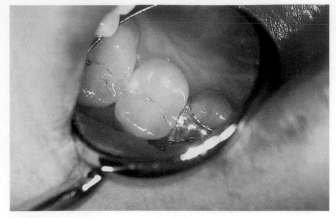

FIGURE 32-6
Endogenous stain. Secondary caries. (Courtesy Dr. George Taybos, Jackson, Miss.)

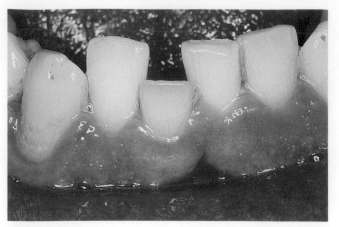

FIGURE 32-8
Endogenous stain. Pulpal necrosis. (Courtesy Dr. George Taybos, Jackson, Miss.)

from the pigments of restorative material containing metal seeping into the dentinal tubules often reveal a gray shadow adjacent to the restoration (Figure 32-7). Similar staining can occur as a result of leakage between the restoration and the tooth, which allows saliva and bacteria to penetrate and begin the process of recurrent caries. Recurring caries will appear as a gray or brown area adjacent to the margin of a defective restoration. Endodontically involved teeth often appear darker clinically (Figures 32-8 and 32-9), whereas internal resorption often manifests as the classic "pink tooth" (Figures 32-10 and 32-11). Careful inspection of the area with supportive radiographic diagnostic information is essential to determine the appropriate source of the staining.

All the endogenous stains previously discussed cannot be removed by simple polishing procedures. These stains are imbedded in the enamel and dentin matrix and require more complex restorative and cosmetic procedures to treat the affected areas. Methods for the cosmetic improvement of teeth affected by endogenous or intrinsic stains include enamel microabrasion, vital and nonvital tooth bleaching, composite restorative materials bonded as overlays, laminate veneers, and

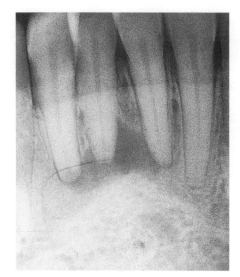

FIGURE 32-9
Endogenous stain. Radiograph of pulpal necrosis of Figure 32-8. (Courtesy Dr. George Taybos, Jackson, Miss.)

combination treatments. Chapters 35 and 36 provide specific information on these procedures.

Exogenous stains

Stains that can be removed are most commonly categorized as *environmental exogenous* and *extrinsic* stains. These stains are associated with exposure to the following:

- Certain foods
- Tobacco
- Tea
- Coffee
- Airborne particles

Exogenous stains can be identified by color, distribution, and tenacity.[54] Individuals vary widely in the rate and amount of accumulated extrinsic stains. Certain factors are known to predispose a person to the accumulation of both dental deposits and stains; these include the following:

- Enamel roughness
- Organic salts in saliva

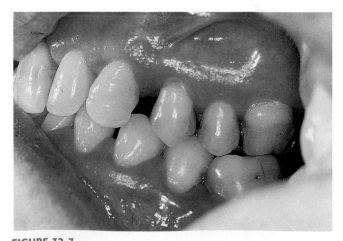

FIGURE 32-7
Endogenous stain. Amalgam restoration. (Courtesy Dr. George Taybos, Jackson, Miss.)

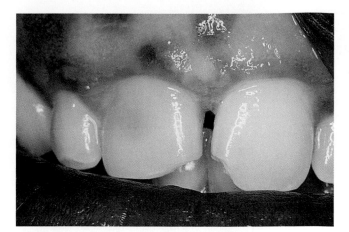

FIGURE 32-10
Endogenous stain. Internal resorption (i.e., pink tooth). (Courtesy Dr. George Taybos, Jackson, Miss.)

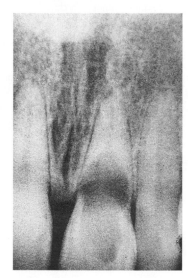

FIGURE 32-11
Endogenous stain. Radiograph of Figure 32-10. (Courtesy Dr. George Taybos, Jackson, Miss.)

- Increased or decreased salivary flow
- Poor oral hygiene

Scaling and polishing procedures can remove most extrinsic stains (discussed later in this chapter). Some of the more common extrinsic stains are summarized in Tables 32-5 and 32-6. In the tables, stains are categorized by *exposure elements* and by *color of appearance*.

The most common extrinsic stains by an exposure element are tobacco and food stains. Tobacco stains range in appearance from tan to dark brown or black and cover approximately the cervical one third to one half of most affected teeth (Figure 32-12). This type of staining occurs mostly on lingual and palatal surfaces and is commonly found in pits and fissures and other enamel irregularities. Tobacco staining has been found to be directly proportional to the number of cigarettes smoked per day.[49] Staining also may be found in individuals who smoke pipes or cigars and those who use smokeless tobacco (snuff or chewing; Figure 32-13).

DENTAL CONSIDERATIONS

Tobacco stains may, over time, penetrate the enamel and become intrinsic.

Food staining is common in individuals who frequently drink coffee and tea. Other categories of food that may contribute to stain include the following:

- Cola drinks
- Red wine
- Berries such as raspberries and blueberries
- Spices
- Leaves and nuts of the betel plant
- Licorice
- Candy containing coloring agents

Stains resulting from ingestion of these foods range from tan to dark brown in color and occur over broad, smooth tooth surfaces and in pits and fissures (Figure 32-14).

Table 32-5	Extrinsic Stains: Categorized by Exposure		
CATEGORY	**PRIMARY SITES**	**COMPOSITION AND APPEARANCE**	**ETIOLOGY**
Tobacco	Cervical one third to one half of lingual surfaces; pits and fissures	• Tars, pigments • Light brown to dark-leathery, brownish-black	Smoking
Food	Cervical one third to one half of lingual surfaces; pits and fissures	• Food pigments • Brownish-pellicle–type stain	Consumption of tea, coffee, cola, red wine, berries, spices, betel leaves, nuts, and candy
Metallic Materials	Cervical one third; primarily anterior teeth affected but possibly occurring on random surfaces	Associated with specific metals: • Copper or brass exhibiting bluish-green • Iron and nickel showing greenish-brown	Environmental, food, water
Drug, Therapeutic Intervention	Cervical one third; pits and fissures	• Plaque bacteria, tin, reactions with food colors • Usually brown in color	Extended antibiotic use, stannous fluoride, chlorhexidine

Table 32-6		Extrinsic Stains: Categorized by Color	
CATEGORY	**PRIMARY SITES**	**COMPOSITION AND APPEARANCE**	**ETIOLOGY/PREVALENCE**
Black Line	Thin band along gingival margin on buccal or lingual surfaces; most common on posterior palatal	• Ferric sulfide fine line following contour of gingival crest with no apparent thickness	• Iron in saliva or gingival fluid, plaque biofilm, or bacteria • Affecting all ages • Most common in women
Green	Cervical one third to one half of facial surfaces of maxillary anteriors	• Inorganic elements, chromogenic bacteria • Light to dark green • Embedded in bacterial plaque	• Poor oral hygiene, surface irregularities • Most common in children
Gray Green	Cervical one third of labial surfaces	• Oils, resin, and pigments • Embedded in pellicle and bacterial plaque	• Poor oral hygiene, marijuana smoking
Orange	Thin line; cervical one third of incisors	• Chromogenic bacteria • Usually orange or red stain on facial and lingual surfaces of anterior teeth	• Poor oral hygiene • Most common in children

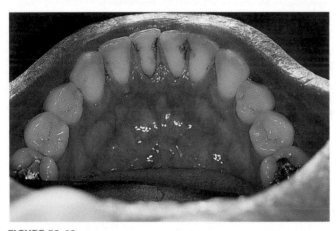

FIGURE 32-12
Extrinsic stain. Tobacco smoking. (Courtesy Dr. George Taybos, Jackson, Miss.)

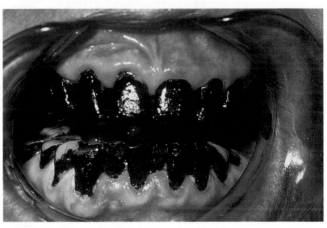

FIGURE 32-14
Extrinsic stain. Betel nut stain. (Courtesy Dr. George Taybos, Jackson, Miss.)

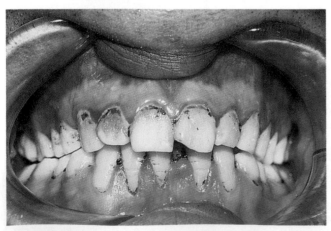

FIGURE 32-13
Extrinsic stain. Tobacco snuff. (Courtesy Dr. George Taybos, Jackson, Miss.)

Stains associated with metal exposure or drugs and therapeutic agents also have been identified. Metallic stains vary in color depending on the metal or the metallic salt that is ingested or inhaled. Green or blue-green colors result from copper or brass, whereas brown colors may result from an ingestion of materials or dust particles containing iron (Figure 32-15). The majority of these stains have been attributed to industrial dust, but they may also be found in various foods and water.

Many drugs or therapeutic agents may cause tooth stains, only a few of which are described here. Surface discolorations and staining have occurred after extended topical or systemic antibiotic use or in studies of antibacterial agents with anti–plaque biofilm activity.[45,59] These stains have been attributed to the direct effects of the agent on bacterial plaque biofilm. The most common and well-known antibacterial agent attributed to staining is chlorhexidine. A dark-brown stain beginning at the gingival margin can be noted shortly after beginning the daily use of a chlorhexidine regimen (Figure 32-16). A brown- to

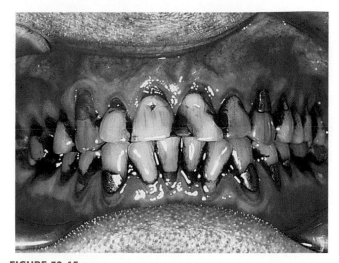

FIGURE 32-15
Extrinsic metallic stain. **Topical iron.** (Courtesy Dr. George Taybos, Jackson, Miss.)

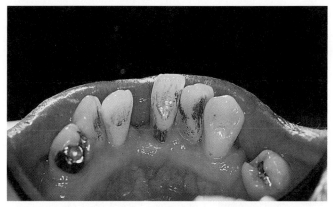

FIGURE 32-16
Extrinsic stain. **Chlorhexidine.** (Courtesy Dr. George Taybos, Jackson, Miss.)

black-pigmented stain in plaque biofilm–associated areas also has been reported in several clinical studies and is attributed to dentifrices containing stannous fluoride.[76] A summary of extrinsic exposure stains is shown in Table 32-5.

Stains categorized by color include black-line stain, green stain, gray-green stain, and orange stain, summarized in Table 32-6. Black-line stain usually occurs as a continuous thin band along the gingival margin and follows the crestal contour on lingual palatal or proximal surfaces (or on both) (Figure 32-17). It occurs at all ages and is found more often in women. The primary cause of this deposit is iron compounds in saliva or gingival circular fluid that become embedded in the dental pellicle, the plaque biofilm, the bacteria in plaque biofilm, or a combination of these locations. This stain is a ferric sulfide compound and is most often found in a relatively clean mouth.[54]

Green stain occurs primarily on cervical areas of the maxillary anterior teeth and is associated with the primary dental cuticle. The stain is usually crescent shaped, close to the gingival margin, and colored light green to yellow-green to dark green. Green stains are usually a result of poor oral hygiene and are associated with chromogenic bacteria and gingival hemorrhage. The enamel beneath a green stain may become demineralized or carious as a

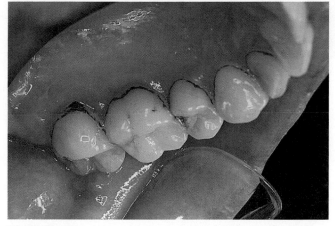

FIGURE 32-17
Extrinsic stain. **Black line.** (Courtesy Dr. George Taybos, Jackson, Miss.)

result of cariogenic plaque biofilm accumulations. The roughened surface then encourages reaccumulation of plaque biofilm and recurrence of green stain. This stain is often difficult to remove with polishing agents. If the patient is not allergic to iodine, then including a small amount of it in the **polishing agent** can aid in the removal of the green stain. Gray-green stain occurs around the gingival one third of teeth as a result of marijuana use. The stain is caused from oils, resin, and pigments found in marijuana. Orange stain is fairly rare. It occurs at the cervical third of incisor teeth and may be attributed to chromogenic bacteria.

STAIN EVALUATION

Clinically, stains are evaluated by severity and location. Light, moderate, or heavy stains may be generalized or localized in specific areas. Because these categories are simply observations and have no specific scientific guidelines, variations of conclusions between practitioners often result. Attempts have been made to develop scoring procedures to evaluate the extent of intrinsic and extrinsic staining for research purposes. One of the first attempts to evaluate stain clinically was the categorization of both the *intensity* and the *severity* of the stain, as well as the *specific tooth area* covered.[38] Other approaches attempted to quantify tooth stain by the use of plastic chips of various standardized colors[77] or grading stain on a *stain–to–no stain basis*.[58] These measurements are commonly used in research to compare stain development or removal among treatment groups in clinical trials.

PROFESSIONAL TREATMENT OF EXTRINSIC STAINS

32-2 to 32-8

As part of the dental prophylaxis regimen, areas of stained enamel and dentin are professionally polished with an abrasive agent after the appropriate debridement or scaling procedures.

DENTAL CONSIDERATIONS

Polishing coronal surfaces includes the removal of stain and soft debris, acquired pellicle, and a small portion of fluoride-rich outer layer of enamel. This is an especially important factor to recall when polishing teeth in children because of the incomplete enamel mineralization of newly erupted teeth.

During treatment planning, the dental hygienist must keep the following factors in mind:

- Selection of the least-abrasive polishing agent possible that will thoroughly remove plaque biofilm and stain

> **Note**
>
> The clinician must have a thorough understanding of the basic principles and correct techniques that relate to selection of the abrasive agent, mechanical devices, and the specific procedures involved.

- Use of proper techniques to reduce unnecessary iatrogenic **abrasion** on exposed enamel and dentinal surfaces during the procedure

Varying factors of time, speed, and pressure (load) use also contribute to the clinical outcome.

Abrasive Agents

Abrasive agents are incorporated into prophylaxis pastes for the purpose of cleaning and polishing. A dental abrasive changes the surface of the tooth by frictional grinding, rubbing, scraping, and abrading any surface irregularities. As this process proceeds from coarse abrasion (cleaning) to fine abrasion (polishing) the surface to be polished is approached with a series of finer and finer abrasives, until the scratches are smaller than the wavelength of visible light, which is 0.5 mcm.[23] When scratches are created that are this size, the surface appears smooth and shiny—the smaller the scratches, the more shiny the surface (which places a large emphasis on the size [grit] of the polishing agent particle selected). During polishing the surface of the tooth passes through various stages—from irregular to grooved to finely abraded—with a concomitant increase in smoothness and light reflectance. The last stage is regarded as the *polished surface*.

Many prophylaxis pastes are available, each brand varying considerably in abrasiveness. The abrasives contained in these commercially available products are similar to those in dentifrice products.[14,50] The major difference is that the abrasive levels in professional products are much higher. Factors determining the abrasiveness and polishing potential of an agent include particle hardness, shape, size, and concentration. Abrasives vary markedly in inherent hardness and shape. Within the same polishing product, abrasive particle sizes are graded from fine to coarse. Harder, rough-shaped, large, particle-size compounds produce more abrasive action than particles that are soft, smooth shaped, and small. Polishing products are also available that claim to change from a coarse polishing agent to a fine paste during use. The basic concept behind polishing is that as each of these factors (i.e., particle size, shape, hardness) decrease, surface abrasion is lessened and the surface becomes smooth or polished.

To select the appropriate polishing agent for the surface or restorative material to be polished, dental hygienists must recognize that the most abrasive agents should not be used on materials that are softer than the abrasive particle. It cannot be overemphasized that the selection of the prophylaxis paste should be intentional and part of the treatment planning. One polishing agent is not meant for all tooth surfaces or all types of restorative materials![6,33] Table 32-7 has a list of the Knoop hardness numbers for tooth structures, restorative materials, and abrasive agents. Many of the abrasives used in prophylaxis polishing paste are 10 times (or more) harder than the material they are used to polish!

Polishing Agents

The two main abrasive polishing agents used in dental prophylaxis products or available as chemical compounds are (1) **pumice** and (2) **calcium carbonate.** Calcium carbonate may be purchased as chalk or whiting, is manufactured in several particle shapes and sizes, and is less abrasive than pumice. Calcium carbonate produces minimal scratches and results in a smooth polished surface that reflects light. Pumice is also manufactured in a wide variety of particle sizes, and its use ranges from an abrasive stain-removal agent to fine polishing of acrylic dentures. Other polishing agents that are found in oral prophylaxis polishing pastes include silica, tin oxide, silex, and zirconium silicate. Diamond and aluminum oxide polishing paste, rubber polishing cups, disks, or points are also available for polishing and maintaining esthetic restorations.[41,43]

Most professional dental abrasive or polishing products have been categorized as *fine, medium,* or *coarse,* although no standardized definitions exist for these terms. One manufacturer's

Table 32-7	**Knoop Hardness Values of Esthetic Restorative Materials, Abrasive Agents, and Tooth Structures**
	KNOOP HARDNESS NUMBER

Tooth Structures	
ENAMEL	355-461
DENTIN	68
CEMENTUM	40

Resin Composites	
ANTERIOR	46-48
POSTERIOR	45-64
MICROFILLED	18.7-57.6
HYBRID	51.1-64.8
GLASS IONOMER	18-31
METAL REINFORCED	14-24
PORCELAIN	14

Abrasive Agents Used in Prophylaxis Pastes and Toothpastes	
CALCIUM CARBONATE	135
PUMICE	590
ALUMINUM OXIDE	2100
SILICON CARBIDE	2780

fine prophylaxis paste may be more abrasive than another manufacturer's medium paste. As a result, clinicians should use the least-abrasive paste in the product line first. If more abrasive is needed to remove a particular stain, then the clinician should start the process with a medium or coarse paste, followed by the finer abrasive to finish the polishing. Additional factors must also be considered in the polishing procedure. These include the mechanical device used for polishing, indications and contraindications for use, and specific technique functions.

MECHANICAL DEVICES FOR POLISHING

Porte Polishers

The **Porte polisher** is a simple, hand-held device featuring a tapered orangewood point. This manual instrument may be adapted to the various aspects of the teeth and rubs the abrasive agent against the tooth surface with a wedge-shaped, tapered, or pointed wooden point (Figure 32-18).

This technique requires considerable hand strength and control, but the advantages of portability, ability to access obscured malpositioned tooth surfaces, generation of minimal frictional heat, lack of engine noise, and minimal bacterial aerosol offer a valuable adjunctive instrument that should be the method of choice for selected patients. A more common device for polishing is the engine-driven polisher.

Engine-Driven Polishers

Engine-driven polishing is widely used in clinical practice because of its efficiency and efficacy. The power for engine-driven polishing may be derived from an electric motor or compressed air, which is the power source for most of today's dental units. A slow-speed hand piece is attached to the appropriate dental tubing unit. The hand piece selected for use should be specifically designed for the system being used; it may screw, snap, lock, or clip onto the power source. Attached to the hand piece is the prophylaxis angle (or prophy angle).

Prophy angles are designed with either straight or contraangled shanks. They can be either reusable after sterilization or disposable (Figure 32-19). It has been shown that the disposable prophy angle works as effectively as the autoclavable angle, with the added benefit of eliminating any potential for cross-contamination between patients.[15] A rubber cup or brush is then attached to the prophy angle. A sterilized hand piece and prophy angle (or disposable prophy angle) should be used for each patient. Disposable prophy angles are not sterilizable.

Prophy cups are designed with varying degrees of flexibility. The interior walls may have a ribbed-open, ribbed-webbed, or ribbed-turbine configuration. These ribs and webs permit retention of the prophy paste. Those cups without webs allow for greater flexibility of the rim. Brushes are designed with different shapes and degrees of flexibility. Most commonly, the cup or brush comes prepackaged and attached to the disposable prophy angle. If a sterilizable prophy angle is used, then the cup or brush attaches by means of a mandrel that latches, screw, or snaps into place. Equipment and procedure preparation are summarized in Table 32-8.

Whatever mechanism or power source is used in any given clinical setting, the dental hygienist should become familiar with the operation and maintenance of the system and the knowledge to troubleshoot if the polishing instrument fails to properly function. The hand piece and the prophylaxis angle require proper care and maintenance, especially because they should be autoclaved after each use. The clinician should refer to specific manufacturer recommendations for such maintenance procedures, because some warranties on equipment become void if the manufacturer's instructions have not been followed.

Indications for use

The engine-driven polisher is indicated for most clinical applications in which the operator has access to a slow-speed hand piece. Patient compliance and acceptance are high; engine-driven polishers are regarded as the instrument of choice for many patients and operators.

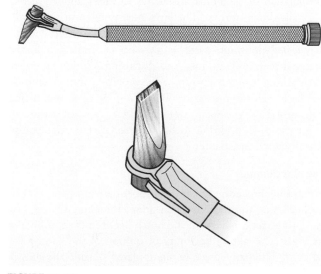

FIGURE 32-18
Wooden point on Porte polisher.

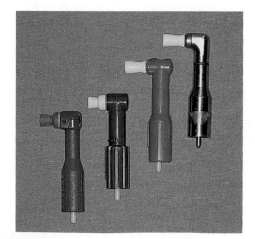

FIGURE 32-19
Prophy angles. Sterilizable *(right)* and disposable *(first through third from left)*.

Table 32-8	Engine-Driven Polishing: Equipment and Procedure Preparation	
EQUIPMENT PIECE	**USE**	**FEATURES**
Hand Piece	• Low (or slow) speed: 6000 to 10,000 rpm • Must supply adequate torque	• Requires routine maintenance
Prophylaxis Angle	• Contra-angle or right-angle attachment	• Disposable or reusable and sterilizable
Attachments *RUBBER CUP* **RIBBED AND WEBBED** **HARD OR SOFT** **LATEX FREE**	• Ribbing: Facilitates holding of polishing agent • Soft rubber cup: More flexibility	• Rubber cup on all exposed tooth surfaces
OCCLUSAL BRUSH **HARD OR SOFT**	• Soft brush: Usually adequate for occlusal stain removal	• Brush only on occlusal surfaces
Abrasive Agent	• Least-abrasive agent used to sufficiently remove stain	• Fine grit or toothpaste agent should be used (If medium or coarse grit is needed for heavy stain removal, then fine grit should follow its use.)
Protective Equipment	• Safety glasses for patient • Personal protective wear for operator	• Protection from aerosol splatter to eyes • Protection from aerosols generated from procedure
Aerosol Control	• Saliva ejector, high-speed suction, or both • Air/water syringe	• Excessive saliva produced during procedure • Periodic rinsing of area completed

rpm, Revolutions per minute.

Distinct Care Modifications
Because of the hand piece's association with "the drill," a thorough explanation of the procedure is warranted for apprehensive patients, first-time patients, and especially young children. A simple "show-and-tell" technique is generally sufficient to introduce the patient to the rotating action of the soft rubber cup and the sound produced by the hand piece.

Distinct Care Modifications
Contraindications for the rubber-cup polishing procedure include allergies to latex or fluoride.

The guidelines for engine-driven polishing include patient selection and preparation, unit and operator preparation, and actual clinical technique.

Patient selection and preparation

Patient medical history and treatment plan should always be reviewed for any possible contraindications to the procedure.

In such instances, the following are available: rubber-cup latex-free products, prophy pastes, and pumice slurry without fluoride. Safety glasses for the patient are recommended to ensure that pumice, aerosols, or both do not contaminate the patient's eyes.

Offering the patient a tissue or wipe is appreciated, as is the option to manage the saliva ejector during the procedure. A thorough explanation of the procedure allows young children and those new to the engine-polishing method an idea of what to expect from the procedure. Children and some adults may be intimidated by the sound of the hand piece, and a simple explanation or demonstration usually eases the apprehensions associated with the sound of the drill.

Unit and operator preparation

Unit preparation includes obtaining the necessary equipment: hand piece and prophy angle with specific attachment (brush or cup) desired. The engine-polishing procedure requires adequate evacuation, because the polishing agent and the mechanical manipulation in the mouth stimulates salivary glands to secrete more saliva than normal. The air/water syringe must be available to rinse the area as each arch segment is completed. Finally, the selected polishing paste or abrasive (as indicated in the treatment plan), dental floss, and disclosing solution complete the polishing armamentarium. Operator preparation emphasizes basic aerosol protection barriers such as a well-fitting mask, protective eye wear, a face shield, or a combination of these barriers, in addition to basic personal protective equipment discussed in Chapter 7.

Clinical technique

All polishing procedures mandate proper patient-operator positioning. Using the modified pen grasp, the clinician rests the hand piece over the hand in the notch between the thumb and forefinger. This allows flexibility of motion of the hand piece and cord. The hand piece is manipulated outside the mouth first, by the application of light, steady pressure on the rheostat to evaluate speed and proper function of the device. The clinician fills the rubber cup with polishing paste by slowly running the hand piece in the polishing agent or by dipping the rubber cup or brush into the abrasive-filled Dappen dish or small-prepackaged container. The stable fulcrum is established and the rheostat slowly activated so that the applicator rotates at a slow, steady speed just before the cup or brush is placed against the tooth surface. The hand piece and angle must supply adequate torque to maintain the abrasive against the tooth for polishing. The rubber cup is refilled with abrasive paste as necessary. The abrasive-filled container or Dappen dish may be held in the nondominant hand for ready access. In addition, the abrasive may be applied directly to the teeth just ahead of the path of the rubber cup or brush.

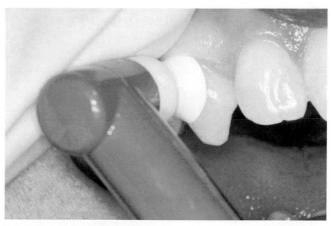

FIGURE 32-20
Rubber cup. Subgingival application.

> ### Prevention
> A bare or saliva-laden cup void of polishing agent does not polish the teeth and generates heat.[60]

Regardless of how the abrasive is placed on the tooth, adequate amounts must be used. Usually a full rubber cup of abrasive is sufficient for two to three teeth.

The rubber cup is refilled as necessary, a stable fulcrum reestablished, the hand piece activated slowly, and the rubber cup placed on the tooth surface before polishing procedures continue.

> ### Note
> The lip of the cup can be flared and slipped slightly subgingival so that the most coronal aspects of the sulcus may be cleaned for therapeutic effects on the root surface (Figure 32-20).

A systematic approach increases efficiency and ensures all surfaces are adequately polished. Most surfaces can be polished in 2 to 5 seconds with the use of a light, steady speed in a patting motion, adapting the rubber cup smoothly to cover all exposed tooth surfaces.

The clinician should apply the rubber cup to proximal surfaces by sliding the lip of the cup as far proximally as possible and slightly under the contact point area (Figure 32-21). Vertical, oblique, or horizontal stroke direction is used as the rim of the cup is moved across the tooth surface. Adapting the lip of the cup into the occlusal grooves often suffices for stain removal from these difficult areas.

When the rubber cup does not remove occlusal stain adequately, the brush attachment should be considered. Brush attachments should be used *only* on occlusal surfaces and should not be used on any other tooth surfaces because they are highly abrasive, especially to soft tissues,[64] and difficult to control. Brushes are available with soft or firm bristles. The softer bristles are usually adequate for stain removal, and they hold an abrasive agent more readily. Clinical procedures are summarized in Tables 32-9 and 32-10.

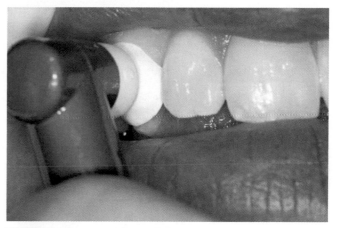

FIGURE 32-21
Rubber cup. Interproximal application.

the tooth builds up frictional heat that may cause discomfort, pain, and possible pulpal damage.

This is especially critical for anterior teeth, which provide minimal insulation for the pulp because of the lesser amount of dentin and enamel compared with that on posterior teeth. Clinicians may also observe the patient's facial expression carefully to detect signs of discomfort from heat. Patients apparently in pain should be asked whether they sense heat. If so, then the polishing procedure should be adjusted to reduce heat by the reduction of the duration of each application, by the pressure of the cup or brush on the tooth, or by both.

The speed of the cup is critical both in minimizing frictional heat and in ensuring effective polishing. Operating the cup at high speeds is both harmful and ineffective.[60] Because determining the exact **revolutions per minute** (rpm) rarely is possible during operation, using the lowest possible speed that moves the

> ### Prevention
> Using intermittent pressure on the tooth allows the heat generated to dissipate between each stroke.

Whether a cup or brush is being used, the attachment and abrasive should be used with moderate intermittent pressure.[65] Constant pressure of the rubber cup or brush on

cup or brush against the tooth without stalling is recommended. Sound also may provide a clue for determining whether the cup is rotating too rapidly.

> ### Note
> A high whine or whistle in the hand piece usually indicates excessive speed.

Table 32-9	Engine-Driven Polishing: Procedures	
POLISHING CONSIDERATIONS	**CONCERNS**	**RECOMMENDED ACTIONS**
Health History	• Latex allergy • Fluoride allergy • Children	• Use latex-free rubber cup. • Use nonfluoridated paste. • Do not use pumice slurry on primary teeth.
Treatment Plan	• Contraindication immediately after root-planing procedure	
Grasp	• Use of modified pen grasp	• Rest hand piece and cord over outreached hand to ease manipulation.
Hand Piece Control	• Establishment of stable fulcrum • Use of lowest possible speed to reduce frictional heat	• Use either external or internal fulcrum (wide fulcrum provides increased stability). • Never use fulcrum on loose teeth. • Use light, steady pressure on rheostat to produce even, low speed.
Rubber Cup and Abrasive	• Gentle activation of rubber cup in polishing agent • Dipping into polishing agent to fill rubber cup	• Adequately fill rubber cup with polishing paste. • Refill rubber cup after completion of every two to three teeth; use adequate amount.
Systematic Approach	• Polishing of all exposed tooth surfaces	• Place lip of cup slightly subgingivally and into interproximal spaces; rubber cup is usually adequate for occlusal surfaces. • A brush may be used for heavily stained occlusal surfaces.

Table 32-10	Engine-Driven Polishing: Procedures Control	
POLISHING CONSIDERATIONS	**CONCERNS**	**RECOMMENDED ACTIONS**
Polishing Agent	An empty cup generates more heat.	One rubber cupful of polishing agent should be used to polish only two to three teeth.
Pressure	Moderate intermittent pressure is preferred; heavy pressure creates more heat and more abrasive action.	Intermittent pressure permits heat dissipation.
Engine Speed	Speed used should be the lowest possible hand piece speed that will move the cup or brush against the tooth without stalling; consistent, low speed is recommended.	Observe the whine of the engine; usually 20 psi is adequate.
Abrasion Control	Increased time spent polishing a tooth surface increases abrasive effect.	Polish approximately 2 to 5 seconds per tooth, which is usually adequate to remove stain and soft deposit. Reinstrumentation may be necessary to remove residual stains or deposit.

psi, Pounds per square inch.

To achieve the lowest possible speed, the rheostat may need to be activated to a high or medium speed and then backed down to a low speed before the tooth is touched with the attachment. Most dental units have a gauge that measures air pressure for each hand piece connector in **pounds per square inch** (psi). Operating the hand piece at approximately 20 psi seems to be sufficient for stain removal. Table 32-9 provides a summary of factors to consider in controlling the negative aspects of the polishing procedure.

At the completion of the polishing procedure, the patient's dentition should be rinsed thoroughly to remove all residual polishing agent. Proximal areas should then be flossed with either dental floss or dental tape. Inspection for remaining stain should be performed with good intraoral light, compressed air, mouth mirror, and a disclosing solution. The clinician should remove any remaining plaque biofilm or stain by either reinstrumenting the area or repolishing the surface. Finishing strips or dental tape rubbed with a small amount of prophy paste before flossing assists in the removal of residual interproximal stain. The type of deposit remaining determines which procedure is indicated.

Precautions and safety issues

Several fundamental principles are important in rubber-cup polishing (Box 32-2). Cosmetic polishing with the rubber cup immediately after scaling and root planing on patients with deep periodontal pockets is contraindicated and should be scheduled for a separate appointment. The polishing agent may be pushed into the pocket and result in increased gingival inflammation.

Air-Powder Polishers

Air-powder polishing is a mechanism for polishing the teeth that propels a slurry of water and sodium bicarbonate under air and water pressure. The psi produced depends on the type of **air-powder polisher** being used. The hand piece has a nozzle through which the slurry is propelled when a foot control is activated. Air-powder polishers are manufactured hand piece units that attach directly to the air/water connector on the dental unit (Figure 32-22), as separate units, or in combination with an ultrasonic scaler (Figure 32-23).

Indications for use

The air-powder polisher has been shown to be a safe, efficient, and effective means of removing extrinsic stain and plaque biofilm from tooth surfaces.[8,9] The air-powder polisher was reported to remove plaque biofilm and stain as effectively as a

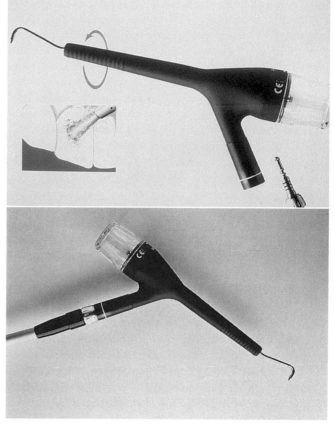

FIGURE 32-22
PROPHYflex unit. (Courtesy KaVo America, Lake Zurich, Ill.)

BOX 32-2

PRINCIPLES FOR RUBBER-CUP POLISHING

- Review medical history and treatment plan for any possible contraindications to the procedure.
- Determine whether the patient has a history of allergy of toxic reaction to fluoride or latex and adjust equipment (prophy cup or paste) as necessary.
- Use a stable fulcrum (absolutely essential) to provide the patient with a sense of confidence in the technique and avoid slippage and possible damage to the tissues.
- Use intermittent pressure against the tooth in a gentle patting or sweeping motion.
- Apply even pressure when polishing cemental surfaces to prevent ditching.
- Maintain a slow, consistent engine speed (desirable at approximately 20 pounds per square inch [psi]).
- Keep the rubber cup filled with abrasive to prevent frictional heat buildup in the tooth.
- Use brush attachments on occlusal surfaces only.
- Start with the least-abrasive agent to prevent unnecessary removal of tooth structure, moving to the next abrasive if the first fails to remove the stain.
- Do not use pumice slurry on primary dentition because of the resulting abrasion.[29]

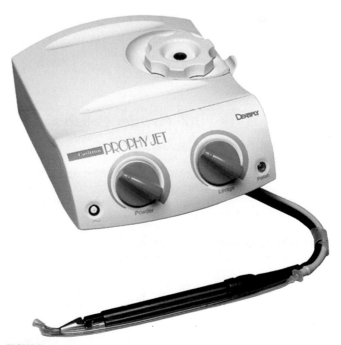

FIGURE 32-23
Prophy-Jet and ultrasonic scaler combination. (Courtesy DENTSPLY Professional, York, Pa.)

rubber cup and does so in less time.[72] It has also shown equal effectiveness in decreasing root surface roughness after instrumentation.[37] Exposed cementum and dentin structures are more vulnerable to abrasion, and the loss of these structures because of air-powder polishing has been reported in the literature.[9,19,34] However, these same reports indicate no negative effect from using the air-powder polisher on intact enamel surfaces (air-powder polishing is less abrasive than most polishing pastes[26]). A summary of indications is found in Table 32-11.

Some patients exhibit extensive staining on root structures, particularly at the cementoenamel junction (CEJ) or on areas with extensive recession. If these stains are removed with a curet, then the root structure will be reduced over the years, particularly if those patients are on a frequent supportive care interval. One option for stained root surfaces that presents no esthetic concern is to leave the stain on the exposed surface and explain to the patient that stain will not harm the teeth or gingiva and is not related to oral disease. For instances when stain removal is necessary for esthetic concerns, the air-powder polisher is preferable to the curet. The air-powder polisher has been shown to remove less root structure than the curet in simulated 3-month recalls for 3 years. In addition, stain was removed more than three times faster with the air-powder polisher.[8] Caution is recommended whenever root surface polishing is necessary. Any method capable of removing stain from the root surface will also remove cementum and dentin. Manufacturers and researchers agree that prolonged use of the air-powder polisher on these surfaces is not advised.[9,19]

The air-powder polisher has also been used for debridement of Class V abraded areas before placement of glass ionomer cements. A comparison of the enamel-cement interface of a glass ionomer cement placed in Class V abrasions cleaned by a rubber-cup polish and an air-powder polisher was conducted. Results indicated the air-polished tooth had less microleakage around the enamel-cement interface than the tooth prepared with the rubber-cup polisher.[11] Similar results were noted when using the air-powder polisher before sealant application. The air-powder polisher was reported to be superior to rubber-cup polishing in preparing enamel for etching and sealants.[20,62] Deeper resin penetration into enamel and increased sealant bond strength was also reported in comparison with traditional polishing with pumice and water.[10,56]

Many operators prefer using the air-powder polisher on orthodontic patients, and researchers support this application.

In addition, no contraindications exist regarding orthodontic bracket adhesive systems used with the air-powder polisher. The guidelines for air-powder polishing include patient selection and preparation, unit and operator preparation, and actual clinical technique.

Type of powder

Everything stated in this chapter regarding air-powder polishing refers to use of the air-powder polisher using the traditional polishing agent—a specially prepared sodium bicarbonate. This is not the type of sodium bicarbonate consumers can purchase. Instead, it has been treated to be free-flowing with calcium phosphate and silica; this polishing agent is a food grade material—each particle is approximately 74 mcm in size.[5] Air-power polishing with sodium bicarbonate is safe for enamel, amalgam, gold, porcelain, implants (titanium), and orthodontic materials.

Recently a new powder has been developed for air-powder polishing that is sodium free (Jet Fresh from DENTSPLY, York, Pa.). It was developed for patients who cannot tolerate sodium bicarbonate for health or taste reasons. This sodium-free powder is made of aluminum trihydroxide, which is much more abrasive than sodium bicarbonate. Research indicates that the aluminum trihydroxide powder is safe for enamel; however, the powder is too abrasive for use on other tooth structures, and its use should be avoided on all dental materials.[33]

> *Distinct Care Modifications*
>
> Air-powder polishing has been found to be more efficient than rubber-cup polishing and appears to be the most effective method of plaque biofilm removal for treating orthodontic patients.[9,21]

Table 32-11	**Air-Powder Polishing: Indications for Use**	
PROCEDURE	**ADVANTAGES**	**DISADVANTAGES**
Plaque Biofilm and Stain Removal	• Works as well as rubber cup but in less time • Decreases root surface roughness after instrumentation • Produces no negative effect on intact enamel surfaces	• May not prevent plaque biofilm reaccumulation better than rubber cup • Reports of loss of exposed cementum and dentin in literature
Class V Restorations Preparation	• Produces less microleakage at enamel and bonding interface	
Sealant Preparation	• Produces deeper resin penetration into enamel • Increases sealant bond strength	• Can abrade existing sealants
Orthodontics	• Polishes more efficiently than rubber cup • Increases bonding strength if used before bonding • Not contraindicated on orthodontic bracket adhesive systems	

Patient selection and preparation

Because of the various indications and contraindications for air-powder use, patient selection and treatment planning are critical. Patient selection should include a thorough health history review to screen out patients on sodium-restricted diets, as well as those with respiratory illnesses, hypertension, and certain infectious or systemic diseases. Caution or complete avoidance of the air-powder polisher is also advised on patients with composite or cosmetic restorations. (Extensive discussion on maintaining esthetic restorations is provided later in this chapter.)

Patient preparation should include a thorough explanation of the procedure, removal of contact lenses, antimicrobial prerinse, and application of a lubricant to the lips. A damp gauze pad may be placed on the patient's tongue to help absorb the powder that accumulates in the patient's mouth. Because of the excessive aerosols produced, additional patient preparation includes protective apparel such as safety glasses or a drape over the nose and eyes and placement of a plastic or disposable drape over the patient's clothing. Patient considerations for air-powder polishing are summarized in Table 32-12.

Unit and operator preparation

Unit preparation includes obtaining all the necessary equipment: air polisher, abrasive powder, floss, disclosing solution, high-speed evacuation system, and preprocedural antimicrobial rinse. Ideally the unit should be placed on the opposite side of the dental chair within comfortable reach of the clinician. Water lines should be flushed before use, according to the recommendations of the Centers for Disease Control and Prevention (CDC). The hand piece nozzle is prepared according to manufacturer's suggestions and the powder compartment filled with abrasive suggested for the machine being used. Because of the excessive aerosols produced, operators are advised to add a face shield and a well-fitting mask with high-filtration capabilities[46] to their already existing personal protective equipment. An aerosol-reduction device that connects the suction to the air-polisher hand piece has been shown to be effective in controlling and reducing air-powder aerosols, thus decreasing the potential for disease transmission[47] (Figure 32-24).

Clinical technique

Positioning of the patient and operator are basically unchanged, although direct vision and access become elementally important when the polisher is active. Raising the back on the patient's

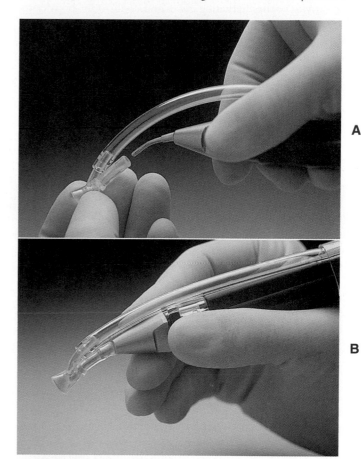

A

B

FIGURE 32-24
A, Jet shield assembly. **B,** Jet shield. (Courtesy DENTSPLY Professional, York, Pa.)

Table 32-12	Air-Powder Polishing: Patient Considerations	
POLISHING CONSIDERATIONS	**CONCERNS**	**RECOMMENDED ACTIONS**
Health History Review	• Review for contraindications	• Health contraindications: Sodium-restricted diet, respiratory illness, hypertension, infectious diseases • Dental contraindications: Composite or esthetic restorations, crown margins, existing sealants, minimal abrasive effects on porcelain or gold
Patient Preparation	• Thorough explanation of procedure	• Ask patient to remove contact lenses • Prerinse with antimicrobial agent • Apply lubricant to lips
Aerosol Protection	• Both patient and operator protected from aerosol	• Patient: Safety glasses, drape over nose and eyes, drape over clothing, preprocedural mouthrinse • Operator: PPE, face shield, well-fitting high-filtration mask

PPE, Personal protective equipment.

chair up to a 45-degree angle may provide a better field of vision and increase patient comfort. The rheostat has two compression levels. Full compression releases the aerosol powder-abrasive from the tip. Pressing the foot pedal halfway produces a stream of water useful for rinsing and cleaning. The clinician should check the amount of water and powder coming from the unit before activation in patients' mouths to test the sensitivity of the alternating cycles and confirm the powder-to-water ratio. The procedure requires adequate evacuation; use of a high-speed suction with an assistant is optimal. When the clinician is performing air polishing without the aid of a dental assistant, the use of a saliva ejector or an aerosol-reduction device (or both) is suggested.

The patient's head is turned slightly toward the clinician, who uses direct vision as much as possible. An external soft tissue fulcrum is established and a modified pen grasp is used with the hand piece and cord resting gently on the hand. Properly managed, the cord supports the necessary light grasp and instrument balance.

The nozzle should be held 3 to 4 mm from the tooth surface. Holding the nozzle farther from the tooth surface minimizes the abrasive action and increases the aerosol. The tip should be angled diagonally, with the spray directed toward the middle one third of the exposed tooth, using a constant circular motion, interproximal to interproximal (sweeping or paintbrush motion). A systematic approach ensures all tooth surfaces are adequately polished. The clinician should alternate cycles of full-compression powder-spray and half-compression rinse every two or three teeth to increase efficiency and patient comfort. For anterior teeth, the tip should be directed at a 60-degree angle to the tooth (Figure 32-25). For posterior teeth an 80-degree angle should be used (Figure 32-26), and for occlusal surfaces a 90-degree angle is appropriate (Figure 32-27). The stream should *not* be aimed at the soft tissue but toward the occlusal or incisal surfaces. Using correct angulation of the hand piece nozzle reduces the amount of aerosolized spray.[3] The suction device should be held as close as possible to the tip of the air-powder polisher (following the tip as it moves in a rapid, sweeping motion from surface to surface). The clinician

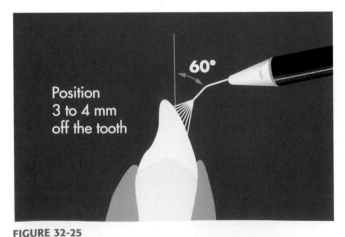

FIGURE 32-25
Air-powder polishing anterior 60-degree angle. (Courtesy DENTSPLY Professional, York, Pa.)

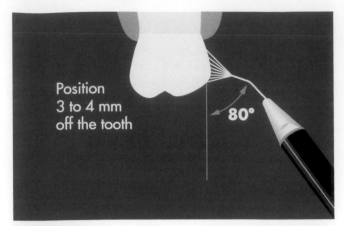

FIGURE 32-26
Air-powder polishing posterior 80-degree angle. (Courtesy DENTSPLY Professional, York, Pa.)

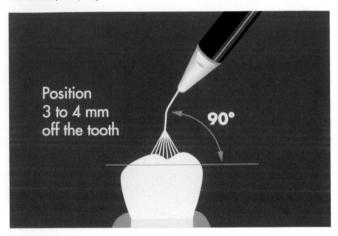

FIGURE 32-27
Air-powder polishing occlusal 90-degree angle. (Courtesy DENTSPLY Professional, York, Pa.)

should use the hand and the patient's cheeks or lips to help contain aerosols. When an aerosol-reduction device is used with the air-powder polisher, the clinician should follow the manufacturer's recommendations for variations to adaptation and angulation.

Clinicians should rinse excessive slurry from the patient's mouth often. In the case of normal soft deposit and stain debridement, the tip should be kept in constant circular motion with an exposure time of ½ to 1 second on each surface.[1,67] Approximately 5 seconds or less on each tooth is generally more than adequate to remove even the most difficult stains. Root surfaces abrade more quickly than enamel surfaces, and less time should be used in these areas. Technique recommendations for the air-powder polisher are summarized in Box 32-3.

The finishing steps that were mentioned with the engine polishing, such as rinsing, flossing, and inspection for remaining stain, should be accomplished at the completion of the air-powder polishing procedure (Table 32-13). Thorough rinsing is essential after air-powder polishing because of the basic nature of the sodium bicarbonate. Often the patient appreciates additional steps, such as allowing the patient to help wipe away the debris from the face with a moist towel and offering lip balm (see Table 32-12).

BOX 32-3

EQUIPMENT AND ACTIONS ASSOCIATED WITH AIR-POWDER POLISHING

Armamentarium
Air-powder polishing unit
Hand piece and nozzle or necessary attachments
Abrasive powder
Evacuation system (high or low speed)
Aerosol-reduction device (optional)
Air/water syringe
Floss
Disclosing solution
Preprocedural antimicrobial rinse

Aerosol-Reduction Strategies
Use hand and patient's cheeks or lips to contain aerosols.
Hold nozzle 3 to 4 mm from tooth surface.
Use proper tip angles for various areas of mouth.
Angle nozzle diagonally toward incisal to middle one third of tooth.
Use constant circular motion.
Hold suction device as close as possible to movement of working tip.
Use aerosol-reduction device.

Nozzle Angulation
Posterior: 80 degrees
Anterior: 60 degrees
Occlusal: 90 degrees

Sequence
Follow systematic approach.
Keep tip in constant circular motion.
Maintain sweeping motion from interproximal to interproximal.
Allow ½ to 1 full second on each tooth surface.
Alternate cycles of full-compression powder spray and half-compression rinsing every 1 to 3 teeth or 1 to 3 seconds.
Rinse excessive slurry from patient's mouth thoroughly and often.
Finishing steps similar to engine-driven polishing.
Perform additional rinsing and provide patients with wipes to help them clean up after procedure.

Considerations
Transient soft tissue abrasion should heal with no long-term effects.
Bacteremia may be created when gingival inflammation is present (similar to rubber-cup polishing).
The serum pH can rise; therefore air-powder polishing is contraindicated on patients with sodium-restricted diets, hypertension, or respiratory or infectious diseases.

Precautions and safety issues

When the clinician performs air-powder polishing, aerosols of microorganisms that contaminate surfaces several feet from the operative site have been reported.[24] Gloves; masks; protective lenses for patient, operator, and assistants; high-volume evacuation; and a laminar airflow to reduce airborne bacteria are important to minimize this problem. Some researchers suggest using a preprocedural rinse with 0.2% chlorhexidine for 2 minutes helped reduce bacterial counts in aerosols[74]; others have reported no significant reduction of bacteria-laden aerosols with prerinsing.[7] Use of an aerosol-reduction device is also suggested. Surface areas require thorough disinfection after this procedure.

Because of these and other concerns, researchers have suggested that use of the air-powder polisher should be avoided on patients with respiratory or infectious diseases, on those who are on sodium-restricted diets, and on those who have hypertension.[3] Some soft tissue abrasion of a transient nature can be expected when using the air-powder polisher; however, it returns to a normal state very quickly. Small blood clots at the margin of the gingiva immediately after use of the air-powder polisher have been noted, with no signs of abrasion or long-term irritation.[35,44] Another study compared the development of bacteremia in subjects receiving a rubber-cup polish and those who were air-powder polished. Although not statistically significant, more subjects receiving a rubber-cup polish

---

Table 32-13	**Finishing and Evaluating the Polishing Procedure**	
POLISHING CONSIDERATIONS	**CONCERNS**	**RECOMMENDED ACTIONS**
Finishing Steps	• Thorough removal of remaining interproximal stain • Flossing of interproximal surfaces • Flossing of surfaces adjacent to edentulous areas	• Remove interproximal stains; use fine sandpaper strips to help remove interproximal stains. • Wipe polishing paste on floss before flossing. • Use regular floss or dental tape.
Follow-Up Evaluation	• Use of disclosing solution, compressed air, and light	• If plaque biofilm or calculus is still present, then reinstrument. • If the stain is still present, then reinstrument, repolish, or both.

developed bacteremias than those who were air-powder polished. If gingivitis is not present, then the likelihood of a patient developing a bacteremia from air-powder polishing is no greater than if he or she were to receive a rubber-cup polish.[31]

MAINTAINING ESTHETIC RESTORATIONS

Esthetic dentistry has become an integral part of today's dental practice. Patients that have crown and bridge restorations and are having cosmetic resin, composite bonding, and veneers placed to enhance their smiles. Because improper oral care can quickly destroy many of these types of restorations, dental hygienists must understand maintenance requirements associated with esthetic dentistry. Dental hygienists are ethically obligated to care for esthetic restorations. The adaptation of polishing procedures to protect the integrity of esthetic restorations requires time and planning and should be a part of treatment planning. The first step before polishing restorations is to identify the location of the restorations and determine the type of material of which they are made. Some esthetic restorations, such as hybrid composites or microfilled composites, will develop a more highly polished surface than glass ionomers. Having the knowledge of how these materials respond to polishing and what types of polishing agents should be used is essential. Table 32-14 presents different types of restorative materials and suggests agents that are safe to maintain the integrity of the surface characterization of these esthetic restorations.

The prophy pastes used for polishing are not compatible with various types of esthetic restorative materials (e.g., microfilled composites, hybrids, glass ionomers, porcelain, veneers).[6] As stated previously, no prophylaxis polishing paste was ever intended for use with esthetic restorative materials. If only one polishing agent is to be used in a dental hygiene practice, then it should be a cleaning agent, such as Pro Care (Young Dental Manufacturing, Earth City, Mo.). Pro Care does not scratch tooth surfaces or restorative materials.

Coarse polishing paste, air-powder polishers,[53] use of acidulated phosphate fluorides,[13,25] and even hard toothbrushing with abrasive toothpaste[63] have been shown to be abrasive and destructive to the surface characteristics of restorative material. One study demonstrated that polishing pastes roughen the surface of composite resins; thus their use should be avoided at

those sites.[57] Another short-term study demonstrated that polishing after root planing improved the smoothness of the marginal portion of cast gold crowns more than simple root planing alone.[75]

Application of the air-powder polisher on most restorative materials should be carefully managed. Esthetic restorations (i.e., composites, veneers, porcelain) have exhibited wear and surface roughness when exposed to the air-powder polisher,[5,12,39,53] although in 1984 Patterson and McLundie reported minimal in vitro effects on porcelain and hard gold alloy.[52] Care is recommended around crown margins because cement may be eroded[5] and loss of marginal integrity on porcelain restorations has been identified.[18,68] Air-powder polishing also has been shown to abrade dental sealants.[30] Table 32-15 presents recommendations regarding the use of air-powder polishing with esthetic materials. Essentially, air-powder polishing and agents intended for use on tooth structures are not compatible with esthetic restorations.

Polishing Restorative Materials

Basic guidelines for esthetic dentistry start with careful instrumentation with a curet to debride around the restoration. Scalers or powered scalers (sonic or ultrasonic) should not be used because they can scratch the surface and break down the filler particles.[78] The next step is to apply a diamond, aluminum oxide, or low-abrasive toothpaste directly to the restoration and then polish thoroughly using a rubber cup for 30 seconds. Diamond polishing paste is suggested when only porcelain is exposed. Aluminum oxide paste is recommended for use on highly filled hybrid composites[32] and resin or porcelain restorations when resin cement or cementum is exposed.[41,43] It has also been suggested that low-abrasive toothpaste also may be used for the polishing agent, but no research has documented this suggestion.

Clinicians should floss while the paste is still on the restoration to carry the paste interproximally. When all surfaces have been polished, the restoration is rinsed and inspected for further stain.[41,43] If stain remains after initial polishing procedures, then aluminum oxide discs, points, and strips of varying **grit** level may be used. These steps are followed by aluminum oxide polishing paste to leave an esthetic, final polish.[48] Esthetic and

Table 32-14	Compatibility of Prophylaxis Paste, Sodium Bicarbonate, and Aluminum Trihydroxide (Jet Fresh) with Esthetic Dental Restorative Materials		
RESTORATIVE MATERIAL	**PROPHYLAXIS PASTE**	**SODIUM BICARBONATE**	**ALUMINUM TRIHYDROXIDE**
Porcelain	Not advised	No*	Not advised
Hybrid Composite	No	No	No
Microfill Composite	No	No	No
Glass Ionomer	No	No	No

*Produces rapid loss of cements and jeopardizes restoration.

Table 32-15			**Recommendations for Polishing Esthetic Restorative Materials**[4]		
MATERIAL	**PORCELAIN**	**PORCELAIN AND RESIN CEMENT INTERFACE**	**GLASS, RESIN IONOMERS**	**MICROFILLED COMPOSITES**	**HYBRID COMPOSITES**
Suggestions for Polishing Techniques I	Proxyt (Ivoclar Vivadent) Coarse ↓ Medium ↓ Fine	Finishing diamond (Use finest grit and water spray)	PoGo polishing disc (DENTSPLY Caulk)	PoGo polishing disc	PoGo polishing disc
Suggestions for Polishing Techniques II	D◆FINE porcelain polishers (Clinician's Choice) (Use dry and at low speed, with moderate pressure)	Rubber finisher, polisher Coarse ↓ Medium ↓ Fine (Finish with diamond paste on a felt wheel)	Proxyt (Use petroleum jelly or water to prevent desiccation)	Rubber polisher (designed for microfilled composites) ↓ Prisma Gloss (DENTSPLY Caulk)	Rubber finisher ↓ D◆FINE rubber polishing points for hybrids (Clinician's Choice) ↓ Prisma Gloss (aluminum oxide paste, prophy cup, and water) ↓ Prisma Gloss Extrafine
Suggestions for Polishing Techniques III	Shimmer	Shimmer	Shimmer	Shimmer	Shimmer or Porcelize diamond paste

porcelain restorations always should be polished first, following the guidelines mentioned previously. The remaining teeth may then be polished using the appropriate methods for the clinical situation. This is to reduce the possibility of having a coarse abrasive (that can scratch the esthetic surface) remain in the rubber cup or the mouth when esthetic maintenance is being rendered.

Implant Polishing

Air-powder polishing can be safely used on implants and has been reported to remove 100% of bacteria in the presence of periimplantitis.[1,4,51] Figure 32-28 is scanning electron microscope (SEM) photograph of implant material before and after treatment with air-powder polishing for 5 seconds, which represents approximately 10 years of recare visits. Research suggests minimal to no alteration or damage to implant surfaces from air-powder polishing, which leaves the surfaces smooth and bacteria free.[2,4,27] Many implants have fixed porcelain crowns or bridges with limited access to the actual titanium implant, and esthetic restorative materials placed on implants should not be polished with air polishing. Those restorations should be polished with the appropriate agent for that particular esthetic material. Professional, clinical decision-making skills are necessary in these situations to achieve the desired clinical outcome. Guidelines used to maintain esthetic restorations are found in Table 32-16.

THERAPEUTIC POLISHING

Therapeutic polishing is the removal of toxins from the unexposed root surfaces, which results in a decrease in disease parameters. Polishing root surfaces is possible with both the rubber-cup or air-powder polisher; however, the evidence indicates the use of the air-powder polisher for this purpose. The rationale for this selection may be the result of the effectiveness and efficiency of this device. Root surfaces also may be polished with an air-powder polisher when exposed during a surgical procedure.

The air-powder polisher works well in removing plaque biofilm, endotoxins, and stain from root concavities and furcations as an adjunct to periodontal surgery,[28] but it may offer no measurable benefit beyond ultrasonic debridement.[36] One *in vitro* study suggests that using an ultrasonic scaler followed by air-powder polishing creates an environment in which fibroblast growth and vitality is greater than for either teeth that were ultrasonically scaled without polishing or control teeth with remaining calculus.[22] Whether used as a follow-up to ultrasonic scaling or on calculus-free root surfaces, the air-powder polisher may play a significant role in the future in the removal of endotoxins on exposed root surfaces during surgery.

When polishing for therapeutic benefits with the air-powder polisher, the hygienist should follow the precautions and considerations presented previously. Most importantly, the

Table 32-16	Guidelines Used to Maintain Esthetic Restorations*	
POLISHING CONSIDERATIONS	**CONCERNS**	**RECOMMENDED ACTIONS**
Instrumentation	Improper instrumentation can scratch surface and break down filler particles.	Carefully debride area with curet (scalers and powered scalers are contraindicated).
Thorough Polishing with Rubber Cup	Diamond polishing paste should be used when only porcelain is exposed. Aluminum oxide should be used for highly filled hybrid composites, resin, or porcelain restorations when resin cements or cementum is exposed.	Apply a diamond, aluminum oxide, or low-abrasive toothpaste directly to restoration.
Floss	Proximal stain should be thoroughly removed.	Perform flossing while the paste is still on restoration to carry paste interproximally.
Rinsing and Evaluation	Remaining pumice particles should be thoroughly removed.	If the stain remains, use aluminum oxide discs, points, and strips of varying grits from coarse to fine; follow this step with aluminum oxide polishing paste for a final polish.

*The clinician should remember to *always* polish esthetic and porcelain restorations *first;* then polish the remaining teeth using appropriate methods indicated by the clinical situation and treatment plan.

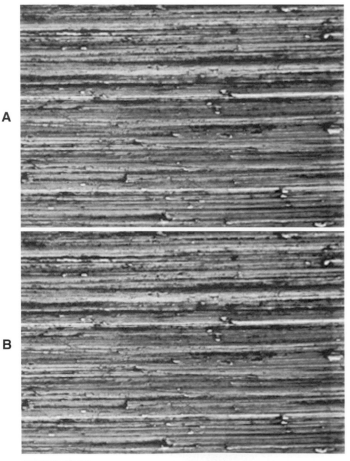

A

B

FIGURE 32-28
Scanning electron microscope (SEM) photographs (150×) of IMX titanium implant material untreated **(A)** and treated **(B)** with an airpowder polisher for 5 seconds. Reader should note no changes in the surface characterization.

clinician should take care to direct the air-powder spray against the root surface, not the exposed soft tissues.

ROLE OF POLISHING IN DENTAL HYGIENE CARE

Professionals should consider all of the options available in treatment planing for the polishing procedure. As with any other procedure, clinicians must consider esthetic, therapeutic, and patient goals to design the treatment plan that meets each patient's specific needs. Applying these concepts allows the hygienist to accomplish a safe, effective, and thorough polishing procedure for cosmetic and therapeutic treatment.

References

1. Atkinson DR, Cobb CM, Killoy WJ: The effect of an airpowder abrasive system on in vitro root surfaces, *J Periodontol* 55(1):13-8, 1984.
2. Augthun M, Tinschert J, Huber A: In vitro studies on the effect of cleaning methods on different implant surfaces, *J Periodontol* 69(8):857-864, 1998.
3. Barnes CM: The management of aerosols with airpolishing delivery systems, *J Dent Hyg* 65(6):280-282, 1991.
4. Barnes CM, Fleming LS, Meuninghoff LA: An SEM evaluation of the in-vitro effects of an air-abrasive system on various implant surfaces, *Int J Oral Maxillofac Implants* 6:463-469, 1991.
5. Barnes CM, Hayes EF, Leinfelder KF: Effects of an airabrasive polishing system on restored surfaces, *General Dentistry* 35(3): 186-189, 1987.
6. Barnes CM et al: Essential selective polishing: the maintenance of esthetic restorations, *J Dent Hyg* 12:18-24, 2003.
7. Bay NL et al: Effectiveness of antimicrobial mouthrinses on aerosols produced by an air polisher, *J Dent Hyg* 67:312-317, 1993.
8. Berkstein S et al: Supragingival root surface removal during maintenance procedures utilizing an air-powder abrasive system or hand scaling, *J Periodontol* 58:327-330, 1987.

9. Boyde A: Airpolishing effects on enamel, dentine and cementum, *Br Dent J* 55:486-488, 1984.

10. Brocklehurst PR, Joshi RI, Northeast SE: The effect of air-polishing occlusal surfaces on the penetration of fissures by a sealant, *Int J Paediatr Dent* 2:157-162, 1992.

11. Cooley RL, Lubow RM, Patrissi GA: The effect of an air-powder abrasive on glass ionomer microleakage, *General Dentistry* 37(1):16-18, 1989.

12. Cooley RL, Lubow RM, Atrissi GA: The effect of an airpowder abrasive instrument on composite resin, *J Am Dent Assoc* 112(3):362-364, 1986.

13. Council on Dental Materials, Instruments and Equipment: Effect of acidulated phosphate fluoride on porcelain and composite restorations (status report), *J Am Dent Assoc* 116:115, 1988.

14. Davis WR: Cleaning, polishing and abrasion of teeth by dental products, *J Cosmet Sci* 1:38, 1978.

15. Dean MC, Douglas MB, Blank LW: A comparison of two prophylaxis angles: disposable and autoclavable, *J Am Dent Assoc* 128(4);444-452, 1997.

16. Dunipace AJ et al: An in situ interproximal model for studying the effect of fluoride on enamel, *Caries Res* 31(1):60-70, 1997.

17. Featherstone JD: Prevention and reversal of dental caries: role of low level fluoride, *Community Dent Oral Epidemiol* 27(1):31-40, 1999.

18. Felton DA et al: Effect of air-powder abrasives on marginal configurations of porcelain-fused-to-metal alloys: an SEM analysis, *J Prosthet Dent* 65:38-43, 1991.

19. Galloway SE, Pashley DH: Rate of removal of root structure by the use of the prophy-jet device, *J Periodontol* 58(7):464-469, 1987.

20. Garcia-Godoy F, Medlock JW: An SEM study of the effects of air-polishing on fissure surfaces, *Quintessence Int* 7:465-7, 1988.

21. Gerbo LR, Barnes CM, Leinfelder KF: Applications of the air-powder polisher in clinical orthodontics, *Am J Orthod Dentofacial Orthop* 103:71-3, 1993.

22. Gilman RS, Maxey BR: The effect of root detoxification on human gingival fibroblasts, *J Periodontol* 57(7):436-440, 1986.

23. Gladwin M, Bagby M: *Clinical aspects of dental Materials,* Philadelphia, 2000, Lippincott Williams & Wilkins.

24. Glenwright HD, Knibbs PJ, Burdon DW: Atmospheric contamination during use of an air polisher, *Br Dent J* 159(9):294-297, 1985.

25. Gonzalez E et al: Decrease in reflectance of porcelains treated with APF gels, *Dent Mater* 4(5):289-295, 1988.

26. Gutmann ME: Air polishing: a comprehensive review of the literature, *J Dent Hyg* 72:47-56, 1998.

27. Homiak AW, Cook PA, DeBoer J: Effect of hygiene instrumentation on titanium abutments: a scanning electron microscopy study, *J Prosthet Dent* 67:364-369, 1992.

28. Horning GM, Cobb CM, Killoy WI: Effect of an air-powder abrasive system on root surfaces in periodontal surgery, *J Clin Periodontol* 14(4):213-220, 1987.

29. Hosoya Y, Johnston JW: Evaluation of various cleaning and polishing methods on primary enamel, *J Periodontol* 13(3):253-269, 1989.

30. Huennekens SC, Daniel SC, Bayne SC: Effects of air polishing on the abrasion of occlusal sealants, *Quintessence Int* 22(7):581-585, 1991.

31. Hunter KM, Ferguson MM et al: Bacteraemia and tissue damage resulting from air polishing, *Br Dent J* 167(8):275-278, 1989.

32. Jefferies SR: The art and science of abrasive finishing and polishing in restorative dentistry, *Dent Clin North Am* 42(4):613-627, 1998.

33. Johnson WW et al: An in vitro investigation of the effects of an aluminum air polishing powder delivered via the Prophy Jet on dental restorative materials, *J Prosthodont* 13:1-7, 2004.

34. Kee A, Allen DS: Effects of air and rubber cup polishing on enamel abrasion, *Dent Hyg* 62:55, 1988 (abstract).

35. Konturri-Nahri V, Markkanen S, Markkanen H: Gingival effects of dental airpolishing as evaluated by scanning electron microscopy, *J Periodontol* 60:19-22, 1989.

36. Krupa CM et al: In vitro evaluation of air-powder polishing as an adjunct to ultrasonic scaling on periodontally involved root surfaces, *Dent Hyg* 62:55, 1988.

37. Leknes KN, Lie T: Influence of polishing procedures on sonic scaling root surface roughness, *J Periodontol* 62:659-662, 1991.

38. Lobene RR: Effects of dentifrices on tooth stains with controlled brushing, *J Am Dent Assoc* 77(4):849-855, 1968.

39. Lubow RM, Cooley RL: Effect of air-powder abrasive instrument on restorative materials, *J Prosthet Dent* 55(4):462-465, 1986.

40. Marinelli CB et al: An in vitro comparison of three fluoride regimens on enamel remineralization, *Caries Res* 31(6):418-422, 1997.

41. McGuire MK, Miller LM: Maintaining esthetic restorations in the periodontal practice, *J Periodontal Res* 16(3):230-239, 1996.

42. Mellberg JR: Enamel fluoride and its anti-caries effects, *J Prev Dent* 4(1):8-20, 1977.

43. Miller LM: Porcelain veneer protection plan: maintenance procedures for all porcelain restorations, *J Esthet Dent* 2(3):63-66, 1990.

44. Mishkin DJ et al: A clinical comparison of the effect on the gingiva of the Prophy-Jet and the rubber cup and paste techniques, *J Periodontol* 57(3):151-154, 1986.

45. Moffitt JM et al: Prediction of tetracycline-induced tooth discoloration, *J Am Dent Assoc* 88(3):547-552, 1974.

46. Molinari JA: Face masks: effective personal protection, *Compend Cont Educ Dent* 17(9):818-21, 1996.

47. Muzzin KB, King TB, Berry CW: Assessing the clinical effectiveness of an aerosol reduction device for the air polisher, *J Am Dent Assoc* 130(9):1354-1359, 1999.

48. Nash LB: Maximizing esthetic restorations: the hygienist's role, *Pract Procedures Aesthet Dent* 3(3):17-18, 1991.

49. Ness L, Rosekrans DL, Welford JF: An epidemiologic study of factors affecting extrinsic staining of teeth in an English population, *Community Dent Oral Epidemiol* 5(1):55-60, 1977.

50. O'Brien W, Ryge G: *An outline of dental materials and their selection,* Philadelphia, 1978, WB Saunders.

51. Parha PL et al: Effects of an air-powder abrasive system on plasma-sprayed titanium implant surfaces: an in vitro evaluation, *J Oral Implantol* 15:78-86, 1989.

52. Patterson CJ, McLundie AC: A comparison of the effects of two different prophylaxis regimes in vitro on some restorative dental materials: a preliminary SEM study, *Br Dent J* 157(5):166-170, 1984.

53. Reel DC et al: Effect of a hydraulic jet prophylaxis system on composites, *J Prosthet Dent* 61(4):441-445, 1989.

54. Reid JS, Beeley JA, MacDonald DG: Investigation into black extrinsic tooth stain, *J Dent Res* 56(8):895-899, 1977.

55. Retief DH et al: In vitro fluoride uptake distribution and retention by human enamel after 1- and 24-hour application of various topical fluoride agents, *J Dent Res* 59(3):573-582, 1980.

56. Scott L, Greer D: The effect of an airpolishing device on sealant bond strength, *J Prosthet Dent* 58:384-387, 1987.

57. Serio FG et al: The effect of polishing pastes on composite resin surfaces: a SEM study, *J Periodontol* 59(12):837-840, 1988.

58. Shaw L, Murray JJ: A new index for measuring extrinsic stain in clinical trials, *Community Dent Oral Epidemiol* 5(3):116-120, 1977.

59. Solheim H, Eriksen HM, Nordbo H: Chemical plaque control and extrinsic discoloration of teeth, *Acta Odontol Scand* 38(5): 303-309, 1980.

60. Spierings TA, Peters MC, Plasschaert AJ: Thermal trauma to teeth, *Endod Dent Traumatol* 1(4):123-129, 1985.

61. Steele RC et al: The effect of tooth cleaning procedures on fluoride uptake in enamel, *Pediatr Dent* 4(3):228-233, 1982.

62. Strand GV, Raadel M: The efficiency of cleaning fissures with an air-polishing instrument, *Acta Odontol Scand* 46:113-117, 1988.

63. Strassler HE, Moffitt W: The surface texture of composite resin after polishing with commercially available toothpastes, *Compend Cont Educ Dent* 88:26-30, 1987.

64. Thompson RE, Way DC: Enamel loss due to prophylaxis and multiple bonding debonding of orthodontic attachments, *Am J Orthod* 79(3):282-295, 1981.

65. Tilliss TS, Hicks MJ: Enamel surface morphology comparison. Polishing with a toothpaste and a prophylaxis paste, *Dent Hyg* 61(3):112-115, 1987.

66. Tinanoff N et al: Effect of a pumice prophylaxis on fluorite uptake in tooth enamel, *J Am Dent Assoc* 88(2):384-389, 1974.

67. Toevs SE: Root topography following instrumentation, *J Dent Hyg* 59(8):350-354, 1985.

68. Vermilyea SG, Prasanna MK, Agar JR: Effect of ultrasonic cleaning and air polishing on porcelain labial margin restorations, *J Prosthet Dent* 71:447-452, 1994.

69. Vogel RJ: Intrinsic and extrinsic discoloration of the dentition (a literature review), *J Oral Med* 30(4):99, 1975.

70. Walsh MM et al: Effect of a rubber cup polish after scaling, *J Dent Hyg* 59(11):494-498, 1985.

71. Waring MB et al: A comparison of engine polishing and toothbrushing in minimizing dental plaque reaccumulation, *J Dent Hyg* 56(12):25-30, 1982.

72. Weaks LM et al: Clinical evaluation of the Prophy-jet as an instrument for routine removal of tooth stain and plaque, *J Periodontol* 55:486-488, 1984.

73. White DJ, Chen WC, Nancollas GH: Kinetics and physical aspects of enamel remineralization—a constant composition study, *Caries Res* 22:11-19, 1988.

74. Worral SF, Knibbs PJ, Gelenwrikght HD: Methods of reducing bacterial contamination of the atmosphere arising from use of an air-polisher, *Br Dent J* 163:118-119, 1987.

75. Yagi H et al: Effects of repeated hand instrumentation on the marginal portion of a cast gold crown, *J Periodontol* 69(1):41-46, 1998.

76. Yankell S, Emling RC: Understanding dental products: what you should know and what your patient should know, *Comp Cont Dent Educ* 1:7, 1978.

77. Yankell SL et al: Effects of chlorhexidine and four antimicrobial compounds on plaque, gingivitis, and staining in beagle dogs, *J Dent Res* 61(9):1089-1093, 1982.

78. Zitterbart PA: Effectiveness of ultrasonic scalers: a literature review, *Gen Dent* 35(4):295-297, 1987.

Dentinal Hypersensitivity

Martin Addy • Nicola X. West

INSIGHT

One of the most common, yet misunderstood, challenges within the dental office is dentinal hypersensitivity. A myriad of over-the-counter (OTC) home care products (as well as professionally applied, in-office treatment options) is available to the dental hygienist to recommend and use for this condition. Understanding the various functions and applications of each product and treatment option is essential to make effective clinical decisions.

✦✦ CASE STUDY 33-1 Treatment of Dentinal Hypersensitivity to Cold Stimuli

Ms. Suki Yamagashi, a 28-year-old Asian woman, arrives for a supportive care appointment and appears to be in good physical health. Her health history reveals she is single, an attorney at one of the town's law firms, and has no contraindications to dental treatment. The clinical examination reveals all extraoral conditions are within normal limits. All intraoral findings are also within normal limits, except for two areas of localized 3-mm recession on the facial surfaces of teeth #6 and #12. While probing these areas, Ms. Yamagashi asks the hygienist to stop because of the pain from the cold metal probe. On questioning about these areas, she says they have been sensitive to cold for several years; however, in the past few months she has noticed pain in these areas even if something is slightly cold. Ms. Yamagashi has stopped eating ice cream and does not have ice in beverages.

KEY TERMS

burnishing	efficacy	intratubular	pulpitis
causation	Hawthorn effect	osmotic	regression to the mode
control product effect	hydrodynamic theory	oxalates	reactionary dentin
dentin hypersensitivity	*in situ*	peritubular	reparative tertiary dentin
dentinal tubules	*in vitro*	placebo effect	smear layer

LEARNING OUTCOMES

After reading this chapter the student will be able to:

1. Understand the hydrodynamic theory of pain conduction.
2. Describe the three main categories of stimuli that elicit a pain response and give examples of each.
3. Describe desensitizing agents and products available for self-care.
4. Select office procedures for the treatment of sensitivity based on patient needs and evaluate the response to agents.
5. Evaluate the literature on desensitizing agents to determine the most effective products for self-care and professional use.

Teeth, dentistry, and pain are frequently linked in the minds of the general public. This is perhaps not surprising given that the majority of the sensory nerves in the dental pulp are pain receptors supplied via the maxillary and mandibular branches of the trigeminal nerve. Depending on the stimulus and the condition of the pulp, dental pain can represent various proportional combinations of nerve responses. However, research has revealed that the status of the dental pulp cannot be determined by the characteristics of the painful response.[150] High on the list of painful dental conditions is **dentin hypersensitivity.**

The pain receptors are mainly of two types: (1) the A beta and A delta fibers triggered physically to give a short, sharp pain and (2) the C fibers stimulated chemically to give a protracted dull ache or throbbing sensation.[117] The characteristic short, sharp pain of dentinal hypersensitivity reported by a majority of sufferers suggests the A beta and delta receptors are usually involved alone.

Dentin hypersensitivity, a common occurrence, is poorly understood and led one author to characterize it as a mystery.[100] Twenty years after that remark, and after many research studies, the cause of dentinal hypersensitivity is still unknown. Prevention is often difficult, and management strategies are not always evidence based.

This chapter presents what is known about dentin hypersensitivity and application of knowledge to plan management rather than just treatment strategies for sufferers. The emphasis is to discuss whether dentinal hypersensitivity is a tooth wear phenomenon.[45]

Terminology

Dentin or dentinal hypersensitivity is a common, painful condition of the teeth characterized by short, sharp pain in response to certain stimuli. At a macroscopic level, sensitive dentin appears the same as nonsensitive dentin (although differences exist at the microscopic level).[3,96] The condition of the pulp in dentinal hypersensitivity is not known, although the history of the condition does not suggest inflamed pulp. Therefore the term *dentinal sensitivity* is somewhat inaccurate and inappropriate. Dentin cannot itself be sensitive; therefore the term *dentin hypersensitivity* would more closely describe the condition observed clinically. Many terms have been used to describe this condition:

- Dentinal hypersensitivity
- Dentin sensitivity
- Cervical dentinal sensitivity
- Sensitivity
- Root sensitivity
- Cemental hypersensitivity and sensitivity
  - Dentinal sensitivity
  - Root or cervical sensitivity

The term *root sensitivity* has recently been suggested by the European Federation of Periodontology as the term to describe the sensitivity of

> **Note**
> These terms are misleading, because dentinal hypersensitivity can occur at any tooth surface, even though the facial cervical site is the most common area.

teeth arising from periodontal disease or periodontal treatments.[146] The term was adopted because of the uncertainty of whether this type of sensitivity was truly dentin hypersensitivity: having a prevalence of more than 80% in periodontal patients.[34] Certainly it does not fit the definition of dentin hypersensitivity because microorganisms invade the root **dentinal tubules** of periodontally involved teeth and for considerable distances toward the pulp.[15] *Cemental hypersensitivity and sensitivity* is a totally inappropriate term (not the least because cementum is rapidly lost from root surfaces once exposed).[23] The fact that the term *dentin sensitivity* is not an accurate descriptor for the condition does not mean it should be dropped. The term has been in widespread use for many decades and identifies to the clinician a specific condition distinct from other painful dental problems. Given that the condition was given a definition at an international meeting, it would seem sensible to universally recommend the term *dentin sensitivity* and discourage the use of other terminology.

Definition

An international workshop on the design and conduct of clinical trials for dentin hypersensitivity published a definition in 1997[89] largely based on one suggested in 1983.[50] Dentin hypersensitivity is characterized by short, sharp pain arising from exposed dentin in response to stimuli from the following causes:

- Thermal (occurs most often)
- Evaporative
- Tactile
- Osmotic or chemical (used when no other form of dental defect or pathologic condition can be determined)

The Canadian Advisory Board on Dentin Hypersensitivity suggested a further small modification in 2003, namely that *disease* should be substituted for *pathologic condition*.[31] On close inspection, the definition makes three specific but associated statements:

1. An assumption of exposed dentin (This requirement can create clinical difficulties for two reasons. The first reason is that dentin may be exposed but not clinically evident. A scanning electron microscopy [SEM] study of impressions of the buccal cervical area of teeth revealed a significant underdiagnosis of exposed dentin.[23] The second reason is that symptoms may be caused by another condition rather than dentinal hypersensitivity.)

2. A clinical descriptor of the condition highlighting the classical symptoms and the various stimuli that can evoke the response (The short, sharp nature of the pain is also most important, because evidence indicates that in some cases the pain may persist as a dull ache for variable time periods after removal of the stimulus. In these rare cases evidence indicates an associated **pulpitis**[46] and suggests the need for a management strategy focusing on the pulpitis [e.g., endodontics] rather than the dentin hypersensitivity.)

3. Invites, even recommends, the clinician to consider a differential diagnosis before concluding the symptoms are, indeed, caused by dentin hypersensitivity alone[51]

Differential Diagnosis

Short, sharp pain on appropriate stimulation characterizes a number of dental conditions other than dentinal hypersensitivity, including all of those associated with dentinal hypersensitivity. These causes of "dentinal" pain have exposed dentin although, in some cases, this is not visible to the clinician and may be via an enamel defect. Other causes of short, sharp dentinal pain include the following:

- Dental caries
- Chipped teeth
- Fractured teeth
- Fractured restorations
- Marginal leakage around restorations
- Cracked tooth syndrome
- Palatogingival grooves
- Other development defects of enamel

In addition to the stimuli producing pain in dentinal hypersensitivity, biting or chewing may be the more common stimulus inducing sensitivity in cracked tooth syndrome.

DENTAL CONSIDERATIONS

Another diagnostic issue concerning dentinal hypersensitivity is a growing problem, namely the hypersensitivity sometimes associated with vital bleaching using peroxides.[84] The symptoms are identical to dentinal hypersensitivity; however, researchers are still unclear whether the bleach or the vehicle in which the bleach resides acts as the stimulus through an **osmotic** process, or if the bleach directly affects pulpal nerves. To confound the problem, whether the bleach, the vehicle, or both are stimulating exposed dentin or dentin by way of the overlying enamel is not clear. More clinical research is urgently needed before inroads to preventing this problem can be made.

The need for a differential diagnosis in cases of possible dentinal hypersensitivity is twofold. The management and treatment of the other causes of dental pain is usually completely different from that of dentinal hypersensitivity.[51] More than one cause for dental pain in the same mouth is possible. In summary, essentially the diagnosis of dentinal hypersensitivity should be based on exclusion (this is discussed further in Management Strategies for Dentinal Hypersensitivity).

Mechanism Theories

How an appropriate stimulus applied to exposed dentin could evoke an essentially instantaneous painful response has been the subject of debate for many decades. Three hypotheses have been presented over the years[14,81]:

1. Direct innervation of the dentin
2. Odontoblast transducer mechanism (odontoblast extended the full length of the tubule)
3. Hydrodynamic theory

DIRECT INNERVATION

One of the most obvious hypotheses was that dentin was innervated and therefore nerves were directly triggered. Some histologic techniques using stains that proved not totally specific for nerve fibers lent credence to this idea. Later evidence from electron microscopy revealed that nerve fibers did, indeed, penetrate the dentinal tubules but only for a very short distance into the inner dentin. Any clinician could further convince himself or herself of the invalidity of this hypothesis by applying topical anesthetic to exposed dentin without reducing sensitivity.

ODONTOBLAST EXTENSION IN TUBULE

The odontoblast transducer mechanism was thought responsible because the odontoblast embryologically originates from the neural crest. Direct microscopic techniques again proved the odontoblast process did not extend the full length of the tubules. In addition, although cavity preparation destroys or disrupts the odontoblast layer below, every clinician knows—as do patients—that the dentin remains sensitive.

HYDRODYNAMIC THEORY

This leaves the **hydrodynamic theory.** In the middle to late nineteenth century, it was determined that an outward flow of fluid along the dentinal tubules exists. Based on this (and without research evidence), in 1900, Gysi[79] proposed the hypothesis that appropriate stimuli applied to dentin increased this fluid flow that, in turn, triggered the pulpal nerves (Figure 33-1). The scientific community had to wait another 60 years before Brännström and colleagues[27-30] published eloquent studies to elevate the hypothesis to the hydrodynamic theory that has remained unchallenged to this day.

The principle of the mechanism remains the same—that most stimuli cause an increased outward fluid flow and therefore a pressure change across the dentin. This is thought to distort the A beta and delta fibers by a mechanoreceptor action to cause pain. This is not unlike gently applying fingertip pressure just above the skin to the skin hair, which relays a touch sensation. An additional process may be involved, because when fluid flow changes rate in a tubule, an electrical discharge occurs (called *streaming potential*) across the dentin. Whether this can reach proportions to electrically stimulate nerves is not known but is possible.[17,76]

DENTAL CONSIDERATIONS

The definition of dentinal hypersensitivity highlights a number of stimuli that can evoke a response. Of these, cold is reported as most problematic and is fairly commonly used in clinical trials.[131] Lesser cited is heat, perhaps because heat is the exception causing an inward flow of fluid such that the response time is longer.[118]

All of the research by Brännström and colleagues[27-30] investigated the sensitivity of dentin with dentinal hypersensitivity not considered. Nevertheless, it would not be unreasonable to expect the same hydrodynamic mechanism to operate. For this

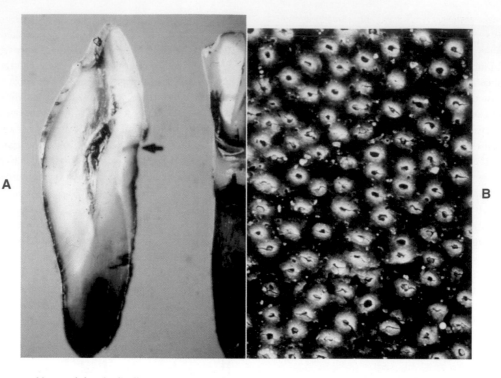

FIGURE 33-1
A, Lateral view of hypersensitive tooth longitudinally sectioned through cervical abrasion cavity. Methylene blue dye penetration can be seen *(arrow).* **B,** Scanning electron microscopy (SEM) of the same abrasion cavity, showing large numbers of open tubules (×1000). (Courtesy Absi EG et al, Dental hypersensitivity—the effect of toothbrushing and dietary compounds on dentine in vitro: an SEM study, *J Oral Rehabil* 19(2):101-110, 1992.)

to occur, lesions of dentinal hypersensitivity would require tubules open at the dentin surface and unobstructed to the pulp. Studies of extracted teeth provided compelling evidence for this requirement,[2,3,96] with sensitive teeth having many more (8×) and wider (2×) tubules at the buccal cervical area compared with nonsensitive teeth[3] (Figure 33-2). Additionally, dye penetration to the pulp was seen only in sensitive teeth.[3] Although

number and radius of tubules are relevant to fluid flow and therefore sensitivity, tubule radius is probably more important because fluid flow is proportional to the fourth power of the radius.[132] As an example, doubling the diameter of a tubule increases fluid flow sixteenfold. These characteristics of lesions of dentinal hypersensitivity clearly have important implications to the causative factors involved, as well as to the development of preventive and management strategies for the condition.

Epidemiologic Considerations and Distribution

Prevalence and incidence figures for dentinal hypersensitivity have been drawn for the most part from studies that do not conform to conventional epidemiologic designs. True randomized selection of subjects for the studies has not been used; population sizes have been relatively small and variable, and inappropriate diagnostic methods sometimes have been used. The result has been figures that vary at the extreme (3% to 60%),[4,141] particularly if the data from periodontal patients are included (where 70% to almost 100% figures are reported). As discussed, however, these latter percentages should be considered for root sensitivity and not dentinal hypersensitivity. In those surveys in which subjects were diagnosed through examination, the figures are surprisingly consistent (around 15% of adults have one or more teeth with dentinal hypersensitivity).[4]

The demographics of the sufferers are perhaps more interesting, because they provide some evidence, albeit circumstantial,

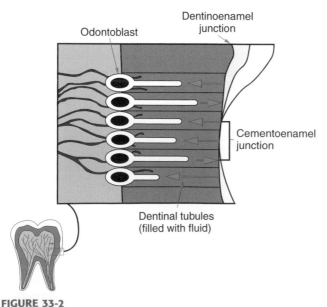

FIGURE 33-2
Hydrodynamic theory of dentinal sensation, as described by Brännström.[29]

about possible causative factors (Box 33-1). Thus although the age range for the condition is wide (namely teenage to the seventh decade), the peak incidence appears between 20 to 40 years.[14,61,72] Additionally, women are more frequently affected and at a younger mean age.[61,72] The relative young age for the condition suggests that age changes may progressively reduce the hydraulic conductance of dentin. The increased predilection in women may hint at an oral hygiene and dietary influence (discussed later in the chapter). Interestingly, in 2002 a global survey of 11,000 male and female subjects was conducted by the Research Quorum in Basingstroke, Hampshire, U.K. (survey unpublished). The study was based on individual perception of sensitivity, and it found 37% to 52% of subjects reporting sensitivity, suggesting other causes for the condition. Women again reported a higher prevalence than men. Professionals have also reported varying perceived levels of dentinal hypersensitivity in their patients. Dental hygienists reported twice the number of patients with perceived hypersensitivity as that reported by dentists.

DENTAL CONSIDERATIONS

Virtually all studies that reported the distribution of dentinal hypersensitivity found that the canines and first premolars were most commonly affected; next, the incisors and second premolars; and least, the molars.[12,72,131] By the nature of the studies, these data related only to the facial cervical sites. Again, these data provide some insight into the cause of the condition.

Etiology

One review article questioned whether dentinal hypersensitivity was a tooth wear phenomenon.[45] Because exposure of dentin commonly occurs as a result of gingival recession, the authors wondered whether dentinal hypersensitivity may be a product of the wear phenomenon of the hard and soft dental tissues. As stated in the definition of dentinal hypersensitivity and demanded by the hydrodynamic mechanism, dentin has to become exposed and the tubule system opened. These apparently different processes may be considered under the headings of *lesion localization* and *lesion initiation*.[4] Dentin exposure, le-

---

BOX 33-1

DEMOGRAPHICS OF DENTINAL HYPERSENSITIVITY

- Fifteen percent of individuals will have one or more episodes of dentinal hypersensitivity.
- The peak incidence for dentinal hypersensitivity is 20 to 40 years.
- The incidence of dentinal hypersensitivity is greater in women.
- Dental hygienists report twice the level of dentinal hypersensitivity in patients than is reported by dentists.
- Canines and first premolars are most often affected; the next most affected teeth are the incisors and second premolars, with molars being least affected by dentinal hypersensitivity.

---

sion localization, and dentinal hypersensitivity can occur only through loss of periodontal tissues, gingival recession, or loss of enamel and tooth wear.

GINGIVAL RECESSION

Apical migration of the gingival margin along the root surface is one of the least understood and least researched areas of dentistry.[157,170] This is particularly the case in the most common type of recession, in which the gingival tissues are otherwise healthy. Indeed, it would appear that healthy recession is most commonly associated with true dentinal hypersensitivity. This lack of knowledge led one author to describe gingival recession like dentinal hypersensitivity had been previously—as an enigmatic condition.[157]

Of course, other types of gingival recession are described (and at least some evidence exists regarding their cause). These include recession associated with acute and chronic periodontal diseases, periodontal treatments, and factitious injury. The few reviews on the subject of gingival recession and numerous statements made in other publications identify toothbrushing as an causative factor.[157,170] The supportive data comes from epidemiologic studies, case reports, and anecdote—making the evidence circumstantial rather than factual. Much of the epidemiologic data are similar for dentinal hypersensitivity, gingival recession, and plaque biofilm scores (particularly in respect to distribution).

> **Note**
> Teeth and tooth surfaces that receive most attention during the brushing cycle overall show the highest predilection for recession, with a more common incidence on the left side in societies where a majority is right handed.

Healthy gingival recession thus shows side, site, and tooth number distributions that coincide with toothbrushing habits and handedness.[12]

Plaque biofilm scores derived from epidemiologic and clinical studies also correlate with sites of gingival recession and, for that matter, dentinal hypersensitivity, coinciding with the lowest plaque biofilm scores.[12-14] In some individuals and at some sites, some predisposing factors for recession must be anatomical and related to missing or fenestration of facial and lingual alveolar bone. Although circumstantial, the evidence that toothbrushing is involved in gingival recession is compelling; however, randomized controlled clinical data are needed to prove a causal relationship. The mechanism of healthy gingival recession as a result of chronic trauma has only been hypothesized, with the exception of the questionable value of animal research data.

Much is made of the features of toothbrushing habits, such as frequency, method, and force, as well as the characteristics of the toothbrush used. These observations appear to be total conjecture and are based on logical rather than biological premises. Two notable omissions from the debate are (1) the role of toothpaste in

> **Note**
> The type of gingival recession most commonly associated with dentinal hypersensitivity appears also to be associated with good oral hygiene.[12]

gingival recession and (2) the relationship of recording gingival excoriation after toothbrushing and possible relevance to recession. In conclusion, the type of gingival recession most commonly associated with dentinal hypersensitivity appears also to be associated with good oral hygiene.[12]

★ CASE APPLICATION 33-1.1

Etiology of Dentinal Hypersensitivity

Ms. Yamagashi's clinical findings would lead one to investigate the gingival recession and health of the gingival tissues. What might be the cause of Ms. Yamagashi's pain?

Should the hygienist review toothbrushing habits with Ms. Yamagashi?

TOOTH WEAR

Exposure of dentin through loss of enamel means the lesions of dentinal hypersensitivity could be localized at any tooth surface; however, by virtue of enamel thickness, the cervical areas should show the highest predilection.* *Tooth wear* is a composite term encompassing the three processes by which hard dental tissue may be lost:

1. Abrasion
2. Attrition
3. Erosion[22,112,113]

The tooth wear observed on any one tooth may be a combination of two or more of the wear processes, even though in a particular individual one may dominate. Several lengthy texts are available on tooth wear and its individual facets. Much of the data are derived from epidemiologic surveys,[104,128] a large and increasing number of studies *in vitro,* and a smaller number of studies (at present) *in situ.*† From this large and expanding database on tooth wear, this chapter concentrates on evidence concerned with localization and initiation of lesions of dentinal hypersensitivity.

Clearly, attrition can expose dentin at occlusal and incisal surfaces, particularly in individuals with parafunctional habits such as bruxism.[122] Furthermore, case reports of dentinal hypersensitivity at occlusal surfaces are available. However, the role of attrition alone or combined with abrasion or erosion has received little research attention; therefore wear of facial cervical enamel by abrasion (toothbrushing) and erosion alone or combined is discussed in this chapter.

Toothbrushes alone have no effect on enamel. The majority of toothpastes contain abrasives, which are softer than enamel and therefore cause minute amounts of enamel wear in a lifetime's use.[6] The very rare exceptions are toothpastes that contain nonhydrated alumina that can abrade enamel (although few data are available to support this theory). Enamel is, however, very susceptible to acid erosion where the acids can be derived from intrinsic (gastric) or, more often, extrinsic (dietary)

sources.[177,178] Evidence drawn from studies *in situ* reveal that individuals who consume 1 L of soft drinks per day, which is not uncommon, can lose 1 mm of enamel in 2 to 20 years.[90] The range is large because individual susceptibility to erosion varies considerably.[90] Such a rate of enamel loss at the facial cervical area means that dentin can readily become exposed.

The erosion process has two parts:

1. Irreversible loss of enamel by acid dissolution
2. Enamel softening to a depth of several microns[58]

DENTAL CONSIDERATIONS

Softened enamel is extremely fragile and can be removed by minor physical traumas, including toothbrushing even without toothpaste.[55,56] Indeed one study *in vitro* showed that softened enamel can be removed by licking action of the tongue.[75]

In summary, erosion and toothbrush-toothpaste abrasion can cooperate additively, even synergistically,[47,56] to remove enamel to expose dentin (particularly at the facial cervical area). This raises the question concerning the timing of toothbrushing following meals.

> **Prevention**
>
> Given the preventive rather than therapeutic action of toothpaste, the logical, if not biological, regimen must be to brush before meals.[16] The idea of delaying toothbrushing after meals to allow rehardening of the softened enamel has also been suggested, but this may take several hours.[57]

OPENING OF TUBULES

The initiation of dentinal hypsersensitivity lesions by exposing the dentin tubule network could occur by physical or chemical means (or by both), which essentially represent tooth wear processes applied to dentin. What attrition produces on dentin is not known; the possible effects of toothbrushing and erosion alone, and combined on dentin, is discussed here. The majority of conclusions are drawn from studies *in vitro,* with some from studies *in situ.* The research relevant to dentinal hypersensitivity considers the effect of wear on the **smear layer** that, in experimental models, covers the tubules and is about 1 mcm thick. The smear layer is produced by abrasion of the plastic dentin and consists of hydroxyapatite and collagen. Whether the same or a similar layer is present *in vivo* is not known; however, as stated previously, nonsensitive, exposed dentin surfaces have very few exposed tubules[2] and, presumably, a calcified covering layer must be derived from the dentin itself or from saliva.

A toothbrush alone causes minimal wear to dentin, and a study *in vitro* demonstrated that removal of the smear layer to open tubules took several hours of constant brushing (equivalent to several years of normal toothbrushing).[1] These data essentially rule out the toothbrush alone as a causative factor in dentinal hypersensitivity. When toothpaste enters the scenario, the outcome is markedly and variably changed, depending on the toothpaste used. Studies *in vitro* and *in situ* indicate that most toothpastes readily

> **Note**
>
> A toothbrush alone causes minimal wear to dentin.[1]

---

*References 22, 91, 112, 113, 122, 128, 177, 178.
†References 22, 91, 112, 113, 122, 128, 177, 178.

remove the smear layer to initially open tubules and in a time frame equivalent to a few days of normal toothbrushing.[21,172] This can be explained by the action of both the abrasives and the detergents. Some narrowing of the tubule orifices may occur with more brushing; however, essentially, most products expose tubules. Some formulations, notably those containing artificial silicas with nonionic detergents, occlude the tubules with a plug of the contained silica.[21] Most conventional toothpastes contain the anionic detergent, sodium lauryl sulfate, which appears to prevent the uptake of silicas to the dentin surface. Some desensitizing toothpastes contain active ingredients to occlude tubules, such as strontium. Unfortunately, no direct evidence indicates that strontium salts directly occlude tubules. In fact, the available evidence contradicts such an effect.[10,106]

Dentin is more susceptible to erosion than enamel but also shows the same irreversible loss and surface softening.[92,168] The softened zone of dentin is similarly weak to that of enamel and easily removed physically.[75] Soft drinks; some alcoholic beverages; and acidic foods, including yogurt, readily dissolve the smear layer to expose tubules and in a very short time[1] (Figure 33-3). In addition, some mouthrinses with pH levels below 5 remove the smear layer, again in a short time frame.[7,21,139] Because of the softened zone, erosion and toothbrush-toothpaste abrasion clearly can interact to remove dentin and expose tubules.

> **Note**
> Erosion and toothbrush-toothpaste abrasion can interact to remove dentin and expose tubules.

> **Note**
> Unfortunately, what little evidence is available suggests softened dentin is slow to remineralize, if at all.[168]

Evidence is available that strongly suggests that dentinal hypersensitivity lesions can be localized through dentin exposure by the effects of toothbrushing and erosion alone or combined, causing gingival recession or loss of enamel. Gingival recession is probably the more important factor in the exposure of dentin. Similarly, the initiation of dentinal hypersensitivity, through tubule opening, can occur through toothbrushing with toothpaste and erosion, again alone or combined. Available data suggest that erosion is the more dominant factor. The overall conclusion must therefore be that dentinal hypersensitivity results from the wear of dental and gingival tissues.

> **Note**
> Dentinal hypersensitivity results from the wear of dental and gingival tissues.

Management Strategies for Dentinal Hypersensitivity

An ideal treatment for dentinal hypersensitivity would be one that provides immediate and lasting relief of pain.[5] Clinical experience suggests that the professional approach to dentinal hypersensitivity has been heavily treatment based, with little regard for the control of the causative and predisposing factors that created the problem. This is perhaps not surprising because sufferers and practitioners are virtually bombarded with a vast array of products formulated to treat dentinal hypersensitivity. The global sensitivity survey[31] indicated that dental professionals were confident concerning the diagnosis of dentinal hypersensitivity but not in its management.

Reviewing dentinal hypersensitivity clinical trials helps explain this conundrum. The literature contains evidence for the apparent **efficacy** of a wide range of quite different, if not bizarre, agents for the treatment of dentinal hypersensitivity. In explanation, the protocols for comparing different agents are not standardized, resulting in numerous variables to be compared. A paste with an active agent may be tested against its base paste, a conventional fluoride paste, or another paste with an active agent. Treatments rarely take into account causative factors, and the measurement of pain is difficult to standardize between individuals because of its subjective nature. Other complicating factors in research studies, such as the **placebo effect, Hawthorn effect, regression to the mode,** and **control product effect,** compound the interpretation of clinical findings and hide the true effect of the treatment. For example, in one study[174] the placebo effect was shown to reduce the possibility of identifying whether the agent being tested was effective by 40%.

The clinical efficacy of many of the current products tested also appears to be at the lower end of the therapeutic range. This may be because of any of the following conditions:

- Low success rate of the agent reaching the target site
- Lack of sensitivity of the clinical trial
- Lack of understanding of the patients' interpretation of the pain-evoking stimuli
- Recovery time between repeated stimulation
- Clinician-patient relationship
- Potency of the active agent

As with all conditions or diseases, management strategies, which include treatment, are usually more successful than treatment alone.[130] Failure to consider **causation** in the management of dentinal hypersensitivity (as is the case with dental

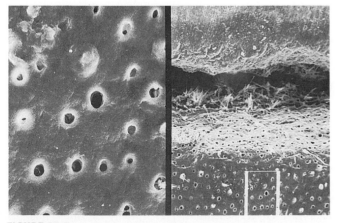

FIGURE 33-3
Sensitive dentin under high magnification. Reader should note the open tubules. (From Addy M: Etiology and clinical implications of dentine hypersensitivity, *Dent Clin North Am* 34[3]:150, 1990.)

caries and periodontal disease) may result in recurrence or failure of treatment. Unfortunately, unlike management strategies for dental caries and periodontal disease, management strategies for dentinal hypersensitivity are not based on clinical data but on the logic derived from the current understanding of the nature of the cause and risk factors for the condition.

Logic-based strategies (based on what seems to be appropriated based on one's senses) and biology-based strategies (based on information obtained from the body's response) are often not the same. With that in mind, proposed management strategy for dentin hypersensitivity can be found in Box 33-2.

ALTERATION OF FLUID FLOW IN DENTINAL TUBULES

Obturation of Dentinal Tubules with Toothpastes or Restorations

Current evidence indicates individuals with dentinal hypersensitivity have dentinal tubules that are patent from the pulp to the oral environment. Clinical evidence shows that dentin surfaces have more and wider tubules than nonsensitive dentin.[3] Based on the hydrodynamic theory, if the tubules are occluded anywhere along their length, then hydraulic conductance will be reduced.[27,79,99]

> *Prevention*
> If the tubules are blocked, then the sharp, shooting dentinal pain symptoms should stop.

The most direct approach to desensitizing dentin is occlusion of the tubule opening. Toothpastes components, such as silica abrasives[6,9,13] or active agents, have been proposed to occlude tubules. Surface barriers can also be professionally applied in many forms:

- Varnishes
- Dentin-bonding agents
- Composite resins
- Glass ionomer cements and compomers

The effectiveness of the tubular occluding agents will depend on their resistance to removal. *In vitro* results demonstrate a number of agents can occlude tubules, but this does not necessarily correlate to the *in vivo* situation in which they must be resistant to the oral challenges of day-to-day activity. Occluding materials can easily be washed from the tubule or may be dissolved by acid. Wear can also occur (e.g., abrading the surface of a dentin-bonding agent or glass ionomer).

Other methods of reducing tubule diameter are stimulation of **intratubular (peritubular)** dentin and the production of **reactionary dentin** and **reparative tertiary dentin.** Tubular occlusion may also be achieved by coagulating the tubular protoplasm with a chemical treatment or a chemical ion, resulting in precipitation of a component in the protoplasmic fluid that creates a tubular plug.

MODIFICATION OR BLOCKING OF PULPAL NERVE RESPONSE

Chemically with Potassium Ions

Potassium ions may reduce the excitability of the intradental nerve by spreading out along the tubules and raising the concentration of extracellular potassium ions blocking the intradental nerve function.[114] This hypothesis is based on animal experiments and has not been confirmed on human teeth (in which the diffusion distances are greater[136] and a continual outward flow of dentinal fluid to the oral environment occurs[169] that tends to oppose any inward diffusion).[135]

Physically with Endodontics or Extraction

Obviously, these methods are permanently effective at stopping pain from dentin hypersensitivity by removing the nerve or tooth.

Any treatment will not be optimal if these factors are not considered and modified accordingly. Various ideal features have been suggested in an attempt to clarify the requirements necessary for a satisfactory treatment material.[40,78] Recommendations for an ideal dentin hypersensitivity treatment material are as follows:

- Easy to administer
- Requires minimal number of dental appointments

BOX 33-2

DIFFERENTIAL DIAGNOSIS OF DENTINAL HYPERSENSITIVITY

- Ensure the correct diagnosis of dentinal hypersensitivity is based on a history and examination, which is compatible with the clinical descriptor contained in the definition.
- Consider a differential diagnosis as suggested by the definition of dentinal hypersensitivity, which may alone explain the symptoms or identify the presence of other conditions contributing to the pain of dentinal hypersensitivity.
- If present, treat all secondary conditions, which are contributing symptoms similar to dentinal hypersensitivity.
- Identify causative and predisposing factors, particularly in respect to erosion and abrasion. Detailed dietary histories, in writing, should be considered. Oral hygiene habits should form part of the history, including frequency, duration, and timing of brushing; brushing technique; estimation of brushing force; frequency of brush change; and appearance of brush at change. A medium brush is recommended, because a soft head can hold more toothpaste and cause greater abrasion.[53] Toothbrushing behavior is often best appraised by observing the patient brushing.
- Remove or modify identified causative or predisposing factors. In particular, offer dietary advice to minimize erosion and oral hygiene instruction to minimize abrasion, as well as to separate abrasion from erosion.
- Recommend or provide treatments that relate to the individual needs of the sufferer. The number of teeth involved and the severity of the pain are important variables, which should influence the treatment options.
     Two treatment approaches exist:
     1. Alteration of fluid flow in dentinal tubules
        - Obturation of dentinal tubules with toothpastes or restorations
     2. Modification or blocking of pulpal nerve response
        - Chemically with potassium ions
        - Physically with endodontics or extraction

- Requires shortest possible time per application
- Presents no danger to teeth, soft tissues, or system
- Causes no discoloration of teeth or soft tissues
- Gives the greatest assurance of success in the total eradication of pain and discomfort
- Results in the greatest permanence of relief
- Requires minimum expense

Although no material has yet met these proposals, prevention and relief of dentinal hypersensitivity has been accomplished by various methods.

Administration of Treatment

Treatment for dentinal hypersensitivity can be accomplished in the clinic or at home, depending on the degree of the problem and the dentist-patient preference. Home treatment usually involves toothpastes and mouthwashes, is by far the easiest method of administering treatment, and is fairly inexpensive.

Professional treatment includes the following:

- Application of sealants and restorations
- Laser treatment
- Endodontics
- Periodontal surgery such as gingival grafting to cover exposed root surfaces
- Prevention advice

The dental professional must choose which treatment option is best suited to each circumstance, with the possibility of more than one treatment method being used at any one time.

Similarly, stabilizing the sensory nerve membrane with potassium ions also can be effective. Obviously the clinician's aim is to alleviate and prevent pain, but treatment options will be influenced by the severity of the condition and the number of teeth involved.

Note

The more satisfactory treatments are those that permanently seal off the tubules without damaging the pulp and tooth or dampening neural impulses. By reducing the number of open tubules or their orifice diameter, dentin becomes less permeable and fluid flow is less marked; therefore the sensory nerves will not be activated and no pain will be perceived.

OVER-THE-COUNTER PRODUCTS USED IN THE MANAGEMENT OF DENTINAL HYPERSENSITIVITY

A wide range of commercially available products is manufactured for self-treatment. Products in the marketplace such as toothpastes, gels, and mouthrinses include components to reduce dentinal hypersensitivity:

- Potassium
- Strontium
- Oxalate
- Fluoride salts

One of the difficulties in the interpretation of the data for the efficacy (i.e., effectiveness) of agents and products must be the quality of earlier studies. Newer study protocols have improved with the introduction of *Guidelines for Good Clinical Practice* for clinical trials.[94]

Strontium Salts

Toothpastes containing strontium salts have dominated the market of desensitizing pastes for the last 30 years and have therefore been subjected to most methods of testing for efficacy.[103] Studies conducted in the late 1990s reported on the product's use in treating dentinal hypersensitivity and indicated that repeated use increased its effectiveness. It was concluded that strontium salts have equivocal beneficial effects at reducing dentinal hypersensitivity under numerous trial designs.[97,137,174]

The theory behind incorporating strontium salts in toothpastes comes from the ability of the salt to have a considerable affinity for dentin because of the high permeability and possibility for absorption into or onto the organic connective tissues and the odontoblast processes.[143] Researchers have proposed that strontium combines with dentin to form a strontium-apatite complex, with a significantly higher radiodensity than hydroxyapatite.[66]

Note

Strontium salts have equivocal beneficial effects at reducing dentinal hypersensitivity.

Note

Strontium combines with dentin to form a strontium-apatite complex that has a significantly higher radiodensity than hydroxyapatite.[66]

Strontium chloride

A review of strontium chloride studies found in the literature* indicated no definite conclusion as to the efficacy of strontium chloride for the management of dentin hypersensitivity. Some studies found a significant reduction in dentinal hypersensitivity,† whereas other studies reported no significant differences between groups using other ingredients.‡ Many factors within the studies and subjects affected the outcomes of these studies, and study protocols varied considerably, making complete comparisons difficult.

Strontium acetate

Several studies investigating the efficacy of strontium acetate compared with other desensitizing agents have been conducted with varying results.[11,97,137,174]

Work in vitro with the strontium acetate toothpaste has been very promising, achieving good tubule occlusion of etched dentin (but because of the silica abrasive).[9,21,173] Even more exciting was the finding that the silica layer was not removed when rinsed.[9] Unfortunately, these properties have not been demonstrated with the same success in the treatment of dentinal hypersensitivity clinically (Figure 33-4).

---

*References 16, 20, 24, 33, 41, 70, 86, 100, 137, 152, 154, 156, 160, 166, 180.
†References 24, 33, 41, 86, 100, 160, 166.
‡References 16, 20, 70, 137, 152, 156, 180.

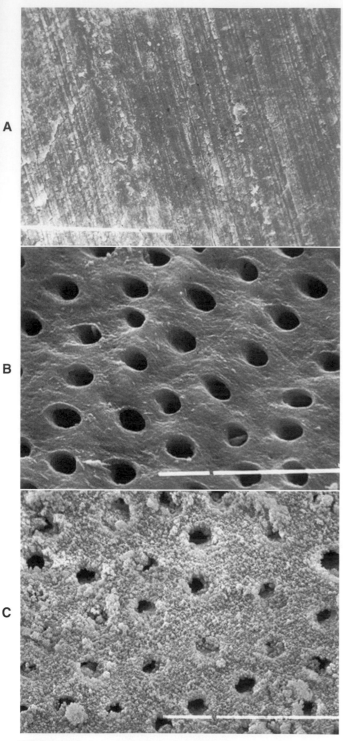

FIGURE 33-4
A, Smear layer of dentin. **B,** Open dentinal tubules. **C,** Silica occluding open dentin tubules.

Potassium Salts

The most frequently used potassium salts are nitrates, chloride, citrates, and oxalates. A number of studies have investigated potassium salts, with results showing an improvement in the patients' perceived symptoms of dentinal hypersensitivity.[161,176] Furthermore, and more importantly, studies on toothpastes by a number of authors have demonstrated a significant or favorable benefit from a potassium-based paste over a control paste,* although other studies failed to show these beneficial effects.[69,174]

Particular attention has been focused on potassium nitrate, resulting in a Cochrane review.[140] Because of the rigors of this type of analysis (a meta-analysis), very few of all the papers in this field could be incorporated (indeed only four). Subsequently the conclusion published was that no strong evidence supports the efficacy of potassium nitrate for the treatment of dentinal hypersensitivity. This again reiterates the need to look carefully at trial design for future studies to try to achieve more meaningful data.

> **Note**
> Potassium salts are now the most commonly used agents for the treatment of dentinal hypersensitivity being incorporated into toothpastes and mouthrinses.

Oxalates

The idea of **oxalates** acting as desensitizing agents has gained popularity. The mode of action has been proposed as tubule occlusion by oxalate ions reacting with calcium ions in the dentinal fluid to form insoluble calcium oxalate crystals, 1 to 2 mcm in diameter, deposited in the tubule apertures.[74] This was confirmed with x-ray diffractometer analysis.[126] A recent in vitro study[158] evaluated the effects of preapplication or postapplication of calcium chloride on occluding ability of potassium oxalate—the calcium potentially enhancing uptake. However, results showed no significant difference between the treatments. In vitro work has shown that although oxalates result in good tubule occlusion, they can be easily washed from the surface of dentin from acids in the oral environment.[10,21]

The following oxalate salts are used in commercially available products:

- Potassium
- Citrate
- Ferric
- Dipotassium
- Monohydrogen-monopotassium

Dipotassium oxalate produced fewer but significantly larger calcium oxalate crystals than monohydrogen-monopotassium oxalate; however, the larger crystals were not as effective at occluding the open tubules.[133] Monohydrogen-monopotassium oxalate also had a pH lower than dipotassium oxalate, 3.0 and 5.6, respectively; therefore the former released a much higher concentration of calcium ions from dentin and accelerated crystal formation. In summary, oxalates appear to have limited ability to reduce the pain from dentinal hypersensitivity.

> **Note**
> Oxalates appear to have limited ability to reduce the pain from dentinal hypersensitivity.

Fluorides

Incorporation of fluoride in the majority of toothpastes is now favored by most pharmaceutical companies because of its proven beneficial effects on reduction of dental caries. Various

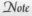

---

*References 36, 129, 145, 148, 153-154.

fluoride compounds have been documented for the treatment of dentinal hypersensitivity:

- Sodium fluoride
- Sodium silicofluoride
- Stannous fluoride
- Sodium monofluorophosphate

Sodium fluoride and silicofluoride

Many investigators have found fluoride toothpaste and high concentrations of fluoride solutions highly effective in the treatment of dentinal hypersensitivity.[11,38,66,125,162] In today's market, toothpastes are produced with very high sodium fluoride, 2800 ppm, and marketed for the treatment of dentinal hypersensitivity. A combination of products has sometimes appeared of value. The addition of 2% sodium fluoride solution, applied after the individual was pretreated with 10% strontium chloride solution, produced greater reduction in sensitivity than fluoride alone.[66] This, however, was demonstrated for only one parameter (cold air), and no placebo or control was used in the investigation. Fluoride treatment alone resulted in a considerable reduction in sensitivity. The placebo effect may explain this result.

In explanation of the effects of sodium fluoride on tooth sensitivity, SEM with x-ray diffraction analysis revealed that deposition of precipitated calcium fluoride occurred in the peritubular dentin after 2% sodium fluoride solution administration. This was thought to be the result of the interaction of fluoride ions with dentinal fluid that is saturated with calcium and phosphate ions.[54] This concept was also supported in another study in which calcium fluoride or fluorapatite was reported to reduce the functional radius of the dentinal tubules.[159] However, calcium fluoride crystals are very small and do not totally occlude tubules. This may explain why a single dose was not particularly effective compared with oxalates.[133] Fluoride salts possess a considerable affinity for the dentin surface but do not occlude the tubules.[10] It has been suggested that fluoride may eventually mechanically block the tubules or that fluoride in the organic matrix of the dentin blocks the transmission of stimuli. The former view would support Brännström's hydrodynamic theory[27] and is favored by others.[74]

Stannous fluoride

The efficacy of aqueous stannous fluoride has been documented with regards to reducing dentinal hypersensitivity.[100,123] Immediate relief with topical stannous fluoride had been demonstrated.[163] In contrast, other studies could not demonstrate a positive result with a 0.4% stannous fluoride with 0.76% sodium monofluorophosphate toothpaste.[26,85]

Various concepts have been suggested for the mechanism of stannous fluoride in the management of dentinal hypersensitivity. First, it acts as an enzyme poison to inactivate the odontoblast processes.[64] This seems unlikely because the odontoblast is believed to play no role in the transmission of the stimuli.[30] Second, it may just precipitate on the dentin surface to occlude the tubules.[25]

Using SEM with microprobe analysis, tin and fluoride have been identified on the dentin surface after treatment with stannous fluoride.[59] A heavy deposit of tin salts on the dentin surface, that could not be removed by rinsing, has been observed.[10] Furthermore, a more recent in situ report[124] demonstrated a tin-rich surface deposit occluding nearly all open tubules in a dentin disc after 2 weeks of brushing with an anhydrous stannous fluoride gel. Substantial structural fluoride was also deposited in this dentin.

Sodium monofluorophosphate

Sodium monofluorophosphate has been incorporated in toothpastes for many years to reduce the incidence of dental caries. It may also aid the reduction of dentinal hypersensitivity.[26,60,86,121] Higher concentrations of fluoride, however, were not shown to be any more effective.[83] In contrast, another study found no significant difference between sodium monofluorophosphate, strontium chloride, and placebo toothpastes.[152]

As with many of these compounds, the exact mechanism of action is unknown. Interaction of fluoride with enamel is thought to result in the formation of fluoroapatite.[77] Further evidence has shown sodium monofluorophosphate to have a protective effect on the dentin surface against acid attack, reducing enamel solubility.[48,63] SEM data *in vitro* showed sodium monofluorophosphate had no effect on the dentin surface after treatment, leaving the tubules patent.[25] An increased resistance of dentin to electrical stimuli was found with the use of sodium monofluorophosphate.[8]

More recent findings suggest that sodium fluoride is superior to sodium monofluorophosphate regarding fluoride deposition on the teeth.[52] The fact that dentinal hypersensitivity is still a large problem in populations that use a fluoridated toothpaste and live in fluoridated-water regions is interesting; this may be caused by the delivery system.[50] The majority of toothpastes now contain fluoride in some form, as do many mouthwashes. In addition, specifically designed mouthwashes for high fluoride uptake are available; however, the incidence of dentinal hypersensitivity remains high.

Sodium Citrate Pluronic F-127 Gel

Sodium citrate pluronic F-127 gel has been shown to significantly reduce the hydraulic conductance of dentin *in vitro*.[42,74] Researchers have proposed that the polyglycol found in this compound may decrease dentinal hypersensitivity by protein precipitation in the tubular contents, or that mucins from saliva may precipitate out and reduce tubular size by adhering to the dentin surface.[120,171] The combined activity of the ingredients seems to result in the production of citrate anions derived from sodium citrate and citric acid complexing with calcium on the surface of the dentin to form a nonionized complex.[119] As for the action of sodium citrate, only a weak reduction in sensory nerve activity was achieved in an animal model.[105]

Other Agents

The effectiveness of a home-use dental rinse containing aluminum lactate was compared with a control rinse. Sensitivity decreased significantly at weeks 4 and 6, compared with the baseline for both agents. More importantly, the hypersensitivity scores for tactile, cold-air, and cold-water stimuli in the test group were significantly lower at weeks 4 or 6 (or at both), compared with those in the control group.[88] This trial suggests that daily home use of a dental rinse containing aluminum lactate may be effective for treatment of dentinal hypersensitivity. However, more research is needed.

PROFESSIONALLY APPLIED PRODUCTS USED IN THE MANAGEMENT OF DENTINAL HYPERSENSITIVITY

Again a wide range of commercially available products is available for professional treatment. In-office treatments tend to be reserved for the individuals who have received preventive advice and have tried at-home products but found them ineffective (Box 33-3).

BOX 33-3

PROFESSIONALLY APPLIED AGENTS FOR DENTINAL HYPERSENSITIVITY

- Two-percent acidulated sodium fluoride
- Fluoride varnish
- Oxalates
- Alternative Chinese traditional medicine (brushing with a mixture of Dahurian angelica root, the root of Chinese wild ginger, puncture vine, the rhizome of *Davallia,* peppermint, and gallnut)[179]
- Burnishing alone
- Burnishing with hydrogen phosphate or 33% sodium fluoride
- Calcium-fluoride varnish solution

Varnishes and Precipitants

Professionally applied sodium fluoride has been used to treat dentinal hypersensitivity.[39]

A crossover study was conducted in which patients were first treated with fluoride and, if unsuccessful, glass ionomer was used—the latter being significantly more effective.[82]

Another way of applying fluoride is in the form of a varnish. A varnish can set by releasing ethanol and taking up moisture. In this way the insoluble resins, in the shape of a sticky-plastic congealing film, gradually fall out (e.g., sodium fluoride is thought to dissolve and deposit on the tooth). Observation shows that this methodology reduces pain of dentinal hypersensitivity for as long as the film is on the tooth. Although several authors demonstrate a distinct enrichment of the surface enamel with such a varnish,[19,138] the varnish may be effective because of occlusion of the tubules by the resin rather than by the effect of the fluoride.

Oxalates such as fluoride have also been professionally applied; however, success rates for efficacy are uncertain. A recent clinical trial investigated a 1-minute application of ferric oxalate versus placebo treatment.[67] However, no significant differences were noted. After 4 weeks, one study found benefit with potassium oxalate,[127] yet another could not show efficacy over an adhesive primer.[68]

Other Treatment Modalities

Alternative treatment regimens are those of Chinese traditional medicine, which are becoming more and more popular in the Western world, particularly when treatment fails by orthodox methods. Dentinal hypersensitivity has been treated successfully in China by brushing on a mixture of the root of Dahurian angelica, the root of Chinese wild ginger, puncture vine, the rhizome of *Davallia,* peppermint, and gallnut.[179] Unfortunately no clinical trials have yet been undertaken.

In the past, calcium hydroxide was a popular agent for the treatment of dentinal hypersensitivity.[73,101,108] Calcium hydroxide can cause hypermineralization of cementum and increased mineralization of peritubular dentin, thus decreasing the radius of the dentinal tubule and fluid flow,[74] as well as creating tubular occlusion, by binding to the protein radicals.[119] Researchers have noted that calcium ions may decrease nerve excitability; however, at least one study failed to come to this conclusion when testing cat canine teeth. Calcium hydroxide is insoluble and unable to release many free calcium ions.[164] This agent is rarely used today.

Burnishing dentin, particularly with an orangewood stick, has been advocated for alleviating the symptoms of sensitivity, resulting in the formation of a smear layer that partially occludes opened tubules.[134] Second, it may cause the odontoblasts to produce tertiary dentin, although this hypothesis seems less plausible.[134] Root surfaces burnished with calcium hydrogen phosphate were relieved of hypersensitivity, whereas

---

Note
A calcium-fluoride varnish solution is currently marketed that also contains silica, giving good clinical results.

Prevention
Presently an oxalate solution has shown some effectiveness in treating dentinal hypersensitivity.[144]

Prevention
Burnishing dentin with an orangewood stick has been advocated for alleviating the symptoms of sensitivity.

Prevention
The effectiveness of a single application of 2% acidulated sodium fluoride produced fluoride levels detectable for 14 days and general improvement for 6 months.[54]

those treated without the mineral paste did not benefit.[87] Burnishing 33% sodium fluoride on the root surface was superior to plain burnishing.[162] The addition of multiple compounds (glycerin, sodium fluoride, and kaolin) was tried but did not improve dentinal hypersensitivity.[134] Glycerin alone was as effective as the combination of the ingredients.

Studies involving the use of corticosteroids have provided little evidence of efficacy, and their use is based on the assumption that hypersensitivity is linked to pulpal inflammation, which has not been proven. Other outdated forms of treatment for dentinal hypersensitivity include application of silver nitrate, zinc chloride, and formalin.

Restorative Materials

Glass ionomer, resin-reinforced glass ionomer and compomers, adhesive resin primers, and adhesive resin–bonding systems have been used successfully for the treatment of dentinal hypersensitivity. Treatment can be problematic if little tissue loss has occurred, and overcontouring can lead to plaque biofilm–retentive sites and gingival inflammation.[165] Furthermore, sufferers of dentinal hypersensitivity tend to be meticulous at cleaning their teeth, often using excessive brushing force on frequent occasions. Unless the toothbrushing habits are corrected, materials will be easily abraded and lost.

Glass ionomers have been used in the treatment of dentin hypersensitivity with good success.[82,110] Glass ionomer restorations are very effective because they bond to unprepared dentin and appear to have a good clinical life.[82,167] Some researchers have suggested that glass ionomer restorations release sufficient fluoride ions to aid in the treatment of sensitivity; however, this is not the case.

Cavity varnish can give temporary relief of symptoms when applied in a thin film on open dentinal tubules. Advances with cavity varnish have met with great success[80]; however, the smear layer must be modified or removed before application (to occlude the tubules and make the surface resistant to acidic attack).

The use of adhesive resin primer products *in vitro* is well documented in vitro to occlude tubules[155] and has been reported to be clinically effective.[93] However, this too has not been demonstrated clinically.[18] In theory, the concept is clear and practical, with the thin films occluding the tubules. However, sometimes failure of polymerization occurs, and the films can be easily abraded.

As resin-bonding systems have improved, success of treatment has improved from mechanical retention of tags in the tubules to chemically cured bonding agents. After the testing of a primer and conditioner, it was concluded that both were highly effective in reducing or eliminating dentin hypersensitivity for periods up to 6 months.[49] This finding was supported by the outcomes of another study.[115] Once the seal between the material and the root surface has broken down, dentin hypersensitivity may reoccur. The systems incorporating the primer and adhesive components together produce a thicker film and have been used with success.[144] A well-controlled study using another commercially available system again showed efficacy—

the surface not being etched before application of material.[95] The latest bonding systems are hydrophilic, designed to provide a better bond in a wet environment; however, the fluid should be water rather than other liquids.[175]

These materials are frequently used by clinicians for the treatment of dentinal hypersensitivity. Few well-controlled trials support their efficacy, but those that have been reported together with clinical experience support the use of these materials after use of preventive advice and home-use treatment, particularly for isolated teeth that are nonresponsive to other chemicals (Box 33-4).

BOX 33-4

AGGRESSIVE AND IRREVERSIBLE TREATMENTS FOR DENTINAL HYPERSENSITIVITY

- Restorative materials
  Glass ionomer
  Resin-reinforced glass ionomer and compomers
  Adhesive resin primers
  Adhesive resin–bonding systems
- Lasers
- Iontophoresis
- Periodontal surgery (gingival grafting or root coverage procedures)
- Endodontics
- Extractions

LASERS

Neodymium:yttrium-aluminum-garnet (Nd:YAG) laser irradiation has been advocated for the alleviation of symptoms from dentinal hypersensitivity and is thought to work by coagulation of proteins in the dentinal fluid (reducing permeability).[71] It is also believed to create an amorphous sealed layer on the dentin surface that appears to be caused by partial meltdown of the surface.[116] However, open peripheral tubules are possible, negating any benefit. The Nd:YAG (erbium) laser has been used with encouraging results.[107,142] Other clinical studies do not support this finding,[109] with the laser treatment reducing the pain sensation but not significantly different from the placebo treatment.

Recently the GaAlAs laser was compared with a fluoride varnish in a clinical trial,[43] with no significant differences found; an Er:YAG (erbium) laser[149] showed some effect compared with the control at low setting.

> *Note*
> The clinical results obtained from laser therapy do not seem to justify the high cost of the equipment needed for this purpose.

IONTOPHORESIS

Iontophoresis is another method that has been investigated for the treatment of dentinal hypersensitivity.

The mechanism is a negatively charged fluoride applicator on the tooth surface and the positive potential designed to facilitate entry of negative fluoride ions into the dentin.[98]

Iontophoresis is technically difficult and very operator sensitive, because the electric current can easily pass through the gingivae instead of the dentin.[37] Excellent results were found using an iontophoretic toothbrush with a toothpaste containing 2000 ppm of sodium fluoride.[98] Double-blind trials have been conducted[65,111] (as have open trials using iontophoresis with topical application of 2% sodium fluoride), with immediate success.[32] Open trials must be viewed with skepticism; the very act of using a different type of equipment to impart treatment often leads to a high placebo effect. The significant success of iontophoresis was conducted with neutral 2% sodium fluoride solution; out of 160 teeth, 134 displayed immediate desensitization, 16 displayed partial desensitization, and 10 displayed no effect at all. However, no controls were used in this investigation.[35] In another recent study, iontophoresis of fluoride and strontium ions were superior in their overall effects to potassium ions.[102] Different clinical trials have evaluated iontophoresis.* However, no substantial explanation has been found for the effect (if any) of iontophoresis.

PERIODONTAL SURGERY

Coronally repositioning periodontal flaps or gingival grafting procedures to cover areas of exposed dentin have been advocated as treatment regimens for dentinal hypersensitivity. Compared with the other modalities of treatment for this condition, periodontal surgery is an invasive procedure and results can be unpredictable because further recession is always possible.

ENDODONTICS AND EXTRACTION OF TEETH

As a last resort, endodontics and extraction of teeth have been used to alleviate the pain of dentinal hypersensitivity when all other methods of pain relief have failed.

Summary

Clinically, many treatment modalities are available for dentinal hypersensitivity that the clinician may find successful to alleviate this episodic condition. If one toothpaste is not found to be effective, then another may be used with success. The patient needs to try a number of different approaches. Unfortunately no one treatment seems to suit all patients. The least-invasive home care treatments are usually advocated first, followed by professional in-clinic treatment.

In recent years the standard of reporting in clinical trials has improved, particularly with the advent of Good Clinical Practice.[94] However, unequivocal data on efficacy of treatments for dentinal hypersensitivity have not been produced, despite good theory, in vitro data, and supporting clinical trials. Therefore attention must be focused on the design of the clinical trial to perfect a model that can differentiate among products and accommodate challenges such as the placebo effect.

Interestingly, surveys[62] and market research would suggest that a high proportion of individuals with dentinal hypersensitivity do not seek or receive treatment or take advantage of accessible home care products such as toothpastes medicated for the treatment of dentinal hypersensitivity. Because life expectancy has increased in the Western society and clearly includes the retention of a functional natural dentition prone to tooth wear,[104] we can expect that in the future more adults will report dentinal hypersensitivity and request treatment.

References

1. Absi EG, Addy M, Adams D: Dentinal sensitivity: the effects of toothbrushing and dietary compounds on dentin in vitro—a SEM study, *J Oral Rehabil* 19:101-110, 1992.
2. Absi EG, Addy M, Adams D: Dentinal sensitivity: the development and evaluation of a replica technique to study sensitive and nonsensitive cervical dentin, *J Clin Periodontol* 16:190, 1989.
3. Absi EG, Addy M, Adams D: Dentinal sensitivity: a study of the patency of dentinal tubules in sensitive and non-sensitive cervical dentin, *J Clin Periodontol* 14:280-284, 1987.
4. Addy M: Dentinal sensitivity: new perspectives on an old problem, *Int Dent J* 52(suppl):367-375, 2002.
5. Addy M: Clinical aspects of dentinal sensitivity, *Clin Mater* 7: 219-225, 1991.
6. Addy M, Hunter ML: Can tooth brushing damage your health? Effects on oral and dental tissues, *Int Dent J* 53:177-186, 2003.
7. Addy M, Loyn T, Adams D: Dentinal sensitivity-effects of some proprietary mouthwashes on the dentin smear layer: a SEM study, *J Dent* 19:145-152, 1991.
8. Addy M, Morgan T: The effect of toothpaste on the electrical resistance and scanning electron microscopic appearance of dentin, *J Dent Res* 102(61), 1982 (abstract).
9. Addy M, Mostafa P: Dentinal sensitivity II. Effects produced by the uptake in vitro of toothpastes onto dentin, *J Oral Rehabil* 16:35-48, 1989.
10. Addy M, Mostafa P: Dentinal sensitivity I. Effects produced by the uptake in vitro of metal ions, fluoride and formaldehyde onto dentin, *J Oral Rehabil* 15:575-585, 1988.
11. Addy M, Mostafa P, Newcombe RG: Dentinal sensitivity: a comparison of five toothpastes used during a 6-week period, *Br Dent J* 163:45-50, 1987.
12. Addy M, Mostafa P, Newcombe RG: Dentinal sensitivity: the distribution of recession, sensitivity and plaque, *J Dent* 15: 242-248, 1987.
13. Addy M et al: The effect of toothbrushing frequency, toothbrushing hand, sex and social class on the incidence of plaque, gingivitis and pocketing in adolescents: a longitudinal cohort study, *Community Dent Health* 7:237-247, 1990.
14. Addy M et al: The distribution of plaque and gingivitis and the influence of brushing hand in a group of 11-12 year old school children, *J Clin Periodontol* 14:564-572, 1987.
15. Adriaens PA, DeBoever JA, Loesche WJ: Bacterial invasion in root, cementum and radicular dentin of periodontally diseased teeth in humans—a reservoir of periodontopathic bacteria, *J Periodontol* 59:222-230, 1988.

*References 32, 65, 98, 102, 112.

16. Anderson DJ, Matthews B: An investigation into the reputed desensitizing effect of applying silver nitrate and strontium chloride to human dentin, *Arch Oral Biol* 11:1129-1135, 1966.

17. Anderson DJ, Ronning GA: Osmotic excitants of pain in human dentin, *Arch Oral Biol* 7:513-523, 1962.

18. Anderson MH, Powell LV: Desensitization of exposed dentin using a dentin bonding system, *J Dent Res* 73:297, 1994 (abstract).

19. Arends J, Lodding A, Petersson LG: Fluoride uptake in enamel, *Caries Res* 14:403, 1980.

20. Auvenshine RC, Eames WB: The biological effects of a desensitizing solution of the gingival and pulp tissues, *J Ala Dent Assoc* 56:17, 1972.

21. Banfield N, Addy M: Dentinal sensitivity: development and evaluation of a model in situ to study tubule patency, *J Clin Periodontol* 31:325-335, 2004.

22. Bartlett D, Smith BGN: Definition, classification, and clinical assessment of attrition, erosion and abrasion of enamel and dentin. In Addy M et al, eds: *Tooth wear and sensitivity,* Martin Dunitz, 2000, London.

23. Bevenius J, Lindskog S, Hultenby K: The micromorphology in vivo of the buccocervical region of premolar teeth in young adults. A replica study by scanning electron microscopy, *Acta Odontol Scand* 52:323-334, 1994.

24. Blitzer B: A consideration of the possible causes of dental hypersensitivity: treatment by a strontium dentifrice, *Periodontics* 5:318-321, 1967.

25. Blunden R et al: The effects of compounds used clinically in the management of dentinal sensitivity on some physical properties of dentin, *J Dent Res* 60:1981 (abstract).

26. Bolden TE, Volpe AR, King WJ: The desensitizing effect of a sodium monofluorophosphate dentifrice, *Periodontics* 6:112-114, 1968.

27. Brännström M: A hydrodynamic mechanism in the transmission of pain-produced stimuli through the dentin. In Anderson DJ, ed: *Sensory mechanisms in dentin,* Oxford, 1963, Pergamon Press.

28. Brännström M: The elicitation of pain in human dentin and pulp by chemical stimuli, *Arch Oral Biol* 7:59-62, 1962.

29. Brännström M, Aström A: The hydrodynamics of the dentin: its possible relationship to dentinal pain, *Int Dent J* 22:219-227, 1972.

30. Brännström M, Lindén L-Å, Johnson G: Movement of dentinal and pulp fluid caused by clinical procedures, *J Dent Res* 47:679-682, 1968.

31. Canadian Advisory Board on Dentinal Sensitivity: Consensus-based recommendations for the diagnosis and management of dentinal sensitivity, *J Can Dent Assoc* 69:221-228, 2003.

32. Carlo GT, Ciancio SG, Seyrek SK: An evaluation of iontophoretic application of fluoride for tooth desensitization, *J Am Dent Assoc* 105:452-454, 1982.

33. Carrasco PH: Strontium chloride toothpaste effectiveness as related to duration of use, *Pharmacol Ther Dent* 1:209-215, 1971.

34. Chabanski M et al: Prevalence of cervical dentin sensitivity in a population of patients referred to a specialist periodontology department, *J Clin Periodontol* 23:989-992, 1996.

35. Chen X, Morihana T, Gangarosa LP: Four year summary of dentinal sensitivity incidence and treatment by iontophoresis in dental students, *Arch Oral Biol* 39(suppl):125, 1994.

36. Chesters R et al: Use of multiple sensitivity measurements and logic statistical analysis to assess the effectiveness of a potassium-citrate-containing dentifrice in reducing dentinal hypersensitivity, *J Clin Periodontol* 19:256-261, 1992.

37. Ciancio SG: Delivery systems and clinical significance of available agents for dentinal hypersensitivity, *Endod Dent Traumatol* 2:150-152, 1986.

38. Clark DC, Al-Joburi W, Chan ECS: The efficacy of a new dentifrice in treating dentin sensitivity: effects of sodium citrate and sodium fluoride as active ingredients, *J Periodontal Res* 22:89-93, 1987.

39. Clark DC et al: The effectiveness of a fluoride varnish and a desensitizing toothpaste in treating dentinal sensitivity, *J Dent Res* 20:212, 1985.

40. Colaneri JN: A simple treatment of hypersensitive cervical dentin, *Oral Surg Oral Med Oral Pathol* 5:276-279, 1952.

41. Collaert B, Speelman J: The treatment of dentinal sensitivity, *Rev Belge Med Dent* 46(2):63-73, 1991.

42. Collins JF, Perkins L: Clinical evaluation of the effectiveness of three dentifrices in relieving dentin sensitivity, *J Periodontol* 55:720, 1984.

43. Corona SA et al: Clinical evaluation of low-level therapy and fluoride varnish for treating cervical dentinal hypersensitivity, *J Oral Rehabil* 30(12):1183-1189, 2003.

44. Council on Dental Therapeutics: *Accepted dental therapeutics,* ed 40, Chicago, 1984, American Dental Association.

45. Dababneh RH, Khouri AT, Addy M: Dentinal sensitivity-an enigma? A review of terminology, epidemiology, mechanisms, aetiology and management, *Br Dent J* 187:606-611, 1999.

46. Dachi SF: The relationship of pulpitis and hyperaemia to thermal sensitivity, *Oral Surg Oral Med Oral Pathol* 19:776-785, 1965.

47. Davis WB, Winter PJ: The effect of abrasion on enamel and dentin after exposure to dietary acid, *Br Dent J* 148:253, 1980.

48. Davis WB, Winter PJ: Dietary erosion of adult dentin and enamel protection with a fluoride toothpaste, *Br Dent J* 143:116-119, 1977.

49. Dondi Dall'orologio G et al: Clinical evaluation of Gluma and Gluma 2000 for treatment of hypersensitive dentin, *Arch Oral Biol* 39(suppl):126, 1994.

50. Dowell P, Addy M: Dentinal sensitivity—a review, aetiology, symptoms and theories of pain production, *J Clin Periodontol* 10:341-350, 1983.

51. Dowell P, Addy M, Dummer P: Dentinal sensitivity: aetiology, differential diagnosis and management, *Br Dent J* 158:92-96, 1985.

52. Duckworth RM, Moore SS: Salivary fluoride clearance after use of NaF dentifrices: a dose response study, *J Dent Res* 73(4):1994 (abstract).

53. Dyer D, Addy M, Newcombe RG: Studies in vitro of abrasion by different manual toothbrush heads and a standard toothpaste, *J Clin Periodontol* 27(2):99-103, 2000.

54. Ehrlich J et al: Residual fluoride concentrations and scanning electron microscopic examination of root surfaces of human teeth after topical application of fluoride in vivo, *J Dent Res* 54:897, 1975.

55. Eisenburger M, Shellis P, Addy M: Scanning electron microscopy of softened enamel, *Caries Res* 38(1):67-74, 2004.

56. Eisenburger M, Shellis P, Addy M: Comparative study of wear of enamel by alternating and simultaneous combinations of abrasion and erosion in vitro, *Caries Res* 37:450-455, 2003.

57. Eisenburger M et al: The use of ultrasonication to study remineralization of eroded enamel, *Caries Res* 35:61-66, 2001.

58. Eisenburger M et al: Ultrasonication as a method to study enamel demineralization during acid erosion, *Caries Res* 34:289-294, 2000.

59. Ellingsen JE, Rölla G: Treatment of dentin with stannous fluoride: SEM and electron microprobe study, *Scand J Dent Res* 15:281-286, 1987.

60. Ericcson Y: Fluoride in denitrifies—investigations using radioactive fluoride, *Acta Odontol Scand* 19:41-75, 1961.

61. Fischer C, Fischer RG, Wennberg A: Prevalence and distribution of cervical dentinal sensitivity in a population in Rio de Janeiro, Brazil, *J Dent* 20:272-276, 1992.

62. Flynn N, Galloway R, Orchardson R: The incidence of hypersensitive teeth in the West of Scotland, *J Dent* 13:230-236, 1985.

63. Forward GC: A new method of measuring hydroxyapatite dissolution rate, *Caries Res* 11:9-5, 1977.

64. Furseth R: A study of experimentally exposed and fluoride treated dental cementum in pigs, *Acta Odontol Scand* 28:833-850, 1970.

65. Gangarosa LP et al: Double-blind evaluation of duration of dentin sensitivity reduction by iontophoresis, *J Acad Gen Dent* 37:316-319, 1989.

66. Gedalia I, Brayer L, Kalter N: The effect of fluoride and strontium application on dentin: in vivo and in vitro studies, *J Periodontol* 49:269-272, 1978.

67. Gillam DG et al: Clinical evaluation of ferric oxalate in relieving dentinal sensitivity, *J Oral Rehabil* 31:245-250, 2004.

68. Gillam DG et al: Comparison of two desensitizing agents for the treatment of cervical dentin sensitivity, *Endod Dent Traumatol* 13:36-39, 1997.

69. Gillam DG et al: Efficacy of a potassium nitrate mouthwash in alleviating cervical dentinal sensitivity, *J Clin Periodontol* 23:993-997, 1996.

70. Gillam DG et al: Clinical efficacy of a low abrasive dentifrice for the relief of cervical dentinal hypersensitivity, *J Clin Periodontol* 19:197-201, 1992.

71. Goodis HE et al: Laser treatment of sensitive dentin, *Arch Oral Biol* 39(suppl):128, 1994.

72. Graf HE, Galasse R: Morbidity, prevalence and intra-oral distribution of hypersensitive teeth, *J Dent Res* 56(spec issue):1977.

73. Green BL, Green ML, McFall WT: Calcium hydroxide and potassium nitrate as desensitizing agents for hypersensitive root surfaces, *J Periodontol* 48:667-672, 1977.

74. Greenhill JD, Pashley DH: Effects of desensitizing agents on the hydraulic conductance of human dentin in vitro, *J Dent* 60:686-698, 1981.

75. Gregg T et al: A study in vitro of the abrasive effect of the tongue on enamel and dentin softened by acid erosion, *Caries Res* 38(6):557-560, 2004.

76. Griffiths H et al: The measurement in vitro of streaming potentials with fluids flow across dentin and hydroxyapatite, *J Periodontal Res* 28:59-65, 1993.

77. Grøn PG, Caslavska V: Fluoride deposition in enamel from monofluorophosphate application, *Caries Res* 15:90-97, 1981.

78. Grossman LE: A systematic method for the treatment of hypersensitive dentin, *J Am Dent Assoc* 22:592-602, 1935.

79. Gysi A: An attempt to explain the sensitiveness of dentin, *Br J Dent Sci* 43:865-868, 1900.

80. Hack GH, Thompson VP: Cavity varnishes: their ability to occlude dentinal tubules—hypersensitive dentin: biological basis of therapy, IADR/AADR satellite symposium, 1993, *Arch Oral Biol* 39:149S, 1994.

81. Hall RC, Embery G, Shellis RP: Biological and structural features of enamel and dentin: current concepts relevant to erosion and dentinal sensitivity. In Addy M et al eds: *Tooth wear and sensitivity*, London, 2000, Martin Dunitz.

82. Hansen EK: Dentinal sensitivity treated with a fluoride containing varnish or a light cures glass ionomer liner, *Scand J Dent Res* 100:305-309, 1992.

83. Hargreaves JA, Chester CG: Clinical trial among Scottish children of an anticaries dentifrice containing 2% sodium monofluorophosphate, *Community Dent Oral Epidemiol* 1:47-57, 1973.

84. Haywood VB: Dentinal sensitivity: bleaching and restorative considerations for successful management, *Int Dent J* 52(suppl):376-385, 2002.

85. Hazen SP, Volpe AR, King WJ: Comparative desensitizing effect of dentifrices containing sodium monofluorophosphate, stannous fluoride and formalin, *Periodontics* 6:230-232, 1968.

86. Hernandez F et al: Clinical study evaluating the desensitizing effect and duration of two commercially available dentifrices, *J Periodontol* 3:367-372, 1972.

87. Hiatt WH, Johansen E: Root preparation: obturation of dentinal tubules in the treatment of root hypersensitivity, *J Periodontol* 43:373-380, 1972.

88. Higuchi Y et al: Clinical evaluation of a dental rinse containing aluminum lactate for the treatment of dentinal sensitivity, *J Clin Dent* 7:9-12, 1996.

89. Holland G et al: Guidelines for the design and conduct of clinical trials on dentin sensitivity, *J Clin Periodontol* 24:808-813, 1997.

90. Hughes JA et al: Development and evaluation of a low erosive blackcurrant juice drink 3: final drink and concentrate, formulae comparisons in situ and overview of the concept, *J Dent* 27:345-350, 1999.

91. Hunter ML, West NX: Mechanical tooth wear: the role of individual toothbrushing variables and toothpaste abrasivity. In Addy M et al eds: *Tooth wear and sensitivity*, London, 2000, Martin Dunitz.

92. Hunter ML et al: Erosion of deciduous and permanent dental hard tissues in the oral environment, *J Dent* 28:257-264, 2000.

93. Ianzano JA, Gwinnet AJ, Westbay G: Polymeric sealing of dentinal tubules to control sensitivity: preliminary observations, *Periodontal Clin Investig* 15:13-16, 1993.

94. ICH Topic 6 Guideline for Good Clinical Practice: CPMP/ICH/135/95 17th July 1996.

95. Ide M et al: The role of a dentin bonding agent in reducing cervical dentin sensitivity, *J Clin Periodontol* 25:286-290, 1998.

96. Ishikawa S: A clinico-histological study on the hypersensitivity of dentin, *Kokubyo Gakkai Zasshi* 36:68-88, 1969.

97. Jackson RJ, McDonald FE: A comparison of dentifrices for the treatment of dentinal sensitivity, *Arch Oral Biol* 39(suppl):133, 1994.

98. Jensen AL: Hypersensitivity controlled by iontophoresis: double blind clinical investigation, *J Am Dent Assoc* 68:216-225, 1964.

99. Johnson G, Brännström M: Outward fluid flow in dentin under a physiologic pressure gradient: experiments in vitro, *Oral Surg Oral Med Oral Pathol* 35:238-248, 1973.

100. Johnson RH, Zulgar-Nairn BJ, Kovall J: The effectiveness of an electro-ionizing toothbrush in the control of dentinal hypersensitivity, *J Periodontol* 53:353-359, 1982.

101. Jorkjend L, Tronstad L: Treatment of hypersensitive root surfaces by calcium hydroxide, *Scand J Dent Res* 80:264-266, 1972.

102. Kalsi DS, Gill AS: Iontophoresis of KNO_3, $SrCl_2$ in dental hypersensitivity, *Arch Oral Biol* 39(suppl):128, 1994.

103. Kanapka JA: Over the counter dentifrices in the treatment of tooth hypersensitivity: review of clinical studies, *Dent Clin North Am* 34(3):545-560, 1990.

104. Kelly M: *Adult dental health survey: oral health in the United Kingdom 1998,* London, 2000, Office for National Statistics.

105. Kim S: Hypersensitive teeth: desensitization of pulpal sensory nerves, *J Endod* 12:482, 1986.

106. Kun L: Etude biophysique des modifications des tissues dentaires prevoquees par l'application totale de Strontium, *Schweiz Monatsschr Zahnheilkd* 86(7):661-676, 1976.

107. Lan WH, Lui HC: Treatment of dentinal sensitivity by Nd:YAG laser, *J Clin Laser Med Surg* 14:89-92, 1996.

108. Levin MP, Yearwood LL, Carpenter WN: The desensitizing effect of calcium hydroxide and magnesium hydroxide on hypersensitive dentin, *Oral Surg Oral Med Oral Pathol* 35:741-746, 1973.

109. Lier BB et al: Treatment of dentinal sensitivity by Nd:YAG laser, *J Clin Periodontol* 29:501-506, 2002.

110. Low T: The treatment of hypersensitive cervical abrasion cavities using ASPA cement, *J Oral Rehabil* 8:81-89, 1981.

111. Lutins ND, Greco GW, McFall WT: Effectiveness of sodium fluoride on tooth hypersensitivity with and without ionophoresis, *J Periodontol* 55:285, 1984.

112. Mair LH: Wear in the mouth: the tribological dimension. In Addy M et al eds: *Tooth wear and sensitivity,* London, 2000, Martin Dunitz.

113. Mair LH et al: Wear: mechanisms, manifestations and measurement—report of a workshop, *J Dent* 24:141-148, 1996.

114. Markowitz K, Bilotto G, Kim S: Decreasing intradental nerve activity in the cat with potassium and divalent cations, *Arch Oral Biol* 36:1-7, 1991.

115. Martens LC: Effects of anti-sensitive toothpaste on opened dentinal tubules and on two dentin-bonded resins, *Clin Prev Dent* 13(2):23-28, 1991.

116. Matsumoto K et al: Study of the treatment of hypersensitive dentin by GaAlAs laser diode, *Japan J Conserv Dent* 28:54, 1985.

117. Matthews B, Andrew D, Wanachantararak S: Biology of the dental pulp with special reference to its vasculature and innervation. In Addy M et al eds: *Tooth wear and sensitivity,* London, 2000, Martin Dunitz.

118. Matthews B, Vongsavan N: Interactions between neural and hydrodynamic mechanisms in dentin and pulp, *Arch Oral Biol* 39(suppl):S87-S95, 1994.

119. McFall WT Jr: A review of the active agents available for treatment of dentinal hypersensitivity, *Endod Dent Traumatol* 2: 141-149, 1986.

120. McFall WT Jr, Hamrick SW: Clinical effectiveness of a dentifrice containing fluoride and a citrate buffer system for treatment of dentinal sensitivity, *J Periodontol* 58(10):701-705, 1987.

121. McFall WT Jr, Morgan WC Jr: Effectiveness of a dentifrice containing formalin and sodium monofluorophosphate, *J Periodontol* 56:288-292, 1985.

122. Meurman JH, Sorvari R: Interplay of erosion attrition and abrasion in toothwear and possible approaches to prevention. In Addy M et al eds: *Tooth wear and sensitivity,* London, 2000, Martin Dunitz.

123. Miller JT et al: Use of water free stannous fluoride containing gel in the control of dental hypersensitivity, *J Periodontol* 40: 490-491, 1969.

124. Miller S et al: Effects of treating human dentin in vivo and in situ with an anhydrous stannous fluoride preparation, *Arch Oral Biol* 39(suppl):151, 1994.

125. Minkov B et al: The effectiveness of sodium fluoride treatment with and without ionophoresis on the reduction of hypersensitive dentin, *J Periodontol* 46:246-249, 1975.

126. Mongiorgi R, Prati C: Mineralogical and crystallographical study of γ-calcium oxalate on dentin surfaces in vitro, *Arch Oral Biol* 39(suppl):152, 1994.

127. Muzzin KB, Johnson R: Effects of potassium oxalate on dentin hypersensitivity in vivo, *J Periodontol* 60:151-157, 1989.

128. Nunn JH: Prevalence and distribution of tooth wear. In Addy M et al eds: *Tooth wear and sensitivity,* London, 2000, Martin Dunitz.

129. Ong G, Strahan JD: Effects of a desensitizing dentifrice on dentinal hypersensitivity, *Endod Dent Traumatol* 5:213-218, 1989.

130. Orchardson R: Strategies for the management of dentinal sensitivity. In Addy M et al eds: *Tooth wear and sensitivity,* London, 2000, Martin Dunitz.

131. Orchardson R, Collins WJN: Clinical features of hypersensitive teeth, *Br Dent J* 162:253-256, 1987.

132. Pashley DH: Mechanisms of dentin sensitivity, *Dent Clin North Am* 34(3):449-474, 1990.

133. Pashley DH, Galloway SE: The effects of oxalate treatment on the smear layer of ground surfaces of human dentin, *Arch Oral Biol* 30(10):731-737, 1985.

134. Pashley DH, Leibach JG, Horner J: The effects of burnishing NaF/kaolin/glycerin paste on dentin permeability, *J Periodontol* 58:19-23, 1987.

135. Pashley DH, Matthews WG: The effects of outward forced connective flow on inward diffusion in human dentin in vitro, *Arch Oral Biol* 38:557-582, 1993.

136. Peacock JM, Orchardson R: Effects of potassium ions on action potential conduction in A- and C-fibers of rat spinal nerves, *J Dent Res* 74:634-641, 1995.

137. Pearce NX, Addy M, Newcombe RG: Dentin hypersensitivity: a clinical trial to compare 2 strontium desensitizing toothpastes with conventional fluoride toothpaste, *J Periodontol* 65:113-119, 1994.

138. Petersson LG: Fluoride gradients outermost surface enamel after varied forms of topical application of fluorides in vivo, *Odontol Rev* 27:25, 1976.

139. Pontefract HH et al: Erosive effects of some mouthrinses on enamel: a study in situ, *J Clin Periodontol* 28,319-324, 2002.

140. Poulsen S et al: Potassium nitrate toothpaste for dentinal sensitivity. In *The Cochrane library,* issue 2, Chichester, UK, 2005, John Wiley & Sons.

141. Rees J, Addy M: A cross sectional study of dentinal sensitivity: the effect of age, gender, periodontal disease, smoking and social class, *J Clin Periodontol* 29:997-1003, 2002.

142. Renton-Harper P, Midda M: Nd:YAG laser treatment of dentinal hypersensitivity, *Br Dent J* 172:13-26, 1992.

143. Ross MR: Hypersensitive teeth: effect of strontium chloride in a compatible dentifrice, *J Periodontol* 32:49-53, 1961.

144. Russell CM, Dickinson GL, Downey MC: One-step versus Protect in the treatment of dentinal hypersensitivity, *J Dent Res* 77:199, 1997 (abstract).

145. Salvato AR et al: Clinical effectiveness of a dentifrice containing potassium chloride as a desensitizing agent, *Am J Dent* 5: 303-306, 1994.

146. Sanz M, Addy M: Group D summary, *J Clin Periodontol* 29(suppl 3):195-196, 2002.

147. Schaeffer ML, Bixler D, Pao-Lo Y: The effectiveness of iontophoresis in reducing cervical hypersensitivity, *J Periodontol* 42:695, 1971.

148. Schiff T et al: Efficacy of a dentifrice containing potassium nitrate, soluble pyrophosphate, PVM/MA copolymer, and sodium fluoride on dentinal hypersensitivity: a twelve week clinical study, *J Clin Dent* 5:87-92, 1994.

149. Schwartz F et al: Desensitizing effects of an Er:YAG laser on hypersensitive dentin, *J Clin Periodontol* 29(3):211-215, 2002.

150. Seltzer S, Bender IB, Ziantz M: The dynamics of pulp inflammation: correlation between diagnostic data and actual histological findings in the pulp, *Oral Surg Oral Med Oral Pathol* 16:846-969, 1963.

151. Selvig KA: Ultrasonic changes in human dentin exposed to weak acid, *Arch Oral Biol* 13:719-734, 1968.

152. Shapiro WB et al: Controlled clinical comparison between a strontium chloride and sodium monofluorophosphate toothpaste in diminishing root hypersensitivity, *J Periodontol* 41:523-525, 1970.

153. Silverman G, Gingold J, Curro FA: Desensitizing effect of a potassium chloride dentifrice, *Am J Dent* 7:9-12, 1994.

154. Silverman G et al: Assessing the efficacy of three dentifrices in the treatment of dentinal hypersensitivity, *J Am Dent Assoc* 127:191-201, 1996.

155. Simpson ME, Ciarlone AE, Pashley DH: Effects of dentin primers on dentin permeability, *J Dent Res* 72:127, 1993 (abstract).

156. Smith BA, Ash MM Jr: Study of a desensitizing dentifrice and cervical hypersensitivity, *J Periodontol* 35:222-231, 1964.

157. Smith RG: Gingival recession: reappraisal of an enigmatic condition and a new index for monitoring, *J Clin Periodontol* 24:201-205, 1997.

158. Suge I et al: Effects pre- or post application of calcium chloride on occluding ability of potassium oxalate for the treatment of dentinal sensitivity, *Am J Dent* 18(2):121-125, 2005.

159. Tal M et al: X-ray diffraction and scanning electron microscopic investigations of fluoride treated dentin in man, *Arch Oral Biol* 21:285-290, 1976.

160. Tarbet W et al: Home treatment for dentinal hypersensitivity: a comparative study, *J Am Dent Assoc* 105:227-230, 1982.

161. Tarbet WJ et al: Clinical evaluation of a new treatment for dentinal hypersensitivity, *J Periodontol* 51:535-540, 1980.

162. Tarbet WJ et al: An evaluation of two methods for the quantitation of dentinal hypersensitivity, *J Am Dent Assoc* 98:914-918, 1979.

163. Thrash WJ, Dorman LH, Smith DF: A method to measure pain associated with hypersensitive dentin, *J Periodontol* 54(3):160-162, 1983.

164. Trowbridge HO: Mechanism of pain induction in hypersensitive teeth. In Rowe NH, ed: *Proceedings of symposium on hypersensitive dentin: origin and management,* Edinburgh and London, 1985, E & S Livingston Ltd.

165. Trowbridge HO, Silver DR: A review of current approaches to in-office management of tooth hypersensitivity, *Dent Clin North Am* 34(3):561-582, 1990.

166. Uchida A et al: Controlled clinical evaluation of a 10% strontium chloride dentifrice in the treatment of dentinal sensitivity following periodontal surgery, *J Periodontol* 51:578-581, 1980.

167. Van Dijken J: Three year evaluation of the effect of surface conditioning on bonding of glass ionomer cement in cervical abrasion lesions, *Scand J Dent Res* 100:133-135, 1992.

168. Vanuspong W, Eisenburger M, Addy M: Cervical tooth wear and sensitivity: erosion, softening and rehardening of dentin: effects of pH, time and ultrasonication, *J Clin Periodontol* 29:351-357, 2002.

169. Vongsavan N, Matthews B: Fluid flow through cat dentin in vivo, *Arch Oral Biol* 37:175-185, 1992.

170. Watson PJC: Gingival recession, *J Dent* 12:29-35, 1984.

171. Wei SHY et al: Evaluation of dentifrices for the relief of hypersensitive tooth surfaces, *Quintessence Int* 11:67-73, 1980.

172. West N, Addy M, Hughes J: Dentinal sensitivity: the effects of brushing desensitizing toothpastes, their solid and liquid phases and detergents on dentin and acrylic—studies in vitro, *J Oral Rehabil* 25:885-895, 1998.

173. West NX: *Dentinal sensitivity: clinical and laboratory studies of toothpastes, their ingredients and acids,* doctoral dissertation, Wales, 1995, University of Wales.

174. West NX et al: Dentin hypersensitivity and the placebo response: a comparison of the effect of strontium acetate, potassium nitrate and fluoride toothpastes, *J Clin Periodontol* 24:209-215, 1997.

175. Xie J, Power JM, McGuckin RS: In vitro bond strength of two adhesives to enamel and dentin surfaces under normal and contaminated conditions, *Dent Mater* 9:295-299, 1993.

176. Yates R et al: The effects of a potassium citrate, cetylpyridium chloride, sodium fluoride mouthrinse on dentin hypersensitivity, plaque and gingivitis, *J Clin Periodontol* 25:813-820, 1998.

177. Zero DT: Etiology of enamel erosion: intrinsic and extrinsic factors—etiology of dental erosion-extrinsic factors, *Eur J Oral Sci* 104:162-171, 1996.

178. Zero DT, Lussi A: Etiology of enamel erosion: intrinsic and extrinsic factors. In Addy M et al, eds: *Tooth wear and sensitivity,* London, 2000, Martin Dunitz.

179. Zhang H-Q, Wu XB: Treatment of dentin hypersensitivity with Chinese traditional medicines, hypersensitive dentin: biological basis of therapy, IADR/AADR satellite symposium, 1993, *Arch Oral Biol* 39:136S, 1994.

180. Zinner DD, Duany LF, Lutz HJ: A new desensitizing dentifrice: preliminary report, *J Am Dent Assoc* 95(5):982-985, 1977.

Periodontal Dressings and Suturing

Katherine Karpinia

INSIGHT

Dental hygienists seldom have an opportunity to place sutures, but they may have the need to remove sutures, to place and remove periodontal dressings, and to provide postoperative instructions to patients. With the knowledge of wound healing and dental materials, the dental hygienist is in a position to provide patients with an understanding of expectations after surgery and to assess surgical sites when dressings and sutures are removed.

✦ CASE STUDY 34-1   Suturing: Three Specific Procedures

Case 1: Esthetic Treatment for a Lost Tooth

Henry Augsberger, a 21-year-old male patient, came to the clinic seeking esthetic treatment for a lost tooth. At age 8 he experienced trauma to the anterior maxilla while playing baseball. Subsequently, the maxillary left central incisor was lost and the underlying bone was resorbed, leaving an obvious concavity. Mr. Augsberger requested esthetic recontouring of the facial maxilla adjacent to the tooth loss site. After considering the treatment options, he chose a **free soft tissue graft** procedure.

Black silk sutures (size 4-0) were used for the procedure. The graft was stabilized with interrupted sutures at the inferior lateral borders, and overlapping figure-X periosteal sutures were placed across the graft's surface (Figure 34-1). A surgical dressing was not used after suturing was completed.

Case 2: Suturing for a Periodontal Flap Procedure

A periodontal flap procedure and **osseous surgery** were performed on a systemically healthy 58-year-old female patient, Marti Martinez, after the completion of initial periodontal therapy. The goals of the surgical treatment were to reduce the pocket depth, **debride** root surfaces, and recontour **osseous** defects, thereby improving the long-term prognosis for tooth retention. A **full-thickness periodontal flap (mucoperiosteal flap)** procedure was the surgical method chosen.

A continuous interlocking suture technique was used to approximate facial and lingual soft tissue flaps. The continuous interlocking suture was also used to obtain primary flap closure over the mesial and distal edentulous ridge adjacent to the remaining molar tooth (Figure 34-2). The entire surgical area was covered with a **periodontal dressing** after the procedure.

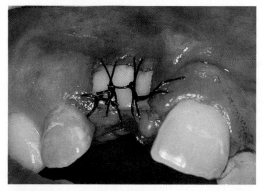

FIGURE 34-1
Periosteal suture (silk) secures a free soft tissue graft.

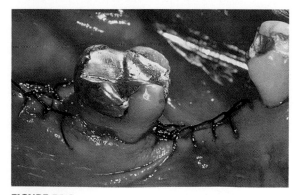

FIGURE 34-2
Continuous locking sutures (silk) approximate a facial and lingual periodontal flap.

✦ CASE STUDY 34-1 | Suturing: Three Specific Procedures—cont'd

Case 3: Suturing after Frenum Removal

Before orthodontic closure of a diastema between the maxillary central incisor teeth, a 33-year-old male patient, Cary Fienstra, was advised to have a large maxillary anterior frenum (Figure 34-3) surgically removed. Excessive musculature and interproximal penetration of the frenum inhibited mesial tooth movement and would have impaired long-term retention after orthodontic treatment. A **frenectomy** was the surgical treatment selected.

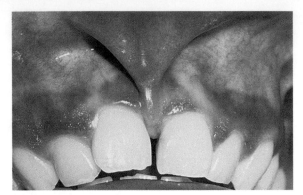

FIGURE 34-3
Large maxillary anterior frenum. (Courtesy Dr. Frederic Brown, Gainesville, Fla.)

Simple interrupted sutures of 4-0 chromic gut were used to approximate the soft tissue borders (Figure 34-4). A periodontal dressing was not used after the procedure.

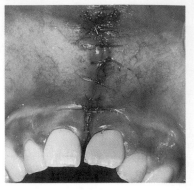

FIGURE 34-4
After a frenectomy is performed, simple interrupted sutures (chromic gut) approximate the soft tissue borders. (Courtesy of Dr. Frederic Brown, Gainesville, Fla.)

KEY TERMS

asbestosis	full-thickness periodontal flap	multifilament	periodontal flap
debride	(mucoperiosteal flap)	osseous	periodontal surgery
free soft tissue graft	mesothelioma	osseous surgery	surgical flap
frenectomy	monofilament	periodontal dressing	suture material

LEARNING OUTCOMES

After reading this chapter the student will be able to:

1. Understand the basic concepts of suture materials, suture design, and suturing techniques.
2. List the available periodontal dressings, and state the rationale for their use.
3. Describe the characteristics of the ideal suture material and the ideal periodontal dressing.

4. Discuss the uses, advantages, and limitations of suture materials and periodontal dressings.
5. Assist healthcare professionals in the selection, use, and removal of periodontal sutures and dressings, and explain the use of these materials to patients.

After periodontal surgery, periodontal sutures are used to approximate or bring together soft tissues and to stabilize the closure. Clinicians use a surgical needle to guide **suture material** through oral soft tissues, thereby approximating a **surgical flap** and increasing the chances of optimal healing. Suture materials vary widely in composition and type and are selected according to the preference of the clinician and the requirements of the procedure. Ideally, sutures function as passive tools; they exert no active control over the **periodontal flap.**

In most cases, traumatized tissues have a higher risk of compromised wound healing[5]; therefore the surgical technique is a more important factor than the type of suture selected. A flap

that is accurately designed, gently handled, and carefully positioned will keep its position independent of the suture material or suturing technique. The dental suture and suture knots should be positioned to prevent irritation and should be tied snugly, not tightly, to ensure minimal tissue tension.

Suture Materials

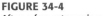

34-1

Suture materials are classified as absorbable or nonabsorbable and natural or synthetic (Box 34-1). Absorbable sutures are often selected when suture removal is uncertain or undesirable (e.g., as with small children, sensitive area, placement beneath

BOX 34-1

COMMON SUTURE MATERIALS

Nonabsorbable Sutures
Natural material
Silk
Plain collagen
Chromic collagen

Synthetic material
Polypropylene
Polyester
Nylon
Polytetrafluoroethylene (PTFE)

Absorbable Sutures
Natural material
Plain gut
Chromic gut
Catgut

Synthetic material
Polyglycolic acid
Polyglactin 910
Poliglecaprone 25

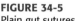

Absorbable Sutures		
Type	Size	Needle
Plain gut	4-0	3/8 Circle, reverse-cutting
Plain gut	5-0	3/8 Circle, reverse-cutting

FIGURE 34-5
Plain gut sutures.

Absorbable Sutures		
Type	Size	Needle
Chromic gut	3-0	3/8 Circle, reverse-cutting
Chromic gut	4-0	3/8 Circle, reverse-cutting
Chromic gut	5-0	3/8 Circle, reverse-cutting
Chromic gut	6-0	3/8 Circle, reverse-cutting

FIGURE 34-6
Chromic gut sutures.

Absorbable Sutures		
Type	Size	Needle
Coated Vicryl (Polyglactin 910)	4-0	3/8 Circle, reverse-cutting
Coated Vicryl (Polyglactin 910)	5-0	3/8 Circle, reverse-cutting
Coated Vicryl Rapide (Polyglactin 910)	5-0	3/8 Circle, reverse-cutting

FIGURE 34-7
Examples of absorbable suture materials are shown.

an external flap) or when the difficulty of suture removal outweighs the advantage (e.g., limited access, patient anxiety, postoperative discomfort). Absorbable sutures are manufactured from the collagen of healthy mammals or from synthetic polymers. Absorbable types of suture include plain gut, chromic gut, catgut, polyglycolic acid (Dexon), polyglactin 910 (coated Vicryl), and poliglecaprone 25 (Monocryl) (Figures 34-5 through 34-7).

Nonabsorbable sutures improve suture retention over a long period. This type of suture characteristically retains its tensile strength longer, giving the wound sufficient time to heal. Nonabsorbable sutures are especially useful in implant and regenerative procedures. Types of nonabsorbable sutures include silk, plain and chromic collagen, polypropylene, polyester, nylon (Ethilon), and polytetrafluoroethylene (Gore) (Figure 34-8).

The suture material most often used in dentistry is silk.[4] However, no single suture material is recommended by every surgeon within a specialty. Silk sutures are specially processed to provide optimal handling and knot security without excessive capillarity. **Multifilament** sutures, especially silk, have exceptional handling characteristics: flexibility, pliability, ease of manipulation, and superior knot holding. **Monofilament** sutures (e.g., nylon, polypropylene, gut) are generally stronger and more durable than multifilament sutures and cause less tissue inflammation. However, monofilament sutures are more difficult to manipulate and have inferior knot security. When the reactions of oral tissues to polytetrafluoroethylene (PTFE) sutures and silk sutures were compared, inflammatory infiltrate increased over a 7-day period for both types of suture. The inflammation appeared more intense with the silk suture.[6] In a

comparison of silk, chromic gut, PTFE, and polyglactin 910 suture materials, silk sutures seemed to allow the greatest bacterial migration.[9] PTFE sutures appeared to be the most tissue friendly.

Unfortunately, the ideal suture material does not exist. However, many types of suture material offer outstanding characteristics and are relatively close to the ideal (Box 34-2).

Body enzymes and macrophages digest natural absorbable sutures (gut). These sutures are made of highly purified collagen from sheep, cattle, or feline intestines. Synthetic absorbable

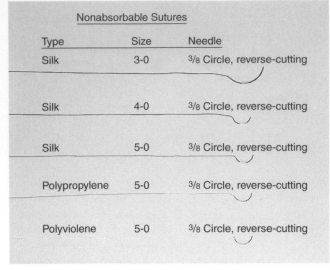

FIGURE 34-8
Examples of nonabsorbable suture material are shown.

BOX 34-2

CHARACTERISTICS OF THE IDEAL SUTURE MATERIAL

- Comfortable to use and easy to manipulate
- Not likely to cause any adverse tissue reactions
- Able to inhibit bacterial growth
- Very strong, even in the suture's smallest diameter
- Easy to tie in knots, remains tied, and will not injure adjacent tissues
- Sterile and conveniently packaged
- Not adversely affected by products or contaminants in the oral cavity
- Noncarcinogenic and nonallergenic

---

sutures are hydrophobic and are eventually broken down by hydrolysis, a process during which water penetrates the suture material and breaks down its polymer chain. This process correlates with a leukocytic cellular response that removes suture material and cellular debris from the wound area. Some absorbable sutures are chemically structured or manipulated to lengthen the absorption time. For example, chromic gut suture is treated with a chromium salt solution that enhances its resistance to proteolytic enzymes.[4]

Suture Needles

Because of the restricted access in the oral cavity, suture needles have a rounded shape. The needle is composed of a point, a body, and an attachment end for the suture material. Most attachment ends are swaged; that is, the suture material is press-fit or fused to the metal needle, resulting in less tissue trauma when the needle pulls the suture through tissue. The needle's point is generally sharp and may be standard or taper cut. Standard points are sharp at the tip, with the cutting ability blending with the needle body as it is engaged. Taper-cut points ex-

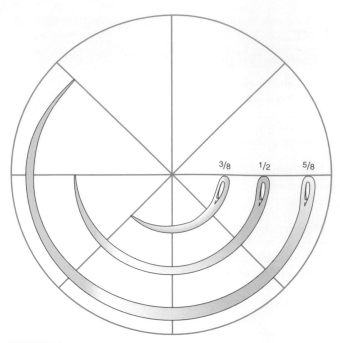

FIGURE 34-9
Suture needles are measured as a portion of a complete circle.

tend farther along the needle body and offer a more tapered, sharp, and delicate penetration through the tissue. They are commonly used for mucogingival procedures.

The body of the needle is measured in metric units or inches as a portion of a complete circle. The more commonly used needles measure ⅜ inch, ½ inch, or ⅝ inch[5] (Figure 34-9).

The three types of suture needles are available (1) conventional cutting suture needles, (2) reverse cutting suture needles, and (3) taper-cut suture needles. A reverse cutting suture needle is triangular in cross-section (similar to a sickle scaler), has three cutting edges, and is drawn through the tissue with the base of the triangle facing the coronal aspect of the soft tissue. The broad triangular base creates a wide area of enhanced tissue resistance, reducing the risk of the suture material tearing soft tissue as pressure is applied to move and tie the suture. Conversely, conventional cutting suture needles are passed through the soft tissue with the base of the triangular needle facing the apical aspect of the soft tissue. As a result, a narrow V is created at the point where the greatest pressure is exerted when the suture is pulled and tied. This configuration poses a greater risk of tissue tearing and suture loss than would occur as a result of using reverse cutting suture needles (Figure 34-10).

Suture Size

Suture size is classified by the diameter of the suture's surface material and is stated numerically by the number of zeros. Size is measured in decreasing diameter from 1-0 (pronounced *one-oh*), the largest suture, to 11-0, the smallest suture. For example, 5-0 (00000) sutures are smaller in diameter than 4-0 (0000) sutures. The smaller the suture size, the less tensile strength the suture material has. The suture size most commonly used in

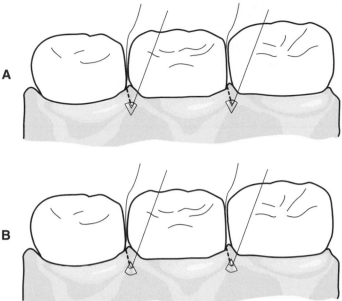

FIGURE 34-10
Triangular cross-section of a needle. **A,** Reverse cutting needle with a broad triangular base faces the coronal aspect of the soft tissue. **B,** Conventional cutting needle with a narrow V faces the coronal aspect of the soft tissue.

dentistry is 4-0, although 5-0 sutures are often used for mucogingival procedures (see Figures 34-5 through 34-8).

Suture Packaging

Manufacturers package sutures in two covers. The inside sealed sterile cover holds the suture needle and material; this inner package is then placed into an outer, nonsterile covering (Figure 34-11). This packaging technique makes it easier to maintain a sterile surgical field. Nonsterile hands may grasp the outer covering and carefully open the package, allowing the inside sterile package to contact (drop into) the surgical instrument field

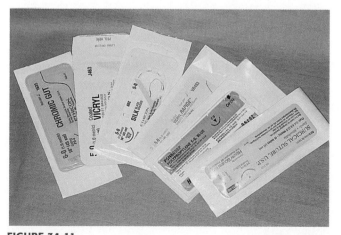

FIGURE 34-11
Suture packaging has a sterile inner package and a nonsterile outer wrapping.

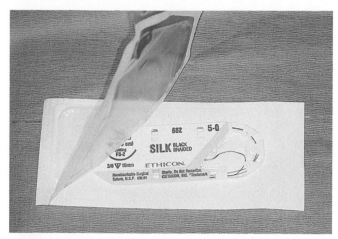

FIGURE 34-12
The outer, nonsterile suture wrapping can be opened, and the inner, sterile package can be allowed to drop onto the surgical instrument tray.

(Figure 34-12). Dual packaging is convenient and helps prevent cross-contamination.

Suturing Techniques

When suturing periodontal flaps, the clinician inserts the needle through the soft tissue flap approximately 3 mm from the gingival margin. Care must be taken not to drag the suture material through the flap or exert excessive pressure on the wound edge, thereby injuring the flap or tearing through the wound margin. Once the suture has been tied, suture scissors are used to cut the ends to a comfortable length, leaving approximately 2 mm of free suture adjacent to the knot.

Several different techniques can be used to place sutures. Some commonly used suturing techniques are described in the following sections.

INTERRUPTED SUTURES

The simple interrupted loop suture technique and the simple interrupted figure-8 modification of that technique are the methods most commonly used to close flaps. For a simple interrupted loop pattern, the needle enters through the facial flap from the outer epithelial surface toward the underlying bone; it passes through the interdental area, penetrates the lingual flap from its inner osseous undersurface, and then exits the outer epithelial surface. The clinician ends the loop by passing the needle back through the interdental area and tying a knot on the facial surface (Figure 34-13), creating a suture circle or loop.

✦ CASE APPLICATION 34-1.1

Case 3: Suturing after Frenum Removal
In Case 3, a simple interrupted loop suture technique was used to approximate the wound margins after removing the maxillary anterior frenum.

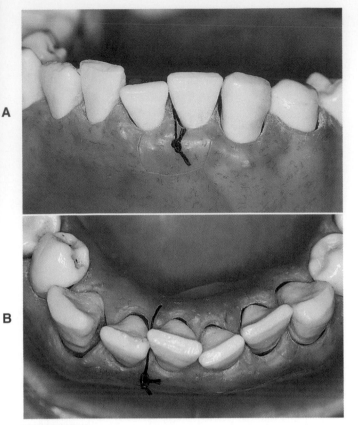

FIGURE 34-13
Simple interrupted loop suture. **A,** Facial view. **B,** Incisal view.

SLING SUTURES

The single interproximal sling suture technique is used to secure a facial or lingual flap and involves only two papillae. The needle penetrates the outer surface of the distal papilla, passes under the distal contact area, goes around the tooth and under the distal contact area, captures the mesial papilla, and returns by the aforementioned route; the suture then is tied on the facial surface (Figure 34-14). The continuous independent sling suture technique, which is used for a facial or lingual flap, functions in a similar manner. It captures the adjacent facial or lingual papilla, respectively, as it *slings* individual teeth until the suture is knotted at its termination (Figure 34-15). The continuous double sling suture technique involves both a facial and a lingual flap. One of the flaps, either the facial or the lingual,

For the figure 8 modification of the simple interrupted loop suture pattern, the steps are the same as those used for the simple loop pattern with one exception: the needle penetrates the lingual flap from its outer epithelial surface and exits the flap's inner osseous surface before being returned to the facial area to be tied. Completion of the suture knot creates the figure-8 form.

CONTINUOUS SUTURES

Continuous sutures join multiple papillae on one flap to an adjacent flap in an uninterrupted fashion, or they allow independent suturing of a periodontal flap. The continuous simple loop suture pattern may be extended to include many adjacent interdental spaces. The needle penetrates the facial flap and passes through the lingual flap, and the pattern continues in this manner until a knot is tied at the termination of the suture. The continuous locking suture technique uses a single interrupted suture first. Subsequently, the needle is passed through the outer surface of the facial flap and the inner surface of the lingual flap, forming a loop. The needle then is passed through the loop, and the suture is snugly pulled. This pattern of locking each loop is continued until a knot is tied at the termination of the suture.

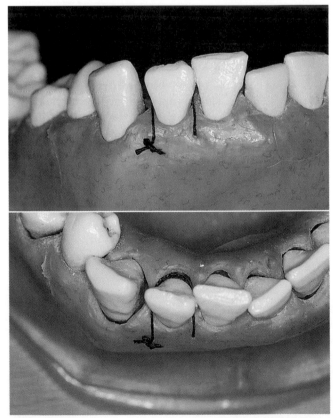

FIGURE 34-14
Single interproximal sling suture. **A,** Facial view. **B,** Incisal view.

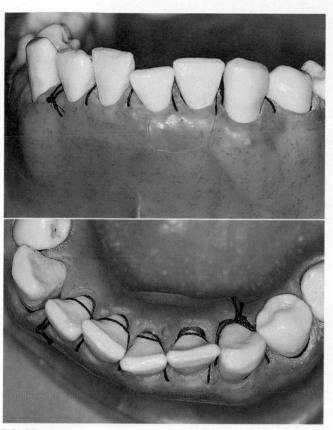

FIGURE 34-15
Continuous independent sling suture. **A,** Facial view. **B,** Incisal view.

is secured first. The opposite flap then is sutured identically (Figure 34-16). The continuous double sling suture requires two knots: (1) initial loop and (2) final tie. Both knots are usually located near the original insertion. The continuous double sling suture allows a facial flap to be positioned independently of a lingual flap.

MATTRESS SUTURES

The vertical mattress and horizontal mattress suture techniques permit precise flap placement, adapt flaps to underlying bone, resist muscle pull, and aid adaptation of wound margins. For the vertical mattress suture pattern, the first puncture is placed more apically, and the suture emerges more coronally. The suture is passed through the interproximal area, and a similar technique is used in the opposing flap. The suture is knotted near its origin (Figure 34-17). The horizontal mattress suture pattern is similar except that the suture runs beneath the flap in a horizontal direction, and the emerging parallel strands cross over the interdental papillae (Figure 34-18). Both techniques provide unequivocal flap control.

PERIOSTEAL SUTURES

The periosteal suture technique permits involvement of the periosteum and superficial bony surface as an option to soft

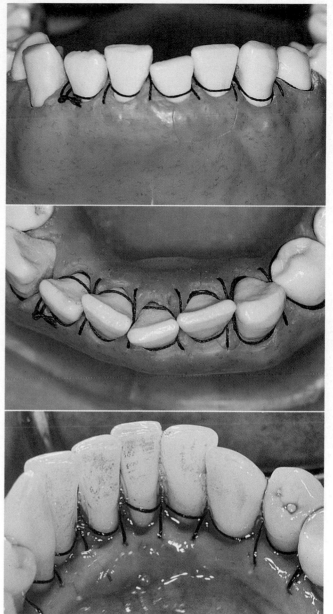

FIGURE 34-16
Continuous double sling suture. **A,** Facial view. **B,** Incisal view. **C,** Lingual view.

tissue suturing. The needle penetrates the periosteal surface at a 90-degree angle and, under gentle pressure, glides along the surface of the bone. It exits the periosteum without elevating or tearing the structure.

> ### ✺ CASE APPLICATION 34-1.3
>
> ## Case 1: Esthetic Treatment for a Lost Tooth
> In Case 1, a periosteal suture was used to secure placement of a free soft tissue graft.

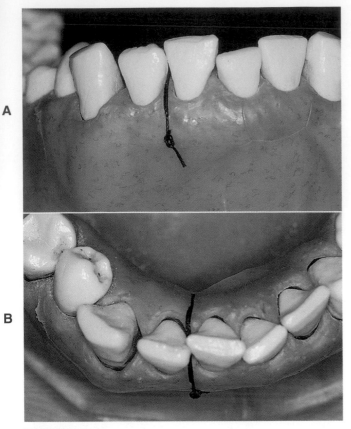

FIGURE 34-17
Vertical mattress suture. **A,** Facial view. **B,** Incisal view.

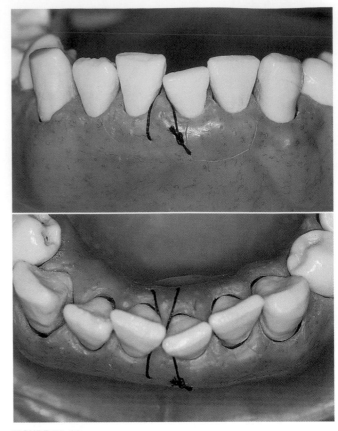

FIGURE 34-18
Horizontal mattress suture. **A,** Facial view. **B,** Incisal view.

Postoperative Instructions

- Explain and provide a written copy of postoperative care instructions to the patient that includes an emergency contact telephone number (Box 34-3).
- Provide the patient with a prescription for an analgesic and possibly an antibiotic.
- Discuss with the patient instructions for taking the medications, and provide these instructions in writing.
- Ensure that the patient has someone to drive him or her home, depending on the type of anesthesia and medications administered.
- Provide self-care instructions to the patient.
- Schedule a postoperative appointment approximately 1 week after surgery.

34-2
34-3

Suture Removal

Suture materials become contaminated as they pass through the periodontal flap during initial placement and while they remain in the oral environment. Most sutures are removed 7 to 10 days after placement.

Steps involved in suture removal are the following:
- Irrigate the surgical site with an antimicrobial solution such as chlorhexidine gluconate before removing sutures.

BOX 34-3

POSTOPERATIVE CARE AND PROCEDURES

- Use an ice pack intermittently (5 to 10 minutes at a time) for the first few hours after surgery to reduce swelling.
- Limit physical activity while healing.
- Control bleeding with light finger pressure on gauze or a tea bag placed over the area.
- Do not rinse while bleeding; rinsing will prolong the bleeding.
- Eat a well-balanced soft diet for the first several days to promote healing.
- Do not be alarmed if portions of the periodontal dressing break off before the postoperative appointment. Notify the office to find out whether the dressing should be replaced.
- Avoid smoking; smoking interferes with the wound healing process.
- Use a disinfectant rinse twice a day to assist in the control of plaque biofilm. (Chlorhexidine or essential oil mouthwash may be used.)
- Use an extra-soft toothbrush and warm water to gently clean interproximally where accessible once or twice a day. Areas of the mouth not affected by surgery can be cared for as normal.
- Call the office if questions or a problem should arise.

- Carefully remove any remaining periodontal dressing to ensure that the healing gingival tissues are not disrupted.
- Carefully lift suture knots, and cut the suture strand close to the gingival soft tissue.
- When removing continuous sutures, cut each section individually to prevent the dragging of lengthy, contaminated sutures through healing tissue.
- Secure and gently pull each knot away from the surgical flap, allowing short segments of suture to be guided from the surgical site with minimal discomfort to the patient.
- Place each knot on gauze as it is removed.
- Count all knots to ensure complete removal of the suture material.
- Record in the patient file the appearance of the tissue, healing characteristics, and number of knots removed.

Prevention
Irrigate surgical site with an antimicrobial before suture removal.

Periodontal Dressings

Periodontal dressings were first introduced in 1923 by Dr. A.W. Ward.[8] Dr. Ward's Wondr-Pak consisted of zinc oxide–eugenol (ZOE) mixed with pine oil, asbestos, and alcohol.

The use of periodontal dressings arose from a desire to:
- Protect surgical sites from trauma
- Increase patient comfort
- Prevent wound contamination by oral debris
- Stabilize periodontal flaps
- Immobilize soft tissue grafts

Other advantages include the following:
- Tooth desensitization
- Tooth splinting
- Attempts to prevent excessive proliferation of granulation tissues

Tannic acid was added to periodontal dressings to facilitate hemostasis[3] but was later removed because of the possible risk of liver damage if it were to be absorbed systemically. Asbestos was removed because of the risk of **asbestosis,** lung cancer, and **mesothelioma.**

ZOE dressings contain approximately 40% to 50% eugenol and were popular in the past because of their anodyne effects on sensitive dentin and gingival soft tissues.[10] However, eugenol, which increases in amount as zinc eugenate decomposes, has been shown to contribute to delayed healing, inflammatory or allergic reactions, and tissue necrosis.[8,10] When set, eugenol dressings have a hard, brittle consistency, with sharp edges and minimal flexibility. Most modern periodontal dressings are formulated without eugenol.[7]

The characteristics of an ideal periodontal dressing are listed in Box 34-4.

Some widely used dressings that do not contain eugenol are the following:
- Coe-Pak Periodontal Dressing (GC America, Inc., Alsip, Ill.) (Figure 34-19)
- Zone Periodontal Pak (DUX Dental, Oxnard, Calif.) (Figure 34-20)

BOX 34-4

IDEAL PROPERTIES OF A PERIODONTAL DRESSING

- Sets slowly enough to allow adequate manipulation
- Is firm enough to maintain the required shape
- Has smooth, nonirritating surfaces
- Maintains its flexibility to withstand distortion and displacement without fracturing
- Holds its dimensional stability to prevent leakage and the accumulation of debris
- Inhibits bacterial growth
- Is nonallergenic
- Has an acceptable taste

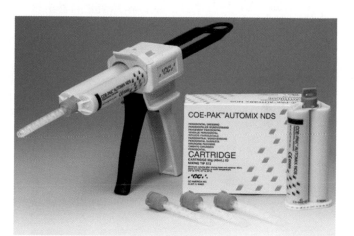

FIGURE 34-19
Coe-Pak Periodontal Dressing. (GC America, Inc., Alsip, Ill.)

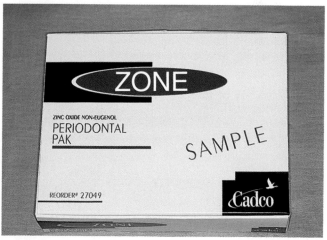

FIGURE 34-20
Zone Periodontal Pak. (DUX Dental, Oxnard, Calif.)

- Periocare Periodontal Dressing (Pulpdent Corp., Watertown, Mass.)
- Peripac Periodontal Pac (DENTSPLY Preventive Care, York, Pa.)
- Barricaid Visible-Light-Cure Periodontal Dressing (DENTSPLY Preventive Care, York, Pa.)

PROCEDURE FOR MIXING AND PLACING PERIODONTAL DRESSINGS

The following procedure for mixing and placing Zone Periodontal Pak, Coe-Pak, and Periocare is provided:

- Extrude equal lengths of paste (catalyst) and a gel (base) from each tube onto a mixing pad (Figures 34-21 and 34-22).
- Thoroughly spatulate the paste and gel on a special mixing pad.
  - Shape the cohesive product into a cylindrical rope or log form.
  - Carefully mold the product to fit the surgical site (Figures 34-23 and 34-24).

Peripac is distributed in a ready-to-use form that does not require mixing before placement.

Prevention

During placement of any periodontal dressing, care should be taken to prevent the dressing from extending onto occlusal or incisal surfaces (interfering with occlusion) or from projecting apically, past the mucogingival junction, possibly leading to mucosal irritation.

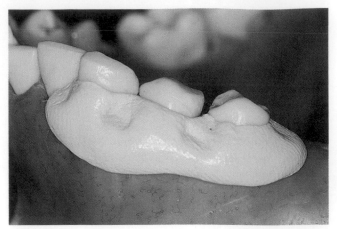

FIGURE 34-23
Intraoral placement of a Coe-Pak Periodontal Dressing.

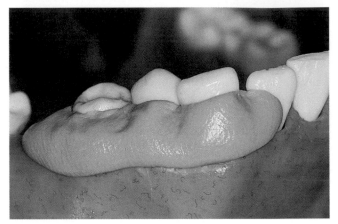

FIGURE 34-24
Intraoral placement of a Zone Periodontal Pak.

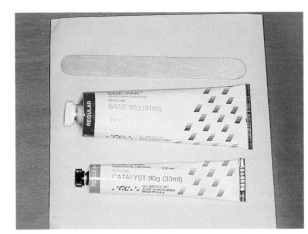

FIGURE 34-21
Coe-Pak Periodontal Dressing tubes separate the base *(top)* and the catalyst *(bottom)* before a periodontal dressing is mixed.

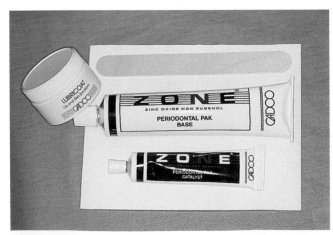

FIGURE 34-22
The Zone Periodontal Pak includes a base *(top tube)*, a catalyst *(bottom tube)*, and a lip and skin emollient *(jar at left)*. (DUX Dental, Oxnard, Calif.)

Barricaid is a single-component, light-activated periodontal dressing supplied in a syringe that can be used outside the mouth as a wound dressing or as a disposable dispenser for intraoral application of material directly onto the wound site.

Whether to use a dressing after **periodontal surgery** is a choice made by the individual clinician.[1,2]

Patient Education Opportunity

Periodontal dressings become semirigid after setting and can withstand some chewing forces without fracturing. Patients should be instructed to eat semisolid foods (e.g., cooked vegetables, pasta, soft meats, fish) and generally to avoid eating or toothbrushing on the side where the dressing is located. Many clinicians prescribe an antimicrobial rinse (chlorhexidine gluconate) for the patient to use while the dressing is in place.

✦ CASE APPLICATION 34-1.4

Types of Dressings Used

No periodontal dressings were used for either Mr. Augsberger or Mr. Fienstra. However, a surgical dressing was used for Mrs. Martinez after the procedure.

Most periodontal dressings are removed from the oral cavity within 5 to 10 days of placement. The procedure for removing a periodontal dressing is as follows:

- Dislodge the dressing from the surgical area using a sterile instrument (e.g., cotton forceps) by placing the tip of the instrument under the dressing and lifting.
- Take care to ensure that the sutures are not caught in the dressing.
- Remove the dressing in one large piece or in large individual sections. The surgical site should be clean, and the dressing should come off neatly.
- Remove the sutures after the dressing has been removed. (See the previous section on suture removal.)

References

1. Allen D, Caffesse R: Comparison of results following modified Widman flap surgery with and without surgical dressing, *J Periodontol* 54:470, 1983.
2. Jones D, Cassingham R: Comparison of healing following periodontal surgery with and without dressings in humans, *J Periodontol* 50:387, 1979.
3. Levin M: Periodontal suture materials and surgical dressings, *Dent Clin North Am* 24:767, 1980.
4. Lilly G: Reaction of oral tissues to suture materials, *Oral Surg Oral Med Oral Pathol* 26:128, 1968.
5. Meyer R, Antonini C: A review of suture materials, *Compend Cont Dent Educ* (part I) 1:260, 1989; (part II) 10:360, 1989.
6. Rivera-Hildago F et al: Tissue reaction to silk and Gore-Tex sutures in dogs, *J Periodontal Res* 70:508, 1991.
7. Rubinoff CH, Greener EH, Robinson PJ: Physical properties of periodontal dressing materials, *J Oral Rehabil* 13:575, 1986.
8. Sachs H et al: Current status of periodontal dressings, *J Periodontol* 55:689, 1984.
9. Selvig D et al: Oral tissue reactions to suture materials, *Int J Periodontol Rest Dent* 18:474, 1998.
10. von Fraunhofer J, Argyropoulos D: Properties of periodontal dressings, *Dent Mater* 6:51, 1990.

Operative Procedures

Peter T. Triolo • William H. Tate

INSIGHT

The dental hygienist can perform simple operative dentistry procedures in selected states within the United States, as well as in other countries around the world. As access to care needs expand in the future, the dental hygienist may play an important role in performing operative dentistry procedures in certain situations. In addition, patients often rely on the dental hygienist to answer questions regarding operative procedures. Every dental hygienist must have an understanding of operative dentistry and how to assist the patient in understanding his or her treatment needs.

⚜ CASE STUDY 35-1   Application of Operative Therapies

The dental hygienist greets a 53-year-old woman, Mrs. Daniella Dixon, in the waiting room. She is 10 to 20 pounds overweight and well dressed. She is married and has two children. When the hygienist calls her name, Mrs. Dixon responds immediately by standing and beginning to smile but not broadly. She moves quickly and follows the hygienist into the treatment room.

A review of Mrs. Dixon's medical history reveals the following:

Age 15: Hospitalized after a severe automobile accident; thrown into dashboard and windshield; spent 2 days in the hospital with moderate head injuries, including a concussion; lost consciousness for a few minutes after accident

Age 27: Gave birth to female infant

Age 30: Gave birth to male infant

Age 50: Postmenopausal, prescribed hormone supplement

No other significant medical problems

Social history: Mrs. Dixon is somewhat reserved and rarely smiles. Both children have finished college, have good jobs, and live away from home. Her husband has a management position with a successful company and has just been transferred to the area. Mrs. Dixon drinks both coffee and tea throughout the day. Generally she drinks wine with her dinner.

Dental status: Interproximal enamel lesions, root caries, Class V lesions, restored anterior teeth, and multiple posterior restorations

Periodontal disease: Gingival recession, increased probing depths with spontaneous bleeding, marginal inflammation, and edematous gingival tissue

Missing teeth: All third molars extracted at age 21; all other teeth intact and moderately stained

Oral soft tissues:
- Palate—Presence of small (3 mm) ulcerated areas just palatal to the maxillary incisors
- Lips—Raised vesicles (3 mm) on lower lip near the right angular border

General comments: Mrs. Dixon states that she brushes twice a day. She normally uses Crest toothpaste but may buy another product on sale if she has seen it advertised on television. She flosses a couple of times a week and generally goes to the dentist once a year. However, because of the recent move and her son finishing college, she has not been to a dentist in more than 2 years.

KEY TERMS

amalgam
cavity bases
cavity liners
cavity sealers
cavosurface
composite
convenience form

corrosion
extension for prevention
galvanic reaction
glass ionomers
line angle
marginal breakdown

microleakage
outline form
point angle
polymerization shrinkage
resistance form
retention form

rubber dam
rubber dam clamp
submargination
Tofflemire universal matrix
   system
wall

The dental hygienist serves as an important member of the oral healthcare team, evaluating all surfaces of teeth and the periodontium in the patient's oral cavity using both visual and tactile senses. For many patients the dental hygienist is his or her most regular healthcare provider. The dentist relies on the hygienist to provide important assessment information to develop proper preventive and therapeutic strategies. Because the dental hygienist frequently observes the patient's condition before the dentist does, mental and written documentation of findings is important to assist with any subsequent oral health care.

Operative dentistry is defined as the diagnosis, prevention, and treatment of diseases, developmental defects, and traumatic injuries of hard tissues of individual teeth.[15,16] To ensure proper treatment of an individual tooth, the correct diagnosis must be made. The first step in the diagnosis of a patient is a proper medical and dental history (see Chapter 12). Prevention has both primary and secondary components. *Primary prevention* is to prevent the disease before evidence of its occurrence. *Secondary prevention* is to prevent a recurrence of the disease or an incipient (i.e., initial, just beginning) case from progressing to a more severe state.

Classification and Nomenclature

BLACK'S RESTORATIVE LESION CLASSIFICATION

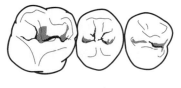

Until recently, most dental restorations were based on the designs of G.V. Black, often referred to as the "father of modern restorative dentistry."[5,15] Dr. Black's classifications and principles were based on the restorative materials of his time, which were primarily dental **amalgam** and gold. Black did not have the benefit of modern bonding systems and restorative materials. His initial classifications are as follows:

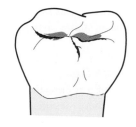

FIGURE 35-1
Class I lesion.

Class I lesion—Occurs in pits and fissures of a tooth (Figure 35-1)

Class II lesion—Occurs on the proximal surface of a posterior tooth (Figure 35-2)

Class III lesion—Occurs on the proximal surface of an anterior tooth (Figure 35-3)

Class IV lesion—Occurs on the proximal surface of an anterior tooth from which the incisal angle is missing (Figure 35-4)

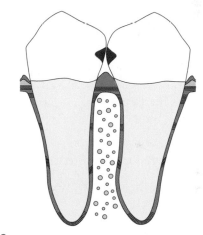

FIGURE 35-2
Class II lesion.

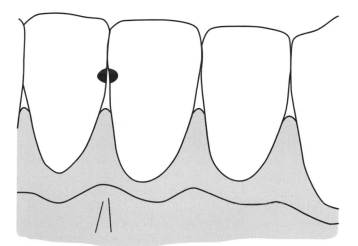

FIGURE 35-3
Class III lesion.

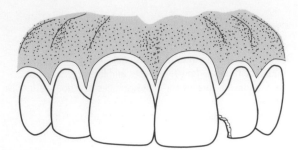

FIGURE 35-4
Class IV lesion.

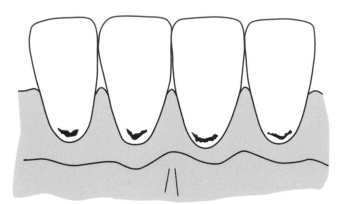

FIGURE 35-5
Class V lesion.

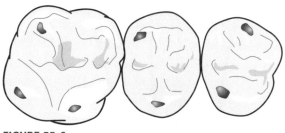

FIGURE 35-6
Class VI lesion.

Class V lesion—Occurs on the gingival third of the labial, buccal, or lingual smooth surfaces of the tooth (Figure 35-5)

Eventually a sixth category was added, although not by Dr. Black, as follows:

Class VI lesion—Occurs on the tips of the cusps or the biting surfaces of the incisors (Figure 35-6)

BLACK'S PRINCIPLES FOR SURGICAL REPAIR OF A DISEASED TOOTH

Black also developed a series of principles to be followed when surgically repairing a diseased tooth.

Outline Form

This process involves placement of the cavity margins (cavosurface) in the position on the tooth that they will occupy in the completed restoration. The **outline form** should encompass the carious lesion and may include portions of dental caries–susceptible areas on the tooth being restored. The outline form should follow a smooth, gentle, sweeping curve, especially on the occlusal surface. Clinicians should visualize this form before any tooth reduction (i.e., instrumentation) occurs to prevent overcutting of tissue. Outline form is determined by many factors, including location and size of the lesion, anatomy of the tooth, type of restorative material, esthetic requirements of the situation, relative position of adjacent structures, functional requirements, and retentive factors.

Black proposed two general principles to guide the establishment of outline form: (1) removal of all enamel not supported by dentin (undermined enamel) and (2) placement of margins in areas of low dental caries susceptibility, often referred to as **extension for prevention.**

Resistance Form

Resistance form is the design and position of the cavity walls that best enable the tooth and the restoration to withstand forces and avoid fracture or breakage of the tooth or the restoration (filling material). Fundamental principles of resistance form include the following:

- Flat floors prepared at right angles to the forces of mastication
- Restriction of preparation extensions to allow strong cuspal and marginal ridges
- Removal of weakened tooth tissue in the preparation design to prevent future tooth fracture
- Consideration of the properties of the restorative materials

Retention Form

Retention form is that shape of the cavity preparation that permits the restoration to resist displacement (or dislodgment) through sliding, tipping, or lifting forces. Factors that enhance retention form include *occlusal dovetails,* converging walls, defined internal line angles, grooves, pins, frictional resistance of walls, and acid etching (used with bonding agents and bonded restorative materials).

Convenience Form

Convenience form is that shape of the preparation that allows adequate observation, accessibility, and ease of operation during the preparation and restorative phases of treatment. Inadequate convenience form prevents proper instrumentation of the cavity preparation. Factors that enhance convenience form include extension of the cavity preparation (taking care to limit excessive extension because of its negative effect on resistance form), a change in the line of approach, and a change in the operating instrument.

Removal of Remaining Carious Dentin

This process involves the excavation of any infectious tooth structure remaining after the basic cavity design has been completed. Incipient lesions, which penetrate the dentinoenamel junction (DEJ) no more than 0.5 mm, generally are removed at the completion of outline, resistance, retention, and convenience form sequence. Extensive lesions, which penetrate the DEJ more than 0.5 mm, will be subjected to further surgical extension until all diseased tissue is removed (or medicated).

Finishing of Enamel Walls

The finishing process involves the smoothing or refinement of the walls of the cavity preparation and cavosurface angles. This step helps to do the following:

- Create an optimal marginal seal between the restorative material and the tooth
- Allow for optimal marginal adaptation (which is less noticeable to the patient and is less plaque biofilm retentive)
- Provide maximal strength to the restorative material and to the tooth at the margin

Cleansing and Medicating of Preparation

This process includes removal of all debris, drying of the preparation (preparation is left slightly damp for increased bonding strength with current bonding systems[10]), inspection for decay and unsound tooth tissue, and placement of medication if indicated.

35-2   COMPONENTS OF PREPARED CAVITIES

Prepared cavities have walls, line angles, and point angles just as the crown of the tooth has surfaces, line angles, and point angles. The nomenclature involved is quite similar in both cases. Most cavity preparations are considered to have a *box* form, and these components are most easily visualized in this form.

Wall

A vertical or horizontal surface within the cavity preparation is called a **wall** and is named according to the closest external surface (e.g., facial, mesial, or lingual wall), for the structure that it approximates (e.g., pulpal wall), or for its relationship to the long axis of the tooth (e.g., axial wall).

Cavosurface

The uncut tooth tissue adjacent to the cavity preparation is the **cavosurface.**

Line Angle

A **line angle** is formed along the junctions of two walls or the junction of one wall and the cavosurface (i.e., cavosurface margin). Line angles are named according to the walls and surfaces involved.

Point Angle

A **point angle** is formed by the junction of three walls within a cavity preparation and is named according to the walls involved.

CLASS I CAVITY PREPARATIONS

A Class I cavity preparation on a molar is used to illustrate the derivation of the nomenclature (Figure 35-7).

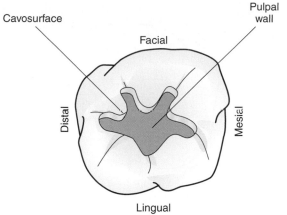

FIGURE 35-7
Class I cavity preparation. Outer surfaces of tooth are designated *mesial, lingual, distal,* and *facial.* Wall at the bottom of the cavity is the pulpal wall. Unprepared external surface of the tooth adjacent to the preparation is the cavosurface.

Walls

A Class I molar preparation normally has curving walls along the facial and lingual sides that blend with the mesial and distal walls. These vertical walls end at a horizontal wall called the *pulpal wall* or *pulpal floor.* Figure 35-8 presents the preparation as a box to assist the dental hygienist in learning the nomenclature.

Line Angles

The three sets of line angles in the Class I preparation are named according to the walls involved (Figures 35-9 through 35-11).

Rule 1

When the name of a line angle or point angle is being developed, the *al* should be dropped and *o* substituted at the end of all words in the name, except the last one (e.g., the line angle formed by the facial wall intersecting the pulpal wall is the

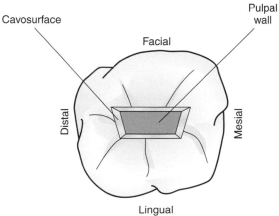

FIGURE 35-8
Reader should compare with Figure 35-7. Preparation is a box with four walls and bottom. Walls of the preparation are named for external surfaces to which they are adjacent; the bottom is called the *pulpal wall* because of its proximity to the pulp.

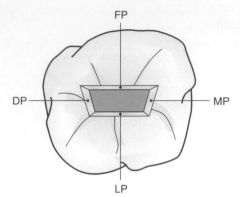

FIGURE 35-9
The four line angles formed at the intersections of the vertical walls with the pulpal wall are the mesiopulpal *(MP)*, lingopulpal *(LP)*, distopulpal *(DP)*, and faciopulpal *(FP)*.

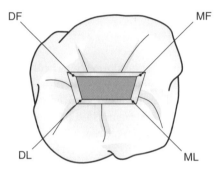

FIGURE 35-10
The four line angles formed where the vertical walls intersect one another are the mesiolingual *(ML)*, distolingual *(DL)*, distofacial *(DF)*, and mesiofacial *(MF)*.

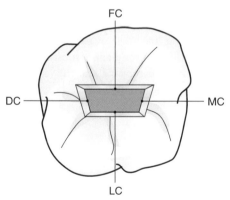

FIGURE 35-11
The four cavosurface line angles formed where the vertical walls intersect the uncut tooth surface are the mesiocavosurface *(MC)*, linguocavosurface *(LC)*, distocavosurface *(DC)*, and faciocavosurface *(FC)*.

faciopulpal line angle). Figure 35-9 shows the remaining line angles formed by the pulpal wall. These line angles are not straight but follow the outline form of the preparation. Figure 35-10 shows the line angles formed by the intersection of one vertical wall with another. In the actual cavity preparation, these are not sharp corners but curves. Figure 35-11 illustrates the four line angles formed by the intersection of the vertical walls with the cavosurface.

Rule 2

When *cavosurface* is one of the words used in the description of a line angle, this word is placed last (e.g., the intersection of the facial wall with the cavosurface is the *faciocavosurface* line angle). The other three cavosurface line angles are named in a similar manner.

Point Angles

Four internal point angles constitute a Class I occlusal preparation (Figure 35-12). The name of each is derived by combining the names of the involved walls using rule 1.

CLASS II CAVITY PREPARATIONS

The Class II cavity preparation removes the proximal surface (Figure 35-13). The occlusal portion is prepared similar to a Class I preparation, but the marginal ridge is involved to allow

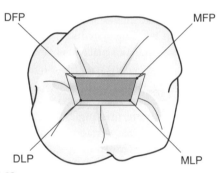

FIGURE 35-12
The four point angles formed at the intersection of three internal walls. Intersection of three walls at lower left, for example, is the mesiolinguopulpal *(MLP)* point angle. *DLP,* Distolinguopulpal; *DFP,* distofaciopulpal; *MFP,* mesiofaciopulpal.

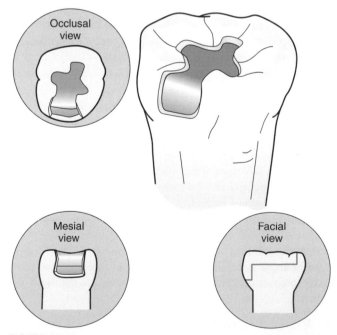

FIGURE 35-13
Class II mesioocclusal cavity preparation on tooth #19. Reader should compare with the occlusal view in Figure 35-7.

access to the proximal surface. A Class II preparation is an extension of the Class I into the proximal area.

Walls and Cavosurface

The occlusal walls are identical to those of the Class I preparation. The proximal portion includes an axial wall parallel to the long axis of the tooth and a gingival wall (floor) adjacent to the gingival tissues (Figure 35-14). The facial and lingual walls of the proximal portion are termed the *facioproximal* and *linguoproximal* walls.

Line Angles

In the proximal portion the internal line angles (Figure 35-15) are the following:
- Axiopulpal
- Axiogingival
- Axiolinguoproximal
- Axiofacioproximal

- Gingivolinguoproximal
- Gingivofacioproximal

In the proximal portion the external line angles (Figure 35-16) are the following:
- Linguoproximocavosurface
- Facioproximocavosurface
- Gingivocavosurface

Point Angles

The intersection of the gingival and axial walls with each of the proximal walls forms two point angles: (1) axiogingivo*linguo*proximal and (2) axiogingivo*facio*proximal (Figure 35-17).

CLASS III CAVITY PREPARATIONS

Dental caries on the proximal surface of anterior teeth may be removed by either a facial or a lingual approach. Figure 35-18 illustrates the cavity outlines resulting from each approach, as well as the walls resulting from the preparations. The dental practitioner can identify line angles and point angles for each of the preparations.

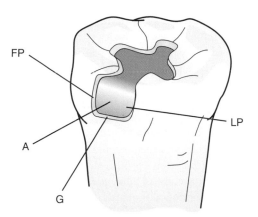

FIGURE 35-14
The walls of the proximal portion of the preparation are the gingival (G), linguoproximal (LP), axial (A), and facioproximal (FP).

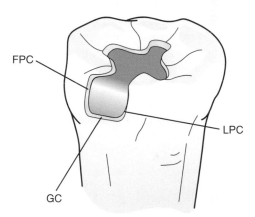

FIGURE 35-16
The cavosurface line angles of the proximal portion of Class II preparation are the gingivocavosurface (GC), linguoproximocavosurface (LPC), and facioproximocavosurface (FPC).

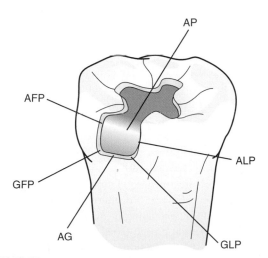

FIGURE 35-15
The line angles of the proximal portion of Class II mesioocclusal preparation are the gingivolinguoproximal (GLP), axiolinguoproximal (ALP), axiopulpal (AP), axiogingival (AG), axiofacioproximal (AFP), and gingivofacioproximal (GFP).

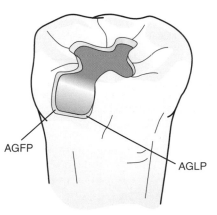

FIGURE 35-17
The internal point angles of the mesioproximal portion of Class II mesioocclusal preparation are the axiogingivolinguoproximal (AGLP) and axiogingivofacioproximal (AGFP).

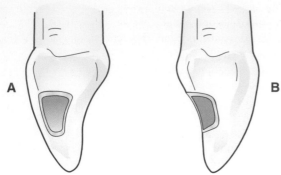

FIGURE 35-18
Walls of Class III cavity preparation. **A,** Labial access. **B,** Lingual slot access.

CLASS IV CAVITY PREPARATIONS

Figure 35-19 is a proximal view of a Class IV restoration to help develop the nomenclature for this preparation.

CLASS V CAVITY PREPARATIONS

The Class V preparation is similar to a Class I preparation except for its location in the gingival one third of the facial or lingual surface. Class V also may be viewed as a box with four sides and a bottom (Figure 35-20). On an anterior tooth the occlusal wall is called the *incisal wall.*

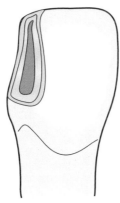

FIGURE 35-19
Proximal view of Class IV cavity preparation walls.

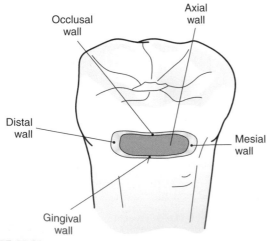

Occlusal wall
Axial wall
Distal wall
Mesial wall
Gingival wall

FIGURE 35-20
Walls of Class V cavity preparation on posterior tooth.

Minimally Invasive Dentistry

The traditional treatment for the carious lesion has remained essentially the same since G.V. Black introduced his principles more than a century ago. As stated, his *extension for prevention* has been an important tenet for every dentist educated in the twentieth century; however, some have challenged Black's ideas. Bronner[6] and Markley[11] published works on more conservative cavity design in the first half of the twentieth century. Osborne, Hoffman, and Ferguson[13] and Sigurjons[18] addressed these issues in the 1970s and 1980s.

AMALGAM-SEALANT COMBINATIONS

The advent of adhesive dentistry began in the 1950s, when Buonocore[7] discovered that acid etching of tooth enamel increased the retention of restorative materials. With subsequent advances in bonding systems[20] and resin **composite** materials, prevention of dental caries and greater conservation of tooth structure became possible. These advances initiated the era of minimally invasive dentistry.

A 10-year clinical study by Mertz-Fairhurst and colleagues[12] compared traditional Class I amalgam restorations to Class I amalgams placed only in areas of the fissure systems where actual dental caries had been diagnosed. In the latter group the fissures remaining after the placement of those smaller restorations were sealed with a resin fissure sealant. At 10 years, 7 of the 79 traditional amalgam restorations had failed, and only 1 of the 77 amalgam-sealant combination restorations had failed. This definitive study provided excellent support for dentists limiting the size of cavity preparations to the decayed area (i.e., dental caries–directed preparations) and addressing the principle of extension for prevention with materials such as fissure sealants.

The clinician can establish outline form using these parameters simply by removing carious dentin and the overlying unsupported enamel. Osborne and Summitt[14] state that this allows for conservation and maintenance of tooth structure and leaves more occlusal enamel, which is better suited for occlusal function and resistance to occlusal wear than restorative materials. These concepts, along with surgical treatment of only active dental caries (observed radiographically to have penetrated the dentin) and with use of all available means to stop and reverse dental caries, represent truly minimal intervention and the current state of the art in operative dentistry.

With the advent of adhesive dentistry, prevention of dental caries and greater conservation of tooth structure are possible. In addition, evidence indicates a possible shift in philosophy from the traditional surgical model of excision to a more modern medical model of treatment.[2,8] Hume[9] stated that dentists should modify their 200-year-old philosophy of treating dental caries like gangrene by extracting or excavating and filling. He advocated a treatment approach based on the structure and behavior of the lesion. Carious lesions in dentin and cementum are reversible to some degree, and Hume further recommended that clinicians consider including nonsurgical healing of these lesions in the treatment plan. As a result, more and more of today's oral healthcare teams are developing their treatment strategies based on the consideration of dental caries as an infectious disease.

CASE APPLICATION 35-1.1

Conservative Extension for Prevention

Mrs. Dixon's treatment plan called for a number of small occlusal restorations, which would be opportune situations for minimally invasive procedures. Rather than the standard Black style of outline form on the occlusal surface of her mandibular molar, the outline could be confined to the area of localized dental caries in the central pit. The dental caries would be surgically excised in this area only, and a small esthetic composite (or small amalgam) suitable for the posterior teeth could be bonded in place. The adjacent grooves could then be treated with a fissure sealant (Figure 35-21). In essence, Black's extension for prevention would be obtained not by the outline of the preparation but rather by the conservative treatment of the adjacent fissures with proven sealants.

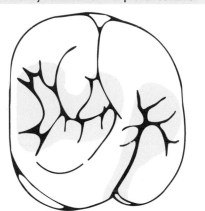

FIGURE 35-21
Occlusal view of molar for sealant application. Shaded area is etched, and a pit fissure sealant or flowable resin composite is bonded in place.

Esthetic Dentistry

Since the introduction of the acid-etch technique,[7] dental manufacturers have developed numerous generations of restorative tooth-colored materials. Patients are becoming more informed on the availability of these esthetic materials and are demanding their use by the dental profession. Many are aware of the option of treating stained teeth with a bleaching or whitening technique (see Chapter 39) or coverage by direct or indirect resin composite or porcelain veneers and crowns. Patients may also have spaces (i.e., diastematas) that can be closed with the same materials. Some patients, however, are not educated about the availability of these products and techniques.

CASE APPLICATION 35-1.2

Tooth Discoloration

Mrs. Dixon does not smile often, primarily because she is self-conscious about the discoloration of her maxillary anterior teeth. With proper education from the dental team, she can be made aware of esthetic interventions for the treatment of her dentition.

The patient's personality change after esthetic treatment is one of the most rewarding accomplishments for the dental team. Many new materials have been developed, and many traditional ones have been substantially improved to add to the dental team's armamentarium for the treatment of these cases.

Isolation of Teeth

A proper operating field is necessary to perform operative procedures with optimal results. Isolating the field does the following:

- Prevents moisture contamination of the operating field and of the restorative materials, a situation that could lead to failure of the restoration
- Retracts and controls the soft tissues
- Protects the patient against aspiration of instruments and materials
- Provides optimal visibility of the operating site
- Provides an effective infection control barrier for the dental operatory

While isolating the operative field, the clinician should not interfere with visual or mechanical access to the operating (i.e., surgical) site, injure soft or hard tissues, or cause discomfort.

The type of isolation required depends on the duration of the procedure and the degree of dryness necessary. For some procedures, cotton roll isolation can be accomplished with a saliva ejector and a high-volume oral evacuation system. Cotton roll holders can be used in the mandibular arch. Absorbent triangles over the parotid duct can be used with cotton rolls for increased moisture control. Cotton roll isolation offers ease and speed of application. However, risks include contamination of the operating field, limited retraction of soft tissues, and no protection against the patient aspirating debris or objects.

The **rubber dam** (i.e., dental dam) meets the criteria listed for proper isolation. Disadvantages are that the clamp can irritate and even lacerate the gingival tissues, placement of the dam can be time-consuming for the beginning clinician, and some patients are sensitive to the latex of the rubber dam (although nonlatex rubber dams are available). Overall, however, the advantages of using a rubber dam outweigh the disadvantages.

Distinct Care Modifications
Rubber dam application may not be possible with teeth that have not erupted sufficiently, with some third molars, or with extremely malpositioned teeth. In addition, patients with asthma may find breathing difficult. Patients with a latex allergy should have latex-free rubber dam material used for application.

ARMAMENTARIUM

Figure 35-22 illustrates the necessary armamentarium for rubber dam placement. The Young's frame is a common type of rubber dam holder. This metal or plastic U-shaped frame holds the dam away from the patient's face. The Woodbury holder is an elastic band that fits around the back of the patient's head and is attached to the sides of the dam with three clips on each side. It provides excellent lip and cheek retraction.

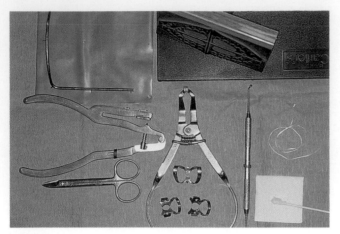

FIGURE 35-22
Tray setup for rubber dam application.

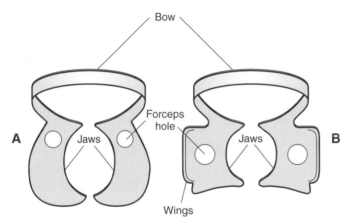

FIGURE 35-23
Rubber dam clamps. **A,** Wingless. **B,** Winged.

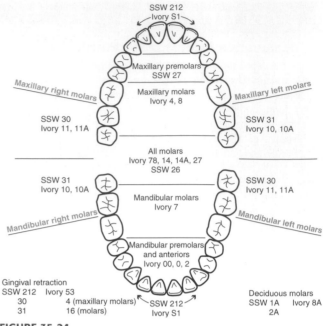

FIGURE 35-24
Chart of suggested clamps to be used in various areas of mouth.

PREPARATION OF PATIENT

If the patient has never experienced placement of a rubber dam, then the clinician should explain the benefits, such as elimination of debris in the mouth (which could be swallowed) and prevention of a contaminated restorative site. The procedure also should be explained briefly so that the patient knows what to expect. Because the patient will not be able to talk with the dam in place, the clinician may suggest signals to be used if the patient should need to communicate.

EXAMINATION OF MOUTH

The clinician should examine the site where the dam is to be placed and floss the teeth to determine whether passing the dam between any of the teeth will be difficult. If floss cannot be passed through the contact, then the reason should be determined. Calculus, restoration overhangs, and rough proximal surfaces should be removed. Teeth with very tight contacts may need to be wedged apart before dam placement. If needed, then a wooden wedge may be placed into the involved proximal space for 1 to 2 minutes, then the contact checked again with dental floss. The clinician also must check the patient's occlusion to determine whether any unusual anatomical parts may interfere with

> **Patient Education Opportunity**
>
> Before placing a rubber dam, the clinician should always explain the rationale for the isolation procedure and what the patient might expect. Some patients may be fearful of having the rubber dam placed over the mouth. The patient should be assured that breathing will not be affected. In addition, the clinician can suggest signals to be used if the patient needs to communicate during the appointment.

The **rubber dam clamp** anchors the dam to the tooth (Figure 35-23); therefore this tooth is referred to as the *anchor tooth*. Clamps may be winged or wingless. The jaws of the winged clamp have small projections (i.e., wings) that allow the clamp to be mounted on the dam before the dam is placed on the teeth. The dental chart is helpful in the determination of which clamps are most likely to fit particular teeth (Figure 35-24).

The dam material is available in several weights (thicknesses) and in various colors. Heavier material is typically used for restorative procedures, because the added weight provides better retraction of the gingivae, lips, and cheeks and because the material does not tear easily. Lightweight material is used more often during endodontic procedures, because only one tooth is isolated, tearing is less of a problem, and the lighter material is easier to manipulate.

> **Prevention**
>
> The bow of the clamp is applied with the rubber dam or after the rubber dam is in place. With the exception of the no. 212 anterior clamp, each clamp should be tied with dental floss approximately 12 inches in length before the clamp is placed on the tooth. For maximal protection, the floss may be threaded through both holes in the jaws of the clamp in case the clamp breaks in two pieces. The purpose of the floss is to allow retrieval of the clamp or the broken pieces should it break or be accidentally swallowed or aspirated.[23]

the restoration. The shape and size of the arch, position of the teeth, edentulous spaces, and fixed prostheses must be noted. This information will be needed to punch the rubber dam holes correctly.

SELECTION OF CLAMP

The rubber dam clamp is selected on the basis of the anatomy of the anchor tooth (see Figure 35-24). The location and number of the involved teeth will determine which teeth are to be isolated. Minimal access is obtained by isolation of one tooth distal and two teeth mesial to the teeth being restored. The most distal tooth in the quadrant should be clamped and isolation extended to the opposite lateral incisor to obtain the following:

- Greater access
- Maximal retraction of the lips, cheeks, and tongue
- More teeth for a finger rest

If only the anterior teeth are involved, then the clinician may isolate from the first premolar to the contralateral first premolar. Both premolars may be clamped or ligated (i.e., tied) with dental floss or a small piece of rubber dam used to wedge the dam in the interproximal areas.

PLACEMENT OF CLAMP

Box 35-1 provides a list of steps used to place the clamp. When properly placed, all four prongs should contact the tooth near its line angles at a position cervical to the height of contour (Figures 35-25 and 35-26). The clamp should be stable when rocked gently from side to side with light finger pressure and should not impinge on the soft tissue. If these criteria are not met, then the clamp should be repositioned or, if necessary, another clamp selected. If the clamp rotates or slides off the tooth or rests on the papilla, then the clamp is too large. If the clamp does not fit over the height of contour or pops off the tooth, then the clamp is too small. Because the prongs are pointed and can cut the

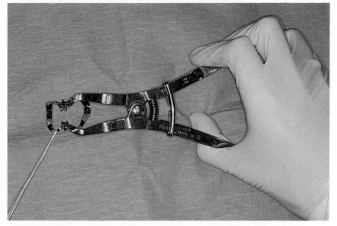

FIGURE 35-25
Clinician engages the locking ring by pointing forceps upward, then squeezing and releasing (see Box 35-1).

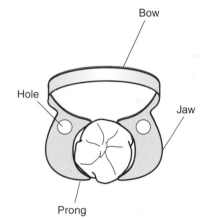

FIGURE 35-26
All four prongs of clamps should be in contact with tooth.

gingiva or gouge the root surface, forceps should always be used to disengage or reposition the clamp.

PREPARATION OF RUBBER DAM (DENTAL DAM)

The rubber dam is punched to suit each clinical situation. The number, size, and location of the holes are determined by the following:

- Location and size of the teeth to be isolated
- Shape and size of the arch
- Position and spacing of the teeth
- Type of preparation

A template or rubber dam stamp can be used as a guide to mark the location of the holes to be punched (Figure 35-27). If this is not available, then the dam can be punched according to a mandibular and maxillary chart (Figure 35-28).

- The clinician should mark the central incisors near the midline of the dam, allowing 4 mm of rubber between anterior holes and 5 mm of rubber between posterior holes.
- The holes for Class V restorations should be marked 1 mm to the facial side for facial lesions or 1 mm to the

---

BOX 35-1

STEPS FOR CLAMP PLACEMENT

1. Determine the anchor tooth and select the appropriate clamp.
2. Tie floss around the bow of the clamp to permit retrieval if the clamp slips off the tooth.
3. Place the clamp on the forceps.
4. Squeeze the handles together to open the jaws of the clamp.
5. With the tips of the forceps upward, the locking ring will slide toward the handle of the forceps holding the jaws of the clamp open (see Figure 35-25).
6. Position the clamp over the tooth.
7. Rotate it lingually to seat the lingual jaw first, because vision is more restricted in this area.
8. Rotate the clamp facially to seat the facial jaw. Be certain that the jaws do not drag across the tooth, scarring the cementum.
9. Squeeze the handles of the forceps to release the locking ring and allow the jaws of the clamp to engage the tooth.

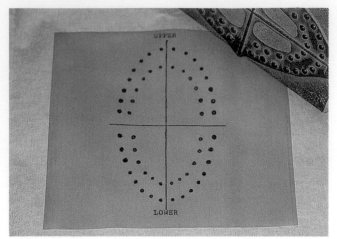

FIGURE 35-27
Rubber dam stamp.

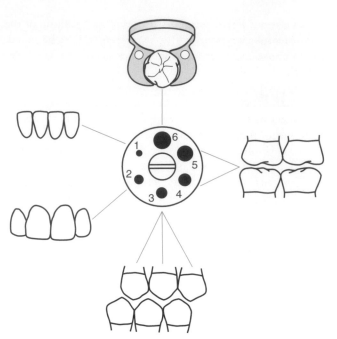

FIGURE 35-29
Suggested sizes of holes to be punched in dam for various teeth.

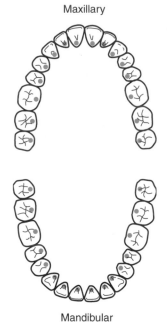

Maxillary

Mandibular

FIGURE 35-28
For the average-sized arch, the clinician should punch the central incisors approximately 1½ inches from the edge of the dam near the midline. Additional holes should be punched using guidelines in text.

lingual side for lingual lesions. An additional 1 mm of rubber between adjacent teeth should be allotted for the gingival retraction needed for access to the Class V lesion.

- The size of the hole to be punched depends on the size of the tooth. For a six-hole punch, the smaller size 2 hole is used for all mandibular incisors and maxillary lateral incisors; the medium size 3 hole for premolars, canines, and maxillary central incisors; the size 5 hole for molars; and the size 6 hole for the anchor tooth and clamp (Figure 35-29).
- As the hole is punched, the clinician should pull the dam up the punch spike to be certain it has cut completely through the dam.

- A water-soluble lubricant may be applied in the area of the punched holes to aid the passing of the rubber dam through the proximal contacts of the teeth.

PLACEMENT OF RUBBER DAM AND FRAME

Before rubber dam placement, the clinician should take the following preparatory steps:

- Lubricate the patient's lips with petroleum jelly to protect them against dryness and irritation from the dam. A rubber dam napkin may also be placed to increase patient comfort during the procedure. The napkin will absorb

any fluids seeping from the corners of the patient's mouth and act as a cushion between the patient's skin and the rubber dam.

- Place the powdered side of the dam facing the clinician to reduce light reflection.
- Choose one of two alternative methods of placing the clamp and dam on the tooth based on the clinical situation, clinician's preference, and availability of clamps.
- If a wingless clamp is used, then place the clamp on the tooth and recheck its stability.
- Orient the rubber dam, and place the index finger of each hand on opposing sides of the hole to be placed over the clamped tooth.
- Stretch the dam to enlarge the hole, and slide the dam over the bow and under each of the jaws.
- When the tooth and clamp are fully exposed with the rubber dam against the gingiva, use a T-ball burnisher blade to pull the floss tied to the clamp through the hole.

The dam may also be placed on the bow of the wingless clamp before placement on the tooth, which may be easier for the inexperienced clinician. This allows maximum access and visibility while applying the clamp. Care must be exercised to avoid placement of excess pressure on the clamp, thus traumatizing the tooth or surrounding gingiva as the dam is seated.

To use a winged clamp, the clinician should orient it to the correct hole in the dam, and proceed as follows:

- Lubricate the patient's lips with petroleum jelly to protect them against dryness and irritation from the dam. A rubber dam napkin may also be placed to increase patient comfort during the procedure.
- Place the powdered side of the dam facing the clinician to reduce light reflection.

- Engage the clamp onto the forceps.
- Slide one wing into the hole, then stretch the dam toward and over the opposite wing (Figure 35-30). The dam may be placed on the frame at this stage, if desired.
- Place the clamp on the anchor tooth as described previously, looking through the opening and under the dam to check the position of the clamp relative to the gingiva before releasing the forceps.
- Pull the rubber dam off the wings, and allow it to slide against the tooth and rest under the clamp. Vision is more limited with this method, but placement is faster because the clamp, dam, and frame are placed simultaneously. After the clamp and approximating dam are positioned properly, isolate the most anterior tooth. Then place the frame, if not already carried into position with the clamp, to hold the dam away from the patient's face and to provide access to the working area.
- Position the base of the U-shaped frame downward, with the concave side of the frame toward the patient.
- Gently pull the rubber dam over the small metal protrusions on the frame to hold the dam in place.
- Stretch the dam to open the holes over the remaining teeth, one at a time.
- Pass the dam through the contact areas. This is more easily done with an assistant, who stretches the dam over each contact area.
- Push the rubber through the contact areas by using waxed floss or tape to engage the leading edge of the rubber and carrying it first against one proximal surface and then the other (Figure 35-31). Do not try to force the whole width of the septum through at once; this is difficult to accomplish and may result in tearing of the dam. If the dam is not fully through the contact areas, then it will be difficult to tuck it into the facial and lingual sulci. Repeat the flossing procedure if needed.
- After the dam is through the contact areas, readjust the frame to hold the dam more tightly.

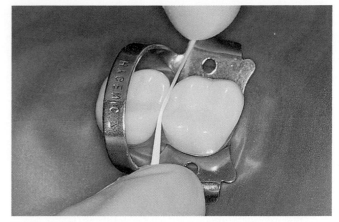

FIGURE 35-31
When necessary, the clinician should push the interseptal rubber through the contacts with dental floss.

- Center the frame to avoid endangering the patient (i.e., the ends of the frame should be away from the patient's eyes).
- Tie the floss attached to the clamp to the frame so that the floss is out of the operating field.
- Tuck (invert) the dam into the sulcus around each tooth to prevent seepage of sulcular fluid and saliva. Starting at the distal, position the blade of a plastic instrument or T-ball burnisher parallel to the distofacial line angle of the tooth, directed slightly into the sulcus. Slide it to the mesial line angle, using the edge of the blade to push the rubber into the gingival sulcus (Figure 35-32). Simultaneously, direct a stream of air into the sulcus to dry the tooth, rubber dam, and soft tissue to prevent the rubber dam from sliding back out of the sulcus. Repeat this step for each tooth on both the facial and the lingual surfaces.

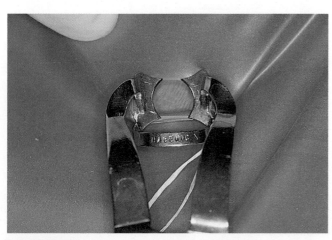

FIGURE 35-30
Winged clamp being held by dam before placement on tooth.

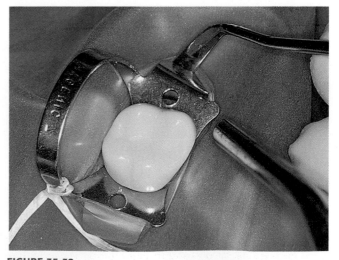

FIGURE 35-32
The clinician should invert the dam into the sulcus using a thin (not sharp) blade. Air helps dry the tooth and dam and creates a seal.

- Stabilize the rubber dam by ligating a piece of dental floss around the most anterior tooth (Figure 35-33) or by wedging a small piece of rubber into the embrasure between the last exposed tooth and the rubber dam (Figure 35-34). For dam applications isolating the teeth from first premolar to first premolar, the ligature or rubber dam wedge method of stabilization may be used instead of clamps.
- After the dam is correctly placed, insert a saliva ejector under the rubber dam onto the floor of the mouth.

A properly applied rubber dam should do the following:
- Isolate the working area with no moisture present
- Expose the teeth to be treated and provide sufficient visual access and finger rests for the clinician
- Be stable and secure, with no potential damage to the hard and soft tissues
- Be inverted into the gingival sulcus
- Be comfortable (Figure 35-35)

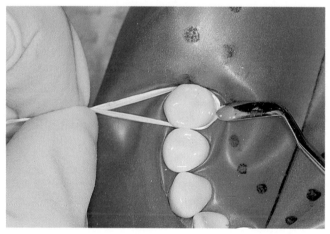

FIGURE 35-33
The loop of ligature is pushed below the cingulum with the blade while pulling the ends in an apical direction.

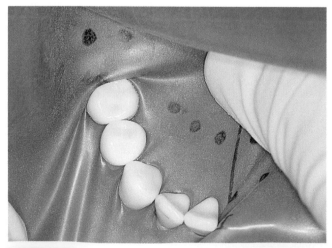

FIGURE 35-34
The piece of rubber dam is stretched and pushed into the contact area.

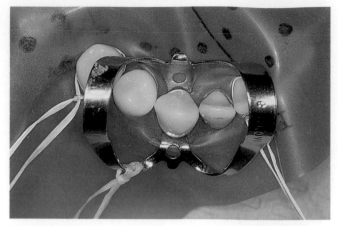

FIGURE 35-35
Isolation achieved through properly mounted rubber dam.

APPLICATION OF GINGIVAL RETRACTOR CLAMP

The gingival retractor clamp pushes the gingival tissue and rubber dam material away from the site of the Class V preparation (Box 35-2). This retractor has two jaws (with prongs), two bows, and notches for the clamp forceps. The bows have different lengths, which provide this clamp with specific lingual and facial sides (Figure 35-36). When the retractor is oriented to the tooth, the flat portion of the bow will be to the facial lesion side of the tooth. The gingival retractor clamp should be stabilized with low-fusing compound (Figure 35-37).

REMOVAL OF RUBBER DAM

Before removing the dam, high-volume evacuation should be used to remove all debris from the operating field. If a gingival retractor has been used, then the clinician should remove it first

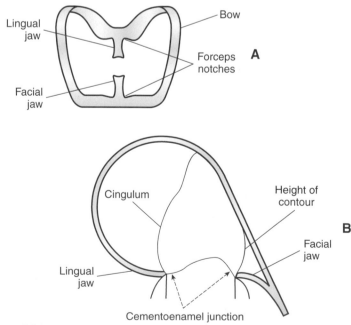

FIGURE 35-36
A, Parts of gingival retractor. **B,** Relationship of gingival retractor jaws to landmarks on anterior tooth.

BOX 35-2

STEPS FOR APPLICATION OF GINGIVAL RETRACTOR CLAMP FOR CLASS V RESTORATIONS

1. Insert the forceps into the notches and expand the jaws of the retractor. For greater access and visibility, seat the lingual jaw first.
2. Slide it gently against the lingual surface until the clamp is apical to the height of contour and flush with, but not impinging on, the gingival tissue.
3. Use the opposite hand to stabilize the lingual jaw.
4. At the same time, rotate the forceps to move the facial jaw apically along the facial surface until the facial jaw is apical to the height of contour and contacts the dam overlying the gingiva.
5. Using the jaws of the clamp, gently retract the gingiva and dam to expose the gingival extent of the carious lesion.
6. Spread the jaws wide enough to avoid scraping against the tooth as the jaws are seated. This would scar the tooth, making it more susceptible to plaque biofilm accumulation and dental caries. If possible, then retract the gingiva until the gingiva is at least 0.5 to 1.0 mm apical to the gingival margin of the lesion. The bows of the clamp should be parallel to the tooth's occlusal plane to ensure even retraction of the gingiva.
7. Remove the forceps from the retractor while continuing to support the lingual and facial aspects of the retractor with the other hand.
8. Continue the support until dental compound has been placed under the bows and onto the occlusal and incisal surfaces of the surrounding teeth (see Figure 35-37). Dental compound stabilizes the gingival retractor to avoid slippage during the procedure. Trauma to tooth structure and damage to the preparation or restorative material may occur if the clamp slips.
9. Warm the compound stick over a flame until the end begins to sag.
10. Temper it in warm water until the material is warm and malleable but not hot.
11. Mold the compound over the top of one retractor bow and the occlusal and incisal surface.
12. Continue molding the compound until it fills the space between the bow and the tooth. Repeat the procedure for the other bow.
13. Check the retractor with light finger pressure to make sure that it resists movement, is stable, and evenly retracts the gingiva and rubber dam.

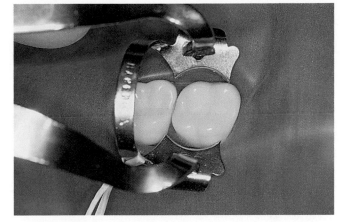

FIGURE 35-37
Mounting and placement of gingival retractor (see Box 35-2).

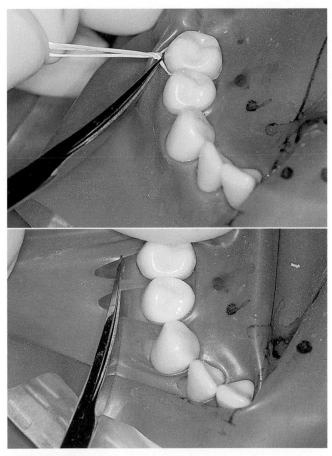

FIGURE 35-38
Rubber dam removal. The tip of the lower scissors blade extends well beyond the rubber to ensure complete cutting of the septum each time.

and apply the forceps in an occlusolingual direction to break the compound off the teeth. The retractor then is removed carefully in an occlusal direction without touching the newly placed restoration or the tooth surface. The clinician then must remove any remaining compound with a sharp instrument and remove the ligature or rubber dam wedge from the most anterior tooth. The dam should be stretched to the facial side, away from the teeth, and one finger placed under the stretched dam to protect the patient's lips and cheeks while the interdental areas of the dam are cut (Figure 35-38). The clinician should cut the entire septum with one stroke from the facial aspect and pull the dam in a lingual direction.

Pulling an uncut dam up through the contacts or snipping the interproximal areas in stages may cause thin pieces of dam to tear or remain around the tooth. A ring of rubber dam material remaining around a tooth would tend to migrate apically, because the apex is the most constricted area of the tooth. This could cause a gingival abscess, bone destruction, or even loss of the tooth.[1]

The clinician must remove the clamp, dam, and frame at the same time, laying the dam on a light-colored surface and checking to ensure that no small pieces of rubber are missing and still in the patient's mouth. Except for the severed interdental pieces, the dam should appear as it did before placement (Figure 35-39). Any piece that is left in the mouth should be removed with dental floss or an explorer. The clinician then must rinse and evacuate the oral cavity, examining the soft tissue for any trauma. The patient should be informed that some discomfort might occur after the anesthetic wears off.

Evaluation Criteria

APPLICATION OF RUBBER DAM

- Isolated area is clean and dry
- Number of teeth exposed provides visual access and finger rests
- Clamp is stable and secure and does not impinge on gingiva
- Dam is held securely by ligature or wedges
- Dam is inverted into the gingival sulcus
- Patient is comfortable
- If used, gingival retractor is stable and retracts the gingiva and dam

REMOVAL OF RUBBER DAM

- All rubber dam material, ligatures, and other debris have been removed.
- No significant soft tissue injury is present.

Restorative Materials

Four primary materials are used in the restoration of teeth: (1) dental amalgam and (2) resin composite (or **glass ionomers** and combinations or modifications), (3) gold or other precious or nonprecious metals, and (4) porcelain or other ceramic materials. Dental amalgam, resin composite, and gold foil

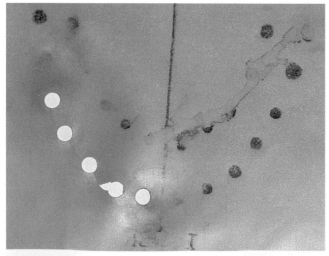

FIGURE 35-39
Clamp, dam, and frame removal. A piece of rubber dam is missing next to the fourth hole from the bottom.

materials can be placed *directly* in one appointment. Laboratory-processed resin composite, cast gold, and porcelain are generally considered *indirect* restorative materials and are placed in two separate dental appointments. This discussion focuses on the directly placed materials.

AMALGAM

35-3

Amalgam, by definition, is an alloy of mercury with any other metal. Dental amalgam is made by vigorously mixing mercury with a silver-tin alloy for a few seconds. The plastic mass is then placed into a cavity preparation, with the mixture compressed (condensation) to remove the excess mercury-rich phase. The hardening mass is then carved and finished to restore tooth form and function.

Advantages

- *Durable.* When properly placed under ideal conditions (dry field) and in conservative cavity preparations, amalgam has a long service life.
- *Economic.* Amalgam is the least expensive of the restorative materials and usually can be placed in the least amount of time.
- *Low technique sensitivity.* Amalgam is less affected by clinician error and nonideal placement conditions.
- *Broad applicability.* Amalgam can be used routinely in Class I, II, V, and VI lesions and also in certain Class III situations.
- *Easy.* Amalgam is easily manipulated.
- *Quick.* Amalgam requires less placement time.
- *Sealant capability.* **Corrosion** products seal the tooth-restoration interface, which can reduce **microleakage.**
- *Direct placement.* Amalgam is placed in a single appointment, although certain physical properties may be improved by polishing, which would be accomplished at a subsequent appointment. No interim restoration is normally required.

Disadvantages

- **Marginal breakdown.** Amalgam is a brittle material with poor edge strength.
- *Nonesthetic.* Amalgam has a silver-gray shade.
- *Potential* **galvanic reaction.** If it comes into contact with dissimilar metals, then amalgam may cause the patient to experience a tingling or shocklike feeling.
- *Public perception.* The general public has a poor perception of mercury toxicity.

Patient Education Opportunity

Patients may have questions regarding the safety of amalgam restorations. As stated on the American Dental Association (ADA) web site in 2006, "Dental amalgam is considered a safe, affordable and durable material that has been used to restore the teeth of more than 100 million Americans. Dental amalgam has been studied and reviewed extensively, and has established a record of safety and effectiveness" (http://www.ada.org/prof/resources/topics/amalgam.asp). Although dental amalgam is only one of several materials available for patients' restorative treatment needs, clinicians consider it to be safe and effective.

CAVITY SEALERS, LINERS, AND BASES

After a cavity preparation has been completed, the cut tooth surface should be treated before the placement of the amalgam restoration. The three principal options are cavity sealers, liners, and bases. **Cavity sealers** include (1) resins dissolved in a volatile solvent that leaves a resin layer after evaporation that is 2- to 5-microns thick and (2) resin bonding agents. **Cavity liners** are thin (less than 1 micron) resin or cement coating materials used to provide a barrier for protection of the pulp from restoration by-products and oral fluids. Liners can also be used to provide a therapeutic effect. **Cavity bases** are thicker (greater than 1 micron) cement filler materials used to provide thermal protection for the pulp or to provide a strong replacement material for missing dentinal tooth structure (Figure 35-40).

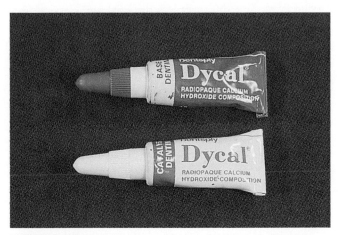

FIGURE 35-40
Calcium hydroxide liner.

Restorative Procedures

AMALGAM PLACEMENT TECHNIQUES

Class I, V, and VI Preparations

Once the tooth has been prepared and the freshly exposed surface has been treated with a cavity sealer, liner, or base, the clinician can begin placing the restorative material. Most amalgam delivery systems are capsule based. Some require activation of the capsule before mixing. *Activating* is essentially breaking the barrier that exists in the capsule that prevents the mixing of the silver-tin alloy with the mercury during storage (Figure 35-41). Usually this procedure consists of pressing the two halves of the capsule together or twisting them in opposite directions. This will vary according to manufacturer.

The clinician should set the controls on the amalgamator (i.e., amalgam mixer) to the manufacturer's recommended settings, place the activated capsule in the triturator, and turn it on; when it shuts off, the capsule may be removed. With some products the recommendation may be to remove the pestle from the capsule and triturate again for a short time. This process is known as *mulling* and may improve the plasticity of the mix.

Once mixed, the amalgam must be placed (Figures 35-42 and 35-43), condensed, and carved in a limited period. This *working time* varies by manufacturer and product (Box 35-3).

The following are the three objectives of condensation:

- Removal of excess mercury from the mix to obtain minimal mercury in the final restoration
- Compaction of the plastic mass to increase the density of the restoration by reducing voids

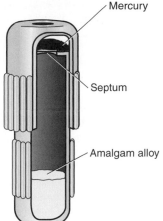

FIGURE 35-41
Preproportioned capsule showing mercury and powder separated by septum that must be perforated before mixing.

- Adaptation of the amalgam as closely as possible to the preparation walls and angles

A condenser should be selected that will fit all areas of the preparation. A small nib (i.e., the working end of the instrument) imparts more pressure than a larger nib, assuming that a constant load is applied. The technique for condensation of the amalgam should be in an orderly, stepwise, and overlapping pattern (Figure 35-44).

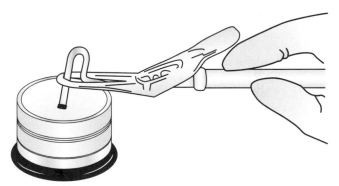

FIGURE 35-42
An amalgam well is used to hold the amalgam after trituration (see Box 35-3).

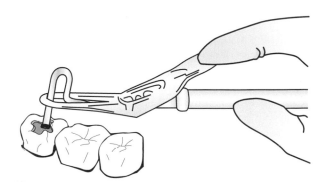

FIGURE 35-43
Amalgam is transported from the amalgam well to the cavity preparation with an amalgam carrier (see Box 35-3).

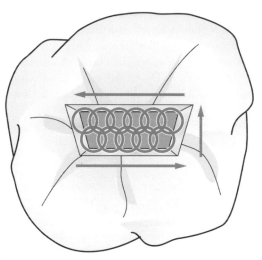

FIGURE 35-44
The pattern of condensation should be continuous overlapping strokes.

Multiple increments of amalgam are almost always required to restore a tooth. In these cases the clinician should use a series of smaller mixes rather than one large mix, because the last portion of a large mix has often lost much of its plasticity and will not be able to be condensed and carved properly. Each individual placement of the amalgam must be completely condensed before an additional increment is placed. The clinician *should not fill the cavity with multiple increments of amalgam and then condense all at one time.* Instead, the clinician should continue adding and condensing the material incrementally until the cavity is moderately overfilled. This is done to ensure that the mercury-rich surface layer is removed from the area that will become the surface of the restoration and all cavosurface margins are covered with the restorative material.

Once the cavity has been overfilled and condensed, limited time is available to carve the restoration. The objective of carving the amalgam is to reproduce the desired dental anatomy and thus ensure a proper harmony of form and function. Carving should be performed with sharp instruments to eliminate thin overextensions of material beyond the preparation margins. These overextensions, termed *flash,* are very thin and brittle, which makes them susceptible to fracture, resulting in rough or open margins. The initial phase of carving, or formation of the restoration anatomy and contours, should be accomplished before the amalgam has reached its initial set.

For the Class I and Class VI restorations, the clinician should begin carving by using an instrument such as a Walls, Hollenback, or cleoid-discoid carver or a large burnisher to remove the excess amalgam and to locate the restoration margins. An amalgam carver of choice is used to remove the remainder of the excess by placement of the carver on the tooth surface and carving parallel to the located margin (Figure 35-45). Correct carving technique for placement of tooth anatomy requires carving from the tooth surface to the amalgam. Carving from amalgam to tooth can result in gouging or ditching the restoration at its margin. The clinician should place cuspal inclines by carving perpendicular to the margins, with a portion of the blade resting on sound tooth structure (Figure 35-46). If the blade of the carver is not resting on the tooth (i.e., freefloating), then it can easily overcarve or gouge the restoration (Figure 35-47). Care must be taken to avoid carving grooves that are too deep and that tend to leave thin margins susceptible to fracture. These deep grooves may expose preparation walls as the clinician removes amalgam from the cavosurface margin while attempting to form cuspal anatomy in harmony with the deep grooves. Deep grooves are also more difficult to polish during finishing procedures.

The Class V restoration is a much easier restoration to carve. An explorer or other instrument of choice generally is used to remove the excess amalgam and to obtain the proper inciso-(occluso)gingival and mesiodistal contours of the tooth (Figure 35-48). Allowing part of the instrument tip to remain on the tooth structure (as with the Class I) is also important so that the restoration borders are not submarginated or gouged. **Submargination** is the exposure of a portion of the prepared cavity wall caused by underfilling the preparation with the restorative material or by removal of the restorative material from the cavity wall during the carving procedure.

After the appropriate anatomy and contours have been created and the restoration has reached its initial set, the final step of carving, known as *burnishing,* can be performed. Burnishing is a process of smoothing or polishing and is accomplished by lightly rubbing the surface of the amalgam after it has reached its initial set. This process affects only the surface, not the amalgam in the deeper aspects of the restoration. Burnishing removes pits and scratches left by the carving process, improves margins by increasing the density of the restorative material, and expresses more free mercury to make the surface of the restoration stronger. Burnishing should not produce an exceptionally shiny surface. If it does, the surface has been overburnished. Overburnishing increases the risk of surface corrosion because an excessive amount of mercury was brought to the surface, where it oxidizes and corrodes.

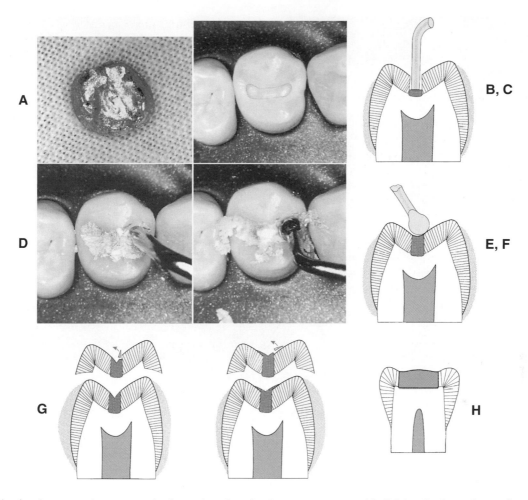

FIGURE 35-45
Restoration of occlusal cavity preparation. **A,** Properly triturated amalgam is a homogenous mass with slightly reflective surface. It flattens slightly if dropped on a tabletop. **B,** Clinician should have a mental image of outline form of preparation before condensing amalgam to assist in locating cavo-surface margins during carving procedure. **C,** Amalgam should be inserted incrementally and condensed with overlapping strokes. **D,** Cavity preparation should be overpacked to ensure well-condensed marginal amalgam that is not mercury rich. **E,** Before carving procedure, burnishing with a large burnisher is a form of condensation. **F,** Carver should rest partially on external tooth surface adjacent to margins to prevent overcarving. **G,** Deep occlusal grooves invite chipping of amalgam at margins. Thin portions of amalgam left on external surfaces soon break away, giving the appearance that amalgam has grown out of cavity. **H,** Fossae should be carved slightly deeper than proximal marginal ridges. (From Roberson TM, Heymann HO, Swift EJ Jr: *Sturdevant's art and science of operative dentistry,* ed 5, St Louis, 2006, Mosby.)

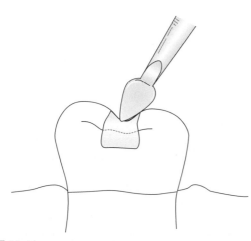

FIGURE 35-46
Correct vertical angulation of cleoid carver.

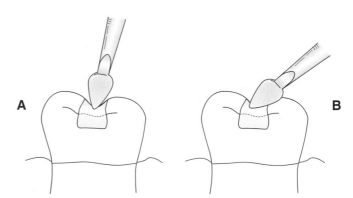

FIGURE 35-47
A, Vertical angulation of cleoid is too steep. **B,** Vertical angulation of cleoid is too flat, and tip is displaced too far toward the opposite cavo-surface margin.

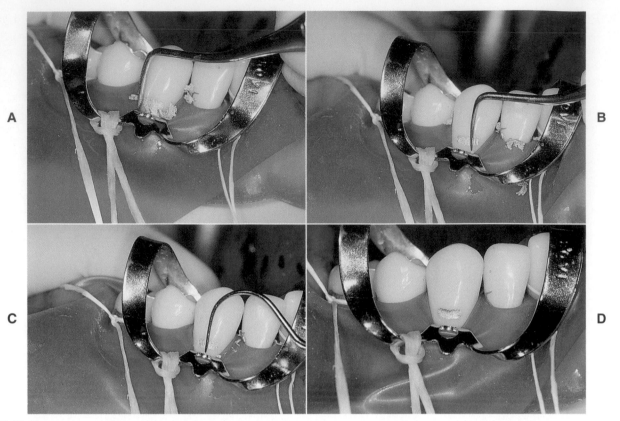

FIGURE 35-48
Carving and contouring of restoration. **A,** Clinician begins the carving procedure by removing excess and locating the incisal margin. **B** and **C,** Explorer is used to remove excess and locate mesial and distal margins. **D,** Finally, excess is removed and gingival margin located.

When the clinician finishes the procedure, any residual amalgam should be expressed from the amalgam carrier. This residue and all amalgam remaining in the well, as well as any scraps remaining from the carving process, should be placed into storage containers designated for this purpose.

Class II Preparations

Class II preparations present an additional challenge in restorations because they are missing one of the confining walls that exist in a Class I, V, or VI preparation. A Class II lesion, by definition, extends onto either the mesial or distal surfaces (or onto both) (see Figure 35-13). Placement and condensation of amalgam into such a cavity preparation will result in the restorative material being expressed out of the cavity because of the missing wall.

To compensate for this lack of natural confinement, a matrix system is used. This system provides a temporary surface to confine the placement and condensation of amalgam. Desirable characteristics of a matrix system include ease of application, convenience of use, easy removal, sufficient rigidity to withstand condensation forces, sufficient versatility to accommo-

date differently sized and shaped teeth, proper height so as not to obstruct the clinician's view, and ability to contour to replicate natural tooth structure.

No matrix system meets all required criteria for all needs. The most popular system is the **Tofflemire universal matrix system** (Figure 35-49). This system is composed of two major components:

1. A retainer, which holds the band in close approximation to the tooth
2. A band, which supplies the missing wall

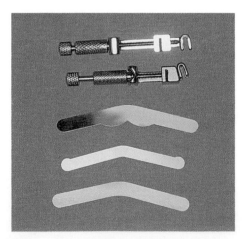

FIGURE 35-49
Straight-angled and contraangled universal (Tofflemire) retainers. Bands are available with varying occlusogingival measurements.

CASE APPLICATION 35-1.3

Class II Preparations
Included in Mrs. Dixon's treatment plan was the need to replace one of the existing Class II amalgam restorations on tooth #19.

The Tofflemire retainer is versatile in that it can be placed on either the facial or the lingual side of the tooth to be restored. The retainer and band generally are stable when placed properly. The retainer is easily separated from the band when finished. Bands with varying occlusogingival widths are available, although they are flat and need to be individually contoured. The band is placed on a paper pad (or other resilient surface) and burnished to achieve the desired contour. If a bonding system is to be used as the cavity sealer, then a light coating of wax or petroleum jelly may be used to reduce adhesion of the amalgam to the matrix band.

Placement of Matrix

When using the Tofflemire system, the clinician should place the band into the retainer so that the narrow end of the formed loop is directed toward the gingiva (Figure 35-50). The slot openings in the retainer also must be directed toward the gingiva. This will allow for easy removal of the retainer after the placement process. In most cases the retainer will be placed on the facial side of the tooth. If lingual placement is required, then a contraangled retainer is recommended. For facial placement, the proper orientation of the band (when the retainer is sitting on the counter with the slot opening downward in the gingival direction) will have it exiting the end of the retainer to the *left* for placement in the mandibular left and maxillary right quadrants and exiting to the *right* for the mandibular right and maxillary left quadrants.

The clinician places the two ends of the band into the retainer's angled slit and tightens the outer knurled knob. The band then is slipped over the tooth and pushed gently into place. The clinician should inspect for correct placement. The

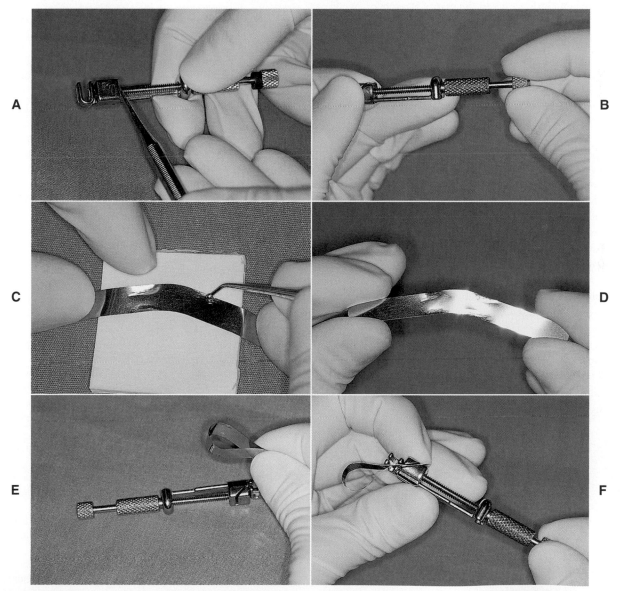

FIGURE 35-50
Positioning band in universal retainer. **A,** Explorer pointing to locking vise. View is showing gingival side of vise. **B,** Pointed spindle is released from locking vise by turning small knurled nut counterclockwise. **C.** Contour band with egg-shaped burnisher. **D,** Contoured band. **E,** Clinician folds band to form loop and positions in retainer, with occlusal edge of band first. **F,** Spindle is tightened against band in locking vise.

band should extend beyond the gingival seat. No rubber dam material should be caught between the band and the tooth. The cavosurface margin also must be inspected to ensure that all enamel is sound and intact. The band should extend slightly above the occlusal border of the preparation. The clinician tightens the band by turning the long inner knurled knob.

The band should be sealed at the gingival margin by the use of a wooden wedge. The wedge will adapt the band against the tooth to prevent any amalgam from being condensed out of the preparation into the gingival sulcus, creating an overhang of amalgam. Such an overhang can have deleterious effects on the health of the periodontal tissue.[1] The wedge also provides some separation of the teeth, which will help compensate for the thickness of the matrix band so that proximal contact can be properly restored when the band is removed. Placement of the wedge creates gingival tissue retraction, which will assist the clinician in exposing, visualizing, and carving the amalgam in the area of the gingival seat when the matrix is removed. Wedge placement will also aid in the development of the proximal contour and will prevent or diminish seepage of fluid at the gingival margin of the preparation.

Placement of Wedge

The clinician should select a wedge of the proper height, width, and contour. If the wedges available are not the proper size, then they can be modified with a sharp blade. The wedge should be placed from the embrasure that allows the closest adaptation of the band to the tooth, usually into the embrasure from the side opposite the retainer. Most of the wedge should be located gingival to the gingival cavosurface margin of the preparation (Figure 35-51). After insertion, the clinician applies moderate pressure with an amalgam condenser, the handle of a mirror, or the handle of cotton pliers to drive the wedge into the gingival embrasure and create tight adaptation of the band and slight separation of the teeth. The position of the wedge should be checked routinely, because the rubber dam tends to push the wedge out of the embrasure. The clinician reapplies pressure as needed to reinsert the wedge.

The technique for placement of amalgam into a Class II preparation is similar to that for the Class I, with additional consideration to the proximal box (Figure 35-52). The amalgam is triturated and carried to the preparation in the manner described previously (Box 35-4).

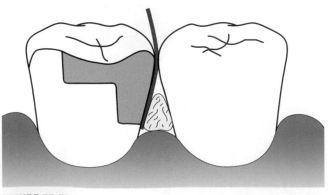

FIGURE 35-51
Wedge placement.

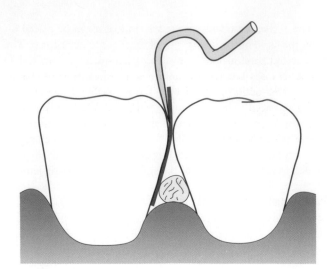

FIGURE 35-52
Excess amalgam is carved to free the matrix band and form the occlusal embrasure. This reduces the risk of an amalgam fracture in the area of the marginal ridge during matrix band removal (see Box 35-4).

BOX 35-4

AMALGAM PLACEMENT FOR CLASS II PREPARATIONS

1. In a Class II situation, the initial placement of amalgam should be on the gingival floor of the proximal box. To obtain proper adaptation to the gingival floor, the small end of the amalgam carrier and the small amalgam condenser should be used.
2. Condense the amalgam first into the proximal point and line angles.
3. Use lateral condensation against the matrix band and against the proximal walls.
4. Continue to add amalgam and to condense into the proximal box until the axiopulpal line angle is reached.
5. At this point, add and condense amalgam to the occlusal and proximal portions of the preparation concurrently until a moderate overfill condition exists.
6. Carve back to locate margins as in the Class I situation.
7. Free the occlusal surface of the band in the area of the marginal ridge by carving the occlusal embrasure with the tip of an explorer (see Figure 35-52). This will allow smooth removal of the band without fracturing the amalgam in the proximal box.
8. Remove the wedge with cotton pliers. Stabilize the matrix band and amalgam with an index finger.
9. Loosen both nuts on the retainer and remove it from the band.
10. Remove the band from the uninvolved contact (if only one proximal surface is being restored) while stabilizing the restoration with the index finger.
11. Remove the band from between the restoration and adjacent tooth by gently pulling in an oblique direction (45 degrees occlusofacially).
12. Carve the gingival seat area with an interproximal carver or explorer and then carve the proximal margin walls before finishing the occlusal carving as described earlier.
13. Check proximal contour and contact.

35-3 DIRECT RESIN COMPOSITE RESTORATIONS

The term *composite* refers to the fact that inorganic filler has been added to an organic resin matrix. Modern dental resin composites have been designed for use in all areas of the dentition, with anterior composites, posterior composites, universal composites, and composites specially designed to imitate multiple shades and opacities of enamel and dentin. Each of these various types of composite has its own peculiar advantages and disadvantages.[15]

Advantages

- *Esthetic considerations.* Resin composites are much more natural appearing than metals.
- *Economic considerations.* Composites are slightly more expensive than amalgam but are less expensive than ceramics or metals.
- *Broad applicability.*
- *Direct placement.* Resin composite restorations can be applied in a single appointment.
- *Ability to set on demand.* Resins are light polymerized, so material sets only when exposed to a particular type of light.
- *Low marginal leakage on enamel.* When placed properly, margins are bonded.
- *No galvanic response.* Resins are nonmetallic.
- *No mercury.* Public perceptions are positive regarding composite restorations.

Disadvantages

- *Polymerization shrinkage.* Material shrinks as it polymerizes.
- *Durability.* Life expectancy is less than for amalgam, metal, or ceramic. Wear is greater.
- *High technique sensitivity.* As a bonded restoration, appropriate isolation and tooth conditioning are vital.
- *Variable handling.* Products vary as to stiffness, slumping, and packing. New packable composites do not handle as well as amalgam.
- *Time requirements.* Generally, resin takes more time to set than amalgam.

PLACEMENT OF COMPOSITE RESTORATIONS

All composite restorations must have the tooth surface acid conditioned or acid etched before placement of the restoration. The use of 30% to 40% phosphoric acid has been the material of choice for many resin composite-bonding procedures.

However, some bonding systems contain self-etching primers.[4,22] These types of bonding systems do not require a separate acid-etching step.

⚡ CASE APPLICATION 35-1.4

Class III and IV Restorations

Mrs. Dixon also has Class III and Class V restorations included in her treatment plan.

The use of acid to etch the tooth decalcifies the enamel, leaving microscopic irregularities that increase the surface area and provide for mechanical interlocking of the resin with the tooth. Acid also cleans the surface, which decreases the contact angle between the enamel and the adhesive and permits increased wetting of the surface. The etched enamel has a very high surface energy—more than twice that of untreated enamel. This causes a low-viscosity resin to be drawn into these surface irregularities by capillary action, resulting in improved adaptation to the tooth and thus improved marginal seal of the restoration.

Shade must be obtained before the placement of the rubber dam. After rubber dam placement, the teeth reversibly dehydrate, which causes them temporarily to appear lighter. If obtained at this time, then the shade will not match that obtained after the rubber dam is removed and the teeth rehydrate to their normal state; the new restoration will appear lighter.

Next, the rubber dam should be placed. After the dentist has prepared the cavity, the clinician should apply the phosphoric acid etchant to the tooth for 10 to 30 seconds[3] and rinse thoroughly with water for at least 10 seconds. Many bonding systems have different application procedures. The clinician must follow each system's requirements precisely. The steps that can be used with one system cannot be used with another. Currently, products are available from seven generations of development. These systems may vary from one to eight different components in a kit but generally include a primer (sometimes provided in two bottles to be mixed immediately before use) and a relatively low-viscosity resin as the bonding agent.

Class III Preparations

A Class III preparation poses a similar problem to the Class II preparation in that a proximal wall is missing to confine the restorative material. The same solution, the matrix band, is used. Because composites are light-polymerized materials, a clear Mylar matrix band without a retainer generally is used. After preparation the clear matrix is placed between the preparation and the adjacent tooth. A wedge is placed in a manner similar to the Class II situation. The matrix should extend beyond the gingival wall and beyond the incisal wall of the preparation. It should be long enough to wrap around the tooth so that it can be grasped with the fingers and adapted to the surface of the tooth being restored.

The clinician must place the bonding agent as directed by the manufacturer, limiting its placement to those areas in need of restoration. Excess bonding agent smeared beyond the extent of etching will not bond to the tooth and may entrap oral fluids, which will lead to staining. After placement of the bonding agent, light polymerization should be performed as recommended by the manufacturer. The clinician should ensure that the polymerization unit is in proper working order and check it regularly with a radiometer to ensure that it has sufficient output (300 mW/cm^2).[17,19]

The composite of choice then should be placed into the preparation and pushed into position. Resin composite handles much differently than amalgam. It cannot be condensed with much pressure because the composite is essentially a liquid; attempts to do so will result in the condenser being pushed through it. Composites also cannot be carved in the same way, so little need exists to overfill. The clinician must take care to adapt the composite to the walls and especially into retention divots or grooves to improve retention. Increments should not be greater than 2 mm thick, because evidence indicates that such thickness may not be adequately polymerized internally.[16]

After slightly overfilling the preparation, the clinician may sculpt the material to proper form. The matrix band then is pulled around the tooth to condense the composite, and the material is light polymerized. All margin seals should be checked, and no voids, pits, or submarginal areas should exist. If such defects occur, then material can be added at this time if the surface has remained uncontaminated.

Class I, II, and VI Preparations

The Class I, II, or VI composite restoration is placed similar to the amalgam restorations of the same class. The major difference is in the handling characteristics of the materials. The Class II posterior composite restoration must use a matrix band, which can be of the Tofflemire style or a system designed specifically for use with resin composite.

FINISHING OF COMPOSITE RESTORATIONS

The primary objective of finishing the composite restoration is to obtain the smoothest surface possible. The smoother the surface, the lower is the possibility of plaque biofilm accumulation and staining and the greater is the possibility of an acceptable esthetic result. The smoothest surface is that obtained by the tight adaptation of a matrix band to the restorative material.[21] Therefore the clinician should attempt to use only the amount of material necessary to fill the cavity. Any excess needs to be removed, which will necessitate additional finishing and polishing procedures and will reduce the smoothness of the surface.

Gauging the precise amount of restorative material needed to fill the preparation exactly so that no finishing is necessary is extremely difficult. Therefore the removal of excess material is almost always required, as is the need to modify restoration contours so that they are compatible with tooth form. In short, composite resin finishing procedures are typically required.

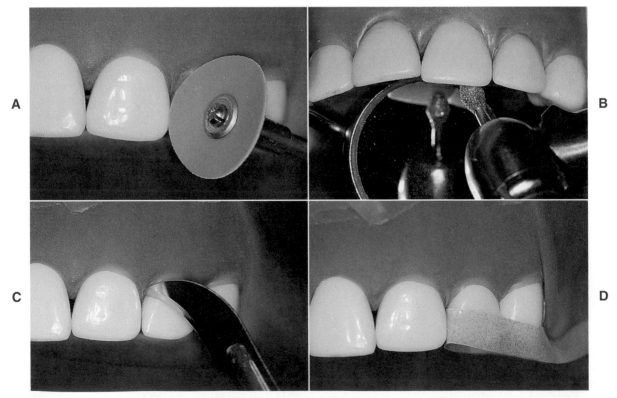

FIGURE 35-53
Finishing composites. **A,** Abrasive disc mounted on mandrel can be used for finishing when access permits. **B,** Round carbide finishing bur is well suited for finishing lingual surfaces. **C,** No. 2 surgical blade in Bard-Parker handle can be used for removing interproximal excess. **D,** Abrasive strip should be curved over area to be finished.

All contouring, finishing, and polishing techniques and associated systems use the principle of sequential removal of various amounts of material. These techniques begin with the coarsest abrasive necessary to accomplish removal of a defect or unwanted contour, followed by the use of finer abrasives until the required surface smoothness is obtained. This process is begun by removal of the gross excess material at the gingival margin with a sharp blade (i.e., no. 12 scalpel, composite blade, gold knife). Carbide or diamond composite finishing burs then are used to contour surfaces and refine marginal areas. Abrasive impregnated discs are available in various thicknesses and grits for facial, lingual, incisal, and some proximal areas. Composite finishing strips can be used in areas where the discs are not accessible. Final polishing can be accomplished with the use of fine abrasive rubber rotary instruments and polishing pastes (Figure 35-53; see also Chapter 32).

References

1. Abrams H et al: Gingival sequelae from a retained piece of rubber dam: a report of a case, *J Ky Dent Assoc* 30:21, 1978.

2. Anderson MH, Bales DJ, Omnell K: Modern management of dental caries: the cutting edge is not the dental bur, *J Am Dent Assoc* 124:37-44, 1993.

3. Barkmeier WW, Los SA, Triolo PT: Bond strengths and SEM evaluation of Clearfil Liner Bond 2, *Am J Dent* 8:289-293, 1995.

4. Barkmeier WW, Shaffer SE, Gwinnett AJ: Effects of 15 vs 60 second enamel acid conditioning on adhesion and morphology, *Oper Dent* 11:111-116, 1986.

5. Black GV: *The technical procedures in filling teeth,* Chicago, 1903, Blakely Printing.

6. Bronner FJ: Engineering principles applied to class II cavities, *J Dent Res* 10:115-119, 1930.

7. Buonocore MG: A simple method of increasing the adhesion of acrylic filling materials to enamel surfaces, *J Dent Res* 34:849-853, 1955.

8. Elderton RJ: Variability on the decision-making process and implications for change toward a preventive philosophy. In Anusavice KJ, ed: *Quality evaluation of dental restorations: criteria for placement and replacement,* Chicago, 1989, Quintessence.

9. Hume WR: Need for change in standards of caries diagnosis: perspective based on the structure and behavior of the caries lesion, *J Dent Educ* 57:439-443, 1993.

10. Kanca J III: Effects of resin primer solvents and surface wetness on resin composite bond strength to dentin, *Am J Dent* 5:213-215, 1992.

11. Markley M: Restorations of silver amalgam, *J Am Dent Assoc* 43:133-146, 1951.

12. Mertz-Fairhurst EJ et al: Ultraconservative and cariostatic sealed restorations: results at year 10, *J Am Dent Assoc* 128:55-66, 1998.

13. Osborne JW, Hoffman R, Ferguson GW: Conservation of tooth structure, *J Ala Dent Assoc* 56:24-26, 1972.

14. Osborne JW, Summit JB: Extension for prevention: is it relevant today? *Am J Dent* 11:189-196, 1998.

15. Roberson TM, Heymann HO, Swift EJ Jr: *Sturdevant's art and science of operative dentistry,* ed 5, St Louis, 2006, Mosby.

16. Rueggeberg FA, Caughman WF, Curtis JW Jr: Factors affecting cure at depths within light-activated composite resins, *Am J Dent* 6:91-95, 1993.

17. Rueggeberg FA, Caughman WF, Curtis JW Jr: Effect of light intensity and exposure duration on cure of resin composite, *Oper Dent* 6:91-95, 1994.

18. Sigurjons H: Extension for prevention: historical development and current status of GV Black's concept, *Oper Dent* 8:57-63, 1983.

19. Tate WH, Porter KH, Dosch RO: Successful photocuring: don't restore without it, *Oper Dent* 24:109-114, 1999.

20. Triolo PT, Swift EJ, Barkmeier WW: Shear bond strengths of composite to dentin using six dental adhesive systems, *Oper Dent* 20:46-50, 1995.

21. Trushowsky RD: Use of a clear matrix to minimize finishing of a posterior composite, *Am J Dent* 10:111, 1997.

22. Vargas MA, Cobb DS, Denehy GE: Evaluation of adhesive systems using acidic primers, *Am J Dent* 10:219-223, 1997.

23. Wilder AD, May, KN, Studevant CM: Preliminary considerations for operative dentistry. In Robertson TM et al, eds: *Sturdevant's art and science of operative dentistry,* ed 5, St Louis, 2006, Mosby.

Esthetics

Kristine A. Hodsdon

INSIGHT

Dental hygienists need only consider the driving forces of the population demographics, advances in material science and technologies, and pop culture trends such as makeover television programs to understand the esthetic revolution. Esthetic dentistry and whitening is now synonymous with patients who desire not only healthy mouths but also attractive smiles. Getting involved in esthetic and whitening services increases a dental hygienists' value to the dental office team. Many dental hygienists take on the role of in-office whitening coordinator, developing restorative maintenance programs or becoming patient advocates for restorative home care regimens. Esthetics and whitening are challenging ways to expand dental hygienists' careers and bring new dimensions to their diagnostic skills.

✶ CASE STUDY 36-1   Direct Composite Placement by the Dental Hygienist

Patient profile: Lexie Miller, a 17-year-old young woman, came to the office as new patient and was unhappy with her previous dentist. She had been seen on a regular 6-month recare schedule but was now overdue by 4 months.

Chief complaint: Nothing specific was bothering her; she needed an examination and preventive care.

Health history: The patient had no contraindications to treatment. She has seasonal hay fever and takes cetirizine (Zyrtec) as needed.

Dental history: No significant findings exist. She has been seen on a fairly regular basis. Existing restorations: tooth #30, occlusal amalgam. The patient has generalized gingivitis and moderate bleeding—especially interproximally. She does not floss regularly but does brush daily. The dental hygienist has stressed the importance of efficient home cares techniques, with emphasis on daily interproximal plaque biofilm removal. DIAGNOdent was used to check occlusal and buccal surfaces. Findings are within normal limits (WNL). The clinician will treat her with fluoride varnish and home fluoride (1.1% neutral sodium). Some chemical and acid erosion also is evident. The hygienist discussed the patient's diet and beverage consumption.

Radiographic findings: Four bite-wing and three periapical radiographs were taken to check the bone level and decay. Interproximal decay was evident on radiographs:

- Tooth #13, distoocclusal
- Tooth #14, mesioocclusal
- Tooth #18, mesioocclusal
- Tooth #20, distoocclusal

Diagnosis: The parent and patient chose to do composite resins on teeth #13 and #14. The dentist will prepare the cavity preparations, and the expanded function restorative hygienist will complete the restorative and polishing services (Figure 36-1).

✶ CASE STUDY 36-2   Cosmetic Whitening for Fluorosis

Patient profile: Jimmy Rogers, a 13-year-old boy, has relocated to the Southeast after living in Colorado since birth. He is healthy and participates in sports.

Chief complaint: Jimmy exhibits brown discoloration on the right central incisor (Figure 36-2). The cause is unknown.

Health history: WNL

Dental history: No significant findings exist. Jimmy has maintained routine dental treatment on a 6-month basis since age 3. The brown discoloration has been present since eruption, and no evidence of similar discoloration is noted on other teeth. Neither the patient nor his parents mentioned any history of trauma to the primary and permanent teeth. Generalized hypocalcification is present.

Radiographic findings: No radiographic pathologic condition exists.

Diagnosis: No disease is documented; treatment recommendation is cosmetic whitening.

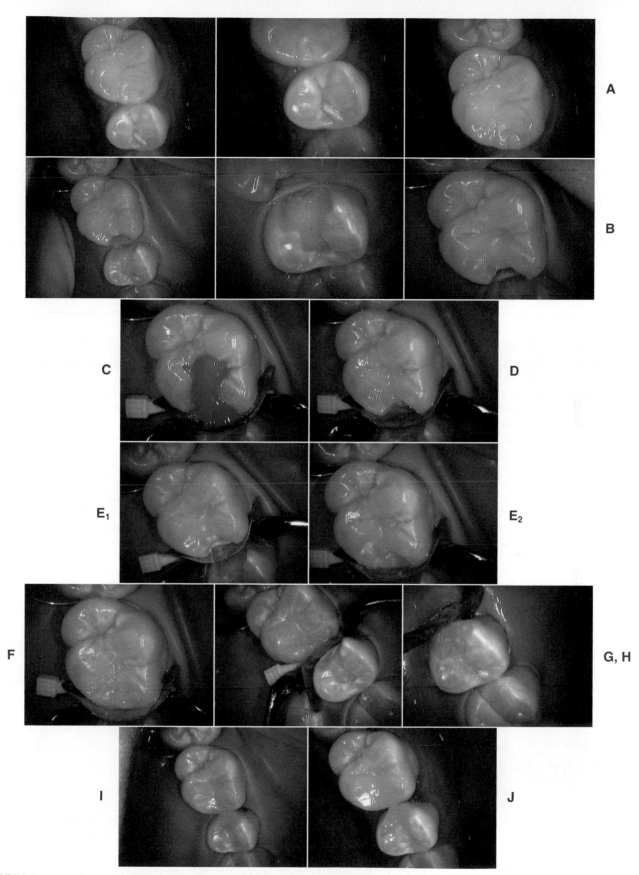

FIGURE 36-1

Case Study 36-1. **A,** Teeth #13 and #14—clinically, only radiographic decay was detected. Because of size and location of the incipient decay, composite restorative bonding was material of choice. **B,** Teeth prepared and the decay removed. Conservative cavity preparation was #13 (distoocclusal) and #14 (mesioocclusal). **C,** Pink-colored rubber dam is used to isolate the teeth. Interproximal band and wedges are used to ensure marginal contour. Picture shows tooth #14 (etched with 37% phosphoric acid solution). **D,** Tooth #14 (bonding agent after etch). **E,** Layering technique for the composite material was planned because of the depth of the preparation. Picture shows tooth #14 with the first layer of flowable filler composite. **F,** Tooth #14 with the final layer of flowable filler composite. **G,** Tooth #13 banded and wedged before filling the preparation cavity. **H,** Tooth #13 completely filled with composite material but has not been polished. **I,** Teeth #13 and #14 are completely restored and polished. Reader should note the rubber dam is still in place and the teeth, because of the isolation techniques, are dehydrated. **J,** Rubber dam has been removed. Teeth are more hydrated, and final intraoral picture is taken.

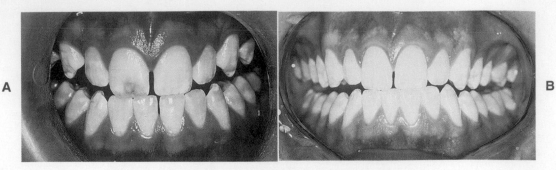

FIGURE 36-2
Case Study 36-2. **A,** Right central incisor of 13-year-old Jimmy Rogers exhibits brown discoloration of unknown cause. **B,** At the 7-year recall appointment, with no interim treatment, brown discoloration has not returned. (From Haywood VB, Leonard RH: Nightguard vital bleaching removes brown discoloration for 7 years: a case report, *Quintessence Int* 29[7]:450-451, 1998.)

✦ CASE STUDY 36-3   Cosmetic Whitening for Tetracycline Stain

Patient profile: Kathleen O'Bryan is a 43-year-old white woman; she is 5-feet 8-inches tall and weighs 145 pounds. She works in manufacturing and currently lives in the southeastern portion of the United States. Mrs. O'Bryan's family relocated from Denver 5 years ago. She is married and has two children, ages 17 and 21.

Chief complaint: Ms. O'Bryan states that she never smiles widely enough to show her teeth in a photograph because of the color of her teeth. She has not previously had any treatment for the discoloration, except for a whitening dentifrice.

Health history: The patient's mother has insulin-dependent diabetes mellitus (IDDM). Mrs. O'Bryan was tested for diabetes 10 years ago, and normal blood sugar levels were found. She reports allergies to sulfonamides and aspirin. She also reports frequent headaches (one to two times a week). She took tetracycline as a young child but cannot recall her exact age at the time.

Dental history: Mrs. O'Bryan has a history of trauma to the maxillary left central tooth #9, which was subsequently treated endodontically. An incisal chip was repaired with a mesioincisal composite.

Radiographic findings: Radiographs of anterior teeth revealed a periapical lesion on her mandibular left lateral tooth #23. The maxillary left central tooth #9 requires restorative treatment.

Diagnosis: Mrs. O'Bryan has experienced moderate tetracycline staining and requires restoration (Figure 36-3).

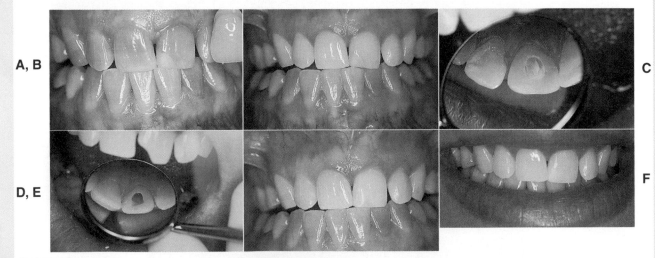

FIGURE 36-3
Case Study 36-3. **A,** Intraoral photograph of 43-year-old Kathleen O'Bryan showing moderate tetracycline (TCN) stain. Maxillary left central incisor has undergone endodontic therapy. **B,** 12-month bleaching recall. Maxillary left central incisor retained discoloration. **C,** Old discolored composite is removed from the nonvital maxillary left central incisor. **D,** Results after an in-office application of 35% hydrogen peroxide (H₂O₂). **E,** Results after restorative placement of white composite core in pulp chamber. **F,** Patient at 13-month recall. Whitening effects were successfully achieved. (From Haywood VB: *Contemp Esthet* and *Restor Pract* 15, 1997.)

⚡ CASE STUDY 36-4   Cosmetic Whitening for Yellowing

Patient profile: Margo Randall is a 29-year-old singer who belongs to a local repertory theater. Mrs. Randall is currently in a production of the musical *Carousel.* Because of her full-time employment as a medical receptionist to support her husband through law school and her busy rehearsal schedule for the upcoming production, Mrs. Randall says she feels that she has little time for herself.

Chief complaint: Ms. Randall has noticed a slight yellow cast to her teeth and wonders whether she could do something to make her smile brighter.

Health history: Noncontributory

Dental history: Mrs. Randall has received regular, routine dental care since early childhood. Her oral hygiene is remarkable, with no bleeding on probing at any previous dental examination. She has benefited from a fluoridated water supply and fluoridated dentifrice all her life. Except for the slight yellow color apparent in her anterior teeth, she is not experiencing any dental problems at this time.

Radiographic findings: No radiographic pathologic condition exists.

Extraoral findings: A 3-mm round, elevated, pigmented nevus is evident on her left cheek, just inferior to the zygoma.

Diagnosis: No restorative needs exist; the patient has a cosmetic need for whiter teeth (Figure 36-4).

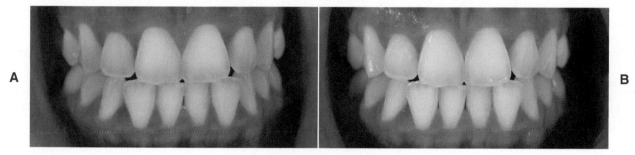

A   B

FIGURE 36-4
Case Study 36-4. **A,** Intraoral photograph of Margo Randall before tooth-whitening procedures. **B,** Patient at 2-week recall showing results of simultaneous treatment of the maxillary and mandibular arches. (From Sagel PA et al: Vital tooth whitening with a novel hydrogen peroxide strip system: design, kinetics, and clinical response, *Compend Contin Educ Dent* 21[suppl 29]:S15, 2000.)

KEY TERMS

anterior guidance	composites	indirect restorations	potassium nitrate
block-out resins	desensitizers	in-office bleaching	preformed dual-tray systems
canine guidance	direct restorations	laser bleaching	resin cements
carbamide peroxide	extrinsic stains	light-assisted bleaching	restorative polishing systems
ceramic	fluorosis	magnification	tetracycline
compomers	hydrogen peroxide	minocycline	ultraviolet-light systems
composite resin	hygiene smile assessment	night guard vital bleaching	vertical dimension
composite sealant	indirect resin systems	over-the-counter product	wear facets

LEARNING OUTCOMES

After reading this chapter the student will be able to:

1. Discuss the validation of the psychologic and sociologic effects of physical attractiveness on human self-esteem.
2. Generate an understanding of esthetic dentistry and dental hygiene and its value to dental hygienists and their patients.
3. Establish a process for designing effective "smile assessments."
4. Review evidence-based dental and dental hygiene techniques that preserve a patient's restored smile while maintaining oral health.
5. Discuss methods of identifying and documenting esthetic restorations, preventive maintenance, and home care solutions that are currently available.
6. Select appropriate professional, supportive care measures and recommend home self-care techniques for various esthetic restorations.
7. Assist the patient in understanding the importance of his or her role in preserving and maintaining restorative dentistry and oral health.
8. Assist the patient in becoming proficient in maintaining healthy gingival tissue, emphasizing the importance of daily dental plaque biofilm elimination and commitment to supportive care.
9. List tolerability issues regarding the use of tooth-whitening agents that contain peroxide.
10. Discuss the advantages, disadvantages, clinical indications, and contraindications for tooth whitening.
11. List the common side effects of dental whitening and their contributing factors.
12. Explain the importance of dental professional and patient communication throughout the bleaching process, as well as the role of the dental hygienist in dental-whitening therapy.
13. Demonstrate and describe the clinical techniques used for fabrication of a night guard.
14. Compare and contrast the whitening effect of in-office and home-applied vital tooth bleaching and how these two systems might be used in conjunction with one another.
15. Discuss the effects of whitening agents on enamel, dentin, pulp, and restorative materials.
16. Investigate products currently available for cosmetic whitening, including professional, over-the-counter, in-office, and home-applied whiteners.
17. Describe the role of dental hygienists in planning, implementing, and evaluating cosmetic-whitening procedures.

Overview of Esthetics

Beauty and the emotional response to it are important aspects of esthetic and restorative dentistry.[15] People choose to wear a certain outfit or wear their hair straight or curly hair based on personal taste (i.e., what they believe to be attractive). Just as taste in clothing and hairstyles vary from person to person, so does the meaning of what constitutes a beautiful or perfect smile. It may mean a disease-free smile, a Hollywood-white smile, or an amalgam-free smile.

Oral healthcare professionals have the chance to offer esthetic treatment options (or *smile designs*) that can, in some cases, be life altering. Many consumer magazines have published articles and surveys that underscore the public's emphasis on looking good and feeling good. According to a 2004 independent study conducted on behalf of the American Association of Cosmetic Dentistry,[2] the following is true:

- A smile is considered to be an important social asset by 99.7% of Americans.
- A majority of adults (96%) believe an attractive smile makes a person more appealing to members of the opposite sex.
- A strong percentage (74%) of adults feel an unattractive smile can hurt a person's chances for career success.

When people were asked what they would most like to improve about their smiles, the most common response was, "Whiter and brighter teeth." Additionally, growing evidence addresses esthetic restorative treatment and its positive effect on patients' self-esteem and sense of well-being.[14]

Types of Tooth-Colored and Esthetic Restorations

RESTORATIVE OPTIONS

The search for restorations that reproduce natural dentition has changed operative dentistry and dental hygiene.[51] The explosion in the field of material technology and adhesion is revolutionizing the way dentistry is delivered. The emphasis on conservation of tooth structure, biocompatibility with gingival tissue, dental implants, improved bonding with natural teeth, and cosmetic improvements has ignited this rapid development. These definitive restorations fall under two categories: (1) **direct restorations** and (2) **indirect restorations**. **Indirect resin systems** are laboratory-fabricated restorations that share the same advantages of being part of the composite resin category. Their indications may be anterior veneers, posterior restorations, or both. With an indirect restoration (indirect bonding), the dentist prepares a tooth (teeth), and an impression is taken. This impression is sent to a laboratory. The dental laboratory, in partnership with the dentist, fabricates the restoration on a stone model made from the impression. Direct systems are composed of **composite resin** and indirect or laboratory-fabricated restorations that include composite resin and porcelain. When either category is completed and meticulously polished, these restorations can be virtually impossible to tell apart from adjacent natural dentition.[20,46]

Restoring a decayed tooth or replacing a defective filling can create a myriad of confusion concerning the best restorative products and techniques. No absolutes or best ways to treat restorative patients exist, and one material does not serve all needs. The following are general guidelines for the hygienist to consider when assessing esthetic treatment options:

- Material selected (should be based on individual patient situation and location in mouth)
- Technique modality used (for the tooth preparation)
- Restoration fabrication used
- Luting and bonding agent used
- Restorative hygienist's or dentist's skill, judgment, and expertise
- Laboratory technician's skill, judgment, and expertise (in situations involving indirect restorative systems)[8,46,47]

Because restorative products can change rapidly, dental hygienists should continually research and learn about the newest advances in restorative and esthetic dentistry. This in turn will allow the dental hygienist to guide the patient to the best services for his or her clinical needs and goals regarding the smile.

DIRECT MATERIALS AND PROPERTIES

Composite-based resin material contains an organic resin base and inorganic glass filler particles. Composite resins are usually classified according to the filler particle size, such as microfill composites; hybrid **composites;** and glass- or resin-modified ionomers, **compomers,** and nanomers. Macrofill composites have a particle size ranging between 10 and 100 mcm; microfills can range from 0.04 to 1.0 mcm. Hybrid composites exhibit a combination of particle sizes from minifill to microfill. Compomers are a combination of glass ionomers and composite material that can release fluoride. Nanomers', or nanocomposites', particle size are 0.0001 mcm.[16,38]

Composite resin systems can be used in the restoration of anterior or posterior teeth. Anterior composite materials that have a high shine (microfill, nanomers) can mimic enamel, are highly polishable, and leave the control and artistry of the restoration to the restoring dentist or dental hygienist. Microfills are usually used in Class III and Class V restorations or veneers. Hybrid composites are often used in posterior teeth because of their strength and polishability; examples are Class I or Class II restorations and Class IV anterior restorations.[16,38,39]

Clinical examination will show that microfill composites, when finished and polished precisely, are very glossy and feel smooth to the tip of an applied explorer. Hybrids may cause more of a drag when an explorer is drawn across the surface. Glass- or resin-modified ionomers tend to have a moderately rough surface that attracts stain more readily than composites. When these materials are polished, a smooth surface is achievable. Nanomer particles polish well and have a luster similar to a microfill, but they have the strength and wear properties of a hybrid.[21,34,35,39]

INDIRECT MATERIALS AND PROPERTIES

Indirect restorative systems (porcelain and **ceramic**) continually increase in options and popularity. Indirect restorations are fabricated in a laboratory and cemented or bonded to natural tooth surfaces. This procedure requires excellent communication and collaboration between the restoring dentist and the laboratory technician fabricating the restoration. Porcelain and ceramic materials are the foundation for indirect esthetic options. They are used for inlays, onlays, veneers, metal-free crowns, and crowns with metal substructures. Pressed ceramic, which is fabricated according to the lost wax technique, offers marginal integrity, strength, and wear consistent with enamel. It consists of Lucite-reinforced, low- to medium-fusing, fine-grain glass particles. Pressed porcelain restorations are bonded to the tooth structure, as are traditional, buildup, porcelain (stackable) restorations. As long as these restorations are properly maintained, they have the ability to last 10 years or more (Box 36-1). The glaze on ceramic restorations will retain its gloss for many years, unless the surface is removed during insertion, finishing, or polishing. If the glaze is compromised, then more aggressive techniques may be used to restore luster.[37,38,39,46,47]

Resin cements or adhesives used to bond the indirect restoration may abrade more easily than composites, because they do not have as much filler loading or particles. Resin agents also may have a tendency to stain because of a higher water adsorption compared with that of restorative composite materials. The porcelain-resin cement interface may present roughness, which may accumulate stain and plaque biofilm, initiating an inflammatory response.[38,39]

As stated earlier, indirect restorations are laboratory fabricated, with the exception of computer-aided design/computer-aided manufacturing (CAD/CAM), which can be a chairside option, and should follow the same maintenance regimen as porcelain.

BOX 36-1

REASONS FOR MAINTAINING ESTHETIC RESTORATIONS

- Lessens plaque biofilm retention and improves gingival health
- Improves the compatibility of the restorative material, oral soft tissues, and shade coordination to surrounding dentition
- Improves marginal adaptation and integrity, longevity, and esthetics
- Improves cleansing by the patient
- Increases symmetrical surface texture to adjacent or opposing teeth
- Increases or preserves the luster or beauty of the restoration (i.e., shape, color, glaze)
- Establishes a practice's long-term commitment to restorative maintenance
- Provides anatomical form for occlusal harmony
- Protects surface glaze and material luster

Dental Hygienist Role as an Esthetic Therapist

IDENTIFYING AND RECORDING ESTHETIC MATERIALS

Visual examination and identification of esthetic materials is facilitated with proper instrument selection. This includes a sharp explorer; a mirror; dental floss; a small surgical air tip; **magnification** loupes; illumination; and radiographs, digital photography, or both. Radiographic images can aid in the identification because of the varying radiopacities of esthetic materials.[31,33] The most radiopaque shades are from metal (e.g., amalgam, gold). Composite resins containing filler particles, and ceramic materials have varying radiopacities. Microfill composite resins contain only small silica particles and appear radiolucent. Conventional radiography generally shows 16 shades of gray but still may limit the ability to determine the restoration and tooth interface. However, newer digital imagery can show several hundred variations of color and may further aid dentists and dental hygienists in radiographic identification of esthetic restorations.[31]

Clinical identification begins by applying air to clear debris or to dry tooth surfaces. Because most composite and ceramic materials reflect, refract, absorb, or transmit light rays differently than enamel and dentin, a method known as *transillumination* can be used to visually distinguish restorations.[33,42] This is achieved by reflecting light through the tooth from the lingual surface using a mouth mirror and a specialty or dental unit light. The light source illuminates the tooth and restorative materials differently for visual recognition. A simple technique to check margins can be achieved with the use of a small surgical suction tip (preferably plastic.) The tip can dry an area and lightly pulls the tissue back so that the hygienist can inspect the margins. This skill of detecting marginal discrepancies is greatly enhanced when the clinician uses magnification loupes and illumination.[33]

Distinct Care Modifications
Poorly finished and polished margins may retain stains and dental plaque biofilm, resulting in localized inflammation of surrounding gingival tissue.

Careful tactile sensitivity is essential to distinguish the restorative material and tooth structure margin. The clinician should use gentle pressure with exploratory stokes. If the margin is incorrectly identified as calcified deposit and aggressively scaled, then damage to the esthetic filling and possible tooth structure may occur.[33] Delicately examining and exploring the integrity of the restoration margins allows the dental hygienist to assess the integrity of the restoration.[39,45]

HYGIENE SMILE ASSESSMENTS

A **hygiene smile assessment** involves subjective, objective, and clinical considerations. A dental hygienist can develop the skills needed to look at the clinical variables of the smile and the intangible reasons patients seek care. Patients seek esthetic treatments for a variety of reasons ranging from economic and social to psychologic and egoistic. They may choose to restore teeth damaged by traumatic injury, developmental anomalies, and oral disease. From the esthetic assessment of the patient, the dental hygienist may determine that the patient wants changes to the smile purely for cosmetic reasons.[31] When no clinical need-based indication for a restoration exists and the patient insists on smile design, he or she must be made aware of the biological price that is paid when the natural tooth-tissue interface is violated, as well as when tooth structure is unnecessarily removed. Elective contemporary procedures require that the patient be completely informed about all benefits and risks of treatments, and this recognition should be documented in writing before therapy begins. (See Chapter 3 for information on informed consent.)

Dental hygienists can begin to develop smile assessments that can augment the dental hygiene clinical assessment. By developing a checklist for a comprehensive review of the patient's smile, the dental hygienist can assess and document all supporting structures, facial abbreviations, lips, gingival tissue, osseous tissue, and teeth (Box 36-2). Generally, the teeth should be in the center of the mouth with no distractions. The upper lip should fall near the maxillary gingival line, and the lower lip should cradle the maxillary incisal plane. If the teeth are not in the middle of the smile, then excessive gingival display may occur when smiling. This gingival-to-lip relationship is often termed a *gummy smile,* which can be defined as any patient who shows more than 2 mm of gingival tissue during a smile. The causes of such conditions are beyond the scope of this chapter; however, they are part of the dental hygienists' smile assessment.[13]

The smile assessment can uncover the integrity of previous restorations, dark lines in the gingival margin, breakdown of previous tooth-colored restoration, opaque

Note
Beautiful smile designs must be in harmony with posterior anatomy.[57]

BOX 36-2

ESTHETIC DISCREPANCIES CHECKLIST

- Midline discrepancy
- Diastema
- Axial alignments (tooth inclination) (all upper teeth should point toward navel)
- Gingival margin (anterior to posterior progression)
- Excess gingival display (gummy smile)
- Abrasion and abfraction (site specific or generalized)
- Incline of incisal plane
- Crown length (70/30; should look like a rectangle, not a square)
- Open gingival embrasures (black triangles)
- Gingiva to lip distance (1 mm from incisal edge of upper centrals to incisal edge of lower lip)
- Color
- Cervical margin recession

crowns, missing teeth, and occlusions. **Wear facets** or flat chewing surfaces could place abnormal stress on the anterior teeth.[57] Without correction in the posterior, the anterior esthetics will be out of synch with the posterior function. Understanding the essentials of occlusal and functional concepts allows the dental hygienist to customize education for the patient as it relates to the longevity of the esthetic dentistry. Areas to consider when assessing and discussing smile design options with patients include the following:

- Loss of **vertical dimension** (vertical height or distance between maxillary and mandibular teeth)
- Lack of **canine guidance** (the movement of the maxillary canine and the incisal edge of the manibular canine)
- Lack of **anterior guidance** (the most anterior contact and the first occlusal contact to occur on one or more teeth when closing the mandible against the maxilla)

Each of these can be a symptom of bruxism, clenching, or faulty occlusion. Looking at general facial features can identify heavy bruxers.[49,50] During the examination the clinician should ask himself or herself the following:

- Has the distance between the tip of the nose and chin shortened over time?
- Have the muscles of mastication thickened?
- Is there a loss, in excess of 20%, of the natural tooth surface on the anterior teeth?
- Are the canines flat?

Often the patient's perceived need and ideal care are not in alignment. Patients may have a chief complaint of a rotated incisor (or chipped central incisor). Not understanding the pathologic reasons for these occurrences, the patient may seek treatment for one or two teeth. Proper examination will assist the clinician in determining the origin of a pathologic condition, the current situation, and the ideal restorative plan[50] (Box 36-3).

A separate esthetic form or clinical software may be used to record the completed esthetic dentistry treatment and future treatment plans. Additional charting symbols may be developed for esthetic materials and included in the record. Auditing the esthetic treatment form before the hygiene appointment, as well as making necessary preparations, allows the clinician to work seamlessly while adding value for the patient.

PROTECTING THE ESTHETIC RESULT

Because improper professional and patient self-care can adversely affect the longevity and appearance of cosmetic and esthetic restorations, some basic principles should be followed to preserve the substance and beauty of the service.[31] Once the dental hygienist has distinguished natural enamel from restored tooth surface and an evaluation of the condition of the restoration has been made, appropriate instruments and polishing mediums can be selected[6-8,31] (Box 36-4).

Aggressive scaling with hand instruments can chip, mar, or damage the delicate edges of esthetic restoration.[7] Dull curettes may ditch or scratch the surface of a tooth-colored restoration and compromise the surface characteristics. The majority of information concerning hand instrumentation of tooth-

---

BOX 36-3

HYGIENE OCCLUSAL ANALYSIS AND CLINICAL SIGNS: OBSERVE AND RECORD STANDARDS AND DEVIATIONS

- Normal unworn teeth without dentin showing (whenever dentin visible, loss of enamel occurs [through ongoing damage or damage that has been restored])
- Class V noncarious lesions (wedge defects at cervical third usually found on facial surface, rarely on lingual)
- Parafunctional habits (clenching; grinding; biting on pens, pins, nails; unusual postural habits)
- Premature occlusal contacts or functional interferences (can result in avoidance patterns and wear that can affect the anterior teeth)
- Cuspid contact (with lateral excursion, canines should stay in contact and posterior teeth separate [i.e., cuspid and canine guidance, cuspid protection]; malpositioning or worn canines can cause stress in posterior teeth)
- Anterior contact of four incisors (creates anterior guidance allowing posterior teeth to separate; anterior coupling [contact] should be present; lack of anterior guidance causes group function in posterior)
- Changes in radiographic anatomy (site-specific variation of the lamina duras, variations of the periodontal space, root fractures, root resorption, hypercementosis, and pupal calcifications)
- Localized soft tissue inflammation

---

colored restorations concludes sharp curettes offer the tactile sensitivity necessary to debride without scratching the esthetic materials.[31,42] A gentle, horizontal stroke rather than a heavy, up-and-down stroke should be applied to safeguard the integrity of a bonded margin. Some of the newer plastic instruments with streamlined shanks and blades may also be considered for debriding. These can be sharpened with material-specific sharpening stones.[31]

The same care must be taken with air-powered polishers as with the selection of instruments. Two types of powder are available for use in air-powered polishers: (1) sodium bicarbonate and (2) aluminum trihydroxide. The use of aluminum trihydroxide polishing powder should be avoided on all restorative materials. Sodium bicarbonate can be used on porcelain, but it should be avoided on composites, glass ionomers, and cement-margin interfaces.[6,21]

Ultrasonic and sonic powered instruments should not be used on or around a tooth with a tooth-colored restoration. Ultrasonic and sonic scalers damage the surface or margin of composite restorations, fracture porcelain, scratch gold, and debond the adhesive properties.[6,7]

Acidulated phosphate fluoride and stannous fluoride should not be used in patients with tooth-colored restorations. Acidulated phosphate fluoride has been shown to etch porcelain and may affect the filler particles in composite resins. Stannous fluoride may also cause discoloration of the restorations. Sodium fluoride treatments delivered after esthetic recare, after

BOX 36-4

TECHNIQUE GUIDE FOR POLISHING ESTHETIC RESTORATIONS

Step One: Identify

Begin by identifying between natural tooth structure and the type of restorations:

- Microhybrid, hybrid, microfill

Step Two: Evaluate

Determine the extent of polishing necessary, as well as renewing or replacement needed, using a checklist for evaluating definitive restorations:

- Plaque biofilm accumulation
- Calculus accumulation
- Color match and discoloration
- Staining
- Loss of surface glaze
- Labial and palatal restorations, margins, integrity
- Intact margin
- Visible crevice at margin (e.g., cracks visible on transillumination, fracture present, debonded or lost, overcontour, secondary caries, marginal leakage, microcracks, overhangs, open margins, undercontour margins, overcontour margins, ditches, grooves)

Step Three:

Plaque Biofilm or Light Stain Removal:

- A tooth or restoration that exhibits little to no stain, and the only goal is minimal stain or plaque biofilm removal, can be polished with nonabrasive toothpaste or composite paste on a soft prophy cup, polishing points, cups, or bristles.

Medium to Heavy Stain Removal:

- Begin to polish with extrafine composite paste, in a wet environment.
- Distribute polish adequately over the entire surface and use a light intermittent stroke contacting the restorative and tooth surface for no more than 15 to 30 seconds each. (The goal is for restoration polishing, not recontouring or margin obliteration.)
- Carry paste interproximally with floss and rinse to clear area before reexamining.
- If stain removal and high shine (leaving the desired surface texture on) is the goal, and a paste alone did not achieve the desired results, then it may be necessary to move on to more aggressive techniques in a progressional process.
- Selections include higher-grit pastes, impregnated rubber polishing instruments, cups, discs, silicone points, goal hair wheels, strips, carbide burs (all in grades ranging from extrafine through coarse).
- Rinse away the polishing agents and particles between the levels of coarseness to avoid continually abrading the surface.
- Once stain removal is achieved, reverse the process and finish polishing with the least-abrasive composite polish and instrument to achieve the desired high shine and surface texture.
- Remember to continually add water to the buffing cup, point, or brush.

Interproximal Stain:

- Interproximal stain removal and surface preservation can be achieved universally with aluminum oxide polishing strips.

- Start at the "safety center," with the finest grade and graduate to the next coarsest grade until the stain is gone.
- Complete the process by reversing the sequence and graduate to the finest grade until the restoration is smooth.

Step Four: Renewing Composites

- Stain at the margins, visual crevice <60 mcm, or "the little black line" that sometimes appears after placement, may need additional care and renewal services.
- Depending on state, practice acts and allowable functions will determine the choice of instrumentation for this step.
- Severe microleakage and open margins may require restoration replacement and a doctor's evaluation.
- Start with either a coarse point, diamond-impregnated rubber polishing points, slow-speed hand piece with a polishing and finishing bur, air abrasion (aluminum oxide), or high-speed (carbide finishing bur, fissure preparation bur).
- Gently roughen the restoration to minimally open the margins and remove the irregular marginal staining or black line.
- Once the marginal stain is removed, scrub area clean by using a mixture of a cleaner and disinfectant and pumice with a brush applicator (or use a chlorhexidine antibacterial scrub and a bristle brush in a slow-speed hand piece).
- Wash and dry the area.
- Etch the discrepancy several millimeters past the previously stained area. Use a disposable brush or applicator tip to agitate the etchant for 15 to 20 seconds. When renewing a composite restoration, the clinician may choose to use a plastic strip or guard interproximally to preserve the adjacent tooth.
- Rinse off the etchant for 5 seconds with an air/water spray.
- Apply enamel-bonding agent (follow the manufacturers directions).
- Apply the composite material. A sable brush, small soft paintbrush, or applicator brush can be used to manipulate the renewal sealant.
- Cure for 40 seconds.
- Remove Mylar strip or guard if used.
- Smooth and polish the area with composite polishing paste.

Step Five: Increasing Vitality and Longevity

- Once either the stain removal procedures or the renewal services are complete, follow the final steps to further preserve the integrity of the restoration.
- After polishing the renewed restoration and enamel, use a disposable brush or applicator tip to agitate the etchant for 5 seconds. When applying a composite sealant, the clinician may choose to use a plastic strip or guard interproximally to preserve the adjacent tooth.
- Rinse off the etchant for 5 seconds with an air/water spray.
- Once this has dried, apply a composite surface sealant vigorously into the entire restoration, including margins, with a small brush tip.
- Gently blow off any excess.
- Cure the composite surface sealant for 20 seconds.
- Administer a tray and neutral sodium fluoride application or fluoride varnish application.

definitive restorative placement, and as part of self-care should be a component of all self-care education.[54,55]

Occlusal integrity of the restoration also needs to be considered after the definitive restoration is placed. Protecting the end result may require fitting the patient for a protective night guard or traditional acrylic guard; parafunctional habits (e.g., grinding, clenching, occlusal interferences, fingernail biting, chewing on a pen or pin) can damage or dislodge restorations and natural teeth. Additions to this field for esthetic protection include Nociceptive Trigeminal Inhibition Tension Suppression System (NTI-TSS) appliances and BruxGuard.

ADAPTING POLISHING PROCEDURES TO MAINTAIN ESTHETIC RESTORATIONS

Properly polishing and maintaining restorative treatments is a service that can preserve and prolong longevity of the restoration. Selecting **restorative polishing systems,** polishing pastes, or rubber polishing instruments for either composite or ceramic restorations can be difficult because of the differences in the size, shape, and number of filler particles, as well as the type of resin, the varying porcelain or ceramic materials, and the adhesion to natural tooth structure. One system may be incapable of creating a high shine on all esthetic solutions.[6]

Recognition of the different restorative options will determine what polishing agents to use and what results can be expected. Studies suggest that pairing a specific restorative material with a matching polishing system produced the smoothest surface. Many manufacturers recommend their own products for polishing their restorative materials.[35] Dental hygienists should refer to recommendations for specific products and polishing techniques that can be used for esthetic materials.[6,8]

Traditional prophylaxis (prophy) pastes were never created for polishing esthetic restorations. Prophy paste may roughen, scratch, and dull the surface of tooth-colored restorative material. Coarse prophy paste may also cause premature plucking of glass or silica filler particles from the resin matrix (organic paste) of composites, leaving a porous surface. This may cause

excessive wear, staining, and premature breakdown of the restoration[5-7] (Figure 36-5).

Slight modification of current polishing techniques is required when polishing esthetic restorations with the properly indicated polishing paste.[39] The following points should be considered:

- Hand pieces should be operated at 3000 rpm.[34]
- Adaptation of a soft cup (disposable prophy angle [DPA] or latch type) is preferred because of the fact that the lip of the cup can be flared slightly into the marginal areas.
- The cup should be adequately filled with the paste and held at a 90-degree angle against the tooth.[46] If more than one grit is to be used, then the rubber cup or soft-cupped disposable prophy angle should be changed with each new grit size.
- Using intermittent pressure stokes on the tooth and keeping sufficient paste in the cup will help avoid any frictional heat.
- A limited number of teeth (two to three) should be treated at a time.
- The clinician should begin the process by determining the extent of polishing necessary (i.e., evaluating the restoration and tooth stain accumulation).[7,39]
- A nonabrasive toothpaste and a slow-speed hand piece or soft manual toothbrush can be used for plaque biofilm removal on a tooth or restoration that exhibits no stain yet retains its luster.[6,31]
- Aluminum oxide paste can be used on composite resins, gold, and tooth structure.
- The clinician should begin to polish with extrafine composite paste in a wet environment for best results.
- Water should be continually added to the buffing cup.
- The polish should be distributed adequately over the entire surface and light, intermittent pressure should be used, with the cup contacting the restorative or tooth surface for no more than 15 to 30 seconds.
- The goal is to renew the restoration's surface, not recontour or change the margin integrity.
- The clinician should carry paste interproximally with floss and rinse to clear the area before evaluating the polishing procedure[33] (see Table 36-1).
- If stain removal is the goal, and a paste alone did not achieve the desired results, then it may be necessary to move on to more aggressive techniques in a progressive process from most to least abrasive. Selections include varying paste grits, rotary rubber polishing instruments, and strips, all in grades ranging from coarse to extrafine.
- The clinician should rinse away the polishing agents and particles from the teeth or restoration, as well as change

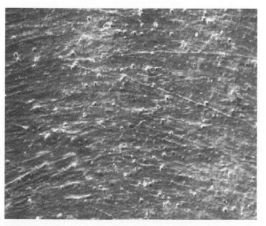

FIGURE 36-5
Scanning electron microscopy (×150) of Durafil composite material polished with coarse prophylaxis paste. Circular pattern of deep, irregular scratches is noted. (Courtesy Caren M. Barnes, RDH, MS Professor, Dental Hygiene Coordinator of Clinical Research UNMC College of Dentistry.)

Table 36-1   Comparison of Available Polishing Products

PRODUCT NAME	MANUFACTURER	MATERIAL INDICATIONS	APPLICATORS	POLISHING AGENT
Cosmetic Polishing Restorative (CPR)	IC Care	Natural tooth structures, porcelain, and composite materials	Occlusal brush, soft cup, polishers, discs	Aluminum oxide
Climpro	3M ESPE	Natural tooth structures, porcelain, and composite materials	Occlusal brush, soft cup, polishers, discs	Perlite
Diamond Glaze Polish	Western Coast	Ceramics and composite	Felt wheel	Diamond
Diamond Polish	Ultradent	Porcelain and ceramic materials	Felt wheel	Diamond
Diamond Polishing Paste	Ivoclar Vivadent	Porcelain	Felt wheel	Diamond
Enamelize	Cosmedent	Natural tooth structures, porcelain, and composite materials	Occlusal brush, soft cup, polishers, discs	Aluminum oxide
Insta-Glaze HYB	George Taub	Natural tooth structures, porcelain, and composite materials	Felt wheel	Diamond
Luminescence	Premier	Porcelain and ceramic material	Felt wheel	Diamond
Next Prophy Paste-Fine	Preventive Technologies Inc.	Natural tooth structures, porcelain, and composite materials	Occlusal brush, soft cup, polishers	Diatomaceous earth (jeweler's rouge)
Nupro Shimmer	DENTSPLY	Natural tooth structures, porcelain, and composite materials	Occlusal brush, soft cup, polishers, discs	Aluminum oxide
Porcelite	Matech	Porcelain and ceramic material	Occlusal brush, soft cup, polishers, discs	Aluminum oxide
Porcelize	Cosmedent	Porcelain	Felt wheel	Diamond
Prisma Gloss	DENTSPLY	Composite	Occlusal brush, soft cup, polishers, discs	Aluminum oxide
Proxyt Fine	Ivoclar Vivadent	Natural tooth structures, porcelain, and composite materials	Occlusal brush, soft cup, polishers, discs	Silicon dioxide
Supersmile Toothpaste	Supersmile	Natural tooth structures, porcelain, and composite materials	Occlusal brush, soft cup, polishers, discs	Silica
Ultra II Polishing Paste	Shofu	Porcelain and ceramic material	Felt wheel	Diamond

Adapted with permission from Vicki McManus, RDH.

the rubber cup between the levels of coarseness, to avoid continually abrading the surface.
- Once stain removal is achieved, the final stage should be reversing the process and finish polishing with the least abrasive polish and instrument.
- At the conclusion of each esthetic management session, the clinician should place a **composite sealant** over the definitive restorations and a neutral sodium fluoride tray or varnish application should be conducted.[6,33]

- Porcelain and ceramic restorations keep their gloss indefinitely, as long as the material was glazed or properly polished before it was seated.[39]
- The clinician should polish with an aluminum oxide paste on porcelain or ceramic restorations when resin cement or cementum is exposed.[7,8]
- If the gloss is gone and only porcelain or ceramic is exposed, then a diamond polishing paste on felt wheels or a Robinson wheel can be used.

- Diamond paste is best used in a dry environment, so use of cotton rolls, dry angles, or bite block is essential.[33]
- With the appropriate polishing system, the clinician should follow the same protocol and instrument sequence as outlined in Chapter 9.

Interproximal stain removal can be universally achieved with aluminum oxide polishing strips. The clinician should begin with the finest grade and graduate to the next coarsest grade until the stain is gone. Then he or she should complete the process by reversing the sequence and graduate to the finest grade until the restoration is smooth.

What clinicians must also keep in mind is that some of these treatments may never provide the restoration with the same luster it had the day it was placed. Depending on the restorative material, some types may appear esthetically unpleasing after appropriate renewing and polishing techniques but remain functional. In other instances, the restoration may require replacing. It becomes effective dental hygiene management when the difference between the need for renewing and polishing or the need for replacement of the restoration can be determined.[31,37]

Self-Care Instructions for Esthetic Restorations

Patients must be proficient in maintaining healthy gingival tissue, with the emphasis placed on the importance of daily elimination of plaque biofilm.[23] Improper brushing techniques, such as scrubbing, excessive speed or pressure, and ineffective plaque biofilm removal may affect the longevity of the esthetic restoration and irritate gingival margins. Clinical studies show that powered toothbrushing demonstrates significant improvement in reducing plaque biofilm and gingivitis over manual toothbrushing, while not causing increased gingival abrasion. Power toothbrushes can minimize challenges imposed by improper brushing techniques and dexterity problems, while ultimately securing health through effective plaque biofilm and stain removal (while respecting the surface characterizations of the esthetic material).[43,52]

Loss of surface luster can also be attributed to abrasive toothpaste, alcohol, and acidulated fluorides. Because the hardness of esthetic restorations mirrors the hardness of dentin and cementum (not enamel), patients need to be aware that abrasive toothpaste (or specifically the abrasive particles in the toothpaste) can adversely affect the restoration. Patients need to be instructed to use the least-abrasive toothpaste.[6]

Alcohol is a solvent of bisphenol-α-glycidyl methacrylate (bis-GMA) resin. The result is a softening of the composite matrix, which in turn may increase the patient's ability to abrade the resin material, making it rougher and possibly causing increased staining and early breakdown. Acidulated phosphate fluoride and stannous fluoride should not be used in patients with tooth-colored restorations. Acidulated phosphate fluoride has been shown to etch porcelain and may affect the filler particles in composite resins. Stannous fluoride may also cause discoloration of the restorations (Box 36-5).[10,54,55,56]

BOX 36-5

SELF-CARE OF ESTHETIC RESTORATIONS

- Neutral sodium fluoride to prevent recurrent caries, decrease sensitivity on root surfaces and at cementoenamel junction
- Alcohol-free products to prevent dehydration of materials and mucosa
- Nonabrasive toothpastes to prevent scratching of porcelain and composite material
- Power-assisted brushing (Oscillating rotating technology or sonic brushes may eliminate any challenges related to improper brushing techniques [e.g., scrubbing, excessive speed or pressure] or dexterity issues, while respecting the luster of the restorative systems and safely removing extrinsic stain.)
- A rubber-tipped stimulator (Use this device by rocking it in the interdental space 10 times between each tooth. In addition, run the stimulator along the contours of the gum line a few times.)
- Water irrigation (Use this to massage the gingival tissues and keep the bioburden under control, which can lead to an inflammatory response.)
- Daily tongue plaque biofilm removal
- Sugar free, alcohol-free, and xylitol-containing gum or fresh breath–related products
- Tobacco cessation
- Evaluate for parafunctional habits and bitegaurds (e.g., grinding, clenching, occlusal interferences, fingernail biting, chewing on pens or pins) (These habits can damage or dislodge restorations and natural teeth.)

Evolution of Bleaching

36-1

"His eyes will be darker than wine, his teeth whiter than milk."[4] This Biblical reference illustrates the idea that teeth should be at their whitest. Then and now, the whiteness of teeth is equated to success and beauty. As time goes on, the appearance of teeth will have a continued effect on the psychologic and sociologic aspects of physical attractiveness.

To appreciate research contributions, the clinician should understand the evolution of dental-bleaching (whitening) practices. In-office tooth bleaching was first documented in the dental literature around 1872, using oxalic acid to lighten nonvital teeth. However, it was not until 1937 that conventional bleaching of vital teeth with heat and strong chemical oxidizing agents was introduced.[16] Many subtle improvements occurred in the basic bleaching procedures throughout the following decades. The first documented attempt at in-office vital tooth bleaching is attributed to Dr. Abbott, who in 1918 determined that high-intensity light would elevate temperature and increase the efficiency of the procedure. In 1965, a rubber dam was introduced and used in combination with **hydrogen peroxide** (H_2O_2) and a heat lamp to whiten teeth.[60] Then, the most notable improvement in dental bleaching occurred in 1968. Klusmier, an orthodontist, and Wagner, a periodontist, independently used Proxigel, an **over-the-counter** (OTC) **product** with 10% **carbamide peroxide** that was indicated for the healing of canker sores and wounds. In addition to promoting wound healing, they also noticed that the material lightened the color of the teeth. With favorable results, Klusmier and Wagner continued to use Proxigel as a bleaching agent.[26,29]

In 1988 Haywood and Heymann conducted a formal clinical and laboratory bleaching study. Their research led to the first published article in dental literature that detailed the first "night guard" bleaching procedure, now known as **night guard vital bleaching** (NVB).[27] NVB involves the fabrication of a custom-fitted tray in which the bleaching solution is applied. The introduction of bleaching raised concerns about the efficacy and safety of bleaching ingredients. The U.S. Food and Drug Administration (FDA) and the American Dental Association (ADA) addressed these concerns.[11,61]

Safety and Efficacy

The efficacy of H_2O_2-based tooth whitening has rarely been questioned. H_2O_2 has generally been regarded as a safe food substance and has long been used for oral wound healing. When used as an oral wound–healing agent, up to 5.3% H_2O_2 is considered effective.[28,61] (This translates into a carbamide peroxide solution of approximately 15%.)

Safety concerns have been raised with the use of H_2O_2 since the introduction of at-home whiteners. Because peroxides are capable of producing free radicals, researchers are concerned with their carcinogenicity (cancer causing) and genotoxicity (gene altering) potential. Thus far no published research has found any statistically significant links.[30,61]

When compared with nonbleached teeth, the amount of enamel removed using a 10% carbamide peroxide solution is equivalent to that lost during a 2½-minute exposure to a cola beverage.[45] Bleaching agents have also been shown to have no or minimal effect on the surface texture, hardness, and wear resistance of enamel. Various studies have shown no indication of either etching or significant changes in the surface morphology of enamel when evaluated under a scanning electron microscope (SEM).[28] The aforementioned confocal laser scanning microscopy study showed that bleached teeth had no micromorphologic changes in the subsurface enamel, dentinoenamel junction (DEJ), or dentin.[58]

In 1972 a research team studied the effects of the penetration of bleaching solution into the pulp chamber and canals. It was found that penetrating solution created the potential for irreversible pulp damage—but only in the presence of excessive heat or trauma. The passage of some of the bleaching material to the pulp occurs within 15 minutes.[12] No difference was found in the pulpal reading before the bleaching process or at any point during the study. Pulpal necrosis occurred during conventional bleaching only when excessive heat or trauma existed. It should be noted that the relationship between exposure time and pulpal necrosis has not been substantiated.[53] Bleaching agents can also permeate nonvital teeth that have lost their nutrient supply as a result of damage (i.e., trauma) or removal of the pulp (i.e., endodontic therapy). Over time the loss of nutrients will result in a darkened tooth. In contrast to vital bleaching, which works

through the outer surface of the tooth and is heat and technique sensitive, nonvital bleaching is either applied within the pulp chamber or applied to the tooth surface without concern for damaging the pulp. Traditionally, treatment options for nonvital teeth sacrificed tooth structure (e.g., crowns, veneers, bonding). An alternative for such teeth is nonvital bleaching, which is a more conservative treatment option.

> ### ★ CASE APPLICATION 36-3.1
> #### Bleaching Nonvital Teeth
> Mrs. O'Bryan had an endodontically treated maxillary left incisor before completing cosmetic whitening. Nonvital bleaching was indicated for her (see Figure 36-3). Accelerated in-office bleaching supplemented by dentist-prescribed, home-applied whitening is a treatment option for her.

Ongoing research is being conducted on the technique, ingredients, efficacy, and safety; however, since the early 1990s tooth bleaching has been generally regarded as one of the safest procedures the dental team can provide to patients. As of this writing, no significant health risks associated with in-office and dentist-dispensed at-home bleaching have been reported (outside of transient tooth sensitivity and gingival irritation).

In one clinical study, 66% of patients reported occasional short-duration side effects of thermal tooth sensitivity, gingival irritation, or both when using a tray system.[47] Thermal sensitivity is thought to be a result of the permeation of peroxide into dentin tubules. This is especially a concern for patients with exposed root surfaces and a history of hypersensitivity. Sensitivity can have various manifestations. Some patients report sensitivity while wearing the tray; others report a residual sensitivity 1 hour after removing the loaded tray. To reduce sensitivity while wearing the tray, the practitioner may recommend decreasing the wear time, decreasing the solution concentration, or alternating the use of the bleaching solution with 5% **potassium nitrate** (a desensitizing agent)[1,56] or fluoride.

Chronic sensitivity may occur immediately after the removal of the loaded tray or after completing the process. This type of sensitivity is attributed to the freely diffusible nature of the peroxide gel rather than the pH and may be treated with the desensitization techniques previously described. Clinical studies have confirmed that discontinuing the bleaching process will stop sensitivity. Haywood showed that an average duration of the side effects was 4.8 days during 42 days of 7-hour treatments.[24] Potential sensitivity issues should be disclosed to the patient before the bleaching process is started. Initial disclosure prepares the patient for any negative side effects and helps ensure overall compliance.

Some manufacturers are making advances in research and patient acceptance in the area of sensitivity. A 2005 study reported that patients who brushed with a desensitizing toothpaste that contained fluoride and the maximum amount of potassium nitrate allowed by the FDA (two times daily, 2 weeks before and during professionally supervised at-home whitening treatment) experienced less sensitivity and generally were more satisfied with their whitening treatment compared with a control group using regular toothpaste.[1]

One study showed that patients who used a whitener that included amorphous calcium phosphate (ACP) were 50% less likely to report sensitivity after the treatment compared with formulations without ACP.[18] ACP was added to a 16% carbamide peroxide gel in a parallel, double-blinded, two-cell, randomized, clinical study design that compared tooth color changes and the difference in transient dentinal hypersensitivity. ACP is a compound originally developed by the American Dental Association Foundation (ADAF) to remineralize teeth and reverse early enamel carious lesions. A 1999 ADAF study performed at the National Institute of Standards showed that ACP also can make teeth less sensitive to hot, cold, air pressure, and tactile stimulation when applied topically either by dental professionals or patients. The study noted that the extra calcium and phosphorus do not appear to alter the effectiveness of the whitener or affect its taste. The same researcher conducted a second study with ACP added to a carbamide peroxide whitening product and determined that ACP products offer 10% better long-term whitening efficacy. Long-term safety of the product has also been demonstrated—no gingival or other effects were observed in the study at day 90 or 180.[19]

Another reported side effect of tooth whitening is gingival irritation.[25] Gingival irritation could be a result of contact with the bleaching solution or an ill-fitting bleaching tray. Various adjustment appointments may be necessary to trim the tray for a better fit.

When proper application techniques were followed, no nonresolving detrimental effects on teeth, existing restorations, or oral tissues were reported. One study researched the use of a 10% carbamide peroxide solution worn for 8 hours a day. After 2 weeks, no detrimental effects were found on oral tissues.[25] Another researcher used confocal laser scanning microscopy to show that even in exaggerated-use conditions, bleaching with H_2O_2 or carbamide peroxide gels results in no changes to the enamel or dentin ultrastructure.[58] However, continual research is being conducted, particularly on the response of resin composite restorative materials to bleaching agents.

In 1994 the ADA Council on Dental Therapeutics published criteria for whitening in its *Acceptance Program for Home-Use Tooth Whitening Products.* The guidelines were intended to document the safety and efficacy levels of whitening products. The ADA recognized that whitening products can be administered or dispensed by dentists, purchased OTC, and categorized into two major groups:

1. Peroxide-containing whiteners or bleaching agents
2. Whitening toothpastes (dentifrices)

Before gels can be awarded the ADA Seal of Acceptance, the program requires manufacturers to determine the degradation of bleaching gels in trays during use. For the whitening gel to be judged efficacious, the guidelines specify that results must indicate a tooth shade change of at least two shades according to a value-oriented Vita shade guide.[61] The guidelines were re-vised in 1995 and 1998 and are again under review for revision. So far, all of the products in the dentist-dispensed or OTC category that bear the ADA Seal of Acceptance contain 10% carbamide peroxide; however, participation in the program is not limited to products of this concentration. Although bleaching agents are available OTC, only those dispensed through the dental office are considered for the Seal, because professional consultation is important to the procedure's safety and effectiveness.

In the category of professionally applied in-office, all products that have the ADA Seal of Acceptance contain 35% H_2O_2, although this concentration is not a requirement of the program. In regard to whitening toothpastes (dentifrices), all of the products in the ADA Seal of Acceptance program contain polishing or chemical agents to improve tooth appearance by removing surface stains through gentle polishing, chemical chelation, or some other nonbleaching action. Several whitening toothpastes that are available OTC have received the ADA Seal of Acceptance (http://www.ada.org/ada/seal/index.asp).[11,61]

Dental Bleaching Agents: Composition and Mode of Action

The two major tooth-bleaching or whitening chemicals are carbamide peroxide and H_2O_2. Although the exact mechanisms of the dental-bleaching process are still being studied, oxidation is believed primarily to be responsible for the observed whitening. During oxidation, the active bleaching ingredient, H_2O_2, typically generates short-lived oxygen intermediates, such as the hydroxyl radical, that enter the enamel or dentin of the discolored teeth and diffuse to areas containing the discoloration. The hydroxyl radicals then break down some of the double bonds in the organic stains, making them more soluble and resulting in notable changes in the refractory index of the enamel. Lighter color at the dentinal level and opaqueness of the enamel layer make teeth appear whiter and brighter. Makers of first-generation whitening agents added glycerin to their products as a thickening and stabilizing agent.[26] Glycerin kept the carbamide peroxide localized to the area of treatment. Newer generations of bleaching agents do not contain glycerin, because it dries the tooth by leaching water from it, dehydrating the tooth surface. Many manufactures have replaced glycerin with glycol or water.

The critical difference between carbamide peroxide and H_2O_2 is in the oxidation process. Carbamide peroxide is a sustained-release agent with greater substantivity and retention rates. It whitens by breaking down urea and H_2O_2. These substances are well tolerated and excreted by the body. Carbamide peroxide has a slower rate of reaction than H_2O_2. Carbamide peroxide is usually delivered using a custom-made tray (NVB) worn from 1 hour to overnight in concentrations ranging from 5% to 40%.[29] A general rule is that a carbamide peroxide concentration is equivalent to approximately three times the comparable H_2O_2 concentration. Therefore a 10% carbamide peroxide gel is roughly equivalent to a 3% H_2O_2 gel. Other possible ingredients of tooth-bleaching gels are Carbopol (slow oxygen releasing), sodium hydroxide, potassium nitrate, flavoring agents, and fluoride.[47] H_2O_2, an immediate-release agent, breaks down into water and oxygen (often accelerated by enzymes such as peroxides). H_2O_2 releases oxygen within the first few seconds of contacting tooth surfaces, and its substantivity can last up to 30 minutes. H_2O_2 concentrations range from 5.5% to 38%.[47]

Patient Selection: Indications and Contraindications

In any discussion of the patient selection criteria for potential bleaching therapy, the clinician should begin with a thorough diagnosis, which has been described as "the single most important determinant of the success of bleaching for any discoloration."[22] Components of this phase include a thorough medical-dental history and clinical examination.

Before looking at what causes teeth to become discolored, the clinician should review natural tooth structure and its subsequent colors. Enamel is composed of millions of rods (also called *prisms*), forming a crystalline lattice structure (also known as *hydroxyapatite*). In general, clinicians refer to these as the *enamel matrix*. Dentin is the underlying layer of each tooth and makes up the largest part of the tooth. Therefore natural tooth color, whether yellowish white to grayish white, depends primarily on two things:

1. Thickness of enamel
2. Underlying dentin color

Natural tooth color can be affected by both extrinsic (outside) and intrinsic (inside) color changes.[60] Two of most commonly used shade guides to determine the shade of a tooth are called (1) *value-oriented Vita shade guide* (Figure 36-6) and (2)

Chromosome by Ivoclar Vivadent (Table 36-2). Coffee, tea, tobacco, berries, plaque biofilm, accumulation, red wine and other substances that contain pigment can cause **extrinsic stains.** These stains occur on the surface of the tooth.

Generally the clinician can remove extrinsic stains by a thorough mechanical scaling and polishing of the tooth (i.e., professional prophylaxis).[31] Toothpaste in conjunction with toothbrushes has an effect on tooth color by preventing and removing stain and plaque biofilm. If cracks in the enamel exist or if the enamel surface is highly porous (demineralized), then extrinsic stains have the potential to penetrate the enamel matrix. In these instances the stain cannot be mechanically removed and must be treated chemically.

Intrinsic stains refer to stains that occur within the tooth structure.[60] The stain can be either embedded into the enamel

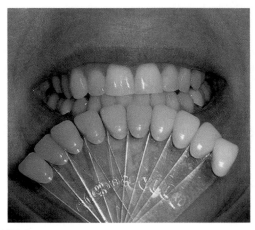

FIGURE 36-6
Value-oriented Vita shade guide.

Table 36-2	Shade Guide Selection and Setup

Chromosome by Ivoclar Vivadent					
This is a shade guide set up by color groups and then arranged by hues—light to dark.					
BLEACH	**WHITE**	**YELLOW**	**ORANGE**	**GRAY**	**BROWN**
010	110	210	310	410	510
020	120	220	320	420	520
030	130	230	330	430	530
040	140	240	340	440	540

Vita Shade Guide				
This is a standard shade guide and the most popular. Clinicians can put this into any order, either by letter or by groups lightest to darkest.				
WHITE	**YELLOW**	**ORANGE**	**GRAY**	**BROWN**
B1	B2	A3	A4	D6
A1	D1	B5	B6	C4
A2	E1	E2	B4	C3
C1	C2	E3	C6	D4

or the dentin. Some of the primary sources of intrinsic stains are the following:

- Aging
- Trauma
- Certain medications
- Chromgenic foodstuffs

Intrinsic stains cannot be removed with mechanical cleaning. They must be whitened via chemical bleaching.[31] Considering this, pertinent medical history questions should address systemic medications, such as **tetracycline** (TCN), minocycline, and fluoride that cause intrinsic tooth discoloration.

Although rare, other conditions, such as jaundice and amelogenesis imperfecta, may also contribute to tooth discoloration. Dental conditions such as dental caries or faulty restorations may contribute to tooth discolorations and should be identified before bleaching therapy is prescribed. Conditions such as erosion, large pulp chambers, exposed root surfaces, hypersensitivity, white or opaque spots, dark stains, and esthetic restorations should be considered for bleaching patients.

A thorough health history would reveal previous ingestion of TCN or a derivative of TCN. For example, the patient may have cystic fibrosis and use TCN, a common treatment for this disease. Teeth are most susceptible to TCN discolorations during formation, beginning the second trimester *in utero* and continuing to approximately 8 years of age.

★ CASE APPLICATION 36-3.2

Tetracycline Stain and Tooth Whitening

Mrs. O'Bryan's case illustrates TCN staining (see Figure 36-3).

Researchers believe that TCN particles incorporate in the dentin during calcification of the teeth through chelation with calcium, which forms TCN orthophosphate.[44] The result is the discoloration of the dentin. The process displays itself as a result from exposure to sunlight. Because the labial surfaces of the incisors are more prone to sunlight exposure, they tend to darken faster and more intensely than their molar counterparts.

The dentist should identify the severity and type of discoloration. Some patients respond favorably to the bleaching process, whereas others do not. TCN stains have four degrees:

- First degree is a light-yellow to light-gray stain that is uniformly distributed in localized areas and is amenable to bleaching techniques.
- Second degree is a darker and more extensive yellow-gray hue. This degree is also amenable to the bleaching techniques.
- Third and fourth degrees are more intense dark gray-blue, banding stains. Favorable results have been achieved with third-degree stains by lengthening the bleaching duration.
- Fourth-degree stains may never completely lose their gray color.[22]

A derivative of TCN is **minocycline,** which is a routine prescription for adolescent and adult treatment of acne, as well as a variety of other infections. This medication may cause a sudden appearance of a ringlike stain. Although TCN use results in dentin discoloration during calcification of the teeth, minocycline use leads to discolorations in already erupted and formed teeth. Unfortunately, adults are also at risk for this stain because minocycline is absorbed in the gastrointestinal tract. The tooth pigmentation results from minocycline's ability to chelate with iron and form insoluble complexes. Like TCN staining, minocycline stains have degrees of severity and distribution. The mild cases are amenable to bleaching, whereas more severe cases (i.e., heavier banding) may require porcelain lamination.[9,22]

The medical-dental history may also reveal whether fluoride has been ingested. An excessive amount of fluoride ingestion results in **fluorosis.** The fluorosis stain exhibits itself as brown or flat gray pigmentation on smooth enamel or as white spots.[60] The teeth most commonly affected are the maxillary premolar and molar regions. The bleaching process does not remove the white spots; however, it lightens the background crown area, creating less contrast. Bleaching is contraindicated for fluorosis conditions with severe enamel loss.

Age, as mentioned earlier, is another factor that affects the coloration of teeth. Studies have confirmed that teeth darken and become more yellow as age increases. With age, teeth may appear darker as a result of lifelong consumption of chromogenic foods. For example, years of coffee drinking and smoking can have a cumulative and drastic effect on the appearance of the teeth. These stains readily adhere to tiny cracks and fractures on the enamel surface. Fortunately, these types of stains respond favorably to bleaching. Teeth (vital or nonvital) discolored from trauma also respond well to bleaching.[22,23,48,52]

Dental implications of aging include a gradual thinning of enamel that is caused by natural occlusal forces. As a response to these forces, reparative or secondary dentin forms as a natural protective mechanism of the tooth. This secondary dentin is more translucent and appears darker in color. Unfortunately, this natural occurrence is more difficult to bleach. Other conditions that should be considered for patient selection include erosion, large pulp chambers, exposed root surfaces, hypersensitivity, white or opaque spots, dark stains, and esthetic restorations.[31,32]

Although the success of bleaching has been widely documented, some patients may not benefit from the bleaching process. Therefore the clinician should not to encourage unrealistic expectations. A thorough clinical examination can be helpful in the determination of the appropriateness of bleaching and in the projection of realistic bleaching outcomes.

Data Collection: The Clinical Examination

Evaluating the need for tooth whitening can occur at various points in the patient's course of dental care. After periodontal debridement, some patients may be satisfied with the appearance of their teeth, and tooth-whitening procedures are not necessary. Likewise, after use of the air-powered polishers for removing extrinsic stain from smooth and fissured enamel surfaces, the need for whitening procedures may be eliminated.

A radiographic evaluation rules out potential acute problems such as abscesses, internal resorption, and caries, which can cause tooth discoloration. If any of theses problems exist, then they should be treated before any whitening procedure. Radiographs are also used to assess the pulp size. Enlarged pulp chambers may increase the potential for hypersensitivity. Specific teeth may require pulp vitality testing. These conditions may require additional restorative treatment or extended time with whitening treatments.[31]

Dental and periodontal charting are other components of the clinical examination performed before whitening. The dental charting exhibits caries, faulty restorations, and other restorative needs.[31,32] Dental hygienists should identify existing restorations in the esthetic zone and inform the patient that those restorations will not change color with whitening. This information may affect the patient's desire to bleach or confirm the need for postwhitening dental procedures, such as replacing composites, veneers, or crowns if these restorations do not blend with the new tooth color. Shade selection with the use of a shade guide should be documented at every hygiene session. Tooth whitening should be considered before porcelain veneer placement either to eliminate the need for veneers, to reduce the amount of opacifiers needed to mask discolorations, or to give the patient the option of attempting a less expensive and less invasive treatment. After veneer placement, bleaching may be used to relighten teeth if they relapse, to further lighten the apparent color of existing veneers by bleaching the underlying nonbleached tooth structure from the lingual, or to clean stained margins on existing veneers. The hygienist should identify older amalgam restorations in need of replacing before initiating whitening procedures to avoid any greening or discoloration of the teeth around the restoration from the procedure or from resultant translucency of teeth.[31,61]

The periodontal charting records areas of attachment loss. Additional information such as the patient's history of bruxism, sensitivity, and dental injuries should be collected. Before initiating tooth whitening, the hygienist and dentist should address and treat all of these potential problems.[31,32]

After the clinical examination, the dentist can then develop a treatment plan and the dental hygienist can present whitening options to the patient, time commitment required for the procedure, potential side effects, anticipated cost, and predicted outcomes. It should be stressed that the whitening process may involve periodic reevaluations to monitor progress.

Patient Instructions

Patients need to understand that whitening is never 100% guaranteed, and observed tooth color change can be dependent on the following factors:

- Whitening agent (concentration)
- Type of service
- Whitening time (daily and totality)

- Initial tooth color
- Specific tooth region
- Etiology of stain
- Accuracy of tray fabrication (if NVB)

Instruction for NVB may include the following:

- Emphasis on effectively removing plaque biofilm and bacteria from the surfaces and between teeth before inserting the whitening tray

> **Patient Education Opportunity**
>
> As with any dental procedure, the clinician should provide the patient with written instructions. Specific patient instructions should be given to the patient both orally and in writing. The patient should be given well-written and easy-to-follow instructions. Many ADA-approved bleaching systems have the appropriate patient education instructions in the kit.[46]

- Use of a nonabrasive whitening dentifrice before, during, and after the bleaching regimen is completed to help fortify the achieved cosmetic results
- Removal of excess whitening material that may migrate on the gingival tissue after placement of the tray
- Cessation of smoking and drinking any dark-pigmented liquid during the process (and instructions to minimize these habits after treatment)
- Instructions to contact the office if mild tooth sensitivity or gum irritation occurs
- Scheduling of a follow-up appointment 1 to 2 weeks after the whitening kit is received to voice concerns and share successes[32]

Modes of Delivery: Bleaching Techniques

IN-OFFICE AND LIGHT-ASSISTED BLEACHING

Administering tooth-bleaching services through dental practices benefits the patient and the professional by the following:

- Improving patient compliance
- Getting rapid results
- Eliminating costly OTC options or repeat options
- Representing a viable option for handling patent's extreme sensitivity
- Generating practice income
- Properly assessing of the patient's teeth and shade

In-office bleaching, also known as *power bleaching,* is a technique used by dental professionals. Currently three options are available for full-mouth whitening: (1) chemically activated systems, (2) light systems, and (3) laser-activated systems.[46] Chemically activated systems use carbamide peroxide, calcium peroxide, and H_2O_2 without a light to bleach teeth. The concentration of the bleaching agent varies in each gel. The **light-assisted bleaching** systems use an ultraviolet (UV) or visible (blue source) light, not a laser. The light activates the gel to imitate the bleaching process. The exact mechanism of action this option provides is unclear, yet it yields similar results as *take-home* whitening options. **Laser bleaching** and **ultraviolet-light systems** use light-absorbed H_2O_2, along with laser energy to accelerate the bleaching process.[15]

These application techniques use a higher concentration of H_2O_2 than NVB (typically 35% or greater) and require precision isolation and close patient monitoring throughout the procedure. Local anesthetics are contraindicated because they hinder patient communication about procedural discomforts (e.g., gingival burning, improper rubber dam clamp placement). These systems are ideal for patients who need quick results and for those who have stubborn, unresolved stains. Today most systems do not rely on heat but rather concentrated halogen, plasma arc, xenon arc, or metal haloid to activate the bleaching process.[16,46]

In-office bleaching has advantages and disadvantages. The procedure is the most expensive bleaching choice for the patient. A large percentage of the cost of the procedure is the result of the chair time needed. Many office protocols include from one to three whitening sessions, with 30 to 60 minutes contact time for whitening. Because some manufacturers recommend agitation of the bleach while on teeth, dental team members need to be available so that the patient is not left alone with active gel on the teeth. Because of their high chemical concentrations, these whitening agents have a potential to cause significant soft tissue irritation and damage. A properly placed and seated rubber dam or block-out resin provides an appropriate barrier. **Block-out resins** are light-cured resin materials that can be used as a rubber dam substitute during whitening procedures and when fabricating whitening trays. Many manufacturers incorporate fluoride ions and potassium nitrate to help minimize or eliminate sensitivity. Studies have shown that when using higher concentrations of whitening solutions, the shade change is less stable.[31] This problem can be managed with application of take-home whitening trays after the in-office procedure. In-office whitening is great for patients who seek immediate bleaching results or who are scheduled for additional esthetic restorative options. This whitening method is also used for patients who show poor compliance with at-home whitening or who have difficulty with trays. Most insurance policies do not cover bleaching administered solely for esthetic purposes.

LASER BLEACHING AND ULTRAVIOLET-LIGHT SYSTEMS

The term *laser whitening,* as used in this chapter, refers to professionally controlled, in-office services using a high concentration of H_2O_2 and an added energy source to excite the process of tooth bleaching. Laser whitening is believed to accelerate the H_2O_2 particles (15% to 38%) to enhance whitening results. Laser whitening may require additional training and certification for the dental hygienist.

A few laser manufacturers have received FDA clearance to use laser energy (gallium-aluminum-arsenide or diode) to whiten teeth. This type of laser is easily switched from periodontal therapy to a laser "smile instrument" by simply removing the soft tissue headpiece and replacing it with the whitening wand.

A properly placed rubber dam or a protective light-cured resin on the soft tissue provides an appropriate barrier from the lasers. The products are usually premixed and are dispensed directly from their syringe onto the teeth.

The following are a few additional safety concerns for both the clinician and the patient:
- Laser-safe eye protection for everyone in the treatment room
- First-aid kit containing vitamin E, aloe vera, and zinc oxide or propylene glycol
- Concerns based on patient data and need

When choosing a suitable laser, areas for the clinician to evaluate include efficacy of each laser and its wavelength, thermal effects, and pulpal response.[32]

DENTIST-PRESCRIBED, SELF-APPLIED SYSTEMS

Tray Method

NVB is one of the *dentist-prescribed, self-applied* methods. This technique is initiated in the dental office after the data collection phase has been completed and informed consent has been obtained. This supervised at-home tray method has proven to be the most accessible and acceptable option for the majority of dental offices and patients. It treats all the surfaces of the teeth and may be more advantageous in delivering low concentrations over a longer time period versus intermittent high doses.

These products contain various percentages of carbamide peroxide and H_2O_2. Other differences include viscosity, flavoring agents, packaging, whitening tray material, **desensitizers,** and fluoride ingredients.

The first step in preparing for the NVB technique is to complete an initial examination of tooth discoloration or stains. Once diagnosis is complete, the clinician should replicate the patient's oral cavity (alginate impression) to form a study cast. From the study cast, a custom-fit plastic night guard (bleaching tray) is fabricated with a vacuum-forming machine (Figure 36-7). The tray is then trimmed. Tray design is dependent on the viscosity of the bleaching material and the individual manufacturer suggestions.[29]

★ CASE APPLICATION 36-3.3

At-Home Tray-Based Tooth Whitening Systems

Tray designs can vary, depending on individual patient indications. For example, a scalloped reservoir tray was used initially for Mrs. O'Bryan. However, when she returned 7 months later, a nonscalloped, nonreservoir tray was indicated (see Figure 36-9), because it can seal the environment and hold the bleaching agent against the neck of the tooth. This second tray provided the supply of material needed to whiten the challenging gingival third of the tooth.

The self-applied bleaching process usually takes 2 to 6 weeks. Additional time may be indicated for slow-responding discolorations such as TCN, brown fluorosis, or inherent discolorations. Although retreatment is typically not indicated for several years, patients are told to expect stable results for 1 to 3 years with cosmetic whitening. Some color changes may be permanent or longer lasting.

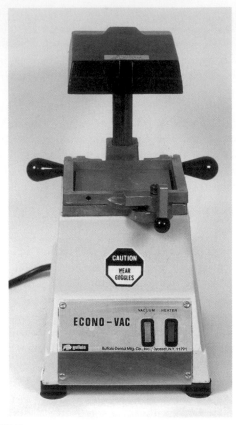

FIGURE 36-7
Vacuum-forming machine used for fabrication of night guard. (From Bird DL, Robinson DS: *Torres and Ehrlich modern dental assisting,* ed 8, St Louis, Saunders, 2005.)

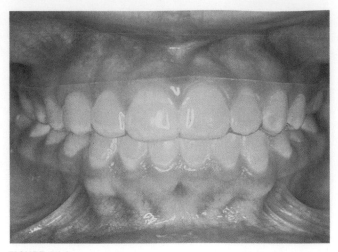

FIGURE 36-9
Nonscalloped and nonreservoir custom-fitted bleaching tray design. (Courtesy Van B. Haywood, DMD, Augusta, Ga.)

spacer on the facial aspect of each tooth on the dental cast. Recent studies and manufacturers' instructions concur that reservoirs are not needed for whitening to occur and may not affect the clinical rate that whitening takes place or the efficacy of the gel. As always, one should follow the specific manufacturer's instructions.[32]

Scalloped trays are trimmed after the tooth is contoured at the gingival-tooth interface, as illustrated in Figure 36-8. A nonscalloped tray, pictured in Figure 36-9, is evenly trimmed approximately 2 mm from the gingival crest onto the gingival tissue.

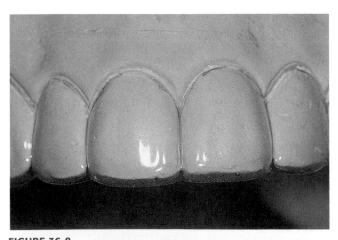

FIGURE 36-8
Scalloped tray design. (From Haywood VB, *Contemp Esthet and Restor Pract* 9, 1999.)

Tray design and fabrication options include soft or rigid, reservoir or nonreservoir, and scalloped or nonscalloped trays. Soft trays are now preferred to the original rigid trays for ease of fabrication and patient comfort. Reservoirs are used with the more highly viscous bleaching materials. The reservoirs are formed with the addition of 0.5 mm of light-cured resin or

> ### ✸ CASE APPLICATION 36-2.1
> #### Posttreatment Follow-Up
> Jimmy showed stabilization for 7 years without requiring interim or touch-up bleaching treatments. The posttreatment photograph is shown in Figure 36-2, *B*.

The patient should wear the night guard for 2 to 6 hours a day. Initially, when NVB was first introduced, treatments were scheduled for 1 to 2 hours. It has been suggested though that more than 60% of the peroxide remains active in the tray—even after 4 hours of use. Therefore patients may obtain better whitening results with a specified amount of gel if they can wear the tray overnight.[50] Thus nighttime bleaching is the method most often preferred.

Patients should be informed that teeth might appear "splotchy" during the early stages of tooth whitening procedures. This is a result of the individual tooth's response or is caused by the varying amounts of whitening agent on the tooth. Reassuring patients that a more homogeneous appearance can be expected with continued treatment is important.

PREFORMED DUAL-TRAY SYSTEMS

Another advance recently introduced into the whitening market is the **preformed dual-tray system,** which includes a non-custom or prefilled, adaptable, disposable tooth-whitening tray that eliminates the need to take alginate impressions and pour and trim models, using laboratory time, or to create boil-and-bite trays. A kit includes a gingival barrier, and the product is a reloaded 9% H_2O_2 tray. The patient simply places the trays on the upper and lower arches, gently presses, and removes the outer tray. The patient is then left with a clear polypropylene tray covering each arch. The trays are worn for 30 minutes and discarded after use.

OVER-THE-COUNTER OPTIONS

Various forms of application of OTC whiteners include preformed trays, strips, pens, applicator brushes, liquids, and paint-on options. The H_2O_2 concentrations found in OTC products range from 3.5% to 12%. The increase in popularity of "trayless whitening" technology provides the consumer with application choices ranging from once or twice a day to nighttime application. Many manufacturers are spending millions of dollars advertising their OTC whitening products, resulting in increased patient awareness of tooth whitening. These direct-to-consumer whitening products have provided a gateway for patients and dental hygienists to discuss esthetics.

Several OTC dental-bleaching systems contain ingredients similar to professional bleaching products. However, at the time of this publication, the ADA has not approved any of these systems unless they are also dispensed in dental offices. Dental professionals should be aware that OTC products achieve some lightening effect. The following are some anecdotal disadvantages to OTC whitening products:

- Ill-fitting mouthguard trays
- Tissue irritation
- Low percentage of peroxide, undisclosed percentage of peroxide, or both
- Low viscosity
- Varying pH levels
- No professional supervision during use

Dental hygienists should educate their patients that the results may vary using OTC products.[32,61]

Adverse effects associated with the use of OTC whiteners appear to be rare; however, systematic collection of such data is difficult.

⚡ CASE APPLICATION 36-4.1

Matching Patient Need with Whitening System or Product

Given Mrs. Randall's lack of personal time and her desire for a whiter-appearing smile, she is an excellent candidate for OTC technology.

Role of the Dental Hygienist

The dental hygienist will encounter patients seeking advice about cosmetic whitening. Some patients will not be satisfied with the results of their OTC whitening products and will ask for advice. During the debridement appointment, patients often disclose concerns about the color of their teeth to the dental hygienist, and inquiring and new patients often ask the dental hygienist about whitening options. After completion of clinical and radiographic assessment, a color assessment for each patient can be performed. To perform a "color assessment," the hygienist should have the patient look into a mirror. He or she should then say, "We now know that teeth can change color over time. What I'd like to do now is to assess the current color of your teeth. I'll need your help with this part." This immediately gets the patient involved in the care and gives the dental hygienist an opportunity to comfortably discuss noninvasive cosmetic procedures.

Each dental hygiene operatory should be equipped with shade guides. Shade guides should be set up from lightest to darkest, making sure that the guide also includes newer "whitening" colors. The hygienist should hold the shade guide so that the patient can see the colors and have the patient help select the appropriate shade (Box 36-6). If the patient is interested in whitening, then he or she will naturally bring up the topic with the dental hygienist (and the hygienist will be able to ask other questions). These questions might include the following: "Other than the color shifts, is there anything else that you notice about your smile?"

With the advent of computer-imaging systems that provide photographic images of patients' teeth, dental hygienists have the opportunity to discuss esthetics with patients. Attractive posters and current brochures describing dental whitening should be located in patient reception areas. Having sample

---

BOX 36-6

TIPS FOR SHADE SELECTION AT HYGIENE SESSIONS

- For most accurate results, the colors in the room and patient clothes should be neutral.
- Cover colored clothes with a neutral (gray) cloth, and have female patients remove their lipstick.
- Wet the teeth before taking an impression to ensure that they will not be dehydrated.
- The patient's mouth should be at eye level.
- Determine the *amber* or *gray* color type of the patient.
- Determine the base shade of the patient, and remove the corresponding shade group.
- Determine the shade intensity within the shade group.
- Compare the selected shade once again with the natural tooth.
- When taking a smile shade during the comprehensive examination, use the canine tooth for the base shade when possible.
- Note the range of shade, striations, and color banding or mottling. Close inspection will reveal a blending of several colors.[46]

trays, whitening strips, and prebleaching and postbleaching photographs available for patient education is also helpful. After the dental examination, diagnosis, and treatment planning phase, the dental hygienist can initiate treatment for patients interested in cosmetic whitening. Cosmetic whitening is a service that brings great pleasure, boosts confidence, and improves the quality of patients' lives. At the same time, knowledge of cosmetic-whitening procedures can make the dental hygienist a more effective team member in the changing dental care environment.

Many OTC preventive products include whitening agents, including whitening floss, dentifrices, chewing gum, and mouthrinses. As new whitening products are introduced, the dental hygienist should critically review evidence-based research that evaluates their safety and efficacy.

References

1. Alexander D: *Sensodyne helps make whitening patients more comfortable.* Available at http://www.dental-professional.com. Accessed on August 1, 2005.
2. American Academy of Cosmetic Dentistry: *Cosmetic dentistry consumer stats.* Available at http://www.aacd.com/media/market_research_data.aspx. Accessed July 1, 2005.
3. Ames G: Removing stains from mottled enamel, *Dent Cosmos* 24:1674-1677, 1937.
4. Barker et al, editors: *The NIV Study Bible, Genesis* 49:12, Grand Rapids, Mich., 1995, Zondervan Publishing.
5. Barnes C: Adapting polishing procedures to maintain esthetic restorations, *J Dent Hyg* 4:22-24, 2005.
6. Barnes C, Covey D, Walker M: Maintenance of the esthetic integrity of dental restorations, *RDH* 23(3):74, 2003.
7. Barnes C et al: Essential selective polishing: the maintenance of esthetic restorations, *J Pract Hyg* 5:18-24, 2003.
8. Blitz N: *Diagnosis and treatment evaluation in cosmetic dentistry: a guide to accreditation criteria,* Madison, Wis., 2000, American Academy of Cosmetic Dentistry.
9. Bowles WH, Bokemeyer TJ: Staining of adult teeth by minocycline by septic proteins, *J Esthet Dent* 9(1):30-34, 1997.
10. Burchard HH: *A textbook of dental pathology and therapeutics,* Philadelphia, 1998, Lea & Febiger.
11. Burrell KH: ADA supports vital tooth bleaching—but look for the seal, *J Am Dent Assoc* 128(suppl):3S-5S, 1997.
12. Cooper JS, Bokmeyer TJ, Bowles WH: Penetration of the pulp chamber by carbamide peroxide bleaching agents, *J Endod* 18(7):315-317, 1992.
13. Curtis JW et al: Assessing the effects of 10% carbamide peroxide on oral soft tissue, *J Am Dent Assoc* 127(8):1218-1223, 1996.
14. Davis LG, Ashworth PD, Spriggs LS: Psychological effects of esthetic dental treatment, *J Dent Res* 26(7):547-554, 1998.
15. Dorfman W: In-office and light assisted tooth whitening: current trends and practice growth potential, *AACD Monograph* 203:33-35, 2004.
16. Fortin D, Vargas MA: The spectrum of composites: new techniques and materials, *J Am Dent Assoc* 131:6:26S-30S, 2000.
17. Gerlach RW et al: A randomized clinical trial comparing a novel 5.3% hydrogen peroxide whitening strip to 10%, 15% and 20% carbamide peroxide tray-based bleaching systems, *Compend Cont Educ Dent* 29(suppl):S22-28, 2000.
18. Giniger M: A 180-day clinical investigation of the tooth-whitening efficacy of a bleaching gel with added amorphous calcium phosphate, *J Clin Dent* 16(1):11-16, 2005.
19. Giniger M et al: The clinical performance of professionally dispensed bleaching gel with added amorphous calcium phosphate, *J Am Dent Assoc* 3(136):383-392, 2005.
20. Gladwin M, Bagby M: *Clinical aspects of dental materials,* Philadelphia, 2000, Lippincott Williams & Wilkins.
21. Goldstein RE: Maintenance of esthetic restoration, *Contemp Esthet Restor Pract* 6:2:10-15, 2002.
22. Goldstein RE et al: Bleaching of vital and pulpless teeth. In Cohen S, Burns RC, eds: *Pathways of the pulp,* ed 6, St Louis, 1994, Mosby.
23. Haywood VB: Tooth bleaching: commentary in current concepts, *AACD Monograph* 42-43, 2003.
24. Haywood VB: Nightguard vital bleaching: current concepts and research, *J Am Dent Assoc* 128(suppl):19-25, 1997.
25. Haywood VB: The Food and Drug Administration and its influence on home bleaching, *Curr Opin Cosmet Dent* 12-18, 1993.
26. Haywood VB: Nightguard vital bleaching: a history and products update: I, *Esthet Dent Update* 2(4):63-66, 1991.
27. Haywood VB, Heymann HO: Nightguard vital bleaching, *Quintessence Int* 20(3):173-176, 1989.
28. Haywood VB, Houck VM, Heymann HO: Nightguard vital bleaching: effects of varying pH solutions on enamel surface texture and color change, *Quintessence Int* 22(7):775-782, 1991.
29. Haywood VB, Leonard RH: Nightguard vital bleaching removes brown discoloration for 7 years: a case report, *Quintessence Int* 29(7):450-451, 1998.
30. Haywood VB et al: Effectiveness, side effects, and long-term status of nightguard vital bleaching, *J Am Dent Assoc* 125(9):1219-1226, 1994.
31. Hodsdon KA: What color is your DPA? *RDH* 8, 2005. Available at http://rdh.pennnet.com. Accessed September 1, 2005.
32. Hodsdon KA: *Demystifying smile: strategies for the dental team,* Tulsa, 2003, PennWell Corporation.
33. Hodsdon KA: Postoperative care for esthetic restoration: a challenge to dental hygienists, *J Pract Hyg* 7:19-24, 1998.
34. Hoel DC et al: The effect of these finishing systems on four esthetic restorative materials, *Oper Dent* 23:36-42, 1998
35. Hondrum So, Fernandex R Jr: Contouring, finishing, and polishing class V restorative materials, *Oper Dent* 22:30-36, 1997.
36. Jay AT: Tooth whitening: the financial rewards, *Dent Manag* 30(12):28-31, 1990.
37. Jones LA: Comparative indications for esthetic indirect restorations: a dentist's guide, *Contemp Esthet and Restor Pract* 2:56-61, 2004.
38. Jones T: Caring for composites: a prophy paste story, *RDH* 5:59-61, 2005.
39. Mange P: Conservative restoration of compromised posterior teeth with direct composite: a seven-year report, *Prac Perio Esth Dent* 12(8):747-749, 2000.
40. McCracken MS, Haywood VB: Demineralization effects of 10 percent carbamide peroxide, *J Dent* 24(6):395-398, 1996.
41. McGuire MK, Miller L: Maintaining esthetic restorations in the periodontal practice, *Int J Periodontics Restorative Dent* 16(3):231-239, 1996.
42. McInnes C et al: Stain removal ability of the sonicare electric toothbrush, *J Clin Dent* 5:13-18, 1994.
43. McManus V: Beauty and the dental hygienist, *Contemp Oral Hyg* 6:30-32, 2005.

44. Mello HS: The mechanism of tetracycline staining in primary and permanent teeth, *J Dent Child* 34(6):478-487, 1967.

45. Miller M: *2003 Reality,* Houston, 2003, Reality Publishing Company.

46. Narcisi EM, Diperna JA: Multidisciplinary full-mouth restoration with porcelain veneers and laboratory-fabricated resin inlays, *Pract Periodontics Aesthet Dent* 11(6):721-728, 1999.

47. Nathoo SA et al: Kinetics of carbamide peroxide degradation in bleaching trays, *J Dent Res* 75(2149):286, 1996 (IADR abstracts).

48. Odioso LL et al: Impact of demographic, behavioral, and dental care utilization parameters on tooth color and personal satisfaction, *Compend Cont Educ Dent* 29(suppl):S35-41, 2000.

49. Okeson J: *Management of temporomandibular disorders and occlusion,* ed 5, St Louis, 2003, Mosby.

50. Reis-Schmidt T: Cosmetic demands drive development of material and applications, *Dent Prod Rep* 12:46-51, 1996.

51. Robinson PG et al: Manual versus powered toothbrushing for oral health, *Cochrane Database Syst Rev* Apr 18(2):CD002281, 2005.

52. Sagel PA et al: Vital tooth whitening with a novel hydrogen peroxide strip system: design, kinetics, and clinical response, *Compend Cont Educ Dent* 29(suppl):S10-S15, 2000.

53. Schulte JR et al: The effects of bleaching application time on the dental pulp, *J Am Dent Assoc* 125(10):1330-1335, 1994.

54. Soeno K et al: Effect of acidulated phosphate fluoride agents and effectiveness of subsequent polishing on composite material surfaces, *Oper Dent* 27:3005-3010, 2002.

55. Soeno K et al: Effect of acidulated phosphate fluoride agents on the surface characteristics of composite restorative materials, *Am J Dent* 13(6):297-300, 2000.

56. Tam L: Effect of potassium nitrate and fluoride on carbamide peroxide bleaching, *Quintessence Int* 32(10):766-770, 2001.

57. Touati B: Defining form and position, *Pract Periodon Aesthet Dent* 10:(7):800-807, 1998.

58. White DJ et al: Effects of tooth whitening gels on enamel and dentin ultrastructure: a confocal laser scanning microscopy pilot study, *Compend Cont Educ Dent* 29(suppl):S29-S34, 2000.

59. Wilkins EM: *Clinical practice of the dental hygienist,* ed 9, Philadelphia, 2006, Lippincott Williams & Wilkins.

60. Yiming L: Quest for whiter teeth: a continued demand in esthetic dentistry, *AACD Monograph* 11:41-43, 2005.

61. Yiming I.: Tooth bleaching using peroxide-containing agents: current status of safety issues, *Compend Cont Educ Dent* 19(8):783-794, 1998.

Orthodontics

Sylvia Frazier-Bowers • Elizabeth Maxbauer

INSIGHT

Dental hygienists have a vital role to play in the diverse and dynamic field of orthodontics, whether they are employed in a general practice environment or in an orthodontic office. Patients often ask dental hygienists questions regarding orthodontic treatment and options. This chapter provides an overview of orthodontic treatments available to consumers.

KEY TERMS

ankylosis	interdisciplinary patient care	orthopedics	root resorption
diastema	malocclusion	overbite	serial extraction
frenectomy	microimplants	overjet	stability
frontal resorption	orthognathic	retention	undermining resorption

LEARNING OUTCOMES

After reading this chapter the student will be able to:

1. Relate the history and biology of the specialty of orthodontics to dental professionals.
2. Classify malocclusion according to Angle's system.
3. Be aware of the dental hygienist's role in patient selection and referral for orthodontic treatment.
4. Identify normal ranges of dental development, and recognize deviations from this range.
5. Discuss the three dimensions of the facial structure, and recognize normal and abnormal skeletal structure.
6. Recognize the role of different specialties in interdisciplinary orthodontic treatment.
7. Discuss third molar considerations for postorthodontic recommendations.
8. Instruct orthodontic patients in proper oral hygiene management.
9. Demonstrate knowledge of orthodontic terms by using them in written and verbal communication.
10. Recognize basic types of treatment components, including those for space management, detrimental oral habits, orthopedic development problems, and orthodontic correction.
11. Recognize general retention devices and guidelines.

A 58-year-old woman comes into the general dental practice where you work for her first regularly scheduled supportive care visit. During the interview, you learn that Mrs. Jones has been placed on a 2- to 3-month supportive care recall schedule because of her history of periodontal disease. Previously, Mrs. Jones was treated for active periodontal disease, requiring flap curettage in all posterior segments. Your review of her records reveals that, before periodontal therapy, the prognosis for her mandibular incisors was poor (Class II mobility) and that she is missing several posterior teeth. When presented with the option of extracting the mandibular anterior teeth and prosthetic replacement, she insisted on maintaining these teeth for as long as possible.

A review of her medical history reveals a *family history* of diabetes and hypertension, but she is currently healthy and has no history of any medical problems. At the conclusion of her periodontal therapy, a complete radiographic series was taken, which she has brought with her to the appointment (Figure A). During her visit with you, Mrs. Jones states that she is now interested in orthodontic treatment to fix the *gaps* in her teeth (Figure B). Your advice to Mrs. Jones should be that orthodontic care is appropriate for a woman of her age and dental history as long as she maintains supportive care visits and practices excellent oral hygiene.

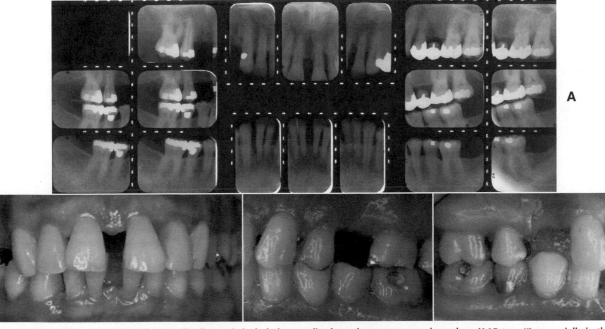

A, Complete radiographic series. The specific diagnosis included generalized, moderate to severe bone loss (AAP type II), especially in the mandibular anterior, with several missing teeth including #1, #2, #5, #13, #16, #17, #18, #31, and #32. (Courtesy Dr. R.A. Beane.)
B, Clinical photos (frontal, left, and right facial) taken during the intraoral examination reveals that dental midlines are coincident with midsagittal plane; molar relationship is end to end (not quite a full-cusp Class II); canine relationship is Class II; overjet = 8 mm and overbite = 4 mm. (Courtesy Dr. R.A. Beane, UNC School of Dentistry.)

According to the National Health and Nutritional Examination Survey (NHANES III) study, it has been estimated that, in the United States, more than one half of the population has some sort of malocclusion. Depending on the geographic region and socioeconomic background, up to 50% of U.S. children receive some type of orthodontic care.[5,15,23] The benefits of orthodontics include improving long-term stability of the dentition (discussed later), esthetics, and in some cases, function. Whether orthodontic correction improves long-term periodontal health remains controversial.[27] Nonetheless, an important goal for the dental hygienist is to be aware of common orthodontic problems and to be familiar with the basic treatment approaches that exist to correct these problems.

Orthodontics was the first specialty formed in dentistry and the third specialty in dentistry and medicine. The first textbooks describing the orthodontic specialty were written by Norman Kingsley, circa 1850, but much of today's practice of orthodontics is based on the teachings of Edward Angle beginning in the early 1880s. Angle, who is also thought to be the father of orthodontics, established the three classes of **malocclusion** as we know them today (discussed later). These classifications are based on the occlusal relationships of the first molars and should be well known by all members of the oral healthcare team.[2]

Components of the Orthodontic Assessment

ANGLE'S CLASSIFICATION

When the dental hygienist examines a patient for the first time during routine care, he or she will make an assessment of the condition of the teeth and periodontium. Part of the examination should include specific aspects of the occlusion. As mentioned earlier, Angle's classification of malocclusion serves as an excellent reference for evaluation and diagnosis (see Figure 17-27). This classification is stated in the box to the side.

Although this classification of malocclusion was established in the early 1900s, it still largely exists today but with notable modifications. With the introduction of cephalometric radiography in the late 1940s, more attention is paid to the skeletal relationships of the jaws and their effect on the dental relationships of the teeth (Figure 37-1). Moreover, with the introduction and continued development of digital records, advanced imaging capabilities, and advances in soft tissue esthetics and surgical stability, the specialty has adopted a contemporary classification system, including the skeletal, dental, and soft tissue considerations.

> *Angle's Classification*
>
> Class I: represented by a normal relationship of the molars but characterized by malposed, rotated, or otherwise incorrect line of occlusion
>
> Class II: represented by the distally positioned lower molar relative to the upper molar and may be present with or without rotated or malposed teeth
>
> Class III: represented by mesially positioned lower molar relative to the upper molar and may be present with or without rotated or malposed teeth

ANTEROPOSTERIOR RELATIONSHIPS

Skeletal Evaluation

In a dental hygiene practice, orthodontic problems resulting from *anteroposterior discrepancies* or *crowding* and alignment issues will probably be the most readily observed. During the examination, the dental hygienist should pay special attention to the relative relationship of the lower jaw to the upper jaw (Figure 37-2). While observing the patient's profile, whether the lower jaw is significantly deficient or retrusive should be noted, which is termed *retrognathic* (skeletal Class II). Conversely, whether the opposite relationship exists where the lower jaw is significantly protruded should also be noted, which is termed *prognathic*

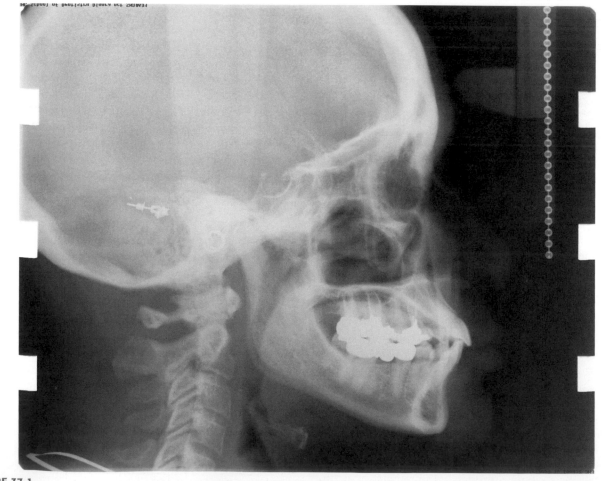

FIGURE 37-1
Pretreatment cephalometric radiograph of patient indicating a skeletal Class I relationship. (Courtesy Dr. S.A. Frazier-Bowers, UNC School of Dentistry).

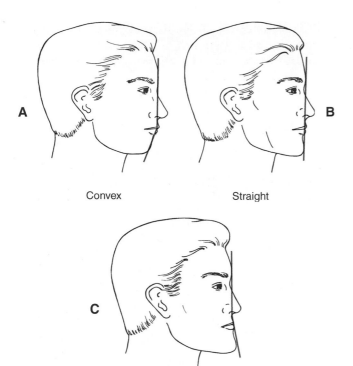

Convex

Straight

Concave

FIGURE 37-2
Profile convexity or concavity results from a disproportion in the size of the jaws but does not by itself indicate which jaw is at fault. A convex facial profile **(A)** indicates a Class II jaw relationship, which can result from either a maxilla that projects too far forward or a mandible too far back. **B,** An example of a straight facial profile. A concave profile **(C)** indicates a Class III relationship, which can result from either a maxilla that is too far back or a mandible that protrudes forward. (From Proffit WR, Fields HW, Sarver DM: *Contemporary orthodontics,* ed 4, St Louis, 2007, Mosby.)

(skeletal Class III). Alternatively, these same relationships can result from a protrusive upper jaw–normal lower jaw (Class II) and from a retrusive upper jaw–normal lower jaw (Class III). Careful clinical observation is often a good indicator of the skeletal relationships described previously but is not a substitute for a cephalometric radiograph (see Figure 37-1). The cephalometric radiograph not only provides the proper record to document the patient's pretreatment facial proportions but also allows for evaluating treatment response after orthodontic treatment.

Soft Tissue Evaluation

Although the skeletal relationship of the jaws is important in determining the nature of the orthodontic problem, another equally important factor, the *soft tissue,* has reemerged. In the 1950s and 1960s, the use of cephalometrics in treatment planning was a routine part of the diagnostic workup. As a result, the orthodontist typically paid more attention to the patient profile as compared with other components of facial balance, such as the soft tissue and the smile. A shift in focus toward a *soft tissue paradigm* in orthodontics today has led to an increased awareness of improved diagnostic and treatment strategies to correct these problems.[28] A proper evaluation of the soft tissue is similar to the skeletal and dental evaluation and should include clinical observation from the frontal (with and without

smile) and profile views. In addition to the clinical examination, diagnostic tools include extraoral photos on frontal (with and without smile) and on profile and digital videography to capture the dynamic smile.[28] Some important soft tissue considerations include the soft tissue profile, interlabial gap (distance between the lips at rest) and incisor show at rest, gingival display on smile, lip fullness, nasolabial angle (angle formed by the nose and the upper lip), and chin projection. Evaluation of the soft tissue should answer questions such as the following:

- Is the soft tissue profile balanced, concave, or convex?
- Is lip strain present at rest?
- Are the lips protrusive or retrusive?
- Is the face height shortened, normal, or long when viewed from a frontal or profile view?
- Is the *mentalis muscle* (chin) strained?

Although these soft tissue relationships are important to consider during the examination, the focus will be the dental relationships discussed later.

Dental Evaluation

In many cases, the Class II or Class III relationships of the jaws as discussed previously occur with the corresponding Angle's molar relationships. However, observing a patient with a Class II skeletal relationship without the corresponding Class II dental relationship is possible. The reverse situation is also possible, that is, a Class II dental relationship superimposed on a well-balanced Class I skeletal pattern. Regardless of the situation, observing the overjet relationship of the anterior teeth is important because it is often a direct consequence of the molar relationship. **Overjet** is defined as horizontal overlap of the incisors measured in millimeters (see Figure 17-28). An *increased overjet* or protrusion of the teeth is usually associated with a Class II malocclusion, whereas a *reverse overjet* corresponds with a Class III malocclusion. Reverse overjet is also referred to as an *anterior crossbite* relationship. The dental hygienist should recognize these relationships not only to determine when to refer, but also to monitor potential gingival problems that may occur as a result. For instance, severely protrusive maxillary incisors in young children can often occur with chronically inflamed gingiva surrounding the maxillary incisors (Figure 37-3). In this

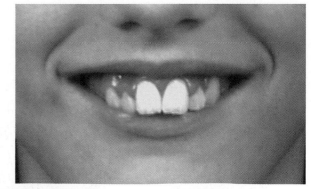

FIGURE 37-3
Clinical photograph of a 9-year-old girl with protrusive maxillary incisors and an increased interlabial gap. Note the exposed maxillary teeth and resultant inflamed and edematous gingiva. (Courtesy Dr. S.A. Frazier-Bowers, UNC School of Dentistry.)

case, orthodontic treatment may be justified not only to help resolve the irritated gingiva, but also to improve self-esteem.

CROWDING AND ALIGNMENT

Crowding of the teeth is perhaps the easiest orthodontic problem to recognize because it represents the most common diagnosis.[12,24] Crowding can occur as a mild, moderate, or severe problem. The dental hygienist should be familiar with how to identify these three categories of severity with the following guidelines:

- Mild crowding: 2 to 3 mm of space deficiency
- Moderate crowding: 4 to 6 mm of space deficiency
- Severe crowding: 7 to 10 mm of space deficiency

Whether the crowding problem is mild, moderate, or severe, it is often caused by *arch-length discrepancies,* or an inadequate amount of space available for the erupting permanent dentition. In young children, incisor crowding is somewhat acceptable because of the following:

- An expected increase exists in arch length resulting from growth.
- A gain of leeway space exists resulting from the difference in tooth size from the deciduous molars to the permanent premolars.

Alignment problems may also exhibit as an excess of space. This problem may be the result of a tooth-size discrepancy or a single or multiple **diastema** (Figure 37-4, *A*). A diastema is simply an area of excess space between two or more teeth. This excess space can occur as a result of a tooth-size discrepancy or secondary to significant protrusion and overjet. The most common isolated diastema occurs in the maxillary midline and is more prevalent in blacks than other racial groups. In some cases, a maxillary midline diastema is accompanied by a low attached frenum. Management of this clinical situation may require a **frenectomy** procedure, which cuts the frenum to reposition it apically (Figure 37-4, *B*).

VERTICAL DIMENSION

This section discusses vertical relationships of the teeth, or **overbite** (see Figure 17-29). A normal overbite (amount of vertical overlap between the anterior maxillary and mandibular teeth) is roughly defined as a 2-mm overlap of the maxillary central incisors to the mandibular central incisors. This relationship can also be represented as a percentage of maxillary coverage of the mandibular incisors. For instance, one half of the mandibular incisors that are covered by the maxillary incisors can be referred to as a 50% overbite. Interestingly, one example of a problem resulting from malocclusion is seen in a patient with Class II deep bite (Figure 37-5). Impingement of the lower teeth on the palatal gingiva not only creates discomfort to the patient but also propagates an unstable periodontal condition. A significant overbite relationship can cause impingement of the lower teeth into the soft tissue of the palate. When the reverse relationship occurs and *no vertical overlap* exists, this is referred to as an *openbite*. An openbite malocclusion may be caused by a thumb-sucking habit or result from a tendency toward this type of growth pattern. In fact, the

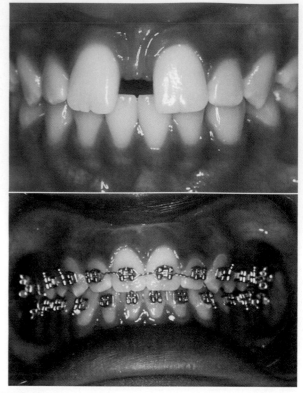

FIGURE 37-4
A, Maxillary midline diastema and low attached frenum in a black patient before orthodontic treatment. **B,** After initial space closure with braces, a frenectomy was performed to apically reposition the frenum and to help prevent the reopening of the maxillary diastema. (Courtesy Dr. R.A. Beane, UNC School of Dentistry.)

occurrence of an openbite greater than 2 mm is five times more prevalent in blacks than in other racial groups, whereas a severe deep bite is two times as prevalent in whites as compared with blacks or Hispanics.[24]

TRANSVERSE RELATIONSHIP

The dental hygienist should also be aware of posterior *crossbite* relationships that may exist. A posterior crossbite exists when the maxillary posterior teeth are lingually positioned relative to the mandibular teeth. This relationship may result from skeletal asymmetry or a functional shift caused by a constricted maxillary arch. A posterior crossbite relationship rarely spontaneously corrects itself and therefore requires an orthodontic consultation and treatment (see the discussion under Treatment Components later in this chapter). As a result of this transverse problem, the *dental midlines* do not coincide with the midsagittal plane.

Biological Tooth Movement: Orthodontic Treatment Effects on the Periodontium

Once the dental hygienist is able to recognize the broad categories of orthodontic problems, he or she can begin to explore how these problems are corrected from a biological perspective. The biology of tooth movement relies heavily on a healthy

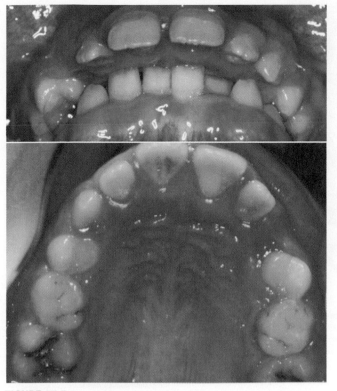

FIGURE 37-5
A, A 10-year-old patient with a *deep bite* into palatal gingiva. **B,** Occlusal photo of maxillary arch shows inflamed palatal gingiva caused by palatal impingement of lower incisors. (Courtesy Dr. R.A. Beane, UNC School of Dentistry.)

periodontium in addition to controlled orthodontic forces. The same components that make up the dental structures are also responsible for the successful movement through bone in response to orthodontic forces. Orthodontic tooth movement results in the gradual movement of teeth through the bone in response to a prolonged, but controlled, force. This principle is based on the fact that, as the tooth moves in response to a force, the bone remodels around it.

The biological details of this process are heavily dependent on the periodontal ligament (PDL) (see Chapter 16). The PDL is compressed in response to orthodontic pressure, and the fluid within the space is *squeezed out,* causing the PDL to be compressed against the bone. This immediate reaction to force of the PDL occurs within a minute,[6] but the maximal compression of the PDL occurs within hours. Forces that are light and prolonged result in the remodeling of the adjacent bone by a process called **frontal resorption** (Figure 37-6). In this paralleled process, bone is resorbed on one front (pressure side) and is laid down on the opposite side (tension side). Force that is too heavy causes remodeling to occur but only after necrosis has occurred to the PDL on the pressure side. This remodeling initiates a cascade of events that subsequently results in **undermining resorption.** Histologically, undermining resorption is seen as a compressed and avascular PDL that, after several days of excessive force, has recruited osteoclasts from the adjacent marrow spaces to resorb the underside of the lamina dura (Figure 37-7). Clinically, the result of undermining resorption is that the patient experiences more pain than when a lighter force is used. This circumstance ultimately results in less efficient tooth movement, requiring up to twice as long for the tooth to move the same distance under ideal circumstances.

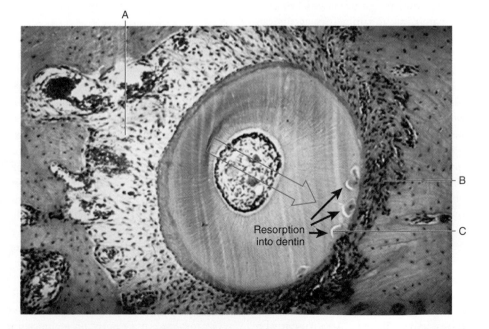

Resorption into dentin

FIGURE 37-6
Coronal section through the root of a premolar being moved to the right *(arrow).* Note the zone of periodontal ligament compression to the right and tension to the left. Dilation of blood vessels and osteoblastic activity *(A)* can be seen on the left. Osteoclasts removing bone are present on the right *(B).* Areas of beginning root resorption that will be repaired by later deposition of cementum also can be seen on the right *(C).* (From Proffit WR, Fields HW, Sarver DM: *Contemporary orthodontics,* ed 4, St Louis, 2007, Mosby.)

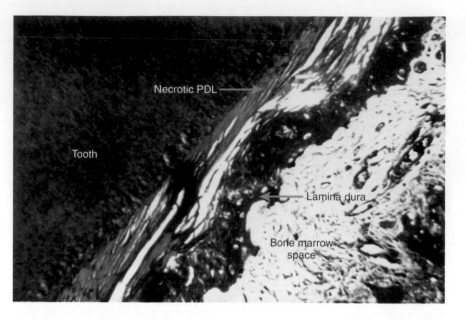

FIGURE 37-7
Histologic specimen of compressed periodontal ligament (PDL) area after several days. When the PDL is compressed to the point that blood flow is totally cut off, differentiating osteoclasts within the PDL space is not possible. After a delay of several days, osteoclasts within adjacent marrow spaces attack the underside of the lamina dura in the process called *undermining resorption*. (From Proffit WR, Fields HW, Sarver DM: *Contemporary orthodontics,* ed 4, St Louis, 2007, Mosby.)

ALVEOLAR BONE

The dental hygienist must understand the basics of orthodontic tooth movement because adding periodontal disease to this equation might cause undesired effects. Normally, the response of the periodontium to orthodontic movement is unremarkable. Evidence suggests that the alveolar bone height in response to prolonged orthodontic forces remains stable, with an average of 0.5-mm bone loss.[16] In the presence of periodontal disease, however, the presence of pathologic inflammatory agents can cause a net loss of alveolar bone height. However, an important point to note is that, in an individual with controlled periodontal disease, the effects on the alveolar bone and PDL are similar to that of a normal patient. In fact, the use of orthodontics to increase bony support around periodontally involved teeth has been reported.[20] The clinician must distinguish in these cases that the bony support has not extensively increased, but instead a long junctional epithelium is formed. In any case, the patient with controlled periodontal disease who initiates orthodontic treatment is advised to maintain more frequent supportive care intervals (every 3 to 4 months) as compared with the average patient.

GINGIVA

Although the effect of orthodontic treatment on the patient's alveolar bone may not be immediately perceptible without a radiograph, the effects on the gingiva are obvious. Orthodontic treatment does not intrinsically cause gingivitis, but it does certainly make cleaning the teeth challenging. In a patient who is already experiencing difficulty maintaining proper oral hygiene, this situation may worsen with braces. Particularly in young patients who have not yet mastered toothbrushing skills,

noticing increased plaque biofilm accumulation and acute gingivitis during orthodontic treatment is common. These patients can benefit from additional instruction during orthodontic visits from the pediatric dentist or dental hygienist. In young patients, progressing into attachment loss is unusual for this situation, but progression is a possibility for the adult patient, especially persons 30 years of age and older.[21] Younger patients, conversely, are likely to show an increase in problems with *attached gingiva* or mucogingival problems.[21]

ROOT STRUCTURE

As part of the routine examination, past or present radiographic records will be reviewed. In addition to noting alveolar bone height, the root structure should be assessed. Roots that appear unusually shortened should be documented and brought to the attention of the treating orthodontist, as well as the patient. This pathologic process, termed **root resorption,** occurs when the normal remodeling process required to move teeth causes an unbalanced attack on the cementum of the root. Normally, the coupled resorptive and appositional process occurs without creating clinically significant loss of root structure. In fact, estimates suggest that 90% of maxillary teeth and more than one half of all teeth experience some root resorption but that this phenomenon is usually clinically imperceptible.[23] Fewer than 20% of patients experience a clinically significant permanent loss of root structure. Severe root resorption can be a problem in *rare* cases, when forces are extreme, or as a result of a genetic predisposition toward this problem.[11] The more likely cause of severe localized root resorption includes, for example, instances when maxillary incisors are forced against the lingual cortical plate.[14] Fortunately, as a routine part of orthodontic treatment, the orthodontist will take a progress radiograph to detect this potential problem. In the event that the dental hygienist detects this condition first, the orthodontist should be notified immediately. If a patient develops severe root resorption, then orthodontic treatment should be ended as soon as possible. Similarly, if a patient exhibits severe root resorption before orthodontic treatment, then proceeding with orthodontic treatment may be contraindicated, and continuation will depend on the duration and type of orthodontic treatment planned.

Referral

The dental hygienist is in a unique position to observe a wide spectrum of occlusal problems. He or she may be the first person to inform the patient that these problems exist. Using the information discussed previously, the dental hygienist should carefully evaluate the patient in the three planes of space (anteroposterior, vertical, and transverse), as well as for alignment irregularities to determine whether a problem exists. In some cases, the patient may actually solicit advice of the dental hygienist. Most orthodontists use a system of numbering teeth, called the *Palmer notation method* (Figure 37-8). In this method, the mouth is divided into four quadrants, upper left, upper right, lower left, and lower right. The designation of the teeth in each quadrant is constant, with the centrals always being numbered *1,* laterals are number *2,* and this sequence continues until the third molar in each quadrant being designated as number *8.* This numbering system is quite different from the *universal numbering system* that most general dentists use whereby the upper right third is designated number *1,* and this sequence continues, with each tooth having a unique number through number *32* (see Figure 37-8). Finally, the dental hygienist may encounter a system that is common outside of the United States, called the *Federation Dental International (FDI).* This system is similar to the Palmer notation but uses a two-digit system whereby the first number represents the quadrant of the mouth (1 through 4), with the first quadrant being the maxillary right. The second number of this system represents the specific tooth type in each quadrant, similar to the Palmer notation (i.e., centrals are number *1,* laterals number *2,* and so on).

According to the American Association of Orthodontists, a checkup by an orthodontic specialist for a patient who is no older than age 7 years is ideal because it enables the orthodontist to determine whether any problems exist and to advise further whether treatment will be necessary. At this screening appointment, if the orthodontist discovers orthodontic problems that are significant, he or she will also determine the best time for the patient to be treated. Although determining whether a patient should initiate treatment will be the decision of the orthodontist, the dental hygienist should be familiar with contraindications to treatment, such as severe root resorption and periodontal disease. In the case of root resorption, the orthodontist must weigh the treatment benefits against the risk of creating more root resorption. In many cases, this risk may result in deferring or limiting treatment. If periodontal disease is well controlled and the patient agrees to more frequent periodontal maintenance visits, then beginning orthodontic treatment is reasonable. However, for patients with active disease, necessary periodontal therapy, including scaling, root planing, and surgery, must be completed, and the patient must be reevaluated before orthodontic treatment can proceed.

Numbering System

R									L						
1	2	3	4	5	6	7	8	9	10	11	12	13	14	15	16
18	17	16	15	14	13	12	11	21	22	23	24	25	26	27	28
8	7	6	5	4	3	2	1	1	2	3	4	5	6	7	8
8	7	6	5	4	3	2	1	1	2	3	4	5	6	7	8
48	47	46	45	44	43	42	41	31	32	33	34	35	36	37	38
32	31	30	29	28	27	26	25	24	23	22	21	20	19	18	17

FIGURE 37-8
Diagrammatic representation of tooth numbering systems commonly used today. Diagram indicates four quadrants, with the top left representing the patient's right maxillary quadrant, top right is the patient's left maxillary quadrant, bottom left is the patient's right mandibular quadrant, and the bottom right represents the patient's left mandibular quadrant. The system commonly used by orthodontists, the *Palmer notation*, is shaded in peach; the Federation Dental International (FDI), used in many foreign (non-U.S.) countries is shaded in turquoise; and the universal numbering system, used by most American general dentists, is shaded in yellow.

Seeking orthodontic treatment with symptoms of temporomandibular joint disorder (TMD) is not unusual for a patient. The determination of whether to delay treatment while addressing the TMD concerns depends on the nature and the intensity of the problem. A *clicking* joint is not always associated with pain and is rather common in adolescents.[17] In some cases, however, clicking may represent a more significant *internal derangement* (the articulating disk or ligament become displaced) and thus requires therapy. For TMD problems that are caused by an internal derangement of the joint, (e.g., dislocated jaw, displaced disk, injury to the condyle) or degenerative joint disease (e.g., osteoarthritis, rheumatoid arthritis), orthodontic treatment should not be initiated until the pathologic process is addressed and resolved. However, if the problem is determined as being muscular in origin, then the appropriate nonsteroidal antiinflammatory drug, muscle relaxant, stress-reduction plan, or any combination can be prescribed for the patient. Depending on the intensity of the pain, the orthodontist may also prescribe an acrylic *bite-guard* appliance to be worn before starting orthodontic treatment.

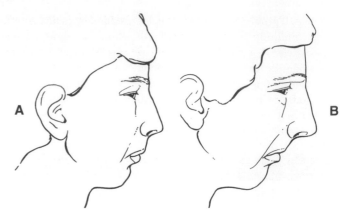

FIGURE 37-9
Facial outline of a patient with a Class II malocclusion who was treated with four premolar extractions and extraoral traction. Note the negative changes in the profile as the mandible has retruded further after orthodontic treatment. **A,** Before treatment. **B,** After treatment. (McNamara JA: *Orthodontics and dentofacial orthopedics,* Ann Arbor, Mich, 2001, Needham Press.)

Treatment Phase Options

ONE-PHASE (COMPREHENSIVE) AND TWO-PHASE TREATMENT METHODS

Although the American Association of Orthodontists recommends that children be examined by an orthodontist by age 7 for initial screening, the question remains, when should patients *start* orthodontic treatment? No one answer exists to this question. Instead, the decision to start treatment should be based on the individual patient's needs and concerns. Orthodontics may start at any age. One in five orthodontic patients is an adult.[1] However, many orthodontic problems are easier to correct if detected at an early age before jaw growth has slowed.

The orthodontist should choose the mode of treatment best suited for each patient. In the earlier days of orthodontics, treatment options from which to choose were limited. Orthodontists often waited until patients had their permanent dentition to begin treatment. If a crowding problem or large overjet was found, a serial extraction protocol most often solved the problem. **Serial extraction** is the sequential removal of the deciduous teeth such that enough space is gained in the front portion of the mouth for the permanent teeth to erupt. The sequential removal of deciduous teeth was often followed by premolar extraction to gain additional space. This *one-phase* or *comprehensive* treatment plan was considered the norm. Although this method is still valid today, it may not address facial or profile concerns for all patients with a Class II malocclusion. In patients who have a Class II malocclusion characterized by maxillary skeletal protrusion, a retrusive mandible, and severe overbite, this method might adversely affect the patient's profile (Figure 37-9).

TWO-PHASE TREATMENT

During the last two decades, early intervention (often called *two-phase treatment*) has become an acceptable option for many patients. Two-phase treatment involves early interceptive treatment during the patient's mixed dentition and is typically performed on patients who have a moderate to severe malocclusion to reduce its severity before brace placement. Phase I (of the two-phase treatment) is typically of short duration (commonly 6 to 14 months). At the end of this phase of treatment, the patient may or may not be required to wear a retainer during the transition to the permanent dentition. Once the permanent teeth have erupted, the orthodontic appliances would then be placed to align and detail the permanent dentition in phase II. This second phase of braces often will be of shorter duration because of the phase I treatment.

The goal of phase I intervention is to provide specific patients with early correction for a large number of existing or developing factors. These conditions include anteroposterior or transverse skeletal imbalances, oral neuromuscular problems, dental crowding, space management caused by premature loss, or overretention of primary teeth, as well as therapy for deleterious oral habits, such as thumb sucking. A variety of appliances can be used during phase I. These appliances will be described later in this chapter.

Advantages of Early Treatment

A variety of treatment options is now available that can be used successfully in the mixed dentition to produce significant changes in the dental, skeletal, and musculature structures.[18]

Physiologic advantages of early treatment include the following:

- Patients in this age range (7 to 10 years) are typically cooperative and excited about starting early treatment.
- During this developmental stage, children

> *Prevention*
>
> Early intervention in orthodontics may correct a developing problem before it has progressed significantly, either lessen or avoid the need for more extensive treatment in the future, and reduce the total time that full braces are needed.

generally become more aware of their physical appearance and exhibit the desire to *fit in.*

- Early correction of a skeletal imbalance such as a large overjet *(buck teeth)* might play an important role in the establishment of a healthy self-image.[1]

Disadvantages of Early Treatment

Not all patients benefit from early intervention. If the treatment plan's steps and objectives are not defined clearly and the interceptive treatment continues over an extended period, then such treatment can lead to patient noncompliance and dissonance. Not all orthodontists are trained in early or two-phase treatment.

Although phase I treatment may lessen the amount of time the patient is in full braces (phase II), this mode of treatment also requires more patient time and more visits in total. This situation can sometimes lead to patient *burnout* and compliance problems (although compliance problems can be an issue in any aspect of patient care).

ONE-PHASE (COMPREHENSIVE) TREATMENT FOR ADOLESCENTS OR ADULTS

The one-phase method of treatment typically begins no sooner than the late mixed dentition and would more likely start when the patient has his or her permanent dentition. Additional orthodontic appliances, such as a palatal expander or quad helix (examples to follow), might be used just before or during the placement of full braces. If the treatment plan is not overly complex, such as that involving orthognathic surgery, then treatment time is typically between 24 and 36 months, if the patient is cooperative.

Advantages of One-Phase Treatment

In many patients, allowing the eruption of all permanent teeth (except for third molars) before initiating orthodontic treatment is best. If all of the permanent teeth are allowed to erupt before the initiation of orthodontic treatment, then the treatment can proceed in a straightforward and predictable manner.[22] In addition, the growth potential of the patients can be predicted more clearly. This concern would be an issue especially in older adolescent patients with a Class III malocclusion who may require surgical correction, when growth should cease before any surgical intervention.

Disadvantages of One-Phase Treatment

If the assumption is made that orthodontic treatment does not start until the loss of all primary teeth, then leeway space might be lost during the exfoliation of the primary second molars. A loss of leeway space might influence directly the decision for an extraction verses a nonextraction course of treatment. If a skeletal imbalance is present in the anteroposterior dimension, then the beginning functional appliance therapy while the patient is actively growing is crucial. Intervention in late adolescence might significantly lessen the chance for ideal treatment outcome without surgical intervention.

Finally, the period of adolescence to adulthood (ages 13 to 20 years) is a period of major physiologic and hormonal transition, which can lead to social and cooperation challenges. Adolescents often go through a rebellious or defiant period during this time, and cooperation may be an issue.[7] Additionally, scheduling adolescent patients for regular orthodontic visits once they enter high school is typically difficult. If treatment is begun early enough, then a worthy goal to consider is to plan to complete the orthodontic treatment before the high school years.

Treatment Components

COMMON ORTHODONTIC APPLIANCES USED IN BOTH ONE-PHASE AND TWO-PHASE TREATMENT   `37-2`

Recent advances in orthodontic technology over the last few decades have led to notable improvements in treatment.[8] Interest in preserving a balanced face and profile in addition to developing a functional occlusion has increased. Nonextraction treatment protocols have become more prevalent as bonded appliances, interproximal reduction *(stripping),* and rapid maxillary expansion have become routine parts of the orthodontist's armamentarium. The following sections describe common phase I appliances.

Rapid Maxillary Expansion

Rapid maxillary expansion (RME) appliances (Figure 37-10) are used to correct posterior crossbites and increase the arch perimeter to alleviate modest tooth-size–arch-length discrepancies (large teeth–small jaws) and crowding. Typically, these expanders are either a bonded acrylic-type expander used in mixed dentition or a banded expander that is used when the first premolars are present. The appliance has a midpalatal screw that generally is turned or *activated* on a daily basis. The activations open the midpalatal suture, producing an increase in the width of the maxilla.[19] These appliances are typically activated for 20 to 45 turns (0.2 mm per turn) and will then remain fixed in place for an additional period (usually 3 to 5

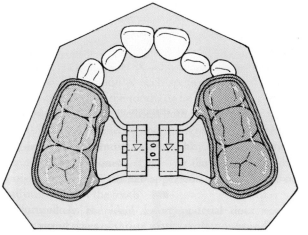

FIGURE 37-10
Bonded acrylic splint rapid maxillary expander. (From McNamara JA: Treatment of patients in the mixed dentition. In Graber TM, Vanarsdall RL, Vig KWL, eds: *Orthodontics: current principles and techniques,* ed 4, St Louis, 2005, Mosby, p 548.)

months) to allow for reossification of the involved sutures (Figure 37-11). Following expander removal, the patient is given a retainer or maintenance plate for **retention,** as well as to allow for the settling of the molars fully into occlusion.

Expanders are easiest to use before the ossification of the involved sutures, which generally occurs between the ages of 18 and 20 years. Although using an RME in adults is possible, it is normally used in conjunction with a surgical procedure, *surgically assisted rapid palatal expansion,* to open the midpalatal suture.

DENTAL CONSIDERATIONS

In many instances, when a bonded expander is removed, the gingival tissue will look very red and hyperplasic for a short time, similar to the condition of the gingival tissue when a periopack is removed postsurgically. This condition, however, is not one of great concern; the tissue redness and hypertrophy will usually resolve within the next several days with proper home care.

Facial Mask

For patients with a Class III malocclusion, a facial mask (Figure 37-12) can be used in conjunction with the RME during phase I treatment. Hooks are incorporated into the design of the RME at the time of fabrication. Elastics connect these hooks to the facial mask. The treatment effects produced by this type of

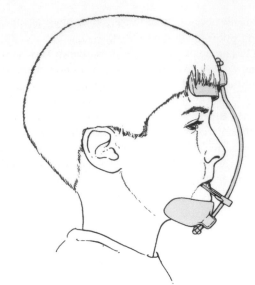

FIGURE 37-12
The orthopedic facial mask of Petit. (From McNamara JA: Treatment of patients in the mixed dentition. In Graber TM, Vanarsdall RL, Vig KWL, eds: *Orthodontics: current principles and techniques,* ed 4, St Louis, 2005, Mosby, p 567.)

appliance include a forward movement of the maxilla and maxillary dentition and downward and backward rotation of the mandible. Because the facial mask intervention is accomplished at an early age, the treatment effects ultimately produced in the face are incorporated into the future craniofacial growth that occurs over a long period. The facial mask can be worn during nonschool hours to create a positive overjet. The facial mask is not effective in a nongrowing patient (adult).

Schwarz Appliance

The Schwarz expander (Figure 37-13) is a removable acrylic appliance with metal clasps. This expansion device can be used in the maxilla or mandible. Typically, the Schwarz expander is used in the mandible to upright the posterior teeth and provide

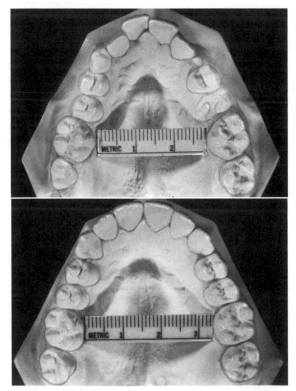

FIGURE 37-11
Maxillary arch width changes associated with rapid maxillary expansion. The pretreatment transpalatal width is 28 mm. After expansion and fixed appliance therapy, the transpalatal width is 33.5 mm. (McNamara JA: *Orthodontics and dentofacial orthopedics,* Ann Arbor, Mich, 2001, Needham Press.)

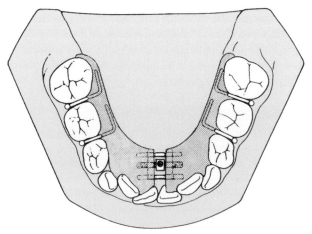

FIGURE 37-13
Mandibular occlusal view of a Schwarz expansion appliance. (From McNamara JA: Treatment of patients in the mixed dentition. In Graber TM, Vanarsdall RL, Vig KWL, eds: *Orthodontics: current principles and techniques,* ed 4, St Louis, 2005, Mosby, p 551.)

additional arch length for the alignment of the anterior teeth. A midline expansion screw is built into the appliance that is activated (turned) typically once or twice per week for a period of 3 to 5 months. The appliance is then worn for an additional period as a retainer to sustain the achieved result. This appliance can be used in both the mixed and the permanent dentition and is almost always used in conjunction with RME.

Quad Helix Appliance

The quad helix (Figure 37-14) is a fixed (cemented) expansion device made from 0.036-inch stainless steel wire. It can be used on the upper or lower teeth for minor expansion of the dental arches. A significant amount of the expansion is derived from the buccal tipping of the posterior teeth and thus is best used when only a modest amount of arch expansion is needed. It can be used in both the mixed and the permanent dentitions.

Transpalatal Arch

The transpalatal arch (Figure 37-15) is also a fixed maxillary-banded appliance consisting of bands on the maxillary permanent first molars with a *transpalatal* bar connecting the two bands. This appliance can be used as both an active appliance (for molar rotation and distalization) and a stabilization appliance used to maintain the position of the permanent first molars, as well as to provide anchorage for counterforces used during active orthodontic treatment. This appliance is effective as a type of *space maintainer* during the loss of the primary second molars to preserve leeway space by maintaining the distal position of the upper first permanent molars.

Lingual Arch

The lingual arch (Figure 37-16) is a fixed appliance that is similar to the transpalatal arch but is fashioned for the mandibular arch, with bands on the permanent first molars and a bar running along the lingual of the lower teeth. This appliance can also be used during the transition to the permanent dentition to prevent the mesial drift of the attached permanent first molars during loss of the primary second molars. The lingual arch is typically removed following the eruption of the second premolars.

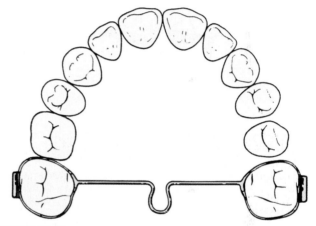

FIGURE 37-15
Occlusal view of a transpalatal arch. (From McNamara JA: Treatment of patients in the mixed dentition. In Graber TM, Vanarsdall RL, Vig KWL, eds: *Orthodontics: current principles and techniques,* ed 4, St Louis, 2005, Mosby, p 546.)

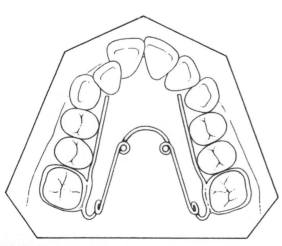

FIGURE 37-14
Occlusal view of a maxillary quad helix. (McNamara JA: *Orthodontics and dentofacial orthopedics,* Ann Arbor, Mich, 2001, Needham Press.)

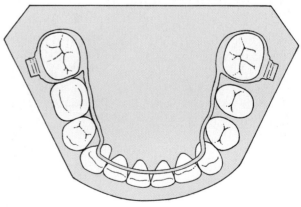

FIGURE 37-16
Occlusal view of a lower lingual arch. (From McNamara JA: Treatment of patients in the mixed dentition. In Graber TM, Vanarsdall RL, Vig KWL, eds: *Orthodontics: current principles and techniques,* ed 4, St Louis, 2005, Mosby, p 546.)

Headgear

Headgear (Figure 37-17) is a generic term for an extraoral traction device that can be used to restrict the downward and forward growth of the maxilla in patients with a Class II malocclusion. These removable appliances are made of two parts: a wire framework and either a *facebow* that attaches posteriorly to fixed structures in the mouth (usually maxillary first molar bands) or so-called J-*hooks* that attach anteriorly to the archwire or to hooks soldered to the maxillary archwire in a patient with upper braces (Figure 37-18). The ends of the facebow or

J-hooks are attached to a type of strap that is worn externally around the head. Depending on the direction of the force desired, the headgears can come in many different styles, such as a cervical pull (neck strap), straight-pull, or high pull, described according the direction of force produced. All extraoral traction appliances require a high level of patient compliance. Recent developments in technology have provided a variety of additional retraction methods that do not require the same level of patient cooperation.

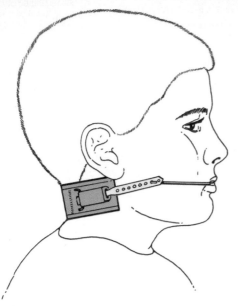

FIGURE 37-17
Lateral view of a headgear consisting of a facebow with cervical neck strap. (From McNamara JA: Treatment of patients in the mixed dentition. In Graber TM, Vanarsdall RL, Vig KWL, eds: *Orthodontics: current principles and techniques,* ed 4, St Louis, 2005, Mosby, p 556.)

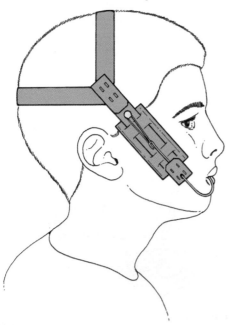

FIGURE 37-18
Lateral view of a high-pull headgear. (From McNamara JA: Treatment of patients in the mixed dentition. In Graber TM, Vanarsdall RL, Vig KWL, eds: *Orthodontics: current principles and techniques,* ed 4, St Louis, 2005, Mosby, p 557.)

> ### Patient Education Opportunity
>
> Patients who wear extraoral traction devices such as the headgear or facial mask should avoid *horseplay* while the appliance is in place. The appliances are fragile, with sharp edges and might easily be pulled out of place. The force of the elastics or head strap might then force the extraoral device to lodge into the patient's cheek or eye. Remind the patient to remove these appliances before physical playtime activities.

Molar Distalizing Appliances

Appliances such as the Pendex (Figure 37-19), Pendulum, Jasper Jumper, Distal Jet, or Wilson mechanics are used primarily for maxillary molar distalization. As with the headgear, these appliances provide the force and movement needed for Class II correction. Unlike the headgear, these fixed appliances require only minimal patient cooperation. Appliance selection is based on the amount and direction of maxillary tooth distalization required, as well as the orthodontist's preference and ease of use. Although these appliances can be used in the late mixed dentition, they are primarily used in the permanent dentition.

Lip Bumper

The lip bumper (Figure 37-20) is an appliance that is typically used on the lower arch of patients who have very tight buccal or labial musculature. This U-shaped appliance attaches to buccal tubes on the molar bands and can be either fixed or

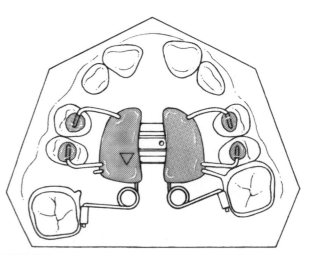

FIGURE 37-19
Occlusal view of a Pendex appliance. This Pendex has been activated unilaterally on the patient's right side by removing the locking wire. Both locking wires can be removed at the same time. (McNamara JA: *Orthodontics and dentofacial orthopedics,* Ann Arbor, Mich, 2001, Needham Press.)

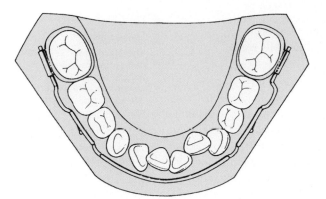

FIGURE 37-20
Occlusal view of a mandibular lip bumper. The wire inserts into tubes on the first molars and is positioned 2 to 3 mm from the tooth surface. (From McNamara JA: Treatment of patients in the mixed dentition. In Graber TM, Vanarsdall RL, Vig KWL, eds: *Orthodontics: current principles and techniques,* ed 4, St Louis, 2005, Mosby, p 553.)

removable. The appliance then lies between the teeth and the lips, shielding the teeth from the forces exerted by the oral musculature. The lip bumper not only provides expansion, but it can also upright the posterior teeth. This appliance is usually worn full time in either the mixed or the permanent dentition.

Functional Orthopedic Appliances

The term **orthopedics** is defined as "functional orthodontic therapy; utilization of muscle forces to effect changes in jaw position and tooth alignment by removable appliances."[29] This classification of appliances works to correct skeletal imbalances both in the transverse dimension (e.g., the RME) or in the anteroposterior dimension (functional jaw) orthopedic appliances (e.g., Herbst, FR 2 of Fränkel, Twin Block, Bionator). These types of appliances can be both fixed and removable.

A plethora of functional jaw orthopedic appliances is available; Figures 37-21 and 37-22 list two examples. The important fact to remember is that all functional jaw orthopedic appliances work to position the mandible forward. This forward posturing leads to changes in the dental and skeletal relationships in a growing individual. Functional jaw orthopedic appliances are not effective in adults.

ORTHODONTIC TREATMENT MODALITIES COMMONLY USED FOR ONE-PHASE (COMPREHENSIVE) TREATMENT

Components of Braces

The term *braces* is a generic term that includes the appliances in the mouth used for tooth movement. The usual complement of braces can include the following parts (Figure 37-23).

Brackets

Brackets are small fixtures that are bonded to the tooth surface. These appliances are often *preadjusted,* with the required torque and angulation specific to a given tooth built into the structure of the brace. The brackets are usually bonded to the facial or buccal surfaces of the teeth. A treatment alternative is available, termed *lingual* braces, which are bonded on the lingual surfaces

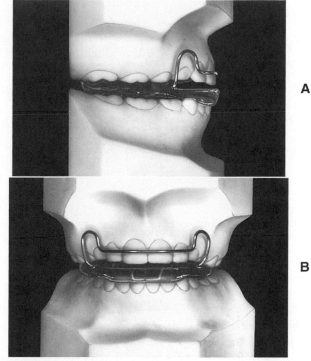

FIGURE 37-21
Lateral **(A)** and frontal views **(B)** of a bionator. (McNamara JA: *Orthodontics and dentofacial orthopedics,* Ann Arbor, Mich, 2001, Needham Press.)

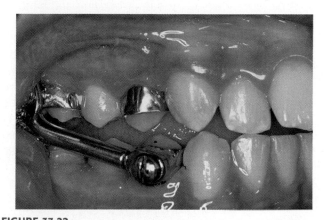
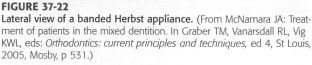

FIGURE 37-22
Lateral view of a banded Herbst appliance. (From McNamara JA: Treatment of patients in the mixed dentition. In Graber TM, Vanarsdall RL, Vig KWL, eds: *Orthodontics: current principles and techniques,* ed 4, St Louis, 2005, Mosby, p 531.)

of the teeth. This practice is not common. Technology in bracket design continues to evolve and improve, with countless variations that include ceramic or *clear* brackets, gold brackets, and self-ligating brackets that do not require an elastic tie or ligature to engage the wire.

Bands

These braces consist of a thin band of stainless steel or titanium metal that is preformed and to which a bracket or tube is attached. Bands encircle the tooth and usually have attachments that are fixed or soldered to the buccal or lingual surfaces (or both) of the bands to accommodate the archwire, an elastic tie,

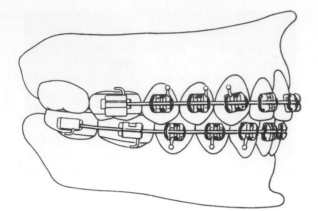

FIGURE 37-23
Example showing a dentition with full fixed appliances. In this instance, brackets are placed premolar to premolar, and the braces on the molars are bands. The archwire, as well as the elastic ties, can be seen.
(McNamara JA: *Orthodontics and dentofacial orthopedics,* Ann Arbor, Mich, 2001, Needham Press.)

and a headgear or lip bumper. Although some orthodontists choose to use brackets exclusively, the use of bands on the posterior teeth often decreases the chance of braces loosened in this area caused by the forces of mastication. Bands are usually cemented using resin cement with high cohesive strength.

DENTAL CONSIDERATIONS

Before the advancements made in bonding and banding cement technology, experiencing decalcification during orthodontic treatment was commonplace for an orthodontic patient. Although not totally eradicated, decalcification can be controlled with proper monitoring, diet, and oral hygiene instructions, as well as by using the new fluoride-releasing varnishes, sealants, and cements that can be applied to the tooth during brace placement procedures. In addition, the proper use of prescription-level, one-step 1.1% fluoride gel-toothpaste combinations or fluoride rinses further helps prevent decalcification. With today's advancements in products and technology, decalcification should be the exception rather than the rule.

Separators

Before placing orthodontic bands, a separator may be needed to open slightly the mesial and distal contacts of the banded tooth. The placement of separators increases the ease of proper band placement for the orthodontist and comfort for the patient during the banding procedure. These separators come in a variety of materials, including elastic (elastomeric), metal spring, and brass wire (the elastomeric being the most common one you may encounter). Even though all separators can be placed with specific orthodontic pliers, the elastomeric separator can also be inserted by *flossing* the separator down between the teeth, using two pieces of floss through the separator to stretch it open. An important point to note is that all separators encircle the contact area; thus they should be visible from the occlusal surface. Separators are usually in place 1 to 2 weeks. During this time, patients are advised to avoid flossing in that area and to avoid eating sticky food.

Orthodontic wires

Orthodontic wires engage in the horizontal slot in the brace; and the archwire, tied in to the bracket with some type of ligature, actually provides the energy or action needed to move the teeth. Without an archwire or tie in place, the brace would be inactive. Archwires come in many different sizes, dimensions, strengths, and metal alloys. In the early years of orthodontics, precious metals such as gold were used routinely. Stainless steel replaced these metals in the middle of the twentieth century and is still in use today. In the last few decades, significant advances have been made in fabricating orthodontic wires. Before this time, using wires that provided a high force over a short period was common, thus causing greater levels of patient discomfort. New alloys such as titanium molybdenum alloy (TMA) or nickel titanium (NiTi) can provide a lower force that acts consistently over a longer period. In the near future, dentistry is likely to see the introduction of *composite plastics* that will potentially provide comparable strength and springiness with nonsuperelastic wires.[23] Because of these advances in wire technology, patient discomfort is lessened, the time between orthodontic appointments can be lengthened, and fewer visits in total are required. Progress in tooth movement is achieved in treatment by progressing size, strength, stiffness, and resilience of the wires during the subsequent orthodontic visits.

Brace ligation

The wire must be held in place to remain engaged tightly in the horizontal slot of the braces for full movement to occur. This task is often accomplished by using elastic ties (often called *Os* or *donuts*) or metal ligature wire ties, which are changed or tightened during the orthodontic appointments. Elastics ties that are formed in a chain (power chain), elastic (power) thread, or coil springs can be used for space closure and pressure for lateral tooth movement.

In the last several years, several types of *self-ligating* brackets have been developed. These brackets have a metal shield or slide incorporated into the brace that holds the orthodontic wire firmly in position. The orthodontic team can open this device for wire changes and then close it to engage the wire fully, a procedure that often requires special training to manage efficiently.

Intraoral elastics

To provide an additional force either within the arch or between the arches for tooth movement, intraoral elastics (rubber bands) can be used. Patients can place these elastics, and they

Prevention
The elastomeric separators can sometimes become lodged subgingivally if the patient forgets and flosses the separator into the adjacent gingiva or chews something especially resilient. Most elastomeric separators are now radiopaque. If the patient has separators in place, then make certain that a portion of the separator is positioned above the occlusal surface. If not, then the separator should be removed and replaced. In addition, check radiographs carefully for any subgingival artifacts indicating separator displacement.

are usually directed to change them daily. The elastics come in a variety of sizes and strengths, usually described as *diameter* (in inches) and *ounce strength* (e.g., ¼ inch, 6 ounce), and can be worn in a multitude of ways, depending on the desired tooth movement. The orthodontist determines the amount of wear needed per day. Patient compliance is a necessary element in elastic wear to achieve a successful outcome.

Alternative to Braces

A number of new treatment approaches have been developed in the last several years that use a series of removable, clear, retainer-like appliances (or aligners) to move the teeth in a sequential manner. One such method, The Invisalign System, became available commercially in June 1999 (Figure 37-24). Thin and flexible, each aligner is worn for a period of at least 2 weeks and provides minute movements throughout the mouth. Patient discomfort is minimal.

Even though the desired outcome can often be accomplished, limitations in tooth movement are inherent with this method. Perhaps the criterion most important to achieve the desired treatment outcome is patient selection. Generally, patients with mild to moderate spacing, rotations, and crowding are good candidates. Patients with complex malocclusions involving a significantly deep bite, large openbites, or severely tipped teeth may not be good candidates for this type of treatment. As with all removable appliances, patient compliance is an important factor in treatment success.

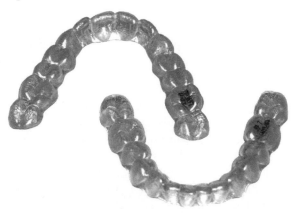

FIGURE 37-24
Maxillary and mandibular aligners. A patient identifier number is incorporated into the aligner in the first molar region. (McNamara JA: *Orthodontics and dentofacial orthopedics*, Ann Arbor, Mich, 2001, Needham Press.)

DEBONDING AND DEBANDING

The dental hygienist may be involved in removing orthodontic appliances or scaling the teeth following appliance removal. This process, commonly referred to as *debonding and debanding*,

can be relatively straightforward with the appropriate armamentarium of instruments. Today, even ceramic brackets are easier to remove thanks to technical improvements in adhesives and bracket design that allow for easy removal. The instrument most commonly used is special *bracket-removing* pliers that, when squeezed onto the bracket, causes the base to be distorted and subsequently debonded (Figure 37-25). Similarly, the process of band removal requires *band-removing* pliers that dislodge the stainless steel band from the tooth (Figure 37-26). After completing both arches, excess bonding resin will always need to be removed because the debonding process separates the base of the bracket from the resin. Removing excess resin can be accomplished with a number 12 fluted carbide bur (finishing bur) using sweeping motions until the teeth are smooth (Figure 37-27). Immediately after removing the braces, the gingiva may appear inflamed and edematous. With proper oral hygiene and a thorough cleaning, this condition should be temporary. In some cases, a rubber *tooth positioner* may be used to help massage the gingival (Figure 37-28). This appliance is used primarily for accomplishing minor finishing that may not otherwise occur. The patient is instructed to wear the positioner full time for several days and 12 hours a day for 2 to 4 weeks thereafter. This appliance, similar to other removable appliances, has great benefits when used properly but is of little use if worn minimally or not at all.

RETENTION AND STABILITY

One of the most frequently asked questions of the orthodontist, even before braces are worn, is, "How long will I have to wear a retainer?" The answer to this question may vary, depending on the orthodontist, but the fact remains that relapse of orthodontic correction may occur at any time; therefore the longer

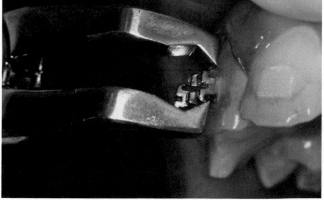

FIGURE 37-25
Removal of bonded brackets. A special pliers can be used to fracture the bonding resin, which usually results in much of the resin left on the tooth surface. This works particularly well with twin brackets. The advantage of this method is that the bracket usually is undamaged; the disadvantage is heavy force that may cause enamel damage. The alternative is to use a cutter to distort the bracket base. The first approach is more compatible with recycling of brackets, but the second is safer and usually leaves less resin to remove from the tooth surface. (From Proffit WR, Fields HW, Sarver DM: *Contemporary orthodontics*, ed 4, St Louis, 2007, Mosby.)

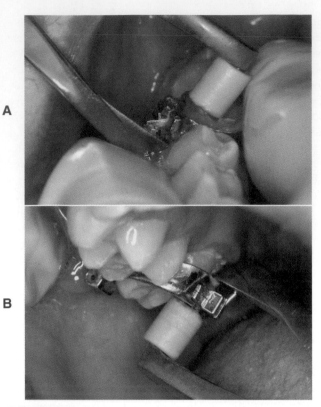

FIGURE 37-26
Removal of molar bands with a band-removing pliers. **A,** Lower posterior bands are removed primarily with pressure from the buccal surface. **B,** Upper posterior bands are removed from the lingual surface using a lingual attachment welded to the band. (From Proffit WR, Fields HW, Sarver DM: *Contemporary orthodontics,* ed 4, St Louis, 2007, Mosby.)

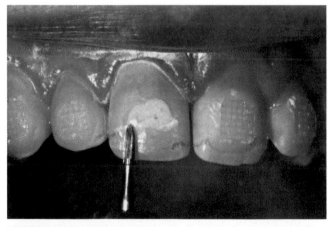

FIGURE 37-27
During debonding, the bond failure usually occurs between the base of the bracket and the resin, leaving excess resin on the tooth. Removing excess bonding resin is best accomplished with a smooth number 12 fluted carbide bur, followed by pumicing. The carbide bur is used with a gentle wiping motion to remove the resin. (From Proffit WR, Fields HW, Sarver DM: *Contemporary orthodontics,* ed 4, St Louis, 2007, Mosby.)

a retainer is worn, the more stable the correction will be. Several factors can influence the **stability** of orthodontically corrected teeth, with the most significant being reorganization of gingival tissues, changes resulting from growth, and pressure from the soft tissue.[4] Once the appliances are removed and the teeth are no longer splinted to their neighbor, each tooth is subsequently

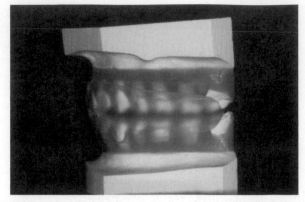

FIGURE 37-28
A tooth positioner, made from a transparent plastic material, placed in the patient's mouth. The patient bites into the positioner, which creates forces to displace the teeth slightly and massages the gingival. A device of this type is most effective in moving teeth if it is placed immediately after the fixed appliance is removed. (From Proffit WR, Fields HW, Sarver DM: *Contemporary orthodontics,* ed 4, St Louis, 2007, Mosby.)

able to respond to the forces of mastication, thus allowing reorganization of the PDL to occur. This reorganization, which occurs over a 3- to 4-month period, necessitates that a retainer be worn full time for at least this time period.[25]

Relapse of the teeth following orthodontic correction may also occur if significant movement is achieved or if the teeth are positioned where the lips exert a great deal of pressure. In this case, a permanent form of retention should be considered (discussed later). Finally, because many orthodontic patients fall into the *growing* category, retaining the position of the teeth will be necessary until growth has ceased. This necessity is particularly important because evidence shows that individuals continue to grow even throughout their adult years.[3] More importantly, for young patients who initially demonstrated an abnormal pattern of growth (Class II or III), this pattern continues during late adolescence even after the braces are removed. For the patient in Class III, for instance, the mandibular growth is likely to continue, possibly enough to require orthodontic retreatment.

Hawley Retainers

One of the hygienist's roles is to recognize a variety of appliances and understand their function. The most common retention appliance is a standard Hawley retainer (Figure 37-29). This appliance is designed with palatal acrylic to help maintain the lingual position of the teeth and with a labial bow from canine to canine to maintain incisor inclination and alignment. In many cases, a *Hawley type* of appliance will be used in the upper arch, although some custom variations may exist to the standard design. The same type of appliance design may be used in the lower arch with the greatest variation being the clasp.

> **Patient Education Opportunity**
> Regardless of the retainer design, to keep the appliances hygienic, the patient is instructed to clean the appliances at the same time that the teeth are cleaned using dentifrices or a retainer cleaning solution that can be purchased at a local drug store.

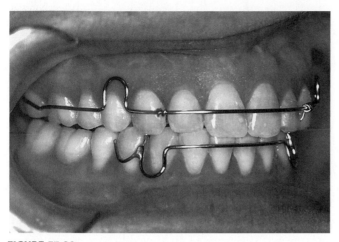

FIGURE 37-29
Hawley retainers. (McNamara JA: *Orthodontics and dentofacial orthopedics*, Ann Arbor, Mich, 2001, Needham Press.)

Thermoplastic Retainers

In recent years, fabricating *thermoplastic* or *invisible* retainers for the upper and lower arches has become more popular for esthetic reasons (Figure 37-30). This appliance is essentially a vacuform appliance that resembles bleaching trays, except that the material is closely adapted to the teeth without additional space (i.e., for bleaching material). With this shift toward a more esthetic look, thermoplastic retainers have become popular. The major disadvantage of this type of retention is that they are less sturdy than their acrylic counterparts and may need to be replaced more frequently.

Fixed Retainers

One common exception to Hawley-type retention can be when the initial orthodontic problem includes a midline diastema (in the maxilla) or multiple areas of spacing. In these cases, a lingual wire bond (between the centrals or from lateral to lateral) is prescribed to prevent relapse of the spaces. Bonding the wire in a position is necessary to avoid the lower teeth from occluding

on the wire and to avoid impinging on the palatal gingiva. Another indication for a fixed retainer in the lower arch is in cases in which a significant amount of expansion was achieved, excessive pressure exists from the lower lip onto the incisors, or both (Figure 37-31). Disadvantages, however, to the fixed-retainer design can be found. It is *not* uncommon for a patient's retainer to *debond* and require

> *Note*
> The inherent difficulty in cleaning the fixed appliance may lead to gingival problems (i.e., gingivitis).

> *Note*
> The decision for removing a fixed retainer should be based on the stability of the appliance, as well as the patient's ability to maintain proper oral hygiene.

the attention of an orthodontist after several years. However, after years and even decades have passed, many individuals lose contact with the orthodontist who treated them and therefore may delay addressing this problem. Alternatively, this situation may require the patient to find a new orthodontist.

RETENTION AND THIRD-MOLAR CONSIDERATIONS

For decades, an active debate has taken place as to whether extraction of third molars helps improve the stability of the orthodontic correction.[10] Many studies have evaluated this question and found both in favor of[9] and against third molar extraction. The best study design to explore this type of question is a *randomized clinical trial* (RCT). One study asked whether the presence of third molar teeth contributed to late incisor crowding. It concluded that no evidence was found that prophylactic extraction of wisdom teeth improved outcomes compared with no extraction.[10] Despite this fact, other factors need to be considered regarding the extraction of third molars. Recent studies have determined that periodontal disease is much more likely in adults with third molars as compared with those without them. This prevalence is thought to be caused primarily by the presence of specific bacteria in recurrent pericoronitis infections that tend to infect the periodontium of the remaining teeth. Hence, although orthodontic stability may not be affected by the presence of third molars, if careful evaluation and

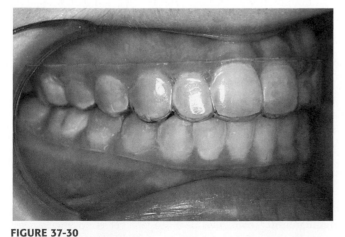

FIGURE 37-30
Invisible retainers. (McNamara JA: *Orthodontics and dentofacial orthopedics*, Ann Arbor, Mich, 2001, Needham Press.)

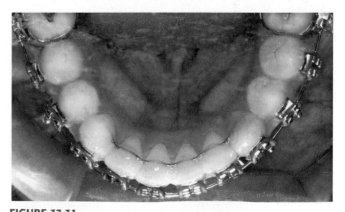

FIGURE 37-31
Bonded Krause retainer. (McNamara JA: *Orthodontics and dentofacial orthopedics*, Ann Arbor, Mich, 2001, Needham Press.)

monitoring of these teeth reveal frequent inflammation, then extraction may be warranted.

Interdisciplinary Patient Care

Advances in every specialty of dentistry have enabled clinicians to expand the options that are available for patient care. Increasingly, interdisciplinary teams composed of practitioners from many different dental disciplines work together to develop a comprehensive treatment plan for patients with complex dental challenges and compromised occlusions. The orthodontist often coordinates the interdisciplinary treatment provided by many dental specialists who work together as a team. The following sections highlight instances in which **interdisciplinary patient care** is a factor.

IMPACTED TEETH

In patients who have permanent teeth that fail to erupt into the arch, two treatment options are available. The impacted tooth can be extracted. This plan, used infrequently, is usually indicated if the tooth is endangering the roots of the surrounding teeth or if the tooth is located in a position deemed too difficult to move into the arch. In many instances, removing this tooth may lead to the need for prosthetic replacement, either by implant or bridgework.

A second option would be to expose the tooth surgically and bring it into the dental arch orthodontically. In this instance, cohesive treatment planning by the general dentist, oral surgeon, and orthodontist should be coordinated to achieve the desired outcome. Typically, the general dentist would perform the initial diagnosis and send the patient for a consultation to the orthodontist and the oral surgeon. If the exposure was appropriate and the treatment was accepted by the patient, then braces would be placed before tooth exposure. Preliminary tooth alignment would be needed to open the space required for the exposed tooth to be brought into the arch. Once this space is created, the surgeon would then expose all or part of the crown tooth. The surgeon may attach a bracket, hook, button, or gold chain to the crown of the exposed tooth. Soon thereafter (usually 5 to 10 days), the orthodontist engages or ties the attachment to the archwire, thus creating the gradual force needed to bring the impacted tooth into occlusion.

ANKYLOSED TEETH

Occasionally, a primary or permanent tooth will become fused to its surrounding bone. This condition is called **ankylosis.** In many cases, a diagnosis of ankylosis is made when the tooth in question appears submerged when compared with the surrounding teeth. Referrals are typically made to the dentist or oral surgeon for extraction (of primary teeth) or luxation (of permanent teeth).

CONGENITALLY MISSING TEETH

In patients who are missing permanent teeth, the decision needs to be made whether to replace the missing tooth prosthodontically or to close the space. Making this decision may require the dentist or orthodontist to order a *diagnostic setup*. This diagnostic tool is used to predict treatment success. To make a diagnostic setup, impressions are taken of the patient's upper and lower teeth. After the impressions are poured in plaster and the casts are trimmed, the proposed treatment plan is carried out on the dental casts by repositioning the teeth and waxing them back onto the cast in their ideal location. Diagnostic setups can be made in-office but are usually fabricated at a qualified dental laboratory. The finished setup then reveals the approximate treatment outcome.

If implant replacement is indicated, then the patient's teeth are orthodontically repositioned and the edentulous space is idealized to the specifications of the oral surgeon, as well as the restoring dentist. The ideal spacing between the adjacent tooth roots, as well as mesiodistal crown width, is of utmost importance in a satisfactory treatment outcome.

If the primary tooth has been retained at that site, the temporary solution may then be to keep the retained primary tooth in place as long as possible to maintain the bony support until replacement is desired. The optimal time for implant placement is after all facial growth has ceased; therefore this procedure would be the treatment plan of choice for growing adolescents. This option, however, has its limitations. If the retained tooth is too large mesiodistally (e.g., a retained primary second molar) or too small (e.g., a retained primary lateral incisor), then the upper and lower arches may be prevented from occluding properly. Adjustments may be made to the existing primary tooth by the general dentist (either tooth-size reduction with a fissure bur or tooth-size enhancement with temporary bonding) to create a retained tooth with the ideal mesiodistal width. The orthodontist can then align the teeth to create a proper occlusion. This type of treatment is not effective, however, if the root structure of the retained tooth is too wide to accommodate space closure, such as in the case of some retained primary second molars.

MALFORMED TEETH

The most common malformed tooth is the maxillary lateral incisor. Commonly referred to as *peg* or *pegged,* its shape can be significantly shorter, narrower, or more tapered than normal. If the tooth-size discrepancy is minor and bilateral in nature, then restoration may not be needed. The orthodontist has several treatment options, including closing the space and making compensations in the opposing arch for proper occlusion. If the space is large or unilateral, the space would then be idealized by the orthodontist to match the other teeth. The patient is then referred back to the referring dentist or prosthodontist for the desired restorative treatment. All final restorative work is completed after active orthodontic treatment is finished.

ORTHOGNATHIC (CORRECTIVE JAW) SURGERY

Orthognathia is "the study of the causes and treatment of conditions related to the malposition of the bones of the jaw."[29] Thus **orthognathic** (corrective jaw) surgery refers to the surgery needed to correct the malalignment or imbalance of the bones of the jaw. In adults, facial growth has virtually ceased. Thus the orthodontic and orthopedic options available to promote facial balance and skeletal growth in children or adolescents are not available for adults. Significant skeletal imbalances, such as a severe Class II or III malocclusions or severe skeletal openbites, may require surgical intervention in one or both jaws.

The orthodontist works closely with the oral and maxillofacial surgeon before surgery. The teeth need to be positioned properly and in a stable position with respect to each jaw such that the jaws can be aligned surgically in a stable and balanced relationship. Typically, orthodontic treatment is approximately one half to two thirds completed before surgery. After orthognathic surgery, the orthodontic appliances are left in place an additional 6 to 12 months to allow for fine detailing of the occlusion.

MICROIMPLANTS

"In recent years, endosseous implants have become practical, predictable and reliable adjuncts to dental rehabilitation. The concept of osseointegration can be used innovatively now in orthodontics to provide rigid anchorage for tooth and bone movement. Retromolar implants have been used as orthodontic anchorage for over 20 years."[13] A variety of implant variations have been used to provide the needed anchorage to attain a counterbalance of the forces used to close spaces and distalize the dentition. Although the use of **microimplants** in orthodontics is not currently commonplace, they may arguably be the leading advancement in orthodontic technology in this century.

Role of the Dental Hygienist in Orthodontics

DENTAL HYGIENIST'S ROLE IN A GENERAL DENTAL SETTING

The dental hygienist has a crucial role in the early recognition of a patient's malocclusion and timely referral for orthodontic intervention. The dental hygienist is often the first clinical contact a patient has with the dental office.

> *Note*
>
> The hygienist's role as the primary provider of routine prophylaxis and prevention-oriented oral health instruction lends itself greatly to the early detection and referral of potential orthodontic problems.

As mentioned at the beginning of this chapter, using the components of the orthodontic assessment is important when evaluating patients. For ease of use, the dental hygienist can summarize the components into six quick steps (Box 37-1).

Oral Care Appointments during Orthodontic Treatment

Routine oral care appointments are of utmost importance to the orthodontic patient. For patients with oral hygiene challenges, the orthodontist may request that the dental hygienist place the patient on more frequent supportive intervals than normal. The dental hygienist can provide invaluable counseling

---

> **BOX 37-1**
>
> ## ORTHODONTIC SIX-POINT QUICK CHECK SYSTEM
>
> Begin by examining *each arch separately* and evaluating the following categories:
> 1. Arch width (molar-to-molar transpalatal width of 36 mm is average)
> 2. Excessive spacing or crowding present
> 3. Missing or ankylosed teeth
>   Then note the relationship between the upper and lower teeth in occlusion. Evaluate the following:
> 4. Angle's classification
> 5. The amount of overbite and overjet present
> 6. Any openbite or crossbite present

---

regarding proper home care, dietary instruction, and using oral care products and devices for proper home care. Oral irrigation devices, as well as powered toothbrushes, often greatly aid a patient with home care challenges.

Significant calculus deposits are not typically found on orthodontic bands. Attention, however, should be paid to the cervical and subgingival portions of the teeth. Depending on the orthodontic appliances involved, the dental hygienist may want to supplement the rubber-cup polishing with a soft bristle brush on the rotary hand piece or polish with the air-powder polisher. Flossing should be done routinely and can be aided greatly by using a floss threader. Topical fluoride applications may be applied, although they have been known to possibly inhibit the bonding of brackets if the orthodontic procedure is done within 24 hours after the fluoride application. Tooth whitening products should not be used while fixed orthodontic appliances are in place. The tooth surface under the fixed appliance would not be accessible to the whitening product. Thus the patient might be left with a striated whitened effect.

The orthodontic office should be contacted with any problems or concerns. Loose or leaking bands, brackets, or other fixed appliances that are left unattended over an extended period can lead to tooth damage and decay.

> *Patient Education Opportunity*
>
> During the prophylaxis of an orthodontic patient with fixed appliances, care must be taken with instrumentation along the cemented margins of the appliance. Although checking for voids or leaks in the cement with an explorer is important, you should not attempt to scale around the margins of the appliance except for removing gross debris. Dislodging an appliance with pressure at the cemented margin is quite easy.

DENTAL HYGIENIST IN THE ORTHODONTIC PRACTICE

Many career opportunities are available to the dental hygienist in an orthodontic office. With the dental hygienist's unique background in basic, behavioral, and clinical sciences, he or she can be a great asset in the following areas.

CASE APPLICATION 37-1.1

Dental Hygiene Treatment Plan Needed

Mrs. Jones is back for her 3-month supportive care visit after successfully beginning orthodontic treatment. The orthodontist sent a copy of her case workup and treatment plan for your records. The following orthodontic problem list was provided:

- Pathologic considerations: History of periodontal disease now controlled but with significant generalized attachment loss (4- to 7-mm probing depths); poor prognosis of mandibular incisors with all incisors having Class II mobility
- Alignment: Multiple missing teeth; severe maxillary spacing and mild-to-moderate mandibular spacing
- Anteroposterior: Skeletal Class II with bimaxillary protrusion; flared and bodily protrusive incisors; Class II dentition; overjet: 8 mm
- Vertical: Mild dental deep bite
- Dental protrusion–facial esthetics: Protrusive lips, deep mentolabial fold, and poor throat form

Mrs. Jones's orthodontist also provided her treatment objectives:

- Maintain periodontal condition and continue to improve oral hygiene self-care.
- Maintain present dentition (although prognosis is poor for mandibular anterior teeth).
- Align and reduce spacing in arches, helping decrease overjet and lip protrusion.
- Achieve Class I canines and Class II molars.
- Level arches.

List the important tasks that you must complete during the supportive care visit for Mrs. Jones (who has a history of periodontal disease and is currently in braces).

Treatment Coordinator

The dental hygienist can be used to assist the orthodontist with the initial orthodontic evaluation in the following ways:

- Conduct the patient interview to gather detailed information regarding the patient's health, as well as medical and dental history.
- Identify restorative and periodontal concerns before the initiation of treatment.
- Assist the orthodontist in the case presentation of the orthodontic treatment plan, as well as oral health and home care instruction.

Record Taking

- Take, trace, and analyze cephalometric and panoramic radiographs.
- Take diagnostic photographs and orthodontic impressions.

Clinical Duties

- Perform the trial sizing of orthodontic bands.
- Prepare the tooth surface for bonding (similar to procedures used for placing sealants).

- Assist in the complete removal of banding and bonding adhesives with rotary instruments at the brace removal appointment.

Although not every orthodontic office employs dental hygienists, certainly, most orthodontic offices would benefit greatly from the effective utilization of this position. The field of orthodontics offers dental hygienists an interesting alternative to the traditional position in a general dental office. However, regardless of the practice setting, dental hygienists have a vital role to plan in the field of orthodontics.

References

1. American Association of Orthodontists web site: http://www.braces.org.
2. Angle EH: *Treatment of malocclusion of the teeth and fractures of the maxillae, Angle system,* ed 6, Philadelphia, 1900, SS White Dental Manufacturing.
3. Behrents RG, Johnston LE Jr: The influence of the trigeminal nerve on facial growth and development, *Am J Orthodol* 85:199-206, 1984.
4. Blake M, Bibby K: Retention and stability: a review of the literature, *Am J Orthod Dentofacial Orthop* 114(3):299-306, 1998.
5. Brunelle JA, Bhat M, Lipton JA: Prevalence and distribution of selected occlusal characteristics in the US population, 1988-91, *J Dent Res* 75:706-713, 1996.
6. Burstone CJ, Pryputniewicz RJ, Bowley WW: Holographic measurement of tooth mobility in three dimensions, *J Periodont Res* 13:283-294, 1978.
7. Daniel S, Harfst S: *Mosby's dental hygiene: 2004 update,* St Louis, 2004, Mosby.
8. Elgoyhen JC: Mandibular growth alteration and variable treatment circumstances: contradictions between laboratory and clinical observations. In Hunter WS, Carlson DS, eds: *Essays in honor of Robert E Moyers,* Ann Arbor, Mich, 1991, Center for Human Growth and Development.
9. Elter JR et al: Third molars associated with periodontal pathology in older Americans, *J Oral Maxillofac Surg* 63:179-184, 2005.
10. Harradine NW, Pearson MH, Toth B: The effect of extraction of third molars on late lower incisor crowding: a randomized controlled trial, *Br J Orthod* 25:117-122, 1998.
11. Hartsfield JK Jr, Everett ET, Al-Qawasmi RA: Genetic factors in external apical root resorption and orthodontic treatment, *Crit Rev Oral Biol Med* 15:115-122, 2004.
12. Helm S: Prevalence of malocclusion in relation to development of the dentition, *Acta Odontol Scand* 28(Suppl 58):122, 1970.
13. Huang LH, Shotwell JL, Wang HL: Dental implants for orthodontic anchorage, *Am J Orthod Dentofac Orthop* 127:713-722, 2005.
14. Kaley J, Phillips C: Factors related to root resorption in edgewise practice, *Angle Orthod* 61:125-132, 1991.
15. Kelley J, Harvey C: *An assessment of the teeth of youths 12-17 years,* US Department of Health, Education and Welfare Publication No (HRA) 77-1644, Washington, DC, 1977, National Center for Health Statistics.
16. Kennedy DB et al: The effect of extraction and orthodontic treatment on dentoalveolar support, *Am J Orthod* 84:183-190, 1983.
17. Magnusson T: Five-year longitudinal study of signs and symptoms of mandibular dysfunction in adolescents, *Craniol* 4:338-344, 1986.

18. McNamara JA: *Orthodontics and orthopedic treatment in the mixed dentition,* Ann Arbor, Mich, 1993, Needham Press.

19. McNamara JA: *Orthodontics and dentofacial orthopedics,* Ann Arbor, Mich, 2001, Needham Press.

20. Melsen B, Agerbaek N, Markenstam G: Intrusion of incisors in adult patients with marginal bone loss, *Am J Orthod Dentofacial Orthop* 96(3):232-241, 1989.

21. Moriarty JD; Simpson DM: Incidence of periodontal problems in patients with dentofacial deformities, *J Dent Res* 63(Special Issue A):1249, 1984.

22. Moyers RE: *On the nature of orthodontics,* Ann Arbor, Mich, 1985, Needham Press.

23. Proffit WR, Fields HW Jr: *Contemporary orthodontics,* ed 4, St Louis, 2007, Mosby.

24. Proffit WR, Fields HW, Moray LJ: Prevalence of malocclusion and orthodontic treatment need in the United States: estimates from the NHANES III survey, *Int J Adult Orthodon Orthognath Surg* 13:97-106, 1998.

25. Reitan K: Principles of retention and avoidance of posttreatment relapse, *Am J Orthod* 55:776-790, 1969.

26. Roberts WE, Ferguson DJ: Cell kinetics of the periodontal ligament. In Norton LA, Burstone CJ, eds: *The biology of tooth movement,* Boca Raton, Fla, 1989, CRC Press.

27. Sadowsky C, BeGole EA: Long-term effects of orthodontic treatment on periodontal health, *Am J Orthod* 80:156-172, 1981.

28. Sarver DM, Ackerman MB: Dynamic smile visualization and quantification: part 1—evolution of the concept and dynamic records for smile capture, *Am J Orthod Dentofacial Orthop* 124:4-12, 2003.

29. *Stedman's medical dictionary,* ed 24, Baltimore, Md, 1982, Williams & Wilkins.

Oral Malodor Diagnosis and Management

Kristy Menage Bernie

INSIGHT

Oral malodor is a common condition that will be encountered daily in clinical practice. The dental hygienist must be able to integrate oral malodor management strategies throughout the preventive and therapeutic appointment. In addition to the obvious unpleasantness associated with oral malodor, the connection between oral malodor and periodontal disease may also provide key motivational opportunities to achieve optimal oral health.

✸ CASE STUDY 38-1 | Oral Malodor Management

Karen Miller, a 43-year-old divorced professional, is reentering the workforce and is seeking ways to enhance her appearance. During the hygiene assessment, she discloses her use of the following oral hygiene–related products:
- Breath mints
- Chewing gum
- Manual toothbrush and fluoride toothpaste (used two to three times a day)

Ms. Miller is a patient of record and has a history of localized periodontal pocketing that has remained unresolved. Although she has expressed her understanding of the periodontal disease process, adherence to oral hygiene recommendations is lacking.

Clinical evaluation reveals localized bleeding on probing and pocket depths of 5 to 6 mm in the posterior region. In addition, Ms. Miller's tongue has a thick coating. Even though radiographs do not show significant bone loss, areas of slight bone loss exist in the posterior region.

KEY TERMS

deplaque	halitosis	methyl mercaptan	tonsilloliths
fetor ex ore	hydrogen sulfide	organoleptic	volatile sulfur compounds
fetor oris	gram-negative	oral malodor	

LEARNING OUTCOMES

After reading this chapter the student will be able to:
1. Differentiate among the etiologies associated with malodor.
2. Identify the intraoral niches involved in the production of oral malodor.
3. Explain the relationship between oral malodor and periodontal disease.
4. Establish clinical management protocols for oral malodor.
5. Discriminate among various mechanical and chemotherapeutic methods for oral malodor treatment and prevention.
6. Identify methods to discuss professionally the topic of oral malodor with patients.

Halitosis, or **oral malodor,** has represented a condition that has held age-old interest and remedies. Ancient texts refer to the condition confirming a variety of social stigmas and diseases thought to be associated with oral malodor. The term *halitosis* has been used to describe bad breath, and yet the true meaning of this term is *abnormal odor,* whereas **fetor oris** or **fetor ex ore** are terms that accurately describe what 80% to 90% of individuals with bad breath experience: odor originating and emanating from the oral cavity.[58,63,70] Exact estimates of people who suffer from oral malodor are difficult to determine. However, the billion-dollar cosmetic oral healthcare products industry indicates that people are not only interested in fresh breath, but are also self-diagnosing and treating the condition. Ironically, dental intervention of oral malodor is not part of routine care and ranks behind dental caries and periodontal disease as a chief compliant by patients.[32]

> *Note*
>
> The American Dental Hygienists' Association defines optimal oral health as "A standard of health of the oral and related tissues which enables an individual to eat, speak, and socialize without active disease, discomfort, or embarrassment and which contributes to general well-being and overall total health."[3]

The American Dental Hygienists' Association's definition of optimal oral health reaches beyond disease-based parameters of health and includes a focus on what means the most to patients—social factors. Therefore dental hygienists must incorporate oral malodor discussion and treatment into their clinical protocols. Clinicians who incorporate these strategies will gain patient appreciation and a new method to motivate the patient to optimal oral health while acknowledging that social factors are important to this end. Although bad breath has been viewed as mainly a social embarrassment, disease-related components warrant further concern by the dental community.[75] Dental professionals and especially dental hygienists are in a position to assist patients in assessing oral malodor conditions and addressing the causes while recommending daily intervention for reducing oral malodor.

The exact science behind oral malodor—the causes, effects and treatment—has been established only recently.[1] The complexity of the condition, combined with the discomfort on the part of dental professionals to discuss the topic, has been a barrier to integrating fresh-breath strategies into clinical protocols. In addition, because the U.S. Food and Drug Administration (FDA) considers bad-breath products to be cosmetic versus therapeutic, no regulation or research benchmarks have been established; thus oral malodor treatment remains a condition that has not been given serious consideration. Regardless of the challenge behind diagnostics and lack of science, many patients are interested in methods to prevent and treat the condition.

The role of the dental hygienist in addressing oral malodor is significant and appropriate. New research has also brought to light the role oral malodor plays in the progression of periodontal infections.[38] Incorporating oral malodor treatment into the dental hygiene diagnosis and treatment plan will not only provide an additional motivation for patients but might also affect overall health because many of the fresh breath methods will also improve or maintain oral health. Tying social factors with disease education represents a patient-centered approach that addresses a major condition of concern to millions of patients: bad breath.

Malodor Etiologic Factors

Historically, education has focused on systemic-based malodor conditions. However, 80% to 90% of malodor originates from oral cavity. Classification of oral malodor includes intrinsic and extrinsic pathways. Extrinsic causes include substances such as tobacco or certain foods that are absorbed into the circulatory system and released through the pulmonary respiration or saliva. Intrinsic factors are divided into systemic origin and represent 10% of malodor, whereas 90% is directly related to intraoral sources.[1,58,63,70]

> *Extrinsic and Intrinsic Malodor Sources*
>
> - Extrinsic: Food, medications, alcohol, tobacco—substances absorbed via the circulatory system
> - Intrinsic: Systemic based—10% oral based; 90% bacteria and bacteria by-products

Seven common sources have been identified and include both intrinsic and extrinsic pathways. These sources include the following:
- Mouth and tongue
- Nasal, nasopharyngeal, sinus, and oropharyngeal
- Xerostomia induced
- Primary lower respiratory tract and lung
- Systemic disease
- Gastrointestinal diseases and disorders
- Odiferous ingested foods, fluids, and medications[14]

The dental hygienist should have a basic understanding of these sources to establish clinical and daily management protocols. Dental intervention will affect most of these causes, except those that are systemically induced. The focus of management strategies should be aimed at the particular sources that can be controlled by dental intervention.

MOUTH AND TONGUE

The mouth and tongue account for the majority of malodor sources attributed to bacteria accumulation on the posterior surface of the tongue and in periodontal pockets greater than 4 mm. Food debris around restorations and oral tissue lesions can also contribute to the condition. Research has established that the metabolic activities of anaerobic bacteria are responsible for the odors produced.

DENTAL CONSIDERATIONS

Dental hygiene intervention will be key in treating and preventing oral malodor, with strategies that are consistent with those that achieve optimal oral health. Daily and clinical intervention will be the primary focus of dental strategies.

NASAL, NASOPHARYNGEAL, SINUS, AND OROPHARYNGEAL

Odor emanating from the nose, when the mouth is closed, indicate this source.

> **Note**
> Allergies, common colds, and sinusitis can produce odor.

Conditions can lead to postnasal drip and will contribute to bacteria accumulation on the posterior dorsum of the tongue and back of the throat. Odor-related conditions in this category might require medical intervention, as well as thorough oral hygiene practices. Medications taken to address these conditions often cause xerostomia, another source of oral malodor that increases the risk of dental caries.

XEROSTOMIA INDUCED

Xerostomia affects nearly everyone, whether as a result of diminished salivary flow during sleep or from medications, systemic disease, or tobacco use.

> **Note**
> When salivary flow is diminished, oral malodor increases as a result of increased bacterial growth and activity.

The lack of saliva is tangential with a lack of naturally occurring antibacterial substances that keep bacteria in check. This source of oral malodor will also be a focus of oral malodor–management strategies.

PRIMARY LOWER RESPIRATORY TRACT AND LUNG DISEASE

> **Distinct Care Modifications**
> Dental intervention strategies would be confined to medical referral and thorough oral health assessment and management.

Compromised pulmonary function and related diseases are at the root of this form of malodor. Lung abscesses, lodged foreign bodies, necrotizing pneumonia, pulmonary cancer, and tuberculosis are some of the conditions attributed.

SYSTEMIC DISEASES

Focus on this category of malodor has been mainstay in both medicine and dentistry, and yet systemic disease accounts for only 10% of malodor sources.[58,63,70]

> **Note**
> Hepatic failure, renal failure, and diabetes represent some of the conditions that may result in oral malodor.

Hepatic conditions are associated with sulfur or rotten egg odors, whereas renal failure is characterized by an ammonia odor, with dialysis associated with a fishy odor. Diabetes, particularly uncontrolled or undiagnosed conditions, has an acetone fruity sweet smell. As with pulmonary-related odors, this category requires medical referral and cannot be solved via dental or oral hygiene intervention strategies.

GASTROINTESTINAL DISEASES AND DISORDERS

Odor that is caused by gastrointestinal diseases and disorders is systemically based and can be related to conditions such as heartburn, stomach gas, spontaneous laryngitis, and stomach pain. An inadequate esophageal seal, as well as more serious gastric diseases, can also result in this type of malodor. The associated odor typically resembles the most recently eaten food and is commonly expelled via belching. This category will also benefit from medical evaluation of the underlying cause for treatment and resolution.

ODIFEROUS INGESTED FOODS, FLUIDS, AND MEDICATIONS

The final category of malodor relates directly to an extrinsic source and is controlled by avoiding causative substances that are responsible for the malodor. It is considered transitory and is due to absorption of the substance into the circulatory system. Once in the system, the odors are expelled via respiration and the saliva. The easiest to detect and experienced by all, this type of odor must work its way through the body to be eliminated. Masking odors can provide temporary resolution and, when combined with thorough oral hygiene practices, is the only solution, aside from avoiding the offending substances.

> **Patient Education Opportunity**
> Explain to patients that tobacco and alcohol are examples of agents that elicit strong odors, even hours after exposure.

> **Distinct Care Modifications**
> Considering that most malodor is oral in nature, treatment strategies and protocols should be designed to manage and prevent oral-based malodor and is well within the scope of practice for the dental hygienist.

Each of these categories represents a concise method for assessing oral malodor origins and can be used as a benchmark for dental professionals.

> ✦ **CASE APPLICATION 38-1.1**
>
> **Initiating a Malodor Discussion**
> What additional assessment would you initiate in Ms. Miller's case? What strategies would you use to begin a professional and comfortable discussion of oral malodor as a common side effect of periodontal disease?

Physiologic Factors of Oral-Based Malodor

Oral-based malodor is a direct result of microbial activity and attributed to **gram-negative** anaerobic flora, the same flora that is associated with periodontal infections. Gram-negative, anaerobic bacteria produce odor-related compounds called volatile sulfur compounds (VSCs),[33] which are by-products of bacteria metabolism similar to the more commonly known endotoxins that destroy periodontal tissue. In essence, these bacteria produce both gaseous (VSC) and *solid* (endotoxins) by-products. The primary VSCs produced by flora include **hydrogen sulfide** (H_2S), and **methyl mercaptan** (CH_3SH) and comprise 90% of the VSCs found in expelled air along with cadaverine.[25,32,71] Although hydrogen sulfide is associated with patients who are periodontally healthy, methyl mercaptan is associated with people who have periodontal disease.

Bacteria produce VSCs by degrading sulfur-containing peptides, proteins, and amino acids. Cysteine, methionine, and serum proteins result in large amounts of hydrogen sulfide and methyl mercaptan production. Polyamines, alcohols, phenyl compounds, alkamines, ketones, and nitrogen-containing compounds also contribute to detectable odors. The vast array of malodorous compounds make the task of pinpointing culprits challenging beyond the previously mentioned sulfur compounds and cadaverine, and thus research focuses primarily on the presence of sulfur components. Hydrogen sulfide has a rotten egg odor, whereas methyl mercaptan has the odor of feces, and cadaverine has a corpselike odor, accounting for the differences in odors detected when assessing patients with or without periodontal infection.

ORAL NICHES FOR ODOR-RELATED BIOFILMS

The primary sites of biofilm accumulation have been identified as the posterior dorsum of the tongue, pocket depths greater than 4 mm, and the tonsillar region. Other contributing factors include reduction of salivary flow and an alkaline pH, which creates an ideal environment for bacteria proliferation, purification, and odor production.

The anatomical features of the tongue (Figure 38-1) provide the ideal surface for bacteria and food retention and, without daily cleansing, will be a major source of oral malodor in both healthy and periodontally involved cases. Tongue coating is made up of a complex biofilm containing dead epithelial cells, food debris, blood cells, and bacteria.[23,24]

DENTAL CONSIDERATIONS

The various tongue papillae and crevices, combined with lingual tonsils and mucous glands, increase the accumulation of biofilms and represent an ideal environment for entrapping debris and retaining substrate, both of which favor anaerobic bacteria.

Less associated, but of great interest, is the production of VSCs from periodontal pockets deeper than 4 mm.[34] These sites are secondary to the tongue in terms of odor production and are

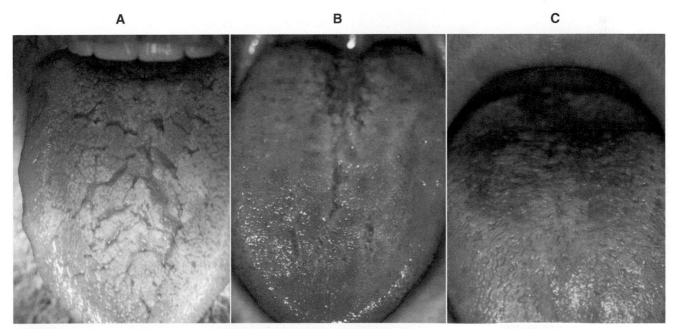

FIGURE 38-1
A, Note fissures trapping bacteria and resulting light coating of the tongue. **B and C,** Different clinical pictures of heavily coated tongues. (A, Courtesy Michelle Hurlbutt, RDH, BS. B and C, From Newman MG et al: *Carranza's Clinical Periodontology,* 10th ed, St Louis, 2006, Saunders.)

obviously associated with periodontal infections. As crevicular fluid flow increases in infected sites, so does methionine and thus the production of methyl mercaptan. Pockets of 5 mm or greater also represent the baseline for sites that are at risk for periodontal infection and sites that qualify for treatment with locally applied chemotherapeutics (see Chapter 27).

The final site of odor-related biofilm collection is the tonsillar area. Palatine tonsils with deep crypts can harbor food and bacteria and lead to the formation of **tonsilloliths,** which are semicalcified masses of bacteria and food that emit odor when air is exhaled[18,49,61] (Figure 38-2). These sources appear as white embedded masses, which may be singular or multiple. The tonsil tissue is also involved in postnasal drip and provides a niche to harbor biofilms that contribute to oral malodor.

Identifying accumulation sites of odor-related biofilms is important for oral malodor assessment and treatment. Additionally, these sites are interconnected and contribute to each other through biofilm translocation, in terms of potential for oral malodor production, as well as periodontal infection progression. Thus considerations for oral malodor will parallel those for periodontal health and management.

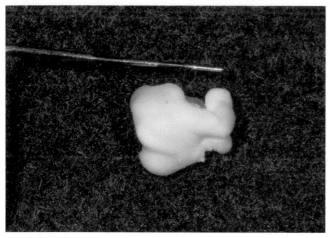

FIGURE 38-2
Tonsilloliths are semicalcified masses that imbed in tonsil and adenoid tissues. These masses can be uncomfortable, have a significant odor component, and are typically benign. (Courtesy Michelle Hurlbutt, RDH, BS.)

Oral Malodor and Periodontal Disease

Historical connections between oral malodor and periodontal disease traces back to ancient times. Hippocrates made the following observation: *"If the gingiva become healthy again, the offensive odor vanishes."*[75] The connection goes far beyond periodontal-infection malodor in that VSCs are toxic metabolites and have been implicated in accelerating the disease process and playing a major role in pathogenesis. Research in the last 60 years has focused on this important relationship, which has demonstrated reduction in oral malodor through

periodontal treatment. This outcome goes beyond disease parameters by addressing patient-centered concerns and needs.

Obviously, periodontal conditions favor the growth of the organisms associated with oral malodor. In fact, periodontal disease–associated biofilms, known as the *orange and red complexes,*[67] produce VSCs as end-products of metabolism and thus increase the presence and severity of oral malodor.

VSCs are produced through microbial putrefaction of food debris, cells, saliva, and blood within the oral cavity. Gram-negative flora is the primary source of this putrefaction process. Through the metabolism of cysteine and methionine, VSC formation occurs. Sources of sulfur-related components include the saliva, plaque biofilm, and gingival crevicular fluid. VSC production is significant in periodontal infection and directly related to subgingival and tongue flora.

VSCs have also been associated with an increase in mucosa permeability, which permits additional bacteria and endotoxin invasion and may lead to the progression of periodontal infections. Most importantly, these compounds have been shown to interfere with collagen and protein synthesis, as well as to suppress deoxyribonucleic acid (DNA) synthesis, thereby impeding wound healing.* Research suggests that the presence of these compounds may accelerate the periodontal infection process.[53]

Additionally, VSCs play a role in penetration of lipopolysaccharides (LPSs) through inflamed and healthy epithelium. Tissue destruction occurs through both direct and indirect pathways, including effects on gingival fibroblasts, decrease in collagenous protein, and suppression of DNA synthesis. These pathways may also affect the immune response and contribute to the production of collagenase, which increases tissue destruction. Research suggests that methyl mercaptan is more deleterious to tissue than hydrogen sulfide and demonstrates an increase in disease severity when the ratio of methyl mercaptan exceeds that of hydrogen sulfide.[54]

In addition to pockets deeper than 4 mm, the tongue contributes significantly to both odor and potential disease progression. The coating in periodontally involved cases is estimated to be four to six times greater than in healthy individuals.[29,34,75] The combination of tongue- and pocket-produced odors leads to a more severe condition and requires clinical management considerations. Both gingival inflammation and the tongue are the main contributors to oral malodor in periodontal cases.[39] Box 38-1 summarizes of the relationship between oral malodor and periodontal disease.[42]

✪ CASE APPLICATION 38-1.2

Correlation of Malodor to Oral Disease

How would you relate Ms. Miller's oral malodor and periodontal condition? What other areas of the mouth would you bring to her attention?

*References 9, 26, 43, 75-76.

BOX 38-1

PERIODONTAL INFECTION AND ORAL MALODOR

1. Periodontal disease is caused by anaerobic and facultative protein–utilizing bacteria.
2. Bacteria are located in periodontal pockets, deeper than 4 mm, and older established plaque biofilm where sulfur-containing substrates are available.
3. Subgingival anaerobes, such as *Porphyromonas gingivalis, Prevotella* spp., and many others, reduce sulfur-containing amino acids to hydrogen sulfide (H_2S), methyl mercaptan (CH_3SH), and dimethyl sulfide (CH_3SCH_3), referred to as *volatile sulfur compounds (VSCs)*. VSCs are some of the specific by-products of bacterial metabolism of many different host substrates, including, but not limited to, crevicular fluid constituents, leukocytes, gingival bleeding, epithelial cells, and other bacteria and their constituents.
4. VSCs are released into the oral environment where they mix with expired air and contribute to malodor.
5. VSCs might contribute to the pathogenesis of periodontitis because they have pathogenic potential on a variety of host cells and processes.
6. The plaque biofilm associated with periodontitis lesions lead bacteria to other oral sites, such as the tongue dorsum, where they colonize and contribute to the total oral malodor status.

Adapted from Newman M: The role of periodontitis in oral malodour: clinical perspectives. In van Steenberghe D, Rosenberg M, eds: *Bad breath: a multidisciplinary approach,* Leuven, Belgium, 1996, Leuven University Press, pp 3-14.

Diagnosis

Although nearly everyone experiences this condition at one time or another, the diagnostic science of oral malodor has been elusive. Clinical diagnostic tools are limited, with some of them testing for gram-negative anaerobic bacteria activity. Oral malodor management and detection has been a challenge for a variety of reasons, including lack of odor at the time of assessment. The best detecting *device* is the human nose, and developing a device that is as skilled and sensitive has continued to defy the research community. This type of assessment is subjective and can be uncomfortable for both the examiner and the subject. To complicate matters, self-perception of breath odor is not reliable because of self-odor acclimation.[16] Thus the practicality of chairside diagnostics remains unrealistic.

However, in research, the following diagnostic tools are used to assess treatment outcomes and evaluate products that are designed to eliminate oral malodor, including organoleptic judges, gas chromatography, microbiological assay, and sulfide-detection devices. With each of these methods, baseline measurements are taken and then used throughout the study to determine the effectiveness of a particular oral malodor–controlling agent or protocol.

The gold standard and most reliable oral malodor diagnostic is the **organoleptic** judge. These judges are specialized individuals who can discern the difference and quality of odor, based on an odor-intensity scale (Box 38-2), and who can provide the most consistent measurements and evaluation.[21] Unfortunately, even within this method, limitations exist.

Gas chromatography, a laboratory-based procedure, assesses for the presence of specific VSCs and, although reliable, is very costly[46] and still cannot 100% replicate the ability of the human nose.

Portable sulfide monitors are also available (Figure 38-3). However, these devices are more sensitive to hydrogen sulfide in mouth air than methyl mercaptan from crevicular air.[15,20,77] In addition, patients must refrain from consuming odor-related foods, oral hygiene, and wearing any fragrance before assessment.[14,32] Gas chromatography is more reliable than the sulfide-detecting device in terms of methyl mercaptan detection, the VSCs that are associated with periodontal infection.[20] VSC-detecting technology has also been incorporated into periodontal probes and tongue paddles.[36,73] However, these products did not succeed in the chairside marketplace.

The benzoyl-DL-arginine-naphthylamide (BANA) test evaluates specific sites for by-products from *Treponema denticola,*

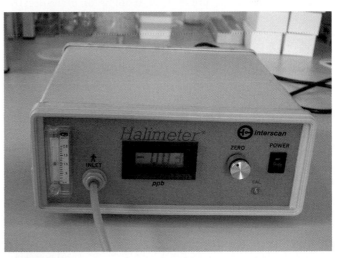

FIGURE 38-3
Portable sulfide monitor. (From Newman MG et al: *Carranza's Clinical Periodontology,* 10th ed, St Louis, 2006, Saunders.)

BOX 38-2

ORGANOLEPTIC INTENSITY SCALE

Rating	Odor Intensity
0	Absence of odor
1	Questionable to slight malodor
2	Slight malodor exceeding the threshold of malodor recognition
3	Moderate malodor; odor is definitely detected
4	Strong malodor
5	Severe malodor

Loesche WJ, Kazor C: Microbiology and treatment of halitosis, *Periodontol 2000* 28:256-279, 2002.

Porphyromonas gingivalis, and *Bacteroides forsythus.* This assay detects the enzymes from these bacteria that degrade BANA, a synthetic trypsin substrate. A positive BANA test determines not only the presence of periodontal associated bacteria but also the presence of VSC-producing flora.[30] This method is easily administered chairside, with the only limitation being the site of bacteria culturing and consistency for future testing.

These options leave little for clinical application, and no diagnostic tool for use by patients currently exists. The most reliable means for daily patient assessment is a trusted family member or friend, in essence, a trusted *nose.* Regardless of the lack of specific diagnostic tools being available for clinical practice, preventing the condition is something in which most dental patients are interested. With this fact in mind, clinicians should not get too discouraged with the lack of diagnostic tools and instead focus on educating patients on how to maintain fresh breath and improve overall oral health.

Clinical Management of Oral Malodor

The primary factors associated with oral malodor production include salivary flow; presence of biofilms or gram-negative anaerobic bacteria; the oral pH; and the presence of cellular protein, food debris, or any combination. These factors are indicative of manifestation of oral infections, particularly periodontal diseases. Therefore patient assessment should include consideration of these factors to develop a clinical protocol.[42] The goals of both clinical and daily management include the following[4]:

> *Note*
>
> The primary factors associated with oral malodor production include salivary flow; presence of biofilms or gram-negative anaerobic bacteria; the oral pH; and the presence of cellular protein, food debris, or any combination.

- Increase in salivary flow
- Elimination of gram-negative bacteria or biofilms from key intraoral niches
  - Posterior dorsum of the tongue
  - Sulcus or periodontal pockets
  - Tonsillar region
- Neutralization of VSCs

Clinical intervention begins with a careful review of the medical and dental history.

> *Note*
>
> Assessment of daily habits, including ingestion or use of fresh-breath–related products, will be essential in determining a patient's interest and awareness of oral malodor.

In many instances, patients treat their condition with sugar-containing products, which might be contributing to other dental disease processes, such as dental caries. Careful evaluation of medications and habits that may contribute to oral malodor via xerostomia and pH imbalance is also warranted.

The process should continue with an examination of oral tissues and a thorough periodontal examination, providing an excellent opportunity to initiate oral malodor education.

Oral lesions, tonsoliths, and restorations that trap food and bacteria are also common sources of oral malodor. The assessment should also include notation of the tongue coating to include the color, texture, and description of the coating. The tongue coating is an excellent example of a complex biofilm that has proven to contribute not only to oral malodor, but to periodontal disease as well.[31]

> *Patient Education Opportunity*
>
> During the periodontal examination, be sure to inform patients that probing depths greater then 4 mm will produce bad breath.

The clinical phase should continue to focus on removing plaque biofilm and bacteria via instrumentation.[37,55] Consideration for using VSC-neutralizing agents will assist in jump-starting the oral malodor–management regimen. Preprocedural and postprocedural rinsing with neutralizing agents will decrease VSCs, and irrigating with these agents will neutralize subgingival VSCs.[71] Irrigation is most effective through a powered scaling device and subgingival inserts. In addition, powered scaling devices will lead to thorough biofilm disruption and removal.

The next phase of clinical intervention involves tongue cleaning or deplaquing. Many clinicians choose to **deplaque** the tongue at the conclusion of the appointment while having patients observe the procedure (Figure 38-4). Although the patient observes the procedure, dialog should take place that emphasizes this oral hygiene method as one of the best to reduce malodor on a daily basis, as well as to reduce flora associated with periodontal infection.[6] Adding this procedure to instrumentation protocols is an important step in clinical management of oral malodor and for daily oral hygiene routines[37] (Figure 38-5).

The final phase of daily and clinical intervention includes neutralization of VSCs through postprocedural rinses. Agents known to neutralize VSCs include chlorhexidine, zinc, and chloride dioxide. Products that contain antimicrobial agents, as well as neutralizers, may be particularly effective in reducing malodor. Postprocedural rinsing is also a welcome finishing

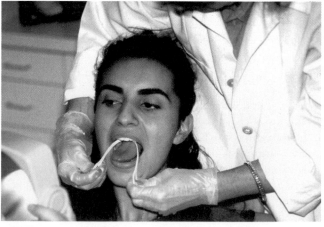

FIGURE 38-4
Clinical tongue deplaquing. The clinician completes the tongue deplaquing procedure while the patient observes. Dialog should include the fact that this procedure is one of the most effective ways to ensure daily fresh breath. (Courtesy Educational Designs.)

touch to the dental hygiene experience and will remove any debris resulting from the instrumentation process.

CLINICAL MANAGEMENT FOR PERIODONTAL DISEASE

For periodontal cases, clinicians should consider implementing full-mouth disinfection (FMD) or accelerated instrumentation-phased appointments, the latter of which is a process of accelerated treatment, which includes full-mouth instrumentation in two visits, within 24 hours, and use of chlorhexidine, which will eliminate malodor and fast-track aesthetic treatment plans, health and healing, and referral for further periodontal treatment, if necessary. Some studies assert that FMD is more effective over time than traditional quadrant scaling and root planing (four appointments with completion in 6 weeks), with the following outcomes:

- Gain in clinical attachment
- Greater reduction in probing depths
- Eradication of *P. gingivalis*
- Greater reduction in spirochetes and motile organisms subgingivally

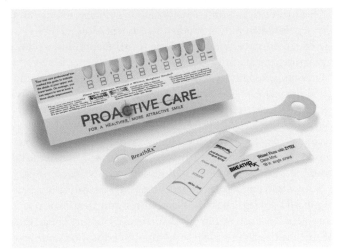

FIGURE 38-5
Clinical tools for chairside tongue deplaquing are an important part of completing the dental hygiene experience. (Courtesy Discus Dental, Culver City, Calif.)

BOX 38-3

PROPOSED CLINICAL PROTOCOL FOR ORAL MALODOR MANAGEMENT

The dental hygienist is in a key position to implement a patient-centered approach that addresses social considerations and ultimately improves oral health. The following represents a suggested process of care that includes integration of oral malodor assessment and treatment with traditional dental hygiene treatment protocols.

Assessment Phase
   I. Review medical history.
      Include questions regarding family history of systemic illnesses, xerostomia, or medications that contribute to oral malodor.
  II. Review current oral hygiene routine.
      Assess *real* time spent and tools used, as well as technique used.
 III. Determine current usage and frequency of usage of oral malodor–related products.
      Toothpaste: Note specific brand and times per day.
      Mouthrinse: Note specific brand, times per day, and amount of time rinsing.
      Breath mints: Note specific brand and times per day.
      Chewing gum: Note specific brand and times per day.
      Other: Note tongue gels, breath sprays, etc.
 IV. Perform oral cancer screening.
      • Note that oral lesions can emit odor.
  V. Perform comprehensive periodontal examination.
      Pocket depths of 4 mm or greater are more likely to produce VSCs.
 VI. Note the condition of the surface of the tongue.
      Tongue coating in periodontal patients is four to six times greater than normal.

 VII. Identify restorations, crowns, and bridges that need replacing. These plaque biofilm–retentive areas can produce oral malodor.
VIII. Note the presence of oral lesions and tonsilloliths.
      Tonsil stones have a malodor component.

Clinical Protocol
   I. Use preprocedural and postprocedural antibacterial mouthrinse to neutralize volatile sulfur compounds.
  II. Eliminate or reduce plaque biofilm and calculus for nonperiodontal cases. (Initiate full-mouth disinfection protocol for periodontal cases.)
     a. Use instrumentation as indicated.
     b. Perform subgingival irrigation to neutralize VSCs via automated scalers or other irrigation device.
     c. Remove remaining plaque biofilm from interproximal regions.
     d. Perform selective polishing as indicated.
     e. Perform tongue biofilm–deplaquing procedure using tongue scraper and antibacterial- or VSC-neutralizing agent.
 III. Evaluate for additional preventive care.
 IV. Instruct patient on daily care for fresh-breath maintenance, and make product recommendations.
  V. Schedule supportive care follow-up as indicated, and evaluate fresh-breath success.

VSCs, Volatile sulfur compounds.

• Greater reduction in oral malodor with the results being maintained 8 months after instrumentation[7,35,51,52]

The theory behind accelerated instrumentation includes preventing translocation of biofilms from sites that have yet to be instrumented or other intraoral niches retaining periopathogenic flora to one that has been instrumented, as well as assisting the immune response and healing.[28] Using chlorhexidine will also have an added benefit of VSC neutralization, which accounts for the immediate reduction in oral malodor. Suggested modifications to the protocol (Box 38-3) include using powered instrumentation and simultaneously administering VSC-neutralizing agents, tongue scraping versus brushing, using locally applied antibacterial agents,[66] and treatment phases completed at least within 1 week versus 24 hours.[5] Regardless of the health of the patient, oral malodor education and intervention is warranted and should be an integral part of every preventive appointment.

✷✷ CASE APPLICATION 38-1.3

Identifying Opportunities to Discuss Oral Malodor

Consider the clinical protocols you would implement in Ms. Miller's case and why. Identify opportunities during the appointment that would be suited for discussion about oral malodor and its origins.

Mechanical and Chemotherapeutic Oral Malodor Management

The cornerstone to reducing oral malodor begins with daily mechanical plaque biofilm control to remove odor-producing biofilms and with chemotherapeutics to affect flora and neutralize VSC odor. This protocol can be easily implemented along with that of general oral health maintenance. It can provide an increased opportunity for patient compliance over the traditional disease motivation model. Recommendations from dental hygienists should include strategies that incorporate daily mechanics combined with use of chemotherapeutics to neutralize VSCs and control gram-negative flora. In addition, patients should be advised of methods to maximize salivary flow.

The simplicity of managing and eliminating oral malodor is directly related to oral hygiene strategies with which many patients are already familiar. Daily use of a toothbrush, interdental cleaning tools, a tongue cleaner, and agents to neutralize VSCs may provide desired results and affect overall oral health.

MODIFYING TRADITIONAL PLAQUE BIOFILM–CONTROL STRATEGIES

Given that the average amount of time that patients spend on oral hygiene routines is 24 to 60 seconds,[11] methods that can be used to be more effective within this span of time are critical for optimal oral health. The opportunity to enhance compliance lies in oral malodor reduction to thorough daily oral hygiene practices with traditional toothbrushing and interdental care. Additionally, consideration should include using automated toothbrushes and flossers. Automated plaque biofilm–removal devices provide a safe and effective means for plaque biofilm removal that does not require much skill on the part of the user (see Chapter 24).

TONGUE CLEANING

Oral malodor reduction includes not only traditional plaque biofilm–removal strategies but tongue cleaning as well. Daily removal of the tongue coating will not only reduce oral malodor and produce a cleaner tongue but may also reduce periodontal-related bacteria[32,72] (see Figure 38-1; Figure 38-6).

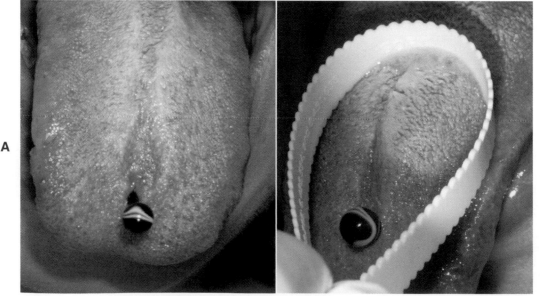

FIGURE 38-6
A, Coating is noted on this pierced tongue. **B,** Gentle scraping of the tongue can remove bacteria and by-products from the oral cavity. Tongue deplaquing is easily accomplished with the appropriate tool. (Courtesy Michelle Hurlbutt, RDH, BS.)

The history of modern tongue-cleaning devices dates back to 1794, and these devices were in great demand. In 1920, researchers recommended that tongue cleaning take place in the morning on an empty stomach and as part of daily oral hygiene practices to reduce oral flora and bad breath.[12] Research today demonstrates that cleaning the surface of the tongue with a tongue scraper is more effective than using a toothbrush. Devices that are specifically designed for deplaquing the tongue have proven effective, easy, and safe for patients to use while eliminating bacteria and by-products from the oral cavity.[13,64,72] A recent study demonstrates that cleaning the tongue with a toothbrush resulted in 45% reduction of VSCs, whereas cleaning with a plastic scraper reduced VSCs by 75%.[47] In addition, recent data show that persons using tongue scrapers have an improvement in taste after 2 weeks.[50]

A combination of tongue cleaning and using VSC-neutralizing agents such as zinc-containing compounds[40,60] may result in extended malodor reduction. Following are special considerations regarding cleaning the tongue:

- Patients should be instructed chairside (Box 38-4) while observing the procedure (Figure 38-7) or the process with the specific device they will be using.

BOX 38-4

TONGUE DEPLAQUING PROCEDURE

1. With the patient observing the procedure, have the patient extend his or her tongue and place an antibacterial agent to the surface of the tongue.
2. Apply light pressure and place the tongue-cleaning device as far posterior on the surface of the tongue as possible.
3. Gently move the cleaning device forward and remove the tongue coating or debris via suction or 2- × 2-inch gauze square. Repeat as needed.
4. Take the opportunity to explain that this process will help reduce oral malodor when implemented on a daily basis.

- Tongue cleaning with a tongue-cleaning device should take place at least daily and even more frequently for people with a heavier tongue coating.
- Morning deplaquing may be easier for patients who are prone to gagging; some patients even complete the procedure in the shower.
- Tongue cleaners come in all shapes and sizes, from simple blade styles to automatic devices (Figure 38-8), and selection should be based on patient need and preference.
- This procedure alone will dramatically improve oral malodor and may generate great interest and motivation for patients.

CHEMOTHERAPEUTIC AGENTS

Active ingredients to reduce oral malodor can be found in mouthrinses, toothpastes, tongue gels and sprays, and chewing gum or mints. Avoiding sugar-containing products will be important for obvious reasons, and avoiding habits that dry the oral cavity will also assist in reducing oral malodor. Chlorhexidine,[56,69,79] chlorine dioxide,[19,65] cetylpyridinium chloride (CPC),[29,44] zinc,[10,64,78-80] essential oils,[17,48] triclosan,[45,68,81] or a combination of these agents[8,56,57] is used to combat oral malodor, as well as to promote gingival health. Zinc is particularly effective in neutralizing VSC because zinc ions have a strong affinity for the thiol groups that are present in VSCs, which render them nonmalodorous by converting them to nonvolatile sulfides.[62,74] Box 38-5 reviews the mechanism of action and the impact on breath odor for each of these agents. Selection of products should be based on patient needs and compliance.

Regardless of agent selection, patients will be interested in the various *vehicle* options, such as toothpaste, tongue sprays, and mouthrinses. Pairing the patient with the appropriate agent and delivery option will lead to successful treatment (Figure 38-9).

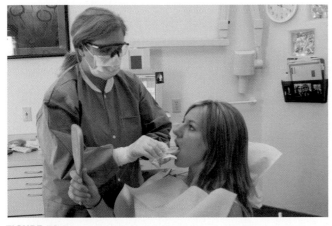

FIGURE 38-7
An alternative method for tongue deplaquing procedure—regardless of the method used, the patient observes the process. (Courtesy Michelle Hurlbutt, RDH, BS.)

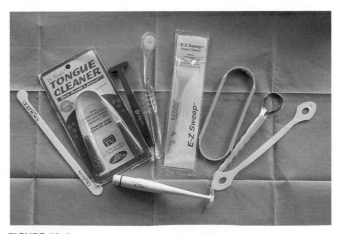

FIGURE 38-8
Various tongue-cleaning oral hygiene aids are available and more effective in reducing oral flora and malodor than toothbrushes. (Courtesy Educational Designs, San Ramon, Calif.)

BOX 38-5

ACTIVE AGENTS FOR NEUTRALIZING VOLATILE SULFUR COMPOUNDS AND CONTROLLING GRAM-NEGATIVE ORAL FLORA

- Zinc: recognized and effective VSC-neutralizing agent
- Essential oils: recognized antimicrobial agents affecting VSC-producing organisms
- Chlorhexidine gluconate: broad-spectrum antimicrobial agent that also neutralizes VSCs
- Chlorine dioxide: recognized VSC-neutralizing agent
- Cetylpyridinium chloride: recognized mild antimicrobial agent affecting VSC-producing organisms
- Triclosan: recognized mild antimicrobial agent affecting VSC-producing organisms
- Combination of these agents to achieve antimicrobial and VSC-neutralizing results (i.e., for oral malodor control, an antimicrobial agent and neutralizing agent; products that combine agents for optimal oral malodor control)

VSCs, Volatile sulfur compounds.

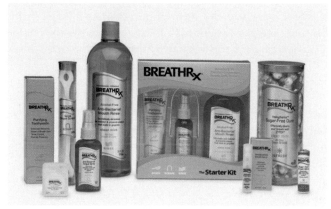

FIGURE 38-9
The BreathRx product line combines mechanical tools with chemotherapeutics. This alcohol-free system uses cetylpyridinium chloride to affect odor-producing bacteria and zinc to neutralize VSCs. (Courtesy Discus Dental, Culver City, Calif.)

METHODS TO INCREASE SALIVARY FLOW

Many situations can cause decreased salivary flow, which results in xerostomia and an increase in oral malodor.[27] Medications, medical conditions, and various oral habits can lead to dry mouth or reduced salivary flow.[25] Not only will oral malodor be more prevalent in this population but also other oral health concerns arise, including the potential for an increase in decay. As a result, methods to increase salivary flow warrant consideration and include recommending use of saliva substitutes, in-creasing intake of water, and chewing sugar-free gum or mints. Chewing gum or mints should be sugar free and preferably contain xylitol, which is known to affect bacteria associated with dental caries. In addition, products containing zinc will be beneficial in neutralizing VSC.[74] Avoiding alcohol-based mouthrinses is recommended to circumvent potential increase in oral malodor conditions.[40] In addition, alcohol-based mouthrinses have been reported to desiccate the oral mucosa and worsen xerostomic symptoms.[22] Alcohol-free mouthrinses, which also include active ingredients to neutralize VSCs and combat bacteria growth, are readily available and indicated for people who should avoid alcohol-containing products or those who prefer these formulations (go to the Evolve site http://evolve.elsevier.com/Daniel/ to see Table 38-1).

Patient Education

Integration of oral malodor education and management into the dental hygiene appointment is an integral part of overall oral health and addresses patient-centered concerns. Although this condition can be uncomfortable to discuss for both the dental hygienist and the patient, simple strategies are available that, when used, provide a professional method for frank discussion. Box 38-6 outlines the various opportunities for oral malodor education and discussion.

Additionally, patients rely on clinicians for clear and concise information and suggestions for reducing oral malodor. Box 38-7 outlines the basic oral hygiene strategies and recommendations that can be suggested. These suggestions, combined with basic oral malodor facts as outlined in Box 38-8, will provide clinicians ample justification and resources to discuss oral malodor effectively and comfortably. Figure 38-10 is a diagram of a tongue cleaner used to remove oral debris. This can be used as an educational tool to demonstrate the efficacy of tongue deplaquing to patients.

BOX 38-6

DISCUSSING ORAL MALODOR DURING THE DENTAL HYGIENE EXPERIENCE

- Assess use of oral malodor–related products.
- Correlate probing depth of more than 4 mm with oral malodor.
- Deplaque the tongue, and *show* patients the biofilm or tongue coating substance.
- Use positive dialog (maintain fresh breath versus eliminate bad breath).

BOX 38-7

ORAL HYGIENE RECOMMENDATIONS FOR REDUCTION OF ORAL MALODOR

- Use automated toothbrushes.
- Use automated interdental devices.
- Use active agent–impregnated floss.
- Use tongue scrapers and deplaquing devices combined with antibacterial tongue gels or sprays.
- Use neutralizing agent–containing toothpastes; also mouthrinses, mints, chewing gum, and other vehicle options.
- Avoid sugar-containing chewing gum, mints, or lozenges; instead, use items containing xylitol or other active ingredients such as zinc.
- Maintain regular professional dental hygiene care and intervention.

✴ CASE APPLICATION 38-1.4

Self-Care Oral Hygiene Strategies

What oral hygiene strategies would you recommend for Ms. Miller, and why? How would you use these recommendations to improve Ms. Miller's oral hygiene compliance? What terminology would you incorporate to convey a positive message regarding oral malodor management?

BOX 38-8

ORAL MALODOR FACTS

- You get to wear a mask at work; your patients do not!
- The billion-dollar bad-breath industry is an indicator that patients are self-diagnosing, self-treating, and willing to spend money for fresh breath.
- Tongue deplaquing at every dental hygiene visit is the most effective means to *show* patients their bad breath and involve them in their oral care.
- Probing depths greater than 4 mm produce VSCs or bad breath.
- More than 80% of malodor is oral in nature.
- Patients *accept* oral malodor assessment by the dental profession.
- Social factors are the primary motivation behind all successful hygiene routines.
- Many breath control products contain sugar and may increase the chance for other oral diseases.
- Daily tongue deplaquing is one of the most effective means to maintain fresh breath.
- Full-mouth disinfection protocol reduces bad breath over standard scaling and root planing protocols.

VSCs, Volatile sulfur compounds.

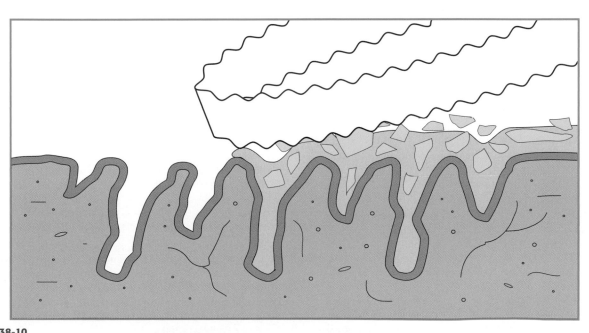

FIGURE 38-10
Illustrates the anatomical structures on the dorsum of the tongue and the removal of debris using a tongue scraper.

Considerations and Future Trends

Dental hygienists must focus on methods to improve oral health via patient-centered approaches. Considering quality-of-life parameters will empower dental hygienists in assisting patients in achieving optimal oral health.[41] Studies have begun to evaluate the correlation between successful oral hygiene routines and social-related factors such as oral malodor. Although challenging to establish through long-term research, patient-centered approaches will undoubtedly result in higher success rates in periodontal therapy and ultimately overall well-being.

The considerable impact of oral malodor on daily life has been acknowledged by many sources, and, as evidenced by the clinics specifically designed to treat the condition, interest exists on the part of consumers. Oral malodor can be treated in traditional practice settings, and the process begins with frank discussion, education, and correlation with existing oral conditions. Thus dental hygienists who incorporate oral malodor strategies are meeting a long-unmet need by consumers.

Because oral malodor has proven to be an elusive condition to research and a topic that is uncomfortable for clinicians to broach, few credible resources exist on which to rely. Nonetheless, in 2003, the American Dental Association (ADA) established research guidelines to provide a structure on which products used in the management of oral malodor can be considered for ADA acceptance.[2] As such, future research will undoubtedly continue and has finally garnered the appropriate professional acknowledgement as a condition that is important to oral health. However, current evidence is sufficient to warrant clinical integration of oral malodor management. This concept represents a patient-centered approach that will provide new motivation for thorough daily oral hygiene routines. Additionally, science has supported these methods as a means to prevent oral malodor and promote oral health. Prevention is the cornerstone of dental hygiene practice, and integration of oral malodor strategies complements traditional clinical protocols.[1,59]

References

1. American Dental Association, Council on Scientific Affairs: Association report: oral malodor, *J Am Dent Assoc* 134:209-214, 2003.
2. American Dental Association, Council on Scientific Affairs: *Acceptance program guidelines—products used in the management of oral malodor,* Chicago, 2003, The Association, pp 1-11.
3. American Dental Hygienists' Association, policy glossary definition, pp 1-99.
4. Bernie KM: Continuing education: advancing the art and science of dental hygiene through oral malodor management, *Contemporary Oral Hyg* 4(4):20-26, 2004.
5. Bernie KM: Full-mouth disinfection: an overview of research and clinical application, *Hygiene Report* May 2001, pp 10-13.
6. Bernie KM: Marketing memo tips for success: oral malodor assessment and management: a patient-centered approach, *J Pract Hyg* 8(2):9, 1999.
7. Bollen CML et al: The effect of a one stage full-mouth disinfection on different intra-oral niches—clinical and microbiological observations, *J Clin Periodontol* 25:56-66, 1998.
8. Borden L et al: The effect of four mouthrinses on oral malodor, *Compendium* 23(6):531-546, 2002.
9. Bosy A et al: Relationship of oral malodor to periodontitis: evidence of independence in discrete subpopulations, *J Peridontal* 65(1):37-46, 1994.
10. Bruette DM et al: Effects of methyl mercaptan on human gingival fibroblast shape, cytoskeleton and protein synthesis and the inhibition of its effect by zinc. In van Steenberghe D, Rosenberg M, eds: *Bad breath: a multidisciplinary approach,* Leuven, Belgium, 1996, Leuvan University Press.
11. Cancro LP, Fischman SL: The expected effect on oral health of dental plaque control through mechanical removal, *Periodontal 2000* 8:60-74, 1995.
12. Christen AG, Swanson BZ: Oral hygiene: a history of tongue scraping and brushing, *J Am Dent Assoc* 96:215-219, 1978.
13. Christensen G: Why clean your tongue? *J Am Dent Assoc* 129(11):1605-1607, 1998.
14. Clark GT, Nachnani S, Messagi DV: Detecting and treating oral and non-oral malodors, *J Calif Dent Assoc* 25(2):133-145, 1997.
15. Coil JM: Characterization of volatile sulphur compounds production at individual crevicular sites. In van Steenberghe D, Rosenberg M, eds: *Bad breath: a multidisciplinary approach,* Leuven, Belgium, 1996, Leuven University Press, pp 29-34.
16. Eli I et al: Self-perception of breath odor, *J Am Dent Assoc* 132:621-626, 2001.
17. Fine DH et al: In vivo antimicrobial effectiveness of an essential oil-containing mouth rinse 12 h after a single use and 14 days' use, *J Clin Periodontol* 32:335-340, 2005.
18. Finkelstein Y: The otolaryngologist and the patient with halitosis. In Rosenberg M, ed: *Bad breath: research perspectives,* Tel Aviv, Israel, 1995, Ramot Publishing, Tel Aviv University.
19. Frascella J, Gilbert R, Fernandex P: Odor reduction potential of a chlorine dioxide mouthrinse, *J Clin Dent* 11(2):39-42, 1998.
20. Furne J et al: Comparison of volatile sulfur compounds concentrations measured with a sulfide detector vs gas chromatography, *J Dent Res* 81:140-143, 2002.
21. Greenman J et al: Assessing the relationship between concentrations of malodor compounds and odor scores from judges, *J Am Dent Assoc* 136:749-757, 2005.
22. Guggenheimer J, Moore, PA: Xerostomia: etiology, recognition and treatment, *J Am Dent Assoc* 134:61-69, 2003.
23. Hinode D et al: Relationship between tongue coating and secretory-immunoglobulin A level in saliva obtained from patients complaining of oral malodor, *J Clin Periodontol* 30(12):1017-1023, 2003.
24. Kazro CE, Mitchell PM, Lee AM: Diversity of bacterial populations on the tongue dorsa of patients with halitosis and healthy patients, *J Clin Micro* 41:558-563, 2003.
25. Kleinberg I, Codipilly M: The biological basis of oral malodor formation. In Rosenberg M, ed: *Bad breath: research perspectives,* Tel Aviv, Israel, 1995, Ramot Publishing, Tel Aviv University.
26. Klokkevold P: Oral malodor: a periodontal perspective *J Calif Dent Assoc* 24(2):153-159, 1997.
27. Koshimune S et al: Low salivary flow and volatile sulfur compounds in mouth air, *Oral Surg Oral Med Oral Pathol Oral Radiol Endod* 96:38-41, 2003.
28. Koshy G, Esmonde F, Ishikawa C: A full-mouth disinfection approach to nonsurgical periodontal therapy—prevention of rein-

fection from bacterial reservoirs, *Periodontol 2000* 36:166-178, 2004.

29. Kozlovsky A et al: Efficacy of a 2-phase oil:water mouthrinse in controlling oral malodor, gingivitis, and plaque, *J Periodontal* 67:577-582, 1996.

30. Kozlovsky A et al: Correlation between BANA test and oral malodor parameters, *J Dent Res* 73:1036-1042, 1994.

31. Loesche W, De Boever E: Strategies to identify the main microbial contributors to oral malodor. In van Steenberghe D, Rosenberg M, eds: *Bad breath: research perspectives,* Tel Aviv, Israel, 1995, Ramot Publishing, Tel Aviv University, pp 41-54.

32. Loesche WJ, Kazor C: Microbiology and treatment of halitosis, *Periodontol 2000* 28:256-279, 2002.

33. McNamara TF, Alexander JF, Lee M: The role of microorganisms in the production of oral malodor, *Oral Surg Oral Med Oral Pathol Oral Radiol Endod* 34:41-48, 1972.

34. Miyazaki H, Fujita IS, Takehara T: Relationship between volatile sulphur compounds and oral conditions in the general Japanese population. In van Steenberghe D, Rosenberg M, eds: *Bad breath: a multidisciplinary approach,* Leuven, Belgium, 1996, Leuven University Press, pp 165-178.

35. Mongardidi C et al: One stage full- versus partial-mouth disinfection in the treatment of chronic adult or early-onset periodontitis: I—long term clinical observations. *J Periodontol* 70:632-645, 1999.

36. Morita M, Musinski DL, Wang HL: Assessment of newly developed tongue sulfide probe for detecting oral malodor, *J Clin Periodontol* 28:494-496, 2001.

37. Morita M, Wang HL: Effects of periodontal therapy on sulcular/tongue sulfide level: a pilot study, *J Clin Periodontol* 29:844-847, 2002.

38. Morita M, Wang HL: Association between oral malodor and adult periodontitis: a review, *J Clin Periodontol* 28:813-819, 2001.

39. Morita M, Wang HL: Relationship between sulcular sulfide level and oral malodor in subjects with periodontal disease, *J Periodonol* 72(1):79-84, 2001.

40. Nacnani S: The effects of oral rinses on halitosis, *J Calif Dent Assoc* 24(2):145-150, 1997.

41. Needleman I et al: Impact of oral health of the life quality of periodontal patients, *J Clin Periodontol* 31:454-457, 2004.

42. Newman M: The role of periodontitis in oral malodour: clinical perspectives. In van Steenberghe D, Rosenberg M, eds: *Bad breath: a multidisciplinary approach,* Leuven, Belgium, 1996, Leuven University Press, pp 3-14.

43. Ng W, Tonzetich J: Effect of hydrogen sulfide and methyl mercaptan on the permeability of oral mucosa, *J Dent Res* 63(7):37-46, 1984.

44. Niles HP, Gaffar A: Advances in mouth odor research. In van Steenberghe D, Rosenberg M, eds: *Bad breath: research perspectives,* Tel Aviv, Israel, 1995, Ramot Publishing, Tel Aviv University.

45. Nogueria-Filho GR et al: Effect of triclosan dentifrices on mouth volatile sulphur compounds and dental plaque trypsin-like activity during experimental gingivitis development, *J Clin Periodontol* 29:1059-1064, 2002.

46. Oho T et al: Characteristics of patients complaining of halitosis and the usefulness of gas chromatography for diagnosing halitosis, *Oral Surg Oral Med Oral Pathol Oral Radiol Endod* 91:531-534, 2001.

47. Pedrazzi V et al: Tongue-cleaning methods: a comparative clinical trial employing a toothbrush and tongue scraper, *J Periodontol* 75(7):1009-1012, 2001.

48. Pitts G et al: Mechanism of action of antiseptic, anti-odor mouthwash, *J Dent Res* 62(6):738-742, 1983.

49. Pruet CW, Duplan DA: Tonsil concretions and tonsilloliths, *Otolaryngol Clin North Am* 20:305-309, 1987.

50. Quirynen M et al: Impact of tongue cleansers on microbial load and taste, *J Clin Periodontol* 31:506-510, 2004.

51. Quirynen M et al: The role of chlorhexidine in the one-stage full-mouth disinfection treatment of patients with advanced adult periodontitis: long-term clinical and microbiological observations, *J Clin Periodontol* 27:578-589, 2000.

52. Quirynen M et al: Full-mouth versus partial-mouth disinfection in the treatment of periodontal infections, *J Dent Res* 74: 1459-1467, 1995.

53 Ratcliff PA, Johnson P: The relationship between oral malodor, gingivitis, and periodontitis: a review, *J Periodontol* 70(5): 485-489, 1999.

54. Ratkay LG, Tonzeitich J, Waterfield JD: The effect of methyl mercaptan on enzymatic and immunological activity leading to periodontal tissue destruction. In van Steenberghe D, Rosenberg M, eds: *Bad breath: a multidisciplinary approach,* Leuven, Belgium, 1996, Leuven University Press, pp 35-45.

55. Roldan S et al: A combined therapeutic approach to manage oral halitosis: a 3-month prospective case series, *J Periodontol* 76(6):1025-1033, 2005.

56. Roldan S et al: Comparative effects of different chlorhexidine mouth-rinse formulations of volatile sulphur compounds and salivary bacterial counts, *J Clin Periodontol* 31:1128-1134, 2004.

57. Roldan S, Winkel EG, Herrera D: The effects of a new mouthrinse containing chlorhexidine, cetylpyridinium chloride and zinc lactate on the microflora of oral halitosis patients: a dual-centre, double-blind placebo-controlled study, *J Clin Periodontol* 30: 427-434, 2003.

58 Rosenberg M: The science of bad breath, *Sci Am* 286(4):72-79, 2002.

59. Rosenberg M: Consensus report 1: the clinical approach to breath malodour. In van Steenberghe D, Rosenberg M, eds: *Bad breath: a multidisciplinary approach,* Leuven, Belgium, 1996, Leuvan University Press, p 285.

60. Rosenberg M et al: Bad breath: research perspectives. In *Advances in mouth odor research,* Tel Aviv, Israel, 1995, Ramot Publishing, Tel Aviv University, pp 55-69.

61. Rosenberg M, Leib E: Experiences of an Israeli malodor clinic. In van Steenberghe D, Rosenberg M, eds: *Bad breath: research perspectives,* Tel Aviv, Israel, 1995, Ramot Publishing, Tel Aviv University.

62. Schmidt NF, Missan SR, Target WJ: The correlation between organoleptic mouth-odor ratings and levels of volatile sulfur compounds, *Oral Surg Oral Med Oral Pathol Oral Radiol Endod* 45:560-567, 1978.

63. Scully G et al: Breath odor: etiopathogenesis, assessment and management, *Euro J Oral Sci* 105:287-293, 1997.

64. Seemann R et al: Effectiveness of mechanical tongue cleaning on oral levels of volatile sulfur compounds, *J Am Dent Assoc* 132: 1263-1267, 2001.

65. Silwood CJL, Grootveld MC, Lynch E: A multifactorial investigation of the ability of oral health care products to alleviate oral malodour, *J Clin Periodontol* 28:634-641, 2001.

66. Slots J, Jorgensen MG: Effective, safe, practical and affordably periodontal antimicrobial therapy: where are we going, and are we there yet? *Periodontal 2000* 28:106-176, 2002.

67. Socransky SS et al: Checkerboard DNA-DNA hybridization, *Biotechniques* 17:789-792, 1994.
68. Sreenivasan P: The effects of a triclosan/copolymer dentifrice on oral bacteria including those producing hydrogen sulfide, *Eur J Oral Sci* 111:223-227, 2003.
69. Sreenivasan PK, Gittins E: Effects of low dose chlorhexidine mouthrinses on oral bacteria and salivary microflora including those producing hydrogen sulfide, *Oral Microbiol Immunol* 19:309-313, 2004.
70. Tonzetich J: Production and origin of malodor: a review of mechanisms and methods of analysis, *J Periodontol* 48:13-20, 1977.
71. Tonzetich J: Direct gas chromatographic analysis of sulphur compounds in mouth air in man, *Arch Oral Biol* 16:587-597, 1971.
72. Tonzetich J, Ng SK: Reduction of malodor by oral cleansing procedures, *Oral Surg Oral Med Oral Pathol* 42:172-181, 1976.
73. Torresyap G et al: Relationship between periodontal pocket sulfide levels and subgingival species, *J Clin Periodontol* 30:1003-1010, 2003.
74. Waler SM: The effect of zinc-containing chewing gum on volatile sulfur-containing compounds in the oral cavity, *Acta Odontol Scand* 55:198-200, 1997.
75. Yaegaki, K: Oral malodor and periodontal disease. In van Steenberghe D, Rosenberg M, eds: *Bad breath: research perspectives,* Tel Aviv, Israel, 1995, Ramot Publishing, Tel Aviv University.
76. Yaegaki K, Sanada K: Biochemical and clinical factors influencing oral malodor in periodontal patients, *J Periodontol* 63(9):783-789, 1992.
77. Yaegaki K, Sanada K: Volatile sulfur compounds in mouth air from clinically healthy subjects and patients with periodontal disease, *J Periodontol Res* 27:233-238, 1992.
78. Young A et al: Effects of metal salts on the oral production of volatile sulfur containing compounds VSC, *J Clin Periodontol* 28:776-781, 2001.
79. Young A, Jonski G, Rolla G: Inhibition of orally produced volatile sulfur compounds by zinc, chlorhexidine or cetylpyridinium chloride–effect of concentration, *Eur J Oral Sci* 111:400-404, 2003.
80. Young AR, Jonski G, Rolla G: The oral anti-volatile sulfur compound effects of zinc salts and their stability constants, *Eur J Oral Sci* 110:31-34, 2002.
81. Young A, Jonski G, Rolla G: A study of triclosan and its solubilizers as inhibitors of oral malodor, *J Clin Periodontol* 29:1078-1081, 2002.

Emergency Management of Dental Trauma

Dennis N. Ranalli • Deborah Studen-Pavlovich

INSIGHT

Dental hygienists have the knowledge and skill to recognize dental and nondental conditions that place a child or adult at risk for oral trauma. Dental hygienists can help expand the scope of trauma prevention and, through recognition of trauma, can prevent future occurrences to a victim.

CASE STUDY 39-1   Sports-Related Dental Trauma

Tonya Washington, a 16-year-old junior point guard, will be starting in her first high school varsity basketball game. In her excitement about the upcoming competition, Tonya is focused and intense during the last practice before the start of the season. Tonya dribbles the ball down court and sees an opening for a shot. She stops and takes a jump shot from the top of the key. Tonya follows the shot to the basket and leaps for the rebound when the ball glances off the rim. As she comes down with the ball, the elbow of a taller teammate strikes Tonya in the mouth. Tonya is not wearing a mouthguard.

Tonya's right maxillary permanent central incisor is completely knocked out of the socket from the force of the trauma in a lingual to labial direction. The tooth flies out of Tonya's mouth and skids across the floor. Tonya drops down to her knees, hands clutching her mouth, as blood oozes from between her fingers and drips onto the floor. The coach rushes over to Tonya with ice wrapped in a towel and applies the compress over Tonya's mouth. Her teammates search for Tonya's **avulsed tooth** and find it under the team bench. The coach takes Tonya into the locker room and contacts Tonya's mother to inform her about the accident and to advise her to contact Tonya's dentist for an emergency appointment immediately.

KEY TERMS

apexification	child abuse	luxation	orofacial trauma
apexogenesis	crown elongation	mouthguards	prevalence
avulsed tooth	dental neglect	neglect	triage
battered child syndrome	incidence		

LEARNING OUTCOMES

After reading this chapter the student will be able to:
1. Discuss the epidemiologic and etiologic factors of dental trauma.
2. Perform appropriate physical and oral assessments of traumatized dental patients.
3. Describe appropriate protocols for emergency management or referral of patients with dental injuries.
4. Outline proper documentation for traumatized dental patients.
5. Understand strategies for the prevention of orofacial trauma, with particular emphasis on child abuse and sports-related dental injuries.

Dental hygienists have been at the forefront of efforts to promote the prevention of dental caries and periodontal diseases. Despite recent evidence indicating almost one fourth of the U.S. population has experienced a traumatic dental episode to an anterior tooth, prevention of dental trauma has received little emphasis by the dental team. This chapter presents specific concepts to assist the dental hygienist in incorporating strategies for preventing dental trauma into a comprehensive program. The discussion focuses on the diagnosis and emergency management of dental injuries in children and adolescents. The emphasis is on the prevention, recognition, and reporting of **orofacial trauma** associated with child abuse and neglect, as well as the prediction, treatment, and prevention of sports-related dental injuries. Dental hygienists can help expand the scope of trauma prevention from the private-practice setting into community activities to reach larger segments of the at-risk population.

Epidemiology

Traumatic dental injuries pose serious consequences, not only in terms of the pain, suffering, and financial burdens associated with emergency management and long-term treatment, but also as a significant dental public health issue. One study of a large sample population reported that nearly one quarter (24.9%) of the U.S. population between 6 and 50 years of age had experienced dental trauma to one or more anterior teeth. The study confirmed that maxillary anterior teeth were more prone to injury than their mandibular counterparts. In addition, men and boys were more prone to dental injuries than women and girls by a ratio of 1.5 to 1.0. No racial or ethnic factors were found to be significant when considering such injuries.[26]

Evaluating this type of data from the scientific dental literature requires clarification of two terms that are often misused—incidence and prevalence. These terms are sometimes used interchangeably but have different meanings. **Incidence** refers to the number of new cases of trauma that occur during a specific time interval. **Prevalence** refers to the number of cases of trauma that exist at a given moment in time. Thus the information presented in the previous example represents trauma prevalence data.

Developmental Etiology

The developmental etiology of traumatic dental injuries varies according to the patient's chronologic age, level of activity, and state of maturity. For example, the most frequent and often-devastating type of trauma to the primary dentition is the intrusive **luxation** of a primary anterior tooth (Figure 39-1). Toddlers who are learning to walk are especially prone to intrusive luxations because primary anterior teeth are small, and immature alveolar bone is relatively soft. Conversely, the most frequent type of dental injury to the permanent dentition is a crown fracture because permanent anterior teeth are larger, and mature alveolar bone is denser (Figure 39-2). Dental injuries

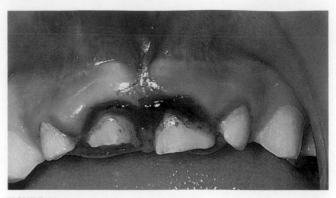

FIGURE 39-1
Intrusive luxation of maxillary primary central incisors.

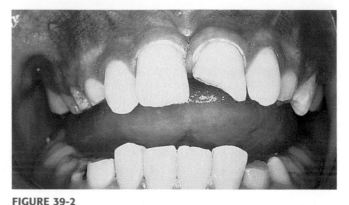

FIGURE 39-2
Enamel-dentin fracture of maxillary left permanent central incisor.

associated with child abuse are more likely in the primary dentition of young children, whereas sports-related trauma is more likely in the mixed or permanent dentitions of adolescents and young adults.

The developmental period between the primary and the permanent dentition phases is a time of significant change as a growing child progresses through the adolescent years toward adulthood. During these developmental periods, the resorption and exfoliation of the primary teeth are accompanied by the timing and sequence of eruption of the permanent teeth until the adult dental occlusion has been established. The child first progresses from the primary dentition to the mixed dentition. The *ugly duckling* stage is the period from the eruption of the permanent lateral incisors to the eruption of the permanent canines (Figure 39-3). During this stage, unesthetic space may develop between the maxillary permanent central incisors, and the crowns of the maxillary permanent lateral incisors may flare. When the maxillary permanent canines do erupt, anterior spacing generally closes, and tooth alignment becomes more esthetic.

Other factors, such as genetics, tooth size, arch length, skeletal growth, and oral habits, also contribute to the ultimate occlusion in the adult permanent dentition. *Occlusion* can be classified broadly as Class I, II, or III based on the molar relationship of the maxillary permanent first molar to the mandibular permanent first molar. *Class I molar relationship* is characterized by the mesial cusp of the maxillary permanent

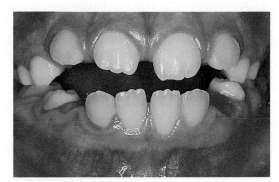

FIGURE 39-3
Ugly duckling stage of mixed dentition.

first molar in occlusal alignment with the buccal groove of the mandibular permanent first molar. *Class II molar relationship* is characterized by the occlusion of the mesial cusp of the maxillary permanent first molar anterior to the buccal groove of the mandibular permanent first molar. This type of molar relationship may be accompanied by protrusion of the maxillary anterior teeth with lack of a protective lip seal. This situation is known as an *accident-prone dental profile* and places the patient at increased risk for dental injury (Figure 39-4). Conversely, *Class III molar relationship* is characterized by the mesial cusp of the maxillary permanent first molar positioned posterior to the buccal groove of the mandibular permanent first molar. When a protruding mandible accompanies a Class III molar relationship, the mandibular arch is increasingly vulnerable to dental trauma.

In summary, a variety of factors place an individual at risk for a traumatic dental injury, including the following:

- Age
- Gender
- Occlusal development
- Vulnerability to abusive behavior
- Level of activity (e.g., learning to walk, participating in sports)

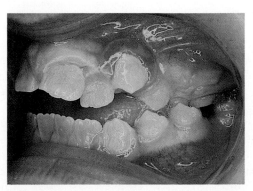

FIGURE 39-4
Accident-prone dental profile of a patient with marked gingival inflammation and dentinogenesis imperfecta.

Sports-Related Injury

39-5
39-6

39-7
39-8

RISK ASSESSMENT

The dental hygienist is in a key position to identify patients who may be at risk for sustaining sports-related dental trauma. In addition to questions related to brushing, flossing, and dietary habits on the dental intake form, the dental hygienist should include the question, "Do you (Does your child) participate in sports?" A positive response allows a detailed discussion of the type of sport, level of participation, and appropriate recommendations for protective athletic equipment.[50]

PREDICTIVE INDEX

To enable clinicians to determine better the likelihood of a patient experiencing a sports-related dental injury, a predictive index has been developed.[22] The predictive index is based on a defined set of risk factors, as discussed previously. The index identifies risk factors in eight categories:

- Demographic information (e.g., age, gender, dental occlusion)
- Type and use of protective equipment
- Velocity and intensity of the sport
- Level of activity and exposure time
- Level of coaching and type of sports organization
- Player position in a contact or noncontact sport
- History of sports-related dental trauma
- Practice or game situation

An analysis of these factors can be used to identify an athlete who is at high risk for an orofacial injury and, more importantly, to recommend specific prevention strategies, such as a properly fitted athletic mouthguard.

ASSESSMENT OF THE TRAUMA PATIENT

Physical Assessment

Before initiating dental treatment, determining the physical status of the trauma victim is essential. The dental injury may be relatively minor compared with a serious head injury. Thus the patient should undergo individual **triage** so that the most serious problems are prioritized for immediate attention. As a first priority, the need for basic life support must be determined. Any life-threatening injury requires activation of the local emergency medical services system. Patients should be observed for signs of shock, and, when required, airway management, breathing, and circulation (*ABCs*) must be maintained until help arrives.[8]

If a *concussion* is thought to have occurred, a rapid neurologic assessment can be performed, including eye opening, verbal response, and motor responses. As with victims who have sustained other serious head injuries, patients with possible concussions must be referred immediately to appropriate medical personnel.[19,27] Trauma patients with *seizure disorders* should be observed carefully before emergency dental treatment is initiated. The most recent dose of antiseizure medication should be determined. For trauma patients with *cardiac disease,* such as rheumatic and valvular conditions, antibiotics are required according to the American Heart Association's guidelines for preventing subacute bacterial (infective) endocarditis.[9] To avoid serious postoperative bleeding episodes or severe infections, patients with bleeding tendencies, those taking anticoagulant medication, and patients who are immunocompromised must be identified so that appropriate preoperative adjustments can be made.

Any drug allergies or current medications should be noted to prevent untoward reactions. Tetanus immunization status should be determined because many dental injuries involve intraoral blood and saliva. Appropriate referral to a physician for a tetanus booster within 48 hours of the accident should be made if the last dose of tetanus toxoid was administered more than 5 years before the accident. Antibiotic coverage and tetanus immunization status are important considerations in this chapter's sports dentistry case study.

Health History

A trauma victim who is new to the dental practice requires a complete health history, including assessment of vital statistics and vital signs. Current patients should already have a completed record and may require only an update of the health history and reassessment of blood pressure and pulse.

Before initiating intraoral trauma evaluation procedures and treatment, *standard precautions* must be implemented to prevent the spread of infectious diseases through blood and body fluids.

DENTAL EVALUATION OF THE TRAUMA PATIENT

Accident History

Trauma is never convenient.

The dental team members should keep in mind that a traumatic episode might be a child's first visit to the dental office. In addition, dental professionals also must recognize their legal and ethical responsibilities to patients of record.

> *Note*
> The dental office should be *trauma-ready* and receptive to patients with emergency dental needs.[2]

The circumstances of the accident are noted, including how, when, and where the accident occurred. The time interval between the accident and the initiation of treatment is especially important; the shorter the interval is, the better the prognosis will be.

DENTAL CONSIDERATIONS

Delays in treatment of traumatic dental injuries will adversely affect long-term outcome.

A previous history of dental trauma can help distinguish between past and recent injuries. This differentiation is an important aspect in establishing an appropriate treatment plan.

> *Note*
> Repetitive patterned injuries also may raise the suspicion of child abuse or other forms of domestic violence.

Subjective symptoms reported by the patient can help the clinician establish a diagnosis. For example, dental sensitivity to touch, air, and cold might indicate a vital tooth with a dentin or pulp exposure. Conversely, sensitivity to percussion, mastication, and heat might indicate a tooth with periapical infection.

Intraoral Examination

The visual examination identifies the type and extent of the injury. *Transillumination* of the tooth can reveal cracks within an intact crown or pulpal hemorrhage into dental tubules. *Palpation* can assist the clinician in determining the degree of mobility of an intact tooth within the socket, the presence of a root fracture, or an alveolar bone segment fracture.

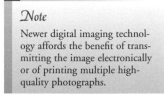

> *Distinct Care Modifications*
> Caution should be exercised when considering palpation of a traumatized tooth.

Percussion of a recently traumatized tooth should be avoided because it adds little diagnostic information and may only exacerbate the existing trauma. *Vitality tests* for teeth are nondefinitive after recent trauma and should be postponed for several weeks to prevent further damage to the traumatized tooth.

Radiographic Examination

The type and extent of the radiographic examination depend on the age of the patient and the severity of the accident. Because of medicolegal and insurance reasons, exposing double-pack film is advisable for practices that use traditional radiography techniques so that an original radiograph may be retained in the patient record.

> *Note*
> Newer digital imaging technology affords the benefit of transmitting the image electronically or of printing multiple high-quality photographs.

The special concern with children's primary dentition is not only the condition of the traumatized primary anterior teeth but also the status of the underlying, developing permanent successors. Radiographic interpretation of trauma to primary teeth should include the presence of crown fractures, root fractures, or displacements, as well as the position and stage of root development of the underlying permanent incisors (Figure 39-5).

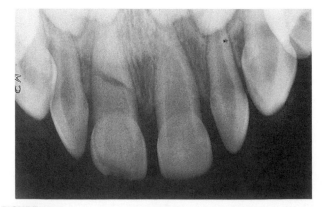

FIGURE 39-5
Middle one third root fracture of maxillary right primary central incisor. The underlying, developing permanent teeth are noted.

In a young patient's permanent dentition, the traumatized area should be evaluated radiographically for the following:

- Crown fractures
- Root fractures
- Displacements
- Degree of root end closure
- Alveolar bone fractures
- Location of tooth fragments or foreign debris

Some patients should have a radiograph of the teeth in the opposing dental arch. Suggested maxillary or mandibular fractures may require panoramic or cephalometric radiographs. Patients also may be referred for computed tomography (CT) scans and magnetic resonance imaging (MRI) as needed.

Treatment Plan

Based on the health history and the clinical and radiographic examinations, the dentist is ready to establish a diagnosis and develop an appropriate treatment plan to maintain the traumatized tooth. Even minor dental trauma, however, may result in pulpal necrosis or tooth loss in the future.

Prevention
From a risk management perspective this information must be explained to the patient (or parent) and documented in the progress notes of the chart to indicate informed consent.

Emergency Management of Dental Trauma

39-9

For the purposes of this chapter, emergency management is described in terms of crown fractures, root fractures, luxation injuries, avulsed teeth, mandibular fractures, and soft tissue trauma. Table 39-1 provides dental treatment codes for procedures related to mouth trauma.

Table 39-1   Procedure Codes Associated with Mouth Trauma

PROCEDURE CODE	DESCRIPTION	PROCEDURE CODE	DESCRIPTION
D0140	Limited oral examination–problem focused	D3351	Apexification–initial visit
D0220	Periapical	D3352	Apexification–interim visit
D0240	Intraoral occlusal film	D3353	Apexification–final visit
D0330	Panoramic radiograph	D4249	Crown elongation
D0340	Cephalometric radiograph	D6292	Maryland lingual wing
D0460	Pulp vitality test	D6293	Maryland pontic
D0471	Diagnostic photographs	D6985	Pediatric partial denture–fixed
D2330	Composite 1 surface–anterior	D7100	Postoperative visit
D2331	Composite 2 surface–anterior	D7110	Simple extraction–single tooth
D2332	Composite 3 surface–anterior	D7111	Coronal remnants–primary tooth
D2334	Composite pin retention per tooth	D7130	Root-tip removal (nonsurgical)
D2335	Composite 4+ or involving incisal	D7273	Stabilization of tooth
D2336	Acid-etched composite crown–primary	D7530	Removal of foreign body
D2337	Acid-etched bandage	D7540	Removal of foreign bodies
D2338	Facing cut into SSC–anterior primary	D7910	Suture small wound
D2390	Resin-based composite crown–anterior	D8003	Root extrusion–fixed appliance
D3110	Pulp cap–direct	D9110	Palliative treatment for dental pain
D3120	Pulp cap–indirect	D9920	Behavior management
D3230	Pulp therapy–anterior primary	C0220	Confirmation periapical
D3310	Root canal–anterior	Y220	Treatment–completed periapical

SSC, Stainless steel crown.

CROWN FRACTURE

Enamel Only

Crown fractures that involve only the enamel are not usually painful and are often unnoticed by the patient. The fractured enamel may feel rough to the tongue. The dental hygienist often discovers enamel-only fractures during a routine dental examination (Figure 39-6). Minimal enamel fractures in both the primary and the permanent incisors may be esthetically recontoured, after which topical fluoride is applied.

Enamel and Dentin

Crown fractures involving the enamel and dentin are sensitive to air, touch, and cold. They have sharp edges and are unesthetic (see Figure 39-6). Emergency management of vital primary and permanent enamel-dentin fractures includes placing a calcium hydroxide pulp-protecting medicament and then an acid-etched composite resin bandage or restoration.

> **Note**
>
> Two other treatment alternatives include composite systems that incorporate dentin bonding agents or the reattachment of the fractured crown fragment.[3]

Enamel, Dentin, and Pulp

Crown fractures that involve the enamel, dentin, and pulpal tissues of vital teeth represent a complex array of diagnostic and treatment possibilities[20] (see Figure 39-6). In the permanent dentition, a vital pulp exposure of a tooth with a closed apex may be treated with a direct pulp cap using calcium hydroxide and then an acid-etched composite resin restoration.

In a vital permanent tooth with an open apex, continued physiologic root formation should be stimulated through **apexogenesis,** a calcium hydroxide pulpotomy technique. For a nonvital permanent tooth with a closed apex, conventional root canal therapy is indicated. A nonvital permanent tooth with an open apex requires **apexification,** a procedure to induce calcific root end closure.

> **Note**
>
> Recently, mineral trioxide aggregate (MTA) has been tested with good results as a pulp-capping agent instead of calcium hydroxide.

DENTAL CONSIDERATIONS

Crown fractures involving the enamel, dentin, and pulp of primary anterior teeth are treated with a formocresol pulpotomy if the primary tooth is vital or with a pulpectomy sealed with resorbable paste if the primary tooth is nonvital. Assessing root resorption is necessary for primary teeth because if less than one half of the root is remaining, then the tooth should be extracted. The final restoration may be either an acid-etched composite resin restoration or an esthetic strip crown in more extensive fractures.

ROOT FRACTURE

Apical One Third

If a root fracture occurs in the apical one third of a primary or permanent anterior tooth and no mobility exists, then the tooth should be observed clinically and radiographically at recall appointments for signs of root healing (Figure 39-7). Adverse sequelae, such as a widening of the periodontal ligament

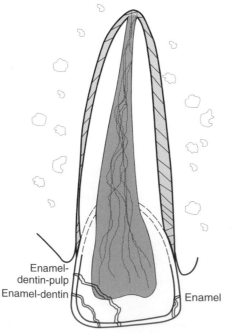

FIGURE 39-6
Crown fractures: enamel only, enamel-dentin, enamel-dentin-pulp.

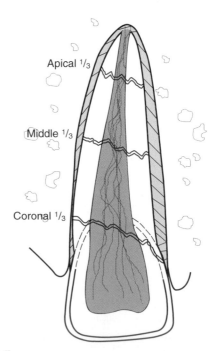

FIGURE 39-7
Root fractures: apical one third, middle one third, coronal one third.

(PDL) space or periapical pathosis, must also be evaluated. In most instances, fractures in the apical one third of a permanent root heal uneventfully and remain vital.

Middle One Third

If the segments of a middle one third root fracture of a permanent tooth are displaced, then the segments should be repositioned and splinted for approximately 12 to 16 weeks (see Figure 39-7). The patient's oral hygiene is critical while the acid-etched composite resin splint is in place. Chlorhexidine gluconate rinses may be beneficial for reducing the oral microflora.[17]

> *Distinct Care Modifications*
>
> The dental hygienist should provide specific home care instructions for proper maintenance of the soft tissues surrounding the injured tooth, as well as tissues in proximity to the splint.

Coronal One Third

Fractures of the root at the coronal one third are the most difficult to manage (see Figure 39-7). Treatment may include root canal therapy, periodontal **crown elongation,** or orthodontic extrusion of the remaining root, then usually a post, core, and crown as a final restoration. Coronal one third root fractures often require extraction and prosthodontic replacement of the lost tooth.

Middle and coronal root fractures in primary teeth should be treated simply. If stable, then the root segment should not be probed because probing may damage the underlying permanent tooth. The primary root fragment should eventually resorb.[37]

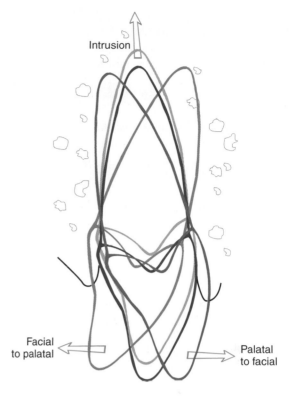

FIGURE 39-8
Luxation injuries: intrusion, facial to palatal, palatal to facial.

DENTAL CONSIDERATIONS

For root fractures with coronal fragment mobility, the tooth should be extracted.

LUXATION INJURY

Primary and permanent teeth may be displaced in a lateral, intrusive, or extrusive direction (Figure 39-8). The major concern with luxated primary teeth is possible damage to the underlying, developing permanent successor.

DENTAL CONSIDERATIONS

Displaced permanent teeth should be repositioned and splinted for approximately 2 weeks.

Antibiotics may be prescribed, and meticulous oral hygiene procedures (as for middle one third root fractures) should be used for displaced, splinted permanent anterior teeth. The major concern with luxated permanent teeth is maintaining the viability of the PDL cells and preventing external root resorption.

AVULSED TEETH

Primary teeth that have been completely luxated out of the alveolar socket should not be reimplanted. Permanent teeth that have been avulsed should be reimplanted as soon as possible to maintain the viability of the PDL cells that remain on the cementum of the root (Figure 39-9). The tooth should be splinted

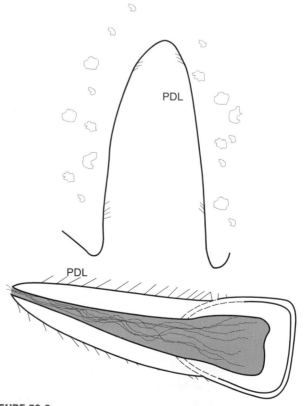

FIGURE 39-9
Avulsed tooth. *PDL,* Periodontal ligament.

in place for approximately 2 weeks, antibiotics prescribed, and meticulous oral hygiene procedures followed. The longer the tooth remains outside the socket, the poorer the prognosis will be because of subsequent external root resorption.

DENTAL CONSIDERATIONS

Reimplant an avulsed tooth as quickly as possible.

⭐ CASE APPLICATION 39-1.1

Prognosis
What do you think might be the prognosis for Miss Washington?

Distinct Care Modifications
The avulsed tooth should be placed in some type of solution for transport to the dental office or hospital emergency room. The tooth should not be transported in a dry gauze or paper towel. Liquids used for tooth transport, from most effective to least effective, include Hank's balanced saline solution, milk, saline, saliva, and water.[4,29]

The patient (or parent), school nurse, or coach should be instructed to reimplant the tooth as quickly as possible at the scene of the accident. However, this expectation can often be unrealistic.

MANDIBULAR FRACTURE

Fracture to the mandible may occur at the condyle, gonial angle, mental foramen region, or mandibular symphysis (Figure 39-10). If the fracture is displaced, the patient will be unable to occlude the teeth in a normal manner. Emergency management includes the removal of any intraoral debris to maintain the airway. The patient should be transported to a hospital emergency room (ER) for further evaluation and treatment.

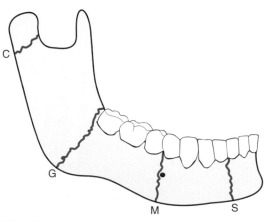

FIGURE 39-10
Mandibular fractures. *C*, Condyle; *G*, gonial angle; *M*, mental foramen; *S*, symphysis.

SOFT TISSUE INJURY

Emergency management for soft tissue lacerations includes hemorrhage control, wound cleansing, suturing, and antibiotics as required. Tetanus immunization status should be reviewed.

Child Abuse and Neglect

HISTORICAL PERSPECTIVE

Child abuse and neglect are not new phenomena but have recently received heightened awareness because of educational programs for healthcare professionals and the general public. Severe punishment of children, infanticide, and ritualistic killings have been reported in many cultures for thousands of years.

The Case of Mary Ellen

The first reported case of child abuse in the United States occurred in 1874 in New York City.[10] Mary Ellen, a 9-year-old girl, was being brutally beaten by her foster parents. At that time, no laws or organizations protected children from parents and guardians or provided removal of children from abusive homes. The social worker who rescued Mary Ellen was forced to have her declared an *animal* so that she could be protected under the auspices of the American Society for the Prevention of Cruelty to Animals (ASPCA). This early effort led to the beginning of the child protection movement in America and the founding of the first Society for the Prevention of Cruelty to Children in 1875 in New York City.

In the early 1900s, activist groups began to condemn many labor practices in factories, textile mills, and coal mines. Through their efforts, the National Children's Bureau (NCB) was established in 1912 to provide information, resources, training, and legislation to child-advocacy organizations. The creation of the NCB was the first time that the federal government officially recognized the need to protect children. Within several years, the bureau succeeded in protecting children working in factories and coal mines by lobbying successfully for the passage of the Keating-Owen Act of 1916.[10]

Battered Child Syndrome

In 1961, Henry Kempe, a Colorado physician, used the term **battered child syndrome** to describe children with numerous unexplained injuries and to characterize child abuse as a diagnosable condition. The term became accepted by the courts as admissible evidence in child abuse cases and strengthened the court's ability to prosecute these cases successfully.[28]

Note
Battered child syndrome describes children with numerous unexplained injuries and characterizes child abuse as a diagnosable condition.

Legislative Efforts

In 1962, states began to mandate child-abuse reporting, and by 1965, all 50 states had some laws for reporting child abuse. During the next decade, additional laws on the reporting of child abuse were developed. These laws defined persons who would be required to report suspected cases of child abuse, designated as *mandated reporters*.[10] In 1974, the Child Abuse Prevention and Treatment Act (CAPTA) addressed many of the previous problems that interfered with protecting children. The Act defined the terms *child abuse* and *neglect* for all states.

Training programs for child welfare professionals were funded and financial incentives provided for states to implement child abuse and neglect awareness programs.

Currently, every state has laws that define child abuse and neglect, reporting mechanisms, and intervention protocols. The states' child protective services are responsible for investigating suspected child maltreatment and providing foster care for child safety.[21] Unfortunately, demand is much greater than the services that can be provided.

DEFINITIONS

Child abuse and neglect include various types of experiences that may be dangerous or life-threatening to the child. The American Academy of Pediatric Dentistry[3] defines **child abuse** as physical or mental injury, sexual abuse, or negligent treatment of a child younger than age 18 by a person responsible for the child's welfare under circumstances that might indicate the child's health or welfare is harmed or threatened. **Neglect** refers to the condition in which any child younger than age 18 lacks adequate food, clothing, medical or dental care, supervision, or other essential care. **Dental neglect** is "willful failure of parent or guardian to seek and follow through with treatment necessary to ensure a level of oral health essential for adequate function and freedom from pain and infection."[3] These three definitions provide the dental team with parameters to identify the different types of child abuse and neglect that may be evident at the dental appointment.

DEMOGRAPHIC FACTORS

Children from all socioeconomic strata may be victims of child abuse or neglect, but the actual incidence remains unknown. Although professionals, as mandated reporters, have an increased awareness of the problem, reluctance to report is still a concern. Approximately 50% to 65% of reported cases are neglect; 25% are physical abuse. Sexual abuse and emotional abuse constitute the majority of the remaining 10% to 25% of cases.[36] In many instances, children who are victims of one type of abuse may also be victims of other forms of abuse.

Although reported at all socioeconomic levels, child abuse and neglect are disproportionately higher among poor families, whether from poverty-related conditions or increased scrutiny by public agencies.[33] No significant correlation between race and the incidence, type, or severity of child abuse and neglect was identified in two national studies.[11] The greater proportion of abused children from minority families may be attributed to a higher rate of investigations in lower-income groups compared with more affluent families.

Children with disabilities are abused at twice the rate as children without disabilities.[49] Disabled children may be more vulnerable to abuse when parents become frustrated with the child's limitations. In addition, the disabled child may be unable to verbalize what happened, thus the details of the abuse remain unknown.

Demographic characteristics vary depending on the type of abuse or neglect. An estimated 906,000 children were reported as abused or neglected in the United States in 2003.[34] The average age of the maltreated child is 7.4 years, although younger children are more susceptible to abuse because of parental reaction to behaviors associated with certain developmental stages, inability to escape from an angry parent, and defenselessness.[44] Girls were slightly more likely to be victims than boys.[34]

Certain family situations also may contribute to child abuse and neglect, including substance abuse, stress, domestic violence, female-headed households, and families without support systems.[10] Estimates suggest that one third of persons who were physically abused or neglected as children will abuse or neglect their own children. Thus child abuse may be a learned behavior that becomes a cycle within a family. Although risk factors must be considered, every child is a potential victim.

EVALUATION OF ABUSE

Because approximately 65% of the cases of physical abuse are associated with craniofacial trauma (head, neck, and mouth), the dental team will likely treat patients who have been abused or currently are victims of abuse.[36]

> *Distinct Care Modifications*
> The dentist and dental hygienist must be receptive to a diagnosis of possible child abuse and neglect for it to be identified, reported, and substantiated properly.

Identification may be aided by the following:
- Obtaining a thorough medical history
- Observing the child's behavior with and without the parent or guardian
- Performing a physical examination

Careful examination of appropriate body surfaces (e.g., head, neck, face, mouth) and documentation with appropriate radiographs and photographs are essential in all cases of sus-

---

BOX 39-1

QUESTIONS TO ASK OR CONSIDER WHILE EXAMINING A SUSPECTED ABUSE VICTIM

- How did the injury occur?
- When did it occur?
- Has the child had similar injuries on several occasions?
- Does the child have a repeated history of hospitalizations, often at different hospitals?
- Has the parent or guardian delayed seeking treatment?
- Does the child act inappropriately to the invasion of personal space by the dental professional?
- Is the parent or guardian hostile or blaming, or is he or she claiming that the child is different or a troublemaker?
- Does a young child accuse someone?
- Does an older child seem reluctant or fearful to say anything when asked what or how the injury occurred?
- Is the child dirty or inappropriately dressed for the season?
- Does evidence exist of old injuries, for example, marks or bruising at various stages of healing?
- Does any evidence exist of burns?
- Does injury exist to the back of the legs, orbital area, mouth, ears, and/or face in general; are frenal attachments torn; are palatal petechiae or fractured or avulsed teeth evident?

pected abuse. Box 39-1 provides questions one can ask or consider while examining an individual to determine whether abuse is suspect.

Health History

The health history will help determine whether the oral condition is the result of abuse or neglect, systemic disease, or accidental injury. Questions should include how and when the injury occurred. The dental team should indicate whether (1) the child has been similarly injured on several occasions in the past, (2) the child has a history of repeated hospitalizations, particularly at different sites, or (3) the parent or guardian has delayed seeking treatment (see Box 39-1). Details regarding any trauma should be complete and obtained from both the child and the parent or guardian. The dental team should be alert to discrepancies in the interview and history when the injury does not match the explanation. For example, an infant who is unable to walk is unlikely to have sustained a fractured femur from crawling.

Behavioral Observations

Specific behavioral changes may be attributed to child abuse and neglect. The child may react inappropriately to stimuli, such as invasion of personal space when the dental hygienist attempts to examine the child's dentition. In addition, the child may not make eye contact and may demonstrate fear of touch. The parent or guardian may be hostile, either blaming or claiming that the child is *different* or is a troublemaker. The child may state that the parent is responsible for an injury. Generally, if younger children accuse someone, then it is usually the truth. In another type of reaction, the child may not volunteer information for fear of repeated injury by the caregiver or separation from the family. Every child is unique, therefore the clinician must evaluate the child's behavior compared with that of children of similar maturity, given a similar set of circumstances. When the dentist or the dental hygienist cannot find an adequate explanation for these types of behavior, child abuse and neglect should be anticipated.

Physical Assessment

The physical status of the child tends to be a more objective measure than behavioral indicators of child abuse and neglect. Factors to consider include whether the child is dirty, is inappropriately dressed for the season, or has unexplained injuries. The child's general appearance may indicate the type of care that the parent or guardian provides. A child with a persistent skin disorder may not be receiving proper hygiene. A child who comes to the dental office wearing a long-sleeved shirt in the summer may be concealing intentional trauma caused by an adult. Children dressed inadequately for cold weather may be victims of neglect at home. An assessment of overall appearance (posture, gait, clothing) should be performed routinely for every child entering the treatment room.

Injury Patterns

Because physical abuse generally leaves noticeable evidence, this form of child abuse is more easily recognized than other forms

of abuse.[46] However, the dentist and the dental hygienist should not assume that all traumatic physical injuries are a result of abuse. Active children do experience normal bruising, and the dental team needs to be familiar with the usual sites of bumps and bruises. Typical sites for bruising are the bony protuberances, including the forehead, chin, elbows, hands, knees, and shins. Because of limited fat available to cushion them, these parts of the body may be more susceptible to injury. On the other hand, if a child exhibits bruising on the backs of the legs, then abuse should be anticipated; children generally injure themselves by running into objects, not backing into them. Similarly, an infant who is brought to the dental office with a hematoma surrounding the eye is most likely a victim of abuse.

In many instances of abuse, children are struck by objects that leave distinctive marks with recognizable injury patterns.[45] For example, a belt will leave a distinct mark where the strap or buckle strikes the skin. Other objects used for discipline, such as hairbrushes, wooden spoons, coat hangers, electrical cords, and rulers, may also leave identifiable marks. The dental professional should examine the shape of the mark to see whether it resembles a known household object that may have been used to inflict the injury (Figure 39-11).

While examining the shape of the mark, the dentist or dental hygienist should observe the color of the bruise to determine its age. Bruises in various stages of healing should alert the dental professional to possible abuse. Rate of healing depends on severity, location, depth, and amount of bleeding into the tissues.[45] Recording information in the progress notes on the color and age of bruises will aid the clinician in documenting a suspicion of child abuse.

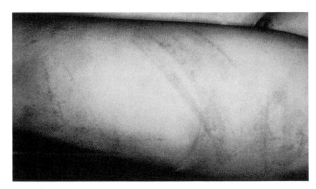

FIGURE 39-11
Physical abuse of child. The injury pattern as a result of using a belt is evident.

Inflicted Burns

Inflicted burns are another manifestation of physical abuse that may be observed during the general assessment of the child. Burns are involved in approximately 10% of physical abuse cases and are classified into three categories: (1) immersion, (2) pattern, and (3) splash. *Immersion burns* are caused by placing a body part, typically the buttocks, feet, or hands, into a very hot liquid.[31] *Pattern burns,* such as cigarette or lighter burns, have an identifying pattern and are usually symmetrical and well defined. *Splash burns* occur when a hot liquid is poured over or thrown at a child. These burns tend to be more severe closer to the craniofacial complex and to become less severe toward the lower body because the liquid loses heat as it runs down the skin.[31] In many instances, splash burns are accidental because curious children may pull hot liquids from a surface and onto themselves. The dental team should question the child on how the burn occurred to determine whether child abuse should be anticipated.

The preceding descriptions of traumatic injuries and conditions are indicators that should alert the dental professional to suspect child abuse. The dental team then must decide whether the injury was accidental, self-inflicted, or an intentional assault by an adult.

Dental Evaluation of Perioral Structures

After completing the general physical assessment, the dental professional should examine the perioral structures. Because most injuries from child abuse cases occur to the region of the head, neck, and mouth, the dental team is ideally suited to detect these cases. A thorough examination of the hard and soft tissues of the perioral structures may help document and substantiate suspected cases of child abuse.

Soft Tissue Assessment

In child abuse, the face is injured more often than any other part of the body.[13] Ready access to the face by the abuser and the psychologic importance of the face and mouth for communication and nutrition are probable reasons. The cheeks are injured most often, followed by the eyes, ears, nose, and lips.[13] Bruises on the ears, especially bilaterally, are rarely accidental. The ears become injured from pinching or pulling, making them bruised or swollen.

The dental team can detect all of these injuries if a thorough general assessment of the child is performed. Clinicians should inquire about any visible wounds, examine any exposed skin, and document the findings of possible traumatic assault in the progress notes of the chart. Identifying these injuries in the office may prevent further harm to the child at home.

Recognizing abusive injuries on the lips is usually easy. Burns may originate from heated objects or cigarettes, and lacerations at the corners of the mouth may be caused by a rope or piece of cloth used as a gag. Injuries to the upper lip and maxillary frenum may result from blunt trauma from an instrument, a finger, or forced feeding. This type of traumatic injury is usually seen in young children 6 to 18 months of age. A lacerated lingual frenum may be indicative of sexual abuse or forced feeding. These types of injuries should be diagnosed and documented during the soft tissue evaluation at the dental appointment.

Examining the gingiva, tongue, and palate may reveal signs of physical and sexual abuse. Identifying sexual abuse in children may be difficult because it is rare and may occur without signs of physical abuse, and the dental team encounters oral sexual lesions infrequently.[18] Oral manifestations of sexual abuse include infections, venereal lesions, and traumatic injuries from oral sex (Figure 39-12). Venereal lesions of gonorrhea, syphilis, herpes, candidiasis, and other viral infections are

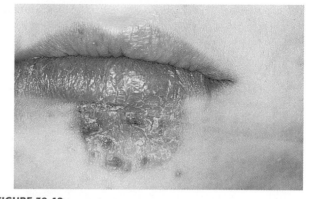

FIGURE 39-12
Four-year-old child with *Candida* infection as a result of sexual abuse.

pathognomonic of sexual abuse in children.[18] The lesions may be sampled, cultured, and identified to substantiate the presence of a sexually transmitted disease. Palatal petechiae or bruising may also indicate sexual abuse by oral penetration. A diagnosis of sexual abuse must be considered when these lesions or injuries are observed at the dental appointment.

Hard Tissue Assessment

Radiographic examination may reveal healing and recurring facial fractures. When facial trauma indicates a possible fracture, the dental team should consider radiographic examination using several different views. Initial management requires attention to basic life support, such as airway maintenance, control of bleeding, and fluid management. A patient with a deviated mandible may have a condylar fracture, which may indicate trauma from child abuse. Nasal and symphyseal fractures may also result from child maltreatment. The dental team should remember that facial fractures are relatively uncommon in children and suggest abuse.[36]

The dentition may be a *permanent register* of child abuse and neglect. Even though abusive parents and guardians may avoid the same hospital or pediatrician's office for emergency care, they generally return to the same dental office. Thus the dental team must be aware of the following:

- Unexplained missing teeth since the previous dental examination
- Any signs of trauma around primary or permanent teeth
- Avulsed, displaced, or mobile teeth
- Fractured teeth or roots[5]

Traumatic injuries in various stages of healing may indicate child abuse and neglect. Delay in seeking care for the traumatized child or a discrepant report of the trauma in addition to the dental injury should arouse suspicion of abuse.

Another aspect of the hard tissue assessment is the evaluation for dental neglect. Dental neglect can be identified by the presence of obvious dental disrepair along with the parents' or guardians' failure to provide adequate dental care. Indicators that may assist in identifying dental neglect in children include the following:

- Untreated, rampant dental caries that can be identified by a layperson

- Untreated pain, infection, bleeding, or trauma affecting the orofacial region
- History of a *lack of continuity of care* in the presence of previously identified dental disease[3]

A complete and accurate dental history is essential in confirming suspicions of neglect. The common factor in dental neglect cases is the failure of the child's caregiver to obtain appropriate care for the child after severe dental pathologic conditions have been identified (Figure 39-13).

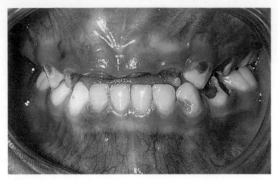

FIGURE 39-13
Three-year-old child with rampant dental caries associated with dental neglect.

The cruelty of physical abuse differs greatly from the debilitation associated with dental neglect. Many caregivers are unaware of the processes and effects of untreated dental disease. However, once the parents or guardians have been informed, the treatment goals explained, and the barriers to care removed, failure to follow through with the treatment plan is considered to be dental neglect. Because optimal oral health is a part of the overall physical health of a child, deliberate dental neglect must be reported because it can cause pain, infection, and possible disability.

> *Note*
> The goal of the evaluation is to document any trauma and then report any suspicion to the appropriate state child protective service agency within the county of residence of the child.

When a child has trauma or dental neglect to the craniofacial complex, the dental team must consider the possibility of child abuse and neglect.

DOCUMENTATION AND REPORTING

Collection of Evidence

One of the most important responsibilities of the dental team in cases of suspected child abuse or neglect is the systematic documentation and collection of physical evidence.[43] This phase is essential for proper identification, diagnosis, and eventual confirmation of abuse or neglect. An examination has little value unless the findings are recorded permanently and accurately in the dental chart for evaluation and comparison at a later date. This information constitutes legal documentation that may be subpoenaed as evidence in a court of law.

All information collected in the medical and dental histories and the physical assessment should be documented in a detailed and objective manner. Positive and negative findings should be recorded, but personal opinions and suppositions should be avoided. Another member of the dental team should be present as a legal witness during the physical assessment and documentation phases of suspected abuse or neglect.

Documentation

Injuries from suspected physical abuse may be documented through the following:

- Written observations
- Photographs
- Radiographs
- Dental casts[43]

Written observations, including detailed descriptions of the injury, should be recorded in the progress notes using black or blue ink or electronically, depending on the type of record system used in the practice. The documentation should include a narrative that indicates the number, type, size, and location of the injury. Diagrams and drawings may be included in the description. Injuries observed on other body surfaces within accepted dental practice should be recorded, with all entries signed and dated by the examiner and recorder.

Photographs are valuable in substantiating child abuse and neglect. Ideally, color photographs should be taken with a 35-mm camera that has a dating option. Digital imaging affords immediate image retrieval to determine image quality and for cataloging. Metric rulers, identification labels, and objects of known dimensions (e.g., coins) may be used to indicate the size of the injury (Figure 39-14). Identification on the back of the photograph should include the name of the patient, date, and film type. Photographs of the patient and the injury should be taken at different angles.

Although the physical injury may not involve hard tissues such as the bones and dentition, a panoramic radiograph or a full-mouth series may be obtained to determine the presence of recent or previous hard tissue injuries to the craniofacial complex. Abnormal tooth development (e.g., dilacerated root, Turner's tooth) indicative of past trauma may be present. These dental anomalies may occur when primary roots are forced into the developing tooth buds from direct blows to the face. The same information that is noted on the photographs should be placed on all properly mounted radiographs.

An impression of the injury can be taken using dental materials such as alginate or compound. The impression should be

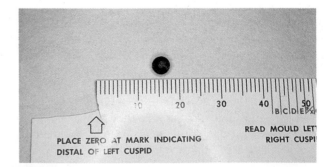

FIGURE 39-14
Documentation of physical evidence (buckshot from buccal mucosa), with use of denture ruler as dimensional guide.

processed as soon as possible and labeled with the same information included on the photographs and radiographs. The impression and cast materials used should also be recorded. Dental casts may be helpful in evaluating and identifying pattern injuries (e.g., bite marks) that involve tissue destruction.

In cases of suspected child abuse and neglect, parent or guardian informed consent is not required for documentation with photographs, radiographs, or dental casts.[43] The general consent obtained before the child's dental examination to perform diagnostic procedures is adequate because all of this documentation is diagnostic in nature. Accuracy and presentation of this evidence are important to substantiate any suspicions of the dental team regarding abuse or neglect.

Professional Responsibilities

Reporting suspected child abuse and neglect to the proper authorities might protect the child from continued pain, suffering, or even death. Dentists are mandated and protected by law in all states to report suspected cases of child abuse and neglect. Presently, dental personnel are mandated reporters in all 50 states.[5] According to the American Dental Association's *Principles of Ethics and Code of Professional Conduct,* the dentist's role in identifying and reporting child abuse and neglect is to:

- Observe and examine suspicious evidence that can be ascertained by the dental team in the office.
- Record, per legal requirements, any evidence that may be helpful in the case review, including the physical evidence and comments from interviews.
- Remain objective toward all parties.
- Treat dental or orofacial injuries.
- Establish or maintain a professional therapeutic relationship with the family.
- Become familiar with the signs of child abuse and neglect, and report suspected cases to the proper authorities consistent with state law.[48]

The American Dental Hygienists' *Code of Ethics** pertaining to the dental hygienist's responsibility in identifying and reporting abuse are to:

- Promote the well-being of individuals and the public by engaging in health-promotion and disease-prevention activities.
- Comply with local, state, and federal statues that promote public health and safety.
- Serve as an advocate for the wellness of patients.

Reporting may result in a positive change in the home environment. By reporting suspicions to the proper agencies, the child may be protected from further abuse. In addition, reporting one child in a family may help protect other children living in the home. In some cases, an agency's investigation of child abuse or neglect may lead to the discovery of other problems within the home, which may enable the agency

> **Note**
> The primary responsibility of the dental team is to identify and report suspected cases of child abuse and neglect.

to provide the family with other appropriate and needed services.

Child abuse and neglect reporting laws may vary from state to state, but all contain specific guidelines for mandated reporters. Initially, an oral report to the child protective agency is made, then a written report is submitted within 36 hours to 5 days, depending on the state where the child resides.[10] State laws define what information the reports must contain, typically the following:

- Name, age, gender, address, and telephone number of the child
- Nature and extent of the suspected abuse or neglect
- Name, address, and telephone number of the parent or guardian
- Mandated reporter's name, address, telephone number, profession, and relationship to the child

Nonmandated reporters may request anonymity. A description of the child's injuries, abuse, or neglect and any indication of prior maltreatment should also be reported.[5]

Once the report has been made, the child protective agency and the judicial system perform all subsequent investigations. This report will result in an investigation if any injury to a child occurs with one or more of the following conditions:

- Explanation of the cause of the injury is inconsistent with the physical findings.
- Injury is incompatible with the child's developmental age.
- Injury seems to be older than the information given by the parent or guardian.
- Appearance of nutritional neglect is evident.[21]

Legal Considerations

When reporting a suspected case of child abuse or neglect, the dental team's ethical obligation is to be consistent with state law. Although all states require reports of suspected child maltreatment, the definitions of abuse vary by state, and not all states mandate the reporting of suspected child neglect. In addition, laws have been enacted that penalize healthcare providers for failure to report suspected cases of child abuse and neglect. These penalties also vary by state.

In general, mandated reporters are protected from legal liability if they make a report in accordance with state laws and in good faith.[14]

With increased public awareness, continuing education courses for the dental team, and lectures on child abuse and neglect in dental and dental hygiene curricula, ignorance in the diagnosis, detection, and reporting of suspected child abuse and neglect is no longer an acceptable reason for failure to report.

> **Note**
> *Good faith* implies that the report was made to protect the child and without malicious intent to do harm.

Strict confidentiality of records must be maintained. Reports and any other information obtained in reference to a report are confidential and are available only to persons authorized by the juvenile courts.[14]

*For the complete *Code of Ethics* document, see Box 3-3 in Chapter 3.

The most important step in reporting and documenting child abuse and neglect is *advance preparation.*

The dental professional must be educated regarding the indicators of child abuse and neglect, understand the legal responsibilities in reporting suspected cases, and know whom to contact when abuse and neglect are suspected. The best action that the dental team can take for an abused or neglected child is to report suspected cases *immediately* to the appropriate agency.

This approach to child abuse prevention is intended to increase awareness among dental professionals regarding the clinical signs and appropriate reporting protocols to break the cycle of abuse. Similarly, prevention of sports-related dental trauma requires enhanced awareness of prevention strategies for patients who participate in competitive sports or vigorous recreational activities.

Prevention of Sports-Related Injuries

Although sports-related traumatic dental injuries continue to occur, reason for optimism exists. Using protective athletic equipment can prevent many of these injuries. Studies demonstrate that in organized sports in which helmets, facemasks, and **mouthguards** are required during practice and in competition, the number and severity of craniofacial and intraoral injuries are reduced significantly.[15-16,24-25,32]

MOUTHGUARDS

At present in most states, rules in five sports at the *amateur* level mandate the use of a mouthguard: boxing, football, ice hockey, men's lacrosse, and women's field hockey. The only sport at the *professional* level that requires a mouthguard is boxing.[40,41]

Athletes for whom mouthguards are recommended include the young soccer player, the high school or college basketball player, and the *weekend warrior* who enjoys a rigorous game of racquetball.[7] This information is especially applicable to the female basketball player with the avulsed tooth in Case Study 39-1.

Although mouthguards offer athletes protection from injury, many athletes choose not to wear them, even in sports that require mouthguards.[23] Some athletes complain that the mouthguard does not fit properly, that it makes them gag, or that it interferes with breathing and speech. All mouthguards are not of equal quality, and complaints are most often attributable to the poor quality of some mouthguards. Recommendations should be made for using a properly fitted mouthguard.[1]

Types

The American Society for Testing and Materials (ASTM) defines three types of mouthguards: type I, or stock; type II, or mouth-formed; and type III, or custom-fabricated.[12]

Stock mouthguards

Stock mouthguards may be purchased at many sporting goods stores. These over-the-counter mouthguards are the least expensive but offer the poorest fit. They must be held in place by clenching the teeth together. Type I mouthguards offer the least protection and interfere most with breathing and speech compared with types II and III. They are not well tolerated by most athletes.[40,41]

Mouth-formed mouthguards

Most mouth-formed mouthguards also may be purchased over the counter. Often referred to as *boil-and-bite* mouthguards, they vary in price, as well as quality. These mouthguards are often formed inadequately by the athlete self-fitting the softened material into the mouth. Retention of type II mouthguards of better quality may be enhanced if the device is properly fitted by a dentist[1,40,41] (Figure 39-15).

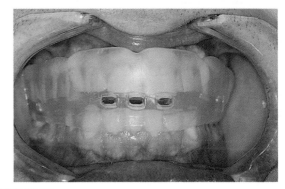

FIGURE 39-15
Properly fitted type II (mouth-formed, *boil-and-bite*) mouthguard.

Custom-fabricated mouthguards

Custom-fabricated mouthguards are made over a stone dental cast of the maxillary arch for athletes with Class I or II malocclusion or over the cast of the mandibular arch for athletes with Class III malocclusion (Figure 39-16). The two most common laboratory methods currently used to custom fabricate a mouthguard are the *vacuum-forming technique* and the *heat-pressure-laminating technique.*[40,41] Because type III mouthguards are made specifically for the individual athlete using an impression, stone cast, and laboratory time and materials, they are the most expensive of the three types of mouthguards. Despite this expense, custom-fabricated mouthguards are superior for protection, comfort, and fit. They interfere least with breathing and speech and generally last longer than either stock or mouth-formed mouthguards.[40,41]

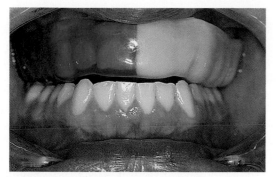

FIGURE 39-16
Properly fitted type III (custom-fabricated) mouthguard.

Inspection, Cleaning, and Storage

Mouthguards should be inspected throughout the course of the season to determine any distortions or bite-through problems, either of which will compromise the mouthguard's ability to protect the athlete. When these problems are detected, a new mouthguard is required for player safety.

Mouthguards should be cleaned and stored properly. They may be brushed with toothpaste and a toothbrush and rinsed with mouthwash or clear water. The water should be cold or lukewarm. Hot water or exposure to direct sunlight will cause the mouthguard to distort. The mouthguard should be stored in a plastic container when not in use.[12,40,41]

Strategies for the Dental Hygienist

A fundamental professional goal for dental hygienists is to preserve the health of the teeth and supporting structures as a significant component of the general health and well-being of the individual patient. Implicit in this goal is active rather than passive daily participation by the patient in preventive practices that will ensure optimal personal health. Furthermore, this goal for the individual may be extended by dental hygienists to larger segments of the general population through dental public health initiatives and community service projects. This broad fundamental goal involves specific patient education objectives and appropriate clinical procedures that dental hygienists use to ensure the prevention of dental caries and periodontal diseases. Dental hygienists also play an important role in preventing traumatic dental injuries.

DOMESTIC VIOLENCE

Although this chapter focuses on issues related to child abuse and neglect, the dental team in the clinical setting may encounter other forms of domestic violence. These forms may include *spousal abuse, elder abuse,* or *date assault.* Dental team members must be aware that any form of domestic violence may be seen in their practice. Similar to child abuse injuries, domestic violence injuries occur generally in the head and neck region. Therefore the dental team will likely observe these injuries.

Public-awareness programs on all forms of domestic violence can be an effective way to publicize availability of services and to provide training programs for healthcare professionals.

The key to prevention is education. The ADA and the American Dental Hygienists' Association have been active in their promotion of programs to educate dental professionals. In 1998, the ADA sponsored the Dentists C.A.R.E. (Child Abuse Recognition and Education) Conference in Chicago. One of the primary goals was to encourage dental professionals, through state and local societies, to form coalitions with public health professionals, child protective services personnel, and advocacy organizations to increase awareness of the incidence of child abuse and other forms of family violence.[6]

Another initiative, the Prevent Abuse and Neglect through Dental Awareness (PANDA) coalition, began in Missouri in 1992. Collaborations with dental professionals, public health agencies, dental insurers, and child protective agencies have made this program effective. Since the inception of this program, reporting rates by dentists have steadily increased.

In addition to the curricular guidelines in the ADA accreditation standards, mandatory continuing education courses in recognizing child abuse and neglect should be recommended for relicensure of dentists and dental hygienists. Education may give professionals the confidence to make reports of suspected child abuse and neglect. Because studies have documented that a lack of knowledge about abuse and neglect resulted in the subsequent lack of reporting, educational efforts should be directed toward breaking the cycle of abuse by enhanced knowledge and active reporting.[13]

Another way to break this cycle of abuse is for the dental team to serve as an example. A *concerned and compassionate* atmosphere in the dental office may offer insight into suitable ways to manage children and adults. The dental professional should counsel patients on primary prevention practices and healthful nutrition habits. Primary prevention efforts should also be directed toward domestic violence.

As in all activities that involve children, some forms of child abuse may occur in youth sports.[35] Long practice hours without adequate rest or refueling, abusive language directed at poor performance, and pressure to win at all costs may be viewed as abusive situations to the child athlete.

The dental professional must demonstrate genuine concern for the patient's total health and show a willingness to help each patient attain this goal.

> *Note*
> The dental team can make a difference in the fight against the escalating public health problem of domestic violence. In addition to protecting children from abuse and neglect, the profession's attitude and actions also may save lives.

MALPRACTICE AND ABUSE ALLEGATIONS

Traditionally, dentists have been protectors of children's health and well-being. Recently, however, this role has been challenged by an increased number of criminal and civil allegations against dentists during conventional patient care. As a result of a lack of parental acceptance of certain behavioral management techniques, dentists are being sued for child abuse, assault, and battery. This litigious behavior appears to reflect two trends in society: (1) an increase in malpractice claims against health professionals and (2) an increase in charges of child abuse against persons who care for children.[47] Hand-over-mouth (HOM) techniques are arguable as assault and battery if used without parental or guardian consent. In addition, physical restraints such as the papoose board may instigate claims of false imprisonment if used without consent.

Prevention is the best defense against potential lawsuits. Communication is the key to prevention. Discussing treatment options and behavioral strategies with the parent or guardian before initiating more invasive care is recommended as an appropriate informed consent procedure and a risk management strategy.

SPORTS DENTISTRY

Trauma-Ready Office

> *Prevention*
>
> One particularly important consideration is to prepare the office and staff to be *trauma-ready* when a patient contacts the practice for an emergency appointment after a traumatic episode.

Several private practice considerations related to sports dentistry are identified previously in this chapter.

Professional responsibility and expeditious scheduling of trauma patients are essential elements to successful patient management.

★ CASE APPLICATION 39-1.2

Preparing for an Emergency Appointment
What steps might Miss Washington's dentist have taken to prepare for an emergency appointment such as hers?

Initial Interview

On most dental history forms, information on participation in organized sports or recreational activities that might place the

> *Prevention*
>
> Include on the dental history form a question related to participation in organized sports or recreational activities that might place the patient at risk for injury.

patient at risk for injury is not solicited, and patients often do not recognize the dentist's need to know unless clinicians ask the question.[39] A positive response allows the dental hygienist to initiate patient-education strategies for preventing sports-related dental injuries.

Congenital Abnormalities and Orthodontic Considerations

Patients with a history of congenital abnormalities, such as the child with cleft lip or palate, the adolescent who is undergoing orthodontic treatment, or the adult who wears prosthetic dental appliances (e.g., implants), must be evaluated thoroughly by the dentist.[1,12] Once this intraoral examination has been completed, the dentist and dental hygienist are better prepared to make an appropriate recommendation for a specific type of mouthguard to meet the individual needs of the patient.

COMMUNITY ACTIVITIES

Dental hygienists have ample opportunities to use their expertise to enhance awareness of trauma prevention in the community by participating in educational activities and public service projects that promote player safety (Figure 39-17). For example, the hygienist can advocate for the use of properly fitted mouthguards for athletes and volunteer for community programs to raise awareness of the benefits of mouthguard use.[1,30,42]

An excellent initial step for the dental hygienist, whether in a private practice, public health, or school-based setting, is to enroll in continuing education courses in sports dentistry and trauma management. The hygienist might participate in the annual symposium sponsored by the Academy for Sports Dentistry. The well-informed dental hygienist will then be in a better position to begin sharing this knowledge with others in the community, such as school nurses, athletic teams and coaches, or governmental agencies. Scouting groups might welcome dental hygiene participation by either providing a forum for a presentation to the group or serving as a mentor for dental health–related projects for scouts to earn merit badges.[42]

Participating in the Special Olympics Special Smiles program provides an excellent opportunity for interested dental hygienists to use a variety of skills.[38] Special Olympic athletes may choose to participate in the Special Smiles program on-site

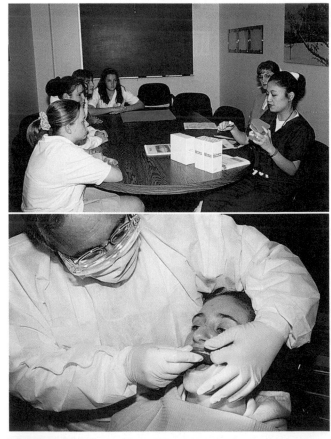

A

B

FIGURE 39-17
A, Dental hygiene students presenting home-care instructions to high school basketball players. **B,** Insertion of custom-fabricated mouthguard.

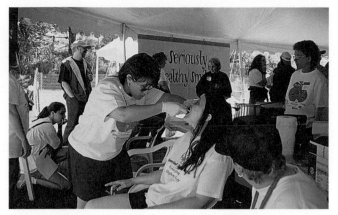

FIGURE 39-18
Fitting of mouth-formed mouthguard in Special Olympics athlete, one of the activities in the Special Smiles program.

at many of their events throughout the United States. Special Smiles includes a dental screening examination, referral for treatment as needed, oral hygiene instruction, and dietary counseling. In 1999, at selected sites, Special Smiles began to offer mouthguards to these special athletes in specified contact sports (Figure 39-18). All participants in the Special Smiles program receive a *goody bag* containing a Special Olympics Special Smiles logo T-shirt and dental hygiene products such as toothpaste, toothbrush, and dental floss. Dental hygienists should use this opportunity to provide community services to an appreciative group of special athletes.

References

1. Academy for Sports Dentistry: *Position statement: a properly fitted mouthguard,* Chicago, 1999, Board of Directors, The Academy.
2. Adair SM, Durr DP: Practical clinical applications of sports dentistry in private practice, *Dent Clin North Am* 35:757-770, 1991.
3. American Academy of Pediatric Dentistry: Reference manual, 2006-2007, *Pediatr Dent* 28:48-50, 2006.
4. American Association of Endodontists: *Recommended guidelines for treatment of the avulsed permanent tooth,* Chicago, 1995, The Association.
5. American Dental Association: *The dentist's responsibility in identifying and reporting child abuse and neglect,* Chicago, 1995, The Association.
6. American Dental Association: *Proceedings of the dentists CARE conference,* Chicago, 1998, The Association.
7. American Dental Association, Academy for Sports Dentistry: *Protect your smile with a mouthguard* (brochure), Chicago, 1999, The Association.
8. American Heart Association: Guidelines for cardiopulmonary resuscitation and emergency cardiac care, *JAMA* 268:2171-2197, 1992.
9. American Heart Association: Prevention of infective endocarditis—Guidelines from the American Heart Association. www.americanheart.org. (Accessed June 4, 2007.)
10. American Humane Association: *Guidebook for the visual assessment of child abuse,* Englewood, Colo, 1996, The Association.
11. American Humane Association: *Trends in child abuse and neglect: a national perspective,* Englewood, Colo, 1984, The Association.
12. American Society for Testing and Materials: *Standard practice for care and use of mouthguards, designation F697-80,* Philadelphia, 1986, The Society.
13. Becker DB et al: Child abuse and dentistry: orofacial trauma and its recognition by dentists, *J Am Dent Assoc* 97:24-28, 1978.
14. Bross DC: Legal aspects of child abuse. In Sanger RE, Bross DC, eds: *Clinical management of child abuse and neglect,* Chicago, 1984, Quintessence.
15. Bureau of Dental Health Education: Mouth protectors for football players: the dentist's role, *J Am Dent Assoc* 64:419-421, 1962.
16. Bureau of Health Education and Audiovisual Services, Council on Dental Materials, Instruments and Equipment: Mouth protectors and sports team dentists, *J Am Dent Assoc* 109:84-87, 1984.
17. Camp JH: Management of sports-related root fractures, *Dent Clin North Am* 44:95-110, 2000.
18. Casamassimo PS: Oral facial lesions in sexual abuse. In Sanger RE, Bross DC, eds: *Clinical management of child abuse and neglect,* Chicago, 1984, Quintessence.
19. Croll TP et al: Rapid neurologic assessment and initial management for the patient with traumatic dental injuries, *J Am Dent Assoc* 100:530-534, 1980.
20. Diangelis AJ, Bakland LK: Traumatic dental injuries: current treatment concepts, *J Am Dent Assoc* 129:1401-1414, 1998.
21. Dubowitz H, Newberger E: Sequelae of reporting child abuse, *Pediatr Dent* 8:88-92, 1986.
22. Fos PJ, Pinkham JR, Ranalli DN: Prediction of sports-related dental traumatic injuries, *Dent Clin North Am* 44:19-34, 2000.
23. Gardiner DM, Ranalli DN: Attitudinal factors influencing mouthguard utilization, *Dent Clin North Am* 44:53-65, 2000.
24. Garon MW, Merkle A, Wright JT: Mouth protectors and oral trauma: a study of adolescent football players, *J Am Dent Assoc* 112:663-665, 1986.
25. Godwin WC et al: The utilization of mouth protectors by freshman football players, *J Public Health Dent* 32:22-24, 1972.
26. Kaste LM et al: Prevalence of incisor trauma in persons 6-50 years of age: United States, 1988-1991, *J Dent Res* 75:696-705, 1996.
27. Kelley JP, Rosenberg JH: Diagnosis and management of concussions in sports, *Neurology* 48:575-580, 1997.
28. Kempe CH et al: The battered child syndrome, *JAMA* 181:17-24, 1962.
29. Krasner P, Rankow HJ: New philosophy for the treatment of avulsed teeth, *Oral Surg Oral Med Oral Pathol* 79:616-623, 1995.
30. Kumamoto DP, Winters JE: Private practice and community activities in sports dentistry, *Dent Clin North Am* 44:209-220, 2000.
31. Lenoski EE, Hunter KA: Specific patterns of inflicted burn injuries, *J Trauma* 17:842-846, 1977.
32. McNutt T et al: Oral trauma in adolescent athletes: a study of mouth protectors, *Pediatr Dent* 11:209-213, 1989.
33. National Clearinghouse on Child Abuse and Neglect Information: *Executive summary: study of national incidence and prevalence of child abuse and neglect,* Washington, DC, 1988, US Government Printing Office.
34. National Clearinghouse on Child Abuse and Neglect Information: *Child maltreatment 2003: summary of key findings.* Available at: www.acf.hhs.gov/programs/cb/pubs/cm03/index.htm. (Accessed June 17, 2005.)
35. National Institute for Youth Sports Administration: *Child abuse and youth sports: a comprehensive risk management program,* Palm Beach, Fla, 1996, The Institute.

36. Needleman HL: Orofacial trauma in child abuse: types, prevalence, management, and the dental profession's involvement, *Pediatr Dent* 8:71-80, 1986.

37. Nowak AJ, ed: *Pediatric dentistry handbook,* ed 2, Chicago, 1999, American Academy of Pediatric Dentistry.

38. Perlman S: Helping Special Olympic athletes sport good smiles: an effort to reach out to people with special needs, *Dent Clin North Am* 44:221-230, 2000.

39. Pollack BR: Legal considerations in sports dentistry, *Dent Clin North Am* 35:809-830, 1991.

40. Ranalli DN: Prevention of craniofacial injuries in football, *Dent Clin North Am* 35:627-646, 1991.

41. Ranalli DN: Prevention of sports-related traumatic dental injuries, *Dent Clin North Am* 44:35-52, 2000.

42. Ranalli DN: Sports dentistry in general practice, *Gen Dent* 48:158-164, 2000.

43. Sanger RG: Documentation and collection of physical evidence. In Sanger RE, Bross DC, eds: *Clinical management of child abuse and neglect,* Chicago, 1984, Quintessence.

44. Sanger RG: Oral facial injuries in physical abuse. In Sanger RE, Bross DC, eds: *Clinical management of child abuse and neglect,* Chicago, 1984, Quintessence.

45. Schmitt BD: Physical abuse: specifics of clinical diagnosis, *Pediatr Dent* 8:83-87, 1986.

46. Schmitt BD: Types of child abuse and neglect: an overview for dentists, *Pediatr Dent* 8:67-71, 1986.

47. Schumann NJ: Child abuse and the dental practitioner: discussion and case reports, *Quintessence Int* 18:619-622, 1987.

48. Sfikas PM: Reporting abuse and neglect, *J Am Dent Assoc* 130:1797-1799, 1999.

49. Waldman HB: Your next pediatric dental patient may have been physically or sexually abused, *J Dent Child* 60:325-329, 1993.

50. Winters JE: Sports dentistry: the profession's role in athletics, *J Am Dent Assoc* 127:810-811, 1996.

Anxiety Control

Lynne Carol Hunt

INSIGHT

The dental hygienist is in a key position to affect the oral health of all patients positively by helping them cope with their anxieties regarding dental treatment.

✷ CASE STUDY 40-1 | Identification and Management of Dental Anxiety

A 47-year-old female patient, Sasha Uri, has arrived for a dental hygiene appointment. This appointment is her second scheduled visit. An hour before her first appointment, she telephoned to cancel. During the initial conversation, Ms. Uri seems to the hygienist to be aloof, distracted, and in a hurry. The hygienist attempts to build a rapport with Ms. Uri, but most of her questions are met with a curt *yes* or *no.* The dental history shows that the last dental visit was approximately 2 years ago, for extraction of an abscessed tooth. Ms. Uri could not recall the date of her last prophylaxis appointment, only that "It was several years ago." Questions related to previous unpleasant dental experiences and anxiety associated with dental care elicit *yes* responses.

With sensitivity and concern, the hygienist inquires about the circumstances of the patient's anxiety. Visibly relieved to be broaching the subject, Ms. Uri reveals that unpleasant childhood dental experiences have left her fearful of oral care. She says that she must force herself to go to the dental office, and she usually goes only for immediate *pain* relief. The inherently unpleasant nature of emergency treatment has further reinforced her aversion to dental care. Because of this lack of care, her oral health has deteriorated, resulting in missing teeth, unrestored carious lesions, and early periodontal disease. Ms. Uri wants to achieve good dental health, but she is anxious and unsure whether she will be able to tolerate or follow through with treatment recommendations. How can the hygienist help this patient successfully manage her anxiety and fear that will allow for a positive oral care experience?

KEY TERMS

anxiety	fear	phobia	spa dentistry
biofeedback	hypnosis	rapport	systemic desensitization
Corah's dental anxiety scale	modeling	relaxation training	
distraction	pain perception		

LEARNING OUTCOMES

After reading this chapter the student will be able to:
1. Differentiate the terms *phobia, fear,* and *anxiety.*
2. Analyze patient responses to questions in the dental history designed to detect anxiety about treatment.
3. Identify the origin of a patient's anxiety through questioning during the initial assessment phase of treatment.
4. Identify and evaluate fear-provoking situations with a patient.
5. Recognize the signs and behaviors that indicate dental anxiety.
6. Evaluate the reliability of tools used to assess dental anxiety.
7. Understand nonpharmacologic strategies that can help patients of all ages develop coping skills for handling their anxiety.
8. Formulate a personalized treatment plan for an anxious patient based on his or her particular circumstances, goals, and level and type of anxiety.

Anxiety toward dental care continues to affect between 10% and 20% of the general population despite advances in pain control.[18,37] Although dental anxiety has been the subject of research for decades, anxiety associated with dental hygiene treatment is just recently being explored. In one of the first studies to examine dental hygiene treatment fear exclusively, de Jongh and colleagues found that only 15% of subjects surveyed experienced no anxiety during dental hygiene treatment and another 15% believed that dental hygiene treatment was more anxiety producing than dental treatment.[12] Treating an anxious patient is also stressful for the clinician.[7]

Levels and types of anxiety are strongly correlated with **pain perception** during dental hygiene treatment.[12,52] Both dwelling on catastrophe (excessive worrying about painful or potentially painful situations of all types) and dental anxiety are also associated with higher levels of pain perception during dental hygiene procedures.[52] In addition, anticipating pain during treatment, feelings of unpredictability, and feelings of no control can all raise anxiety levels among patients.[12]

Gender differences in pain perception and dental anxiety have been widely studied and add yet another dimension to the assessment of patients. Women tend to respond more negatively to stimuli associated with dental care (i.e., chair position, feel of the drill in the mouth), remember their painful experiences, and report more anxiety associated with dental treatment than men.[13,47] Although dental anxiety spreads across all age boundaries, young adults tend to have more fear associated with dental care than older adults.[24,33]

> ### Note
> Levels and types of anxiety are strongly correlated with pain perception during dental hygiene treatment.[12,52] Although dental anxiety spreads across all age boundaries, young adults tend to have more fear associated with dental care than older adults.[24,33]

Even without the effects of gender differences, age variables, or psychologic factors that can contribute to increased anxiety, dental hygiene treatment can be a painful experience. Probing and scaling using mechanical and ultrasonic tools caused mild to moderate pain in patients participating in a study designed to examine the levels of pain associated with seven aspects of dental hygiene treatment:

- Head-and-neck examination
- Hard tissue examination
- Probing
- Scaling with hand instruments
- Scaling with sonic and ultrasonic instruments
- Polishing
- Flossing[56]

Almost 25% of the patients studied claimed to have experienced severe to extreme pain at some point during the appointment, with high scores on the catastrophic feelings scale correlating with higher pain perception scores.[56]

Dental anxiety has been shown to be a contributing factor in dental avoidance, or the failure of patients to seek dental care.* Avoiding care can lead to deteriorating dental health or

*References 14, 18, 37, 51, 56, 61.

exacerbate an existing diseased dental status.[14] Dental anxiety can also lead to increased frequently cancelled or broken appointments in patients actively receiving dental care.[51] Interrupted or failed completion of treatment can adversely affect a patient's oral status, and the vicious circle of dental anxiety, dental avoidance, and deteriorating dental health is reactivated (Figure 40-1). By the time the patient returns for treatment, added invasive and extreme measures might be needed to return the patient to health.

Dental hygienists are often the dental team members who spend the most time with patients and are in a unique position to help patients who have fear of dental treatment. This chapter focuses on behavioral strategies geared toward reducing and controlling anxiety.

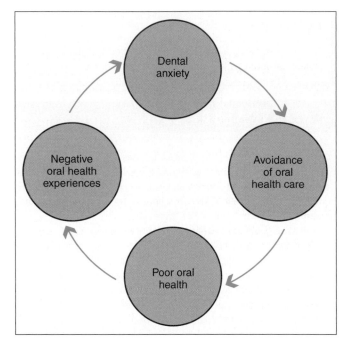

FIGURE 40-1
Negative cyclical pattern of dental anxiety. (Modified from Ronis DL: Updating a measure of dental anxiety: reliability, validity, and norms, *J Dent Hyg* 68:228-233, 1994.)

Definition

Anxiety, fear, and phobia are related terms but are conceptually different.[17,58] All of these feelings generate cognitive and physiologic changes in the body, including emotional upset, with catastrophic feelings, tachycardia, perspiration, muscle tension, gastrointestinal upset, and shaking. Although used interchangeably in the research literature, **fear** is the appropriate term to describe the body's response to an immediate threat, whereas **anxiety** is the appropriate term to describe the body's response to a threat that is not immediate. For example, anxiety is the patient's reaction when thinking about having the teeth probed, whereas fear is the patient's reaction during probing. Fear or anxiety that is irrational, persistent, and unreasonable in relation to the actual threat is a **phobia.** In such cases, the fear or anxiety is so extreme that it causes a person to go to such lengths to avoid situations or objects to the extent that it disrupts normal life. A patient with a true phobia will most likely need referral to a mental health professional for further assessment and treatment before undergoing dental care.

Etiology of Anxiety

Past unpleasant dental experiences are cited most often as the causative factor in anxiety about and avoidance of oral health care. For many anxious individuals, this fear originated from traumatic dental experiences in childhood.[28] Evidence in the research suggests that this anxiety is the *reaction* to those painful memories (or the degree of continued intrusive recollection of the events) that determines whether an individual develops dental anxiety and that nonanxious patients cite terrible dental experiences with equal frequency.[11] In examining the onset of dental anxiety in young adults (18 to 26 years of age), Thomson and colleagues found that the particular temperament and psychologic makeup of the individual was more predictive of anxiety than early trauma.[54] In patients with high dental anxiety, the prevalence of other psychologic disorders is much higher than normal, and they are more likely to maintain their anxiety over time.[32]

Some individuals who have never received dental care are also fearful about dental treatment. Vicarious learning or stimulus generalization might explain this phenomenon. Vicarious learning occurs when anxiety is acquired by watching, listening to, or reading about the experiences of others.[38] Many fearful children have fearful parents. Parents give their children powerful messages consciously and unconsciously about events they find distressing. In studying fearful children, researchers study the parents to determine how closely parental conditioning plays a role in the child's anxiety.[55]

CASE APPLICATION 40-1.1

Diagnosis and Etiology

From Ms. Uri's case study, can you determine whether she is experiencing anxiety or fear or has a dental phobia? What do you suspect is the etiology of her condition?

Treatment Planning

INITIAL ASSESSMENT

Initially, front-office employees should screen for anxiety-related behaviors (e.g., pacing, frequent changes in sitting position, repetitious hand or leg movements) while the patient is in the reception area[39,57,58] (Box 40-1). A history of frequent or broken appointments can also be a red flag for dental anxiety. In addition, the medical history will provide clues to past or present conditions that can affect the emotional stability of patients (current prescription medications used for the treatment of depression or anxiety and substance abuse).[6] Most medical histories in dental offices have one or two broad questions regarding dental treatment fears, but having the patient complete a comprehensive dental history that includes questions designed to identify anxiety can further aid the hygienist in determining a truly effective course of action (Box 40-2). The hygienist should be aware that not all patients, because of embarrassment or denial, will be honest and open about their feelings regarding dental treatment.

If dental anxiety is known or though to be present, the hygienist should determine the degree of anxiety by administering

---

BOX 40-1

ANXIOUS BEHAVIORS IN THE RECEPTION AREA

Fidgeting
Repetitious hand or leg movements
Sitting on the edge of the chair
Pacing
Frequent changes in sitting position
Frequent visits to the restroom
Rapid turning of magazine pages
Startled reaction to office noises

BOX 40-2

SAMPLE DENTAL HISTORY QUESTIONS DESIGNED TO IDENTIFY ANXIETY

1. Did your parents have a positive attitude about dental care?
2. Do you recall any past unpleasant dental experiences?
3. Do you have your teeth cleaned at least once a year?
4. How long has it been since your last dental visit?
5. What kind of treatment did you receive? How did it feel?
6. Do you have concerns about your oral health or about receiving treatment?
7. Have you been satisfied with your dental providers?
8. Have you been satisfied with previous dental work?
9. What dental procedures have you received in the past?
10. Are you anxious about receiving care? If so, what is your level of anxiety?

a dental anxiety questionnaire. One of the more popular and widely used instruments is **Corah's dental anxiety scale** (DAS), which consists of four multiple-choice questions related to dental treatment scenarios.[8] Points are given to correspond with the response selected. For example, one point is given for selecting a response to question #1, two points for a response to question #2, and so on. A patient's cumulative DAS score, which can range from 4 (no anxiety) to 20 (severe anxiety), represents anticipatory anxiety before treatment. A score of 13 or 14 indicates moderate anxiety, and a score of 15 or more indicates high dental anxiety. A modification of the DAS, called the *dental anxiety scale—revised (DAS-R),* has eliminated gender-specific terminology and recognizes dental hygienists, as well as dentists, as oral care providers (Figure 40-2).[44]

During the initial interview with the patient, the hygienist should sensitively ask questions directed toward discovering the circumstances of the patient's anxiety and determining which strategies might be helpful in reducing the discomfort[58] (Box 40-3).

PLAN OF ACTION

Constructing a treatment plan that gives the hygienist maximal control over the patient's treatment experience is crucial to a successful outcome. Dental anxiety has been compared with other medical conditions that require modification of the course of treatment. Less difficult and intensive treatments should be performed first because this tactic increases the patient's tolerance and trust. The treatment plan should include pharmacologic and nonpharmacologic therapies, alone or in combination, to alleviate pain and anxiety. If discomfort is expected during periodontal debridement procedures, both topical and local forms of anesthesia should be used. Depending on

---

Item 1

If you had to go to the dentist tomorrow for a checkup, how would you feel about it?

1.   I would look forward to it as a reasonably enjoyable experience.

2.   I wouldn't care one way or the other.

3.   I would be a little uneasy about it.

4.   I would be afraid that it would be unpleasant and painful.

5.   I would be very frightened of what the dentist would do.

Item 2

When you are waiting in the dentist's office for your turn in the chair, how do you feel?

1.   Relaxed

2.   A little uneasy

3.   Tense

4.   Anxious

5.   So anxious that I sometimes break out in a sweat or almost feel physically sick

Item 3

When you are in the dentist's chair waiting while the dentist gets the drill ready to begin working on your teeth, how do you feel?

1.   Relaxed

2.   A little uneasy

3.   Tense

4.   Anxious

5.   So anxious that I sometimes break out in a sweat or almost feel physically sick

Item 4

Imagine that you are in the dentist's chair to have your teeth cleaned. While you are waiting and the dentist or hygienist is getting out the instruments that will be used to scrape your teeth around the gums how do you feel?

1.   Relaxed

2.   A little uneasy

3.   Tense

4.   Anxious

5.   So anxious that I sometimes break out in a sweat or almost feel physically sick

FIGURE 40-2
Dental anxiety scale—revised (DAS-R). (From Ronis DL: Updating a measure of dental anxiety: reliability, validity, and norms, *J Dent Hyg* 68:228-33, 1994.)

40-1
to
40-4

BOX 40-3

SAMPLE INITIAL INTERVIEW QUESTIONS RELATED TO DENTAL ANXIETY

1. Did your previous hygienist cause you anxiety? If so, what did the hygienist do that made you anxious?
2. What dental hygiene procedures make you feel anxious?
3. What can I do as a hygienist to ease your anxiety?
4. What coping techniques have previously helped you feel more relaxed?
5. Are you currently anxious?

Distinct Care Modifications

Pharmacologic agents are required for painful procedures; however, a purely pharmacologic approach may not help patients overcome their own anxiety. A nonpharmacologic approach may be a more effective long-term strategy because it addresses the psychologic aspects of patients' anxiety.

the invasiveness of the treatment and the patient's pain threshold and level of anxiety, the dentist may prescribe other pharmacologic agents, such as sedatives, nitrous oxide–oxygen analgesia, and oral analgesics. These pharmaceuticals are discussed in other chapters.

Pharmacologic agents are required for painful procedures; however, a purely pharmacologic approach may not help patients overcome their own anxiety. They may credit the drug, rather than their own coping mechanisms, with enabling them to tolerate treatment. A nonpharmacologic approach may be a more effective long-term strategy because it addresses the psychologic aspects of patients' anxiety.*

BUILDING RAPPORT

One of the positive outcomes stemming from a sensitively conducted initial interview and assessment is the building of **rapport** between hygienist and patient. The hygienist's interpersonal relationship with patients influences the way patients perceive their dental experience and their satisfaction with the experience.[38,58] Effective two-way communication establishes trust and fosters an environment in which patients believe that their needs and concerns are taken seriously. With anxious patients, the clinician must assume a calm, confident demeanor and avoid appearing impatient or unsympathetic. The dental hygienist should show care, concern, and

Prevention

With anxious patients, the clinician must assume a calm, confident demeanor and avoid appearing impatient or unsympathetic. The dental hygienist should show care, concern, and respect during all interactions. Words should be chosen carefully so as not to belittle, embarrass, or criticize patients. Failing to establish a positive interpersonal relationship at this stage can result in anger, mistrust, increased anxiety, and subsequent dental avoidance (see Chapter 5).

*References 9, 15, 21, 29, 53, 59.

respect during all interactions. Words should be chosen carefully so as not to belittle, embarrass, or criticize patients. Failing to establish a positive interpersonal relationship at this stage can result in anger, mistrust, increased anxiety, and subsequent dental avoidance. (See Chapter 5 for information on effective communication and building rapport.)

Behavioral Management of Anxiety

Research suggests that behavior strategies, such as **relaxation training** and modeling, can be used to manage patient anxiety.[23,50] A 4-hour course in behavioral techniques taught to a class of dental hygiene students was found to be a significant factor in reducing their patients' anxiety levels.[42] In busy practice settings, dental professionals can be hesitant to add another step, and therefore time, to their treatment protocol. Behavior management of dental anxiety can be as simple as paying attention to a patient's feelings about dental treatment and letting him or her know that you are aware of the patient's fear. Just *knowing* the dentist was informed of anxiety concerning dental treatment was enough to significantly lower state anxiety levels (anxiety based on present moment situations) of dentally anxious subjects in a study conducted by Dailey and colleagues.[10]

INFORMATION PROVISION

An important step in preparing anxious patients for dental care is explaining the proposed treatment. For most patients, knowing what to expect during care helps reduce fear. The dental hygienist should describe the various sensations the patient can expect: feelings, smells, sounds, and sights. For example, during ultrasonic scaling, the patient feels vibrations on the tooth and water spray on the face and hears a high-pitched noise. The sequence of the treatment should also be explained so that the patient is not surprised. Clinicians should choose their words carefully to avoid provoking anxiety and should avoid using dental terminology, which the patient might not understand. Telling the patient, "This might hurt!" will only increase his or her focus on potential unpleasant sensations. A better tactic is to ask the patient, periodically, how he or she is doing. Explanations should help the patient expect a positive experience, thereby countering negative expectations that may have resulted from past dental visits or from information provided by alternative sources.

Patient Education Opportunity

For most patients, knowing what to expect during care helps reduce fear. The dental hygienist should describe the various sensations the patient can expect: feelings, smells, sounds, and sights.

PATIENT CONTROL

Control is the power that an individual has to exercise direction in a situation.[38] To lessen anxiety, patients must believe that they have some control over their treatment.[12] After explaining the procedure and specifying the amount of time it will require, the hygienist obtains the patient's permission to start. Before beginning, however, the clinician and patient agree on a *stop* signal that the patient can use when feeling uncomfortable or needing a rest (e.g., raising his or her right hand). In most cases, the interruptions decrease in frequency toward the end of the appointment. Some patients may need to have the chair adjusted to a less vulnerable position (more upright) at the beginning of treatment. As the appointment progresses and a higher degree of trust is slowly established, patients are more likely to tolerate the recommended supine position.

MODELING

Modeling is the act of observing someone else undergoing treatment, either in person or viewed on videotape, such that the aspects of the procedure and sensations that can be expected are clearly visible to the patient. This behavioral strategy is ideal for children because children learn much of their behavior by observation.[2] Children who observed a peer modeling appropriate behavior during oral care had lower anxiety levels.[36] The benefit of modeling is twofold: (1) It provides information about the procedure, and (2) it allows the patient to observe the model receiving positive reinforcement for appropriate behavior. In private-practice settings, observing an older sibling is a convenient and powerful way to reinforce appropriate behavior. If a compliant sibling is not available, then a parent can act as the model, particularly during the intraoral examination and polishing phases of treatment. Watching a parent undergo deep scaling, of course, would not be the ideal modeling scenario.

DISTRACTION

Distraction diminishes the patient's anxiety by means of preoccupation. The most basic form of distraction is engaging the patient in positive and interesting conversation. Other distraction techniques include virtual vision glasses, television, video games, and audio recordings. In one study, patients who used an audiovisual (AV) device that provided virtual vision reported reduced anxiety.[46] AV distraction, however, might not be appropriate for individuals with high dental anxiety who do not want their fears minimized or ignored. Although most of the participants with moderate anxiety responded with less pain and anxiety when distraction techniques were used, Frere and colleagues found that participants with high anxiety found their anxiety unchanged or intensified.[16]

RELAXATION TECHNIQUES

Relaxation techniques that do not require advanced training, unlike biofeedback or hypnosis, most often use progressive muscle relaxation, breathing exercises, guided imagery, or any combination of these techniques. Progressive muscle relaxation involves systematically tensing and relaxing muscles from head to toe and using deep breathing to further relax the body.[25,60] By lessening the tension that exists in the body, the mind also relaxes. The body and the mind work together and cannot be separated. If the body is relaxed, then the mind cannot maintain a state of tension, and vice versa. Herbert Benson, who coined the term *the relaxation response,* defines this state of being as an "inducible, physiologic state of quietude."[3] Visual imagery adds a cognitive aspect to the relaxation training and can take different forms. The clinician can play an *active role* in deciding what type of pleasant, internal scenario on which the patient can focus (guided imagery), or the patient can elicit a personal mental picture that he or she believes is most effective in calming the patient.[26]

Relaxation training that teaches the patient to relax through paced, deep breathing and relaxing key muscle groups in the body has been shown to reduce dental anxiety.[4,62] In a follow-up study 1 year later, patients who received 10 weeks of relaxation training exhibited the largest reduction on dental fear measures compared with a group that received only nitrous oxide sedation and a group that received 10 weeks of cognitive training.[63] Relaxation training for dental anxiety appears to be beneficial in both the short and the long term.

The relaxation training script in Box 40-4 was adapted from a neurolinguistic programming (NLP) training manual.[22] NLP method was developed by linguist John Grinder and computer expert and gestalt therapist Richard Bandler in an effort to build rapport between patient and clinician by matching verbal and nonverbal communication.[40] Although not appreciably different from other types of deep-breathing scripts in the research literature, several important factors should be noted. First, the script *begins* with an exhalation, stimulating a vagus response, before focusing on deep, controlled inhalation and exhalation of the breath combined with gentle, cognitive urgings to help rid the mind of negative thoughts. Second, patients are instructed to do a *body scan* (an internal visual sweep of the body) to note areas of tension. The breathing is then focused on areas of tension still existing in the muscles.[22] Breathing, muscle tension, and thought processes are all targeted. Reading of the script takes just a few minutes from start to finish. This type of behavioral management of dental anxiety can be taught to all dental healthcare providers and represents a noninvasive, gentle approach to a physically and psychologically distressing experience for a significant number of people.

Before implementing a behavior strategy, such as relaxation training, the dental hygienist should ask patients whether they, themselves, have developed any coping mechanisms. Biggs and colleagues found that fearful dental patients often have their own way of coping with stressful events and that learning new coping mechanisms (breathing and focused attention) was an added stress to some of the subjects in their study.[5]

SYSTEMATIC DESENSITIZATION

Systematic desensitization involves the creation of a hierarchy of fear-producing situations related to the specific fear (Box 40-5). Starting with the least-feared stimulus, the patient gradually progresses through all situations in the hierarchy

BOX 40-4

GUIDED RELAXATION

Teaching the Relaxation Breath

"As you begin to relax, bring your attention to your breathing, noticing just the breath, not necessarily changing it at first, but just allowing it to happen."

"When you want to . . . begin the *Relaxation Breath* . . . exhale completely through your mouth. (Pause.) Inhale a long, slow, deep breath through your nose, and exhale slowly through your mouth." (Pause after each suggestion.)

"You can use this breath now, or anytime you wish . . . to enter the relaxed state . . . or go deeper into the relaxed state."

"You may do the *relaxation breath* again now...and imagining that each time you breathe in...you breathe in relaxation . . . breathe in peace and contentment; and each time you breathe out . . . breathing out whatever you want to release."

"Breathing in relaxation, peace and contentment . . . breathing out whatever you want to release."

To Muscle Relaxation

"As you concentrate your attention on your breathing, focus your eyes on an imaginary spot in the center of your forehead . . . looking at the spot as if you are trying to see it from the inside of your head. . . . Raise your eyes way up as you stare at this spot . . . and notice that your eyes may become tense. . . . That's good, we want to teach your body the difference between tension and relaxation. Your eyelids are controlled by some of the smallest muscles in your body and they may become tired as they become more tense." (Pause.)

"When I count to three, we'll demonstrate the difference between tension and relaxation by allowing your eyelids to relax gently, melting the tension away."

"One . . . two . . . three. . . . Relax your eyelids gently, and notice, as they're closed, a soothing feeling of relaxation moves throughout your eyes, all around your eyes, to the top of your head, and throughout your entire head, down your neck and shoulder, and to your fingertips, all the way down your spine, chest, and abdomen, into your pelvis, and the soothing relaxation continues down your legs all the way to your toes."

"Now, take a moment to notice, as you scan your entire body, if you would like to relax any other part of your body even more. If there is any such place, imagine you can breathe soothing, healing oxygen into that area, and exhale, right through the skin, any tension or discomfort. You can continue this process as long as necessary . . . remembering your breathing as each breath soothes and relaxes you even more."

Hamilton D: *Anodyne practitioner training manual*, San Rafael, Calif, 2004, Anodyne Awareness Training.

BOX 40-5

SYSTEMATIC DESENSITIZATION HIERARCHY FOR TOOTH PROBING

Patient thinks about having the teeth probed.
Patient feels the probe on a finger.
Patient watches a videotape of a person having teeth probed.
Patient watches in a mirror while the hygienist probes a tooth.
Hygienist probes one quadrant.
Hygienist probes entire dentition.

sound. The signal helps an individual become aware of the body's response, thereby helping the person eventually achieve relaxation during stressful situations. The goal of this technique is to enable a person to develop control over involuntary bodily functions, such as pulse and blood pressure. In dentistry, biofeedback has been shown to help patients who suffer from temporomandibular joint disorder but is less commonly used for treating dental anxiety because of the length of treatment required and expense. Biofeedback is used, however, for treating general anxiety and is an option for patients who suffer from anxiety in their everyday lives.

HYPNOSIS

Hypnosis is an altered state of mind in which suggestions are accepted more readily and acted on more powerfully than in the fully conscious state.[35] Hypnosis has been used successfully in managing anxious patients.* The technique has not become widely used because it requires additional training and certification.[19] In addition, a considerable amount of time is needed to induce a useful trance, and some public misconceptions exist about exactly what a trance state entails. Many people fear that hypnosis means that the clinician will have undue influence over their thoughts and actions. Such fears are unfounded.

✦ CASE APPLICATION 40-1.2

Behavioral Management Strategy

Which one of the behavioral management strategies would be helpful for Ms. Uri?

Understanding and Managing the Anxious Child

Strategies that are effective with adults may not always be helpful with children.[38] Distraction, rational discussion, and detailed explanations do not work with children younger than 5 years of age. Neither coercion nor coaxing can achieve a positive outcome. Modeling and the *tell, show, do* approach are two

while maintaining a relaxed state. Because a relaxation response has replaced the anxiety response, patients can cope with the previously feared situations.

BIOFEEDBACK

Biofeedback uses sophisticated monitoring equipment to measure physiologic changes in the body during exposure to stressful stimuli. These changes are signaled by a flashing light or

*References 1, 20, 27, 31, 34, 41, 43, 45, 48

Note

Distraction, rational discussion, and detailed explanations do not work with children younger than 5 years of age. Neither coercion nor coaxing can achieve a positive outcome.

commonly used strategies that have proved useful. To encourage cooperative behavior, the clinician should give children specific directions and specific feedback in age-appropriate terms (e.g., "You are doing a great job of holding your head still."). Positive suggestions and praise are important. The hygienist can also foster a sense of control in children by allowing some degree of participation (e.g., letting patients hold and operate the saliva ejector) and by telling them how long the procedure will take.

Spa Dentistry

It is worth mentioning here that, in an effort to further put patients at ease with dental treatment, some dentists are creating **spa dentistry** by incorporating traditional *spa treatments* (i.e., massage therapy, aromatherapy, pedicures, manicures) into their practices. Although services such as manicures and pedicures are purely pleasant and esthetic distractions for patients, studies suggest that massage therapy and aromatherapy can reduce anxiety (especially when used in combination) and are considered alternative and complementary forms of medicine.[30] These added services are considered to be complements or *accessories* to the dental treatment plan, not the focus.[49]

CASE APPLICATION 40-1.3

Selection of Management Strategy

Which one of the behavioral management strategies would be helpful for Ms. Uri?

References

1. Baker SR, Boaz D: The partial reformulation of a traumatic memory of a dental phobic during trance: a case study, *Int J Clin Exp Hypn* 31:14-18, 1983.
2. Bandura A: *Principles of behavior modification,* New York, 1969, Holt, Rinehart & Winston.
3. Benson H: *The relaxation response,* New York, 1975, William Morrow.
4. Berggren U, Hakeverg M, Carlsson SG: Relaxation vs cognitively oriented therapies for dental fear, *J Dent Res* 79:1645-1651, 2000.
5. Biggs QM, Kelly KS, Toney JD: The effects of deep diaphragmatic breathing and focused attention on dental anxiety in a private practice setting, *J Dent Hyg* 77:105-113, 2003,
6. Centore L, Reisner L, Pettengill CA: Better understanding your patient from a psychological perspective: early identification of problem behaviors affecting the dental office, *J Calif Dent Assoc* 30:512-519, 2002.
7. Corah NL: Dental anxiety: assessment, reduction, and increasing patient satisfaction, *Dentistry* 10:5-9, 23-25, 1990.
8. Corah NL: Development of a dental anxiety scale, *J Dent Res* 48:596, 1969.
9. Corah NL, O'Shea RM, Ayer WA: Dentists' management of patients' fear and anxiety, *J Am Dent Assoc* 110:734-736, 1985.
10. Dailey YM, Humphris GM, Lennon MA: Reducing patients' state anxiety in general dental practice: a randomized controlled trial, *J Dent Res* 81:319-322, 2002.
11. de Jongh A, Aartman IH, Brand N: Trauma-related phenomena in anxious dental patients, *Community Dent Oral Epidemiol* 31:52-58, 2003.
12. de Jongh A, Stouthard M: Anxiety about dental hygienist treatment, *Community Dent Oral Epidemiol* 21:91-95, 1998.
13. Eli I et al: Effect of gender on acute pain prediction and memory in periodontal surgery, *Eur J Oral Sci* 108:99-103, 2000.
14. Elter JR, Strauss RP, Beck JD: Assessing dental anxiety, dental care use and oral status in older adults, *J Am Dent Assoc* 128:591-593, 1997.
15. Enneking D et al: Treatment outcomes for specific subtypes of dental fear: preliminary clinical findings, *Spec Care Dent* 12:214-218, 1992.
16. Frere CL et al: Effects of audiovisual distraction during dental prophylaxis, *J Am Dent Assoc* 132:1041-1038, 2000.
17. Gadbury-Amyot CC: Assessing and managing patients with dental fears, *Compend Cont Educ Oral Hyg* 2:3-10, 1995.
18. Gatchel RJ: The prevalence of dental fear and avoidance: expanded adult and recent adolescent surveys, *J Am Dent Assoc* 118:591-593, 1989.
19. Gatchel RJ: Managing anxiety and pain during dental treatment, *J Am Dent Assoc* 123:37-41, 1992.
20. Golan HP: Control of fear reaction in dental patients by hypnosis: three case reports, *Am J Clin Hypn* 13:279-284, 1971.
21. Hakeberg M et al: Long-term effects on dental care behavior and dental health after treatments for dental fear, *Anesth Prog* 40:72-77, 1993.
22. Hamilton D: *Anodyne awareness practitioner training manual,* San Rafael, Calif, 2004, Anodyne Awareness Training.
23. Hammarstrand G, Berggren U, Hakeberg M: Psychophysiological therapy versus hypnotherapy in the treatment of patients with dental phobia, *Eur J Oral Sci* 103:399-404, 1995.
24. Holzman JM et al: The relationship of age and gender to fear and anxiety in response to dental care, *Spec Care Dent* 17:82-87,1997.
25. Jacobsen E: *Progressive relaxation,* Chicago, 1938, University of Chicago Press.
26. Jepsen CH: Neutralize dental fear with neuro-linguistic programming, *J Dent Pract Admin* 5:105-111, 1988.
27. Kleinhauz M, Eli L: When pharmacologic anesthesia is precluded: the value of hypnosis as a sole anesthetic agent in dentistry, *Spec Care Dent* 13:15-18,1993.
28. Klesges RC, Malott JM: The effects of graded exposure and parental modeling on the dental phobias of a four-year-old girl and her mother, *J Behav Ther Exp Psychiatry* 15:164, 1984.
29. Krochak M, Rubin JG: An overview of the treatment of anxious and phobic dental patients, *Compend Cont Educ Dent* 14:604-615, 1993.
30. Kuryama H et al: Immunological and psychological benefits of aromatherapy massage, *Evid Based Complement Alternat Med* 2:179-184, 2005.
31. Lewis RS: Hypnosis provides therapeutic tool for patient management, *J Mass Dent Soc* 45:2023, 1996.

32. Locker D, Poulton R, Thomson WM: Psychological disorders and dental anxiety in a young adult population, *Community Dent Oral Epidemiol* 29:456-463, 2001.

33. Locker D, Thomson WH, Poulton R: Onset of and patterns of change in dental anxiety in adolescence and early adulthood: a birth cohort study, *Community Dent Health* 18(2):99-104, 2001.

34. Lu DP, Lu GP: Hypnosis and pharmacological sedation for medically compromised patients, *Compendium* 1732-1740, 1996.

35. Meechan JG, Robb ND, Seymour RA: *Pain and anxiety control for the conscious dental patient,* Oxford, 1998, Oxford University Press.

36. Melamed B et al: Reduction of fear-related dental management problems with use of filmed modeling, *J Am Dent Assoc* 90:822-826, 1975.

37. Milgrom P et al: The prevalence and practice management consequences of dental fear in a major US city, *J Am Dent Assoc* 116:641-647, 1988.

38. Milgrom P, Weinstein P, Getz T: *Treating fearful dental patients,* ed 2, Seattle, 1995, University of Washington Press.

39. Millar K et al: Helping anxious adult patients, *Dent Update* 18:18, 20-22, 24-25, 1991.

40. Milliner CB, Grinder J, Topel S: *Leaves before the wind: leading edge applications of NLP,* Portland, Ore, 1995, Metamorphosis Publishing.

41. Moore R, Abrahamsen R, Brodsgaard I: Hypnosis compared with group therapy and individual desensitization for dental anxiety, *Eur J Oral Sci* 104:612-618, 1996.

42. Peretz B, Kaplan R, Stabholtz A: The influence of a patient-management course for dental hygiene students on the dental anxiety of their patients, *J Dent Educ* 61:368-373, 1997.

43. Rodolfa E, Kraft W, Reilley R: Etiology and treatment of dental anxiety and phobia, *Am J Clin Hypn* 33:22-29, 1990.

44. Ronis DL: Updating a measure of dental anxiety: reliability, validity, and norms, *J Dent Hyg* 68:228-233, 1994.

45. Rustvold S: Hypnotherapy for treatment of dental phobia in children, *Gen Dent* 42:346-348, 1994.

46. Satoh Y et al: Relaxation effect of an audiovisual system on dental patients: part 2—Palus-amplitude, *J Nihon Univ Sch Dent* 37:138-145, 1995.

47. Settineri S, Tati F, Fanara G: Gender differences in dental anxiety: is the chair position important? *J Contemp Dent Pract* 6:115-122, 2005.

48. Sklar B: Hypnosis as an alternative in dentistry, *Access* 1:34-35, 1993.

49. Smith K: Spa dentistry—an accessory not an identity, *J Indiana Dent Assoc* 83:8-10, 2004.

50. Smith TA: Evaluating a behavioral method to manage dental fear: a two-year study of dental practices, *J Am Dent Assoc* 121:525-530, 1990.

51. Stewart JE et al: Comprehensive treatment among dental school patients with high and low dental anxiety, *J Dent Educ* 58:697-700, 1994.

52. Sullivan MJ, Neish NR: Catastrophizing, anxiety and pain during dental hygiene treatment, *Community Dent Oral Epidemiol* 26:344-349, 1998.

53. Tay K et al: The effect of instruction on dentists' motivation to manage fearful patients, *J Dent Educ* 57:444-448, 1993.

54. Thomson WM, Locker D, Poulton R: Incidence of dental anxiety in young adults in relation to dental treatment experience, *Community Dent Oral Epidemiol* 28:289-294, 2000.

55. Townend E, Dimigen G, Fung D: A clinical study of child dental anxiety, *Behav Res Ther* 38:31-46, 2000.

56. Tripp DA, Neish NR, Sullivan MJ: What hurts during dental hygiene treatment? *J Dent Hyg* 72:25-30, 1998.

57. Weiner AA: Dental anxiety: differentiation, identification, and behavioral management, *J Can Dent Assoc* 58:580-585, 1992.

58. Weiner AA: *The difficult patient: a guide to understanding and managing anxiety,* ed 2, Cambridge, Mass, 1994, Reniew and Associates.

59. Weinstein P: Breaking the worldwide cycle of pain, fear and avoidance: uncovering risk factors and promoting prevention for children, *Ann Behav Med* 12:141-147, 1990.

60. Wolpe J: Behavior therapy in complex neurotic states, *Br J Psychiatr* 110:28-34, 1964.

61. Woolfolk MW et al: Determining dental check-up frequency, *J Am Dent Assoc* 1999 130:715-723, 1999.

62. Willumsen T, Vassend O, Hoffart A: A comparison of cognitive therapy, applied relaxation and nitrous oxide sedation in the treatment of dental fear, *Acta Odontol Scand* 59:290-296, 2001.

63. Willumsen T, Vassend O, Hoffart A: One year follow-up of patients treated for dental fear: effects of cognitive therapy, applied relaxation, and nitrous oxide sedation, *Acta Odontol Scand* 59:335-340, 2001.

Local Anesthetics

Kathy B. Bassett • Arthur C. DiMarco

INSIGHT

Local anesthetics are used in dentistry primarily to manage pain experienced by the patient during treatment procedures. The dental hygienist is responsible for monitoring the status of the patient who has received a local anesthetic agent and is receiving treatment from the hygienist. Where allowed by state law, dental hygienists deliver local anesthetics during patient care, as well as anesthetize a patient in preparation for restorative therapy or surgery as directed by a dentist.

✴ CASE STUDY 41-1   Anesthesia Considerations

Maria Guyegos is a 150-pound, 57-year-old female, with a blood pressure of 118/80 mm Hg, who is being seen for periodontal therapy of the mandibular right quadrant, which requires local anesthesia. She is difficult to anesthetize and "usually takes a lot of Novocain," according to her health history. Ms. Guyegos has type II diabetes and has not responded well to vigorous therapy. Her blood sugar before her appointment today was 135 mg/dl. She is also medicated with a nonselective beta-blocker for hypertension, which, unlike the diabetes, has responded well to therapy.

KEY TERMS

action potential	concentration gradient	infiltration	o-toluidine
afferent	depolarization	infraorbital	para-aminobenzoic acid
alpha receptors	dyclonine	ketone	posterior superior alveolar
amides	efferent	lidocaine	procaine
anion	epinephrine	local infiltration	pseudocholinesterase
anterior superior alveolar	esters	long buccal	repolarization
articaine	firing threshold	mental	resting membrane potential
aspirating syringe	gauge	mepivacaine	scoop technique
aspiration	Gow-Gates	methemoglobinemia	sodium channels
beta receptors	greater palatine	middle superior alveolar	terminal arborization
bupivacaine	hydrophilic	nasopalatine	tetracaine
cation	hydrophobic	nerve block	topical anesthetic agents
cholinesterase	incisive	norepinephrine	vasoconstrictor
cocaine	inferior alveolar and lingual		

Figure 41-9 and Figures 41-13 through 41-25 are provided courtesy K. Bassett.

LEARNING OUTCOMES

After reading this chapter the student will be able to:

1. Describe the uses of local anesthetics in the practice of dental hygiene.
2. Name the first local anesthetic, and explain why it is no longer the drug of choice.
3. Describe the physiologic mechanism of nerve conduction.
4. Explain how local anesthetics block nerve conduction.
5. Describe the chemical classes of local anesthetics.
6. Discuss the effect pH has on local anesthetics.
7. Describe the pharmacokinetics of local anesthetics.
8. Identify the systemic actions of local anesthetics.
9. Discuss the purpose of adding a vasoconstrictor to a local anesthetic solution.
10. Describe the clinical action of specific local anesthetics.
11. Select the correct armamentarium for individual injections.
12. Describe the basic steps involved in the delivery of a local anesthetic injection.
13. Understand the general principles of technique and safety.
14. Recognize the anatomical landmarks associated with the common local anesthetic injections.
15. Describe all major maxillary and mandibular injection techniques used in dental hygiene practice.
16. Discuss the potential local and systemic complications related to the delivery of local anesthetic agents.

The primary benefit of administering a local anesthetic agent is that pain sensation can be suppressed without generalized depression of the entire nervous system, allowing dental procedures to be performed with much less risk than is associated with general anesthesia. Local anesthetics cause a loss of sensation in a circumscribed area of the body. When delivered near a nerve, local anesthetic agents temporally interfere with the conduction of sensory and motor signals to the central nervous system.

The sensations of pain, temperature, touch, pressure, proprioception, and skeletal muscle tone depend on a rapid, complex flow of information between the nervous system and the rest of the body.

History of Anesthetic Agents

The origin of local anesthetic agents is documented as early as 1532 in the ceremonial use of the coca plant by the Incas. **Cocaine** was extracted from the coca leaf in 1860 by Albert Niemann, who noted that it had a peculiar effect on the tongue, leaving it numb and almost devoid of sensation. In 1884, Carl Koller discovered cocaine's potent local anesthetic effects on the eye. It was immediately adopted for use in eye surgery because, for the first time, operations could be performed on the eye while the patient was fully conscious. In 1884, Richard J. Hall introduced the use of local anesthetics for dentistry, and in 1885, Halsted used cocaine as a **nerve block,** which prohibits conduction of sensations to and from the region supplied by the nerve, for general surgery. During this time, Sigmund Freud was experimenting with cocaine and its effects on the central nervous system.[12,13]

The realization that cocaine was addictive and toxic prompted a search for more acceptable local anesthetic agents. In 1905, Albert Einhorn synthesized **procaine,** which became the prototype for local anesthetic drugs for nearly 50 years. **Lidocaine** was approved for use in the United States in 1948 and **mepivacaine** in 1960.[18] Although many local anesthetics are now available for dental use, the search for the ideal local anesthetic continues.

In 1901, Heinrich Braun discovered that adding epinephrine to cocaine decreased its absorption rate and prolonged the effects of anesthesia, allowing lower doses to be administered. Along with the earlier development of syringes in the 1850s, parenteral administration of cocaine became more effective, easier to deliver, and significantly safer than methods used before that time.

Development of specialized armamentarium paralleled the development of safer, nonaddictive local anesthetic drugs. Dr. Harvey Cook, an army surgeon, developed a breech-loading, cartridge-type syringe that held glass cartridges containing local anesthetic drugs. In 1921, the glass cartridge and syringe were introduced. To reduce the risk of intravascular injection, the first **aspirating syringe** was introduced in 1947, the harpoon-type aspirating syringe in 1957, and finally, the self-aspirating syringe in 1970. Disposable stainless steel needles were introduced in 1959 as a result, in large part, of reports of hepatitis transmission through contaminated needles.

Dental hygienists were first licensed to deliver local anesthetic agents in the state of Washington in 1972, and 36 states followed suit through the year 2005. A thorough knowledge of the process of pain sensation and management is an important part of comprehensive patient care for the dental hygienist.

Dental hygienists must be knowledgeable of the state practice acts in effect for their specific practice locations. Not all states allow dental hygienists to administer injectable local anesthetic agents. When the dentist administers anesthetics for dental hygiene services, the hygienist is often responsible for the preliminary evaluation of medical history and the potential for drug interactions for the selected injectable agent; the hygienist must always monitor for any complications the patient may experience after delivery of the drugs.

In states in which dental hygienists are not allowed to administer injectable local anesthetics, noninjectable local anesthetics may be applied, or the hygienist must apply other pain-management strategies. However, when alternatives are not adequate for pain management, a dentist must administer local anesthetics for hygiene procedures. Significant time management and production benefits exist for the hygienist when licensed and able to deliver appropriate local anesthetics for dental hygiene services. These benefits extend to the dentist as well when the delivery of anesthetics for the dentist's procedures may be delegated to a qualified dental hygienist. This licensed duty for dental hygienists is highly valued by dentists and hygienists in states where it is allowed.

The following discussion will introduce the dental hygiene student to the basic concepts of pain management through the use of local anesthetics delivered for dentistry. When the dental hygienist will be delivering these agents, an in-depth course in pain management and local anesthetics is required.

Physiologic Mechanism of Nerve Conduction

To understand the way a local anesthetic works, the dental hygienist should be familiar with the anatomical and physiologic factors of nerve conduction.

NERVE ANATOMY

Nerves in the human body serve either motor or sensory functions. Although these two types of nerves have slightly different structures, the primary components of neurons are the cell body with nucleus, axon, dendritic zone with free nerve endings (where the stimulus is picked up), and the **terminal arborization** (where the impulse is routed toward the central nervous system) (Figure 41-1).

The primary difference between motor (**efferent**) and sensory (**afferent**) neurons is the location of the cell body along the axon. The cell body provides metabolic support to the neuron. In motor neurons, the cell body is located at the terminal arborization and participates in impulse conduction. In sensory

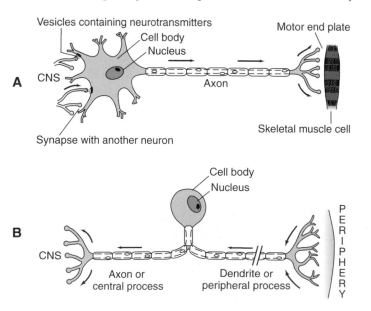

FIGURE 41-1
A, Motor neuron with cell body participating in conduction of impulses. **B,** Sensory neuron with cell body supportive only. *CNS,* Central nervous system. (In Malamed SF: *Handbook of local anesthesia,* ed 5, St Louis, 2004, Mosby. From Liebgott B: *Anatomical basis of dentistry,* ed 2, St Louis, 2001, Mosby.)

neurons, the cell body is located off the axon and does not participate in conducting impulses.

The axon is made up of cytoplasm, called the *axoplasm,* and is surrounded by a multilayer lipid membrane. This membrane plays a key role in the action of local anesthetic drugs on the nerve (Figure 41-2).

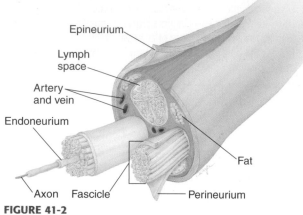

FIGURE 41-2
Diagram of a typical nerve demonstrating the outer layer of tissue or epineurium, the layer surrounding bundles of fiber (fascicles) or perineurium, and the layer surrounding each fiber or endoneurium. (From Thibodeau G, Patton K: *Anatomy & physiology,* ed 5, St Louis, 2003, Mosby.)

BASICS OF NERVE CONDUCTION

The electrical charges of the intracellular and extracellular fluids (fluids inside and outside the nerve cell membrane, respectively) are normally in a state of balance. Intracellular fluids are more negatively charged, whereas the extracellular fluids more positively charged. The relationship between the relative amounts of the ions inside and outside of the nerve membrane is referred to as the **concentration gradient** (Figure 41-3).

The resting state of a nerve is expressed as the **resting membrane potential.** This expression refers to the electrochemical balance between sodium and potassium ions, which is maintained by a process referred to as the *active sodium ion pump.* Sodium and potassium are chemical elements that hold a positive electrical charge. During a resting state, sodium is in greater concentration outside the nerve membrane, at a ratio of 14:1.[18]

In the resting state, the internal environment of the nerve is negatively charged, and the exterior environment is positively charged. To maintain the equilibrium of the nerve membrane, a constant process of ion exchange, referred to as **depolarization** and **repolarization,** occurs.

Nerve conduction depends on the movement of sodium ions through the cell membrane by means of channels that allow the passage of sodium ions through the membrane, referred to as the **sodium channels** (see Figure 41-3).

To elicit a nerve response, a stimulus such as touch or pain must be of sufficient quantity and duration to initiate a significant change in the sodium-potassium balance, expressed as the **firing threshold** (i.e., building to a state of critical mass). Once the firing threshold is met, the sodium ions flood into the nerve

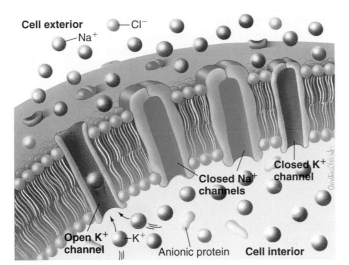

FIGURE 41-3
Role of ion channels in maintaining the resting membrane potential. Some potassium ion (K^+) channels are open in a *resting* membrane, allowing K^+ to diffuse down its concentration gradient (out of the cell) and thus add to the excess of positive ions on the outer surface of the plasma membrane. Diffusion of sodium ions (Na^+) in the opposite direction would counteract this effect but is prevented from doing so by closed Na^+ channels. (From Thibodeau G, Patton K: *Anatomy & physiology*, ed 5, St Louis, 2003, Mosby.)

and potassium ions exit, triggering a transient rapid depolarization of the nerve membrane.

After the rapid depolarization of the membrane, a nerve impulse is generated, sending the sensory touch or pain signal to the central nervous system (Figure 41-4). This nerve impulse

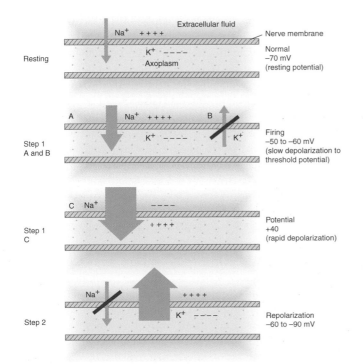

FIGURE 41-4
Top, Resting potential. *Step 1, A and B,* Slow depolarization. *Step 1, C,* Rapid depolarization, nerve impulse conduction initiated. *Step 2,* Repolarization to the resting potential. (From Malamed SF: *Handbook of local anesthesia*, ed 5, St Louis, 2004, Mosby.)

is also known as an **action potential.** After the stimulus is removed, the nerve returns to a resting membrane potential. During the recovery phase, the affected nerve membranes repolarize to their initial electrochemical balance, aided by the reverse action of the active sodium ion pump.[9]

Mechanism of Action of Local Anesthetic Agents

Local anesthetics block the conduction of a nerve impulse by preventing the nerve from reaching its firing potential. Local anesthetics bind to specific receptors in the nerve membrane to prevent the flooding of sodium ions through the cell membrane. As long as the local anesthetic molecules bind to these receptors, the conduction of nerve impulses is prevented (Figure 41-5).

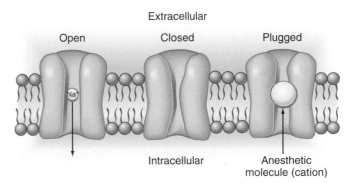

FIGURE 41-5
On the left is an open channel (the usual configuration after a sufficient stimulus has been applied), allowing sodium ion (Na^+) influx through the nerve membrane. The center channel remains closed to sodium ions, which is the usual configuration in the resting state. The right channel, although otherwise in the open configuration, has been closed by an anesthetic cation that is bound to the receptor site in the channel. (Modified from Malamed SF: *Handbook of local anesthesia*, ed 5, St Louis, 2004, Mosby.)

CHEMISTRY

The ability of local anesthetic drugs to block nerve impulse conduction is governed by the acid and base components of each type of drug. The hydrogen ion concentration of a local anesthetic solution determines the pH of the solution—the balance between the available acid and base. This property, in turn, determines how much of the drug is in the acid (**cation**) form and how much is in the base (**anion**) form. The nerve-blocking effects of these agents are thought to be governed by the available base component of the agent. The anion form easily penetrates the membrane carrying the drug inside the nerve, where it is transformed into the cation form, which is key to blocking sensory impulses.

In response to the stimulation of a nerve, the flow of sodium ions through the sodium channels increases. This flow is regulated by specific receptor sites within the channels. When local anesthesia is introduced, the cation form binds to these receptor sites, interfering with the rapid depolarization of the nerve membrane and blocking nerve impulse conduction.

The normal pH of body tissue is 7.4. Local anesthetic solutions available for injection have a pH of 5 to 6. The lower the pH is, the more acidic the solution will be and hence the greater the proportion of drug in the cation form. Once the anesthetic has been injected, the amount of drug in the base (anionic) form increases.

Infection or inflammation in the soft tissues produces an acidic environment, with a pH usually below 6. This acid environment reduces the amount of free base form of the drug available and can make the task of obtaining local anesthesia difficult in areas of the oral cavity that are inflamed or infected (Figure 41-6).

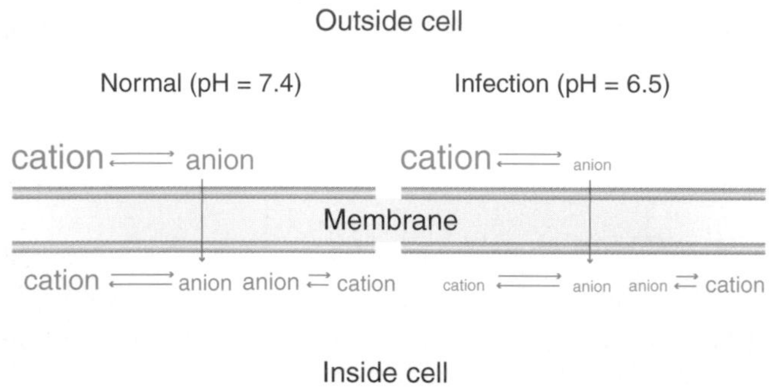

FIGURE 41-6
Effect of hydrogen ion concentration (pH) on local anesthetic drug action. In the normal extracellular environment (pH 7.4, *left side of diagram*), the anion form of the local anesthetic drug exists in sufficient numbers to make anesthesia possible. In infection (pH 6.5, *right side of diagram*), the lower pH reduces the number of anesthetic anions available to penetrate the membrane and the numbers for anesthesia may not be sufficient to be rendered effective.

The clinician should to know the chemical group for local anesthetic drugs used. Local anesthetics used in health care fall into one of two groups: **esters** and **amides.** All local anesthetics packaged for use in dentistry today are in the amide group.

The chemical structure of most local anesthetics includes a **hydrophilic** amino group and a **hydrophobic** aromatic hydrocarbon ring component, separated by an intermediate hydrocarbon chain that contains either an ester or an amide linkage. The hydrophobic group, which has an aromatic nucleus, facilitates the penetration of the anesthetic through the lipid membrane, where the receptor sites for these drugs are located. The more hydrophobic a local anesthetic is, the more potent the drug will be and the longer the duration of action the drug will have. The hydrophilic (water-soluble) component of the local anesthetic agent facilitates diffusion of the drug through the extracellular fluid to the nerve.

Pharmacokinetics

ABSORPTION

The onset of local anesthesia is determined primarily by the molecular properties of the anesthetic. When the anesthetic is injected into the tissues or applied topically, it must diffuse from its site of administration to its sites of action inside the nerve membrane. Anesthetics that have a low molecular weight and a high lipid solubility and that are in the base

form cross the nerve axon membrane with ease. Anesthetics that have a high molecular weight and a low lipid solubility and that are cationic penetrate the axon slowly and have a slow onset of action.

Local anesthetics are absorbed into the bloodstream and distributed to all parts of the body. The rate at which the local anesthetic agent is removed from the site of action, terminating anesthesia, is determined primarily by blood flow at the site of administration. The effects of local anesthetic drugs are reversed as the molecules of anesthetic diffuse out of the axon and are carried away in the bloodstream.

In areas where blood flow is high, anesthetic is rapidly absorbed into the systemic circulation, and anesthesia is terminated. All local anesthetics used in dentistry have vasodilating properties, which increase the systemic absorption of the drug, resulting in a reduced period of anesthesia.

DISTRIBUTION

After absorption into the bloodstream, local anesthetics are distributed throughout the body to all tissues, including the placenta and nerve tissues. Nerve tissues are particularly susceptible to local anesthetic, allowing them to cross the blood-brain barrier easily. The toxicity of a local anesthetic depends on the amount of drug that may accumulate in any tissue, but of particular systemic importance is its accumulation in the brain and cardiac musculature.

METABOLISM

The toxic effects of local anesthetics depend on the balance between the rates of absorption and elimination. The metabolism of these drugs varies greatly and is a major factor in determining the safety of each anesthetic agent. The two major classes of local anesthetics, the amides and esters, are metabolized differently.

The ester local anesthetics are primarily hydrolyzed and inactivated by plasma **cholinesterase** (also known as **pseudocholinesterase**).[14] **Para-aminobenzoic acid** (PABA) is the major metabolic by-product of ester hydrolysis and is excreted in the urine. Most allergic reactions after administration of an ester local anesthetic occur in response to the PABA by-product and not to the anesthetic drug.

Approximately 1 in 2800 individuals has an atypical form of pseudocholinesterase and cannot hydrolyze ester local anesthetics and other chemically related drugs.[5] This form results in higher blood levels in these patients and increases the probability of toxicity. As a partial result of these factors, ester local anesthetic drugs are no longer available for use in dentistry.

The metabolism of amide local anesthetics is more complex than that of esters. In general, the amide local anesthetics are metabolized in the liver by microsomal enzymes.[1] Alcoholics and patients with severe liver disease may accumulate amide local anesthetics, resulting in systemic toxicity.

EXCRETION

The kidneys excrete the metabolic by-products of both esters and amides. A very small amount of the local anesthetic is excreted unchanged in the urine. Only small amounts of esters appear unchanged in the urine because they are almost completely metabolized in the blood. Because the metabolism of amides is more complex, more of the unchanged drug is excreted than with esters. In renal failure, both metabolites and free drug can accumulate.

✦ CASE APPLICATION 41-1.1

Volume of Anesthesia

Considering that Ms. Guyegos has no contraindication to the local anesthetic drugs, no restrictions exist in the volume of the local anesthetic drug that she may have; normal safe volumes may be used.

Pharmacology

OVERVIEW OF COMMONLY USED LOCAL ANESTHETIC AGENTS

41-1

Most local anesthetics agents available today are identified as esters or amides. Only those of greatest significance in dentistry will be discussed here. Table 41-1 lists the local anesthetic drugs currently available in dental cartridges.

Esters

Procaine

Procaine was developed to address the highly addictive and toxic properties of cocaine. Procaine (Novocain) quickly replaced cocaine in both medicine and dentistry.

Procaine causes vasodilation and is quickly removed from the injection site into systemic circulation. It has a relatively short duration of action, unless a **vasoconstrictor** is added. Its slow onset and short duration of action led to its replacement by lidocaine, and it is no longer available in dental cartridges. Procaine is not effective topically. Additionally, procaine was found to be relatively allergenic. It is currently used for patients with documented allergies to amide anesthetic agents and as an antiarrhythmic agent in medicine.

Tetracaine

Tetracaine is 10 times more potent than procaine and more toxic because of its slow metabolism. Tetracaine is rapidly absorbed from the mucous membranes and, if used for topical anesthesia, should be applied to small areas to prevent rapid absorption into the systemic circulation and significant risk of toxic reaction.

For use in dentistry, tetracaine is available as a 2% solution for topical application.

Table 41-1   Local Anesthetic Drugs Available in Dental Cartridges

| GENERIC DRUG | Concentration | | Duration (in minutes) | |
	DRUG (%)	VASOCONSTRICTOR (1:XX)	SOFT TISSUE	PULPAL
Lidocaine	2	None	60-120	5-10
Lidocaine	2	Epinephrine 1:50,000	180-300	60
Lidocaine	2	Epinephrine 1:100,000	180-300	60
Mepivacaine	3	None	120-180	20 (infiltration); 40 (nerve block)
Mepivacaine	2	Levonordefrin 1:20,000	180-300	60
Mepivacaine	2	Epinephrine 1:200,000	120-240	45-60
Mepivacaine	2	Epinephrine 1:200,000	120-300	60
Articaine	4	Epinephrine 1:100,000	180-360	60-75
Articaine	4	Epinephrine 1:200,000 (Canada)	120-300	45-60
Prilocaine	4	None	90-120	10-15 (infiltration); 40-60 (nerve block)
Prilocaine	4	Epinephrine 1:200,000	180-480	60-90
Bupivacaine	0.5	Epinephrine 1:200,000	240-540	90-180

Generic drug names only have been provided; no manufacturer proprietary names are included on this table. For lists of brand names, consult the manufacturers listed on the Evolve site.

Benzocaine

Benzocaine is the most widely used topical anesthetic agent in dentistry. This drug is popular because of its low toxicity and minimal overdose potential. Benzocaine is poorly absorbed through mucous membranes, limiting its field of anesthesia. It is not suitable for use as an injectable agent.[18] For use in dentistry, benzocaine is commonly used in 10% and 20% gel solutions.

Amides

Lidocaine

Lidocaine was the first amide local anesthetic drug distributed for clinical use in dentistry and, within a few years, replaced procaine (commonly known as Novocain) as the drug of choice for pain control in both dentistry and medicine.

> *Note*
>
> Lidocaine is a commonly used local anesthetic in dentistry and is considered the *benchmark* for all new local anesthetics in the United States.

Lidocaine alone possess vasodilating properties, which limit the duration of action. Although lidocaine is effective when used without a vasoconstrictor, adding epinephrine restricts the blood flow into the area of injection and therefore reduces the rate of absorption, thus prolonging the duration of action.

In dentistry, lidocaine 2% is available without a vasoconstrictor or with the vasoconstrictor epinephrine at 1:50,000 and 1:100,000 concentrations. Lidocaine with epinephrine 1:100,000 provides pulpal anesthesia for approximately 1 hour and soft tissue anesthesia for 3 to 5 hours. (For comparison with other related drugs, see Table 41-1.)

Lidocaine is also effective as a topical anesthetic at concentrations ranging from 2% to 10%, available in various ointments, sprays, and viscous solutions and in a *eutectic* mixture (combined with prilocaine). When used topically, the onset of anesthesia occurs within 2 to 3 minutes.

Lidocaine is available in dental cartridges as a 2% solution without vasoconstrictor, 2% with 1:50,000 epinephrine, and 2% with 1:100,000 epinephrine.

Mepivacaine

The onset of action, duration, potency, and toxicity of mepivacaine are similar to lidocaine. Unlike lidocaine, however, mepivacaine produces only slight vasodilation. In a typical dental patient, 2% mepivacaine with a vasoconstrictor provides adequate depth and duration of pain control for most dental procedures. The 3% mepivacaine solution, which is available only without a vasoconstrictor, is often used for short dental procedures and in patients for whom a vasoconstrictor is contraindicated.

Mepivacaine is not effective as a topical anesthetic. Allergic reactions to mepivacaine have not been documented, and the drug shows no cross-allergenicity with the currently available amides.[18]

Mepivacaine is available in dental cartridges as a 3% solution without vasoconstrictor, 2% with 1:20,000 levonordefrin, and 2% with 1:200,000 epinephrine.

Prilocaine

The pharmacologic profile of prilocaine is similar to that of lidocaine and mepivacaine. Similar to mepivacaine, it produces less vasodilation than lidocaine and is available with and without a vasoconstrictor. Unlike mepivacaine, it is significantly less toxic when compared with lidocaine.

Importantly, prilocaine consistently reduces the blood's oxygen-carrying capacity and should not be administered to patients with any condition in which problems of oxygenation may be critical. When used for nerve block anesthesia, prilocaine without a vasoconstrictor produces anesthesia similar in duration to that obtained from lidocaine or mepivacaine administered with or without a vasoconstrictor.

Prilocaine is available in dental cartridges as a 4% solution without vasoconstrictor and 4% with 1:200,000 epinephrine.

Bupivacaine

Bupivacaine also is structurally related to lidocaine and mepivacaine. In contrast, it has stronger vasodilating properties than lidocaine, mepivacaine, and prilocaine.

Bupivacaine is significantly more potent than the other amides and is capable of producing prolonged anesthesia. Bupivacaine is nearly four times more toxic than lidocaine and nearly seven times more toxic than prilocaine. It is used for lengthy dental procedures requiring pulpal anesthesia longer than 90 minutes, for patients who metabolize other drugs quickly, and for managing postoperative pain.

Bupivacaine is available in dental cartridges as a 0.5% solution with 1:200,000 epinephrine.

Articaine

Articaine is the newest amide local anesthetic approved for use in the United States in 2000. Its unique characteristic, compared with other drugs listed previously, is that, although it is an amide, articaine is primarily metabolized as an ester. Articaine is slightly more potent and less toxic than lidocaine.[8]

> *Patient Education Opportunity*
>
> Acetaminophen is a widely used over-the-counter medication that has an independent tendency to induce methemoglobinemia (see Systemic Actions and Complications of Local Anesthetic Agents later in the chapter) in susceptible individuals. Given that the local anesthetic prilocaine also has the same tendency, the clinician should avoid using both at the same time. Therefore, if prilocaine is to be administered as an injectable or topical anesthetic agent during a procedure, the clinician should educate patients about the risks to ensure that they do not take acetaminophen before the procedure or after the procedure, including for postoperative discomfort.

> *Prevention*
>
> Prilocaine has been associated with an increased risk of inducing methemoglobinemia in susceptible individuals. Avoiding its use or using minimal quantities of ingestible or topical prilocaine is important in these individuals. Using benzocaine topical should be avoided as well because it has also been associated with methemoglobinemia.

Notably, articaine is quickly overtaking lidocaine as an anesthetic of choice in countries where it has been available as early as 1976.

Articaine is available in dental cartridges as a 4% solution with 1:100,000 epinephrine; in other countries, it is available as a 4% solution with 1:200,000 epinephrine.

Other Local Anesthetic Agents
Dyclonine

Dyclonine is a **ketone** topical local anesthetic. Cross-sensitivity with other local anesthetics does not occur because dyclonine is chemically different from the ester and amide local anesthetics. It may be used in patients who have a history of allergic or adverse reactions to other chemical groups.

Dyclonine has a slow onset of action, requiring up to 10 minutes to take effect, but the duration of anesthesia may be as long as 1 hour. Systemic toxicity is low because the drug is water insoluble and is not absorbed into the extracellular fluid.

Dyclonine is available in 0.5% and 1% liquid solutions and can be acquired from a compounding pharmacy for use in dentistry. Some on-line buying prescription services list dyclonine products. Dyclonine is not indicated for use by injection or infiltration.

Vasoconstrictors in Anesthetic Solutions

Local anesthetics produce an effect only while bound to receptor sites within the nerve membrane. Most local anesthetics currently used in clinical practice produce some degree of vasodilation. The increased blood flow at the site of injection increases the rate of systemic absorption of the local anesthetic and moves it away from the nerve, which, in turn, shortens the duration of anesthesia. As noted earlier, the degree of vasodilation varies among anesthetic agents.

Any procedure that prevents absorption of the drug prolongs the duration of anesthesia by keeping the anesthetic in contact with the nerve for a longer period. In dentistry, local anesthetics are frequently combined with vasoconstrictors to reduce absorption. The decreased blood flow to the area produced by the vasoconstrictor reduces systemic absorption of the drug. By slowing the rate of absorption of the local anesthetic into the bloodstream, it remains at the injection site longer, and the duration of action is prolonged. The vasoconstrictor also reduces the risks of systemic toxicity from the local anesthetic and bleeding at the site of injection.

The vasoconstrictors used in local anesthetic solutions are identical or similar to the neurotransmitters **epinephrine** and **norepinephrine** released by the sympathetic nervous system. The most common vasoconstrictors available in local anesthetic solutions in the United States are epinephrine and levonordefrin. Epinephrine is the vasoconstrictor most often used and the standard with which other vasoconstrictors are compared.[15]

The concentration of vasoconstrictor in the local anesthetic solution is expressed as a ratio rather than as a percentage, as noted for local anesthetic drugs, representing the amount of vasoconstrictor per milliliter. The most commonly used concentrations of epinephrine for dentistry are 1:50,000 (0.005 mg/ml), 1:100,000 (0.01 mg/ml) and 1:200,000 (0.005 mg/ml). Levonordefrin is only one sixth as effective as epinephrine and is available in a 1:20,000 dilution (0.002 mg/ml).

Epinephrine and levonordefrin cause alpha and beta receptor responses that contract peripheral blood vessels (alpha), relax smooth muscles (beta; for example, bronchodilation and vasodilation), and stimulate the heart (beta). Whereas epinephrine's action is nearly equally divided between alpha and beta influences, levonordefrin is approximately 75% alpha and only approximately 25% beta. By having strong alpha and beta influences, epinephrine is able to constrict peripheral vasculature at the same time it causes bronchodilation, making it useful in emergency situations such as anaphylaxis. With levonordefrin's weak beta stimulation, its effect is primarily peripheral vasoconstriction (alpha), and as such, it is not useful in emergencies because it does not impart significant bronchodilation.[18]

Vasoconstrictors are not ideal drugs. Epinephrine and levonordefrin stimulate **beta receptors** of the myocardium, resulting in an increase in the force of contraction and an increased heart rate. The overall action is direct cardiac stimulation with increased systolic and diastolic pressures, increased cardiac output and stroke volume, increased heart rate, increased strength of contraction, and increased myocardial oxygen consumption. The risks and benefits of using a vasoconstrictor must be assessed for each patient.[12,15]

✦ CASE APPLICATION 41-1.2

Contraindications for Use of Epinephrine

Taking into account Ms. Guyegos' medical history, consider precautions to be taken regarding dental anesthesia. Epinephrine can raise blood sugar levels, which is of particular importance in people with diabetes, especially those not yet under good control despite therapy. In addition, Ms. Guyegos is taking a nonselective beta-blocker. Epinephrine can lead to significant elevations of blood pressure and reflexive bradycardia. Epinephrine is relatively contraindicated for both diabetes and nonselective beta-blockers, which means that it must be given only with caution. Epinephrine should be avoided or used with utmost caution because the risk of adverse reaction is much higher with two separate significant risk factors.

DENTAL CONSIDERATIONS

Another factor of which to be aware is the progression of alpha and beta receptor influences after administering a local anesthetic with epinephrine. The major benefits of using epinephrine in dentistry are from its initial effect on the **alpha receptors** to constrict the peripheral blood vessels. However, over time, the beta effects will predominate. This action can result in postoperative bleeding some time after the procedure is complete and the anesthesia has worn off; thus the drug is acting on the smooth muscles as a vasodilator.

Distinct Care Modifications

Patients who have undergone radiation therapy to the head and neck often sustain damage to the bone in the form of loss of bone-forming and blood-forming tissue. Bone healing is restricted by shortages of bone-forming cells, and the bone is no longer as perfused with blood, which is essential for carrying formative cells, nutrients, and oxygen to the tissues. The already-compromised vascular beds, if compromised further, may lead to what is known as osteonecrosis (ON), a condition caused by any etiology that results in a decrease in oxygenization, cellularity, and vascularity of the bony tissue and actual death of portions of the bone. Osteoradionecrosis refers to a radiation etiology of ON. The death of the bony tissue is considered more a factor of the inability of repair to keep up with the extent of loss than simply the loss itself. It is important to avoid the development of osteonecrosis of the jaws, which are particularly susceptible because of the presence of teeth and periodontium and the availability of teeming colonies of microflora. Vasoconstrictors can result in further injury by constricting the already-compromised vascular beds, increasing the likelihood of osteonecrosis. They should be avoided in these situations.[17]

Most adverse reactions involving epinephrine are short-lived because of epinephrine's rapid metabolism. Some individuals are sensitive to epinephrine and report a sudden increase in heart rate, which is hard to distinguish from a normal reaction to anxiety. If the patient is sensitive to epinephrine or levonordefrin (or both), then local anesthetic drugs without vasoconstrictors can be used safely, or if necessary, doses of vasoconstrictors should be limited. Allergy to epinephrine is impossible.[18]

Administration of Local and Topical Anesthetic Agents

The safe and effective administration of regional or local anesthesia depends on three key factors:

1. Armamentarium-related factors such as equipment and drug selection
2. Patient-related factors such as anatomical variances in skeletal form and nerve innervations
3. Clinician-related factors such as inexperience and poor technique

ARMAMENTARIUM FACTORS

Key components for delivering local anesthetic agents are the needles, cartridges, syringes, and safe-handling practices. Each component has a specific and critical role in the outcome of the safe delivery of these agents to the intended target area. Thoughtful and appropriate selection and use is essential.

Needles

The *single-use* sterile needles for delivery of local anesthetics in dentistry today are the result of research and manufacturing advances. The key characteristics of these needles include a flexible stainless steel shaft, a sharp multilevel beveled point, and a self-threading plastic hub. These design factors enable the clinician to deliver local anesthetics with minimal trauma to the mucosa and subcutaneous tissues. Needles are identified by length and diameter **(gauge),** which must be considered for individual injections.

Length

Needle length varies among manufacturers, but long needles typically average 32 mm, and short needles average 20 mm. The depth of penetration required for successful anesthesia will determine the length of needle. Short needles should be used for injections that do not require significant depth of penetration, such as nerves located a short distance from the penetration site. Long needles should be used when the deposition site is a significant distance from the penetration site, as is the case with mandibular block techniques. Regardless of the type of injection, no needle should be inserted in soft tissue to its hub. Breakage, although rare, is more likely to occur at the hub and is usually the result of lateral pressure exerted against the shank.[5] The clinician should not attempt to change the direction of a needle when it is embedded in tissue. If the needle must be redirected, it should be withdrawn as necessary and redirected.[6]

Gauge

The gauge of the needle refers to the diameter (internal width) of the lumen (hollow portion of the needle). The most common gauges for regional anesthesia of the oral cavity are 25, 27, and 30; the higher the number is, the smaller the opening will be. Current popularity of the smaller-gauge needles (27 and 30) stems from the belief that such needles cause less discomfort during insertion. However, comparisons in clinical studies have shown that patient perception of pain on insertion for a 25-gauge is no different than for a 27- or 30-gauge needle.[3,6] The larger-gauge needles have two advantages over the smaller-gauge needle: (1) less deflection (thus greater accuracy) and (2) ease of positive **aspiration** of blood (thus greater safety). The 25-gauge needle is preferred for all injections posing a high risk of positive aspiration, including inferior alveolar, posterior superior alveolar, and Gow-Gates.

Cartridges

Single-unit, glass cartridges provide a convenient dose form that ensures purity and sterility of the anesthetic solution and permits observation of aspirated blood. The dental cartridge is often called a *Carpule,* which is a trademark name (Carpule is to cartridge as Kleenex is to tissue).

Each year, millions of anesthetic cartridges are used. Based on a complicated manufacturing process that involves many steps and quality control, the contents of these cartridges are reliably sterile and pure for delivery to patients. Cartridges are inspected before shipment, and control samples of each production are set aside for 6 months for continued evaluation.

Although damage to cartridges is rare, it usually occurs during shipment. Before patient use, the cartridges should be visually inspected for the following:

- Signs of breakage (chips, cracks)
- Pea-sized or larger bubbles, which may indicate freezing or contamination
- Extruded plunger, common with freezing

- Altered appearance of the anesthetic solution (cloudiness, sediment), which may indicate overheated or expired solutions

Cartridges have a shelf life of 18 months to 5 years depending on the type of anesthetic, vasoconstrictors, and other chemicals. Solutions with vasoconstrictors have the shortest shelf life. Expiration dates are clearly printed on each cartridge and on the side and bottom of each container. Any anesthetic solution that has passed the expiration date should not be used.

The contents of each anesthetic cartridge are identified by the labeling on the glass tube and include the volume of solution, trade and generic name (identified by a specific color band for each drug) (Figure 41-7, Box 41-1), the concentration of local anesthetic, name and concentration of vasoconstrictor, name and address of supplier, manufacturer's lot number, and expiration date. The dental hygienist should check each cartridge before an injection to confirm that the desired anesthetic and vasoconstrictor are being administered.

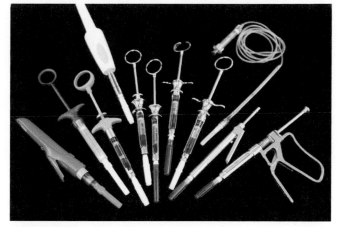

FIGURE 41-8
Local anesthesia delivery syringes. Numerous styles including metal, plastic, safety single use, computerized, pressurized, and a system for subgingival delivery of a specialized topical agent.

Local Anesthetic Solution Band	Color of Cartridge
Articaine HCl 4% with epinephrine 1:100,000	Gold
Bupivacaine 0.5% with epinephrine 1:200,000	Blue
Lidocaine HCl 2%	Light blue
Lidocaine HCl 2% with epinephrine 1:50,000	Green
Lidocaine HCl 2% with epinephrine 1:100,000	Red
Mepivacaine HCl 3%	Tan
Mepivacaine HCl 2% with levonordefrin 1:20,000	Brown
Prilocaine HCl 4%	Black

FIGURE 41-7
Color-coding of local anesthetic cartridges, as per American Dental Association Council on Scientific Affairs. (From Color coding for local anesthesia, *ADA News* 34[8]:28, April 21, 2003. Copyright 2003 American Dental Association. All rights reserved. Reprinted with permission.)

determine which type of syringe is used. Regardless of preference, a syringe should meet the American Dental Association (ADA) standards[6] (Box 41-2).

The most widely used syringe for intraoral anesthesia is the metal, manual-aspiration, cartridge-type syringe. One of the hazards of intraoral anesthesia is the inadvertent intravascular injection. The aspirating syringe allows the practitioner to check for this situation before delivering any drug by creating negative pressure in the cartridge, which provides for visual inspection for any signs of blood or discoloration in the cartridge. The harpoon (hook) on the end of the plunger on an aspirating syringe engages the rubber stopper, allowing the clinician to pull back on the stopper, creating negative pressure inside the cartridge. The incidence of positive aspiration may be as high as 10% to 15% in some injection techniques.[6] The dental professional must purposefully conduct an aspiration test (pull back on the plunger) once the deposition site has been reached and before administering the agent. The gauge of the needle also influences the practitioner's ability to aspirate; the 25-gauge needle is the most appropriate needle for reliable

BOX 41-1

CONTENTS OF A TYPICAL LOCAL ANESTHETIC CARTRIDGE

- Local anesthetic drug
- Vasoconstrictor (if present)
- Sulfite preservative (if vasoconstrictor is present)
- Salt (for isotonicity-tissue compatibility)
- Water (the diluent)

BOX 41-2

AMERICAN DENTAL ASSOCIATION STANDARDS FOR SYRINGES

- Syringe should be durable and able to withstand repeated sterilizations without damage. (If disposable, syringe should then be packaged in a sterile container.)
- Syringe should accommodate a variety of cartridges and needles of different manufacturers and permit repeated use.
- Syringe should be inexpensive, self-contained, lightweight, and simple to use with one hand.
- Syringe should provide for effective aspiration and should be constructed such that blood may be easily observed in the cartridge.

Syringes

Several different types of syringes are available for use in the dental office (Figure 41-8). The most common types are aspirating sterilizable stainless steel syringes and aspirating plastic disposable or sterilizable syringes.[12] Personal preference will

aspiration tests. False-negative aspiration tests have been documented with the use of 27- and 30-gauge needles, the highest incident with the 30-gauge needle; therefore needle selection for use in highly vascular areas should be carefully considered. Self-aspirating syringes are used by some clinicians. When using this type of syringe, careful attention to the manufacturer's instructions is critical to safe use. An extra step is required to confirm aspiration with this type of syringe (Figure 41-9).

New techniques and equipment continue to be introduced for administering local anesthetic agents. The computer-controlled and electronic-induction techniques are gaining in popularity. However, clinical studies indicate that these devices are not likely to replace the standard aspirating syringe.[2,4,13]

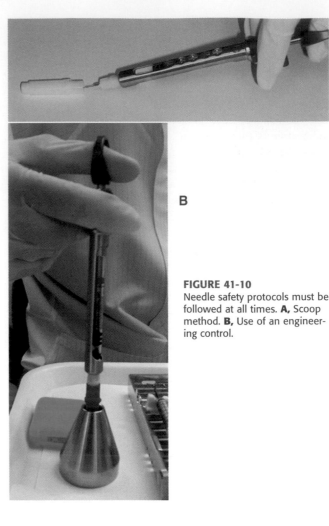

FIGURE 41-10
Needle safety protocols must be followed at all times. **A,** Scoop method. **B,** Use of an engineering control.

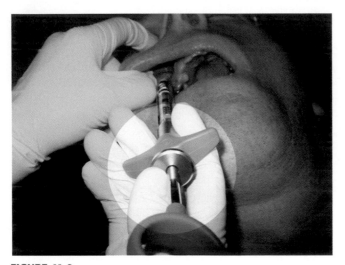

FIGURE 41-9
Self-aspirating syringes must be activated to aspirate.

SAFETY AND HANDLING

Recapping needles presents the greatest risk for occupational injury and the risk for infectious disease transmission to dental health care personnel (HCP). In recent years, HCP have been at risk for contracting hepatitis B and acquired immunodeficiency syndrome (AIDS) through inadvertent needlesticks after an intraoral injection. Numerous techniques (work-practice controls [WPCs]) and devices (engineering controls [ECs]) have been recommended to prevent this potential health hazard. Consensus does not exist for the best solution; however, manual (two-handed) recapping is prohibited. Only one-handed methods of recapping should be used (Figure 41-10). The **scoop technique** is a WPC often recommended by safety and health agencies.[6] This technique requires that the operator slide the uncapped needle into the needle cap (sheath) while it is lying on the instrument tray or table. The cap must not be handled until the point of the needle is protected by the sheath. Care must be taken to avoid contaminating the needle on the instrument tray or outside of the sheath during this process, especially if the needle may be used again for the patient.

Needle guards are ECs designed to provide added protection when handling and recapping needles. The EC should provide a barrier between the tip of the needle and the fingers of HCP throughout the recapping procedure. If a needle is recapped incorrectly when using the needle guard, then the tip of the needle may be contaminated by contact with the guard, or injury may occur to HCP.

Prevention

Needle holders are also available for placement of the needle and syringe after use. The needle is covered, protecting dental health care personnel. Used, recapped needles should be removed from the nondisposable syringe and placed in a sharps container as close to the point of use as possible. Transporting sharps is not recommended. Disposable syringes may also be placed in the sharps container. Both EC safety devices and the scoop technique are effective, and the dental hygienist should determine which method is most appropriate for the work circumstances.

TOPICAL ANESTHETIC AGENTS

Using a topically applied local anesthetic is an important step in the atraumatic process of administering local anesthetic agents. **Topical anesthetic agents** penetrate any mucous membrane approximately 2 to 3 mm (Figure 41-11).

The concentration of agents used for topical anesthesia is typically greater than that for agents administered by injection. The higher concentration facilitates diffusion of the drug through the mucous membrane. Higher concentrations also lead to a greater potential for both local and systemic toxicity.[1] Because topical anesthetics do not contain vasoconstrictors, and because anesthetics are inherently vasodilating agents, vascular absorption of most topical formulations is rapid, and levels in the blood may quickly reach those achieved by parenteral administration.[12] (For specifics on local anesthetic drugs used as topical agents, see the section Overview of Commonly Used Local Anesthetic Agents earlier in the chapter.)

Application

When appropriate, a small quantity of topical anesthetic is applied directly onto a clean, dry area of mucosa at the injection site. A minimal volume of agent is needed to achieve anesthesia at the penetration site. The application of too large a volume of the topical agent can lead to a variety of adverse effects. These effects can be characterized as unpleasantness, local tissue reactions, systemic toxicity, and allergic reactions. Most important,

some topical anesthetics can be rapidly absorbed into the cardiovascular system.

The procedure is most efficiently accomplished by placing a small quantity of topical anesthetic concentrated at the tip of a cotton applicator stick that is applied directly to the prepared penetration site for at least 1 minute.[6]

Topical agents directly applied to the gingiva may be used to control discomfort by means of superficial anesthesia of small areas of tissue during scaling procedures (Figure 41-12). The area needs to be dry, and the selection of topical anesthesic should provide a relatively long anesthetic effect with low toxicity (e.g., benzocaine product, dyclonine). The clinician should avoid swabbing topical anesthetic throughout the mouth instead of using injections. Swabbing does not provide profound anesthesia, and, more important, doses cannot be well documented.[1]

Topical anesthesia for periodontal procedures may be achieved with the subgingival delivery of a eutectic mixture of 2.5% lidocaine and 2.5% prilocaine using a specialized applicator. This method provides approximately 20 minutes of anesthesia at the site following delivery (see Figure 41-12).

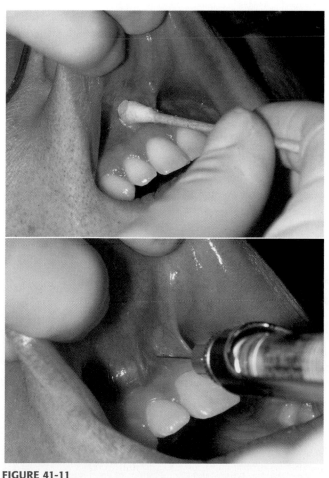

FIGURE 41-11
A, Application of topical anesthetic. **B,** Retraction and penetration for infiltration injection.

⁎ CASE APPLICATION 41-1.3

Anesthesia Selection for Ms. Guyegos

A drug that would work well and pose the least risk for Ms. Guyegos would be a plain solution (i.e., 3% mepivacaine plain), which does not contain vasoconstrictors. Four percent prilocaine plain is also a possibility, although a small but notably higher incidence of paresthesia has been noted with 4% drugs, especially in inferior alveolar nerve blocks. Two percent mepivacaine with 1:200,000 epinephrine is also available and would represent another appropriate choice because of the minimal concentration of epinephrine if duration were insufficient. A combination of 3% mepivacaine along with lesser amounts of 2% mepivacaine with 1:200,000 epinephrine would also be a safe choice for insufficient duration.

Local Anesthesia Techniques

Delivering local anesthetic agents requires the clinician to apply a safe, aseptic approach and to avoid possible complications during the procedure. Safe administration includes a thorough health history review to determine the potential for drug interactions or systemic disease that may require modifications to drug selection or delivery approach. Assessing the patient's blood pressure is important before delivering local anesthetic agents. Safe technique includes the following:

- Stable fulcrum
- Depositing the drug at a slow rate
- Aspiration test before depositing the drug

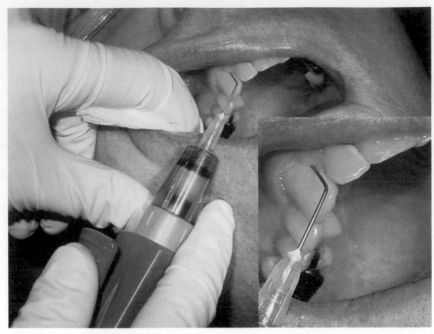

FIGURE 41-12
In Oraqix subgingival gel delivery, solution is placed at depth of pocket and turns to gel at body temperature.

- Appropriate personal protective equipment for both the clinician and the patient
- Close attention to safe handling of a sharp device

Good communication and observation skills are an integral part of pain-management techniques and should be considered a part of the overall process of local anesthesia administration.

INJECTIONS GUIDELINES

Successful safe and repeatable injection technique requires that the clinician apply a basic approach to each injection. Although varying schools of thought exist both regionally and individually, the following steps represent a consistent and safe approach to delivering local anesthetic agents in prescribed locations in the oral cavity. Tables 41-2 and 41-3 provide a summary of the key elements of each injection: penetration point, injection angle, needled gauge, depth of insertion, target structures, drug dose, and the areas effected for maxillary and mandibular injections, respectively. The volumes suggested for each injection are generally adequate for routine dental hygiene procedures. Advanced periodontal scaling procedures often require greater volumes such as are needed for profound pulpal anesthesia when indicated for operative and surgical procedures.

INFORMED CONSENT

Before delivering any anesthetic agents, proper informed consent should be acquired. In addition to discussion about the nature and need for the intended treatment, the patient must be advised of the risks associated with the delivery of injectable local anesthetic agents.

Distinct Care Modifications

Local anesthesia necessary for many dental hygiene procedures may or may not require pulpal anesthesia. Doses for providing soft tissue anesthesia are lower because the duration of anesthesia for soft tissue is longer than for the pulps of the teeth and is easier to achieve. For example, when administering a posterior superior alveolar nerve block for dental hygiene procedures, the recommended volume of 2% lidocaine with 1:100,000 epinephrine is typically 0.9 to 1.5 ml, whereas the volume for restorative procedures is typically 1.2 to 1.8 ml. Some advanced dental hygiene procedures, or lengthy appointments on sensitive teeth, may require more profound anesthesia than minor restorative procedures on teeth, for example, with older, calcified pulps.

Patient Education Opportunity

Important elements in discussing informed consent for local anesthesia delivery begin with a simple definition: "*Local anesthesia* involves receiving an injection *(shot)* that results in temporary numbing of an area with anesthetic solution. Although side effects from receiving local anesthetic are rare, they may include swelling, bruising, temporary muscle tightening, temporary or permanent tingling or numbing of the nerve of the tongue or lip, localized pain or soreness, allergic reaction to the anesthetic solution, or short-term racing of the heart. The dental team needs to be told if you or anyone in your family has ever had difficulty with anesthesia during a surgery." This definition might mean that the patient might have a type of hereditary problem with certain anesthetics (see Systemic Actions and Complications of Local Anesthetic Agents later in the chapter).

Table 41-2 Technique Summary for Maxillary Anesthesia Techniques

NERVE BLOCK	AREAS ANESTHETIZED	NEEDLE (GAUGE AND LENGTH)	PENETRATION SITE	DEPTH AND ANGLE FOR INSERTION	DEPOSITION SITE	DOSE (PULPAL)
Anterior Superior Alveolar (ASA) (Figure 41-13)	*Teeth:* canine, lateral, central *Peridontium and soft tissues:* facial to affected teeth	25-27 G short	Height of mucobuccal fold, slightly mesial to apex of canine	*Depth:* 3-5 mm, to apex of canine *Angle:* approximately 20 degrees to long axis of tooth, slightly mesial to apex of canine, bevel toward bone	Just above periosteum adjacent to apex of canine	0.9-1.2 ml
Middle Superior Alveolar (MSA) (Figure 41-14)	*Teeth:* maxillary premolars and mesiobuccal root of first molar* *Peridontium and soft tissues:* facial to affected teeth	25-27 G short	Height of mucobuccal fold between premolars	*Depth:* 3-5 mm *Angle:* approximately 20 degrees to long axis of tooth, near apex of second premolar, bevel toward bone	Close to bone, above apex of second premolar	0.9-1.2 ml
Infraorbital (IO) (Figure 41-15)	*Teeth:* premolars, canine, lateral, central *Peridontium and soft tissues:* facial to affected teeth	25-27 G short	Height of mucobuccal fold over first premolar	*Depth:* approximately one half length of the needle *Angle:* needle parallel to midsagittal plane aligned with pupil of eye on same side; bevel toward bone	At infraorbital foramen *Note:* Keep pressure over foramen for 1 minute after injection.	0.9-1.2 ml
Posterior Superior Alveolar (PSA) (Figure 41-16)	*Teeth:* maxillary molars except mesiobuccal root of first molar *Periodontal tissues:* buccal to affected teeth	25-27 G short or long	Height of mucobuccal fold lateral to distal-buccal of second molar, posterior to zygomatic arch	*Depth:* approximately two thirds to three quarters length of needle *Angle:* advanced medially along a line 45 degrees to occlusal plane and 45 degrees to midsagittal plane	Posterior surface of the maxilla, superior to the maxillary tuberosity	0.9-1.8 ml
Nasopalatine (NP) (Figure 41-17)	*Teeth:* none *Periodontal tissues:* palatal to incisors and canines bilateral	25-27 G short, 30 G x-short	Just lateral to incisive papilla at widest aspect	*Depth:* 3-5 mm *Angle:* approach at 45 degrees to anterior palate, bevel toward palate	Beneath incisive papilla, at incisive foramen	≤0.4 ml
Palatial Anterior Superior Alveolar (P-ASA) (Figure 41-18)	*Teeth:* canines, laterals, centrals bilateral *Peridontium and soft tissues:* to affected teeth	25-27 G short	Just lateral to the incisive papilla at anterior aspect	*Depth:* 6-10 mm *Angle:* from a 45-degree angle, bevel toward palate	Beneath incisive papilla, slightly into incisive foramen	1.4-1.8 ml
Anterior Middle Superior Alveolar (AMSA) (Figure 41-19)	*Teeth:* premolars, canine, lateral, central *Peridontium and soft tissues:* palatal to affected teeth	25-27 G short	At the junction of the horizontal and vertical aspects of the palate, below a line bisecting the free gingival margin of the premolars	*Depth:* 4-7 mm *Angle:* from opposite side of mouth at right angle to alveolar process, bevel toward palate	Above apex, between premolars on the palatal side	1.4-1.8 ml (0.7-0.9 ml 4% solutions)
Greater Palatine (GP) (Figure 41-20)	*Teeth:* none *Peridontium and soft tissues:* palatal tissues of premolars, molars	25-27 G short, 30 G x-short,	At junction of palatine bone and alveolar process, lingual to second molar, slightly anterior to the greater palatine foramen	*Depth:* 4-6 mm (<10 mm) *Angle:* from opposite side of mouth at right angle to alveolar process, bevel toward palate	At palatine foramina	0.4-0.6 ml

*For most people.
Modified from Malamed SF: *Handbook of local anesthesia,* ed 5, St Louis, 2004, Mosby.

| Table 41-3 | Technique Summary for Mandibular Anesthesia Techniques |

NERVE BLOCK	TISSUES ANESTHETIZED	NEEDLE (GAUGE AND LENGTH)	PENETRA-TION SITE	DEPTH AND ANGLE FOR INSERTION	DEPOSITION SITE	DOSE (PULPAL)
Inferior Alveolar (IA) and Lingual (Figure 41-21)	*Teeth:* all teeth in quadrant *Peridontium and soft tissues:* all peridontium, buccal mucosa premolars to midline, floor of mouth and one half of tongue in quadrant (not soft tissues buccal to molars)	25 G long	Medial to internal oblique ridge, depth of sulcus lateral to pterygomandibular raphe, at or above height of coronoid notch	*Depth:* two thirds to three quarters length of needle, until contact with bone, bevel toward bone *Angle:* barrel of syringe in corner of mouth on opposite side (over bicuspids), parallel to mandibular occlusal plane	On medial surface of ramus, slightly superior to mandibular foramen	1.5-1.8 ml
Buccal (B) (Figure 41-22)	*Teeth:* none *Peridontium and soft tissues:* buccal to molars	25 G long*	Mucous membrane distal and lateral to most posterior molar	*Depth:* ≤4 mm, bevel under tissue, bevel toward bone *Angle:* syringe parallel to occlusal plane, lateral to teeth, bevel toward bone	Supraperiosteal, distal, and buccal to most posterior molar	0.2-0.3 ml (width of rubber stopper)
Mental (M), Incisive (I) (Figure 41-23)	*Teeth:* (M) pulpal limited to tooth at site of infiltration, (I) premolars to midline *Peridontium and soft tissues:* premolars to midline	25-27 G short	Mucobuccal fold at or just anterior to mental foramen	*Depth:* 5-6 mm *Angle:* approximately 20 degrees to long axis of premolars, bevel toward bone	Slightly superior to mental foramen *Note:* (I) Keep pressure over foramen for 1-2 minutes after injection.	0.6 ml
Gow-Gates (G-G) (Figure 41-24)	*Teeth:* all teeth in quadrant *Peridontium and soft tissues:* all peridontium, buccal mucosa premolars to midline, floor of mouth and one half of tongue in quadrant	25 G long	Distal to maxillary second molar at height of mesiolingual cusp	*Depth:* one half to three quarters length of needle; *must* contact bone *Angle:* barrel of syringe in corner of mouth on opposite side; proceed on a parallel line from corner of mouth to tragus	Lateral side of condylar neck *Note:* Patient should keep mouth open for 1-2 minutes after injection.	1.8 ml
Local Infiltration (inf) (Figure 41-11, B); Maxillary or Mandibular	*Teeth:* at site *Peridontium and soft tissues:* at site	25-27 G short	Mucobuccal fold buccal to tooth	*Depth:* 3-5 mm to apex *Angle:* approximately 20 degrees to long axis of tooth, directed toward apex of tooth, bevel toward bone	Apex of tooth	0.6 ml

*Usually given after IA.
Modified from Malamed SF: *Handbook of local anesthesia,* ed 5, St Louis, 2004, Mosby.

BASIC INJECTION TECHNIQUE*

A properly loaded syringe setup will have the cartridge diaphragm toward the needle, with the harpoon firmly seated in the stopper. With the sterile needle attached, the tip of the needle should be checked for any visible barbs before use. The bevel should be oriented to a position that will face the bone during injection. For multiple injections, the needle needs to be changed each three to four penetrations or if it is contaminated by contact with any surface other than the patient's own mucosal tissue.

The thumb ring should be gently pressed to check the flow of anesthetic through the needle. The needle must be recapped by using the one-handed scoop method or a needle holder, without contaminating it on the outside of the cap or other surfaces.

DENTAL CONSIDERATIONS

Orienting the bevel of the needle toward bone lessens the likelihood of discomfort and trauma to the periosteum when bone is contacted. In the event of inadvertent contact, the needle tends to glance off the bone rather than to pierce the periosteum.

Prevention
Position the patient in a semisupine position (to reduce the potential for syncope), and always provide psychologic support for stress reduction. Remember, this point in time is when supportive communication begins. Explain the purpose of topical anesthetic to the patient and that the injection will take some time, stressing the comfort and safety of this technique. Keeping the syringe out of the patient's view is also an important stress-reduction step.

Before approaching with the syringe, establish adequate retraction to visualize the penetration site clearly. Dry the tissue with 2 × 2 gauze before placing a topical anesthetic agent. Using a cotton-tip applicator, an appropriate topical anesthetic agent should be applied at the site of penetration for 1 minute. This point of the procedure can be considered the *rehearsal* for the injection in which the clinician mentally reviews the injection technique and evaluates the patient for anatomical variations that may require adjustment to the planned technique.

To deliver the injection, the clinician should establish a firm, balanced hand rest, avoiding the patient's body as a fulcrum point. The most stable position for the syringe is a *palm-up* grasp, with the index finger extended onto the barrel for support. The large window of the syringe must be facing the clinician, and the length of the cartridge must be visible to evaluate the outcome of the aspiration test and the amount of drug that has been delivered.

The injection is delivered by initially penetrating the tissue 1 to 2 mm (approximately the length of the bevel), with the bevel opening oriented toward bone. A few drops of anesthetic are allowed to be deposited in front of the needle as it is *slowly* advanced. This total volume should be less than 0.2 ml (the width of 1 stopper advanced). The clinician should observe and communicate with the patient throughout the injection, monitoring for signs of discomfort, distress, or adverse reactions.

Prevention
Do not, under any circumstances, deposit the drug if a positive aspiration occurs. This precaution is one of the most important safety steps in delivering local aesthetic agent and prevents the deposition of the drug directly into the bloodstream.

Once the needle is advanced to the appropriate depth and angle for the specific injection, an aspiration test is performed. The best practice is to perform this test twice, rotating the syringe slightly to another position.

The next critical step in delivering a safe and comfortable injection is the pace; slow delivery of the drug reduces the risk of compilations and overdose if the drug is inadvertently injected into the bloodstream and facilitates a comfortable experience for the patient by preventing tearing of tissue from the pressure of the anesthetic solution being injected. A safe injection rate allows for the delivery of a 1.8-ml cartridge of anesthetic over a period of 1 minute. However, some exceptions exist.[18] (See the box feature entitled Distinct Care Modifications on p. 785.)

The clinician should continue monitoring the patient throughout the injection. Reaspirating is important if the clinician believes he or she has changed the depth or angle of the needle during the injection and any time an additional *safety check* is warranted. After completing delivery of the designated dose, the syringe is slowly withdrawn.

The final safety step is to manage and recap the needle properly by using the one-handed scoop method or a needle holder. Preferably, the person delivering the drug should complete the recapping of the needle because this reduces the number of persons who come into contact with the syringe and needle, reducing the accident potential.

After completing the injection, the clinician should observe and communicate with the patient, monitoring for any adverse effects.

SUPRAPERIOSTEAL INJECTION FOR MAXILLARY OR MANDIBULAR ARCHES*

Supraperiosteal injections are indicated for dental procedures that are limited to one or two teeth or for soft tissue anesthesia in a circumscribed area (see Figure 41-11, *B*). Supraperiosteal injection is also referred to as **local infiltration** (inf) or paraperiosteal injection. Anesthesia will affect the large terminal

---

*It is not the intention of the authors for this information to be comprehensive for each injection but rather to serve as an introduction to local anesthesia procedures and to expand the knowledge of the hygienist who will be unable to deliver local aesthetics by nature of their individual state practice act. More comprehensive information for each injection would be included in a full course of study for local anesthesia certification.

*Information in this section is from Malamed SF: *Handbook of local anesthesia,* ed 5, St Louis, 2004, Mosby.

nerve branches of the dental plexus, as well as the entire region innervated by these branches, including the pulp and root area of the tooth, buccal periosteum, connective tissue, and mucous membrane.

Technique Factors

The clinician should apply the basic injection steps previously noted.

- The appropriate armamentarium includes a short needle, gauge 25, 27, or 30 (a 30-gauge needle may be used in areas with limited vascularization).
- A topical anesthetic is applied.
- The penetration site for a supraperiosteal injection is at the height of the mucobuccal fold and above the apex of the tooth to be anaesthetized.
- The insertion angle of the syringe is parallel to the long axis of the tooth and the angle of the maxillary bone.
- To gain access to the site of penetration, the lip is lifted while the tissue is pulled taut with the thumb and index finger.
- The injection is delivered by initially penetrating the tissue a few millimeters and depositing a few drops of anesthetic.
- The deposition site will be close to bone at a depth of 4 to 6 mm. Before depositing the drug, an aspiration test should be performed. *This test is one of the most important safety steps in delivering local anesthetic agents.*
- After a negative aspiration, one-quarter to one-half cartridge (0.4 to 0.9 ml) of an appropriately selected local anesthetic drug is deposited.

MAXILLARY INJECTIONS*

Anterior Superior Alveolar Nerve Block

Anterior superior alveolar (ASA) nerve blocks (Figure 41-13) are indicated for pain management of anterior teeth in one quadrant. Anesthesia will affect the structures innervated by the ASA nerve, including the pulps of the maxillary central incisor through the canine on the injected side.

Technique factors

The clinician should apply the basic injection steps.

- For the ASA nerve block, a 27-gauge short needle is most commonly used.
- To gain access to the site of penetration, the lip is lifted and the tissue is pulled taut with the thumb and index finger.
- The penetration site is at the height of the mucobuccal fold just mesial to the canine, and the angle of insertion is parallel to the long axis of the canine, following the angle of the maxilla.
- The deposition site is at the apex of the canine in the canine fossa at a depth of 4 to 6 mm.

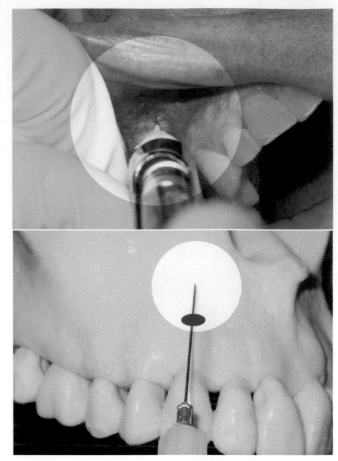

FIGURE 41-13
Anterior superior alveolar (ASA) nerve block. **A,** Penetration site. **B,** Deposition site. The depth of penetration is indicated by the red dot.

- After a negative aspiration, one-half to two-thirds cartridge (0.9 to 1.2 ml) of an appropriately selected local anesthetic drug is deposited.

Middle Superior Alveolar Nerve Block

Middle superior alveolar (MSA) (Figure 41-14) nerve blocks are indicated for pain management of premolars in one quadrant. Anesthesia will affect the structures innervated by the MSA nerve and terminal branches, including the pulps of the maxillary first and second premolars and mesiobuccal root of the first molar on the injected side.

Technique factors

The clinician should apply the basic injection steps.

- For the MSA nerve block, a 27-gauge short needle is most commonly used.
- To gain access to the site of penetration, the lip is lifted and the tissue is pulled taut with the thumb and index finger.
- The penetration site is at the height of the mucobuccal fold between the first and second bicuspids, and the angle of insertion is parallel to the long axis of the bicuspids following the angle of the maxilla.

---

*Information in this section is from Haas DA: An update of local anesthetics in dentistry, *J Can Dent Assoc* 68:546-551, 2002, and Malamed SF: *Handbook of local anesthesia,* ed 5, St Louis, 2004, Mosby.

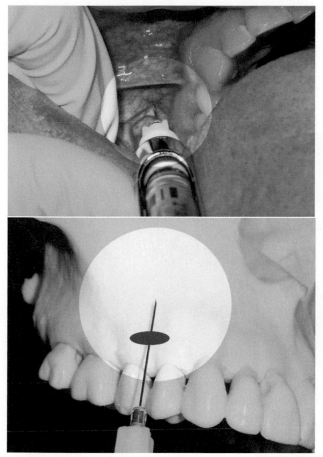

FIGURE 41-14
Middle superior alveolar (MSA) nerve block. **A,** Penetration site. **B,** De-position site. Depth of penetration is indicated by the red dot.

- For the IO nerve block, a 27-gauge short or long needle is used.
- To gain access to the site of penetration, the lip is lifted and the tissue is pulled taut with the thumb and index finger.
- The penetration site is at the height of the mucobuccal fold directly over the first premolar.
- The angle of insertion is oriented toward the IO foramen along a line parallel to the pupil of the eye on the side of injection.
- The deposition site is the area over the IO foramen at a depth adequate to reach the foramen.
- After a negative aspiration, one-half cartridge (0.9 ml) of an appropriately selected local anesthetic drug is deposited.
- To facilitate diffusion of the solution into the foramen, postprocedure finger pressure is maintained over the injection site for 1 to 2 minutes.

Posterior Superior Alveolar Nerve Block

Posterior superior alveolar (PSA) nerve blocks (Figure 41-16) are indicated for pain management of several molar teeth in one quadrant. PSA nerve blocks are also referred to as *tuberosity* or *zygomatic blocks*. Anesthesia will affect the structures innervated by the PSA nerve and terminal branches, including the pulps of the maxillary third, second, and first molars (not complete for some patients) on the injected side. The mesiobuccal root of the maxillary first molar is not anesthetized for most patients.

> *Prevention*
> Special consideration must be given for patients with clotting disorders. The PSA injection has a substantial risk of positive aspiration and hematoma, and therefore it may be contraindicated.

Technique factors

The clinician should apply the basic injection steps.

- For the PSA nerve block, a 27-gauge short needle is commonly used. Some clinicians give this injection with a long needle, whereas others deliver the PSA as a more shallow injection (**infiltration**) with relative success for soft tissue procedures.
- To gain access to the site of penetration, the lip is retracted at a downward angle, lifting the buccal mucosal laterally.
- The penetration site is at the height of the mucobuccal fold, distal to the zygomatic process of the maxilla, and above the distal buccal of the maxillary second molar.
- The angle of needle insertion is upward (at a 45-degree angle to the occlusal plane of the maxillary teeth), inward behind the maxillary tuberosity (45-degree angle to the midsagittal plane), and then must be advance back behind the posterior aspect of the maxilla. To achieve this position, the barrel of the syringe must be angled downward from the occlusal table and outward from the patient's midsagittal plane.
- The deposition site is over the foramen for the PSA nerve on the infratemporal surface of the maxilla.

- The deposition site is above the apex of the second bicuspid at a depth of 5 to 8 mm.
- After a negative aspiration, one-half to two-thirds cartridge (0.9 to 1.2 ml) of an appropriately selected local anesthetic drug is deposited.

Infraorbital Nerve Block

Infraorbital (IO) nerve blocks (Figure 41-15) are indicated for pain management of anterior and premolar teeth in one quadrant, while delivering a smaller volume of local anesthetic than for both the ASA and MSA nerve blocks given for the same area. The IO nerve block is an alternative if both the ASA and the MSA nerve blocks are unsuccessful because of dense cortical bone or local inflammation. The IO nerve block is also referred to as an *ASA nerve block.* Anesthesia will affect the structures innervated by the ASA, MSA, IO nerves, and terminal branches. Areas anaesthetized include the pulps of the maxillary central incisor through the canine, premolars, mesiobuccal root of the first molar (for most patients), buccal periodontium, lower eyelid, lateral aspect of nose, and lip on the injected side.

Technique factors

The clinician should apply the basic injection steps.

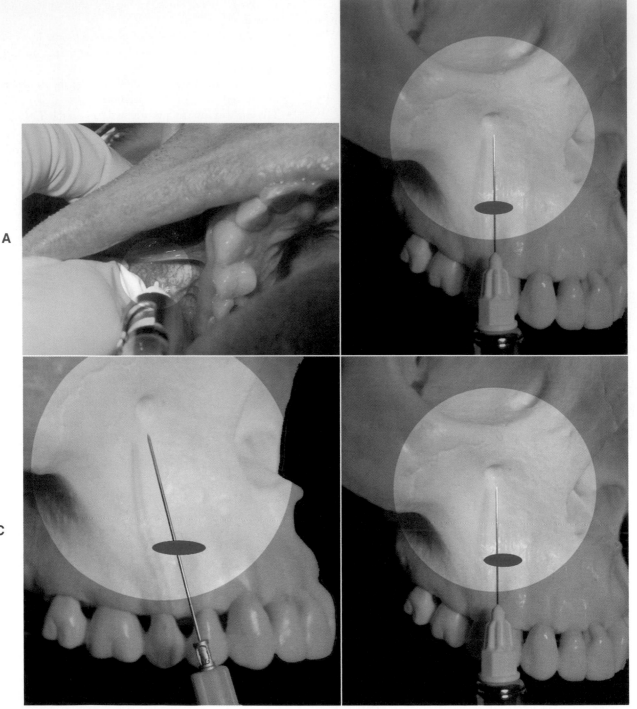

FIGURE 41-15
Infraorbital (IO) nerve block. **A,** Penetration site. **B,** Deposition site. **C,** Penetration depth with long needle. **D,** Penetration depth with short needle. Depth of penetration is indicated by the red dot.

- The depth of insertion is 14 to 16 mm (approximately 4 mm from the hub of a short needle).
- After a negative aspiration, two-thirds to three-quarters cartridge (1.2 to 1.5 ml) of an appropriately selected local anesthetic drug is deposited. To facilitate diffusion of the solution into the foramen, postprocedure finger pressure is maintained over the injection site for 1 to 2 minutes.

Nasopalatine Nerve Block

Nasopalatine (NP) nerve blocks (Figure 41-17) are indicated for pain management of palatal soft and osseous tissue bilaterally from canine to canine. The NP nerve block is also referred to as an *incisive* or *sphenopalatine nerve block*. Anesthesia will affect the structures innervated by the NP nerve bilaterally and terminal branches, including the anterior portion of the hard

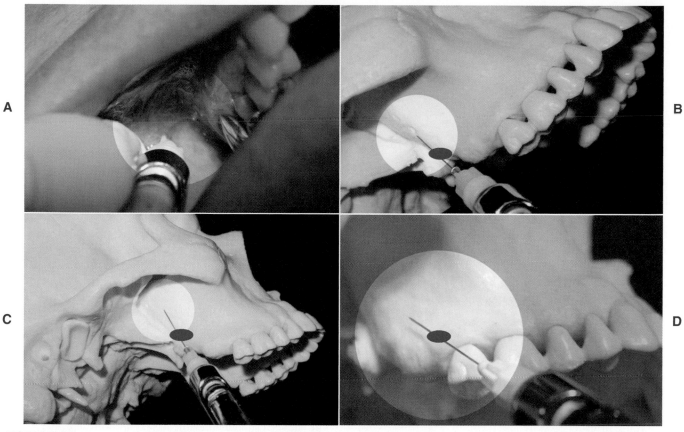

FIGURE 41-16
Posterior superior alveolar (PSA) nerve block. **A,** Penetration site. **B,** Deposition site. **C,** Penetration depth with long needle. **D,** Penetration depth with short needle, given as in infiltration. Depth of penetration is indicated by the red dot.

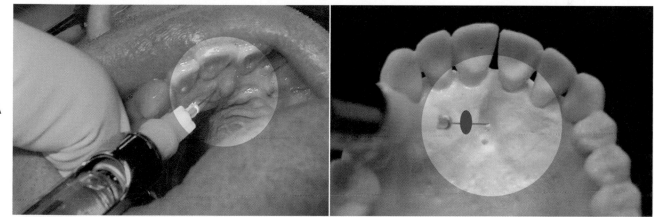

FIGURE 41-17
Nasopalatine (NP) nerve block. **A,** Penetration site. **B,** Deposition site. Depth of penetration is indicated by the red dot.

palate from the mesial of the right first premolar to the mesial of the left first premolar.

Technique factors

The clinician should apply the basic injection steps.
- Topical anesthetic is applied with a 1-minute contact with a topical agent then another 1 minute with pressure applied to the cotton swab (the site will blanch). This pro-

cedure provides *pressure anesthesia* to deeper tissues, enhancing patient comfort.
- For the NP nerve block, a 30-gauge x-short or 27-gauge short is most commonly used. Using a computer-controlled delivery device is ideal for this type of injection.
- The penetration site is the palatal mucosa lateral to the midline of the incisive papilla.

- The angle of insertion is at 45 degrees toward the incisive papilla, with the syringe barrel resting against the lower lip.
- The deposition site is at the incisive foramen, and the insertion depth is 4 to 7 mm. Care is taken to advance slowly until contact with bone is made.
- After a negative aspiration, 1 to 2 stoppers (0.2 to 0.4 ml) of an appropriately selected local anesthetic drug are deposited (the tissue will blanch to a patch extending to the lingual or the anterior teeth).

Palatal Anterior Superior Alveolar Nerve Block

Palatal anterior superior alveolar (P-ASA) nerve blocks (Figure 41-18) are indicated for pain management of the maxillary anterior sextant and are especially helpful for cosmetic procedures that involve assessment of the patient's *smile line*. Anesthesia will affect the structures innervated by the NP nerve and terminal branches and the anterior branches of the ASA nerve, including the facial and palatal periodontium and the pulps of the teeth in the sextant (to a lesser degree for the canines).

Technique factors

The clinician should apply the basic injection steps.

- Topical anesthetic is applied with a 1-minute contact with a topical agent then another 1 minute with pressure applied to the cotton swab (the site will blanch). This procedure provides pressure anesthesia to deeper tissues, enhancing patient comfort.
- For the P-ASA nerve block, a 27-gauge short or 30-gauge x-short needle is most commonly used. Using a computer-controlled delivery device is ideal for this type of injection. To gain access to the site of penetration, the patient is asked to tip the head up and slightly away, opening the mouth wide.
- The penetration site is lateral to the incisive papilla, and the angle of insertion is at 45 degrees to the palate on a line that will enter the NP foramen; the syringe barrel will be coming from in front of the patient.
- The deposition site is in the NP foramen. Care must be taken to advance the needle *slowly* 1 to 2 mm each for 4 to 6 seconds to an insertion depth of 6 to 10 mm.
- Bone is to be contacted at the inner wall of the foramen. Anesthetic is slowly deposited throughout this injection (0.5 ml on insertion).
- After a negative aspiration at the deposition site, the remainder of one cartridge (1.4 to 1.8 ml) of an appropriately selected local anesthetic drug is deposited.

> **Prevention**
> When using a 4% local anesthetic solution, the total volume delivered should be reduced by one half.

Anterior Middle Superior Alveolar Nerve Block

Anterior middle superior alveolar (AMSA) nerve blocks (Figure 41-19) are indicated for pain management of the incisors, canine, and premolars on the side anesthetized, as well as palatal tissue from the midline through the premolars and buccal supporting and overlying tissues of the affected teeth. Anesthesia will affect the structures innervated by the ASA nerve; the MSA nerve, when present; and the subneural plexus of the ASA and MSA nerves and terminal branches, including the pulps of the central and lateral incisors, canine, and premolars on the anesthetized side.

Technique factors

The clinician should apply the basic injection steps.

- Topical anesthetic is applied with a 1-minute contact with a topical agent then another 1 minute with pressure applied to the cotton swab (the site will blanch). This procedure provides pressure anesthesia to deeper tissues, enhancing patient comfort.
- For the AMSA nerve block, a 30-gauge x-short or 27-gauge short needle is most commonly used. Using a computer-controlled delivery device is designed for this type of injection.
- To gain access to the site of penetration, the patient is asked to tip the head up and slightly away, opening the mouth wide.

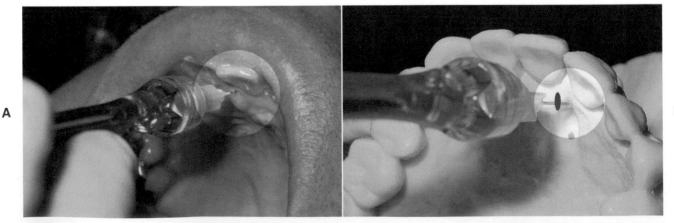

FIGURE 41-18
Palatal anterior superior alveolar (P-ASA) nerve block. **A,** Penetration site. **B,** Deposition site. Depth of penetration is indicated by the red dot.

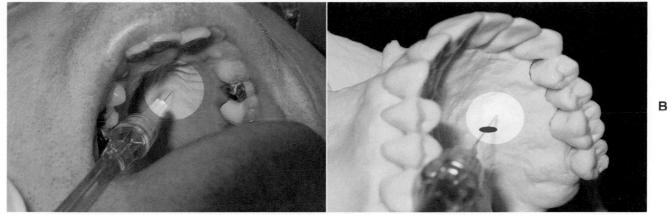

FIGURE 41-19
Anterior middle superior alveolar (AMSA) nerve block. **A,** Penetration site. **B,** Deposition site. Depth of penetration is indicated by the red dot.

- The penetration site is at the junction of the horizontal and vertical aspects of the palate on a line bisecting the gingival margin between the maxillary premolars on that side, and the angle of insertion is at a roughly 45-degree angle to the palate, with the syringe barrel over the opposite side of the mouth.
- The deposition site is approximately halfway between the midpalatal suture and the free gingival margin between the premolars on the side to be anesthetized, and the insertion depth is approximately 4 to 7 mm or to bony resistance. Care is taken to advance slowly until contact with bone is made.
- After a negative aspiration, three-quarters to one cartridge (1.4 to 1.8 ml) of an appropriately selected local anesthetic drug is deposited in a 2% or 3% solution.

Distinct Care Modifications

Modifying deposition rates for administering local anesthetics is not abnormal in certain situations. In the AMSA nerve block, for example, a large volume of solution must be deposited in the palatal tissues, which are often thin and heavily fibrous, resisting the large volumes of anesthetics necessary. A good way to tell whether the deposition is proceeding too quickly is tissue expansion or bulging. If this occurs, the practitioner should stop to allow diffusion and absorption of the solution before continuing. Even though the deposition rate for 1.8 ml of most solutions has been previously described as 1 minute (60 seconds), in the AMSA technique, this time is increased to 3 minutes. If a 4% solution is being used, only one half the volume, or 0.7 ml up to a maximum of 0.9 ml, should be delivered over the same 3-minute time period.[18]

Greater Palatine Nerve Block

Greater palatine (GP) nerve blocks (Figure 41-20) are indicated for pain management of palatal soft and osseous tissue distal to the canine in one quadrant. The GP nerve block is also referred to as the *anterior palatine nerve block*. Anesthesia will affect the structures innervated by the GP nerve and terminal branches, including the posterior portion of the hard palate and its overlying soft tissues, anteriorly as far as the first premolar and medially to the midline.

Technique factors

The clinician should apply the basic injection steps.
- Topical anesthetic is applied with a 1-minute contact with a topical agent then another 1 minute with pressure applied to the cotton swab (the site will blanch). This procedure provides pressure anesthesia to deeper tissues, enhancing patient comfort.
- For the GP nerve block, a 30-gauge x-short or 27-gauge short needle is most commonly used.
- The penetration site is the palatal soft tissue slightly anterior to the GP foramen, and the angle of insertion is perpendicular to the palatal bone at the foramen, with the syringe barrel resting against the lower lip.
- The deposition site is at the GP foramen, and the insertion depth is 6 to 8 mm. Care is taken to advance slowly until contact with bone is made.
- After a negative aspiration, one-quarter to one-third cartridge (0.4 to 0.6 ml) is deposited.

MANDIBULAR INJECTIONS*

Inferior Alveolar and Lingual Nerve Blocks

Inferior alveolar (IA) **and lingual** nerve blocks (Figure 41-21) are indicated for pain management of multiple mandibular teeth in one quadrant. The IA is also referred to as a *mandibular* or *lower block*. Anesthesia will affect the structures innervated by the IA, incisive, and mental and lingual nerves and terminal branches, including the mandibular teeth to midline, anterior two thirds of tongue, and floor of oral cavity.

Technique factors

The clinician should apply the basic injection steps.
- For the IA and long buccal nerve block, a 25-gauge long needle is the appropriate needle to use.

*Information in this section is from Haas DA: An update of local anesthetics in dentistry, *J Can Dent Assoc* 68:546-551, 2002, and Malamed SF: *Handbook of local anesthesia,* ed 5, St Louis, 2004, Mosby.

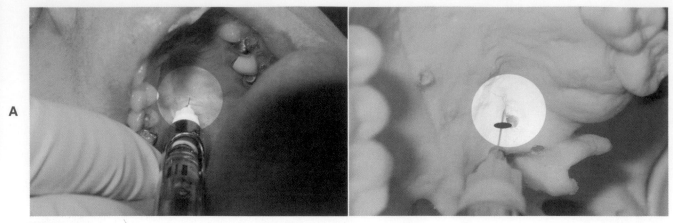

FIGURE 41-20
Greater palatine (GP) nerve block. **A,** Penetration site. **B,** Deposition site. Depth of penetration is indicated by the red dot.

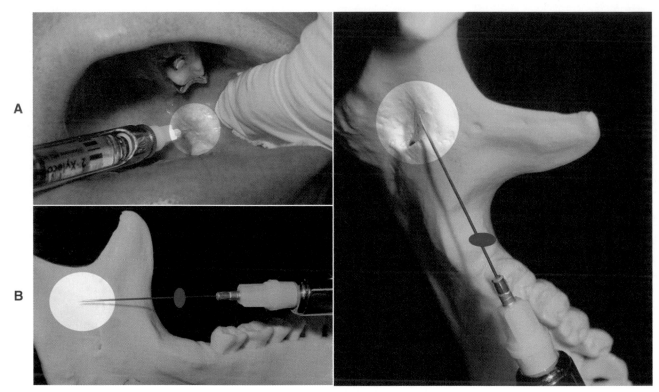

FIGURE 41-21
Inferior alveolar (IA) nerve block. **A,** Penetration site. **B,** Deposition site from medial view. **C,** Deposition site from superior view. Depth of penetration is indicated by the red dot.

- To gain access to the site of penetration, retract the cheek laterally while keeping the finger in the coronoid notch (the greatest concavity on the anterior border of the ramus).
- The penetration site is lateral to the pterygomandibular raphe, and the angle of insertion is with the syringe barrel in the corner of the mouth and over the premolars on the opposite side of the mouth.
- The barrel will be parallel to the occlusal plane of the mandibular molar teeth, and the height of injection will be no less than the height of the coronoid notch.

- The deposition site is at the IA nerve just before it enters the mandibular foramen (on the medial aspect of the ramus) lateral to the medial pterygoid muscle, and the insertion depth is 20 to 25 mm (two-thirds to three-quarters length of long needle). Care is taken to advance slowly until contact with bone is made. Making contact with bone is the *only* way to establish that the needle is at the internal surface of the ramus and *not* in other soft tissue structures.
- One millimeter is withdrawn. After a negative aspiration, three-quarters cartridge (1.5 ml) of an appropriately

selected local anesthetic drug is deposited. The remaining anesthetic is reserved for the lingual and long buccal nerve blocks.

DENTAL CONSIDERATIONS

The lingual nerve travels in close proximity to the IA nerve. Generally, a separate injection is not given for the lingual nerve. If supplemental anesthesia is needed for the lingual nerve, after deposition for the IA nerve block, a small volume of solution is then reserved. The needle is withdrawn halfway, and following negative aspiration the solution is deposited.

Distinct Care Modifications

1. If premature contact with bone occurs, then withdraw needle slightly, and adjust syringe medially over the canine or lateral incisor to increase the depth of insertion to clear premature resistance. Reposition the needle over premolars and advance until contact with bone is made.
2. If no contact with bone is made after readjusting, then withdraw needle to one-half length of needle, and reposition the syringe distally toward the first mandibular molar and advance until contact with bone occurs. If contact with bone is not made completely, then withdraw the needle, and change penetration site 3 mm anteriorly.

Long Buccal Nerve Blocks

Buccal nerve blocks are indicated for pain management of the buccal soft tissue along the molar teeth in the mandibular region. The buccal nerve block is also referred to as a **long buccal** (LB) or *buccinator nerve block* (Figure 41-22). Anesthesia will affect the structures innervated by the buccal nerve and terminal branches to include soft tissues and periosteum buccal to the mandibular molar teeth.

Technique factors

The clinician should apply the basic injection steps.

- For the LB nerve block, a 25-gauge long needle is commonly used after the IA injection.
- To gain access to the site of penetration, the cheek is retracted laterally, pulling the tissue taut.
- The penetration site is in the buccal fold just distal and buccal to the most distal molar tooth in the arch, and the angle of insertion is with the syringe parallel to the occlusal plane on the side of injection and buccal to the mandibular teeth.
- The deposition site is near the buccal nerve as it passes over the anterior border of the ramus. The insertion depth is 2 to 4 mm.

Prevention

It is not uncommon for the tissue to begin *ballooning* slightly at the injection site; slow deposition will minimize this event and allow the solution to diffuse without causing tissue trauma.

Prevention

If the bevel is not fully inserted into the tissue, then the anesthetic solution will be not be deposited under the tissue (and the patient may experience the bitter taste of the solution). Additionally, if resistance is met prematurely, then withdrawing and penetrating more laterally (away from retromolar pad) will allow for better penetration.

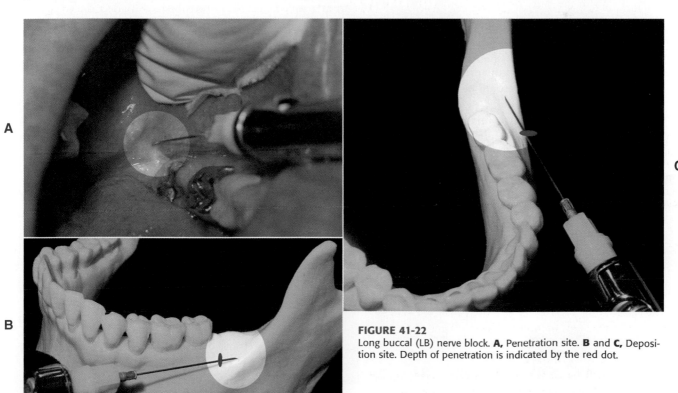

FIGURE 41-22
Long buccal (LB) nerve block. **A,** Penetration site. **B** and **C,** Deposition site. Depth of penetration is indicated by the red dot.

- After a negative aspiration, 1 to 1½ stopper (0.2 to 0.3 ml) of an appropriately selected local anesthetic drug is deposited.

Mental Nerve Block

Mental (M) nerve blocks (Figure 41-23) are indicated for pain management of the buccal soft tissue required for procedures in the mandible anterior to the mental foramen. Anesthesia will affect the structures innervated by the mental nerve, a terminal branch of the IA nerve, to include the buccal mucous membrane anterior to the mental foramen to the midline and skin of the lower lip and chin.

Technique factors

The clinician should apply the basic injection steps.

- For the M nerve block, a 27-gauge short needle is commonly used after the IA injection.
- To gain access to the site of penetration, the lower lip and buccal soft tissue are retracted laterally.
- The penetration site is either (1) at the mucobuccal fold between the premolars, superior to the mental foramen, or (2) at the mucobuccal fold near the apex of the first premolar, just anterior to the mental foramen.
- The deposition site is just above the mental foramen.
- The angle of insertion is either (1) directly vertical to the foramen or (2) at 45 degrees to the long axis of the canine, posteriorly toward the mental foramen, to a depth of 5 to 6 mm.
- After a negative aspiration, one-third cartridge (0.6 ml) of an appropriately selected local anesthetic drug is deposited.

Incisive Nerve Block

Incisive (I) nerve blocks (see Figure 41-23) are indicated for pain management of the pulp for teeth anterior to the mental foramen. This injection is a modification of the mental nerve block and includes the areas innervated by the mental nerve (see Mental Nerve Block). Anesthesia will affect the structures innervated by the mental and incisive terminal branches of the IA nerve, including the buccal mucous membrane anterior to

the mental foramen, usually from the second premolar to the midline and the teeth in that sextant.

Technique factors

The clinician should apply the basic injection steps.

- For the mental nerve block, a 27-gauge short needle is commonly used after the IA injection.
- To gain access to the site of penetration, the lower lip and buccal soft tissue is retracted laterally.
- The penetration site is either (1) at the mucobuccal fold between the premolars, just posterior to the mental foramen, or (2) at the mucobuccal fold near the apex of the first premolar, just anterior to the mental foramen.
- The deposition site is just above the mental foramen. The angle of insertion is either (1) directly vertical to the foramen or (2) at 45 degrees to the long axis of the canine, posteriorly toward the mental foramen to a depth of 5 to 6 mm.
- After a negative aspiration, one-third to one-half cartridge (0.6 to 0.9 ml) of an appropriately selected local anesthetic drug is deposited. Success of this injection for pulpal anesthesia requires the postprocedure step of applying extraoral pressure at the injection site for 1 to 2 minutes to facilitate diffusion of the solution into the foramen.

Gow-Gates Technique

Gow-Gates (G-G) nerve blocks (Figure 41-24) are indicated for pain management of multiple mandibular teeth in one quadrant. The inferior alveolar (IA) nerve block is also referred to as a *mandibular block*. Anesthesia will affect the structures innervated by the IA, mental, incisive, lingual, mylohyoid, auriculotemporal, and buccal nerves and terminal branches, including the mandibular teeth to midline, anterior two thirds of tongue, and floor of oral cavity.

Technique factors

The clinician should apply the basic injection steps.

- For the G-G nerve block, a 25-gauge long needle is the appropriate needle to use.

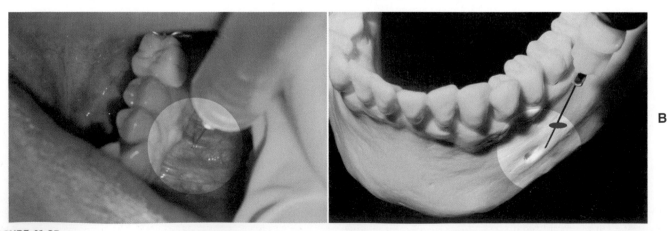

A   **B**

FIGURE 41-23
Mental (M)-incisive (I) nerve block. **A,** Penetration site. **B,** Deposition site. Depth of penetration is indicated by the red dot.

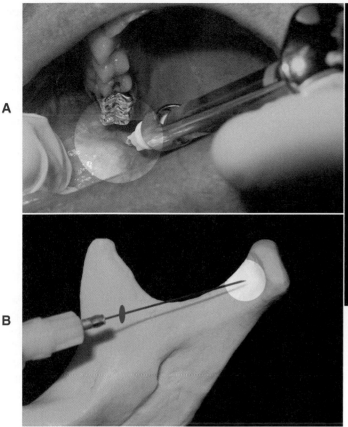

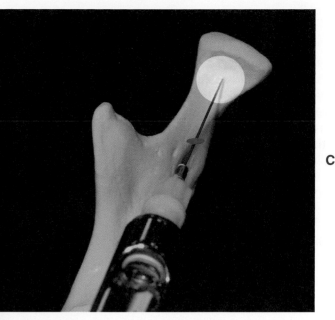

FIGURE 41-24
Gow-Gates (G-G) inferior alveolar nerve block. **A,** Penetration site. **B,** Deposition site from medial view. **C,** Deposition site from superior view. Depth of penetration is indicated by the red dot.

- To gain access to the site of penetration, the cheek is retracted laterally while keeping the finger in the coronoid process (greatest superior and anterior border of the ramus).
- The penetration site is in the mucous membrane just distal to the most posterior molar, on a plane parallel to a line from the intertragic notch to the corner of the mouth at the height of the mesiolingual cusp of the maxillary second molar on the side to be anesthetized. The barrel will be in variable positions from the opposite incisors to the molars, depending on the flare of the ramus.
- The deposition site is at the anterior surface of the neck of the condyle, just below the insertion of the lateral pterygoid muscle, and the insertion depth is 25 mm (three-quarters length of a long needle).
- Care is taken to advance slowly until contact with bone is made. The dental health provider *must* make contact with bone; making contact with bone is the *only* way to establish that the needle is at the neck of the condyle and *not* in the temporomandibular joint capsule, otic ganglion, or too far medial to the deposition site.
- One millimeter is withdrawn. After a negative aspiration, one cartridge (1.8 ml) of an appropriately selected local anesthetic drug is deposited.

Vazirani-Akinosi Nerve Blocks

Vazirani-Akinosi nerve blocks are indicated for pain management of multiple mandibular teeth in one quadrant and when opening and access is limited because of patient factors. The

Vazirani-Akinosi nerve blocks are also referred to as *Akinosi* or *closed-mouth* technique. Anesthesia will affect the structures innervated by the IA, mental, incisive, lingual, mylohyoid, auriculotemporal, and buccal nerves and terminal branches, including the mandibular teeth to midline, anterior two thirds of tongue, and floor of oral cavity.

Technique factors

The clinician should apply the basic injection steps.

- For the Vazirani-Akinosi nerve blocks, a 25-gauge long needle is the appropriate needle to use.
- To gain access to the site of penetration, the cheek is retracted laterally.
- The penetration site is the soft tissue overlying the medial border of the mandibular ramus directly adjacent to the maxillary tuberosity at the height of the mucogingival junction adjacent to the maxillary third molar, and the angle of insertion is with the syringe barrel parallel to the mandible molar teeth.
- The deposition site is on the medial surface of the ramus, superior to the alveolar foramen, and the insertion depth is 25 mm (three-quarters length of a long needle). Care is taken to advance slowly; contact with bone will *not* be made.
- After a negative aspiration, three-quarters to one cartridge (1.5 to 1.8 ml) of an appropriately selected local anesthetic drug is deposited. Notably, some researchers bend the shank of the needle approximately 20 degrees to

facilitate positioning of the needle behind the ligula and near the foramen.[10]

Periodontal Ligament Injection

Periodontal ligament (PDL) injections (Figure 41-25) are indicated for pain management of procedures in which anesthetizing individual teeth is desirable without wide areas of numbness or significant soft tissue anesthesia. Frequently, PDL injections are used to supplement other techniques that have failed to achieve profound anesthesia. PDL injections are also referred to as *intraligamentary* and *peridental injections*. They are a subgroup of what are known as *intraosseous anesthesia techniques* because they work by diffusing through the alveolar bone. Anesthesia will affect the structures innervated by the dental plexus of individual teeth on which the procedure is performed.

Technique factors

The clinician should apply the basic injection steps. Using other techniques to obtain soft tissue anesthesia in the area of PDL injections is often desirable if anesthesia is not already in effect. An example would be to block the buccal nerve before delivering PDL injections on mandibular molar teeth.

If a topical anesthetic is to be used, then it may be applied in one of the following manners. Topical anesthetic is managed with both 1-minute contact with a topical agent then another 1 minute with pressure applied to the cotton swab (the site will blanch). Using a computer-controlled delivery device is helpful in this type of injection, as are several specialized syringes that have been designed to facilitate the deposition of solution against what some researchers consider to be significant back pressure.

- To gain accesses to the site of penetration, the patient is asked to tip the head up and slightly away, opening the mouth wide.
- The penetration site is the depth of the gingival sulcus at the mesial or distal root surface of the tooth to be anesthetized, with the needle oriented toward the long axis of the root of the tooth and the bevel facing the root.
- The optimal depth of penetration is reached when no backflow of solution exists and when blanching occurs when a small amount of solution is deposited. If either is absent, then a deeper penetration and deposit is again made. If unsuccessful, then the needle is withdrawn and another site is selected.
- Once significant blanching and no backflow occur, 0.2 ml or approximately 1 stopper of solution per site (one site is required for single-rooted teeth and two sites for multiple-rooted teeth) is deposited.
- Aspirating is not necessary with this technique because intravascular deposition is not a risk in this location.

DENTAL CONSIDERATIONS

The PDL injection technique is particularly advantageous when IA nerve blocks have been unsuccessful. Individual teeth may be anesthetized with minimal volumes of solution using the PDL injection technique. The most resistant areas for the success of this technique are the maxillary and mandibular canines and in individuals with exceptionally dense alveolar bone. In other instances, an important point to note is that profound anesthesia can be achieved with very small volumes of anesthetic solutions, and the PDL injection technique should be considered whenever the medical status of a patient suggests that profound anesthesia is necessary with minimal volumes of solution.

This technique should *not* be used on primary teeth where permanent teeth exist below them because it may damage the developing teeth. When antibiotic premedication is not ordinarily necessary for anesthesia procedures but is necessary for surgery and periodontal therapy, it *is* necessary if PDL injections will be given. In some instances,

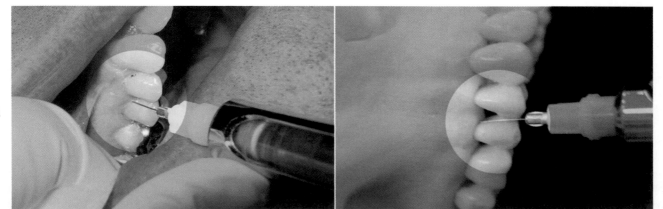

FIGURE 41-25
Periodontal ligament (PDL) infiltration. **A,** Penetration site. **B,** Deposition site.

bending the needle for better access is helpful and even desirable when using this technique.

Documentation of Local Anesthetic Agents

The delivery of any local anesthetic agent must be accurately recorded in the patient's chart for medicolegal documentation. The chart entry must include the following:

- Date of administration
- Type of drug or drugs administered (both topical and injectable)
- Number of injections administered (or area of delivery when topical alone is used)
- Total volume of drug or drugs administered
- Results of aspiration as *positive* (+) or *negative* (−)
- Gauge of the needle or needles used (if it is the policy of the workplace). This information is relevant to the outcome of the aspiration.

In addition to a positive aspiration, any adverse reactions or complications must be recorded. Any first aid that is administered must also be recorded. Box 41-3 presents sample chart entries.

BOX 41-3

SAMPLE CHART DOCUMENTATION FOR LOCAL ANESTHETICS

5/12/07   Benzocaine, R-PSA, MSA, ASA, lidocaine 2% w/ epi 1:100, 2 cart. (−) aspir., no complications.
Name hygienist: RDH

5/14/07   Lidocaine topical, R-IA, LB, mepivacaine 2% w/ levo 1:200, 2.7 ml (+) aspir., visible hematoma, ice 15 minutes, monitor 30 min, no further swelling.
Patient to call if any further problem.
Name hygienist: RDH

Systemic Actions and Complications of Local Anesthetic Agents

All organs with excitable membranes are affected by local anesthetics, including the central nervous system (CNS), cardiovascular system, autonomic ganglia, neuromuscular junctions, and all types of muscle. These agents readily block action potentials in the nervous system and in the cardiovascular system.

Although uncommon, adverse reactions do occur. Syncope is a common adverse reaction in dentistry related to dental anesthesia. Many predisposing factors can increase the possibility of encountering more serious adverse reactions, and these factors must be recognized and noted on health histories before any drugs are administered. Common examples include allergies; the presence of medications that affect the CNS, cardiovascular system, liver, kidneys, or lungs; underlying medical conditions, such as hyperthyroidism, that alter the response to

Distinct Care Modifications

Among other signs and symptoms, individuals with uncontrolled hyperthyroidism typically have increased heart rates and elevated systolic blood pressures stimulated by the excessive release of thyroid hormone. These patients are at risk of developing what is known as a *thyroid crisis* or *thyroid storm*, which is an acute worsening of their signs and symptoms, when vasoconstrictors are administered. This event may happen simply when the stress of an appointment itself causes bodily release of epinephrine on top of already excessive levels. Nonemergent treatment should be postponed until the condition is stabilized, at which time vasoconstrictor-containing local anesthetics may be used when necessary and with caution.[17]

local anesthetic drugs; genetic disorders; psychologic factors; and previous idiosyncratic reactions.

PERIPHERAL NERVE CONDUCTION

The primary clinical function of local anesthetics is a reversible blockade of peripheral nerve conduction. Local anesthetics are nonselective and can block the conduction of action potentials in all neurons to which they gain access. These agents can inhibit the conduction of impulses in motor neurons, at sensory endings, and at synapses.

Although action potentials can be blocked in all types of neurons, some neurons are blocked more readily than others. The loss of nerve function is related to the permeability of the nerve membrane to the anesthetic drugs. As a general rule, local anesthetics block the conduction of action potentials in small, nonmyelinated neurons first.[6] These drugs do not penetrate myelin. Heavily myelinated neurons, such as motor neurons, are affected last.

⋆ CASE APPLICATION 41-1.4

Risk of Peripheral Nerve Damage and Infection

Ms. Guyegos has resisted therapy for control of her diabetes. She remains at risk for infection and worsening disease in her mouth, which is a risk factor for other systemic diseases, especially in patients with diabetes. Denial of treatment based on blood sugar levels in excess of accepted values places her at further risk, especially in light of her dim near-term prospects for achieving normal blood sugar levels after vigorous therapy has failed to achieve them. Treatment with proper precautions and with a clear understanding of the implications of the risk factors is appropriate.

CENTRAL NERVOUS SYSTEM

Local anesthetics are lipid-soluble and cross the blood-brain barrier with ease. At therapeutic blood levels, the CNS effects are not significant. The earliest signs and symptoms of clinical toxicity are CNS excitation and then CNS depression. Convulsions may occur during the excitation phase. CNS depression can range from drowsiness to unconsciousness. Adverse reactions are proportional to the plasma concentration; the higher the plasma level, the greater the danger of adverse effects.

> **Prevention**
>
> Office and clinic personnel must be trained in life support and must be prepared to respond to these signs and symptoms whenever local anesthesia is being used.

The progression of signs and symptoms in toxicity may include anxiety, light-headedness, bilateral circumoral and lingual numbness, dizziness, visual disturbances (diplopia, nystagmus), drowsiness, and disorientation. A temporary loss of consciousness may follow slurred speech, shivering, and tremors, after which a loss of consciousness and a generalized convulsive CNS excitability occurs that is typical of the drug's blockade of inhibitory pathways. Further increases in the local anesthetic dose may progress to cessation of the convulsive state and generalized CNS depression.

An important point to realize is that many signs of local anesthetic drug toxicity also are common manifestations of acute anxiety frequently seen in dental settings. These signs include restlessness, drowsiness, shivering, pallor, and loss of consciousness.

DENTAL CONSIDERATIONS

Lidocaine toxicity, in particular, may not include excitatory signs and symptoms but may proceed directly to the signs and symptoms of CNS depression.

CARDIOVASCULAR SYSTEM

After absorption into the systemic circulation, local anesthetics act on the cardiovascular system. The primary site of action is the myocardium, where the local anesthetic reduces the force of contraction, electrical excitability, and conduction rate. In addition, most local anesthetics cause peripheral vasodilation. Normally, high systemic concentrations are necessary to produce cardiovascular effects. However, cardiovascular collapse and death have been reported with lower doses.[7]

DRUG INTERACTIONS

The CNS depressant effects of local anesthetics are additive

> **Prevention**
>
> The health history review before administering local anesthetic agents must include a *thorough* review of drugs and conditions that compromise or challenge the hepatic microsomal enzyme system.

with other CNS depressants, such as antianxiety drugs, barbiturates, ethanol, and opioids. Drugs that challenge the hepatic microsomal enzyme system or compete with the local anesthetic for the enzymes may delay the metabolism of the local anesthetics, prolonging their systemic effects.

METHEMOGLOBINEMIA

Methemoglobinemia is a condition that binds oxygen in the blood, making it unavailable to the body, and leads to cyanosis. This condition exhibits as anemia and has been associated with a variety of chemicals, including some local anesthetic agents, and is unrelated to either cardiac or respiratory causes.[18]

Several cases of methemoglobinemia have been reported after using prilocaine in particular. This effect is a consequence of the metabolism of the aromatic ring in prilocaine to **o-toluidine.** Benzocaine topical anesthetic has also been implicated, as have several prescription and over-the-counter medications such as acetaminophen. In addition to acetaminophen, patients taking any oxygen-depleting medications are at risk.

The development of methemoglobinemia depends on the total dose of local anesthetic drug administered. This dose may be affected by its combination with drugs or

> **Patient Education Opportunity**
>
> Acetaminophen is a widely used over-the-counter medication that has an independent tendency to induce methemoglobinemia in susceptible individuals. Because the local anesthetic prilocaine also has the same tendency, avoiding the use of both at the same time is prudent. Therefore, if prilocaine is to be administered as an injectable or topical anesthetic agent during a procedure, educating patients about the risks is important to ensure that they do not take acetaminophen before or after the procedure, including for postoperative discomfort.

> **Prevention**
>
> Prilocaine has been associated with an increased risk of inducing methemoglobinemia in susceptible individuals. The clinician should avoid its use or use minimal quantities of injectable or topical prilocaine in these individuals. Benzocaine topical should also be avoided because it has also been associated with methemoglobinemia.

nonpharmaceutical chemicals that independently induce methemoglobinemia in susceptible individuals. The relatively small doses used in dentistry are not likely to present problems in healthy adults. However, in susceptible individuals, lidocaine, mepivacaine, or articaine may be substituted for prilocaine.

ALLERGIC REACTIONS

Allergies to amide local anesthetics are rare, unlike allergies to esters. Fortunately, the primary ester used in dentistry is benzocaine, which is used only as a topical anesthetic. Typical allergic responses to benzocaine exhibit as localized tissue reactions.

Sulfites are used as antioxidant preservatives for the vasoconstrictors used in many of the local anesthetic formulations. Sulfites prolong the otherwise short shelf life of vasoconstrictor-containing cartridges. Unfortunately, sulfite allergies have been increasing, and an individual with a sulfite allergy may not receive any local anesthetic containing a vasoconstrictor. Plain formulations such as 3% mepivacaine and 4% prilocaine without vasoconstrictor are useful substitutions.

MALIGNANT HYPERTHERMIA*

Malignant hyperthermia (MH) occurs more frequently in children (1:15,000 versus 1:50,000 for adults) and is a serious, life-threatening complication encountered with general anesthesia administration. Classified as a syndrome, susceptible individuals have an autosomal-dominant genetic defect. Previously associated with lidocaine and mepivacaine, theories suggest that MH is not likely to occur with the amide local anesthetics. A lack of reports of this adverse reaction, when amide local anesthetic drugs are used in the absence of other known drug associations (succinylcholine and halothane), makes it reasonable to use either amide or ester local anesthetics in these individuals.

Before treating these individuals, however, appropriate consultations with physicians, including the primary care physician; anesthesiology departments of local medical centers; or the Malignant Hyperthermia Association of the United States, should be explored.[18]

ATYPICAL PLASMA CHOLINESTERASE†

Only 1 out of every 2820 individuals is affected by an inherited trait in which the individual's plasma cholinesterase may be unable to metabolize properly succinylcholine and, of particular importance in dentistry, the ester local anesthetics. Normal safe doses of ester drugs in these individuals may result in overdoses, and using amide local anesthetics is indicated.

Local Actions and Complications of Local Anesthetic Agents

LOCAL TISSUE TOXICITY AND SOFT TISSUE INJURY

Tissue in the area of topical and local anesthetic drug placement and through which the needle passes may respond with postoperative inflammation, infection, or both. A topical anesthetic

*Information in this section is from Kalow W: Hydrolysis of local anesthetics by human serum cholinesterase, *J Pharmacol Exp Ther* 104:122-134, 1952.
†Information in this section is from Malamed SF: *Handbook of local anesthesia,* ed 5, St Louis, 2004, Mosby.

that has been placed on the mucosa for too long a period can dry the tissue excessively, leading to redness, pain, swelling, necrosis, and sloughing (Figure 41-26). Delayed hypersensitivities are not uncommon, especially with benzocaine. Passing the needle through mucosa and connective tissue creates reversible damage every time. In such close proximity to bones, nerves, and vessels, a risk of damage exists to one or all with every penetration. Excessive volumes of solution may damage tissue as well. Care must be taken to minimize both the volumes of solution administered and the number of penetrations.

Self-inflicted trauma after local anesthesia, especially in children and in individuals with special needs, is not uncommon (Figures 41-27 and 41-28). Most offices and clinics have systems in place to warn not only the patients but also their care providers regarding avoidance of self-inflicted trauma. Rarely is this complication a significant problem.

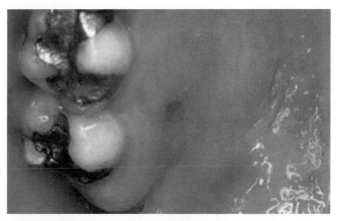

FIGURE 41-26
Anesthetic necrosis following a GP injection.

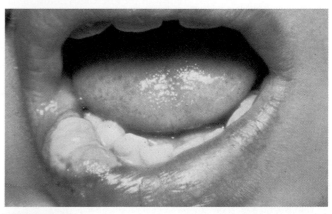

FIGURE 41-27
Lip bite after IA injection. (Courtesy Pierce College Dental Hygiene Program, Lakewood, Wash.)

TRISMUS

Intramuscular and intraoral injections of local anesthetics can cause localized skeletal muscle injury. Affected muscles may include the medial pterygoid, temporalis, and lateral pterygoid. An injury that is of sufficient severity can lead to trismus, which is a prolonged restricted opening of the jaw, commonly known as *tetanus* or *lockjaw*. Trauma to the muscle and vascular tissues from physical, chemical, or microbial origin is the most

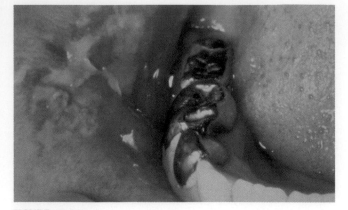

FIGURE 41-28
Cheek bite after IA injection. (Courtesy Pierce College Dental Hygiene Program, Lakewood, Wash.)

common etiologic factor. As might be expected, longer-acting local anesthetics cause a greater degree of skeletal muscle injury than do shorter-acting drugs.[18] Repeated needle penetrations and excessive volumes of solution may unnecessarily damage muscle, vascular tissue, or both and may increase the risk of trismus. The damage is rarely persistent, and muscle regeneration is usually complete within 2 weeks.[16]

PARESTHESIA

Paresthesia is a persistent partial or complete numbness. Associated with trauma during surgical or local anesthesia procedures, in many instances, no explanation can be found for its occurrence because no noted trauma existed before, during, or after the procedure. A neurotoxic effect of the anesthetic solution has also been suspected. Some authorities have suggested a small but more frequent occurrence with 4% solutions, particularly articaine. The clinician must avoid injury to any nerves encountered during local anesthesia procedures and respond appropriately to the development of paresthesias when they do occur.[11]

NEEDLE BREAKAGE

A rare occurrence with today's disposable needles, broken needles occur, most commonly as a result of the fracture of needles at their hubs. Inserting a needle to its hub, bending the needle before insertion, using a gauge that is too small, and using a needle that is only marginally long enough for the procedure all increase the likelihood of needle breakage. Lateral pressure on the needle should be avoided. Needles should not be redirected in tissue; instead, they should be withdrawn all or part of the way out of the tissue before correcting. The direction may be corrected easily if completely withdrawn or the needle tip may be pivoted to correct for the errant direction after appropriate partial withdrawal, before being reinserted to depth. Professional opinions differ as to whether needle bending is ever acceptable.

FACIAL NERVE PARALYSIS

Facial nerve paralysis is a common occurrence when the needle travels too far posteriorly in IA nerve blocks. It may also occur in Vazirani-Akinosi procedures that result from overinserting the needle. In both instances, the needle tips penetrate the parotid gland, which is not innervated by the facial nerve, but the nerve passes through the gland and may be inadvertently anesthetized. The resulting paralysis is transient and will occur only on the affected side. Closing the eye becomes impossible, and facial expression will be lost on the affected side. Adherence to safe technique will reduce the majority of the risk of experiencing this adverse reaction (see the previous sections on injection techniques for the IA nerve block and the Vazirani-Akinosi nerve block).

ULCERATIONS AND EDEMA

Ulcers may form postoperatively after local anesthesia. Patients who are susceptible to herpes simplex outbreaks are at increased risk of the postoperative development of multiple small ulcerations in the area of injection, typically on the palate (Figure 41-29; see also Figure 41-28). As with other oral and circumoral herpetic lesions, they usually resolve uneventfully. Aphthous ulcerations are also seen postoperatively and, similar to

---

Distinct Care Modifications

Even though most paresthesias are transient, if a paresthesia develops after a local anesthetic procedure, consider performing each of the following, once notified of the possible adverse reaction:

Respond: Prompt response by the practitioner is key to continuing a healthy relationship with the patient.

Reassure: Use these contacts as opportunities to educate and reassure the patient on this often unavoidable complication.

Appoint: Schedule the patient for a postoperative examination as soon as possible.

Map: Detail the extent of the paresthesia in diagrams and notes. This step is essential if future reference and comparisons are to be of benefit, including in demonstrating healing or lack of healing.

Refer: Appropriate referrals are sometimes necessary in persistent cases.

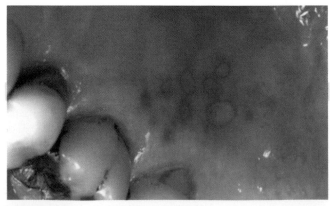

FIGURE 41-29
Postinjection herpetic outbreak.

herpes, outbreaks respond normally. Newer treatments for both conditions provide for substantial improvement in their clinical courses.

Edema is a possible consequence whenever tissue trauma occurs, especially in highly vascularized areas such as the oral cavity. The cause is variable and the treatment is similar to other areas in the body (Figure 41-30 and 41-31).

Special care should be taken when performing the PSA, IA, and M and I nerve blocks in particular. Appropriate-sized needles and careful assessment of anatomy are essential, especially with the PSA nerve block in which overinsertion greatly increases the risk of hematoma formation because of the pterygoid plexus of veins.

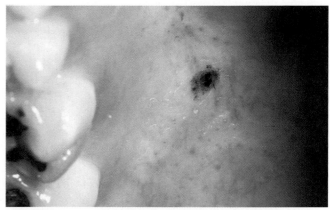

FIGURE 41-32
Hematoma on the palate after GP injection. (Courtesy Pierce College Dental Hygiene Program, Lakewood, Wash.)

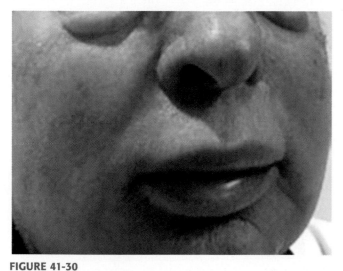

FIGURE 41-30
Angioedema may be seen after topical anesthesia application. (Courtesy Pierce College Dental Hygiene Program, Lakewood, Wash.)

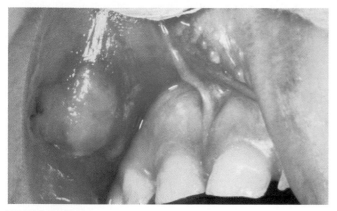

FIGURE 41-31
Localized edema in response to local anesthesia.

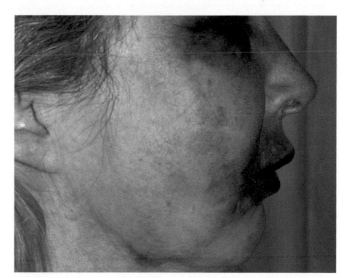

FIGURE 41-33
Bruising after a hematoma.

HEMATOMA

Hematomas may occur, regardless of the efforts taken to prevent them. Rapid hematoma formation during or following an injection is usually the result of the inadvertent nicking of an artery and outflow of blood into adjacent tissues. Nicking a vein may or may not have the same result.[18] Unsightly in certain areas, hematomas are rarely a significant problem, but response should be immediate (Figures 41-32 and 41-33). Swelling ceases when the extravascular pressure equals the intravascular pressure. By quickly placing pressure and ice over the site of swelling (when manageable), decreasing the extent of the hematoma is sometimes possible.

INFECTION

Infection is a rarely encountered postoperative complication after administering local anesthesia today, primarily because of the use of sterile, disposable needles and appropriate infection control guidelines.[18] Patients will typically report pain, an inability to open the jaw easily, or both when postoperative infection is present. Other signs of regional involvement may be present, such as lymphadenopathy. If an area to be treated appears infected before treatment, then using a regional block in which the penetration site is well away from the infected area is recommended. Injection directly into an infected area should be avoided.

References

1. Arthur GR: Pharmacokinetics of local anesthetics. In Strichartz GR, ed: *Local anesthetics: handbook of experimental pharmacology,* vol 81, Berlin, 1987, Springer-Verlag.

2. Bernhard CG, Bohm E: *Local anesthetics as anticonvulsants: a study on experimental and clinical epilepsy,* Stockholm, 1965, Almqvist & Wiksell.

3. Butterworth JF IV, Strichartz GR: Molecular mechanisms of local anesthesia: a review, *Anesthesiology* 72:711-734, 1990.

4. Daly DJ, Davenport J, Newland MC: Methemoglobinemia following the use of prilocaine, *Br J Anaesth* 36:737-739, 1964.

5. Foldes FF et al: The relation between plasma cholinesterase and prolonged apnea caused by pseudocholinesterase, *Anesthesiology* 24:208-216, 1963.

6. Gasser HS, Erlander J: The role of fiber size in the establishment of a nerve block by pressure or cocaine, *Am J Physiol* 88:581-591, 1929.

7. Gettes LS: Physiology and pharmacology of antiarrhythmic drugs, *Hosp Pract* 16:89, 1981.

8. Grossmann M et al: *Pharmacokinetics of articaine hydrochloride in tumescent local anesthesia for liposuction,* Bobenheim, Germany, 1997, Institut für Klinische Pharmakologie.

9. Guyton AC, Hall JE: *Textbook of medical physiology,* ed 10, Philadelphia, 2000, WB Saunders.

10. Haas D: *Techniques for mandible anesthesia* (CD), York, Pa, 2004, DENTSPLY Pharmaceutical.

11. Haas DA: An update of local anesthetics in dentistry, *J Can Dent Assoc* 68:546-551, 2002.

12. Hardman JG et al, eds: *Goodman and Gilman's the pharmacological basis of therapeutics,* ed 9, New York, 1996, McGraw-Hill.

13. Holroyd SV, Wynn RL, Requa-Clark B: *Clinical pharmacology in dental practice,* ed 4, St Louis, 1988, Mosby.

14. Kalow W: Hydrolysis of local anesthetics by human serum cholinesterase, *J Pharmacol Exp Ther* 104:122-134, 1952.

15. Lehne RA: *Pharmacology for nursing care,* ed 4, Philadelphia, 2001, WB Saunders.

16. Libelius R et al: Denervation-like changes in skeletal muscle after treatment with a local anesthetic (Marcaine), *J Anat* 106:297, 1970.

17. Little JW, Falace DA: *Dental management of the medically compromised patient,* ed 5, St Louis, 1997, Mosby.

18. Malamed SF: *Handbook of local anesthesia,* ed 5, St Louis, 2004, Mosby.

Nitrous Oxide and Oxygen Sedation

Ann Brunick

INSIGHT

The dental hygienist will often encounter patients who are anxious about dental treatment. To manage both pain and anxiety effectively, a dental hygienist must have an understanding of the available options. Nitrous oxide (N_2O) and oxygen (O_2) sedation is a safe and effective method proven to be applicable to most patients without any significant side effects. Knowledge of the indications for use, effects, pharmacologic equipment, techniques for administration, and patient responses is critical to the safe use of this form of sedation.

✹ CASE STUDY 42-1 Administration of Nitrous Oxide and Oxygen Sedation

Jacob Gruenwald is a 45-year-old construction worker. Significant items on his health history include a family history of hypertension and cancer. He has had arthroscopic knee surgery after a sports-related injury. Although he has no medication allergies, he is allergic to dust and has seasonal pollen allergies. He ingests prescription antihistamines and decongestants as needed. He carries an inhaler with a bronchodilating drug during "peak season" because he occasionally wheezes on exertion.

Mr. Gruenwald's dental visits have been inconsistent as an adult. He recalls many childhood visits that resulted in at least one restoration. He indicates it "wasn't his favorite place to go." He wants to avoid radiographic (x-ray) procedures because of his intense gag reflex. Toothbrushing and the taste of toothpaste often cause him to gag. His chief complaint at this visit is a lower right molar that throbs at night and has been sensitive to hot, cold, and pressure for several months. He has received no dental care for at least 8 years, and he has made this appointment because he can no longer tolerate the pain.

Mr. Gruenwald has agreed to try nitrous oxide/oxygen (N_2O/O_2) sedation while the radiographs are being taken. The dental hygienist has titrated the N_2O to an appropriate level, and Mr. Gruenwald is relaxed and comfortable.

KEY TERMS

amnesia	anxiolytic	oversedation	scavenging devices
analgesia	biovariability	pain	sedation
analgesic	conscious	pharmacologic sedation	tidal volume
anesthesia	diffusion hypoxia	pulse oximeter	titration
anesthetic	gag reflex	scavenge	unconscious
anxiety	informed consent		

LEARNING OUTCOMES

After reading this chapter the student will be able to:

1. Appreciate the history of N_2O use and its association with the dental profession.
2. Identify the effects of N_2O on pain, anxiety, and the body's systems.
3. Understand the properties of N_2O.
4. Explain indications and relative contraindications for the use of N_2O/O_2 sedation.
5. Identify equipment associated with N_2O/O_2 sedation.
6. Describe the appropriate technique for N_2O/O_2 administration.
7. Recognize the signs and symptoms of ideal sedation and oversedation.
8. Recognize appropriate recovery from N_2O/O_2 sedation.
9. Separate the facts from fallacies associated with chronic exposure to N_2O.
10. Describe methods for the detection and assessment of trace levels of N_2O in the dental setting.
11. Describe methods to minimize trace levels of N_2O in the dental setting.

N_2O/O_2 sedation has enjoyed a long and successful history as an effective method for the management of **pain** and **anxiety.**[23]

In millions of cases documented in the literature, N_2O has been used with no adverse effects.[5,19,28] Thus the safety of the drug is without question. To illustrate its safety further, an allergy to N_2O has never been documented. Few drugs can replicate these statistics.

In 1844, Horace Wells, a Connecticut dentist, discovered that N_2O has **anesthetic** and **analgesic** effects. He used N_2O to anesthetize patients before tooth extractions and other procedures. He taught the technique to medical and dental professionals in the United States and Europe. The American Dental Association (ADA), American Medical Association (AMA), and several other professional societies posthumously recognized him as the "discoverer of **anesthesia.**"[16] Although other anesthetic agents (e.g., ether, cyclopropane) were introduced in the late 1800s and early 1900s, N_2O kept a low profile. Its use began to increase again, however, when dental schools began teaching N_2O/O_2 **sedation** as part of their curricula. Currently, as many as 88% of pediatric dentists use N_2O/O_2, as do most other specialists within dentistry, including dental hygienists.[10] Several states allow dental hygienists to administer and monitor N_2O/O_2 sedation after appropriate education. It is anticipated that many other states will allow this expanded function in the future.

As a discipline, dentistry has historically been a primary user of this type of pain and anxiety management. Procedures performed in periodontics, prosthodontics, orthodontics, dental hygiene, restorative dentistry, oral and maxillofacial surgery, endodontics, and especially pediatric dentistry have been assisted by N_2O/O_2 sedation. However, many other professions have taken advantage of its effectiveness. N_2O/O_2 has been used in emergency medicine and for labor and delivery. The disciplines of podiatry, dermatology, endoscopy, and radiology have cited its use for several procedures. With increasing numbers of outpatient procedures, the use of N_2O/O_2 sedation may increase as well.

N_2O/O_2 sedation is a safe and effective method to assist patients in managing the pain and anxiety associated with many clinical situations. When the educated professional uses the appropriate equipment and techniques for administration and scavenging trace gas, N_2O/O_2 sedation offers many advantages for both the patient and the operator.

Analgesic and Anxiolytic Effects

N_2O has the ability to produce varying degrees of **analgesia** (pain control). The degree of pain reduction depends on a number of factors. Individuals perceive and react to pain differently, and pain is even tolerated differently with the same individual during a variety of different occasions. Stress, age, fatigue, and cultural background are all factors that may influence how a person reacts to pain. N_2O has been shown to reduce mild to severe pain.[6,20]

Many patients postpone or avoid dental care because of their anxiety or fear. N_2O/O_2 sedation is an excellent option for the patient who is anxious or mildly fearful.[15] N_2O is a central nervous system (CNS) depressant that provides a level of sedation in which the patient becomes relaxed and comfortable. This sense of well-being allows the patient to tolerate better the stressful situation and raises the patient's pain threshold. N_2O works well with all age groups; the literature is filled with references of successfully using N_2O/O_2 sedation with children.[13,30]

Patients may indicate an **amnesia** effect associated with N_2O/O_2 use. Their perception of time passage may be slightly altered. Patients may think their office visit was shorter than the actual time elapsed.[32]

N_2O/O_2 may be successfully used in combination with other sedation methods and drugs.[14,31] Effects may be enhanced when words are spoken slowly and soothingly.[2]

DENTAL CONSIDERATIONS

N_2O should not be used as a substitute for local anesthesia when the latter is indicated. Rather, the combination offers excellent results.[3,26]

Edmond Eger II, a prominent anesthesiologist and "adversary-turned-advocate" of N_2O, tested previously reported biological effects. Eger reported that N_2O does not significantly affect the body's systems or adversely affect respiratory, circulatory, cardiovascular, hepatic, or hematopoietic function.[11] Others have supported his claims.[32]

Pharmacology

N_2O is manufactured when the raw ingredient, ammonium nitrate (NH_4NO_3), is heated to approximately 250° C. When heated, NH_4NO_3 decomposes into N_2O, water, and negligible contaminant compounds. The water and contaminants are removed, and the remaining N_2O gas is compressed into a liquid state. The product is refrigerated and stored until transferred to a hospital or distribution center. All manufacturers must comply with the U.S. Food and Drug Administration (FDA) rules and regulations and meet the specifications of the *U.S. Pharmacopeia.*

N_2O, itself, is not flammable; however, it does support combustion. When the gas comes into contact with a substance or flame of 1200° F, it will decompose. If the decomposition occurs under pressure, such as in a high-pressure pipeline or within a cylinder, then a violent explosion will occur. A similar reaction will occur if N_2O comes into contact with a hydrocarbon substance, such as lubricant, grease, or oil. In this scenario the temperature of N_2O is critical. A rapid rise in gas temperature combined with pressure when opening cylinder valves ignites any hydrocarbon contaminant and causes an immediate chemical reaction, resulting in an explosion.

N_2O is one and one-half times heavier than air. Its molecular weight is 44 g/mol. As a gas, N_2O is slightly sweet smelling and colorless and is a relatively insoluble drug. N_2O remains unchanged in the blood, meaning the molecule does not break down. The body absorbs limited amounts of the drug. Because of this property, only small quantities of N_2O are required to reach the required blood concentration levels. Clinical action occurs quickly, usually in 3 to 5 minutes.

N₂O will rapidly replace any nitrogen (N₂) molecule in the body because of a major difference in their pressure gradients. N₂ occupies all air-filled cavities and can be found in areas with rigid or nonrigid boundaries. Pressure may increase temporarily in bony areas such as sinuses and middle ear complexes, and volume may increase in nonrigid areas such as in the bowel or pleural cavity. Therefore in some clinical situations, N₂O/O₂ sedation may be postponed.

Indications

N₂O has **anxiolytic** and analgesic properties. Patients who are mildly anxious for any reason will greatly benefit from this type of sedation. N₂O has the ability to "calm the nerves" or "take the edge off." It produces a relaxed, comfortable feeling. Because fear and anxiety are often associated with pain, N₂O/O₂ sedation is beneficial for managing both.

N₂O/O₂ sedation has a tremendous calming effect on the **gag reflex.**[7] Patients who have difficulty with radiographic procedures, rubber dam placement, taking impressions, or instrumentation are candidates for N₂O/O₂ sedation.

✴ CASE APPLICATION 42-1.1

More Than Antianxiety Use

Mr. Gruenwald, the patient in this chapter's case study, would benefit from N₂O/O₂ sedation not only for pain and anxiety assistance but also for managing his hypersensitive gag reflex during radiography.

N₂O is safe to use in most situations because it does not interact with medications, is nonallergenic, and does not significantly affect body systems. N₂O/O₂ sedation can be used with all age groups. When uncertain about a particular condition, the clinician should consult with the patient's physician before initiating the procedure.

Relative Contraindications

No absolute contraindications exist for N₂O/O₂ sedation. In some situations, however, use of N₂O/O₂ should be postponed or avoided. These situations include the following:

- Patients who have severe phobias or who have strong, controlling personalities generally do not benefit from this procedure. The situation may worsen as the patient resists the drug's calming effects.
- If a patient is inebriated or "high" on drugs, then it is wise to postpone all treatment and avoid N₂O/O₂. Discretion

is key in decisions on use of N₂O/O₂ for a recovering alcoholic or drug addict. The experience may simulate physical and mental sensations previously associated with the addiction.

- Individuals under psychiatric or psychologic care should be carefully evaluated before sedation. Negative aspects of mental disorders could be exacerbated while using N₂O/O₂. Obtaining a physician's recommendation for the use of N₂O/O₂ sedation on patients taking psychotropic drugs is important.
- Persons who do not possess the mental capability of understanding the drug's effects or who cannot communicate signs and symptoms to the operator should not be exposed to N₂O/O₂ sedation. Effective communication is essential to the operator for assessment and monitoring purposes. Therefore discretion is advised for patients with Alzheimer's disease, autism, or other mental deficiencies, as well as someone who cannot understand the language spoken by the clinician.
- Avoiding drug administration for a woman in the first trimester of pregnancy is always recommended because organogenesis during this time is critical. When delivered appropriately, N₂O should not physiologically threaten the fetus; however, similar to radiation, a mother may unfairly blame N₂O if her child is born with a birth defect and she received N₂O/O₂ sedation during the pregnancy. The dental practitioner should consult with the patient's physician and discuss all options before using N₂O/O₂ in any stage of pregnancy.
- N₂O/O₂ sedation should be postponed for patients with a cold, sinus infection, allergy-related symptoms, or other upper respiratory condition that affects airflow through the nasal and bronchial passages. Incomplete or inadequate sedation is likely in these patients.
- Patients who are chronically debilitated and on hypoxic drive because of a respiratory condition should be evaluated before use of N₂O/O₂ sedation. The delivery of supplemental O₂ rather than the N₂O is the concern. In these patients, O₂ is the stimulus for their respiration instead of carbon dioxide. A significant increase in O₂ administration may affect their breathing, and hypoxia could result. Usually these patients are not ambulatory and are not treated in a traditional dental office. Otherwise, however, medical consultation is recommended when a practitioner is unsure of the severity of the patient's condition.
- Because of the expansive nature of the gas, the use of N₂O/O₂ sedation is contraindicated in patients with cystic fibrosis, pneumothorax, recent tympanic membrane surgery or grafting within the ear, and recent ophthalmic surgery in which perfluoropropane or sulfur hexafluoride gas was used.
- N₂O/O₂ sedation should not be used with patients currently taking bleomycin sulfate as treatment for certain cancers. The gas concentrations under certain conditions can increase the incidence of pulmonary fibrosis and other pulmonary diseases.

- Patients who are claustrophobic may be unwilling to use N_2O/O_2 sedation because of the placement of the breathing apparatus over their nose and face.

If, at any time, a patient refuses N_2O/O_2 sedation or does not give informed consent, the clinician must not force the procedure.

Equipment

N_2O/O_2 used in the dental office is stored in metal cylinders (Figure 42-1). The cylinders are typically distributed and exchanged periodically by a distribution company contracted by the office. Depending on the type of N_2O/O_2 sedation system used by the office, the cylinders may be small (*E* size) or larger (*G* and *H* sizes). The company or distributor regularly inspects the cylinders to ensure their integrity. Cylinders are color-coded for correct gas identification. In the United States, N_2O is stored in blue cylinders and O_2 is found in green cylinders.

Safety measures are in place to ensure correct gas identification and cylinder placement on the units. Specific configurations of the cylinder valve stem are present on large tanks, whereas small holes are drilled into the stem of small tanks. These measures ensure the correct gas tank is attached to the correct side of the system, preventing the accidental delivery of 100% N_2O.

A full cylinder of N_2O contains approximately 95% liquid and 5% vapor. When N_2O is being used, ambient air vaporizes the liquid to a gas. The outside of the tank may be cool to the touch during this process. The pressure gauge on the N_2O tank will not drop until most of the liquid is gone. O_2 is compressed into a cylinder as a gas. As O_2 is used, the pressure gauge drops proportionally and accurately reflects the amount of gas available in the tank.

The presence of a fail-safe mechanism means the machine is driven by O_2 flow. If the O_2 tank is depleted during the procedure, then the N_2O flow is terminated. Importantly, additional O_2 should be available at all times to prevent the interruption of ideal sedation.

N_2O/O_2 sedation can be delivered in a dental office through two types of systems: (1) centralized or (2) portable. A *centralized system* uses a mechanism called a *manifold* to connect several large tanks (Figure 42-2). The manifold will automatically activate a full container when one becomes low. This system delivers gas through copper piping to individual treatment rooms and is economically advantageous over a portable system for an office that frequently uses N_2O/O_2 sedation. A *portable system* can also deliver N_2O/O_2 sedation (Figure 42-3). The unit houses smaller cylinders and may be easily moved from one treatment area to another. This type of system may be preferred in offices where N_2O/O_2 sedation is infrequently used.

Both systems have regulators that reduce gas pressure from the tank. Low pressure is necessary for the delivery to a patient. Both systems also have a *flowmeter,* which delivers N_2O/O_2. The amount of each gas being delivered must be visibly monitored on the flowmeter. Knobs, levers, or buttons are used to adjust the gas flow.

A *reservoir bag* hangs from the flowmeter. This bag is used as an extra supply of gas if the patient should need more than the amount being delivered. The bag is also used to monitor the patient's respiration; it slightly inflates and then deflates concomitantly with inhalation and exhalation.

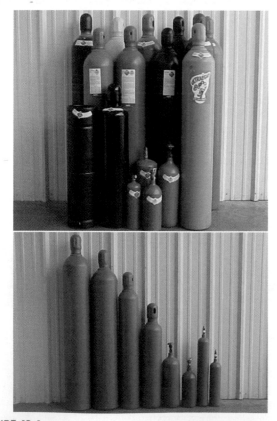

FIGURE 42-1
Variations of gas cylinders. (Courtesy Scott Heppel, nexAir, LLC, Memphis, Tenn.)

Typical System Layout

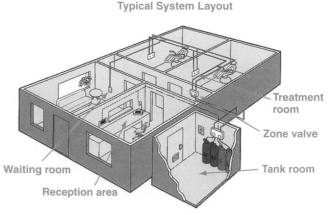

FIGURE 42-2
Centralized nitrous oxide/oxygen (N_2O/O_2) sedation unit. (From Clark MS, Brunick AL: *Handbook of nitrous oxide and oxygen sedation,* St Louis, 1999, Mosby.)

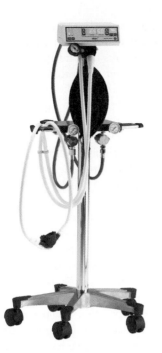

FIGURE 42-3
Portable nitrous oxide/oxygen (N₂O/O₂) sedation unit. (Courtesy Matrx by Midmark, Orchard Park, NY.)

The *conduction tubing* and *nasal hood* are the parts of the unit that bring gas to the patient. All units currently used must have *scavenging capabilities,* which means the devices must have the means to exhaust or vent exhaled gas out of the building. To accomplish this, one hose on the end of the conduction tubing must be inserted into the evacuation system. The nasal hood must have both delivery and scavenging hoses attached to it (Figure 42-4). One or more hoses deliver fresh gas to the patient while other hoses **scavenge** the exhaled gas. Using equipment without these capabilities is practicing below the accepted standard of care, placing the office and practitioners in legal jeopardy or in noncompliance with the U.S. Occupational Safety and Health Administration (OSHA).

Nasal hoods are available in a variety of sizes, both scented and unscented (Figure 42-5). Newer products are designed for single-patient use; however, autoclavable models are still available. Many products are now free of latex.

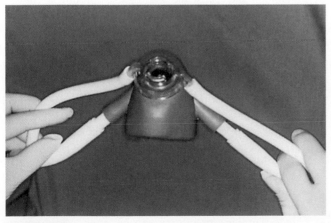

FIGURE 42-4
Scavenging nasal hood.

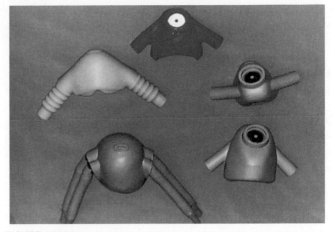

FIGURE 42-5
Variations of scavenging nasal hoods.

All units currently manufactured are designed to deliver a minimum of 30% O₂ at all times. This level ensures that the patient is breathing at least the amount of O₂ in ambient air (21%). The equipment for use in an ambulatory setting is also designed to limit the amount of N₂O that can be delivered to a patient. No more than 70% N₂O can be delivered to a patient when using sedation equipment. N₂O concentrations higher than 70% are unlikely to be used in the dental setting.

Unit features vary according to manufacturer. Some units have lighted electronic displays (LEDs), locks, and audiovisual alarms that indicate low O₂ levels (Figure 42-6). Ergonomics, infection control, ease of portability, and space-saving qualities are considerations of manufacturing design.

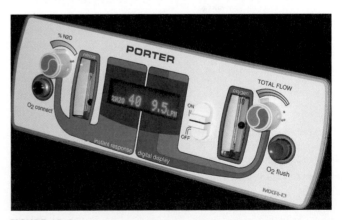

FIGURE 42-6
Variation of flowmeter with lighted electronic display and key lock. (Courtesy Porter Instrument, Hatfield, PA.)

Administration

The success of the N₂O/O₂ experience for both operator and patient largely depends on the technique of administration. Accurate monitoring of the patient for appropriate signs and symptoms of sedation is essential. Healthcare providers must understand the significance of sedation levels and the critical importance of vigilant patient monitoring.

Levels of anesthesia described in the literature pertain primarily to anesthesiologists inducing general anesthesia in a surgical environment. These levels or stages of anesthesia describe various physical and physiologic effects that occur when the CNS is depressed. Consciousness and cognitive awareness leads to unconsciousness, loss of reflexes, and eventually, loss of organ and system function. During ideal N_2O/O_2 sedation in an ambulatory setting, the patient remains in the beginning stage of this progression. Knowing the appropriate signs and symptoms of ideal sedation and oversedation is critical for patient comfort and safety.

IDEAL SEDATION

Patients may experience a variety of signs and symptoms when appropriately sedated. For example, the patient may feel a slight tingling sensation in the extremities or near the mouth. The patient may also sense increased but not uncomfortable body warmth. Some patients feel as if their body has become heavier; some feel lighter.

All patients do not experience the same effects, however, and practitioners must not rely on the presence of these signs and symptoms as indicators of appropriate sedation. With practice the operator will be able to evaluate the patient's body language, facial expression, and eye movement to determine an appropriate sedation level. In ideal sedation the operator may notice that the patient's body is not as rigid. The patient should appear relaxed.

Prevention

In ideal sedation, the patient is relaxed, comfortable, and aware of the surroundings. The patient is always **conscious** and has complete control of gag and cough reflexes. In addition, the patient will always be able to maintain conversation and respond to directions.

Patient Education Opportunity

The patient should be informed that N_2O/O_2 sedation will help him or her feel relaxed and comfortable during dental procedures. The patient should know that he or she will always know the surroundings and what is being done, as well as be able to communicate with the operator.

The patient may also take deep and slow respirations. In most instances the patient's eyes are good indicators of sedation levels. Active blinking and rapid eye movement may suggest the patient is not completely relaxed. When eye movement slows and the patient has a *glazed* look, the sedation level may be more appropriate. Smiles come easily to an ideally sedated patient.

OVERSEDATION

Generally, the oversedated patient is uncomfortable. The patient may rapidly enter the second stage of CNS depression and exhibit only subtle signs. The operator must be cognizant of the signs and symptoms associated with oversedation. Patients should never be left alone when receiving N_2O/O_2 sedation.

Prevention

Oversedation is most often a result of operator error.

When oversedated, the individual may become detached from the environment and indicate an out-of-body or floating experience. Some patients indicate an inability to move or communicate. Some may enter a dreamlike state, whereas others hallucinate. Generally, these feelings are not pleasant, and patients do not want to repeat the experience. Other signs and symptoms of oversedation include drowsiness, dizziness, nausea, or an uncomfortably warm body temperature. When oversedated, the patient may be sluggish, may delay responses, may slur words, and may not make verbal sense. The patient may begin to laugh uncontrollably or may become agitated, violent, or even combative.

Vomiting is associated with oversedation. Vomiting is an especially serious problem if a practitioner is not closely monitoring the patient. *Silent regurgitation* may happen, in which the patient vomits to a point where aspiration of vomitus occurs, which presents a life-threatening situation that may happen quietly and quickly. Preprocedural fasting is recommended to decrease the risk of aspiration should vomiting occur. Patients should avoid heavy meals and fried or fatty foods before sedation; an empty stomach is preferred.[1] Vomiting is also embarrassing for the patient. Most likely, if vomiting occurs during N_2O/O_2 sedation, then the operator oversedated the patient.

A patient may become **unconscious** while using N_2O/O_2 sedation. Unconsciousness is likely to occur when the oversedated patient's head falls forward and the tongue closes off the airway. However, N_2O alone will not likely render a patient unconscious because of the pharmacokinetic properties of the gas. However, the practitioner should always closely monitor a patient and be prepared to activate emergency assistance if necessary.

TECHNIQUE

A major advantage of N_2O/O_2 sedation is that the exact amount of drug may be used to achieve the desired level of sedation. This concept is called **titration.** Most methods of **pharmacologic sedation** do not allow for titration. By titrating N_2O in increments, the operator can accomplish the following:

- Achieve the desired level of sedation
- Assess the current level of sedation
- Maintain and adjust the level of sedation during the appointment
- Terminate the procedure at any point

Components of the Technique for Administering Nitrous Oxide/Oxygen Sedation

- To begin administering, the operator must first have the equipment ready. Machines must be turned on, tanks opened, and **scavenging devices** checked for proper operation.
- **Informed consent** must be obtained before any type of drug is administered for patient treatment. The patient must have a clear understanding of the procedure and its associated effects. If the patient is mentally incapable of understanding this information or cannot communicate during the procedure, N_2O/O_2 sedation is not recom-

mended. Parental or guardian consent for a minor is also required each time N_2O/O_2 sedation is used.

- The patient's health history should be updated at each appointment. Vital signs such as blood pressure, pulse, and respiration should be obtained and recorded as baseline values (Figure 42-7).

- The appropriate size and type of nasal hood should be selected for the patient. Nasal hood size is important because it facilitates gas flow. A poorly fitting hood may block gas flow to the patient or may allow excess gas to contaminate the surrounding air. The clinician secures the hood to the conduction tubing and begins the O_2 flow to the unit, establishing the appropriate flow in liters per minute (L/min). The amount of flow needed largely depends on the patient's **tidal volume** or amount of gas inspired into the lungs. The amount of gas inspired into the lungs per minute is called *minute ventilation*. By multiplying the tidal volume by the person's respiration rate, the operator can determine the appropriate liters per minute. On average,

$$500 \text{ ml (tidal volume)} \times 12 \text{ to } 15 \text{ respirations per minute} = 6 \text{ to } 7 \text{ L/min}$$

Initially, the operator may want to set the O_2 flow slightly higher than this level. Increasing the flow of O_2 at this point eliminates the suffocating or claustrophobic feeling that some patients may experience on initial placement of the nasal hood. Flow may be decreased when the patient has acclimated to the hood.

- The reservoir bag should be observed to confirm the appropriate amount of total gas flow. If the bag is collapsing as the patient is breathing, then he or she is demanding more flow than is being provided. The operator should increase the liters per minute until the bag remains two thirds full during patient respiration. Conversely, if the bag has overinflated, the amount of O_2 should be decreased because the patient is not using as much as is being delivered. Monitoring the reservoir bag constantly for changes in flow amount as required by the patient is important.

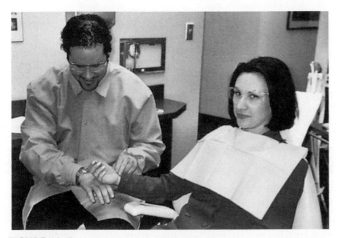

FIGURE 42-7
Preoperative vital signs taken for baseline values.

- Titrating N_2O is begun once the patient is comfortable with the amount of flow being delivered. Knowing the type of delivery system is important. Some machines have separate controls that independently regulate the flow of each gas. With these machines, as N_2O is added, the O_2 flow must be decreased proportionally to maintain the established liters-per-minute flow. For example, if the patient requires a total of 8 L/min, then the addition of 0.5 L N_2O would suggest that the O_2 level must be reduced by 0.5 to 7.5 L. The combined total would then remain at 8 L/min because of the addition of 0.5 L with the reduction to 7.5 L. The separate control system requires adjustment of both gases each time N_2O is added.

> **Prevention**
> To prevent oversedation, using the titration technique for administering N_2O/O_2 sedation is imperative. N_2O must be titrated to the patient slowly and in small amounts.

Other machines automatically adjust the O_2 flow as N_2O is titrated. In this case the established liter-per-minute flow remains constant. Manually adjusting the O_2 level is not necessary with these machines.

The levels of gas depicted by the floating balls or flashing lights do *not* represent the actual percentage of N_2O being delivered, which is calculated by dividing the N_2O L/min by the total liters per minute (Table 42-1).

Some machines do display the amount of O_2 or N_2O being delivered. When N_2O is added, subtracting that amount from the amount of O_2 is necessary. For example, if 70% O_2 were displayed on a dial or LED, then the N_2O percentage being delivered would be 30%.

- The dental hygienist should begin by administering approximately 10% N_2O and then proceed in increments of approximately 5% N_2O. Slow titration allows for maximal clinical effects to occur before additional drug is administered. At least 60 seconds should elapse before more N_2O is added. Additional time should be allowed between increments once signs of sedation are present.

- N_2O delivery or adjustment mandates careful patient monitoring for signs and symptoms of ideal sedation. The patient should be asked to breathe through the

> **Prevention**
> Patient talking is one of the primary sources of trace gas contamination of the air.

nose and should refrain from talking to allow maximum drug effect and to reduce the amount of contaminating trace gas dispersed into the air.

The patient is observed for signs and symptoms of ideal sedation. The patient should be relaxed and comfortable and *never* be uncomfortable. If the patient is dizzy, excessively warm, nauseous, or blacking out or does not respond to inquiries, then the amount of N_2O should be

> **Prevention**
> Never leave a patient alone when N_2O/O_2 sedation is being administered.

Table 42-1	Nitrous Oxide/Oxygen Percentage Chart									
	Liters per Minute Oxygen									
LITERS PER MINUTE NITROUS OXIDE	**1**	**2**	**3**	**4**	**5**	**6**	**7**	**8**	**9**	**10**
1	50	33	25	20	17	14	13	11	10	9
2	67	50	40	33	29	25	22	20	18	17
3	75*	60	50	43	38	33	30	27	25	23
4	80*	67	57	50	44	40	36	33	31	29
5	83*	71*	63	56	50	45	42	38	36	33
6	86*	75*	67	60	55	50	46	43	40	38
7	88*	78*	70*	64	58	54	50	47	44	41
8	89*	80*	73*	67	62	57	53	50	47	44
9	90*	82*	75*	69	64	60	56	53	50	47
10	91*	83*	77*	71*	67	63	59	56	53	50

From Clark MS, Brunick AL: *Handbook of nitrous oxide and oxygen sedation,* ed 2, St Louis, 2003, Mosby.
*Percentage exceeds maximum amount of N_2O needed for the effective management of pain and anxiety in an ambulatory setting and exceeds amounts able to be delivered by analgesic machines.

immediately decreased and the amount of O_2 subsequently increased. The patient should breathe deeply and understand that the uncomfortable feelings will soon disappear. Making the patient comfortable as soon as possible and beginning the process again is preferable, rather than leaving the patient uncomfortable with an insufficient reduction of N_2O. These uncomfortable feelings often explain why patients do not choose N_2O again.

Uncomfortable feelings indicate that the patient is oversedated. The operator must use the appropriate administration technique, constantly monitoring the patient's status. No preset or average percentage of N_2O will achieve optimal sedation. Each individual is unique and requires a different percentage. The N_2O amount used at one visit does not predict the amount needed for the next visit. *Using a prescribed or fixed level of N_2O or an amount based on a previous visit does not reflect the current standard of care for N_2O/O_2 administration.* Oversedation and the resultant negative patient experience are likely when using this approach.

Sedation levels may be intraoperatively adjusted when using N_2O/O_2. Adjustments may be made to increase the level of sedation during difficult or uncomfortable procedures or to reduce the sedation level for finishing or less uncomfortable procedures. This flexibility is one of the many advantages associated with N_2O/O_2 sedation (Figure 42-8).

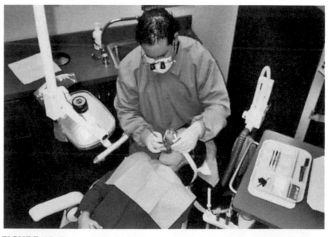

FIGURE 42-8
Operative treatment with patient receiving nitrous oxide/oxygen (N_2O/O_2) sedation.

Recovery

Providing the patient with postoperative O_2 is the final step in the sedation process (Figure 42-9).

As procedures are being completed, N_2O flow may be terminated to begin the required time of postoperative O_2. N_2O exits the body unchanged through the lungs.

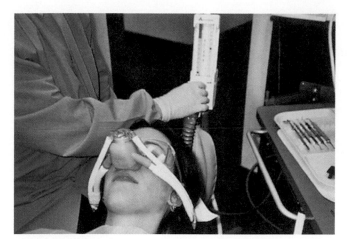

FIGURE 42-9
Postoperative oxygenation.

> **Prevention**
>
> Five minutes of 100% O_2 is considered the minimum time necessary for the patient to recover completely. However, recovery must be assessed before the O_2 is removed. Patients should be asked how they feel, and they should not feel dizzy, lightheaded, lethargic, or groggy. If a patient does not feel completely normal, then 100% O_2 is continued in 5-minute increments. Oxygenating some patients for 15 minutes or more may be appropriate.

DIFFUSION HYPOXIA

Historically associated with N_2O/O_2 sedation, **diffusion hypoxia** is defined as the process by which N_2O exits faster from the body than the O_2 that replaces it. O_2 is slightly diluted and serum O_2 saturation is decreased. These levels return to normal in a short period. This phenomenon has proved to be insignificant clinically.[18,22,24-26] The symptoms of postoperative headache, lethargy, and lightheadedness have been previously associated with diffusion hypoxia. However, because diffusion hypoxia is not clinically significant, the origin of these symptoms is unknown. In most cases, adequate postoperative O_2 eliminates these symptoms for most patients.

VITAL SIGNS

Blood pressure, pulse, and respiration rates should be within a reasonably comparable range of preoperative values. A **pulse oximeter** may be used to monitor serum O_2 saturation levels during N_2O/O_2 administration. Some pulse oximeters simultaneously record blood pressure and pulse as well. Preoperative and postoperative vital signs are required components of the N_2O/O_2 sedation protocol.

> **Prevention**
>
> Postoperative vital signs are an objective measure of recovery.

> **Prevention**
>
> Intraoperative vital signs should be taken if the patient is using 50% or more N_2O.

PSYCHOMOTOR ASSESSMENT

Psychomotor assessments have been made after N_2O/O_2 sedation. Jastak and Orendurff[17] evaluated participants for driving errors and concluded that patients could safely operate motor vehicles after N_2O/O_2 sedation. This study has been the foundation for practitioners dismissing patients without an escort. Others have agreed with this study.[29] However, if the operator believes an escort is necessary, then one should be recommended. Treat each patient individually.

> **Distinct Care Modifications**
>
> The practitioner is always responsible for ensuring adequate recovery before patient dismissal. If it appears that a patient should be escorted home, then the practitioner should recommend one.

RECORD KEEPING

Maintaining complete and accurate records of patient-operator interactions and procedures is important. The same premise is true when using N_2O/O_2 sedation. Several items require documentation after the procedure. Notes can be directly entered on a service record in the patient's chart or on a separate sedation record kept in the chart. If a separate sheet is used, then the patient's name and date must also be included. Including the reason for using this type of sedation would be appropriate. For example, notes would indicate that N_2O/O_2 sedation was used to reduce anxiety or to calm a hypersensitive gag reflex (Box 42-1).

BOX 42-1

DOCUMENTATION AFTER USE OF NITROUS OXIDE/ OXYGEN SEDATION

Maintain complete and accurate records of patient and operator interactions, and record the following procedures:

- Reason for use (e.g., anxiety, to calm a hypersensitive gag reflex)
- Medical consultation with a physician or other healthcare provider
- Preoperative and postoperative vital signs
- Patient's tidal volume or the required liters-per-minute flow (optional)
- Amount of postoperative oxygenation time (in minutes) required for patient recovery
- Negative or adverse reaction to the N_2O/O_2 sedation experience
- Peak amount of N_2O used and duration of sedation

Similar to other clinical situations, medical consultation with a physician or other healthcare providers should be documented in the patient's record. This record serves as legal documentation, as well as a source of information for future practitioners.

Preoperative and postoperative vital signs should also be recorded. Doing so documents prudent recovery assessment. The patient's tidal volume or the required liters-per-minute flow is an optional item. Generally, the *amount* of gas (N_2O and O_2) delivered will not change between visits. This number may be used as a reference point for the next visit.

Dental Considerations

The N_2O percentage used during a patient visit should not be used as a reference for the next visit, and the operator should decide whether this number should be included in the patient record. As previously mentioned, because of individual **biovariability,** the N_2O percentage used in one situation will not be the same on a different occasion. Beginning N_2O/O_2 administration at a fixed point or assuming the percentage will be the same from that of a previous visit is inappropriate.

The operator should record the amount of postoperative oxygenation time (in minutes) required for patient recovery to document an accurate assessment of recovery. Any negative or adverse reaction to the N_2O/O_2 sedation experience should be noted in the patient record to provide other practitioners a history of patient experiences (Figure 42-10).

42-4

Biological Effects and Issues

Since the late 1960s, many references in the literature have implicated N_2O as the causative agent for significant health problems in healthcare personnel chronically exposed to the drug. N_2O has been the common gas delivered by anesthesiologists for most surgical procedures and therefore was initially singled out as the etiologic agent for reproductive problems, spontaneous abortions, cancer, and other conditions. Most research in the 1970s and early 1980s reported similar results. The majority of this research was conducted with a retrospective survey design, which is not proven reliable or valid. From more than 800 articles written on the subject until 1995, fewer than 25 have been shown to merit reliability and validity.[8]

> *Note*
>
> The most significant biological effect linked to N_2O exposure is its ability to inactivate vitamin B_{12}. This inactivation affects the enzyme methionine synthetase, which is essential for deoxyribonucleic acid (DNA) production. Fetal abnormalities in animals and reproductive problems in humans were linked to this DNA effect with chronic exposure to high levels of unscavenged N_2O.[9,12]

These biological effects sensationalized in the literature were noted when high levels of unscavenged trace N_2O amounts were measured.

Since those early studies, equipment and delivery methods have tremendously improved. Using equipment with the capability of scavenging trace gas from the patient is now considered the standard of care. The manufacturers of N_2O/O_2 delivery equipment are continually improving their products and conducting research to ascertain new methods for scavenging trace gas.

Chronic exposure to N_2O has resulted in neurologic signs and symptoms. Individuals acknowledging misuse of N_2O for purposes other than patient treatment have experienced numbness, tingling, and paresthesia in their limbs. They also report impaired dexterity, clumsiness, and a slow or shuffled gait. Some individuals indicate gradual improvement of these symptoms when the abuse is terminated, whereas others note permanent neural injury.[21]

> *Note*
>
> It is important to recognize that no evidence to date indicates a direct causal relationship between reproductive health and scavenged low levels of N_2O for persons chronically exposed to the gas.[27] In addition, no adverse biological effect has been reported in patients receiving N_2O/O_2 sedation for pain and anxiety management in a dental office.

N_2O/O_2 SEDATION RECORD

ASA classification: I II III IV Indications for N_2O/O_2:____________________

Procedural data:	Preoperative	Intraoperative (when >50% N_2O)	Postoperative
Blood pressure:	______	______	______
Pulse:	______	______	______
Respiration:	______	______	______
SpO_2 (>50% / N_2O)	______	______	______

Tidal volume (L/min):____________________

Peak % N_2O admin:____________________ Duration of admin:____________________ minutes

Postop 100% O_2:____________________ minutes

Recovery (pt comments):____________________

Clinician's signature:____________________

FIGURE 42-10
Example of nitrous oxide/oxygen (N_2O/O_2) sedation record.

EXPOSURE LEVELS

The National Institute for Occupational Safety and Health (NIOSH) and the American Conference of Governmental Industrial Hygienists (ACGIH) established exposure recommendations during the administration of N_2O/O_2 over an 8-hour period.[4] These levels, established in 1977, were based on unfounded research and inadequate equipment. The level of N_2O/O_2 is *not* to exceed 50 parts per million (ppm) in a dental office. OSHA still requires that these values be upheld, although at present these limits are being challenged with new research. It is anticipated that these agencies will soon recommend new, accurate, and obtainable limits.

To determine the level of trace N_2O in a dental office, the operator must use a measuring device that detects atmospheric N_2O, such as an infrared spectrophotometer. These machines may be purchased or rented for periodic evaluation. A portable, hand-held device is available that can detect trace gas in the ambient air (Figure 42-11). This option may be advantageous for the office that frequently uses N_2O.

> *Prevention*
> Health practitioners can also determine the amount of their N_2O exposure over a specific period.

A personal monitoring device similar to a radiation dosimetry badge can be worn to determine the amount of N_2O exposure over a specific period (Figure 42-12). The time-weighted average (TWA) device contains an absorbent material that collects N_2O; the device is then returned to the company for

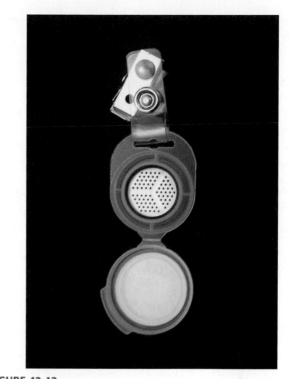

FIGURE 42-12
Nitrous oxide (N_2O) personal monitoring device. (From Clark M and Brunick A: *Handbook of Nitrous Oxide and Oxygen Sedation*, ed 3, St. Louis, Mosby, in press.)

analysis. The company returns a written report to the individual that details exposure levels.

TRACE CONTAMINATION

Dental personnel should use all measures available to minimize the amount of trace N_2O contamination in the office. Potential sources for trace gas leakage exist (Figure 42-13), and several methods are available to scavenge the contaminant.

Baseline values of N_2O contamination should be established for offices that use N_2O/O_2 sedation. A baseline figure documents the amount of trace N_2O in the office when using cur-

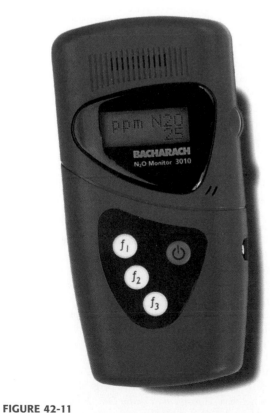

FIGURE 42-11
Hand-held nitrous oxide (N_2O) monitoring system. (Courtesy Bacharach, Inc., Pittsburgh, Penn.)

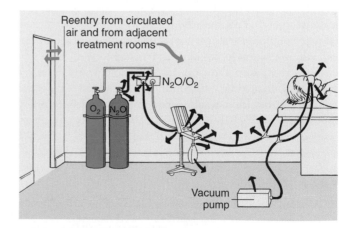

Reentry from circulated air and from adjacent treatment rooms

N_2O/O_2

O_2 N_2O

Vacuum pump

→ = Leak sources

FIGURE 42-13
Sources of potential nitrous oxide (N_2O) leaks.

rent equipment and procedures. From that point, a comparison can be made when additional scavenging methods are used. TWA dosimetry devices may be used if desired. A hand-held device is now available that performs the following:

- Measures the trace gas (ppm) in the air
- Assesses leaks in equipment
- Functions as a personal dosimetry device (see Figure 42-11)

> **Prevention**
> All equipment must have the capability to scavenge exhaled gas from the patient's mask into the evacuation system.

If scavenging equipment is not being used, then the practitioner is practicing below the standard of care and may be subject to legal repercussions. Gas can leak from any portion of the central piping system or through any point of connection with cylinders or valves. A common soap-and-water test can assess the adequacy of fittings and connections. The flowmeter itself can leak. Manufacturers recommend periodic evaluation and routine maintenance of equipment. A maximum of 2 years has been suggested for the period between equipment evaluations. Conduction tubing and reservoir bags should be routinely inspected for cracks and tears. The soap-and-water test can be used for these items as well.

Ensuring the adequacy of the existing evacuation system is important. The system must have sufficient force to evacuate scavenged gas from the nasal hood and must possess properly venting pumps. Office ventilation and air exchange in the ambulatory setting are both being currently investigated for ways to improve the removal of waste N_2O. Air conditioners typically recirculate ambient air rather than provide an air exchange. In this case, N_2O could be circulated throughout the office rather than being removed. Fresh-air vents should be located near the ceiling, whereas exhaust outlets should be near the floor. In addition, open windows are suggested as a method for removing waste gas. Oscillating room fans can assist the gas movement toward an open window or exhaust vent.

The health and safety of the professional dental team is second only to patient safety. All members should be educated on the potential biological effects and issues associated with chronic exposure to N_2O. Personnel should use all available measures to reduce or minimize trace gas contamination. Proper equipment and administration procedures are mandatory. Dental professionals must keep abreast of new technology and reputable research. Participating in continuing education programs that provide the latest recommendations or guidelines is also important.

References

1. ASA Task Force: Practice guidelines for sedation and analgesia by non-anesthesiologists, *Anesthesiology* 96(4):1004, 2002.
2. Barber J et al: The relationship between nitrous oxide conscious sedation and the hypnotic state, *J Am Dent Assoc* 99(4):624-626, 1979.
3. Berge TI: Acceptance and side effects of nitrous oxide-oxygen sedation for oral surgical procedures, *Acta Odontol Scand* 57(4):201-206, 1999.
4. Bruce DL, Bach MJ: *Trace effects of anesthetic gases on behavioral performance of operating room personnel*, HEW Pub No (NIOSH) 76-169, Cincinnati, 1976, US Department of Health, Education, and Welfare.
5. Chancellor JW: Dr Wells' impact on dentistry and medicine, *J Am Dent Assoc* 125:1585-1589, 1994.
6. Chapman WP, Arrowood JG, Beecher HK: The analgesic effects of low concentrations of nitrous oxide compared in man with morphine sulfate, *J Clin Invest* 22:871-875, 1943.
7. Chidiac JJ et al: Gagging prevention using nitrous oxide or table salt: a comparative pilot study, *Int J Prosthodont* 14(4):364-366, 2001.
8. Clark MS, Renehan BW, Jeffers BW: Clinical use and potential biohazards of nitrous oxide/oxygen, *Gen Dent* 45:486-491, 1997.
9. Cohen EN et al: Occupational disease in dentistry and chronic exposure to trace anesthetic gases, *J Am Dent Assoc* 101:21-31, 1980.
10. Davis MJ: Conscious sedation practices in pediatric dentistry: a survey of members of the American Board of Pediatric Dentistry College of Diplomates, *Pediatr Dent* 10:328-329, 1988.
11. Eger E II et al: Clinical pharmacology of nitrous oxide: an argument for its continued use, *Anesth Analg* 71:575-585, 1990.
12. Fujinagra M, Baden JM, Mazze RI: Susceptible period of nitrous oxide teratogenicity in Sprague-Dawley rats, *Teratology* 40:439-444, 1989.
13. Gall O et al: Adverse events of premixed nitrous oxide and oxygen for procedural sedation in children, *Lancet* 358(9292):1514-1515, 2001.
14. Goodall E et al: Self-ratings by phobic patients during dental treatment: greater improvement with nitrous oxide than midazolam, *Hum Psychopharmacol* 9(3):203-209, 1994.
15. Jackson DL, Johnson BS: Inhalational and enteral conscious sedation for the adult dental patient, *Dent Clin North Am* 46(4):781-802, 2002.
16. Jacobsohn PH: What others said about Wells, *J Am Dent Assoc* 125:1583-1584, 1994.
17. Jastak JT, Orendurff D: Recovery from nitrous sedation, *Anesth Prog* 22:113-116, 1975.
18. Jeske AH et al: Noninvasive assessment of diffusion hypoxia following administration of nitrous oxide-oxygen, *Anesth Prog* 51(1):10-13, 2004.
19. Jorgensen NB: *Sedation, local and general anesthesia in dentistry*, ed 2, Philadelphia, 1985, Lea & Febiger.
20. Kanagasundaram SA et al: Efficacy and safety of nitrous oxide in alleviating pain and anxiety during painful procedures, *Arch Dis Child* 84(6):492-495, 2001.
21. Layzer RB: Myeloneuropathy after prolonged exposure to nitrous oxide, *Lancet* 2:1227-1230, 1978.
22. Leelataweewud P et al: The physiological effects of supplemental oxygen versus nitrous oxide/oxygen during conscious sedation of pediatric dental patients, *Pediatr Dent* 22(2):125-133, 2000.
23. Malamed SF, Clark MS: Nitrous oxide-oxygen: a new look at a very old technique, *J Calif Dent Assoc* 31(6):397-403, 2003.
24. Papageorge MB, Noonan LW Jr, Rosenberg M: Diffusion hypoxia: another view, *Anesth Pain Control Dent* 2:143-149, 1993.
25. Primosch RE et al: Effect of nitrous oxide-oxygen inhalation with scavenging on behavioral and physiological parameters during

routine pediatric dental treatment, *Pediatr Dent* 21(7):417-420, 1999.

26. Rodrigo MR: A study of inhalational sedation with nitrous oxide/oxygen for oral surgery in Hong Kong Chinese, *Ann Acad Med Singapore* 15(3):315-319, 1986.

27. Rowland AS et al: Reduced fertility among women employed as dental assistants exposed to high levels of nitrous oxide, *N Engl J Med* 327:993-997, 1992.

28. Ruben H: Nitrous oxide analgesia in dentistry, *Br Dent J* 132:195-196, 1972.

29. Thompson JM et al: Cognitive properties of sedation agents: comparison of the effects of nitrous oxide and midazolam on memory and mood, *Br Dent J* 187(10):557-562, 1999.

30. Veerkamp JS et al: Anxiety reduction with nitrous oxide: a permanent solution? *ASDC J Dent Child* 62(1):44-48, 1995.

31. Veerkamp JS et al: Dental treatment of fearful children using nitrous oxide: part 4—anxiety after two years, *ASDC J Dent Child* 60(4):372-376, 1993.

32. Wang CY et al: A comparative study of sevoflurane sedation with nitrous oxide sedation for dental surgery, *Int J Oral Maxillofac Surg* 31(5):506-510, 2002.

CHAPTER

43

Saliva and Salivary Dysfunction

Francis G. Serio • Mary R. Pfeifer • George M. Taybos

INSIGHT

Saliva is one of the body fluids that provides protection, nutrients, and hydration to the body. The dental hygienist can provide better individualized patient treatment from understanding the functions of saliva and the components that make this fluid unique. Current and future diagnoses of illness are and will continue to be discovered through examination of this fluid.

✸✸ CASE STUDY 43-1 Dental Management of Salivary Gland Dysfunction

Martha Anthony is a 52-year-old white woman. She has not had a supportive dental care visit in more than a year. At this visit, she seems to be blinking her eyes frequently, and when she speaks, it sounds as though her mouth is dry. You question Ms. Anthony about your observations, and she says her eyes have been dry for several months. She purchased some artificial tears from the pharmacy, which work most of the time but only for a few hours. Ms. Anthony did not use the artificial tears this morning because she was in a hurry and did not want to be late for the appointment. She also reports that her mouth has seemed dry during the last several months and that she constantly sips water. These two findings are of concern to you as a dental hygienist because you suspect that Ms. Anthony may have a serious underlying disease. The resulting dry mouth might cause additional oral disease, especially where she has recession.

KEY TERMS

candidiasis	glossitis	pilocarpine (Salagen)	salivary gland acini
cevimeline hydrochloride (Evoxac)	glossodynia	radiation caries	Sjögren's syndrome
dysphagia	keratoconjunctivitis sicca	radiation osteomyelitis and osteo-	xerostomia
exocrine glands	mucositis	necrosis	

LEARNING OUTCOMES

After reading this chapter the student will be able to:
1. Understand the functions of saliva in maintaining oral health.
2. Describe some of the constituents of saliva and their contribution to the oral cavity.
3. Know the classification of the salivary glands according to their type of secretion.
4. Recognize information in a patient's health history that may be related to salivary gland dysfunction.
5. Identify patients with decreased salivary function by (1) asking specific questions, (2) assessing their subjective complaints, and

(3) evaluating abnormal intraoral findings that are consistent with decreased salivary gland function.
6. Manage the oral health problems directly caused by salivary gland dysfunction.
7. Make an overall positive impact in the life of a patient with xerostomia (dry mouth).

Functions of Saliva

Saliva can definitely be described by the old adage that, "You can't tell a book by its cover." Although saliva may appear to be a nondescript liquid, it is actually a complex mixture of water, mucus, proteins, glycoproteins, carbohydrates, antibodies, buffers, fluoride (see Chapter 25), and other substances that provide protection and function in the oral cavity. The functions of saliva are summarized in Box 43-1.

Some salivary glands produce predominantly serous (watery) saliva, whereas others produce a more mucous-type saliva.

Saliva can function only if it is produced. Researchers study both unstimulated salivary flow and stimulated salivary flow. Unstimulated salivary flow in healthy individuals may be affected by the degree of hydration, body position, exposure to light, circadian rhythms, circannual rhythms, and medications. The amount of unstimulated salivary flow varies widely but

BOX 43-1

FUNCTIONS OF SALIVA

- **Fluid or lubricant:** Coats the mucosa and helps protect against mechanical, thermal, and chemical irritation. Assists smooth airflow, speech, and swallowing.
- **Ion reservoir:** Solution is supersaturated with ions (including fluoride) and facilitates remineralization of the teeth.
- **Buffer:** Helps neutralize plaque biofilm pH after eating, thereby reducing the time for remineralization. Root caries are a severe problem in older patients with xerostomia.
- **Cleansing:** Clears food and aids in swallowing.
- **Antimicrobial actions:** Specific (secretory immunoglobulin A) and nonspecific (lysozyme, lactoferrin, and sialoperoxidase) antimicrobial mechanisms help control the oral microflora.
- **Agglutination:** Aggregates and accelerates the clearance of bacterial cells.
- **Pellicle formation:** Protective diffusion barrier is formed on enamel from salivary proteins. Plaque biofilm may adhere to the pellicle.
- **Digestion:** Because of the presence of the enzyme amylase, starchy food debris on the teeth is degraded.
- **Taste:** Saliva acts as a solvent for various spices and other flavoring agents, thus allowing interaction of food with taste buds to facilitate taste. Interestingly, the salt content of saliva is significantly less than plasma, thereby allowing the taste of salt to occur when eating.
- **Excretion:** Because the oral cavity is technically outside the body, substances that are secreted in saliva are excreted. This action is inefficient because excreted material may be reabsorbed farther down the alimentary tract.
- **Water balance:** Under conditions of dehydration, salivary flow is reduced, mouth dryness occurs, a decrease in urine production occurs, and the desire for water consumption increases. These actions are coordinated by the hypothalamus.

From Whelton H: Introduction: the anatomy and physiology of the salivary glands. In Edgar WM, O'Mullane DM, eds: *Saliva and oral health,* ed 2, London, 1996, British Dental Association.

seems to be approximately 0.3 ml/min.[8] Daily volume is approximately 1000 ml. Researchers have suggested that an unstimulated salivary flow rate of 0.1 to 0.3 ml/min may be necessary to avoid xerostomia.[9] Salivary flow is least during sleep, thereby necessitating good nocturnal oral hygiene and not eating any cariogenic substances after brushing for the last time of the day. Stimulated salivary flow may be four to five times greater than unstimulated flow.

> *Note*
>
> Two of the major functions of saliva are to clear foodstuffs from the oral cavity and to buffer any acids produced by cariogenic plaque biofilm.

The capacity to buffer acids caused by cariogenic plaque biofilm is provided primarily by bicarbonate, with phosphate buffers contributing at lower salivary flow rates. The Stephan curve (see Figure 25-1) is a measure of the time required for the mouth to return from an acidic environment to baseline (near neutral, pH 7). The time taken to return to baseline may be affected by the stimulated flow rate of saliva, the buffering capacity, the cariogenicity of the foodstuff consumed, and the aid of food clearance such as rinsing with water.

Salivary proteins serve a variety of functions as well. Sialoperoxidase interferes with bacterial metabolism, and lysozyme attacks the cell wall of susceptible bacteria.[6] Mucins contribute by providing lubrication and aggregation of bacteria. Secretory immunoglobulins such as secretory immunoglobulin A (SIgA) target specific bacterial antigens and contribute to the blockage of bacterial colonization.[11,22] Histidine-rich histatins also have antimicrobial activity and may help neutralize enzymes of bacterial origin.[12] As can be seen by its complexity, creating an artificial saliva that can mimic the many contributions of saliva to oral health and homeostasis is difficult.

> *Note*
>
> Saliva also contributes to the remineralization of teeth.[21]

Calcium and phosphate are found in supersaturated concentrations in saliva. These components may reduce the demineralization of teeth by increasing early remineralization. This remineralization is aided by the presence of fluoride, usually delivered in local form by toothpastes or locally applied fluoride products. Coincident inhibitors of calcification are in saliva to help control the formation of calculus. With plaque biofilm accumulation, these inhibitors are overwhelmed, and calculus will indeed form.

Evidence indicates that in addition to the functional and protective aspects of saliva, saliva may have diagnostic value as well. Theories suggest that proteins originating from cancers may find their way into the saliva.[19,20] To date, extensive work has been done to develop salivary diagnostic tools for cancer proteins, although practical clinical tests have yet to be introduced.[6]

Development of Salivary Glands

The parotid glands are formed by the sixth week of prenatal life, the submandibular glands at the end of the sixth week and beginning of the seventh week, the sublingual glands by the eighth week, and the minor salivary glands after the twelfth week.[2,5] Salivary glands are **exocrine glands,** which have ducts that transport the secretion (saliva) from the glands.

Classification of Salivary Glands

The salivary glands are divided into major glands and minor glands.[2,5] The major salivary glands are the parotid, submandibular, and sublingual glands. These glands are responsible for most of the 0.5 to 0.75 liters of daily saliva production. The minor salivary glands are found throughout the oral cavity and are named according to where they are located (i.e., labial minor, buccal minor, palatal). The salivary glands may also be classified according to their type of secretion: serous, mucous, or mixed. The serous salivary secretion is composed of water, some enzymes (amylase and maltose), salts, and organic ions. The mucous secretion is composed of mucin, which is a lubricating material that aids in chewing, swallowing, and digesting.

Table 43-1 illustrates the three major salivary glands. The *parotid gland,* the largest of the three glands, contributes approximately 25% of the total salivary secretions, produces a serous secretion, and is innervated by the glossopharyngeal nerve (cranial nerve IX). The *submandibular gland,* intermediate in size, contributes approximately 60% of the total salivary secretions, produces a mixed secretion that is predominantly serous, and is innervated by the chorda tympani of the facial nerve (cranial nerve VII). The *sublingual gland,* the smallest of the major salivary glands, contributes only 5% of the salivary secretions, produces a mixed secretion that is predominantly mucus, and is innervated by the chorda tympani of the facial nerve (cranial nerve VII).

The type of secretion can also classify the minor salivary glands. Mucous secretion is found in the glossopalatine, palatine, and posterior lingual minor salivary glands; serous secretion is found only in von Ebner's glands, located on the circumvallate papillae of the tongue; and mixed secretion glands that are predominantly mucus are found on the anterior tongue, buccal mucosa, and labial mucosa. The minor salivary glands collectively contribute 5% to 10% of the total salivary secretion.

Salivary Gland Dysfunction

43-1

The two most common dental complaints from patients are vague tooth pains and dry mouth problems. Determining the underlying cause of the complaints is often difficult and sometimes frustrating. The most common form of salivary gland dysfunction is xerostomia.

DENTAL CONSIDERATIONS

Xerostomia by definition is a dryness of the mouth from a lack of normal salivary gland secretion.[1] Dry mouth is often a subjective complaint by the patient and cannot be correlated to any actual salivary gland dysfunction.[1] In a healthy individual, the saliva lubricates and protects the oral mucosa, aids in cleaning the mouth, regulates the acidity (pH), maintains the integrity of the dentition, and destroys bacteria.[17] Therefore when a decrease in salivary function exists, a predictable sequelae will exist in the oral cavity. The changes in the oral mucosa can range from a dry, smooth-appearing mucosa to ulcerations with secondary infections such as **candidiasis.**[23] The decreased salivary function increases the susceptibility of the dentition to dental caries.[7,13] The patient also may report an altered taste, **glossodynia** or **glossitis,** and difficulty in chewing and swallowing.

The following are the most common causes of xerostomia:

- Medications
- Radiation therapy for head and neck cancers
- Immunologic disease, particularly Sjögren's syndrome

MEDICATIONS

Xerostomia can occur in any age group but is a common complaint in older adults. A long-held belief was that salivary function decreased with age; however, this belief was proven as incorrect.[3,4] However, a decreased stimulated saliva rate appears to exist in individuals who take medications.[3,24]

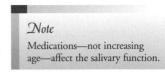

Note
Medications—not increasing age—affect the salivary function.

In one study, a review of the drug intake for a population revealed that 22% take antihypertensive drugs, 20% consume alcohol, 14% take mood-altering drugs, 9% take antihistamines, and 7% take decongestants.[14] Of the 200 most-prescribed medications in 1998, 55 list xerostomia as an expected adverse effect[27] (Boxes 43-2 and 43-3). If age groups are correlated to the use of drugs that can cause xerostomia, the findings then reveal a prevalence of xerostomia in 27% of the

| **Table 43-1** | **Major Salivary Glands: Amounts and Types of Secretions and Innervations** |

SALIVARY GLAND	AMOUNT AND TYPE OF SECRETION*	INNERVATIONS
Parotid Gland	25%; serous secretion	Glossopharyngeal nerve (cranial nerve IX)
Submandibular Gland	60%; mixed secretion but mostly serous	Chorda tympani of the facial nerve (cranial nerve VII)
Sublingual Gland	5%; mixed secretion but mostly mucus	Chorda tympani of the facial nerve (cranial nerve VII)

*Minor salivary glands produce approximately 5% to 10% of the saliva.

BOX 43-2

ORAL SIGNS AND SYMPTOMS OF ADVERSE DRUG REACTIONS

Angioedema	Lichenoid drug reaction
Candidiasis	Mouth ulcerations, stomatitis
Cough	Mouth and jaw discomfort
Dysgeusia	Oral paresthesia
Erythema multiforme	Pharyngitis
Gingival bleeding	Reflux, hyperacidity
Gingival hyperplasia	Tooth disorder
Glossodynia, glossitis	Vomiting
Increased gag reflex	Xerostomia

BOX 43-3

DRUG CATEGORIES THAT CAUSE XEROSTOMIA

Amphetamines: dextroamphetamine and amphetamine (Adderall)
Analgesic agents: nonsteroidal antiinflammatory drugs, narcotics
Antianxiety agents: benzodiazepines
Anticonvulsant drugs: gabapentin (Neurontin)
Antidepressant agents: selective serotonin reuptake inhibitors, tricyclics
Antihistamines
Antimicrobial agents: ciprofloxacin (Cipro)
Antipsychotic agents: risperidone (Risperdal)
Asthma drugs
Cardiovascular agents: angiotensin-converting enzyme inhibitors, calcium-channel blockers, alpha-1 blockers
Decongestants
Gastric acid secretion inhibitors: omeprazole (Prilosec)
Prokinetic gastrointestinal tract agents
Skeletal muscle relaxants: cyclobenzaprine
Tobacco-cessation drugs: bupropion (Zyban)

18-to-34 age group, 35% of the 35-to-54 age group, and 60% of the 55-and-older age group.[18] These findings clearly show that patients of all ages can experience xerostomia from using medications.

RADIATION THERAPY

In 2001, estimates suggested that 30,100 individuals would be diagnosed with cancer of the oral cavity and pharynx. The treatments for head and neck cancer are surgery, radiation therapy, chemotherapy, or a combination of the three modalities. Each modality by itself is wrought with adverse effects. The surgical approach can result in loss of function and disfigurement. Chemotherapy can result in alopecia (hair loss), anorexia, nausea, and immunosuppression with its increased risk for infection. Although chemotherapy can cause a transient salivary gland dysfunction, xerostomia is not generally associated with the chemotherapeutic and surgical modalities, which, unfortunately, is not the case with radiation therapy.

The following are direct effects of radiation therapy to the oral structures:

- **Mucositis**
- **Dysphagia** (difficulty in swallowing)
- Xerostomia
- Candidiasis
- **Radiation caries**
- **Radiation osteomyelitis and osteonecrosis**

The patient who is undergoing radiation therapy will report decreased saliva almost immediately (during the first week of therapy), whereas mucositis generally becomes noticeable after 2 weeks of therapy. Indirect effects of radiation therapy are caused by irreversible changes in the vascular tissue and bone. The most dramatic and dose-limiting effect during radiation therapy is mucositis, which begins in the second week of therapy and then increases in severity as the treatment progresses. Mucositis may become so severe that a nasogastric tube is inserted for feeding, and the radiation therapy regimen is interrupted until the oral signs and symptoms improve. After the radiation therapy is completed, the atrophy and degeneration of the irradiated salivary glands results in little or no salivary gland secretions (see Chapter 48).

SJÖGREN'S SYNDROME

Sjögren's syndrome (SS) (pronounced *show-grens*) is an autoimmune disorder characterized by a classic triad of clinical conditions:

- **Keratoconjunctivitis sicca** (dry eyes)
- Xerostomia
- Connective tissue disease

  SS can occur in two ways:

  - Primary: The primary form of SS is characterized by the presence of only dry eyes and xerostomia.
  - Secondary: The secondary form is characterized by the following:
    - Dry eyes
    - Xerostomia
    - The presence of a systemic connective tissue disorder, such as rheumatoid arthritis (30% to 50%), systemic lupus erythematosus (5%), progressive systemic sclerosis (5%), polymyosilis (4%), or mixed connective disease (3%)

The prevalence of SS is unknown; however, it is estimated to occur in 0.5% of the population, with 80% to 90% of those affected being middle-aged women. The salivary gland dysfunction that occurs with SS is a direct result of the autoimmune lymphocytic infiltration of the salivary gland tissue that destroys the saliva-producing component of the gland. Some evidence exists that viral infections, heredity, and hormones may in some way contribute to SS. Most patients with SS have a reduced resting and stimulated salivary flow rate.[16]

> *Note*
>
> Patients with SS may have an increased risk for lymphoma (non-Hodgkin's B cell)—up to 40 times greater than the normal population.[15]

CASE APPLICATION 43-1.1

Differential Diagnosis

Of the illnesses presented in this chapter, which one seems to fit the symptoms presented by Ms. Anthony?

Dental Management of Salivary Gland Dysfunction

The patient with decreased salivary production creates a unique and often frustrating management problem for the dental hygienist and dentist because no cure is available.

CASE APPLICATION 43-1.2

Management Strategy

Which of the following management strategies would you consider for Ms. Anthony?

DENTAL CARIES

Because of the significant reduction in salivary gland function, the patient is at greater risk for dental caries activity regardless of age. This increased risk requires the patient to have a more serious and meticulous approach to oral hygiene procedures. Patients with salivary gland dysfunction should be treated more frequently than normal, such as every 3 months. The increased dental caries activity can be controlled if the patient improves home care, implements daily use of a focused custom fluoride tray, and rinses with chlorhexidine so that organisms responsible for dental caries are reduced.

ORAL CANDIDIASIS

The increased risk for developing oral candidiasis (erythematous type) is directly related to the decreased salivary function.

Distinct Care Modifications

The patient with oral candidiasis may be better managed with a systemic antifungal agent such as ketoconazole or fluconazole.

For the patient who develops candidiasis, antifungal agents should be prescribed to treat the infection. Oral nystatin preparations can be a problem for the patient with xerostomia. The lozenge and pastilles contain large quantities of sugar, and the suspension may require 2-minute rinses four times a day for 30 days or more.

Throughout the chapter, *Rx* is the prescription; *Disp* is to dispense; and *Sig* is the dosing direction.

Rx: ketoconazole (Nizoral) 200-mg tablets
Disp: tablets no. 15
Sig: Take two tablets on first day at mealtime, then one tablet each day at mealtime, until gone.

Note: Ketoconazole is taken at mealtime because the active antifungal drug requires low gastric pH for maximum systemic absorption.

Rx: fluconazole (Diflucan) 100-mg tablets
Disp: tablets no. 15
Sig: Take two tablets on first day at mealtime, then one tablet each day at mealtime, until gone.

XEROSTOMIA

When evaluating the patient's xerostomia problem, the patient's complaint and the hygienist's concern may be different. Remember to always listen to what patients describe; this description will be their priority. The dental hygienist may focus on the potential for increased dental caries activity, whereas the patient's main concern is the oral dryness that results in difficulty in chewing and swallowing food and even in speaking. The patient's concern is directly related to a decrease in both quantity and quality of the saliva.

For pilocarpine, a prescription medication approved by the U.S. Food and Drug Administration (FDA), to have a positive effect, some residual active salivary gland tissue must be present. The suggested regimen is for the patient to take a 5-mg tablet 30 to 45 minutes before each meal and, if desired, at bedtime. The most frequently noted adverse effect from pilocarpine is perspiration.[26] Evidence exists that using oral pilocarpine during radiation therapy will decrease the severity of salivary gland atrophy and degeneration and decrease the extent and severity of predictable mucositis. If oral pilocarpine is suggested for a patient who is to undergo radiation therapy, a dose of pilocarpine must be taken 1 hour before the radiation treatment. This action results in the degranulation of the secretory granules in the **salivary gland acini.** One of the mechanisms of salivary gland destruction during radiation therapy is the interaction of the ionizing radiation with the granules, which results in the production of destructive free radicals.

Distinct Care Modifications

Relief may be found by treating symptoms with over-the-counter pain relievers, artificial tears, ointments, and saliva substitutes. If the patient's xerostomia is caused by medications, the management is then limited to keeping the mouth moist with plain water or with artificial saliva substitutes such as Oral Balance (Laclede, Inc., Rancho Dominguez, Calif.), Salivart (Gebauer Co., Cleveland, Ohio), or both.

Distinct Care Modifications

If xerostomia is the result of head and neck radiation therapy, then oral **pilocarpine (Salagen)** can be used for treatment.

SJÖGREN'S SYNDROME

Management of the patient with SS should also include care by an ophthalmologist for the dry eyes and by a rheumatologist if arthritis or a connective tissue disorder is present.

Distinct Care Modifications

For patients with SS, pilocarpine and **cevimeline hydrochloride (Evoxac)** is FDA-approved and can be used in the same regimen as with postradiation xerostomia.

Rx: cevimeline HCl (Evoxac) 30 mg
Disp: caps no. 120
Sig: Take one capsule 60 to 90 minutes before meals and at bedtime.
Refills: six (a 6-month supply)
Rx: oral pilocarpine (Salagen) 5-mg tablets
Disp: tablets no. 120
Sig: Take one tablet 30 to 45 minutes before meals and at bedtime.
Refills: six (a 6-month supply)

Note: The patient is directed to take oral pilocarpine 30 to 45 minutes before meals. For most individuals, ingesting the oral tablet will result in maximal salivary gland stimulation within 45 to 60 minutes, which ensures that saliva is present at mealtime. For the patient who takes oral pilocarpine during head and neck radiation therapy, one tablet must be taken 1 hour before the radiation treatment. To obtain the same results with cevimeline, the medication is taken 60 to 90 minutes before meals.

Clues to Determine the Presence of Xerostomia

To assist the dental hygienist in identifying a patient with decreased salivary function, Fox[10] has developed the questions listed in Box 43-4. Box 43-5 lists conditions for which to look in a medical history that might be related to salivary gland dysfunction. Subjective complaints that may be related to salivary gland dysfunction are listed in Box 43-6. Intraoral findings might also indicate decreased salivary function (Box 43-7).

BOX 43-4

QUESTIONS USED TO DETERMINE DECREASED SALIVARY FUNCTION

Do you sip liquids to help swallow dry foods?
Does your mouth feel dry when eating a meal?
Do you have difficulty swallowing any foods?
Does the amount of saliva in your mouth seem to be too little or too much, or is it unnoticeable?

BOX 43-5

MEDICAL HISTORY ITEMS THAT MAY BE RELATED TO SALIVARY GLAND DYSFUNCTION

Atrophic vaginitis
Chronic sinusitis (antihistamines)
Current chemotherapy
Depression (xerostomia-causing medications)
Diabetes
Dry eyes or corneal ulcers and photosensitivity
History of head and neck radiation
Hypertension (xerostomia-causing medications)
Lupus and mixed connective tissue disorders (secondary Sjögren's syndrome)
Recurrent oral candidiasis
Rheumatoid arthritis (secondary Sjögren's syndrome)
Sore muscles and sore joints (analgesic medications)
Other medical conditions involving the heart, lungs, liver, and digestive and gynecologic systems
Other mixed connective tissue disorders (polymyositis, scleroderma, sclerosis)

BOX 43-6

SUBJECTIVE COMPLAINTS THAT MAY BE RELATED TO DECREASED SALIVARY GLAND FUNCTION

Sore or burning sensation in the mouth
Dry, itchy, or tired eyes or feeling of sand in eyes
Continuous cold hands and feet (Raynaud's phenomenon)
General achy muscles and fatigue
History of dry, atrophic vaginitis
Need to suck on candies (e.g., lemon drops) to assist in lubricating mouth throughout the day (also increases the risk of dental decay)
Need to sip water throughout the day and night
Difficulty speaking for more than 10 minutes without drinking water
Difficulty swallowing food at mealtime and need to often drink water to swallow food

---

BOX 43-7

INTRAORAL FINDINGS THAT MAY BE RELATED TO DECREASED SALIVARY GLAND FUNCTION

Atrophic buccal mucosa
Atypical increased activity in dental decay (especially cervical and incisal teeth)
Boggy, smooth, and glassy appearance of the gingival margin (if the gingival sulcus is air dried, decreased, or no gingival crevicular fluid fills the area and the sulcus stays dry and open)
Dental mirror *sticks* to the patient's buccal mucosa
Frothy saliva (thick and bubbly but little or no serous component)
No pooling of saliva in the anterior floor of the mouth
Oral candidiasis
Decreased filiform papilla (glossitis)

References

1. Atkinson JC, Wu AJ: Salivary gland dysfunction: causes, symptoms, treatment, *J Am Dent Assoc* 125:409-415, 1994.
2. Avery JK: *Oral development and histology,* ed 3, New York, 2000, Thieme Medical.
3. Baum BJ: Evaluation of stimulated parotid saliva flow rate in different age groups, *J Dent Res* 60(7):1292-1296, 1981.
4. Ben-Aryeh H et al: The salivary flow rate and composition of whole and parotid resting and stimulated saliva in young and old healthy subjects, *Biochem Med Metab Biol* 36:260-265, 1986.
5. Bhaskar SN: *Orban's oral histology and embryology,* ed 11, St Louis, 1991, Mosby.
6. Bowen WH: Salivary influences on the oral microflora. In Edgar WM, O'Mullane DM, eds: *Saliva and oral health,* ed 2, London, 1996, British Dental Association.
7. Burnett GW: The microbiology of dental infections, *Dent Clin North Am* 14(4):681-695, 1970.
8. Dawes C: Factors influencing salivary flow rate and consumption. In Edgar WM, O'Mullane DM, eds: *Saliva and oral health,* ed 2, London, 1996, British Dental Association.
9. Dawes C: How much saliva is enough for avoidance of xerostomia? *Caries Res* 38:236-240, 2004.
10. Fox PC et al: Sjögren's syndrome: a model for dental care in the 21st century, *J Am Dent Assoc* 129:719-728, 1998.
11. Hay DH, Bowen WH: The functions of salivary proteins. In Edgar WM, O'Mullane DM, eds: *Saliva and oral health,* ed 2, London, 1996, British Dental Association.
12. Lendenmann U, Oppenheim FG: Protein structure and function: histatins. In Guggenheim B, Shapiro S, eds: *Oral biology at the turn of the century,* Basel, Switzerland, 1998, Karger.
13. Mandel ID: The role of saliva in maintaining oral homeostasis, *J Am Dent Assoc* 199:298-394, 1989.
14. Meurmen JH, Rantonen P: Salivary flow rate, buffering capacity and yeast counts in 187 consecutive adult patients from Kuopio, Finland, *Scand J Dent Res* 102(4):229-234, 1994.
15. Neville BW et al: *Oral and maxillofacial pathology,* ed 2, Philadelphia, 2002, WB Saunders.
16. Rhodus NL: Oral pilocarpine HCl stimulates labial (minor) salivary gland flow in patients with Sjögren's syndrome, *Oral Dis* 3:93-98, 1997.
17. Rhodus NL: Xerostomia: an increasingly significant dental management challenge, *NW Dent* 4:14-18, 1997.
18. Sreebny LM, Valdini A, Yu A: Xerostomia: part II—relationship to nonoral symptoms, drugs and disease, *Oral Surg* 68(4):419-427, 1989.
19. Streckfus CF et al: The expression of the c-erbB-2 receptor protein in glandular salivary secretions, *J Oral Pathol Med* 33:595-600, 2004.
20. Streckfus CF, Bigler L: The use of soluble, salivary c-erbB-2 for the detection and post-operative follow-up of breast cancer in women: the results of a five-year translational research study, *Adv Dent Res* 18:17-24, 2005.
21. ten Cate B: The role of saliva in mineral equilibrium-caries and calculus formation. In Edgar WM, O'Mullane DM, eds: *Saliva and oral health,* ed 2, London, 1996, British Dental Association.
22. Walker DM: Oral mucosal immunology: an overview, *Ann Acad Med Singapore* 33(Suppl):27S-30S, 2004.
23. Wolff A et al: Oral mucosal status and major salivary gland function, *Oral Surg* 70:49-54, 1990.
24. Wu AJ, Ship JA: *Characterization of major salivary gland flow rates in the presence of medication and systemic diseases* (abstract), American Academy of Oral Medicine Annual Meeting, 1993.
25. Whelton H: Introduction: the anatomy and physiology of the salivary glands. In Edgar WM, O'Mullane DM, eds: *Saliva and oral health,* ed 2, London, 1996, British Dental Association.
26. Wynn RL: Oral pilocarpine (Salagen): a recently approved salivary stimulant, *Gen Dent* 44(1):22-32, 1996.
27. Zoeller J: The top 200 drugs, *Am Druggist* February:41-48, 1999.

Neurologic and Sensory Impairment

Barbara J. Smith • Robert G. Henry

INSIGHT

Dental hygienists will be caring for an increasingly older patient population with age-associated neurologic disease. In addition, medical science has enabled the survivorship of individuals of all ages with various neurologic diseases and injuries. Understanding the special needs of patients with neurologic disorders will enable the dental hygienist to provide safe, effective care.

CASE STUDY 44-1 | Supportive Care Challenges in the Treatment of the Patient with Quadriplegia

Leo Crosswell is a 53-year-old white man with quadriplegia caused by a high-level *spinal cord injury* (SCI). In 1979, his cervical spine was fractured, with resulting spinal cord damage, as a result of a swimming pool diving accident in Central America. Because of political unrest and a military revolution in the country at the time, his transport to medical attention was delayed for approximately 1 week.

This injury to the cervical vertebrae C2 and C3 left Mr. Crosswell paralyzed below the neck, although basic breathing function remains. He is fitted with an internal urinary catheter with a leg bag and regulates bowel functions with dietary control and assistance. A caregiver helps him with transportation needs and personal hygiene needs, including feeding, dressing, shaving, toothbrushing, and flossing.

Mr. Crosswell is independently mobile with the assistance of a battery-powered wheelchair, which he controls with oral *sip-and-puff* tubes that control the wheelchair's steering and speed mechanisms (Figure 44-1). His torso and extremities rest in custom-fitted cushioned areas and are secured with Velcro straps. He travels to work in a specially modified side-lift van and has a full-time job with a government wildlife and fisheries agency. Mr. Crosswell operates his telephone and computer with the assistance of a custom-fitted *mouthstick,* which is designed to minimize occlusal trauma (Figure 44-2).

On awakening, or after prolonged reclining, Mr. Crosswell's weakened respiratory condition requires initial ventilation with an Ambu bag to reduce the likelihood of orthostatic hypotension. Occasionally, he experiences mild to moderately severe muscle spasms, generally in his extremities, which last from a few seconds to a few minutes. His vital signs fall within normal ranges.

Mr. Crosswell's dental history is unremarkable. He understands the special importance of his teeth, given his dependence on his mouthstick. Accordingly, he brushes twice a day and flosses once a day with caregiver assistance. He has used a variety of manual and electric toothbrushes. Mr. Crosswell uses a fluoridated toothpaste and over-the-counter mouthrinses, some with fluoride. He exhibits good gingival health but has mild recession, toothbrush abrasion and attrition resulting from aggressive toothbrushing, bruxism, and mouthstick use.

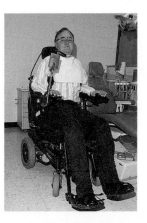

FIGURE 44-1
Oral *sip-and-puff* controlled self-powered wheelchair for patients with quadriplegia.

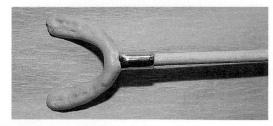

FIGURE 44-2
Custom-fabricated mouthstick for patients with quadriplegia.

Original chapter in previous editions contributed by Kim Curbow Wilcox, PT, MS, NCS and Robert A. DeVille, DMD.

✦ CASE STUDY 44-2 | Supportive Care Challenges in the Treatment of the Patient with Alzheimer's Disease

Denny Walker is an 89-year-old black man who has been diagnosed with Alzheimer's disease. He is married to Nana (nickname for Diana) Walker and has two children and three grandchildren. Before he retired at age 65, he was a high school industrial arts (shop) teacher. He and his wife lived together in their home until 4 years ago (at age 85) when Mr. Walker's memory loss became so severe that Mrs. Walker had to tell him what to do to drive their car, including which gear to put the car into and directions at every crossing. Her concerns resulted in a conversation with her children, who were also concerned. Arrangements were made for Mr. Walker to see a team of memory specialists at the university clinic.

At the university clinic, an **interdisciplinary team** of trained professionals (neurologist, social worker, nurse, and neuropsychiatrist) gave Mr. Walker a series of tests (including laboratory assays, electrocardiogram, and x-ray imaging) and told the family that Mr. Walker met the criteria for the clinical diagnosis of Alzheimer's disease. The team of specialists prepared the Walker family for what to expect in the years to come.

Mr. Walker has progressively declined in both cognitive (capacity to think, learn, and remember) and physical abilities. Two years ago, he became quite angry and violent when Mrs. Walker was trying to bathe

him after he soiled his pants. This episode was the last of many incidents that led Mrs. Walker and her children to find a nursing home, Pleasant Meadows Nursing Home, that could manage his round-the-clock needs. Although she is able to visit her husband regularly (two to three times a week), she feels guilty she was unable to care for him at home. Both of their children live several hours away and do not visit regularly, but they do call Mrs. Walker daily to offer their support.

Mr. Walker sought regular dental care until his diagnosis of Alzheimer's disease 4 years ago. When he was in his 50s, he had all of his upper teeth extracted secondary to periodontal disease and an upper denture constructed. He retained most of his lower teeth until he was 62 when he lost his posterior mandibular molars to periodontal disease and had a lower partial constructed. Since that time, he has retained his remaining 10 natural lower teeth and wears an upper denture and lower partial routinely. Since his diagnosis of Alzheimer's disease, Mrs. Walker has only sporadically taken Mr. Walker to the dentist. During the first visit, Mr. Walker became very agitated in the waiting room and kept repeating that he wanted to go home. At a later visit, he would not sit still for the dental hygienist to provide treatment. Lately, Mrs. Walker thinks that he might need to see a dentist or hygienist because his breath smells so bad.

KEY TERMS

activities of daily living	brain injury	hydrocephalus	musculoskeletal
agnosia	cerebral palsy	hypertonia	neuromuscular
Alzheimer's disease	cerebrovascular accident	hypotonia	paraplegia
amnesia	cognition	infarction	Parkinson's disease
amyotrophic lateral sclerosis	cranial nerve	interdisciplinary team	respiratory
aphasia	degenerative	ischemic	spasticity
apraxia	diplegia	Lou Gehrig's disease	spina bifida
ataxia	dysarthria	mobility	spinal cord injury
athetoid	dysphagia	multiple sclerosis	trauma
athetosis	dystonia	muscle tone	visual deficits
autism	hemiparesis	muscular dystrophies	
Bell's palsy	hemorrhagic		

LEARNING OUTCOMES

After reading this chapter the student will be able to:

1. Describe the prevalence, incidence, and distribution of selected neurologic disorders.
2. Identify the pathologic origin of each selected neurologic disorder.
3. List and describe the specific impairments that may characterize each selected neurologic disorder.
4. Describe the conventional dental treatment modalities for each selected condition, including surgical and nonsurgical approaches such as pharmacologic, behavioral, dietary, interventional, and using assistive devices and special accommodations.

5. Describe modifications the dental hygienist may need to make when providing care to patients with each of the selected neurologic disorders.
6. Describe preventive strategies, including chemotherapeutic agents and caregiver interactions, that may be needed for patients with each of the selected neurologic disorders.
7. Determine the most appropriate method of interacting with a patient who demonstrates a disability.
8. Identify the major legal implications for providing healthcare services to persons with neurologic impairment.

The human nervous system (see Figure 12-11) is made up of the brain, the spinal cord, and spinal and peripheral nerves and directs a vast array of abilities that include thought, movement, language, perception, breathing, emotions, memory, and vision. Because of the enormous role the nervous system plays in day-to-day living, when damage occurs as a result of injury or disease, function and life itself may be lost. The purpose of this chapter is to introduce the reader to a selected variety of neurologic disorders that may affect the provider's ability to deliver routine dental care effectively. Specific techniques that are useful in the care of patients with physical or mental impairments will be included. The chapter is organized by categories of disorders that have similar pathologic origin and occur most often in certain age groups, as laid out in Table 44-1.

> ### Note
> Although this chapter's approach should be helpful, the reader should be cautioned that diseases of the nervous system produce highly specific clinical conditions, and the level of impairment will be determined by the extent and specific location of the disease or disorder. For example, two patients may have the same clinical diagnosis, yet one may have no apparent disability, whereas the other is completely dependent.

Table 44-1	Selected Neurologic Conditions and Disorders
TIME FRAME	**CONDITIONS AND DISORDERS**
Developmental (Early)	• Autism • Cerebral palsy • Hydrocephalus • Spina bifida
Trauma (Early, Middle)	• Brain injury • Spinal cord injury
Cranial Nerve (Middle)	• Bell's palsy
Neuromuscular (Early, Middle)	• Muscular dystrophy
Cerebrovascular (Middle, Late)	• Cerebrovascular accident (stroke)
Degenerative (Middle, Late)	• Alzheimer's disease • Amyotrophic lateral sclerosis • Multiple sclerosis • Parkinson's disease

Early, birth to age 18 years; *middle,* age 19 to 49 years; *late,* age 50+ years.

Although not all conditions are covered here, the cases presented for illustration were chosen to provide the reader with a basic resource database that, with modification and adaptation when appropriate, will allow the reader to understand further a wider range of impairments and deficits.

Selected Neurologic Conditions by Pathologic Origin

DEVELOPMENTAL

Autism

Autism is the third most common developmental disorder in the United States, affecting 3 to 6 per 1000 children. Males are four times more likely to be autistic than females.[19] No common racial, ethnic, or educational characteristics have been found.[3] The disorder is lifelong and characterized by three major symptoms:

- Communication problems
- Repetitive motions
- Problems with social interactions

The behaviors associated with these symptoms can range from mild to disabling. Parents typically detect the disorder before age 3, as the child fails to develop language skills and to interact with others. Children diagnosed with autism typically do not have any significant medical problems and may demonstrate normal to superior intelligence.[10] The cause of autism is unclear, although genetic and environmental factors have been identified. The occurrence of autism is not related to poor parenting practices. No cure currently exists, although early intervention targeted at the core symptoms of the disorder may substantially improve outcomes. Intense behavioral therapy and medications (antidepressants, anticonvulsants, antipsychotics, stimulants, or any combination) may lessen symptoms. Some children with autism grow up to lead near-normal lives, although 80% function at moderately mentally retarded levels.[3]

Of importance to the practitioner are the alterations in communication skills. The autistic individual may not even respond to his or her own name or make eye contact when addressed. In addition, their response to pain may be reduced, but a heightened sensitivity to sound, touch, or other stimulation may be present. Interacting with the caregivers of the autistic individual is essential in mapping out the strategy of interaction. Caregivers can provide critical information that will assist the dental hygienist in identifying useful interaction strategies and avoiding *triggers* toward which the patient reacts negatively.

> ### Autism
> *Description:* developmental disorder described as an emotional disturbance demonstrated by a lack of social interaction with deficits in language, communication, and social skills[8]
> *Clinical presentation:* demonstrated inability to interact with others
> - May exhibit resistive and self-stimulation behaviors such as head banging, rocking, or repeated body movements
> - May also complain of sensitivity to light, sounds, smells, touch, or taste[3]

Cerebral Palsy

Cerebral palsy (CP) affects more than 500,000 Americans.[35] The definition and classification of CP was recently the topic of an international workgroup that proposed the following:

Cerebral palsy describes a group of disorders of the development of movement and posture, causing activity limitation, that are attributed to non-progressive disturbances that occurred in the developing fetal or infant brain. The motor disorders of cerebral palsy are often accompanied by disturbances of sensation, cognition, communication, perception, and/or behaviour, and/or by a seizure disorder.[35]

The signs of CP are usually apparent by 3 years of age, with parents detecting abnormal development of motor skills. CP results from prenatal development abnormalities or perinatal or postnatal damage to the central nervous system before 5 years of age.[10,26] Possible causes of CP include in utero disorders, birth trauma, or neonatal asphyxia.[24] More than 5000 infants and an additional 1200 to 1500 school-age children are diagnosed with CP each year.

The primary characteristic that defines CP is a disorder of movement exhibited in stiffness or rigidity of muscles (**hypertonia**) or low muscle tone (**hypotonia**). Movement disorders may also include **spasticity** (abnormal increase in muscle tone), **ataxia** (inability to coordinate voluntary movement), **dystonia** (sustained muscle contractions resulting in repetitive involuntary twisting motion), or **athetosis** (involuntary, relatively slow writhing movement). Other medical disorders that may accompany CP are mental impairment, seizures, growth problems, impaired vision or hearing, and abnormal sensation and perception.

Several aspects of CP are of importance to the practitioner:

1. Uncontrolled movement can disrupt the provision of care and potentially threaten the safety of the practitioner, as well as the patient.
2. Altered cognitive status and potential sensory deficits may limit the dental hygienist's ability to communicate effectively with the patient.
3. Poor control of the muscles of the throat, mouth, and tongue contribute to drooling, as well as difficulties in eating and swallowing.

Hydrocephalus

Hydrocephalus is a condition that occurs when the amount of cerebrospinal fluid (CSF) produced by the body is greater than that absorbed.[8,10,12] Congenital occurrence accounts for approximately one half of cases. Nearly 80% of patients with congenital hydrocephalus have other defects. In the United States, slightly more than 1 in every 500 children is affected by hydrocephalus.[19] The acquired form of the disorder occurs when the brain is damaged as the result of infection, head trauma, brain tumors, or cysts.[10] Whether congenital or acquired, the accumulation of CSF produces a dilation of the ventricles of the brain, which results in an increase in intracranial pressure and may lead to an enlargement of the cranium if not addressed. A valve or shunt may be placed to control the excessive fluid by diverting it to another part of the body.[10,12] Shunts are subject to blockage and bacterial infection and require surgical revisions over time. With proper treatment, patients with congenital hydrocephalus live productive lives with a normal life span and normal activities. The most common complication of congenital hydrocephalus is learning disability; however, difficulties with visual and motor skills may also be evident. Acquired hydrocephalus may carry additional disabilities, depending on the type and severity of brain damage that accompanies the condition.[26,35]

Spina Bifida

Spina bifida is a neural tube defect occurring in embryologic development and affects approximately 70,000 individuals in the United States.[34] The defect typically involves three to six vertebral segments and may be associated with spinal deformities such as scoliosis.[26] The severity of spina bifida ranges from a completely open spine (rachischisis or spina bifida aperta), which usually results in severe neurologic disturbances and death to spina bifida occulta in which an abnormality exists but results in mild neurologic involvement.[8,26] The defect may include only the sac containing the meninges (meningocele), only the spinal cord (myelocele), or both the meninges and the spinal cord (myelomeningocele).[8,10,15,31] The cause of spina bifida is questionable, with many experts attributing the disorder to environmental factors and maternal vitamin deficiency, specifically folic acid. Spina bifida may occur in conjunction with other congenital defects, such as hydrocephalus.[10]

Approximately 1 of every 1000 newborns is diagnosed with spina bifida.[34] The effects of spina bifida include **neuromuscular** involvement such as paralysis or paresis below the level of the lesion, changes in muscle tone, and sensory deficits. Musculoskeletal complications include scoliosis and other bony deformities as a result of muscle imbalances and changes in muscle tone. The spinal and bony deformities often limit the patient's ability to sit correctly or ambulate and, if severe, may result in respiratory insufficiency. In addition, the sphincters of the bladder and rectum are usually affected, resulting in incontinence or requiring the use of internal or external catheters. The patient's risk of pressure areas and skin breakdown is increased when the musculoskeletal deformities are combined

---

Cerebral Palsy

Description: nonprogressive motor disturbances caused by in utero disorders, birth trauma, or neonatal asphyxia
Clinical presentation: varying degrees of voluntary muscles affected; may demonstrate varying degrees of cognitive involvement
Three main types: Spastic, athetoid, and ataxic

- *Spastic:* most common (70%), with stiffness or rigidity to muscle[10,26]
- *Athetoid:* affects 20%; with low muscle tone, involuntary muscle contraction, and contorted (**athetoid**) movement[26]
- *Ataxic:* affects 10%; wide-based, unsteady gait, with balance, coordination, and speech deficits[10]

Hydrocephalus

Description: when the amount of cerebrospinal fluid produced is greater than that absorbed[8,10]
Clinical presentation: most common complication is a learning disability, although possible difficulty with visual and motor skills
Prognosis: with treatment, people live normal life span and activities

with sensory deficits and bowel and bladder incontinence. Secondary complications of spina bifida include hip dislocation or subluxation and osteoporosis. Each of these deficits contributes to the patient's difficulty in performing mobility activities and **activities of daily living** (ADLs). Because the lesion is typically in the lower one third to one half of the spinal column, the upper extremities are usually not affected. The patient also typically does not exhibit communication, cognitive, or perceptual deficits if spina bifida is the only diagnosis.[10,26,31]

TRAUMA

Brain Injury

Brain injury (BI) is defined as damage to the brain caused by a primary insult such as **trauma** or a secondary insult such as metabolic and physiologic events that occur after the primary damage.[26,28] More than 1.5 million BIs occur in the United States every year, resulting in more than 75,000 deaths per year. BIs can occur at any age. Infants can sustain injuries from being shaken (shaken baby syndrome), and older adults typically sustain brain injuries from falls. However, two thirds of traumatic brain injuries occur in persons younger than the age of 34, with vehicular accidents involving young men ages 16 to 24 accounting for nearly one half.[6,24]

Resultant disabilities from BI depend on the severity of the injury, the location of the injury, and the age and general health of the individual. Some common disabilities include problems with cognition (thinking, memory, and reasoning), sensory processing (sight, hearing, touch, taste, and smell), communication (expression and understanding), and behavior or mental health (depression, anxiety, personality changes, aggression, acting out, and social inappropriateness).[19] The patient may experience unilateral or bilateral paresis or paralysis in addition to changes in muscle tone, sensation, bowel and bladder control, edema, and coordination. The patient may develop contractures, which further hinder mobility activities. Depending on the location of the brain damage, the patient may experience respiratory difficulty. The *Rancho Los Amigos levels of cognitive functioning,* a 7-point scale that describes the cognitive and behavioral recovery sequence, is often used to provide a general description of the patient's abilities.[5-6,24,26,28]

Spinal Cord Injury

Spinal cord injury (SCI) results in a partial or complete loss of neurologic function below the point of the injury. More than 7800 spinal injuries occur in the United States each year, with 250,000 to 400,000 people living with the effects of the injury. Of SCI cases, 80% occur in people younger than 40 years of age, with the highest occurrence between the ages of 16 and 30. Single men are more likely to sustain a SCI than women. More than 44% of all SCIs are caused by motor vehicle accidents, with 24% resulting from violence, 22% from falls, and 8% from sports activities.[22]

If an SCI is complete, the patient will experience no sensation or voluntary movement, and both sides of the body will usually be equally affected. A complete injury can result in the paralysis of all four limbs (quadriplegia) or the lower half of the body (paraplegia). Patients with quadriplegia or quadriparesis may also demonstrate impairment of the respiratory muscles. Depending on the location of the spinal injury, the patient may demonstrate motor and sensory impairments, altered temperature control, impaired respiration, bowel and bladder dysfunction, and changes in muscle tone.[26,30,33]

CRANIAL NERVE

Bell's Palsy

Bell's palsy is a form of temporary facial paralysis caused by damage or trauma to one of the two facial nerves. It typically produces unilateral facial weakness or paralysis. Bilateral involvement may occur but is not common. **Cranial nerve** VII, the facial nerve, innervates the muscles of facial expression (Figure 44-3). The patient typically experiences sensory changes followed by motor deficits. The cause of Bell's palsy is inflammation of the cranial nerve caused by a variety of reasons, including infection of the middle ear, immune disease, and herpes zoster or herpes simplex type 1 of the geniculate ganglion.[4]

Bell's palsy affects 4 of 10,000 people, with no age or race characteristics noted. Between 15 and 40 new cases are diagnosed each year nationwide. The incidence of Bell's palsy increases during pregnancy and with increasing age. Of persons who are diagnosed with the palsy, 50% show spontaneous recovery without medical inter-

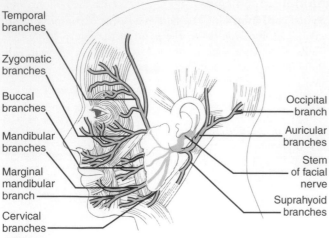

FIGURE 44-3
Facial nerve (cranial nerve VII). Motor branches to muscles of facial expression. (From Liebgott B: *The anatomical basis of dentistry*, ed 2, St Louis, 2001, Mosby.)

vention, 20% recover within 1 to 3 months, and 10% recover within 4 to 6 months.[4,8,26]

Patients with Bell's palsy initially complain of pain posterior to one ear. This episode is later followed by a unilateral facial paralysis, a reduction in the sense of taste, and possibly the inability to blink or close the unilateral eye. The facial paralysis affects the patient's oral motor control, resulting in dysarthria, unilateral drooping of the mouth, difficulty controlling secretions, and an increase in salivation. The patient may also complain of tearing or dryness of the eye along with asymmetrical facial expressions.[26]

NEUROMUSCULAR

Muscular Dystrophy

The **muscular dystrophies** (MDs) are a group of genetic diseases that result in a progressive weakness and degeneration of the skeletal muscles that control movement.[10,18]

The muscular dystrophies have different patterns of inheritance, rates of progression, and distribution of weaknesses, as well as age of onset. Three common types of MD follow:

1. Duchenne, which is most common in boys with an onset between ages 3 and 5 years
2. Facioscapulohumeral, which appears in adolescence
3. Myotonic, which varies in age of onset

The prognosis of MD varies according to the type of MD and the progression of the disorder. Some cases may be mild and progress very slowly over a normal life span, whereas other cases may have more marked progression of muscle weakness, functional disability, and loss of the ability to walk. Skeletal muscle weakness and gait disturbances may make the tasks of getting to the dental office and getting into the dental chair difficult for the patient with MD. The dental hygienist will want to observe whether reduced head control and oral motor control exists. **Dysarthria,** the speech condition resulting from weakened mouth, facial, and respiratory muscles, may make communication difficult for the patient. **Dysphagia,** resulting when weakened muscles in the cheek, tongue, and throat interfere with the swallowing process, places the patient at risk for aspiration. Additional secondary complications include contractures and spinal deformities that may result in skin breakdown. During the later stages of MD, the patient may demonstrate difficulty with opening the mouth. The cranial nerves are not involved in MD.[10,18,26]

The various types of the disease affect more than 50,000 Americans. Although no cure has been found, medications and therapy can slow the course of the disease.[18]

CEREBROVASCULAR

Cerebrovascular Accident

Cerebrovascular accident (CVA) is commonly called *stroke.* CVA is defined as an interruption of the cerebral circulation, resulting in neurologic disability.[26] Strokes, categorized according to the nature of the circulatory disturbance, consist of four general types: arteriovenous malformation (AVM), **ischemic, hemorrhagic,** and **infarction.**[8,15,26] Risk factors for stroke include chronic hypertension, atherosclerosis, tobacco use, heart disease, diabetes, elevated cholesterol and lipid levels, obesity, inactivity, family history of stroke, endocarditis, sleep apnea, sickle cell anemia, and cocaine use. Metabolic syndrome, also known as *syndrome X,* is defined as the presence of three or more of the following five health conditions: obesity, low levels of high-density lipoprotein cholesterol, high triglyceride levels, a blood pressure of 130/85 mm Hg or higher, and diabetes or prediabetes. The risk of CVA doubles with syndrome X. Many of the risk factors may be controlled through medical intervention and pharmacologic measures. Certain risk factors can be modified by lifestyle change.[7]

Stroke is the third leading cause of death and one of the leading causes of disability in the United States. Approximately 730,000 new or recurrent strokes occur each year, which result in 163,000 deaths. Currently more than 4 million people in the United States have survived a stroke and deal with varying degrees of impairment. The risk of stroke increases with age, with more than two thirds of all strokes occurring in persons older than 65 years of age. Additionally, stroke occurs more often in blacks and women than other groups.[23]

A patient who has experienced a stroke may exhibit an especially wide variety of neuromuscular, musculoskeletal, bowel and bladder, integumentary, cognitive, perceptual, visual, behavioral, and communication deficits. The hemisphere of the brain that is affected and the extent of brain damage are key factors in the outcome for the patient. The general neuromuscular deficits may include debilitating impairments of motor control such as *hemiplegia* (complete paralysis on one side of the body) or *hemiparesis* (one-sided weakness), dysarthria, and dysphagia. An increase or decrease in **muscle tone** of the affected side, contractures, edema, decreased tactile and proprioceptive sensations, bowel and bladder dysfunction, and reduced coordination may also be demonstrated. These impairments combine to produce deficits in **mobility,** including the ability to perform bed mobility, transfers, wheelchair propulsion, balance in sitting and standing, and ambulation. Typical cognitive deficits include confusion; lack of orientation to person, place, or time; decreased attention span; inability to process information; and decrease in memory abilities. Patients who have experienced a stroke may also demonstrate perceptual deficits, including unilateral neglect or inattention, distorted body image, or visuospatial distortions. Visual disturbances may include field cuts or problems with depth perception. Many patients who have had a stroke demonstrate changes in behavior including emotional lability and depression. Communication deficits are common when the dominant cerebral hemisphere is involved. These deficits may include expressive or receptive communication and word-finding problems.[24,26,29] Recurrent stroke is frequent; approximately 25% of people who recover from their first stroke will have another stroke within 5 years.[19]

> ## *Distinct Care Modifications*
> - CVA patients are often receiving anticoagulation therapy.
>   - Check medications taken.
>   - Ascertain International Normalized Ratio (INR) (typical therapeutic values are between 2.0 and 3.0, but higher therapeutic ranges may be targeted).
> - Transfers from wheelchair, walker, or other devices to the dental chair are potentially risky for a patient with hemiplegia or hemiparesis.
>   - Position yourself on the patient's affected side when accompanying the patient.
>   - Maintain a protective posture. Stay in close proximity to the patient when the patient is being seated and rising from the chair, even if transfer procedures are not being used.
> - Patients after a CVA are often treated for hypertension.
>   - Check medications that the patient has taken.
>   - Use a 2-minute (or longer) dismissal time to prevent orthostatic hypotension.
> - Patients after a CVA may have visual field cuts. If present, then alert the patient when you are bringing instruments, especially hand pieces, from the affected side.

DEGENERATIVE

Alzheimer's Disease

Alzheimer's disease (AD) is a progressive dementia resulting from the destruction of nerve cells that store information in the brain.[26] More than 4 million Americans have been diagnosed with AD. Estimates suggest that, with a growing number of elderly Americans, up to 10% of those older than 65 years of age and 50% of those older than 85 years of age will be diagnosed with this progressive disease.[1]

Memory loss is the most common initial symptom of AD. As the brain deterioration increases, symptoms progress to multiple medical and motor problems, including deficits in planning motor activities, balance and coordination deficits, difficulty in performing mobility activities and ADLs, and a progressive inability to use assistive devices such as canes and hearing aids.[26] The patient also begins to show cognitive deterioration, including reductions in safety awareness, lack of orientation to place and time, inability to learn or reason, and progressive memory deficits. Secondary problems associated with AD include alterations in sleep patterns, reduction in bowel and bladder control, depression, and oral motor dysfunction that leads to oral neglect.[26]

The hallmark signs of dementia of the Alzheimer's type (DAT) are four traits: **amnesia** (loss of memory), **aphasia** (difficulty with communication), **apraxia** (problems with daily living skills), and **agnosia** (the inability to recognize faces or things). The clinical diagnosis of AD is established using the following six criteria:

1. Clinical examination and documentation by neuropsychologic testing
2. Deficits in two or more areas of cognition
3. Progressive worsening of memory and other cognitive function
4. No disturbance of consciousness
5. Onset between ages 40 and 90 years
6. Absence of systemic disorders or other brain diseases that would explain the cognitive changes[11]

The clinical course of the disease is typically described in three stages: (1) early or mild, (2) middle or moderate, and (3) late or severe. The early stage of the disease is characterized by a steady deterioration of short-term memory, with difficulty in remembering names, losing items, and repeating questions or answers during conversations. Losses in orientation to day, time, and location may also occur. Errors in judgment, getting lost in familiar surroundings, and missing appointments are characteristic of this stage. A blunting of the personality may be observed with diminished emotion and energy. Self-care may diminish. The middle stage of the disease is characterized by a more rapid decline in intellectual capacity. Patients may develop perception problems, experiencing an inability to recognize themselves in a mirror or images on television. A loss of self-care abilities such as bathing, dressing, and eating independently occurs. Oral neglect, first observed in the mild stage of the disease, may become much more

> ## *Alzheimer's Disease*
> *Description:* progressive deterioration of cerebral cortex and other areas of the brain
> *Clinical presentation:* memory loss is the most common initial symptom; symptoms progress as brain deterioration increases, including the following:
> - Difficulty performing ADL
> - Cognitive deterioration
> - Lack of orientation to place and time
>
>   Secondary problems including sleep problems, depression, and oral motor dysfunction.

pronounced and oral self-care habits lost entirely. Restless pacing, agitation, and tearfulness may characterize behavior. Wandering puts the patient at risk of becoming lost if left unsupervised. Family and friends of the patient with AD may no longer be recognized. Personality changes may include being physically or verbally abusive over trivial occurrences. In the late stage of the disease, a person can no longer survive without assistance. Communication ceases to be possible because even simple language is not understood. Patients can no longer answer questions or respond appropriately. Behavioral characteristics include increased anxiety, aggression, and the tendency to touch and examine things with the mouth, as well as a tendency for forced grasping and gripping of objects. Significant body wasting may occur, as well as the development of hallucinations, delusional episodes, or both. Eventually, the patient with AD is totally dependent on others for the basic ADLs, such as dressing, bathing, eating, and using the bathroom.[1,11]

Although the progression is not predictable and varies considerably, the advanced stage of AD may be reached in as little as 2 to 3 years after the initial diagnosis. Although the exact cause of AD is not known, the degeneration of the brain cells may be caused by an abnormality of chromosome 21, or a genetic predisposition to the development of the disease may be present. The risk of AD increases with increasing age and family history.[1,11]

Amyotrophic Lateral Sclerosis

Amyotrophic lateral sclerosis (ALS), also called **Lou Gehrig's disease,** is characterized by degeneration of the cells in the motor neurons of the spinal cord and cerebral cortex. The cell degeneration leads to progressive muscle atrophy and eventually to death within 3 to 5 years in approximately 50% of patients, usually from respiratory failure. The cause of ALS is unknown; however, research is currently directed toward the investigation of gene abnormalities.[2,14,26]

More than 5000 people are diagnosed with ALS yearly, with no trends in racial or ethnic characteristics noted. ALS affects men more often than women and is generally diagnosed after 55 years of age.[2,26]

ALS affects both upper motor neurons and lower motor neurons. Initial symptoms of ALS include muscle cramping, weakness, and atrophy that begin in the small muscles of the hand and forearm. The patient eventually demonstrates dysphagia, dysarthria, muscle atrophy, and paralysis along with changes in muscle tone as a result of the progressive deterioration of the motor neurons. The patient retains all sensory modalities and cognitive capabilities, as well as volitional eye movement and control of the urinary sphincter even during the final stages of ALS.[14,26]

Multiple Sclerosis

Multiple sclerosis (MS) is an autoimmune disorder that results when myelin, the insulating material around nerve cells in the central nervous system, degenerates (demyelinates) in the brain and spinal cord.[10] Damage to myelin results in impaired nerve signaling and may impair normal sensation, movement, and even thinking (cognition) in the late stages (see Chapter 46 for further discussion).

The onset of MS typically occurs between the ages of 20 and 40 years, with an increased incidence in women and whites.[20,26] Although the reason is unknown, the incidence of MS increases as the distance from the equator increases. The cause of MS is largely unknown; however, many theories have been offered, including the presence of a slowly progressing virus, an abnormal immunologic event, a chronic lack of essential fatty acids, and environmental factors. The course of MS is usually exhibited as periods of exacerbation and remission of varying lengths of time.[9-10,13-14,26]

Patients with MS demonstrate varying symptoms, depending on the location and severity of the demyelination. Symptoms typically include fatigue; visual disturbances; bladder and bowel dysfunction; weakness of facial, oral, and body musculature; changes in muscle tone; and deficits in the performance of mobility activities and ADLs. Additionally, the patient may demonstrate numbness or tingling in the hands and feet, which may interfere with oral hygiene self-care. Slurred speech may also interfere with communication between the dental hygienist and the patient. Patients may have reduced respiratory capacity, pressure sores resulting from inactivity and poor positioning, and diminished cognitive functioning in the later stages of the disease.[13,26]

Parkinson's Disease

Parkinson's disease (PD) is a chronic neurologic condition that results in a gradual deterioration of motor control. PD is a slowly progressing disease affecting the substantia nigra in the basal ganglia. PD affects more than 1.5 million Americans. Although the diagnosis is usually made after the age of 50, earlier onset is not uncommon.[21,26]

PD may be seen clinically as changes in movement and functional capabilities caused by a reduction in the production of dopamine. The specific cause of the reduction in dopamine is unknown. Although PD has not been shown to be genetically transmitted, some families exhibit an increased incidence of the disease. No known preventive measures or cures have been found for PD.[21,26]

Parkinson's Disease

Description: progressive **degenerative** disease affecting the substantia nigra in the basal ganglia resulting in the reduction of dopamine

Clinical presentation: wide range of symptoms, including neuromuscular, musculoskeletal, and communication deficits

Three common symptoms:
- *Pill-rolling* tremor of hands (generally happens first)
- Inability to show facial expression
- Festinating gait; *freezing* movement

Patients diagnosed with PD may exhibit a wide range of symptoms, including neuromuscular, musculoskeletal, and communication deficits. The patient may experience bradykinesia, rigidity, or a unilateral resting tremor of the upper or lower extremities, all of which severely impair function. As the disease progresses, the patient may exhibit difficulty maintaining balance during gait and functional activities. The patient with PD may also exhibit an increase in flexion of the neck, trunk, and lower extremities. The facial muscles may be affected, resulting in an inability to show facial expressions. The patient may demonstrate dysphagia, dysarthria, or a reduced speaking volume. A festinating gait, *freezing* in place of movements, and postural ability changes may also be apparent and increase the risk of falls.[16,21,26]

44-2 44-3

Deficits, Dependency, and Effect on Dental Care

Table 44-2 lists many conditions and deficits and their associated effects on the body.

NEUROMUSCULAR DEFICITS

Definition

Motor control is defined as the interaction of neuromuscular, musculoskeletal, cognitive, perceptual, and sensory components to produce functional movement.[24] Deficits in motor control of the trunk, extremities, orofacial musculature, or any combination are common in patients with the diagnoses of stroke, BI, CP, PD, SCI, spina bifida, MS, ALS, hydrocephalus, late-stage AD, Bell's palsy, and MD. These patients may demonstrate difficulty in planning, controlling, and sequencing muscle movements required for efficient functioning.

Deficits in motor control may be exhibited as **hemiparesis, paraplegia, diplegia,** dysarthria, or dysphagia. The patient may also exhibit ataxia of the trunk or extremities or a resting or intention tremor.

Level of Severity

The level of motor control impairment is determined through a wide range of examination tools. The measures include examination of the patient's range of motion, muscle tone, and muscle strength because impairment in these areas will affect motor control. Motor control examination generally includes observation of movement and performance of functional activities.

Treatment Modalities

Patients with motor control deficits generally participate in physical therapy, occupational therapy, speech and language therapy, and therapeutic recreation to improve function. The focus of the therapeutic intervention is the improvement of planning, controlling, and sequencing muscle movement.

DENTAL CONSIDERATIONS

Loss of muscle sequencing and control generally does not significantly restrict the delivery of most dental services. It does, however, often require certain accommodations on the part of the provider. Neuromuscular deficits may interfere with the patient's ambulatory abilities, thus making the tasks of accessing a dental office and sitting down in a dental chair more difficult. The Americans with Disabilities Act of 1990 mandated the removal of many of the physical barriers to access. For example, the addition of handicap parking spaces, handicap access ramps, wider doorways, and handicap accessible restrooms has made most offices reasonably accessible.

Ambulatory problems resulting from neuromuscular deficits may range from dependency on an assistive device such as a cane, crutches, walker, or wheelchair to simply requiring more time to accomplish a specific motor task. In many cases, the provider simply needs to ensure that the office complies with Americans with Disabilities Act of 1990 requirements and to allow sufficient time to get the patient into the office and chair, as well as out of the chair and office after treatment has been completed. The actual treatment time may need little adjustment.

Many wheelchair manufacturers offer both manual and powered wheelchairs that can be tilted and reclined to a variety of positions. Equally crucial to the ability to treat patients in their own chairs is the ability of dental equipment to reach patients. Some equipment delivery systems work exceedingly well, whereas others do not (Figures 44-5 and 44-6). Some manufacturers offer optional air-water-suction-light extensions that are useful when treating patients in wheelchairs.

Although most muscle-control deficits require minimal changes for the dental care provider, some patients with cogni-

Table 44-2 Neurologic Conditions and Deficits

CONDITION OR DEFICIT	NEUROMUSCULAR MOTOR CONTROL	MUSCULOSKELETAL	RESPIRATORY	BOWEL AND BLADDER	INTEGUMENTARY	COGNITION AND PERCEPTION	VISUAL	COMMUNICATION	MOBILITY
Developmental									
Spina bifida	X	X	X	X	X				X
Cerebral palsy	X	X		X	X	X		X	X
Hydrocephalus	X					X			X
Autism						X		X	
Trauma									
Brain injury	X	X	X	X	X	X		X	X
Spinal cord injury	X	X	X	X	X				X
Cranial Nerve VII									
Bell's palsy	X							X	
Neuromuscular									
Muscular dystrophy	X	X	X		X			X	X
Cerebrovascular									
Stroke (cerebrovascular accident)	X	X		X		X	X	X	X
Degenerative									
Multiple sclerosis	X	X	X	X	X*	X*		X	X
Amyotrophic lateral sclerosis	X	X	X		X			X	X
Parkinson's disease	X	X	X	X*	X*			X*	X
Alzheimer's disease	X*	X*	X*	X*	X*	X†		X	X

*Occurs late in the course of the disease.
†Occurs moderate to late in the course of the disease,

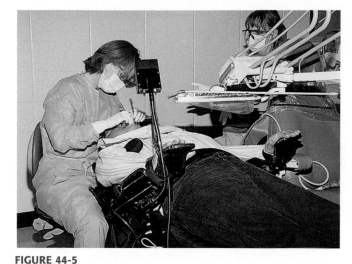

FIGURE 44-5
Patient being treated in his own wheelchair. Note self-contained head-rest.

CASE APPLICATION 44-1.1

Mr. Crosswell: Transportation and Transferring

Mr. Crosswell was transported to the dental office with the assistance of his part-time driver and caregiver, who drives a specially equipped van. He moves his battery-powered wheelchair into the dental operatory using a series of *sip-and-puff* switches that control the speed and direction of the chair, as well as recline it (see Figure 44-1). Once in the treatment room, Mr. Crosswell may be transferred to the dental chair using a standard one- or two-person patient-transfer technique (Figure 44-4). If a transfer is made, care must then be exercised to ensure that any urinary catheter or leg bag remains uncompromised and that gravitational forces are not *working against* normal urinary drainage forces while the patient is positioned in a supine position during lengthy appointments.

However, for patients such as Mr. Crosswell, a transfer is usually not necessary because the patient may be treated in his or her own chair, which is equipped with a headrest and reclines much like a dental chair.

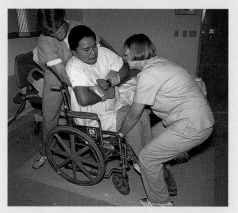

FIGURE 44-4
Two-person transfer technique for immobilized patients. (From Potter P, Perry A: *Fundamentals of nursing,* ed 6, St Louis, 2005, Mosby.)

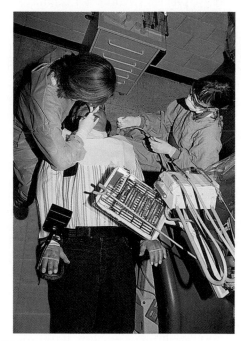

FIGURE 44-6
Over-the-patient delivery system by A-dec (Courtesy A-dec, Inc., Newberg, Ore.)

tive changes (e.g., autism, AD, PD) have problems with motor control. In these cases, protection from inadvertent movements may be needed for the patient and care provider. For minimal movements, caregivers may need to assist by holding one or both hands of the patient and helping with communication during the examination or treatment. If movements cannot be controlled with the caregiver's assistance, then additional measures may be necessary. These measures (restraints and sedation) will need to be determined by the dentist and approved by the caregiver who has power of attorney. If cloth restraints are used to secure arms and legs, then documentation of how, where, how long, and why these restraints were applied and to what areas are required.

For more serious motor-control issues, sedation (either oral or intravenous) may be necessary to prevent the patient from

inadvertent movement during treatment. In these cases, evaluation by a trained dentist or specialist or referral to a practice that can manage these patients in an appropriate setting (either in their office or in a hospital) may be necessary.

Meriting special consideration is the patient with dysphagia. In these cases, special care must be taken to maintain a patent airway. Fortunately, modern high-volume evacuation (HVE) is almost universally available and is invaluable in the rapid removal of saliva, other fluids, and debris from the oral cavity. Use of the rubber dam when possible may prevent accidental aspiration of foreign objects or dropped items. Unfortunately, some patients report increased problems with swallowing while the rubber dam is in place.

When dysphagia is exacerbated by conditions such as rhinitis or upper respiratory tract infections, a simple rescheduling of the appointment may be sufficient. If not, then the patient may better tolerate the appointment in an erect or semierect position.

Another patient meriting special attention is the patient with hemiparesis in which the ability to close one eyelid on the deficit side is impaired. This impairment is common in the patient with Bell's palsy. When this condition occurs, the patient's eye must be protected both from drying and from aerosols and debris. This task can be accomplished by placing damp gauze over the open eye, using care to not touch the eyeball itself. The patient may also have his or her own eye drops or ointment to keep the eye moistened.

When movement of other structures such as the tongue, lips, or jaw is a problem, various devices are available to keep the dental arches open and steady. Bite blocks, or mouth props, or tongue and cheek protectors may be helpful (Figure 44-7). Patients who have problems with motor control also may not be able to hold an intraoral radiograph steady while an operator exposes the film. Even bite-wing or periapical radiographs may be difficult without assistance. For these patients (those with PD, AD, or autism), an additional lead apron for the dental operator to wear along with a set of lead gloves will enable the operator to hold the patient's head still and the x-ray in place while an exposure is made. When using this technique, XCP radiograph holders (Rinn Corporation, Elgin, Ill.) work well to align the x-ray beam in the correct position.

Muscle Tone

Abnormal changes in muscle tone contribute to deficits in motor control. Muscle tone may be increased (hypertonia) or decreased (hypotonia) beyond what is considered normal. An increase in muscle tone with a corresponding increase in reflexes and a velocity-dependent resistance to passive stretch is often referred to clinically as *spasticity*. The type and degree of abnormal muscle tone varies widely among patients with neurologic deficits; however, functional activities are consistently affected by any abnormal changes in tone. Patients with decreased muscle tone are generally not a problem. If spasticity or hyper-

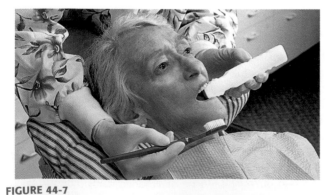

FIGURE 44-7
Open Wide disposable mouth prop on adult. (Reprinted with permission of Specialized Care Company, Hampton, NH.)

✦ CASE APPLICATION 44-2.1

Mr. Walker: Transportation and Transferring

Mr. Walker was transported to the dental office in a wheelchair van from Pleasant Meadows Nursing Home, accompanied by a nurse's aide (NA). He arrived in the dental office stating very loudly, "Where am I?" and calling for his wife, "Where's Nana?" The receptionist, not wanting to call attention to Mr. Walker, quickly took him and the NA to a dental operatory and advised the dental hygienist and dentist of his arrival.

When the hygienist tried to question Mr. Walker about his medical history, the NA interrupted and indicated that all the information she needed was in the paperwork she had brought. The hygienist found the following in the record: DAT diagnosed at age 85, history of stomach ulcers, incontinence of bowel and bladder, aspiration risk and dysphagia, and agitation. Medications that Mr. Walker was taking included galantamine hydrobromide, 8-mg tablets, twice daily for memory; ranitidine hydrochloride, 150 mg, 1 tablet twice daily for stomach ulcers; oxybutynin chloride, 5-mg tablet, 2.5 mg at bedtime for bladder control; and triazolam (Halcion), 5 mg, as needed for agitation. Before proceeding with the dental examination, the dentist asks you to hold one of Mr. Walker's hands and the nurse to hold the other hand so that the dentist can look in the patient's mouth. Should you comply, or should you ask the dentist whether he has consent to do this from the patient's wife?

When you tell the dentist that the patient has a wife, the dentist stops and goes to call her. The dental team must establish who is responsible for Mr. Walker if he is unable to cooperate on his own. Additionally, the information supplied in the paperwork from the NA should have been gathered before the appointment. Knowing in advance that Mr. Walker has a wife should have reduced time and confusion regarding treatment.

Regarding the patient's dysphagia, research has found that the level of severity of dementia correlates with the degree of difficulty of swallowing and increasing risk of aspiration (inhaling food into the lungs). In Mr. Walker's case, he has a moderate risk for aspiration, given that he is moderately demented. In cases in which aspiration poses a risk, the Cavitron (and water spray) should not be used, nor should a three-way syringe be used to wash and clean his mouth out. Other water spray, such as from a hand piece, should be limited or confined to use with a rubber dam if possible. Care should be taken to prevent the patient from swallowing or aspirating any liquid in the mouth, including blood, water, and mouthrinse.

The dentist returns from calling with permission from the patient's wife to perform an examination and x-rays today. When you ask Mr. Walker whether he would let you look in his mouth, he says "OK," but when you put the mirror close to his mouth, he turns his head away and closes his mouth. You decide you may have more luck taking an x-ray, so you wheel him into the radiograph area. He needs some help initially to stand up, but he is able to stand and hold onto the Panorex machine with some reminding. When the Panorex moves approximately halfway around his head, Mr. Walker becomes disoriented and moves his head. Clearly, you will be unable to get a Panorex today without something to help the patient relax. You make another appointment for Mr. Walker to come back for a better examination. You call the patient's wife and let her know that you were unable to get an examination but that the dentist has written a prescription (for a short-term sleeping

CASE APPLICATION 44-2.1–cont'd

medicine: Ativan, 2.0 mg) so that he will relax better and will have him scheduled for the first patient visit in the morning. In addition, you ask Mrs. Walker if she could possibly come to sign a permission form (consent) to have Mr. Walker treated and to be there on the day of his dental visit. Mrs. Walker agrees and makes arrangements for one of her children to bring her to the dental clinic for the next visit you will have with him.

This first appointment with Mr. Walker was not as successful as it might have been. What measures might have been taken before the appointment to ensure a more successful appointment?

tonia is evident, then restraints such as handholding by a caregiver, or using soft restraints, work well.

MUSCULOSKELETAL DEFICITS

Definition

Musculoskeletal refers to the interaction of the muscular and skeletal systems of the body. Because these two systems are intimately related, a deficit or problem in one system directly affects the functioning of the other system. For example, an imbalance in the tone or strength of antagonistic muscles may produce range-of-motion deficits. Musculoskeletal deficits in patients with neurologic diagnoses may be exhibited in a variety of forms, including decreased flexibility, soft tissue contractures, joint contractures, and skeletal deformities such as scoliosis.

Any deficit in the musculoskeletal system affects the ability of the patient to move efficiently and to perform functional activities. A skeletal deficit may also contribute to integumentary complications caused by excessive pressure on the bony prominences as a result of poor positioning or poor posture in the bed or wheelchair.

Deficits in the musculoskeletal system may be observed in patients with the diagnoses of stroke, BI, CP, PD, SCI, spina bifida, MS, ALS, late-stage AD, and MD.

Level of Severity

The level of severity of musculoskeletal dysfunction is assessed through range-of-motion measurements, flexibility tests, radiographs, postural observation, muscle tone evaluation, muscle strength tests, sensory tests, reflex tests, and observation of functional activities.[24,26]

Treatment Modalities

Deficits in the musculoskeletal system may be addressed through therapeutic and medical measures, depending on the specific cause of the problem. For example, an increase in muscle tone as a result of upper motor neuron or lower motor neuron damage may be addressed through medication, range-of-motion exercises, and appropriate positioning.

DENTAL CONSIDERATIONS

Musculoskeletal impairments may occur in such a variety of forms that the dental clinician must carefully assess each patient on an individual basis. In mild cases, the orofacial area may be totally unaffected, in which case the clinician may need to be cognizant only of a patient's other concerns, such as ambulation or the existence of any pressure points.

In cases in which the orofacial area is moderately affected, numerous aids such as bite blocks, props, and positioning devices are available to maintain the jaws in an open and steady position while reducing fatigue of the patient's muscles of mastication. When muscle spasticity is a concern, aspiration devices and retractors are available to protect the patient's tongue, cheeks, and other soft tissues from sharp dental instruments. In more severe cases in which the spasticity is pronounced and constant, a consultation with the patient's physician is needed to determine which, if any, pharmacologic agents (e.g., muscle relaxants) might be safely administered along with their appropriate dosages and sequence.

CASE APPLICATION 44-1.2

Mr. Crosswell: Musculoskeletal Concerns

Mr. Crosswell occasionally experiences muscle spasms in his extremities. These spasms usually last from a few seconds to approximately a minute. He reports that this episode usually occurs when his dietary intake has been altered and his electrolyte balance has been disrupted. The spasms are sometimes sufficient to vibrate his oral cavity area. Whenever this occurs during a dental appointment, a pause in treatment is usually adequate.

CASE APPLICATION 44-2.2

Mr. Walker: Musculoskeletal Concerns

Mr. Walker did not exhibit any musculoskeletal deficits; in fact, he was a strong man.

RESPIRATORY DEFICITS

Definition

Respiration is defined as the process of inspiration, when oxygen is taken into the lungs, and expiration, when carbon dioxide and water is expelled from the lungs. The **respiratory** process is controlled through the diaphragm, which is innervated by cervical spinal segments C3 to C5. Although the diaphragm is the primary respiratory muscle, the abdominal, intercostal, and other accessory muscles also assist in this function.

Level of Severity

Respiratory function is evaluated through pulmonary function tests such as tidal volume, inspiratory reserve volume, and vital capacity. In addition, evaluation of range of motion, muscle strength (especially of the respiratory muscles), posture, and exercise tolerance may be conducted.

A wide range of diagnoses may affect the respiratory function of a patient, including BI, PD, SCI, spina bifida, MS, ALS, late-stage AD, and MD. For example, a patient with a spinal cord lesion above the level of C4 requires the use of mechanical assistance to breathe.

The presence of any respiratory difficulty adversely affects the patient's mobility and ability to perform ADLs. The patient may exhibit shortness of breath, decreased endurance, excessive fatigue, or difficulty with verbal communication. In addition, the patient may complain of difficulty with sleeping, concentrating, or participating in routine activities.[24,26]

Treatment Modalities

Respiratory disorders may be addressed through pharmacologic measures, respiratory therapy, or a combination of both. The diagnoses and the prognosis for recovery determine the treatment of choice. Depending on the diagnosis, the need for continued respiratory care may gradually decline as the patient improves.[24]

DENTAL CONSIDERATIONS

Respiratory problems are common in the dental setting. Even patients with ideal health often experience breathing difficulties that stem from dental anxiety. Elevated respiratory rates, hyperventilation, and other physiologic changes may affect almost anyone. However, this respiratory difficulty may become critical in the patient with existing respiratory problems.

Fortunately, nitrous oxide analgesia will calm the anxious patient, and most modern nitrous oxide systems also deliver a minimum of 30% oxygen (compared with only approximately 21% oxygen in ambient air). This ratio, along with the sedative effect of nitrous oxide, reduces the oxygen demand on the patient and reduces the respiratory rate. Whether coupled with nitrous oxide or not, an emergency oxygen-delivery system should be available in any dental office. An *E*-size cylinder is recommended, which provides 30 minutes of oxygen and is portable.[15] An Ambu bag with a clear mouth and nose mask and linkage to pure oxygen is also recommended because these may affect respiration requirements.

If anesthetic is to be injected in the course of treatment, the clinician should always use care to avoid an intravascular injection and carefully consider the possible consequences of agent or vasoconstrictor overdose. For most patients with respiratory problems, however, the use of a vasoconstrictor is not an absolute contraindication.

If the level of respiratory difficulty is sufficient to require a respirator, then a medical consultation is indicated before the selection and use of a local anesthetic. Some respirator manufacturers supply equipment that is sufficiently portable to allow the patient a fair degree of mobility, in which case the patient may be treated in the dental office. In cases in which the respirator is not portable, several dental specialty companies manufacture dental delivery systems and radiograph equipment that is portable, thus allowing for home or institutional treatment of the patient.[17]

✸ CASE APPLICATION 44-1.3

Mr. Crosswell: Respiratory Concerns

Mr. Crosswell initially depended on a respirator. Over time, and with respiratory therapy and determination, he was able to *wean off* the respirator. Currently, his only assistive respiration requirement is to have his primary caregiver use an Ambu bag to initiate air exchange each morning before the patient arises to a sitting position and is transferred to his wheelchair. This precaution is necessary to avoid orthostatic hypotension or a feeling of *light-headedness*. If dental procedures are prolonged, then a change in position is appropriate every 20 to 30 minutes.

✸ CASE APPLICATION 44-2.3

Mr. Walker: Respiratory Concerns

Mr. Walker had been diagnosed as having an aspiration risk and had previously developed an aspiration pneumonia that was treated with antibiotics 1 year ago. His risk for developing pneumonia is greater than unaffected patients his age because of the degree of severity of his AD.

BOWEL AND BLADDER DYSFUNCTION

Definition

Problems with control of the bladder or bowel are most often referred to as *incontinence*, which is defined as the inability to prevent leakage or excretion of body fluids. Incontinence, although a significant inconvenience that may produce psychosocial disturbances for patients, may also result in serious medical problems. Kidney damage, decubitus ulcers, and autonomic dysreflexia (in persons with SCIs) may result from incontinence.[33]

Level of Severity

The level of severity for bladder or bowel dysfunction may be described in several ways. The number of episodes of urinary or bowel incontinence per day or per hour may be recorded. This documentation allows the patient or caregiver to monitor changes in patient status.

Urinary incontinence may be classified as stress incontinence, urge incontinence, overflow incontinence, or mixed incontinence. Stress incontinence occurs with an increase in intraabdominal pressures such as coughing or laughing, whereas urge incontinence is a strong desire to urinate combined with an uncontrolled release of urine. An overly distended bladder and an inability to prevent urine leakage cause overflow incontinence. Mixed incontinence is a combination of any of the types described.

Treatment Modalities

Deficits in bowel and bladder control may be exhibited in patients with the diagnoses of spina bifida, stroke, BI, CP, SCI, MS, and AD. Patients are given many options for controlling bladder or bowel incontinence. Patients with bladder incontinence may use intermittent catheterization, external catheters, training programs, or as a last resort, padding to prevent medical complications. Patients with bowel dysfunction may use a bowel-management program, digital stimulation, and diet to prevent medical complications. Medications are available to assist in these areas but are usually used when no other means of control has been effective.[14,33]

DENTAL CONSIDERATIONS

A wide variety of conditions may lead to problems with bladder and bowel continence. In more severe cases, the patient may be outfitted with a urinary tract catheter and collection device (usually a leg bag), a colostomy and collection device, or both. In less severe cases, simple absorbent liners within undergarments may suffice. In either case, the patient can generally be treated fairly routinely with attention to a few *common sense* guidelines.

Because bowel and bladder continence problems are often considered somewhat delicate subjects, the provider must approach the subject professionally and maintain a sense of confidentiality. Once a problem is apparent, the provider should determine factors such as the appropriate treatment interval, time of day for the appointment, dietary precautions, and any precipitating factors that might trigger an episode of incontinence. During ambulation or transport, the patient equipped with any collection device or catheter must be kept free of snagging or kinking of lines or tubes.

Furthermore, any collection bags or devices should not be allowed to get into any position (e.g., a leg bag higher than the bladder) that would impede gravitational drainage of urine. This precaution becomes more obvious when—for ergonomic reasons pertaining to the clinician—modern dental treatment often places the patient's head at or even slightly lower than the body and feet (similar to the Trendelenburg position).

Incontinence is surprisingly common among small children who are unimpaired; thus a vinyl type of chair covering is usually preferred to fabric. If fabric is the only material available, then a plastic or vinyl sheet may be placed over the chair before seating the patient. Similarly, the operatory should have noncarpeted floors for ease in cleaning and overall sanitation and disinfection.

★ CASE APPLICATION 44-1.4

Mr. Crosswell: Bowel and Bladder Concerns

Mr. Crosswell wears an internal urinary catheter and a leg bag for collection. Bowel incontinence is almost never a problem. By maintaining the leg bag in a slightly lower position than the bladder and monitoring its contents and collection capacity, routine care is relatively simple. A simple valve allows for draining of the bag. Careful attention is given so that the tubes leading to the bag remain free from any snagging or crimps that would impede drainage.

★ CASE APPLICATION 44-2.4

Mr. Walker: Bowel and Bladder Concerns

Mr. Walker wears an adult diaper (brand name: Depends) and is toilet trained to evacuate before he goes to bed, when he gets up, and twice during the day. When he goes to the dentist, or becomes agitated, he may get off his schedule and have an accident. Having the nurse's aide (or patient's caregiver, if living at home) bring an extra adult diaper to the clinic on the day of the appointment is advisable. Although seldom can a patient make a mess when wearing this protective device, having a wet diaper can be very uncomfortable, may lead to skin breakdown, or may cause agitation or anxiety during the dental procedure. In this case, Mr. Walker did not have any accidents, but the nurse's aide was told to make sure he went to the bathroom before his next appointment, as well as to bring an extra adult diaper on the next visit.

INTEGUMENTARY DEFICITS

Definition

The *integumentary* system functions in the protection of the body, primarily to preserve the necessary fluids required for efficient cellular activity and to protect from the environment. In addition, the skin serves as an organ of excretion through the sebaceous and sweat glands and also assists with temperature regulation and sensation.[8] A lack of skin integrity, also referred to as *skin breakdown*, is a complication of a wide range of diagnoses, including those presented in this chapter.

Level of Severity

A deficit in the integumentary system may be exhibited in a range from a small laceration to a decubitus ulcer. A decubitus ulcer, often called a *pressure sore* or *bedsore*, may be defined as one of four stages or grades. Grade 1 indicates superficial damage to the epidermis and dermal layers, whereas grade 4 refers to damage of the soft tissue to the depth of the bone[26] (Box 44-1).

Because a pressure sore can begin within only a few minutes but requires an extensive amount of time to heal, avoiding prolonged pressure on any bony prominence is important. The patient is at greater risk of developing a decubitus ulcer if tactile, proprioceptive, and pressure sensations are absent or impaired. A reduction in activity and mobility skills and cognitive impairment may also contribute to decubitus ulcer development.[24,26,33]

Treatment Modalities

Prevention may be accomplished through daily, even hourly, skin checks for redness, bruises, or lacerations and through appropriate patient positioning in the bed or wheelchair. Pressure relief, also called *raises,* should be performed every 30 to 60 minutes if the patient is sitting to allow the blood to flow to the areas with increased pressure. Treatment after the development of a reduction in skin integrity may include hydrotherapy with wound care, electrical stimulation, or the administration of hyperbaric oxygen. All effective treatment programs include prevention and positioning.[24,26,33]

> *Prevention*
> The most effective method to treat any deficit in skin integrity is prevention.

DENTAL CONSIDERATIONS

Patients who are confined to a bed or wheelchair are at risk for developing pressure sores. The practitioner should keep this fact in mind because recent dental trends are toward longer dental procedures. Additionally, when treating patients with multiple problems, including difficulty in getting to a dental office, the provider may feel a sense of urgency to accomplish a lot during the patient's scheduled appointment, thus extending the appointment duration. Although unlikely during a dental visit, the provider might thus unwittingly exacerbate an existing or prior condition or even initiate a new one. The patient may be aware of existing pressure point areas that are problematic and thus can inform the provider of positions to avoid.

Treatment is generally practiced through accommodation with special pillows, blankets, or other supports along with frequent position changes (raises) as needed. Occasionally, a patient may require treatment in the semisupine or fully upright position (e.g., some cases of spina bifida). Treatment considerations such as protection of the constantly open eye have been addressed in this chapter's section on neuromuscular deficits.

COGNITIVE AND PERCEPTUAL DEFICITS

Definition

Cognition is defined as the thinking, learning, and memory processes required for knowledge, whereas perception is defined as the ability to recognize and interpret an object. Patients with

cognitive or perceptual deficits may have diagnoses such as stroke, BI, CP, late-stage MS, hydrocephalus, AD, or autism.[8,24]

Patients with cognitive deficits may exhibit confusion; lack of orientation to person, place, or time; and decreased attention span. The patient may also demonstrate difficulty in processing information, which may be further complicated by impaired memory.[6,24,26,32]

Patients with impaired perception may exhibit unilateral neglect or inattention to one side of the body. Deficits in body image and visuospatial orientation are also common, including deficits in right-left discrimination, vertical disorientation, somatagnosia, or ideomotor apraxia.[6,24,26]

Level of Severity

The severity of cognitive or perceptual deficits is usually determined through an evaluation by a team of mental health specialists, including a neurologist or neuropsychologist. The evaluation includes multiple extensive tests to determine the extent of the deficits and how the deficits affect daily functioning. The dental hygienist, however, may perform general testing to determine the patient's short-term memory, attention span, and basic perceptions (Box 41-2).

Treatment Modalities

Occupational therapists, speech-language pathologists, or neuropsychologists, among others, may conduct treatment of cognitive and perceptual deficits.

DENTAL CONSIDERATIONS

Cognitive and perceptual deficits are relatively common in the dental setting. Such deficits may range from the rare cases of severe disorders to the more common cases of patients being unable to accommodate the clinician by complying with simple requests such as *open* and *close* or by confusing *left* and *right.*

In instances when minor problems are evident, patience and empathy on the part of the provider may be all that is required. In severe cases, a consultation with the patient's physician, neurologist, or neuropsychologist may be necessary. In these cases, sedation may be needed. If sedation is unable to be provided by the dentist in his or her office, then referral to a practitioner who is trained in advanced management techniques is indicated.

BOX 44-2

GENERAL TESTING FOR COGNITIVE AND PERCEPTUAL IMPAIRMENTS

Level of alertness
Does patient observe or interact with the environment or other people? Is patient lethargic or agitated?
Level of attention
How long does patient attend to an activity without being easily distracted? Does patient attend to some activities and not to others?
Level of memory
Does patient respond appropriately to biographical questions? Is patient able to recall the steps to a specific activity, such as preparing to brush the teeth?
Level of perception
Does patient ignore one side of the body or any part of the body? Does patient demonstrate awkwardness when performing an activity of which he or she is capable? Does patient confuse directions, such as *left* and *right* or *up* and *down?*

⚝ CASE APPLICATION 44-1.5

Mr. Crosswell: Cognitive Concerns

Mr. Crosswell did not exhibit any cognitive or perceptual deficits.

⚝ CASE APPLICATION 44-2.6

Mr. Walker: Cognitive Concerns

The hygienist can use general questions and observation skills to determine the extent of Mr. Walker's cognitive impairment (see Box 44-2). A simple cognitive test to determine cognition involves three questions, including asking the patient who he is or who is with him, where he is, and what time it is (day, month, and year). Patients who can answer all three questions appropriately are considered oriented to person, place, and time and are called *oriented × 3.* For patients who are more demented, fewer questions can be answered until a patient is not oriented to person, place, or time (oriented × 0). Even severely demented patients are oriented to person (oriented × 1) because they can generally recognize their caregiver.

In this case, Mr. Walker tells you that he is in the dental office and can name the assistant who brought him (oriented × 2). His cognitive-perceptual deficits make it difficult to understand what is being done to him or his teeth. Having his wife there should provide some comfort during treatment, as well as provide passive restraint (holding his hands). She will be your best advocate for helping him with brushing his teeth back at the nursing facility.

VISUAL DEFICITS

Definition

Visual deficits may be caused by damage to the eye, to the pathways from the eye, or to the brain resulting in difficulties in the reception, transmission, and interpretation of the array. Visual deficits may include visual field cuts (i.e., one area of the visual field is no longer seen or recognized), diplopia, double vision, and poor visual acuity (secondary to a reduction in oculomotor control).[24]

Level of Severity

The severity of visual deficits is usually determined through an examination by an occupational therapist or ophthalmologist.

Treatment Modalities

The primary neurologic conditions with visual deficits discussed in this chapter were in patients with BI, SCI, and CVA. The main consideration should be to assess the severity of the visual deficit. An optometrist or ophthalmologist who is knowledgeable of development can provide a diagnosis of visual deficits. Partially sighted or unsighted patients may require assistance in getting to and around the dental office and in being seated.

DENTAL CONSIDERATIONS

The clinician should establish whether the visual deficit involves any special problems such as diplopia, field cuts, or loss of eye movement. This assessment is important for three reasons:

1. The clinician must accommodate certain visual handicaps whenever a demonstration or *show, tell, do* is involved.
2. Home-care instructions may have to be modified so that the patient can adequately administer and modify the home care.
3. If visual field cuts are present (as in patients after a CVA), to prevent injury, the patient must then be alerted when instruments, especially hand pieces, are being brought in from the affected side so that the patient will not suddenly turn into a sharp instrument or hand piece. The patient with visual deficits may also require slightly more time for explanations. In instances in which advanced dental procedures are performed, such as when cosmetic or surgical procedures are planned, caregivers should be present to ensure that patients understand fully.

⚝ CASE APPLICATION 44-2.7

Mr. Walker: Visual and Perceptual Concerns

Mr. Walker had no visual deficits. However, he did have perceptual problems in which he would speak to figures on the television not realizing they were not real people. Similarly, he spoke to his own image in a mirror, not realizing it was his own image.

COMMUNICATION DEFICITS

Definition

Communication is defined as "an exchange of information between individuals using symbol systems such as spoken language or writing."[8] Communication may be accomplished through verbal or written means or through gestures and augmentative communication devices.

A deficit in communication may occur in diagnoses such as stroke, BI, CP, PD, MS, ALS, AD, Bell's palsy, MD, or autism. When damage to the central nervous system occurs, the difficulty in communication is caused by brain damage, which may result in expressive aphasia, receptive aphasia, global aphasia, word-finding deficits, and an overall reduction in language skills. The patient may also demonstrate difficulty with communication caused by oral-motor deficits resulting in dysarthria. Although the mechanism of the deficit varies among the diagnoses, the results are similar. The patient demonstrates difficulty or an inability to understand written or spoken language and is unable to make desires and needs known to others.[16,24]

Level of Severity

The severity of communication deficits is determined through an extensive evaluation by a speech-language pathologist.

Treatment Modalities

Treating a patient with communicative deficits can be challenging. Hopefully, a primary caregiver will be able to provide the clinician with an overview of the nature of the deficit and coping modalities that work best.

DENTAL CONSIDERATIONS

If the problem focuses more on dysarthria (impaired ability to articulate clearly), then the use of pencil and paper, a letter (or picture) board, or a primary caregiver (who is more accustomed to the individual's speech) may be all that is necessary. If, however, the deficit relates to an inability of the patient to receive communication input (e.g., AD, CVA, autism), then more extensive strategies may need to be used. In these more complex situations, the assistance of the primary caregiver, family, or friends may again prove invaluable. These persons may have developed or have access to someone with special communication skills (e.g., *signing*). Consulting with a speech-language pathologist may also be required.

MOBILITY DEFICITS

Definition

Mobility may be defined as functional activities that are used throughout the course of the day. These activities include bed mobility, transfers to all surfaces, wheelchair propulsion, ambulation, and balance in both sitting and standing. Bed mobility includes the ability to roll to either side, come to a sitting position, return to a supine or side-lying position, and assume the

⚜ CASE APPLICATION 44-1.6

Mr. Crosswell: Communication Concerns

Mr. Crosswell has no difficulty with normal verbal communication, although he pauses often to breathe. He signs papers, such as consent forms, with an ordinary ballpoint pen held between his teeth (Figure 44-8). Plastic pens are preferable to metal ones because they presumably cause less occlusal (and subsequent periodontal) trauma in the anterior region of the mouth and are easy to sanitize. The patient is able to communicate with others through the telephone and computer with the use of a custom-fitted mouthstick.

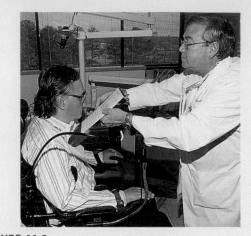

FIGURE 44-8
Patient shown signing consent form using plastic pen held between teeth.

⚜ CASE APPLICATION 44-2.8

Mr. Walker: Communication Concerns

Mr. Walker had a severe problem with agnosia (inability to name people or objects). He would try to appear normal, but he was unable to remember what to call everyday objects such as a hat, pen, pencil, and cup. He was pleasant for the most part, but he could be agitated by having him try to do something he did not want to do: take baths or showers; change clothes; or in this case, go to sit, lie back, and otherwise be in the dental chair. For everyday communication, Mr. Walker seemed to understand, but he was unable to repeat what you said or act on a command such as *open wide*. Although initially he would do as you ask, he would very quickly close his mouth again. Communication is best accomplished for patients with dementia by using the caregiver to get their attention and speaking more slowly, clearly, and directly. Increasing loudness is not usually necessary. Another important reason to keep the caregiver nearby is to have him or her help you with communication. The caregiver may be able to repeat or state more clearly your request when you need to have the patient follow your instructions in the dental chair. In addition, a caregiver such as Mrs. Walker may be the one who will ultimately be responsible for the day-to-day maintenance of his denture or partial and teeth over the coming years and she will need to be shown and educated how best to do this.

prone position. Transfers to the bed, chair, wheelchair, bathtub, toilet, or motor vehicle may be accomplished through a stand pivot, sit pivot, sliding board, or mechanical lift transfer. A patient with a neurologic deficit may use a wheelchair for mobility within the home or community or may be able to ambulate with or without an assistive device. Regardless of the mode of transportation, the patient must be able to negotiate level and unlevel surfaces to be functional. Balance in both the sitting and standing positions is required for safe and efficient performance of ADLs.[24-27,33]

Level of Severity

The level of severity or level of assistance required during mobility activities may be specified on a scale of 1 to 7, ranging from total dependence to total independence. Level 1, total dependence, indicates that the patient requires the assistance of another person to perform mobility activities. Level 7, total independence, indicates that the patient does not require the use of another person nor an assistive device for safe and efficient performance of mobility activities. Each of the levels in between refers to the level of assistance required based on the amount of effort expended by the patient and the caregiver.

Treatment Modalities

The physical therapist and occupational therapist address deficits in mobility activities through functional activity.

DENTAL CONSIDERATIONS

Mobility deficits have been considered throughout this chapter. Mobility impairment has been addressed from the broadest approach possible, such as transport to and from the dental office to mobility issues of getting in and out of the dental chair.

★ CASE APPLICATION 44-1.7

Mr. Crosswell: Mobility Concerns

Mr. Crosswell is an example of a level 1 (totally dependent) mobility deficit. He requires assistance for essentially all functions. Despite these obstacles, his case demonstrates that routine in-office dental care and home hygiene are possible with minimal accommodation on the part of the provider.

★ CASE APPLICATION 44-2.9

Mr. Walker: Mobility Concerns

Mr. Walker did not appear to have mobility problems. He was able to walk and stand in the Panorex machine but needed reminders.

References

1. Alzheimer's Association [Internet], Chicago, 2005, The Association. Available at: http://www.alz.org.
2. Amyotrophic Lateral Sclerosis Association [Internet], Calabasas Hills, Calif, 2005, The Association. Available at: http://www.alsa.org.
3. Autism Society of America [Internet], Bethesda, Md, 2005, The Society. Available at: http://www.autism-society.org.
4. Bell's Palsy Research Foundation [Internet], Montgomery Village, Md, 2005, The Foundation. Available at: http://www.bellspalsy.com.
5. Bouska MJ, Kauffman NA, Marcus SE: Disorders of the visual perceptual system. In Umphred DA, ed: *Neurological rehabilitation*, ed 3, St Louis, 1995, Mosby.
6. Brain Injury Association of America [Internet], McLean, Va, 2005, The Association. Available at: http://www.biausa.org.
7. Brown WV: Metabolic syndrome and risk of stroke, *Clin Cornerstone* 6(Suppl 3):S30-S34, 2004.
8. Dirckx JH, ed: *Stedman's concise medical dictionary for the health professions*, ed 3, Baltimore, 1997, Williams & Wilkins.
9. Frankel D: Multiple sclerosis. In Umphred DA, ed: *Neurological rehabilitation*, ed 3, St Louis, 1995, Mosby.
10. Grundy MC, Shaw L, Hamilton DV: *An illustrated guide to dental care for the medically compromised patient*, Aylesbury, England, 1993, Wolfe Publishing.
11. Henry R, Smith BJ: Treating the Alzheimer's patient. A guide for dental professionals, *J Mich Dent Assoc* 86(10):32-36, 2004.
12. Hydrocephalus Foundation, Inc [Internet], Sangus, Mass, 2005, The Foundation. Available at: http://www.hydrocephalus.org.
13. Joy JE, Johnson RB Jr eds: *Multiple sclerosis: current status and strategies for the future*, Washington, DC, 2001, National Academy Press.
14. Kraft C: Bladder and bowel management. In Buchanan LE, Nawoczenski DA, eds: *Spinal cord injury: concepts and management approaches*, Baltimore, 1987, Williams & Wilkins.
15. Malamed SF: *Medical emergencies in the dental office*, ed 5, St Louis, 2000, Mosby.
16. Melnick ME: Basal ganglia disorders: metabolic, hereditary, and genetic disorders in adults. In Umphred DA, ed: *Neurological rehabilitation*, ed 3, St Louis, 1995, Mosby.
17. Murphy JE: *Mobile dentistry*, Tulsa, Okla, 1996, PennWell.
18. Muscular Dystrophy Association [Internet], Tucson, Ariz, 2005, The Association. Available at: http://www.mdausa.org.
19. National Institute of Neurological Disorders and Stroke [Internet], Bethesda, Md, 2005, The Institute. Available at: http://www.ninds.nih.gov.
20. National Multiple Sclerosis Society [Internet], New York, 2005, The Society. Available at: http://www.nmss.org.
21. National Parkinson Foundation, Inc [Internet], Miami, Fla, 2005, The Foundation. Available at: http://www.parkinson.org.
22. National Spinal Cord Injury Association [Internet], Bethesda, Md, 2005, The Association. Available at: http://www.spinalcord.org.
23. National Stroke Association [Internet], Englewood, Colo, 2005, The Association. Available at: http://www.stroke.org.
24. O'Sullivan SB, Schmitz TJ: *Physical rehabilitation: assessment and treatment*, ed 3, Philadelphia, 2001, FA Davis.
25. Palmer ML, Toms JE: *Manual for functional training*, Philadelphia, 1992, FA Davis.

26. Pauls JA, Reed KL: *Quick reference to physical therapy,* Gaithersburg, Md, 1996, Aspen.

27. Pierson FM: *Principles and techniques of patient care,* Philadelphia, 1994, WB Saunders.

28. Rosenthal M et al: *Rehabilitation of the head injured adult,* Philadelphia, 1985, FA Davis.

29. Ryerson SJ: Hemiplegia resulting from vascular insult or disease. In Umphred DA, ed: *Neurological rehabilitation,* ed 3, St Louis, 1995, Mosby.

30. Schneider FJ: Traumatic spinal cord injury. In Umphred DA, ed: *Neurological rehabilitation,* ed 3, St Louis, 1995, Mosby.

31. Schneider JW: Congenital spinal cord injury. In Umphred DA, ed: *Neurological rehabilitation,* ed 3, St Louis, 1995, Mosby.

32. Simmons NN: Disorders in oral, speech, and language function. In Umphred DA, ed: *Neurological rehabilitation,* ed 3, St Louis, 1995, Mosby.

33. Somers MF: *Spinal cord injury: functional rehabilitation,* Upper Saddle River, NJ, 2001, Prentice Hall.

34. Spina Bifida Association of America [Internet], Washington, DC, 2005, The Association. Available at: http://www.sbaa.org.

35. United Cerebral Palsy [Internet], Washington, DC, 2005, The Association. Available at: http://www.ucp.org.

Mental and Emotional Disorders

Victoria C. Vick

INSIGHT

The dental hygienist will encounter patients with various emotional difficulties and will need to understand the nature of these difficulties to provide appropriate care.

✶✶ CASE STUDY 45-1   Fear and Anxiety in the Dental Patient

The young patient in the reception area, 11-year-old Cissy Holstrom, appears so anxious that the hygienist wonders whether she might leave before her appointment. Her mother is completing Cissy's health history form and is aggravated at or disinterested in her daughter's anxious state. She gives the form to the receptionist and says that this is the third office they have tried in the past year because, "Cissy has just not liked any of the others, and she is afraid of everything. I just hope you can do something with her, because taking her to all these appointments is a real problem." The mother is irritated by the inconvenience to *her.* She says that she has another appointment and will be back to pick up Cissy.

When they hygienist takes Cissy into the treatment room, she is very quiet, almost tearful. She approaches the room cautiously but is trying to cooperate. When she is seated, the hygienist realizes that time with her may be best spent trying to gain the girl's confidence, even if no actual procedures are accomplished. The hygienist would prefer that the mother had stayed so that the hygienist could explain the rationale for proceeding slowly (to develop the trust lacking in her daughter). The hygienist realizes that intervention will be necessary to ensure that Cissy is not blamed for another "inconvenience." The hygienist will also have to be sure the mother understands the importance of building trust and helping Cissy overcome her fear to ensure a successful long-term outcome in dental treatment.

The hygienist begins by asking Cissy general questions to find a nonthreatening area of interest. Such a topic will allow Cissy to feel some control and self-confidence, which are lacking in any anxiety-provoking situation. Once Cissy begins to understand that the hygienist is interested in her as a person and that she has some control, Cissy will likely begin to relax. She may say, "This isn't so bad after all," or "I think I'm going to like it here," or "Nobody has ever listened to me before."

Now both the hygienist and Cissy are in a better position to plan appropriate interventions. Later the hygienist explains the approach to forming a therapeutic alliance with Cissy to her Cissy's mother. The hygienist states that Cissy was *very* cooperative and she is an *excellent* patient. The clinician should reiterate Cissy's cooperation with both Cissy and her mother present so that they hear the same information. Cissy's positive attitude regarding her appointment and her eagerness to return for her next appointment pleasantly surprise her mother.

At her next appointment, Cissy may again appear hesitant. The clinician should reinforce what occurred at the previous appointment. The patient needs time and the practitioner needs patience to help the anxious dental patient overcome the fear and anxiety that have developed over time. Seeing a patient overcome dental fears and anxiety is rewarding.

KEY TERMS

agoraphobia	delusions	major depression	phobia
anorexia nervosa	dependent personality disorder	mania	posttraumatic stress disorder
antisocial personality disorder	depression	narcissistic personality disorder	process schizophrenia
anxiety	disorganized thinking	neuroleptic	reactive schizophrenia
anxiety disorders	fear	obsessions	schizoid personality disorder
avoidant personality disorder	generalized anxiety disorder	obsessive-compulsive disorder	schizotypal personality disorder
bipolar disorder	hallucinations	panic attacks	social phobia
bulimia nervosa	histrionic personality disorder	paranoid personality disorder	stimulus generalization
catatonic behavior	hypomania	personality disorder	worry

LEARNING OUTCOMES

After reading this chapter the student will be able to:

1. Recognize certain behaviors associated with mental and emotional disorders.
2. Understand major classifications of mental illnesses.
3. Identify patients who may be at risk of hurting themselves.
4. Learn appropriate ways of relating to individuals with mental and emotional disturbances.
5. Know where to obtain additional information and make appropriate referrals.
6. Identify specific mental disorders and their relevance to dental treatment.
7. Develop treatment plans that include a mental health assessment.
8. Identify the major oral side effect of antianxiety medications.

> *Note*
>
> Psychologic problems are common today; almost one third of the U.S. population will experience at least one psychiatric disorder in their lifetime.

The dental hygienist must understand the relationship between mental disorders and oral health.

It has been stated that "dental disease and psychiatric disorders are the most prevalent health problems in the United States."[48] This extremely powerful statement should alert dental professionals to the likelihood that they will encounter many psychiatrically troubled individuals and must be knowledgeable and well prepared to treat this segment of the population.

Life actually has two different dimensions: (1) *quantity* of life relates to the life expectancy in terms of years; (2) *quality* of life is a more subjective evaluation of life in general. Assessment of the quality of life should include the following points:

- Physical functioning
- Disease- and treatment-related physical symptoms
- Psychologic functioning
- Social functioning

Mental health is integrated into all four of these domains because it can significantly affect a person's quality of life as defined by these domains. Mental health, in fact, may be the common criterion that allows an individual to live a happy and meaningful life, almost regardless of life circumstances.[33]

Definitions and Classification

The American Psychiatric Association (APA) defines mental disorders as "clusters of persistent, maladaptive behaviors that are associated with personal distress, such as anxiety or depression, or with an impairment in social functioning, such as job performance or personal relationships."[9] The etiology of these disorders is multifactorial, including biological, psychologic, genetic, physical, and neurobiological imbalances.[11,26,37]

A major challenge to mental health professionals has been to develop a medical classification system for abnormal behavior. Many systems have been developed over the years, but professionals in the United States now classify and diagnose abnormal behavior according to one accepted system. The APA system is published as the *Diagnostic and Statistical Manual of Mental Disorders*. The text revision of the fourth edition *(DSM-IV-TR)* provides comprehensive definitions of more than 200 diagnostic categories for identifying and classifying abnormal behavior.

DSM-IV-TR provides a guide to clinical practice for all mental health professionals, facilitates research and education, and improves communication between clinicians and researchers. Psychologists, social workers, and psychiatrists use it for diagnostic purposes and for filing insurance coverage claims.

In *DSM-IV-TR,* each disorder is identified as a clinically significant behavioral or psychologic pattern and is associated with current life problems. *DSM-IV-TR* uses a framework that identifies five separate categories, or *axes,* each referring to a specific set of information (Box 45-1). The first three axes are designed to assess the patient's primary disorder, developmental problems in children and adolescents, and physical illnesses (Boxes 45-2 through 45-4). The last two axes focus on the severity of environmental stressors and the general level of functioning in the past year in social relationships, work, and leisure activities (Box 45-5). The assessment of a person's level of functioning represented on axis V is accomplished using the global assessment of functioning (GAF) (Table 45-1). The GAF scale has 10 divisions of functioning. The GAF assessment is a single number (on a scale of 0 to 100) that the clinician uses to reflect the patient's level of psychologic, social, and occupational functioning.[9]

This chapter addresses the classification and description of mental disorders, symptoms, diagnostic criteria, and treatment strategies, including the implications for treating patients in the dental setting (Box 45-6). Recognition of these disorders by clinicians helps in understanding patients' behavior, motivation, and response to needed and recommended dental treatment.

BOX 45-1

DSM-IV-TR MULTIAXIAL CLASSIFICATION

Axis I: Clinical disorders, other conditions of clinical interest
Axis II: Personality disorders, mental retardation
Axis III: General medical conditions
Axis IV: Psychosocial and environmental problems
Axis V: Global assessment of functioning

Modified from *Diagnostic and statistical manual of mental disorders (DSM-IV-TR),* ed 4 (text revision), Washington, DC, 2000, American Psychiatric Association.

BOX 45-2

DSM-IV-TR Axis I: Clinical Disorders*

Delirium, dementia, amnestic, other cognitive disorders
Mental disorders caused by general medical condition
Substance-related disorders
Schizophrenia and other psychotic disorders
Mood disorders
Anxiety disorders
Somatoform disorders
Factitious disorders
Dissociative disorders
Sexual and gender identity disorders
Eating disorders
Sleep disorders
Impulse control disorders not classified elsewhere
Adjustment disorders
Other conditions of clinical interest

*Disorders usually are first diagnosed in infancy, childhood, or adolescence.

Modified from *Diagnostic and statistical manual of mental disorders (DSM-IV-TR)*, ed 4 (text revision), Washington, DC, 2000, American Psychiatric Association.

BOX 45-4

DSM-IV-TR Axis III: General Medical Conditions

Infectious and parasitic diseases
Neoplasms
Endocrine, nutritional, and metabolic diseases and immunity disorders
Diseases of blood and blood-forming organs
Diseases of nervous system and sense organs
Diseases of respiratory system
Diseases of digestive system
Diseases of genitourinary system
Complications of pregnancy, childbirth, and puerperium
Diseases of skin and subcutaneous tissue
Diseases of musculoskeletal system and connective tissue
Congenital anomalies
Certain conditions originating in perinatal period
Symptoms, signs, and poorly defined conditions
Injury and poisoning

Modified from *Diagnostic and statistical manual of mental disorders (DSM-IV-TR)*, ed 4 (text revision), Washington, DC, 2000, American Psychiatric Association.

BOX 45-3

DSM-IV-TR Axis II: Personality Disorders and Mental Retardation

Paranoid personality disorder
Schizoid personality disorder
Schizotypal personality disorder
Antisocial personality disorder
Borderline personality disorder
Histrionic personality disorder
Narcissistic personality disorder
Avoidant personality disorder
Dependent personality disorder
Obsessive-compulsive personality disorder
Personality disorder not otherwise specified
Mental retardation

Modified from *Diagnostic and statistical manual of mental disorders (DSM-IV-TR)*, ed 4 (text revision), Washington, DC, 2000, American Psychiatric Association.

BOX 45-5

DSM-IV-TR Axis IV: Psychosocial and Environmental Problems

Problems with primary support group
Problems related to social environment
Educational problems
Occupational problems
Housing problems
Economic problems
Problems with access to healthcare services
Legal problems
Other psychosocial or environmental problems

Modified from *Diagnostic and statistical manual of mental disorders (DSM-IV-TR)*, ed 4 (text revision), Washington, DC, 2000, American Psychiatric Association.

Anxiety Disorders

Anxiety disorders have been identified as early as the fourth century BC in the writings of Hippocrates. With the interest in the nineteenth century primarily on psychotic disorders, the study of anxiety disorders was left to internal medicine specialists such as Freud. It was not recognized until the last half of the twentieth century that anxiety disorders could be effectively treated pharmacologically, as well as psychologically.

Rather than focusing on current circumstances, anxiety focuses on *anticipated* outcomes of future events, or "worrying about worry." **Worry,** as related to the person with an anxiety disorder, can be defined as "a relatively uncontrollable sequence of negative, emotional thoughts and images that are concerned with possible future threats or danger."[9]

Note

Anxiety is an irrational emotional response to an imagined threat. **Fear,** on the other hand, is a rational response to a real threat that helps prepare the person to respond to immediate danger.[9,26,37]

Table 45-1	Global Assessment of Functioning (GAF) Scale	
SCORE	**FUNCTIONAL CAPACITY**	**EXAMPLES**
100	Superior functioning in wide ranges of activities, life's problems never seem to get out of hand, sought out by others because of positive qualities	• No symptoms
90	Good functioning in all areas, generally satisfied with all areas of life, normal life concerns	• Mild anxiety before exam • Occasional argument with family members
80	If symptoms present, in response to psychosocial stressors or slight, temporary impairment in social, occupational, or school functioning	• Difficulty concentrating after family argument • Temporarily falling behind in schoolwork
70	Some difficulty with social, occupational, or school functioning, but generally functioning at an adequate level; has some interpersonal relationships	• Depressed mood and mild insomnia • Occasional truancy or theft within household
60	Moderate difficulty with social, occupational, or school functioning	• Flat affect and circumstantial speech, occasional panic attacks • Few friends, conflicts with peers or co-workers
50	Serious difficulty with social, occupational, or school functioning	• Suicidal ideation, severe obsessive rituals, frequent shoplifting • No friends, unable to keep a job
40	Some impairment in reality testing or communication *or* Major impairment in several areas, such as work, school, family relations, judgment, thinking, and mood	• Speech at times illogical, obscure, or irrelevant *or* • *Adult:* avoids social contact, neglect family, unable to work • *Child:* frequently beats up younger children, is defiant at home, failing at school
30	Behavior considerably influenced by delusions or hallucinations or serious impairment in communication or judgment *or* Inability to function in almost all areas	• Sometimes incoherent, actions grossly inappropriate, suicidal preoccupation *or* • Stays in bed all day; no job, home, or friends
20	Some danger of hurting self or others *or* Occasionally fails to maintain minimal personal hygiene *or* Gross impairment in communication	• Suicide attempts without clear expectation of death, frequently violent, manic excitement *or* • Smears feces *or* • Largely incoherent or mute
10	Persistent danger of hurting self or others *or* Persistent inability to maintain minimal personal hygiene *or* Serious suicidal acts with clear expectation of death	• Recurrent violence to self or others

Modified from *Diagnostic and statistical manual of mental disorders,* ed 4 (text revision), Washington, DC, 2000, American Psychiatric Association.

All persons experience anxiety, or a feeling of apprehension, as a reaction to stressful situations. However, some people experience anxiety when no identifiable external cause exists. The anxious person is hypervigilant and displays high levels of diffuse negative emotion, a sense of being out of control, and a state of self-preoccupation relative to what he or she perceives as a threat. If this anxiety occurs without justification and begins to impair the person's ability to function at a normal level, then the problem is considered an anxiety disorder. Along with the feeling of apprehension, the individual may experience predictable physiologic changes, such as increased muscle tension, shallow rapid breathing, increased perspiration, and dry mouth. Anxiety provokes two levels of reaction: (1) subjective feelings (e.g., fear, dread) and (2) physiologic responses (e.g., rapid breathing).[9,11,26,37]

Some anxiety can be an adaptive response because it helps provide motivation to be prepared to meet an upcoming event (e.g., anxiety before examinations), thus providing the initiative and focus to perform well. The other extreme is a prolonged level of high anxiety, not directed at any known upcoming

---

BOX 45-6

DSM-IV-TR CLASSIFICATION

Disorders usually first diagnosed in infancy, childhood, or adolescence

Delirium, dementia, amnestic, and other cognitive disorders

Mental disorders caused by general medical condition not classified elsewhere

Substance-related disorders

Schizophrenia and other psychotic disorders

Mood disorders
  Major depressive disorder
  Bipolar disorders

Anxiety disorders
  Panic disorder
  Agoraphobia
  Specific phobia
  Social phobia
  Obsessive-compulsive disorder (OCD)
  Posttraumatic stress disorder (PTSD)
  Acute stress disorder
  Generalized anxiety disorder (GAD)

Somatoform disorders

Factitious disorders

Dissociative disorders

Sexual and gender identity

Eating disorders
  Anorexia nervosa
  Bulimia nervosa

Sleep disorders

Impulse control disorders not classified elsewhere

Adjustment disorders

Personality disorders

Other

Modified from *Diagnostic and statistical manual of mental disorders (DSM-IV-TR)*, ed 4 (text revision), Washington, DC, 2000, American Psychiatric Association.

BOX 45-7

DSM-IV-TR ANXIETY DISORDERS

Panic disorder

Agoraphobia

Specific phobia

Social phobia

Obsessive-compulsive disorder (OCD)

Posttraumatic stress disorder (PTSD)

Acute stress disorder

Generalized anxiety disorder (GAD)

Anxiety disorder caused by general medical condition

Substance-induced anxiety disorder*

Anxiety disorder not otherwise specified*

Modified from *Diagnostic and statistical manual of mental disorders (DSM-IV-TR)*, ed 4 (text revision), Washington, DC, 2000, American Psychiatric Association.

*Indicates topics not discussed in text.

✯ CASE APPLICATION 45-1.1

Type of Anxiety

Which one of the previous conditions (worry or fear) best describes the type of anxiety presented by Cissy in Case Study 45-1 at the beginning of the chapter?

---

avoidance behavior, or the attempt to avoid the situation that causes or produces the anxiety[9] (Box 45-7).

ETIOLOGY

The etiologic basis for anxiety disorders includes stressful life events and biological components. Neurotransmitters such as serotonin are involved in the etiology of both anxiety disorders and mood disorders (e.g., depression). Similar symptoms in anxiety disorders and mood disorders include guilt, worry, panic, avoidance, and anger, which can lead to a dual diagnosis.[1,9,26,32,37]

The intuitive relationship between stressful life events and onset of anxiety is supported by several studies.[6,35] These studies demonstrate that patients with anxiety disorders are more likely than control subjects to have experienced a negative life event in the months preceding the initial onset of symptoms. The quality or nature of the stressful event may also be important in influencing the type of problem.

In one study, researchers interviewed women attending a general medical clinic to track relative negative life events to specific psychologic outcomes. This study included women who were depressed, those with anxiety disorders, and women who met dual diagnostic criteria. During the year preceding the onset of symptoms, 82% of the depressed women and 93% of the anxious and depressed women reported at least one severe negative life event. Only 34% of the control group reported a similar event. Women with anxiety symptoms were much more

event, which impairs concentration and performance. Prolonged anxiety is nearly an intolerable experience and likely explains why antianxiety medications have become the most popular prescription medications ever developed.[11,32,37]

The Epidemiologic Catchment Area (ECA) study examined the frequency of specific types of anxiety disorders and found that anxiety disorders are more common than any other form of mental disorder. The National Institute of Mental Health (NIMH) reported that within a 6-month period, 7% to 15% of the population (3 to 42 million people) may be diagnosed with one or more of the several anxiety diagnoses. Others have suggested an even higher prevalence of 20%, or approximately 56 million people. One national study found that 17% of U.S. adults have at least one type of anxiety disorder in any given year. These numbers represent a significant portion of the U.S. population, suggesting the enormity of the problem.[40] The major symptom of all 10 anxiety disorders defined by APA is

likely to have experienced an event that involved danger, whereas the women who were depressed were more likely to have experienced a severe loss. The women with mixed symptoms often reported experiencing both types of events. Therefore the type of environmental stress can influence the type of psychologic response the patient may exhibit.[12]

⭐ CASE APPLICATION 45-1.2

Anxiety

From the previous discussion on the etiology of anxiety, what circumstances could have caused Cissy's anxiety?

PANIC ATTACK

Panic attacks can occur alone or with other anxiety disorders, mental disorders, or general medical conditions. **Panic attacks** are experienced as the sudden onset of intense apprehension, often with symptoms such as shortness of breath, palpitations, chest pain, and the sense of losing control. The attack has a sudden onset, usually reaching its peak for fear and apprehension within 10 minutes or less, with the person experiencing a sense of impending doom and the urgent need to flee. To meet diagnostic criteria, at least 4 of 13 symptoms must be present (Box 45-8). The anxiety characteristic of this disorder can be distinguished from generalized anxiety because the anxiety is of greater severity and occurs intermittently. Panic attacks can also occur concurrently with a variety of the other anxiety disorders (e.g., specific, social, posttraumatic stress, acute stress disorder). The following are three types of panic attacks:

1. Unexpected (uncued)
2. Situationally bound (cued)
3. Situationally predisposed

The unexpected attacks happen "out of the blue," whereas situationally bound attacks occur on exposure to or expectation of the situational *cue*, such as speaking in public.[9,11,26,37]

The occurrence of panic attacks is required for a diagnosis of panic disorder (with or without agoraphobia).[9]

PANIC DISORDER

To meet the *DSM-IV-TR* diagnostic criteria for panic disorder, a patient must do the following:

- Experience recurrent unexpected panic attacks, followed by at least 1 month of persistent concern about having another panic attack
- Worry about implications or consequences of the panic attacks
- Exhibit a significant behavioral change related to the attacks (Box 45-9)

Coexistence of a mood disorder such as major depression ranges from 10% to 65% in patients with panic disorder. Comorbid anxiety disorders may be seen. The age of onset varies considerably, but most attacks occur in late adolescence and into the early 30s. Some patients may have no symptoms for years. Most often the condition is chronic, with periods of latency and activity. First-degree relatives are 20 times more likely to experience panic disorder if onset was before age 20. Twin studies have found a genetic component in the development of panic disorder.[9,11,26]

BOX 45-8

DSM-IV-TR DIAGNOSTIC CRITERIA FOR PANIC ATTACK

Discrete period of intense fear or discomfort, in which four or more of the following symptoms developed abruptly and reached a peak within 10 minutes:

1. Palpitations, pounding heart, or accelerated heart rate
2. Sweating
3. Trembling or shaking
4. Sensations of shortness of breath or smothering
5. Feeling of choking
6. Chest pain or discomfort
7. Nausea or abdominal distress
8. Feeling dizzy, unsteady, lightheaded, or faint
9. Derealization (feelings of unreality) or depersonalization (being detached from oneself)
10. Fear of losing control or "going crazy"
11. Fear of dying
12. Paresthesias (numbing or tingling sensations)
13. Chills or hot flashes

Modified from *Diagnostic and statistical manual of mental disorders (DSM-IV-TR)*, ed 4 (text revision), Washington, DC, 2000, American Psychiatric Association.

BOX 45-9

DSM-IV-TR DIAGNOSTIC CRITERIA FOR PANIC DISORDER

1. Both 1 and 2 are present, as follows:
   a. Recurrent unexpected panic attacks
   b. At least one of the attacks followed by at least 1 month of one or more of the following behaviors:
      i. Persistent concern about having additional attacks
      ii. Worry about the implications of the attack or its consequences (e.g., losing control, having a heart attack, going crazy)
      iii. Significant change in behavior related to attacks
2. Panic attacks not caused by direct physiologic effects of a substance (e.g., drug abuse, medication) or a general medical condition (e.g., hyperthyroidism)
3. Panic attacks not better accounted for by another mental disorder (e.g., social phobia, specific phobia, obsessive-compulsive disorder [OCD], posttraumatic stress disorder [PTSD])

Modified from *Diagnostic and statistical manual of mental disorders (DSM-IV-TR)*, ed 4 (text revision), Washington, DC, 2000, American Psychiatric Association.

PHOBIC DISORDER

A **phobia** is defined as "an irrational fear or an obsessive dread."[9] People with a phobic disorder exhibit a fear that is unreasonable, exaggerated, or inappropriate and that leads them to avoid that object, activity, or situation. This avoidance is significant enough that the fear and the response are disruptive to the individual's life. The following are the three basic types of phobias:

1. Agoraphobia
2. Social
3. Specific

Phobias are common and occur in children and adults of either gender, although they are more frequently diagnosed in women. People may be "closet phobics," keeping their fears hidden from others and only pretending to feel better.[26,37]

Many factors can cause a person to have irrational fears such as those found in phobic disorders. Many theorists believe that these fears are conditioned emotional responses to specific circumstances. A classic experiment by John Watson provides an example of the development of a fear based on exposure to a frightening experience. Albert, a toddler, was shown a white rat and expressed no fear of the rat. Then a loud sound was generated behind Albert while he was in the presence of the rat. The loud noise frightened Albert, producing a *startle response,* and the child began to cry. After that experience, when exposed to the rat, Albert would cry and try to avoid it. Albert had acquired a fear of the rat he initially did not have through exposure to a loud and frightening noise, thus developing a *conditioned* fear of the rat. Applying this experiment to common fears, one can see that exposure to a bad experience, whether an object or a situation, can lead to the development of excessive fear. For example, if a child is mocked during a grade-school presentation, then he or she is likely to carry that experience into adulthood and continue to fear speaking in public. Likewise, a person who has a negative dental experience may become a "dental-fears patient."[10]

Watson also discovered that objects similar to the conditioned fear (the white rat), such as Santa Claus, a white rabbit, or crumpled white terrycloth towel, also produced fear in Albert. This **stimulus generalization** is a tendency to display a learned response to situations or objects that are similar to the original feared object or situation. Importantly, parents with irrational fears can "infect" their children with a tendency to develop similar behavioral patterns.[49]

Agoraphobia

Agoraphobia means *fear of open places* and is characterized by a group of related fears: being alone, public places, and traveling away from home (where the person may be unable to escape from an unpleasant or embarrassing situation). The individual with this disorder may avoid stores, crowds, restaurants, and social events; in extreme cases the person becomes housebound, never traveling far from the known safe environment.[9,37]

Social Phobia

Social phobia is a "marked and persistent fear of social or performance situations in which embarrassment may occur."[9] Social phobia affects 3% to 13% of the U.S. population. Patients experience an immediate anxious response to particular social interactions, which often leads to avoidance of the situation or anticipation with a sense of dread. Common features associated include hypersensitivity to criticism, negative evaluation, or rejection; difficulty being assertive; and low self-esteem. Examples of social phobia include the following:

- Fear of public speaking
- Fear of meeting strangers
- Hesitation to accept invitations to social functions
- Embarrassment when eating in public
- Fear of maintaining conversations or eye contact with others in social situations

The diagnosis is made, however, only if the anxiety response interferes with the person's occupational functioning or social life or if the person is significantly distressed about the condition.[9,37]

Adults with social phobia are aware that their fear is excessive. Children, however, may not be aware of the excessive nature of their fears. The onset of social phobia usually is in mid-adolescence, often after a childhood history of shyness. Onset of the condition may immediately follow a stressful or humiliating event. Unlike adults, children are less likely to have the option of avoiding the feared situations or to understand the nature of their intense fear.[9,37]

Specific (Simple) Phobias

In specific, formerly "simple," phobias, the source of fear can be readily identified. The fear is persistent and excessive or unreasonable, cued by the presence or anticipation of a specific object or situation (e.g., flying, heights, animals, dental treatment). Exposure to the phobic cue almost invariably provokes an immediate anxiety response. The phobic situation is either avoided or endured with intense anxiety or distress. The avoidance, anxious anticipation, or distress in the feared situations interferes significantly with the person's normal routine, occupational (or academic) functioning, social activities, or relationships. The person may be greatly distressed about having the phobia.[9,37] These phobias are considered simple only in the sense that the source of the fear is not complex[9] (Box 45-10).

GENERALIZED ANXIETY DISORDER

Generalized anxiety disorder (GAD) is defined in terms of excessive anxiety and worry that the person finds difficult to control and that leads to significant distress or impairment in occupational or social functioning. The following symptoms are often associated with the anxiety:

- Restlessness
- Feeling on edge
- Easy fatigue
- Difficulty concentrating
- Irritability
- Muscle tension
- Sleep difficulties

The intensity, duration, and frequency of the anxiety are greatly exaggerated relative to the likely outcome of the feared situation. The person finds that the thoughts are intrusive and

---

BOX 45-10

FREQUENTLY REPORTED SPECIFIC PHOBIAS

Acrophobia: Fear of heights
Algophobia: Fear of pain
Astraphobia: Fear of thunder, lightning, winds, and heavy rain
Claustrophobia: Fear of confinement or closed areas
Cynophobia: Fear of dogs
Demophobia: Fear of crowds
Haphephobia: Fear of being touched
Monophobia: Fear of being alone
Mysophobia: Fear of germs
Nyctophobia: Fear of darkness or night
Pathophobia: Fear of disease
Pyrophobia: Fear of fire
Zoophobia: Fear of animals

---

that they interfere with normal functioning. Adults with GAD often worry about routine daily responsibilities related to job, finances, or minor activities (e.g., household chores, car repairs). Children with GAD tend to worry about school or athletic performance.[9,37]

Many people with GAD also experience cold and clammy hands, dry mouth, sweating, nausea, trouble swallowing, and an exaggerated startle response. Depression often occurs with GAD, as may other mood disorders. Many people with GAD say that they have been anxious all their lives, but the condition may begin after age 20. The course is chronic and often worsens during or after stressful life events.[9,11,26,37]

OBSESSIVE-COMPULSIVE DISORDER

Obsessive-compulsive disorder (OCD) may be seen as three disorders:

1. Compulsive disorder
2. Obsessive disorder
3. Combination obsessive *and* compulsive disorder

Patients with OCD are plagued with unwanted thoughts (obsessions) and feel that they must take some action (compulsion) that they are not able to control. OCD affects an estimated 1 in 200 teenagers.[9,37]

OCD is characterized by recurrent **obsessions,** ideas, or thoughts that constantly and involuntarily intrude into awareness. These thoughts are generally of a pointless nature, such as continually washing one's hands or checking to make certain the door is locked, over and over again. The person with OCD realizes that these compulsive actions serve no useful purpose but cannot stop them. Theoretically, these obsessive and compulsive actions may be used to prevent other anxiety-producing behaviors or thoughts.[9,37]

POSTTRAUMATIC STRESS DISORDER

The onset of **posttraumatic stress disorder** (PTSD) is preceded by exposure to an extreme traumatic stressor and followed by the development of characteristic symptoms. This stressful event is "outside the normal human experience" or threatens one's basic held values and beliefs. Of those who experience a severely traumatic event, approximately 15% will exhibit symptoms of PTSD. The traumatic event is reexperienced in many ways.

DSM-IV-TR diagnostic criteria include the following:

- Recurrent and intrusive recollections of the event
- Recurrent distressing dreams
- Acting or feeling as if traumatic event were recurring
- Intense psychologic distress on exposure to internal or external cues that symbolize or resemble traumatic event
- Physiologic reactions to these cues

The reexperiencing of the event is often accompanied by persistent avoidance of stimuli associated with the trauma and numbing of general responsiveness (not present before the trauma).

The person may make efforts to avoid thoughts, feelings, or conversations associated with the trauma or avoid activities, places, or people that arouse recollections of the trauma. Patients with PTSD may have greatly diminished interest or participation in significant activities, a feeling of detachment or estrangement from others, and a restricted range of affect. They may sense a "foreshortened future." These patients also often experience persistent symptoms of increased arousal, such as difficulty falling or staying asleep, irritability or outbursts of anger, difficulty concentrating, hypervigilance, or exaggerated startle response.[9,37]

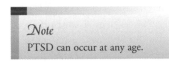

Note
PTSD can occur at any age.

The onset of PTSD symptoms usually occurs within 3 months of the trauma, although symptoms have not appeared until many months or years after the trauma in some cases. The symptoms of the disorder and the level of reexperiencing, avoidance, and hyperarousal symptoms may vary over time. The severity, duration, and proximity of the individual to the event are important in influencing the likelihood of developing PTSD. This disorder can develop in individuals who have no predisposing conditions, especially if the stressor is extreme. Recovery from PTSD is often determined by other complicating factors (e.g., alcoholism, drug abuse, depression), whether the person experienced psychologic problems before the onset of PSTD, and the social support system in place for the patient.[9,37]

TREATMENT

Of the various psychologic treatment strategies to treat anxiety disorders, a cognitive-behavioral approach for phobic disorders, OCD, and PTSD is appropriate.

Pharmacologically these disorders are usually treated with antianxiety medications (Table 45-2). These medications reduce many of the symptoms of anxiety disorders, such as muscle tension, increased vigilance, increased perspiration, palpitations, and gastrointestinal distress. They do,

Note
Treatment of anxiety disorders can be approached psychologically, pharmacologically, or often with both therapies.

Table 45-2	Common Benzodiazepines Used in Treatment of Anxiety Disorders*
GENERIC NAME	**TRADE NAME**
ALPRAZOLAM	Xanax
DIAZEPAM	Valium
LORAZEPAM	Ativan
TEMAZEPAM	Restoril
TRIAZOLAM	Halcion

Modified from Gage TW, Pickett FA: *Mosby's dental drug reference,* ed 7, St Louis, 2005, Mosby.
*All central nervous system (CNS) depressants.

Distinct Care Modifications

A calm, quiet approach should be taken so that the patient is not exposed to stimuli that might trigger the onset of a panic attack or undue anxiety.

however, have several side effects, including daytime sedation, dry mouth, slight impairment in the ability to concentrate, constipation, and (with specific drugs) blurred vision. Withdrawal from these medications can be problematic if the patient has been using the drug for some time, because the original symptoms often return (known as *rebound anxiety*). Equally if not more important than the difficulty patients encounter when they discontinue use of benzodiazepines is their potential for addiction.[1,7,32,37]

DENTAL CONSIDERATIONS

45-2

Patients arriving at the dental office with an anxiety disorder may or may not exhibit signs of the disorder. Given the prevalence of anxiety disorders, many patients are likely to be affected, and the healthcare professional will need to assess the patient's current status at the beginning of the appointment. A sensitive approach enables the dental practitioner to form a clinical judgment as to the patient's mental health status. This assessment is critical to the delivery of care.

Patients with social phobia should have limited interactions during treatment and should receive positive reassurance. If the patient arrives at the office in a state of high anxiety, then medical consultation with his or her psychiatrist or other medical professional may be necessary to determine whether the patient's current condition is stable enough to continue with the dental appointment.*

Patients with anxiety disorders are often taking benzodiazepines or newer medications. The benzodiazepines are

*References 15, 16, 22, 32, 43, 52.

known to cause *xerostomia* (dry mouth), which can exacerbate preexisting periodontal conditions and increase dental caries. Patients may suck hard candy and increase their consumption of cariogenic beverages to alleviate the dry mouth. This can also lead to an increase in dental caries and dental plaque biofilm in general. The patient should be advised of the potential danger of relying on these methods to alleviate dry mouth. Xerostomia reduces the self-cleansing nature of the oral cavity and often leads to increased levels of plaque biofilm with no change in brushing habits.

The clinician should explain the implications of xerostomic changes to patients and inform them of actions to reduce the risks of dental disease. Mouthrinses that contain high levels of alcohol should be avoided because they can cause oral ulcerations to dry mucosal surfaces. Patients should be advised to rinse with water often during the day and to be careful not to brush aggressively if they find their oral tissues are tender and dry from the xerostomia. Vigorous brushing under these conditions can lead to gingival tissue abrasion.[19] Patients with excellent oral hygiene may have difficulty in maintaining their previous level of plaque biofilm control.

Prevention

Patients taking benzodiazepines, as well as many other psychotropic medications, experience xerostomia (dry mouth). Supportive interventions for xerostomia include use of sugarless gum and lozenges to increase salivary flow and help restore the natural cleansing provided by saliva. These patients must understand the reason for their increased plaque biofilm accumulation so as not to worsen their anxiety.

Distinct Care Modifications

- Appointments should be scheduled in the morning.
- Patients should not be kept waiting.
- Length of appointment and amount of work to be done should be minimized to prevent a stressful event.
- Clinician should explain treatment procedures, making certain patient is informed and comfortable with what is to take place.[46,47]

Mood Disorders

Everyone has "bad days," when they feel sad and depressed. Some people, however, experience these "mood swings" for long periods so severely that it significantly interferes with the person's ability to function at acceptable levels. Everyone has experienced one or more significant disappointments in life and the resulting sadness. This reflects a normal period of mourning during which some level of **depression** is to be expected. People who suffer from **major depression** have similar feelings but of much greater severity and duration.

The etiology of mood disorders is controversial. Psychoanalytic theory states that depression results from turning one's anger inward and feeling responsible for all the "bad things." As Maslow suggests, persons might become depressed because they are not able to experience *self-actualization*—the ability to optimize their talents and potential. Others have found convincing evidence that both major depression and **bipolar disorder** are biological in origin, resulting from an imbalance of neurotransmitters in the brain caused by a genetic predisposition or unusually severe stressors. A cognitive approach to causation suggests that depression is *learned helplessness;* people experience stress as inescapable and intolerable. Although no single cause of depression exists, depression clearly results from complex interactions among multiple variables, including biochemical influences, situational stress, and learned experiences.[9,37]

MAJOR DEPRESSIVE DISORDER

Queen Victoria, Lincoln, Moses, and Freud all are thought to have suffered from major depression. Intelligent people who engage in too much self-analysis and self-criticism often experience depression. Although depression receives much publicity when experienced by famous people, many ordinary people suffer from the same condition. Major depression is characterized by at least 2 weeks of depressed mood or loss of interest in otherwise pleasurable activities. At least four additional symptoms must exist (Box 45-11). These symptoms must also be accompanied by impairment in social, occupational, or educational functioning.[9,37]

The incidence of unipolar mood disorder in the U.S. population is 6% to 10%. The cost of depression to society is an astounding $44 billion a year.[27] Women are twice as likely to experience a major depressive episode as men, with 25% of all women likely to have major depression at some point in their lives.[34] Research shows an increase in depression worldwide, as well as earlier onset. Episodes tend to recur in 50% to 80% of patients with a diagnosis of a major depressive disorder. An episode can last from several months to more than 1 year, depending on availability of treatment and the patient's support structure.[11,37,50]

Major stressful life events increase the likelihood of a person developing clinical depression. The events most often associated with increased risk for depression are "major life changes" involving losses of important people or roles.[37]

People experience major depressive episodes in different ways. Patients with major depression find that once-pleasurable activities no longer are important. Families often notice social withdrawal, although depressed individuals may deny feeling sad. Insomnia is the most common sleep disturbance associated with clinical depression. Insomnia can be characterized as *initial* (difficulty falling asleep), *middle* (waking up in the middle of the night and having difficulty falling back to sleep), or *terminal* (waking up early and not being able to go back to sleep).[9,37]

Depressed adults lack motivation, find work and social interactions difficult and exhausting, have marked weight loss or gain, have difficulty sleeping or sleep too much, have a general negative outlook or hopelessness, and possess a sense of worthlessness. The sense of worthlessness or guilt is often exaggerated as trivial day-to-day events are taken as evidence of personal weakness. Many individuals report an impaired ability to think and concentrate and may complain of memory loss. They often blame themselves for being ill and failing to meet interpersonal or occupational responsibilities. Thoughts of death and suicidal ideation are common, with variable frequency, intensity, and lethality.[9,37]

Children and adolescents may manifest an irritable mood rather than a sad or depressed mood. For children, depression can interfere with the development of close relationships and interests in learning and in play. Children and adolescents may exhibit a drop in school achievement as a result of a reduced ability to concentrate. In children, other mental disorders frequently occur in conjunction with a major depressive episode, especially disruptive behavior disorder, attention deficit disorder, and anxiety disorders. In adolescents, disruptive behavior disorders, attention deficit disorder, anxiety disorders, substance-related disorders, and eating disorders are frequently associated with a major depressive disorder.[9,30,37]

Treatment

As with most other mental disorders, treatment of major depressive disorder can be psychologic, pharmacologic, or combination therapy. Research has shown conflicting results in regard to the most effective therapeutic intervention. Most evidence supports a combination of psychotherapeutic and pharmacologic interventions. The two therapies complement each other: one addresses the ability to cope with life events, whereas the other addresses a change in levels of neurotransmitters that control mood.[11,32,37,44]

BOX 45-11

DSM-IV-TR DIAGNOSTIC CRITERIA FOR MAJOR DEPRESSIVE EPISODE

At least one of the symptoms is either (1) depressed mood or (2) loss of interest or pleasure that represents a change from previous functioning for 2 weeks, plus four of the following problems:

1. Depressed mood
2. Loss of interest or pleasure
3. Significant (5% of body weight in a month) weight gain, weight loss, or change in appetite
4. Insomnia or excessive sleep
5. Psychomotor agitation or retardation
6. Fatigue, loss of energy
7. Feelings of worthlessness or excessive guilt
8. Diminished ability to think or concentrate or indecisiveness
9. Recurring thoughts of death or suicidal ideas or attempt
   The following criteria also apply:
- The mood disorder is not caused by bereavement, medical disease, or substance abuse.
- The symptoms cause distress or impair functioning.

Modified from *Diagnostic and statistical manual of mental disorders (DSM-IV-TR)*, ed 4 (text revision), Washington, DC, 2000, American Psychiatric Association.

The first "antidepressant" was a drug originally developed to treat tuberculosis and had side effects of greater optimism and happiness in treated patients. This drug was found to cause irreversible liver damage and was removed from the market, but its introduction dramatically changed the way clinicians viewed treatment of depression. Currently a number of medications are used to treat depression, including monoamine oxidase inhibitors (MAOIs), tricyclics, tetracyclics, selective serotonin reuptake inhibitors (SSRIs), and atypical antidepressants[1,25,32,37,53] (Table 45-3).

Table 45-3	Antidepressants
GENERIC NAME	**TRADE NAME**
Atypical	
BUPROPION	Wellbutrin
NEFAZODONE	Serzone
TRAZODONE	Desyrel
VENLAFAXINE	Effexor
MAOIs	
PHENELZINE	Nardil
TRANYLCYPROMINE	Parnate
SSRIs	
CITALOPRAM	Celexa
ESCITALOPRAM	Lexapro
FLUOXETINE	Prozac
FLUVOXAMINE	Luvox
PAROXETINE	Paxil
SERTRALINE	Zoloft
Tetracyclics	
MAPROTILINE	Ludiomil
MIRTAZAPINE	Remeron
Tricyclics	
AMITRIPTYLINE	Elavil
AMOXAPINE	Asendin
CLOMIPRAMINE	Anafranil
IMIPRAMINE	Tofranil

MAOIs, Monoamine oxidase inhibitors; *SSRIs,* selective serotonin reuptake inhibitors.

Hospitalization is warranted when the patient may be a danger to self or others. Forced hospitalization of a patient jeopardizes the psychotherapeutic relationship and should be done only when no other choice exists.[11,26,37]

DENTAL CONSIDERATIONS

A patient with a major depressive episode may experience feelings of sadness, loss, and rejection. Patients often lose interest and motivation for self-care and may not maintain their previous level of oral hygiene. The clinician should minimize stressful aspects of the appointment for these patients.

The clinician should ensure that the patient receives positive feedback and support relative to oral hygiene habits; patients view negative comments as further examples of their worthlessness. The clinician should be respectful of these patients and their emotional pain and demonstrate sincere interest in their well-being.*

SSRIs, such as escitalopram (Lexapro), citalopram (Celexa), fluoxetine (Prozac), paroxetine (Paxil), and sertaline (Zoloft) are frequently used in the treatment of depression. A common side effect of these medications is xerostomia (see earlier discussion). Preventive dietary and dental hygiene guidance is appropriate for this patient population.†

*References 3, 14, 17, 23-24, 32.
†References 1, 3, 5, 13, 17, 20, 22, 23, 28, 32, 39, 42, 45, 52, 53.

BIPOLAR DISORDER

Bipolar disorder, formerly manic-depressive illness, is a common, recurrent, and severe psychiatric illness that affects 1% to 3% of the U.S. population. The illness is characterized by episodes of mania, depression, and mixed states (i.e., simultaneous manic and depressive symptoms). Bipolar disorder frequently goes unnoticed and untreated for years. The typical onset of a bipolar disorder is between ages 28 and 33 years, with the first set of symptoms equally as likely as manic or depressive. The average manic episode lasts 2 to 3 months; the depressive episode lasts somewhat longer. The long-term outcome of bipolar disorder is mixed, with the majority of individuals experiencing multiple episodes over a lifetime. Both genetic and early environmental factors are associated with the course of bipolar disorder.[9,37]

During their manic episodes, patients display inflated self-esteem, grandiosity, excessive speech, racing and rapidly changing ideas, excessive participation in pleasurable activities, and a decreased need for sleep. **Mania** cannot be maintained for long periods, because the condition is exhausting. Some patients experience increased activity that cannot be considered a full-blown manic episode; this is known as **hypomania.** Hypomanic and manic episodes differ in duration and severity. The hypomanic episode is noticeable to others and lasts at least 4 days (versus 1 week for a full manic episode), without impairment to social or occupational functioning.[9,37]

Treatment

Although psychotherapy is helpful to patients with bipolar disorder, medication is necessary for a successful outcome. The three phases of bipolar disorder need to be addressed in developing a treatment strategy. Active therapies need to be developed for the depressive and manic phases and a maintenance strategy for long-term support. Bipolar disorder can lead to serious personal, interpersonal, and social problems, often accompanied by violence, alcoholism, and sometimes suicide.[37]

Discovered by an Australian psychiatrist, lithium has proved to be an excellent treatment for bipolar patients formerly resistant to treatment. Lithium reduces the recurrence of bipolar disorder when used as a maintenance therapy. The side effect profile includes gastrointestinal irritation, hand tremor, thirst, and muscular weakness. As with any long-term drug therapy, frequent monitoring is required.[14,37]

Carbamazepine and valproate are alternatives to lithium in the treatment of bipolar disorder. Topiramate, a new antiepileptic agent, appears to have efficacy for manic and mixed manic and depressive phases of bipolar disorder. One approach to treatment-resistant patients is to use a combination of mood stabilizers, but this demands knowledge of pharmacokinetic interactions. The effectiveness of psychosocial strategies is under investigation. The current use of psychologic intervention primarily involves identification of stress factors and early signs of recurrence. As with all mental disorders, the patient's social support system is invaluable in the long-term prognosis.[11,37]

DENTAL CONSIDERATIONS

The dental patient with bipolar disorder in its manic phase may report for dental treatment with active symptomatology, including restlessness, aggressiveness, argumentativeness, and irritability. These patients may rapidly switch thought patterns, may be unable to concentrate or focus on topics, and may react unpredictably if pressured.

Distinct Care Modifications
- Ensure that the patient is seen in a quiet and nonstressful clinical environment.
- Approach each procedure with clear, concise explanations.
- Keep a calm yet firm approach to maintain a controlled setting.
- Keep explanations of oral health strategies as concise as possible, because these patients are often not receptive to long descriptive remarks as a result of the bipolar disorder.[32]

Personality Disorders

A **personality disorder** is an "enduring pattern of inner experience that deviates markedly from the expectations of the individual's culture, is pervasive and inflexible, has an onset in adolescence or early adulthood, is stable over time, and leads to distress or impairment."[9] The personality traits that make up these disorders must be present separate from any situational stressor[9,37] (see Box 45-3).

Personality disorders are divided into three clusters in the *DSM-IV-TR*, based on descriptive similarities. *Cluster A* includes the paranoid, schizoid, and schizotypal personality disorders. Individuals with these disorders often appear "odd" or "eccentric." *Cluster B* includes the antisocial, borderline, histrionic, and narcissistic personality disorders. These individuals often appear dramatic, emotional, or erratic. *Cluster C* includes the avoidant, dependent, and obsessive-compulsive personalities. These patients exhibit fear and anxiety.

Individuals with personality disorders do not see their behavior as problematic because of the minimal personal distress associated with the disorder. Many lead normal lives but encounter problems when the personality traits "just below the surface" begin to emerge.

CLUSTER A: DISORDERS OF ODD OR ECCENTRIC BEHAVIOR

Paranoid Personality Disorder

People with **paranoid personality disorder** exhibit unwarranted sensitivity, suspiciousness, envy, and mistrust of others. They show a limited range of emotions and avoid intimacy in interpersonal relationships. These people rarely seek help because of their suspicious nature and thoughts that others' motives are malevolent.[9,37]

Schizoid Personality Disorder

Persons with **schizoid personality disorder** display a marked indifference to the development of interpersonal relationships. They are rarely involved in social events and appear aloof and disinterested in others (i.e., "loners").[9,37]

Schizotypal Personality Disorder

A person with **schizotypal personality disorder** exhibits acute discomfort in close interpersonal relationships and behaves in an eccentric manner.[9,37]

CLUSTER B: DISORDERS OF DRAMATIC, EMOTIONAL, OR ERRATIC BEHAVIOR

Antisocial Personality Disorder

People with **antisocial personality disorder** usually have a history of lying, fighting, stealing, and irresponsibility. They demonstrate a pattern of disregard for the rights of others and manifest impulsive tendencies with little concern of the consequences. These patients seldom seek treatment unless forced to do so, often through the court system, and treatment is often unsuccessful.[9,11,26,37]

Histrionic Personality Disorder

Patients with **histrionic personality disorder** tend to be overdramatic and want to draw attention to themselves and be the center of attention. They have difficulty forming intimate interpersonal relationships but tend to be dependent on others. They often overreact to small matters and seek excitement.[9,11,26,37]

Narcissistic Personality Disorder

People with **narcissistic personality disorder** exhibit a sense of grandiosity and consistent need for admiration. They believe they are superior or unique and are entitled to special treatment, and they expect others to recognize this status. They often believe that they should associate only with people of this same status. Their self-esteem is very fragile, and they are preoccupied with how others view them. They often display great charm and the desire to be pampered. Narcissistic individuals become furious when they do not receive this expected attention. They typically exploit others and display a lack of sensitivity to the needs of others. Those who try to develop close interpersonal relationships with these narcissistic persons are often met with emotional coldness and a lack of reciprocal interest. Disordered narcissists believe that others are envious of them and commonly display arrogant and haughty behaviors (Box 45-12).

Narcissistic traits during adolescence are not necessarily predictive of later narcissistic personality disorder. Men represent 50% to 75% of those diagnosed with this disorder, and less than 1% of the general population is affected. Many highly successful people exhibit narcissistic personality traits, but the diagnosis of narcissistic personality disorder is made only when these traits are inflexible and cause significant impairment or distress.[9,11,26,37]

BOX 45-12

DSM-IV-TR DIAGNOSTIC CRITERIA FOR NARCISSISTIC PERSONALITY DISORDER

A pervasive pattern of grandiosity (in fantasy or behavior), need for admiration, and lack of empathy, beginning in early adulthood and present in a variety of contexts, as indicated by five or more of the following problems:
1. Grandiose sense of self-importance
2. Preoccupation with fantasies of unlimited success, power, brilliance, beauty, or ideal love
3. Belief that he or she is "special" and unique and can be understood only by, or should associate only with, other special or high-status people (or institutions)
4. Need for excessive admiration
5. Sense of entitlement
6. Interpersonally exploitative
7. Lack of empathy
8. Arrogant, haughty behaviors or attitudes

Modified from *Diagnostic and statistical manual of mental disorders (DSM-IV-TR)*, ed 4 (text revision), Washington, DC, 2000, American Psychiatric Association.

CLUSTER C: DISORDERS INVOLVING ANXIETY AND FEARFULNESS

Avoidant Personality Disorder

Patients with **avoidant personality disorder** exhibit a pattern of social inhibition and lack self-esteem. They are afraid that others will criticize their performance or person. These traits are present by early adulthood and cause problems in various situations (Box 45-13). Unlike the schizoid personality, the avoidant personality does *not* want to be alone and wants to enter into social relationships but avoids them because of the fear of failure.[9,11,26,37]

BOX 45-13

DSM-IV-TR DIAGNOSTIC CRITERIA FOR AVOIDANT PERSONALITY DISORDER

A pervasive pattern of social inhibition, feelings of inadequacy, and hypersensitivity to negative evaluation, characterized by four or more of the following problems:
1. Avoids occupational activities that involve significant interpersonal contact because of fears of criticism, disapproval, or rejection
2. Is unwilling to become involved with people unless certain of being liked
3. Shows restraint within intimate relationships because of fear of being shamed or ridiculed
4. Is preoccupied with being criticized or rejected in social situations
5. Inhibited in new interpersonal situations because of feelings of inadequacy
6. Views self as socially inept, personally unappealing, or inferior to others
7. Is unusually reluctant to take personal risks or to engage in any new activities because they may prove embarrassing

Modified from *Diagnostic and statistical manual of mental disorders (DSM-IV-TR)*, ed 4 (text revision), Washington, DC, 2000, American Psychiatric Association.

Dependent Personality Disorder

Persons with **dependent personality disorder** display a "pervasive and excessive need to be taken care of that leads to submission and clinging behavior and fears of separation."[9]

Anger at those they depend on for support is not expressed because of their extreme fear of alienating them. Individuals with this disorder often belittle themselves and their abilities and take criticism as proof of their worthlessness. The initiation of a project is unthinkable because of their lack of self-confidence, and they often present themselves as incompetent. They will make extraordinary self-sacrifices or tolerate verbal, physical, or sexual abuse to maintain an important relationship[9,11,26,37] (Box 45-14).

BOX 45-14

DSM-IV-TR DIAGNOSTIC CRITERIA FOR DEPENDENT PERSONALITY DISORDER

Dependent personality disorder is a pervasive and excessive need to be taken care of, beginning in early adulthood and indicated by five or more of the following problems:

1. Has difficulty making everyday decisions without excessive advice from others
2. Needs others to assume responsibility for most major areas of life
3. Has difficulty expressing disagreement with others because of fear of loss of approval
4. Has difficulty initiating projects or doing things on own
5. Goes to excessive lengths to obtain nurturance and support from others
6. Feels uncomfortable when alone because of fear of being unable to care for self
7. Urgently seeks another relationship as source of support when a close relationship ends
8. Unrealistically preoccupied with fears of being left to care for self

Modified from *Diagnostic and statistical manual of mental disorders (DSM-IV-TR)*, ed 4 (text revision), Washington, DC, 2000, American Psychiatric Association.

BOX 45-15

DSM-IV-TR DIAGNOSTIC CRITERIA FOR OBSESSIVE-COMPULSIVE PERSONALITY DISORDER

Obsessive-compulsive personality disorder is a pervasive pattern of preoccupation with orderliness, perfectionism, and mental and interpersonal control, beginning by early adulthood and indicated by four or more of the following problems:

1. Preoccupation with details, rules, lists, order, organization, or schedules to the extent that the major point of the activity is lost
2. Perfectionism that interferes with task completion
3. Excessive devotion to work and productivity to the exclusion of leisure activities and friendships
4. Overconscientiousness, scrupulousness, and inflexibility about matters of morality, ethics, or values
5. Inability to discard worn-out or worthless objects, even when they have no sentimental value
6. Reluctance to delegate tasks or to work with others unless they submit to his or her rules
7. Adoption of a miserly spending style toward self and others; money hoarded for future catastrophes
8. Rigidity and stubbornness

Modified from *Diagnostic and statistical manual of mental disorders (DSM-IV-TR)*, ed 4 (text revision), Washington, DC, 2000, American Psychiatric Association.

Cultural factors should be considered because some cultures emphasize passivity, politeness, and respectfulness, which may be misinterpreted as traits of dependent personality disorder.

Obsessive-Compulsive Personality Disorder

Persons with obsessive-compulsive personality disorder display "a preoccupation with orderliness, perfectionism, and mental and interpersonal control, at the expense of flexibility, openness, and efficiency."[9] Estimates put the prevalence of obsessive-compulsive personality disorder at approximately 1% of the U.S. population.

People with obsessive-compulsive personality disorder have a need to control and will do so through inordinate attention to details, procedures, lists, or rules to the extent that an important project may never be completed (Box 45-15). They check repeatedly for mistakes, then check again. Perfectionism causes these individuals great distress, because they can never attain their unreasonably high standards.[9,11,26,37]

TREATMENT

Personality disorders are one of the more perplexing groups of mental disorders to treat. These patients rarely appear for treatment of their own volition and are unable to form long-term, stable relationships, such as that needed for successful psychotherapy. They tend to be unaware of their problem. These patients also usually have a coexisting axis I disorder, making it difficult to separate the two in terms of treatment planning.[11,26,37]

Eating Disorders

Dieting is an American obsession, with more than 90 million people in the United States striving to reach their "ideal" weight. Approximately one third of the U.S. population (and increasing) is obese, but these individuals choose weight-loss measures that can be life-threatening. Eating disorders, or their recognition, is a rather recent concern, with few references in the literature before 1960. The increased prevalence of eating disorders in recent decades may be explained by beauty being increasingly equated with thinness, particularly in Western cultures. These disorders are most common in the United States, Canada, Europe, Australia, Japan, New Zealand, and South Africa. In third-world countries, larger body size is seen as beauty and a sign of success.[9,37]

Only anorexia nervosa and bulimia are designated in the *DSM-IV-TR*. However, binge eating is included in "eating disorders otherwise not determined," a classification that includes a number of proposed new categories and disorders.

The cause of eating disorders is not clear but is likely the result of a combination of biological, psychologic, and societal factors. Some suspect a physiologic cause such as a chemical imbalance in the hypothalamus or pituitary gland. Psychologists hypothesize that causes include the societal value on thinness and a negative view of obesity. Others maintain that overly critical parents and the demand for perfectionism in many performance areas lead to eating disorders.[9,11,26,37]

ANOREXIA NERVOSA

Persons with **anorexia nervosa** refuse to maintain a minimal normal weight for their age and height. Anorexia can lead to a life-threatening medical condition. Patients are obsessively concerned with being thin, are intensely afraid of gaining weight, and have a distorted perception of the size and shape of their body (Box 45-16). This disorder is found primarily in women (90%) between the ages of 12 and 40 years. Researchers estimate that 15% to 20% of anorexic persons literally starve themselves to death. Death occurs most often from starvation, suicide, or electrolyte imbalance.[9,11,31,36-37]

Weight loss is attained primarily through the reduction of food intake, with persons initially excluding foods that they consider to be highly caloric. As they lose weight, the fear of weight gain often intensifies. Their self-esteem is highly dependent on their perception of body size and shape. Weight loss is seen as a significant achievement and weight gain as failure. Individuals with this disorder seldom seek treatment because they lack insight or practice denial. Many exhibit coexisting symptoms of OCD and are often preoccupied with thoughts of food. Many individuals with anorexia nervosa exhibit depressive symptoms (e.g., social withdrawal, insomnia, depressed mood) that may meet the diagnostic criteria for major depressive disorder. Other features include a strong need to control one's environment, perfectionism, restrained emotional affect, concerns about eating in public, and inflexible thinking.[9,11,26,37]

During an episode of anorexia nervosa, one of two subtypes can be used in the development of an appropriate treatment plan (see Box 45-16). The *restricting type* describes weight loss accomplished primarily through dieting, fasting, or excessive exercise; in the current episode the patient has not regularly engaged in binge eating or purging. The *binge eating-purging type* describes the individual who regularly engages in binge eating, purging, or both. Most bingers with anorexia practice self-induced vomiting and misuse laxatives or diuretics. Recovering from anorexia nervosa is possible, but some individuals struggle with their fluctuating weight and the resulting deterioration of their health over the course of many years.

BULIMIA NERVOSA

Bulimia nervosa is an eating disorder characterized by repeated episodes of eating abnormally large amounts of food in a short period, often followed by purging. Similar to anorexia nervosa, individuals diagnosed with bulimia nervosa are typically within the normal weight and height range for their age group. This problem usually develops in adolescence or early adulthood. In contrast to the anorexic person, who takes pride in demonstrating self-control, a person who suffers from bulimia feels out of control and ashamed. Bulimia nervosa occurs rarely among moderately or morbidly obese individuals. With both disorders, patients place extraordinary emphasis on body shape and size to determine self-worth and self-esteem.[9,37]

Bulimia is characterized by repeated binge eating episodes followed by extreme efforts to avoid weight gain (Box 45-17). A *binge* is defined as "eating in a discrete period of time an amount of food that is definitely larger than most individuals would eat under similar circumstances."[9] A gallon of ice cream or a whole pie may be consumed at one time, followed by feelings of guilt and depression. Binge eating usually takes place in secrecy, is characterized by rapid consumption, and may or may not be planned. Binge eating episodes are usually triggered by some interpersonal stressor; hunger after a period of fasting; a depressed mood; or unresolved conflicts about body shape,

---

BOX 45-16

DSM-IV-TR DIAGNOSTIC CRITERIA FOR AND TYPES OF ANOREXIA NERVOSA

Criteria
1. Refusal to maintain body weight at or above a minimally normal weight for age and height
2. Intense fear of gaining weight or becoming fat, even though underweight
3. Disturbance in how body weight or shape is experienced, undue influence of body weight or shape on self-evaluation, or denial of the seriousness of the current low body weight
4. In women, absence of at least three consecutive menstrual cycles

Types
1. Restricting: During current episode the person has not regularly engaged in binge eating-purging behavior.
2. Binge eating and purging: During current episode the person has regularly engaged in binge eating or purging.

Modified from *Diagnostic and statistical manual of mental disorders (DSM-IV-TR)*, ed 4 (text revision), Washington, DC, 2000, American Psychiatric Association.

BOX 45-17

DSM-IV-TR DIAGNOSTIC CRITERIA FOR BULIMIA NERVOSA

1. Recurrent episodes of binge eating, as evidenced by the following behaviors:
   a. Eating an amount of food that is definitely larger than most people would eat during a similar period under similar circumstances
   b. Lacking a sense of control over eating during the episode
2. Recurrent inappropriate compensatory behavior to prevent weight gain, such as self-induced vomiting; misuse of laxatives, diuretics, and enemas; fasting; or excessive exercising
3. Binge eating and inappropriate compensatory behaviors at least twice a week for 3 months on average
4. Self-evaluation unduly influenced by body shape and weight
5. Disturbance not occurring exclusively during episodes of anorexia nervosa

Modified from *Diagnostic and statistical manual of mental disorders (DSM-IV-TR)*, ed 4 (text revision), Washington, DC, 2000, American Psychiatric Association.

weight, and size. Bulimic persons may then induce vomiting or take laxatives to rid themselves of the food, a behavior known as *purging*. Vomiting is the most common method used, as practiced by 80% to 90% of bulimic individuals. They use a number of different methods to induce vomiting, such as fingers or instruments to induce their gag reflex. Over time they are able to vomit at will.[9,11,26,37]

The cause of bulimia appears to be both biological and psychologic. Biologically, a chemical imbalance may exist in the hypothalamus or pituitary gland. Bulimic persons may not feel "full" after they have eaten or even binged, which results from a low level of specific hormones that control the feeling of satiety. Psychologically, societal pressures value slenderness, and a negative stigma is associated with obesity. A separate hypothesis suggests that both anorexia nervosa and bulimia are the result of a rigid, rule-governed parental style. Bulimic patients have often experienced an unreasonable amount of rejection and blame during childhood and an inordinate need to strive for perfection to gain positive regard from important figures in their lives.[9,11,26,37]

Two subtypes distinguish bulimia nervosa. Characteristically, the patient with the *purging subtype* is described as "an individual that engages in self-induced vomiting and/or the misuse of laxatives, diuretics, or enemas during the current episode."[9] The *nonpurging subtype* describes the person who uses other methods of inappropriate compensation for the act of overeating; a passive example is fasting, whereas an aggressive method is excessive exercising. Individuals with purging bulimia are more likely to exhibit symptoms of depression and greater preoccupation with body shape and size than individuals with nonpurging bulimia.[9,37]

Individuals with bulimia exhibit an increased frequency of depression and lack of self-esteem. Anxiety disorders are likely to coexist, and at least 30% of these individuals experience a substance-abuse problem. Substance abuse usually stems from initial use of stimulants to control appetite.

DENTAL CONSIDERATIONS

The oral health of patients with bulimia is known to be at risk from the damaging effect on the enamel structure from the intensified acid challenge from regurgitation of gastric contents (Figure 45-1).

Low, unstimulated salivary flow rates and very high counts of *mutans streptococci* and lactobacilli lead to high susceptibility to both dental caries and enamel erosion in patients with diagnosed eating disorders. A significant correlation exists between parotid enlargement and enamel erosion in bulimic patients. Painless enlargement of the parotid salivary glands is common with chronic vomiting. Salivary gland impairment, poor oral hygiene, and poor diet adversely affect dental health.*

Because eating disorders have long-term health effects and can be life-threatening, the manner in which these

*References 29, 31, 36, 41, 51.

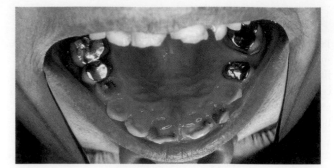

FIGURE 45-1
Tooth erosion caused by bulimia. (From Ibsen OAC, Phelan JA: *Oral pathology for the dental hygienist,* ed 4, St Louis, 2004, Saunders.)

matters are handled can make a significant difference in its outcome. The dental professional who approaches the situation with great sensitivity for the patient and recognizes that intervention is in that patient's best interest can help enable the patient to get the necessary help.

Prevention

Often, generalized destruction of tooth structure directly results from highly acidic stomach contents on the patient's dentition. The damage that follows the binge-and-purge episodes is reduced by meticulous oral hygiene measures, including regular use of fluoride products.

Distinct Care Modifications

- The dental professional is in a unique position among healthcare professionals in identifying patients with eating disorders (because the oral cavity is often a diagnostic feature of the problem).
- Questions regarding diet, eating habits, and exercise may help uncover patterns of an eating disorder.
- If a patient is younger than 18 years of age, then the matter can become a legal and ethical one. In such a case, the dental professional becomes responsible for cautiously advising the parent or legal guardian.

Patient Education Opportunity

The clinician should show the patient any signs of enamel erosion likely caused by bulimic behavior and explain how that process takes place.

Schizophrenia

People with schizophrenia make up most of the patients hospitalized for a mental disorder. A patient with schizophrenia has a mixed set of characteristic symptoms, such as **delusions, hallucinations,** and thought disturbances (Box 45-18). These distortions in thinking, perception, and emotion are often

DSM-IV-TR DIAGNOSTIC CRITERIA FOR SCHIZOPHRENIA

1. Two or more of the following symptoms for at least 1 month:
   • Delusions
   • Hallucinations
   • Disorganized speech
   • Grossly disorganized or catatonic behavior
   • Negative symptoms (e.g., flattened affect, reduced speech)
2. Duration—The patient has shown evidence of the disorder for at least 6 months.
3. Social and occupational dysfunction—The patient has significantly impaired ability to work, study, socialize, or provide self-care.
4. Substance abuse or general medical condition exclusion
5. Schizoaffective or mood disorder exclusion
6. Relationship to a developmental order exclusion

Modified from *Diagnostic and statistical manual of mental disorders (DSM-IV-TR),* ed 4 (text revision), Washington, DC, 2000, American Psychiatric Association.

Table 45-4	Major Types of Schizophrenia
TYPE	**SYMPTOMS**
Disorganized	• Inappropriate laughter and giggling • Silliness • Incoherent speech • Infantile behavior • Strange and sometimes obscene behavior
Paranoid	• Delusions and hallucinations of persecution or of greatness • Loss of judgment • Erratic and unpredictable behavior
Catatonic	• Major disturbances in movement • In some phases, loss of all motion, with patient frozen in a single position and remaining that way for hours or even days • In other phases, hyperactivity and wild, sometimes violent, movement
Undifferentiated	• Variable mixture of major symptoms of schizophrenia • Classification used for patients who cannot be typed into any of the more-specific categories
Residual	• Minor signs of schizophrenia after more serious episode

Modified from Feldman RS: *Understanding psychology,* New York, 1996, McGraw-Hill.

accompanied by social withdrawal and bizarre behavior. Schizophrenia involves a reduced level of functioning in one or more major areas of life, such as work, interpersonal relations, education, and self-care. Probably the most distressing symptom of the disorder is the person's feeling of being out of control regarding thoughts and actions. Along with the dramatic (positive) symptoms are the less dramatic (negative) symptoms, including a flattened affect or apparent absence of emotional expression. Individuals with schizophrenia have poor insight into their illness, which itself is a manifestation of the disorder.[9,11,26,37]

TYPES AND ONSET

The five types of schizophrenia are (1) catatonic, (2) disorganized, (3) paranoid, (4) undifferentiated, and (5) residual[9] (Table 45-4).

Two primary time frames exist for the onset of schizophrenia. In **process schizophrenia** the symptoms begin to develop early in life, with subtle changes becoming more pronounced over time. In **reactive schizophrenia** the onset is dramatic and sudden. Reactive schizophrenia has been shown to respond to treatment more favorably and with a better long-term prognosis than process schizophrenia.[11,26,37,38]

The pattern to the onset of schizophrenia is (1) predromal, (2) active, and (3) residual. The active phase is characterized by either positive or negative symptoms. Positive symptoms include delusions, hallucinations, disorganized speech, catatonia, and disorganized or bizarre behavior. Negative symptoms include flattened or blunted emotions, lack of initiative toward goal-directed behaviors, limited or no verbal communication, and no satisfaction from previously pleasurable activities. The negative symptoms are often difficult to judge because they occur on a continuum and can be attributed to many other factors (e.g., side effect of medication, depression, situational stress).[9,11,26,37]

Schizophrenia is also categorized into positive and negative symptoms. *Negative-symptom schizophrenia* is characterized by a significant reduction in level of functioning, social withdrawal, and a flattened emotional affect. The patient with *positive-symptom schizophrenia* has delusions, hallucinations, and extremes in emotional display.[9,37]

The schizophrenic patient demonstrates an obvious deterioration of functioning in the student, employee, or parent-homemaker role. Disturbances of thought and language are also noted.[9,37]

DELUSIONS

Delusions are bizarre beliefs in spite of their preposterous nature. These patients hold strongly to their beliefs, even when presented with overwhelming evidence to the contrary. They are preoccupied with thoughts about their delusional beliefs during the active phase of the condition. Common delusions include the belief that thoughts are being inserted into one's mind, people are reading the patient's mind, and external forces are exerting control over thoughts and actions.[9,37]

HALLUCINATIONS

Hallucination is defined as "false sensory perception in the absence of an actual external stimulus."[9] Auditory hallucinations are the most common and are most often experienced as voices giving instructions or commenting on behavior. Although these experiences are often frightening to the patient, they may also provide a sense of security and comfort. Hallucinations are very real to the person and persist over time, despite having no basis in reality.[9,37]

DISORGANIZED THINKING

The characteristic of **disorganized thinking** may be the most important diagnostic criterion for schizophrenia. It involves the tendency of a person to say things that make no sense or that are so incoherent that they are regarded as "word salad." Patients with disorganized thinking also tend to answer questions in a very tangential manner and frequently and abruptly shift topics, referred to as *derailment* or *loose associations*.[9,37]

GROSSLY DISORGANIZED BEHAVIOR

Individuals with schizophrenia may have difficulty in daily living activities, such as preparing meals or attending to personal hygiene. They may dress inappropriately for the weather. Aggressive behaviors such as shouting and swearing often occur without external stimulus.[9,37]

CATATONIC BEHAVIOR

Catatonic behavior is seen as an extreme degree of maintaining a rigid posture and resisting efforts to be moved. The other extreme is seen as excessive activity. Catatonic behavior is not specific to schizophrenia and may be seen with other mental disorders.[9,37]

TREATMENT

Neuroleptic Drugs

The most troublesome side effects are called *extrapyramidal symptoms,* including muscular rigidity, tremors, restlessness and agitation, and peculiar postures. Long-term treatment with **neuroleptic** drugs often leads to the development of tardive dyskinesia (TD), which is characterized by involuntary, grotesque movements of the mouth and spasmodic movements of the extremities. This distressing problem is frequently irreversible even after discontinuation of the medication. The incidence of TD increases with length of time taking the medication, with 25% of patients developing the syndrome within 3 months of treatment.[2]

If medication is not continued after recovery from the acute psychotic episode, then as many as 75% of patients will experience another psychotic episode within the first year. Although the continued use of the neuroleptic medication cannot prevent a relapse, it can reduce the recurrence by approximately 60%. Some patients can function at least as well without medication as when taking medication. The difficulty is an inability to distinguish those who *do* from those who *do not* need the continued pharmacologic treatment. Some clinicians choose to prescribe lower doses of neuroleptics to patients with schizophrenia to minimize the potential side effects. Positive aspects of this approach include less-blunted affect, better social psychosocial functioning, and less unusual movement or motor behavior.[37]

Newer forms of antipsychotic medications, known as *atypical antipsychotics,* do not produce extrapyramidal symptoms or TD. These drugs have also proven especially useful for patients who do not respond to the classic neuroleptics, with up to 60% of previous nonresponders showing improvement.

In addition to pharmacologic therapy, psychosocial treatments have been developed for individuals with schizophrenia, including family-oriented aftercare, social skills training, and institutional programs. The aftercare focuses on improving the family's coping skills. Education is probably the most important aspect; the family is informed about what to expect and educated about the nature of the disease. This enables the patient to remain in the home on an outpatient basis and may reduce relapse rates to approximately 20%, compared with 40% of patients not receiving family-oriented aftercare.

Many patients continue to have impaired social and interpersonal skills even when receiving medication. To address these problems, social skills training focuses on role-playing, role-modeling, and reinforcement or social reinforcement for appropriate behaviors. Few data demonstrate improved social adjustment with this approach. In addition to outpatient programs, various types of institutional care continue to be important for the patient with schizophrenia. Most patients experience recurrent phases of the disorder, and brief periods of hospitalization are often beneficial. Some individuals, however, are significantly disturbed and require long-term institutionalized care. Programs are available that reward patients for demonstrating desired behaviors (e.g., grooming, general social courtesies) in an effort to decrease undesirable behaviors (e.g., violence). These positive behaviors are then rewarded with tokens, which can be exchanged for food or privileges. Positive behaviors are rewarded, but inappropriate behaviors are largely ignored. This aspect of treatment has shown outstanding results.[11,26,37]

Schizophrenia affects many areas of a person's ability to function, including cognitive and perceptual, so a multifaceted approach to treatment is required.

Prevention
Caution must be used when working with schizophrenic patients because the potential exists for them to have nonprovoked violent outbursts.

Distinct Care Modifications
- Use of colorful educational materials often helps stimulate and hold these patients' attention.
- Demonstrations of brushing and flossing instructions in front of a mirror may prove helpful.
- Because these patients often have difficulty following the most basic verbal instructions, it may also be helpful for clinicians to demonstrate tasks on themselves.[21,43]

DENTAL CONSIDERATIONS

In providing dental care to schizophrenic patients, the clinician must be aware of the need to alter and adjust treatment approaches for patients who have impaired an ability to think logically. The dental practitioner must also consider the side effects of neuroleptics and the potential for ad verse interactions between medications for schizophrenia and drugs used in dental treatment. These patients often have significant oral disease. A reduced ability to perform adequate self-care is often associated schizophrenia, including preventive oral care. The neuroleptic medications used to treat and maintain these patients may cause bizarre body movements, often in the orofacial region. These spasms can cause the dislocation of the temporomandibular joint, cause difficulty in swallowing, dislodge dentures, and interfere with the natural gag reflex.[2,8] The medications to treat schizophrenia also reduce saliva, resulting in xerostomia. This reduced salivary flow increases the risk of periodontal disease and the onset of rapidly progressive dental caries activity.*

In providing dental treatment to schizophrenic patients, preventive health education is extremely important. Many of these patients, however, do not have the inclination or coordination for routine oral hygiene.

---

*References 1, 4, 8, 16, 17, 21, 48.

References

1. American Dental Association, Council on Scientific Affairs: *American Dental Association guide to dental therapeutics,* Chicago, 1998, ADA Publishing (edited by S Ciancio).
2. Bassett A, Remick RA, Blasberg B: Tardive dyskinesia: an unrecognized cause of orofacial pain, *Oral Surg Oral Med Oral Pathol* 61:570-572, 1986.
3. Beck FM, Kaul TJ: Recognition and management of the depressed dental patient, *J Am Dent Assoc* 99:967-971, 1979.
4. Ben-Aryeh H et al: Salivary flow-rate and composition in schizophrenic patients on clozapine: subjective reports and laboratory data, *Biol Psychiatry* 39:946-949, 1996.
5. Bertram U et al: Saliva secretion following long-term antidepressant treatment with nortriptyline controlled by plasma levels, *Scand J Dent Res* 87:58-64, 1979.
6. Blazer D, Hughes D, George LK: Stressful life events and the onset of a generalized anxiety syndrome, *Am J Psychiatry* 144(9):1178-1183, 1987.
7. Bohn DJ et al: Clonazepam in the treatment of social phobia: a pilot study, *J Clin Psychiatry* 51(5):35-40, 1990.
8. Craig TJ et al: Impairment of the gag reflex in schizophrenia, *Compr Psychiatry* 24:514-520, 1983.
9. *Diagnostic and statistical manual of mental disorders (DSM-IV-TR),* ed 4 (text revision), Washington, DC, 2000, American Psychiatric Association.
10. Doebling S, Rowe MM: Negative perceptions of dental stimuli and their effects on dental fear, *J Dent Hyg* 74(2):110-116, 2000.
11. Feldman RS: *Understanding psychology,* New York, 1996, McGraw-Hill.
12. Findlay-Jones R, Brown GW: Types of stressful life events and the onset of anxiety and depressive disorder, *Psychol Med* 11(4): 803-815, 1981.
13. Fox PC et al: Xerostomia: evaluation of a symptom with increasing significance, *J Am Dent Assoc* 110:519-525, 1985.
14. Friedlander AH, Birch NJ: Dental conditions in patients with bipolar disorder on long-term lithium maintenance therapy, *Spec Care Dentist* 10(5):148-151, 1990.
15. Friedlander AH, Eth S: Dental management considerations in children with obsessive-compulsive disorder, *ASDC J Dent Child* 58(3):217-222, 1991.
16. Friedlander AH, Liberman RP: Oral health care for the patient with schizophrenia, *Spec Care Dentist* 11(5):179-183, 1991.
17. Friedlander AH, Mahler ME: Major depressive disorder: psychopathology, medical management and dental implications, *J Am Dent Assoc* 132(5):629-638, 2001.
18. Friedlander AH, Mills MJ, Wittlin BJ: Dental management considerations for the patients with post-traumatic stress disorder, *Oral Surg Oral Med Oral Pathol* 63(6):669-673, 1987.
19. Friedlander AH, Serafetinides EA: Dental management of the patient with obsessive-compulsive disorder, *Spec Care Dentist* 11(6):238-242, 1991.
20. Friedlander AH, West LJ: Dental management of the patient with major depression, *Oral Surg Oral Med Oral Pathol* 71(5):573-578, 1991.
21. Friedlander AH et al: Dental management of child and adolescent patients with schizophrenia, *ASDC J Dent Child* 60(4):281-287, 1993.
22. Friedlander AH et al: Dental management of the adolescent with panic disorder, *ASDC J Dent Child* 60(4):365-371, 1993.
23. Friedlander AH et al: Dental management of the child and adolescent with major depression, *J Dent Child* 60(2):125-131, 1993.
24. Friedlander AH et al: Dental management of the geriatric patient with major depression, *Spec Care Dentist* 13(6):249-523, 1993.
25. Gage TW, Pickett FA: *Mosby's dental drug reference,* ed 7, St Louis, 2005, Mosby.
26. Gerow JR: *Psychology: an introduction,* ed 3, New York, 1992, HarperCollins.
27. Greenberg PE et al: Depression: a neglected major illness, *J Clin Psychiatry* 54(11):425-426, 1993.
28. Haverman CW, Redding SW: Dental management and treatment of xerostomic patients, *Tex Dent J* June:43-56, 1998.
29. Hellstrom L: Oral complications in anorexia nervosa, *Scand J Dent Res* 85(1):71-86, 1977.
30. Hetherington EM, Parke RD: *Child psychology: a contemporary viewpoint,* New York, 1993, McGraw-Hill.
31. Jensen OE, Featherstone JD, Stege P: Chemical and physical oral findings of anorexia nervosa and bulimia, *J Oral Pathol* 16(8): 399-402, 1987.
32. Little JW, Falace DA: *Dental management of the medically compromised patient,* cd 6, St Louis, 2002, Mosby.
33. Mauro V, Mendloiwuez MV, Stein MB: Quality of life in individuals with anxiety disorders, *Am J Psychiatry* 157:669-682, 2000.
34. McGrath E et al: *Women and depression: risk factors and treatment issues,* Washington, DC, 1990, American Psychological Association.
35. Monroe SM, Simons AD: Diathesis-stress theories in the context of life stress research: implications for depressive disorders, *Psychol Bull* 11(3):406-425, 1991.

36. Ohrn R, Eazeil K, Angmar-Mansson B: Oral status of 81 subjects with eating disorders, *Eur J Oral Sci* 107(3):157-163, 1999.

37. Oltman FO, Emery RE: *Abnormal psychology,* Princeton, NJ, 1995, Prentice Hall.

38. Onstad S et al: Subtypes of schizophrenia: evidence from a twin-family study, *Acta Psychiatr Scand* 84(2):203-206, 1991.

39. Peeters FP, deVries MW, Vissink A: Risks for oral health with the use of antidepressants, *Gen Hosp Psychiatry* 20:150-154, 1998.

40. Reiger DA et al: One-month prevalence of mental disorders in the United States, based on five epidemiologic catchment area sites, *Arch Gen Psychiatry* 45(11):977-986, 1988.

41. Roberts MW, Tylenda CA: Dental aspects of anorexia and bulimia nervosa, *Pediatrician* 16:178-184, 1989.

42. Rundegren J et al: Oral conditions in patients receiving long-term treatment with cyclic antidepressant drugs, *Swed Dent J* 9:55-64, 1985.

43. Shuman SK, Bebeau MJ: Ethical and legal issues in special patient care, *Dent Clin North Am* 38(3):553-575, 1994.

44. Simons AD et al: Toward an integration of psychologic, social and biologic factors in depression effects on outcome and course of cognitive therapy, *J Consult Clin Psychol* 63(3):369-377, 1995.

45. Slome BA: Rampant caries: a side effect of tricyclic antidepressant therapy, *Gen Dent* Nov-Dec:494-496, 1987.

46. Sullivan MJ, Neish N: Catastrophic thinking and the experience of pain during dental procedures, *J Indiana Dent Assoc* 79(4): 16-19, 2001.

47. Sullivan MJ, Neish NR: Psychological predictors of pain during dental hygiene treatment, *Probe* 31(4):123-126, 1997.

48. Thomas A et al: Factors which influence the oral condition of chronic schizophrenia patients, *Spec Care Dentist* 15(2):84-86, 1996.

49. Watson JB, Raynor R: Conditioned emotional reactions, *J Exp Psychol* 3:1-14, 1920.

50. Weisman MM: The changing rates of major depression: cross-national comparisons, *JAMA* 268(21):3098-3105, 1992.

51. Wolcott RB, Yager J, Gordon G: Dental sequelae to the binge-purge syndrome (bulimia): report of cases, *J Am Dent Assoc* 109(5):723-725, 1984.

52. Woodall IJ: *Comprehensive dental hygiene care,* ed 4, St Louis, 1993, Mosby.

53. Wynn RL: New antidepressant medications, *Gen Dent* 45(1): 24-28, 1997.

Immune System Dysfunction

JoAnn R. Gurenlian • Ann Eshenaur Spolarich

INSIGHT

Autoimmune disorders primarily affect women, who often experience one or more of these conditions throughout their lives. Most autoimmune diseases are treated with steroids that pose significant long-term risks to the body, including adrenal suppression. Invasive dental procedures and stress increase the risk for adrenal crisis, and patients may require steroid supplementation as a part of a stress-reduction protocol. Most autoimmune diseases have oral manifestations that require dental hygiene intervention.

✸ CASE STUDY 46-1 Suspicious History of Autoimmune Disease

Sarah Jones is a 34-year-old black woman; she is a new patient and arrives at the clinic for routine dental hygiene treatment. Sarah is a data entry specialist and single mother of two young children. She states that she left her former dental office "because all they ever wanted to do was fill my teeth. I never had any cavities when I was growing up. Why would I have so many cavities now as an adult? Cavities are for kids. I think they were just in it for the money." Sarah tells the hygienist that she is interested in having her teeth cleaned and whitened.

The written medical history form suggests that the patient is in overall good health, with no significant major medical problems indicated. The patient reports taking oral contraceptives and ibuprofen. "My hands are always killing me from spending so much time on the computer, but the ibuprofen doesn't seem to work anymore." She tells you that she has scheduled an appointment with a dermatologist, because she has noticed a rash on her face that does not go away with use of an over-the-counter (OTC) hydrocortisone cream. "I figured that I

should get it checked out. Maybe he can give me something better to use." Other significant findings that emerge from the discussion about Sarah's health include a history of social smoking on weekends and a history of fatigue that increases by the end of the day. "I have a very hectic and demanding job, and two young children. It's probably normal to be this tired. After all, I am getting older."

A visual extraoral and intraoral examination reveals a rash on her face, which is bilateral on either side of the nose; dry patches of skin along the vermillion border of the lower lip; a red, fissured tongue; and dry, friable oral mucosa. The hygienist decides to refer the patient to her general physician for an evaluation before initiating dental hygiene treatment. What condition does the hygienist believe Sarah has? Will any medical tests be required before initiating dental hygiene treatment? How will this patient's medical condition be treated? Are there any important implications for dental hygiene case management that should be taken into consideration? What should the hygienist include in his or her plans for patient education and treatment?

KEY TERMS

acquired immunodeficiency
   syndrome
addisonian crisis
Addison's disease
adrenal crisis
agranulocytosis
allele
anemia
anterior uveitis
antibody
antigens
antiphospholipid antibody
   syndrome
autoantibodies
autoimmune diseases
casts
chronic fatigue syndrome
diabetes mellitus
diffuse scleroderma

discoid lupus
dysarthria
dyspareunia
dysphagia
exocrine gland
exophthalmos
fibromyalgia syndrome
glomerulonephritis
glossodynia
glucosuria
Graves' disease
Hashimoto's thyroiditis
human immunodeficiency virus
human leukocyte antigens
immunologic tolerance
interstitial nephritis
iridocyclitis
keratoconjunctivitis sicca
Libman-Sacks endocarditis

limited scleroderma
linear scleroderma
major histocompatibility complex
   genes
microstomia
monoclonality
monozygotic
morphea scleroderma
multiple sclerosis
myasthenia gravis
nocturia
oligoclonality
pannus
pernicious anemia
polyarthralgia
polydipsia
polyphagia
polyuria

pruritus
psoriasis
Raynaud's phenomenon
rheumatic heart disease
rheumatoid arthritis
scleroderma
secondary adrenal insufficiency
self-tolerance
sine scleroderma
Sjögren's syndrome
systemic lupus erythematosus
systemic scleroderma
telangiectasias
thrombocytopenia
thyrotoxic crisis
thyrotoxicosis
valvular insufficiency
vasculitis

LEARNING OUTCOMES

After reading this chapter the student will be able to:

1. Describe the pathophysiologic nature of immune system dysfunction.
2. Identify common signs and symptoms of various autoimmune diseases.
3. Discuss the classes of drugs that are frequently used to treat autoimmune diseases.
4. Identify oral manifestations of common autoimmune diseases.

5. Recognize the adverse oral complications associated with the classes of drugs used to treat autoimmune diseases.
6. Discuss the effects of chronic steroid use on the human body.
7. Describe risk-reduction strategies used in the dental office to prevent complications associated with adrenal suppression.
8. Implement dental hygiene management considerations for treating patients with autoimmune disease.

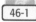

Understanding Immune System Dysfunction

The human immune system reacts to a wide variety of microorganisms, yet it does not react to one's own **antigens.** This ability to discriminate between one's own antigens and nonself (typically microbial) antigens is known as **immunologic tolerance.** Several mechanisms exist by which the immune system prevents immune reactions against self-antigens. When these mechanisms fail, activated T cells and antibodies attack the individual's own cells and tissues. These reactions are known as *autoimmunity,* and result in **autoimmune diseases.**[1]

Immunologic tolerance is "a lack of response to antigens that is induced by exposure of lymphocytes to these antigens."[1] When lymphocytes with receptors for a particular antigen encounter the antigen, one of three responses can occur. First, the lymphocytes may become activated and initiate an immune response. Second, the lymphocytes may be inactivated or killed, resulting in tolerance. Third, antigen-specific lymphocytes may not react at all (and ignore the antigen). The type of reaction is determined by both the nature of the antigen and lym-

phocyte, as well as how the antigen is presented to the immune system.[1]

Understanding how self-antigens induce tolerance is important, because these same mechanisms may be applied to interventions that prevent or control unwanted immune reactions. Methods based on this understanding have been developed to treat autoimmune diseases and allergic reactions, as well as to prevent organ rejection in transplant patients.

Researchers estimate that 2% of the population suffers from autoimmune disease, most of whom are women. Diseases associated with an uncontrolled autoimmune response are often labeled as *autoimmune diseases,* even when little evidence supports an effect on self-antigens.[1]

Two primary factors are necessary for the development of autoimmunity. First, an individual must inherit susceptibility genes that contribute to the failure of immunologic tolerance. Second, environmental triggers must be present to activate self-reactive lymphocytes. A common environmental trigger is infection.[1]

Although multiple genes predispose a person to autoimmune disease, the most important are **major histocompatibility complex** (MHC) **genes**—molecules that encode cytokines and are recognized by T lymphocytes for antigen processing. Many autoimmune diseases are linked to specific MHC alleles. An **allele** is one of several different forms of a gene present on a chromosome. Heterozygous individuals inherit two different alleles: one from the mother and one from the father. Thus the incidence of a particular autoimmune disease is usually greater in someone who inherits a particular allele when compared with others in the general population. This is evident in monozygotic-twin studies that show that when one twin develops an autoimmune disease the other is more likely to develop the same condition when compared with the general population.[1]

Human leukocyte antigens (HLAs) are MHC molecules expressed on the surface of human cells. Although inheriting an HLA allele increases the relative risk of developing an autoimmune disease, the HLA allele itself does not cause the disease; in fact, most will never develop the disease. MHC alleles contribute to the development of autoimmunity because they are inefficient at displaying self-antigens, resulting in defective T-cell response. Non-HLA genes are also associated with autoimmune disease, although their roles are not fully understood.[1]

The manifestation of many autoimmune diseases is often preceded by an infection. An infection triggers a local immune response, causing the release of cytokines and co-stimulators from antigen-presenting cells (APCs). APCs have MHC molecules on their surfaces and activate antigen-specific T cells. Costimulators are molecules necessary to optimally activate T lymphocytes. Tissue-activated APCs stimulate self-reactive T cells that produce an immune attack against self-antigens. Infections also injure tissues and release antigens that are not normally seen by the immune system or are ignored. The presence of these antigens can also initiate an autoimmune reaction.[1]

Antibodies that cause autoimmune diseases are usually **autoantibodies** against self-antigens and are not specific for foreign antigens (i.e., microorganisms). Production of these autoantibodies results from failure of **self-tolerance.** These antibodies bind to self-antigens in tissues or form immune complexes with circulating self-antigens. Bound antibodies deposit in tissues that express self-antigens, which is usually a specific tissue or organ. Conversely, immune complexes are typically deposited in blood vessels, resulting in systemic involvement, which manifests as **vasculitis** and joint and kidney damage.[1]

Autoantibodies can also cause disease without directly causing tissue injury. Some autoantibodies inhibit receptor function, as in **myasthenia gravis** (MG), where acetylcholine receptors (AChRs) are inhibited and neuromuscular transmission fails, causing paralysis. Other antibodies stimulate receptors that would normally be stimulated by a hormone. This is evident in hyperthyroidism, where antibodies against the thyroid-stimulating receptor stimulate thyroid cells directly.[1]

T cells mediate organ-specific autoimmune diseases. Treatment for these disorders is aimed at reducing inflammation with corticosteroids and antagonists to cytokines. Immunosuppressive drugs are used to inhibit T-cell responses and are indicated for many autoimmune conditions.[1] The following is a discussion of common autoimmune disorders and associated treatments, with recommendations for dental hygiene case management.

Sjögren's Syndrome

The triad of **keratoconjunctivitis sicca** (KCS), xerostomia, and a connective tissue disorder characterize **Sjögren's syndrome** (SS). It was first described in 1933 by the Swedish physician Henrik Sjögren. This autoimmune disorder manifests as a wide spectrum of severity and includes primary (SS-1) and secondary (SS-2) forms.

SS is the second most common rheumatologic disorder behind **systemic lupus erythematosus** (SLE). The prevalence of SS in the United States is estimated to be more than 4 million. The female-to-male ratio is 9:1, and the peak incidence occurs in the fourth and fifth decades of life.[59] Isolated cases of SS occurring in children and adolescents have been reported.[81,84,98]

PATHOGENESIS

SS-1 manifests as KCS and salivary gland dysfunction. SS-2 manifests as either KCS or xerostomia in the presence of a diagnosed systemic connective tissue disease.[93] Examples of connective tissue disorders associated with SS-2 include **rheumatoid arthritis** (RA), SLE, scleroderma, fibromyalgia, primary biliary cirrhosis, and **Raynaud's phenomenon.**[93,117] Approximately 15% of patients with rheumatoid arthritis have SS, and secondary SS may develop in 30% of patients with SLE.[79]

SS is characterized by **exocrine gland** dysfunction. Lacrimal glands produce a tear film that lubricates the eyes, whereas salivary glands produce saliva to lubricate the oral mucosa. These lubricants consist of a hydrated gel that contains mucins, water, proteins, and growth factors.[43]

Inadequate volume of tear film leads to keratoconjunctivitis, corneal abrasions, and corneal ulcerations. Salivary gland dysfunction causes xerostomia and enlargement of salivary glands. This enlargement is attributed to infiltrates of lymphocytes and plasma cells.[19] In addition, certain histocompatibility antigens are seen in SS; specifically, HLA-DRw52 is associated with both forms of the disease, and HLA-B8 and HLA-DR3 are seen frequently in SS-1.[79]

International diagnostic criteria are available to assist with diagnosis of the disease, which among others include measures of salivary gland inflammation and the presence of specific autoantibodies in the serum.[111] Biopsy of the labial minor salivary glands demonstrates characteristic focal lymphocytic infiltration.[20] Lymphocytic invasion causing local salivary tissue inflammation and fibrosis combined with autoimmune-mediated interference with neurotransmitter and receptor function appears to be responsible for the clinical manifestations of SS.[112] However, labial salivary gland biopsies taken from patients with severe oral and ocular dryness reveal that as many as 50% of their glandular cells remain intact.[31] This allows SS patients to benefit from saliva-stimulating medications.

Furthermore, chronic inflammation associated with SS can lead to **oligoclonality** (and in some cases **monoclonality**) B cells.[30,53,55] Individuals with SS who have B-cell monoclonality are at increased risk of developing non-Hodgkin's lymphoma.[30,53,73,79]

CLINICAL SIGNS AND SYMPTOMS

Patients with SS develop extraglandular symptoms that include skin changes and musculoskeletal complaints. Dryness, rashes, and Raynaud's phenomenon are common findings. Arthralgia, myalgia, and fatigue with an early onset of aggressive osteoarthritis of the hands and feet are associated with this condition. Common ocular changes in addition to those noted previously include a burning or foreign-body sensation in the eyes, with symptoms seemingly worse at the end of the day.

Internal organ involvement varies considerably in SS-2 and may include pneumonitis, polyneuropathies, **interstitial nephritis, glomerulonephritis,** and vasculitis in addition to the connective tissue disorders noted previously. Blood dyscrasias associated with SS include leukopenia, **thrombocytopenia,** and **anemia**. Individuals with SS have a higher frequency of hypothyroidism. A significant gynecologic problem is vaginal dryness. In pregnant women with SS, an increased risk of recurrent miscarriages or vascular thrombosis exists, and a higher frequency of a fetal complication of congenital heart block is seen.[43]

TREATMENT

Treatment for SS is supportive and focused on palliative measures. Salivary stimulation and replacement therapies are critical to improve patient comfort and function. Salivary stimulation can be achieved mechanically by chewing sugarless gum or sucking on sugarless candies and lozenges that contain xylitol. Sugarless chewing gum containing xylitol has the additional advantages of reducing dental plaque biofilm and dental caries risk.[16,34] Sonic toothbrushing has also been shown to mechanically increase salivary flow in patients with SS.[85]

Stimulation can also be achieved chemically by sucking on sugarless candies or products that contain citric acid, such as vitamin C tablets, sugarless lemon drops, or lozenges. However, caution must be used with citric acid–containing products because of potential adverse effects on tooth enamel.[80,103] Khurshudian reported that oral administration of 150 international units (IU) interferon-α lozenges three times daily improved salivary production and relieved symptoms of xerostomia and xerophthalmia in patients with primary SS. Although more clinical trials are needed, these lozenges appear to be safe and are well tolerated by patients.[57] As of this writing, this product is not available for use in the United States.

The best salivary replacement therapy is to keep the patient hydrated with water. Commercial artificial saliva is available OTC to replace that which is no longer naturally produced. These products contain carboxymethylcellulose to mimic the natural viscosity of saliva; sugar alcohols (e.g., xylitol, sorbitol) as flavoring agents; and parabens, which are preservatives that inhibit bacterial growth. These products provide only short-term relief of symptoms and are inconvenient to use, thus compliance tends to be very poor. Patients who are allergic to paraaminobenzoic acid (PABA) should not use these products.[66,103] Water-based moisturizing gels that can be applied both extraorally and intraorally are excellent artificial saliva products that also provide antimicrobial activity (Biotène Oral Balance gel, Rancho Dominguez, Calif.).

The U.S. Food and Drug Administration (FDA) has approved two cholinergic agonist medications for the treatment of SS: (1) pilocarpine (Salagen) and (2) cevimeline (Evoxac). Cholinergic agonists produce parasympathetic stimulation of the exocrine glands to increase serous secretions. An advantage of these systemic medications is that they stimulate all exocrine glands and relieve multiple symptoms of SS. Given these effects, the most notable adverse side effect is excessive sweating. Another disadvantage is that these drugs work only in patients who still have functional acinar tissue; in patients with extensive glandular destruction from the disease, these drugs may be of little benefit.

Pilocarpine is taken in 5-mg doses, three to four times per day. Efficacy has been established after 6 weeks of use, although the drug must often be taken for 90 days before seeing an optimal effect.[118] A 5-mg daily dose of pilocarpine has been shown to increase both unstimulated whole and stimulated parotid salivary flow in patients with SS over a 6-week study period.[95] Cevimeline is taken in 30-mg doses, three times per day.[118]

Pilocarpine is contraindicated in patients with sensitivity to the drug or its components, uncontrolled asthma, angle-closure glaucoma, or severe liver impairment.

Cevimeline is contraindicated in patients with hypersensitivity to the drug or its components, uncontrolled asthma, narrow-angle glaucoma, acute iritis, or other conditions in which miosis is undesirable.

Caution must be used when prescribing these drugs to patients with heart disease, chronic respiratory disease, and liver or kidney disease. Practitioners should be aware that the excessive sweating caused by these medications may pose a risk of severe dehydration in older patients. Concurrent use of anticholinergic medications may antagonize the effects of cholinergic agonists. Conversely, concurrent use with other cholinergic medications may produce an additive effect.

> *Prevention*
>
> Each of these medications has specific drug interactions, and a drug reference guide should be consulted to ensure compatibility before prescribing these medications.[118]

ORAL SIGNS AND SYMPTOMS

Oral manifestations of SS include enlargement of the major salivary glands, most notably the parotid gland. Other oral signs and symptoms of SS appear in Box 46-1.

For those patients with severe cases of xerostomia, the mucosa may appear very dry and the dorsum of the tongue may be erythematous, fissured, and depapillated. Candidal infections, particularly the erythematous form, are common.[93,94]

Studies of patients with SS have demonstrated that these individuals have significantly higher plaque biofilm index scores, higher dental caries rates (particularly cervical caries), increased alveolar bone loss, deeper clinical attachment levels, and increased distance between the cementoenamel junction (CEJ) and alveolar bone crest.[21,22,73,75] Whether this increased

BOX 46-1

ORAL MANIFESTATIONS OF SJÖGREN'S SYNDROME

Enlargement of salivary glands
Lymphadenopathy
Hyposalivation
Xerostomia
Glossitis
Fissured tongue
Burning mouth syndrome
Mucositis
Angular cheilitis
Candidiasis
Bacterial sialadenitis
Difficulty swallowing, speaking, and singing
Difficulty tasting and tolerating acidic or spicy foods
Difficulty controlling dentures
Increased dental caries, including cervical caries
Periodontal disease with loss of attachment

Modified from Neville BW, Damm DD, Allen CM, Bouqout JE: *Oral & maxillofacial pathology,* ed 2, Philadelphia, 2002, WB Saunders; Rhodus NL: Sjögren's syndrome, *Quintessence Int* 30:689-699, 1999; Wray D et al: *Textbook of general and oral medicine,* Edinburgh, 1999, Churchill Livingstone.

risk is due to hyposalivation or to the presence of an autoimmune disease remains unclear.

DENTAL CONSIDERATIONS

Prevention and maintenance are the key components of dental hygiene intervention for patients with SS. Patients should be counseled to remain hydrated throughout the day and to avoid drinking diuretics such as caffeine and alcoholic beverages. Physician consultations may be warranted to monitor and modify medications that may contribute to xerostomia.[43]

For dental caries prevention, meticulous oral hygiene, daily fluoride therapy, and use of minimally abrasive dentifrices are recommended. Nutrition counseling is recommended to help patients learn to evaluate and limit sucrose intake.[122] Regular use of a preventive mouthrinse and frequent professional debridement appointments are needed to control periodontal disease. Patients who experience **glossodynia** should be counseled to avoid spicy or acidic foods, and topical corticosteroids, analgesics, or anesthetics may be indicated.[43]

Prevention

Individuals with SS who have ocular problems may require assistance to and from the operatory to ensure their safety.

Distinct Care Modifications

As a consideration to SS patients with ocular changes, the clinician should avoid directing the dental light into their eyes and offer them sunglasses during assessment and treatment procedures.

In cases of secondary infections such as bacterial sialadenitis or candidiasis, antibiotic or antifungal therapy, respectively, should be prescribed. Individuals with full or partial appliances should be educated to cleanse them daily to avoid recurrent fungal infections and to leave these appliances out of the mouth for a given period each day.[43,117]

Because patients with SS have an increased risk for non-Hodgkin's lymphoma, they should receive a thorough extraoral and intraoral examination at each appointment. Any changes denoting glandular swelling or lymphadenopathy warrants referral to an oncologist or an oral maxillofacial surgeon for further evaluation.[43]

Rheumatoid Arthritis

RA is a chronic inflammatory disease characterized by pain, swelling, stiffness, and loss of function affecting the joints. It differs from other types of arthritis in that it generally occurs in a symmetrical pattern, often affecting the wrist joints and finger joints closest to the hands. The course of the disease is variable. For many patients, only one or two joints are involved. In 10% of cases, the disease progresses to **polyarthralgia.**[61]

RA occurs in 1% of the population and occurs in all races and ethnic groups. The disease typically begins in older individuals; however, children and adolescents may develop it as well. RA occurs two to three times more often in women than men, although the disorder tends to be diagnosed at a younger age in men than in women.[79]

PATHOGENESIS

RA begins as an attack on the synovium, the inner lining of the joint capsule, triggered by exposure of a genetically susceptible host to an unknown arthritogenic antigen. A chain of events is set up with activation of CD4+ helper T cells and other lymphocytes along with the local release of inflammatory mediators, such as prostaglandins and matrix metalloproteinases, and cytokines that destroy the joint.[29,65] When these cells attack the joint capsule, white blood cells (WBCs) cause a reaction known as *synovitis,* resulting in warmth, redness, swelling, and pain. Cells of the synovium grow and divide abnormally, thickening the synovium and swelling the joint. Granulation tissue, known as **pannus,** forms and produces a sustained, irreversible destruction of cartilage and erosion of subchondral bone.[35,70] Surrounding muscles, ligaments, and tendons that support and stabilize the joint become weak and are unable to function properly. Capsules and ligaments distend and rupture. New bone or fibrous tissue is deposited, causing characteristic deformity of joints, fusion, or loss of mobility. Damage to the bones begins during the first several years of the disease; therefore early diagnosis and treatment is essential.[42,61,67,79]

CLINICAL SIGNS AND SYMPTOMS

Signs and symptoms of RA vary considerably. Classic signs include tenderness, warmth, and joint swelling that typically occur in a symmetrical pattern. The wrists and finger joints closest to the hands are most affected. Other joints affected by RA include the neck, shoulders, elbows, hips, knees, ankles, and feet.

Other signs of RA include occasional fever, malaise, and pain and stiffness that last for more than 30 minutes in the morning or after a period of rest. Symptoms of RA can last for months to years or may resolve spontaneously. One fourth of individuals develop rheumatoid nodules close to the joints. Many individuals with RA will develop anemia. Other conditions associated with RA include KCS, xerostomia, and neck pain. In rare cases, inflammation of the blood vessels, the lining of the lungs, or the pericardium may occur.

TREATMENT

Although no cure exists for RA, treatment is multifaceted. The goal of treatment is designed to relieve pain, reduce inflammation, slow or stop joint damage, and improve ability to function. Treatment consists of lifestyle changes, medications, surgery, and routine evaluations.

Lifestyle changes include periods of rest and exercise. Physical therapy is often used to increase mobility and function. Relaxation therapy and healthful nutrition are important factors in improving a sense of well-being. During periods of exacerbations, some joints may require splinting to provide adequate rest and support.

Multiple medications are available to slow the course of this disease and to reduce inflammation. These medications are listed in Table 46-1.

Nonsteroidal antiinflammatory drugs (NSAIDs) block the synthesis of prostaglandins by inhibiting the enzyme cyclooxy-genase, which reduces the formation of inflammatory mediators that create swelling, fever, and pain. However, blocking cyclooxygenase also blocks the formation of thromboxane A_2, which reduces thrombus formation and prolongs bleeding time (a drug reaction that may be considered an adverse event with long-term NSAID use but is beneficial for patients at risk for thromboembolic conditions). NSAIDs are categorized as either *salicylates* or *nonsalicylates.*

Aspirin and other salicylates are standard, first-line agents for treatment of RA. Although they provide symptomatic relief from pain and joint stiffness, they do not prevent occult joint damage, which often necessitates the addition of a disease-modifying antirheumatic drug (DMARD; see following). Salicylates provide relief from low- to moderate-intensity pain and act peripherally to inhibit the synthesis of prostaglandins in inflamed tissues; they also act centrally by targeting the antipyretic region in the hypothalamus. However, relatively large doses are required for pain relief, which may not be tolerated in some individuals. Diflunisal (Dolobid) is a salicylate that can be taken twice daily and has four times the potency of aspirin when used for the treatment of arthritis and musculoskeletal pain. Salicylates produce many adverse events in multiple body systems, most notably causing gastrointestinal bleeding and ulceration and prolonging bleeding time via irreversible inhibition of platelet aggregation.[51,118]

Acetaminophen (Tylenol) has a similar potency as aspirin and is as effective an analgesic as aspirin. However, acetaminophen has no antiinflammatory activity; thus its usefulness in RA is limited. Most patients who take this medication for arthritis pain relief are either allergic to aspirin and aspirin-containing products or have a history of a disease- or drug-induced bleeding problem (e.g., hemophilia, gastrointestinal ulceration) and are therefore unable to take NSAIDs. Acetaminophen inhibits prostaglandin synthesis in the brain, which accounts for its analgesic and antipyretic activities, but it has limited effects in the periphery.[51]

Indomethacin (Indocin) is a nonsalicylate NSAID that is a more potent antiinflammatory agent than aspirin. It has antiinflammatory, antipyretic, and analgesic activities. Up to 50% of patients taking this medication experience adverse side effects, causing 20% of those affected to discontinue the drug. Adverse events include gastrointestinal complaints; central nervous system (CNS) effects; blood dyscrasias; and hypersensitivity reactions, including itching, rashes, and acute asthma attacks. Aspirin-sensitive patients may show a cross-reactivity with indomethacin. Indomethacin has many drug interactions and is contraindicated in multiple patient populations, which limits its usefulness.[51,118]

Sulindac (Clinoril) is half as potent as and has a lower incidence of toxicity than indomethacin. Tolmetin (Tolectin) is more potent than aspirin but is less potent than indomethacin. Mefenamic acid (Ponstel) is primarily used as an analgesic, but it has no added benefits over other NSAIDs. Toxicity limits its usefulness. Hemolytic anemia is a serious side effect of this drug and may be of autoimmune origin. All of these NSAIDs cause gastrointestinal discomfort, impaired platelet function,

Table 46-1	Drugs Used for the Management of Rheumatoid Arthritis	
SALICYLATES (NSAIDS)	**NONSALICYLATES (NSAIDS)**	**DMARDS**
Aspirin	Acetaminophen	Gold
Diflunisal	Indomethacin	Methotrexate
	Indomethacin and sulindac	Azathioprine and cyclophosphamide
	Mefenamic acid and meclofenamate	Cyclosporine
	Tolmetin	Adalimumab
	Propionic acid derivatives (ibuprofen, naproxen, fenoprofen, ketoprofen, flurbiprofen, oxaprozin)	Etanercept
		Leflunomide
		corticosteroids
		Penicillamine
	Nabumetone	Hydroxychloroquine
	Phenylbutazone	Sulfasalazine
	Diclofenac	Capsaicin

NSAIDs, Nonsteroidal antiinflammatory drugs; *DMARDs,* disease-modifying antirheumatic drugs.
From Jacob LS: *The national medical series for independent study: pharmacology,* ed 4, Philadelphia, 1996, Williams & Wilkins; Wynn RD, Meiller TF, Crossley HL: *Drug information handbook for dentistry,* ed 10, Hudson, Ohio, 2005, Lexi-Comp Inc.

prolonged bleeding time, and a cross-sensitivity reaction with aspirin.[51]

Propionic acid derivatives offer significant advantages over aspirin and indomethacin, because they are better tolerated at antiinflammatory doses. These drugs include ibuprofen (Motrin), naproxen (Aleve, Naprosyn), fenoprofen (Nalfon), ketoprofen (Orudis KT, Oruvail), flurbiprofen (Ansaid), and oxaprozin (Daypro). Each individual agent has unique characteristics and side effects, but all of them are associated with gastrointestinal bleeding, prolonged bleeding time, and renal toxicity. Patients who are allergic to aspirin cannot take these medications. The prolonged half-life of both naproxen and oxaprozin permit twice-a-day and once-a-day dosing, respectively. Piroxicam (Feldene) has similar potency to aspirin and indomethacin, but it has a longer half-life that permits once-a-day dosing. In addition, this drug may inhibit activation of neutrophils, an additional mode of antiinflammatory activity.[51]

DMARDs include a wide range of compounds that are used in conjunction with NSAIDs and that interfere with the pathogenesis of RA. Gold compounds inhibit mononuclear phagocyte maturation and function and may suppress cellular immunity. Parenteral gold is considered to be the most effective second-line drug, but its use continues to decline and its benefits remain controversial. Gold salts have minimal antiinflammatory activity and have little use in mild disease and in advanced cases of RA.[51] Gold compounds are highly toxic and may produce skin and mucosal lesions, as well as neutropenia and thrombocytopenia.[51,67]

Methotrexate (Rheumatrex) is an immunosuppressant that produces antirheumatic effects within 6 weeks of initiating treatment. Aspirin and other NSAIDs increase the risk for methotrexate toxicity by slowing its rate of elimination. Side effects include risk for infection, toxicity, and teratogenicity. Methotrexate is contraindicated in patients with kidney disease. Azathioprine (Imuran) and cyclophosphamide (Cytoxan) are other immunosuppressive drugs that are used to treat refractory RA.[51]

Cyclosporine (Sandimmune) is an immunosuppressant agent that is used for patients with severe, progressive RA. This drug inhibits the production of interleukin-2 (IL-2) by helper T cells and reduces the production and release of other lymphokines in response to an antigenic stimulus. The major side effect is kidney toxicity.[51,118]

Several new DMARDs are on the market for RA. Adalimumab (Humira) and etanercept (Enbrel) are indicated for moderate to severe active RA in patients with inadequate response to one or more other DMARDs. Adalimumab is a recombinant monoclonal **antibody,** and etanercept is a recombinant deoxyribonucleic acid (DNA)–derived protein, both of which bind to tumor necrosis factor-α (TNF-α) receptor sites to decrease the destructive effects of TNF-α activity in the joints. Leflunomide (Arava) is used to reduce the signs and symptoms of RA and produces antiproliferative and antiinflammatory effects.[118]

Patients with severe RA benefit from the use of oral prednisone (Deltasone, Prednisone Intensol, Sterapred). Multiple adverse events associated with steroids limit their long-term use in all but those patients with the most severe forms of RA. Steroids may also be injected directly into an acutely inflamed joint.[51]

Penicillamine (Cuprimine, Depen) is used for patients with refractory RA and is highly toxic and teratogenic. It depresses circulating immunoglobulin M (IgM) rheumatoid factor and depresses T-cell activity. Sulfasalazine (Azulfidine) is as effective as penicillamine but is less toxic and prevents the progression of joint damage. Hydroxychloroquine (Plaquenil) is an antimalarial agent that impairs complement-dependent antigen-antibody reactions. This drug is used to treat both RA and SLE. Antimalarial agents are typically used in combination with aspirin and steroids and produce visual problems and intraoral pigmentation as side effects. Finally, capsaicin, a plant alkaloid derived from hot peppers, is found in many OTC products and is applied topically to relieve arthritic pain.[51,67,118]

When joints become severely deformed and mobility is significantly impaired, surgical therapy may be indicated. Joint replacement, tendon reconstruction, and synovectomy are procedures used to reduce pain, improve the function of the affected joint, and improve the patient's ability to perform activities of daily living (ADLs).

Routine evaluation is another important component of the treatment process. Monitoring the course of the disease and the patient's response to medication, lifestyle changes, or surgical intervention (or a combination of these factors) is an important part of comprehensive care. Routine care typically includes periodic blood and urine analyses, radiographs, and evaluation for signs of osteoporosis. RA increases the risk for osteoporosis, particularly if the patient is taking corticosteroids. Calcium and vitamin D supplements or other medications may be prescribed to treat the osteoporosis.

ORAL SIGNS AND SYMPTOMS

The most common oral manifestation of RA is temporomandibular joint (TMJ) involvement. The TMJ is affected in up to 75% of individuals with this disease.[11,56] Symptoms of RA of the TMJ include bilateral preauricular pain, tenderness, swelling, decreased mobility of the joints, locking of the joints, and crepitus. Radiographic evidence of RA involvement of the TMJ includes erosion of the condyles, reduced translation, and sclerosis of the condyle and eminence.[46,64] An increased incidence of fibrosis and adhesions in the TMJ of individuals with RA exist (compared with those of chronic locking and osteoarthritis).[48]

Another oral condition associated with RA is the development of an anterior open bite, which is attributed to the destruction of the condylar heads and loss of condylar height. This condition may cause obstructive sleep apnea.[105]

DENTAL CONSIDERATIONS

Patients with RA may require medical consultation before treatment depending on the medications prescribed. For those individuals on long-term aspirin or NSAIDs therapy, blood studies may be indicated to detect anemia or changes in platelet function that may prolong bleeding. For those patients who are taking a combination of aspirin and corticosteroids, a pretreatment bleeding time is advisable. Bleeding times greater than 20 minutes should be discussed with the physician and may require modifications before dental care or dental hygiene care (or before both). Individuals receiving long-term corticosteroid therapy may require steroid supplementation before invasive procedures. Patients with RA taking gold salts or immunosuppressives are susceptible to bone marrow suppression, which can result in anemia, **agranulocytosis,** and thrombocytopenia. A complete blood cell count (CBC), differential WBC count, and bleeding time studies are indicated before initiating oral hygiene treatment. In addition, these individuals may develop severe stomatitis from these medications, indicating drug toxicity. In this instance, this finding of stomatitis should be reported to the physician for medication evaluation and modification. The stomatitis itself can be treated with antiseptic mouthrinses, diphenhydramine (Benadryl) elixir, or OTC topical benzocaine ointments.[42,67] Use of penicillamine decreases WBCs and platelets and has been associated with drug-induced pemphigus with oral lesions. Loss of taste has also been reported. Patients taking this medication should also have periodic hematologic evaluation.[38]

Patients with RA and TMJ involvement require palliative measures that include recommendations for a soft diet, moist heat or ice (or both) applied to the face and jaw, and use of an occlusal appliance to decrease joint loading. Individuals severely disabled with RA will have difficulty performing routine oral hygiene.

Distinct Care Modifications

Powered toothbrushes, floss holders, and irrigating devices may be helpful to aid in plaque biofilm removal. Antiseptic mouthrinses and fluoride therapy may be helpful in controlling plaque biofilm and reducing dental caries and periodontal disease. Modifying the schedule of continuing care appointments will be based on clinical findings and the discretion of the dental hygienist.

Distinct Care Modifications

Individuals with RA may have varying degrees of pain and immobility. Sitting for prolonged periods of time in a supine position may be challenging. Scheduling shorter appointments while providing opportunities to change positions frequently may be needed.

Distinct Care Modifications

Use of rolled towels or pillows may be helpful to provide support and relieve painful areas such as the neck, lower back, or joints of the limbs. Some patients may find it more manageable to sit or be placed in a semisupine position, depending on the joints affected by RA and their level of discomfort.

Systemic Lupus Erythematosus

SLE is a chronic inflammatory autoimmune disease that involves multiple organ systems. SLE is characterized by periods of remissions and exacerbations. The disease ranges in severity from mild cases of rash and arthritis to severe illness with renal failure.[41]

Most cases of SLE occur in women, with onset between puberty and the fourth decade of life. The female-to-male ratio is 9:1. After the fourth decade of life, the ratio is approximately 2:1.[61] SLE tends to occur more frequently in blacks, Hispanics, and Asians.

PATHOGENESIS

SLE is an autoimmune disease with a genetic predisposition. Triggers for SLE include infections, exposure to ultraviolet (UV) light, stress, diet, drugs, hormonal changes, and exposure to tobacco and aromatic amines.[2,68,89] Pregnancy can exacerbate the disease.

Patients with SLE produce multiple autoantibodies against normal tissues that are recognized as foreign antigens. These antinuclear autoantibodies (ANAs) are grouped into four categories: (1) antibodies to DNA, (2) antibodies to histones, (3) antibodies to nonhistone proteins bound to ribonucleic acid (RNA), and (4) antibodies to nucleolar antigens. These autoantibodies initiate an inflammatory response and vasculitis and cause deterioration of collagenous connective tissue that can lead to cell death and organ failure.[61,74]

In addition, antiphospholipid antibodies are present in 40% to 50% of lupus patients. These antibodies are referred to as *lupus anticoagulant* and can cause a hypercoagulable state leading to venous and arterial thromboses, recurrent spontaneous miscarriages, and focal cerebral or ocular ischemia. This set of conditions in association with lupus is referred to as *secondary* **antiphospholipid antibody syndrome.**[61]

A genetic predisposition has been supported in SLE, with genes linked to contributions from the MHC and non-MHC genes.[61] Heredity is further supported by the concordance rate in monozygotic twins, which is between 30% and 50%.[2]

CLINICAL SIGNS AND SYMPTOMS

Most patients with SLE have involvement of the skin or joints. The classic presentation is the malar "butterfly" rash that occurs across the nose and cheeks. This photosensitive rash can occur in combination with alopecia. SLE may involve any organ or tissue and can occur in various combinations. An overview of the clinical signs and symptoms of SLE appears in Table 46-2.

TREATMENT

No cure for SLE exists; therefore treatment consists of patient education and medication management for palliative measures or symptom control. Individuals with SLE must be cautioned to limit their exposure to the sun and to use sunscreen regularly. Exposure to UV radiation exacerbates skin conditions (see Table 46-2). Furthermore, they must be encouraged to remain adherent with their medication regimens and follow-up

Table 46-2	Signs and Symptoms of Systemic Lupus Erythematosus
SYSTEM	**FEATURES**
Constitutional	Fatigue, persistent fever in the absence of infection, weight loss
Musculoskeletal	Arthralgia; myalgia; arthritis; Jaccoud's arthropathy with reducible deformities; joint pain and swelling frequently affecting the fingers, hands, wrists, and knees
Skin	Malar butterfly rash, photosensitivity, diffuse rash, skin lesions or nodules, mucous membrane lesions, purpura, alopecia, Raynaud's phenomenon, urticaria, vasculitis
Renal	Hematuria, proteinuria, **casts,** nephritic syndrome, renal failure
Gastrointestinal	Nausea, vomiting, abdominal pain, medical peritonitis with or without ascites, hepatomegaly, pancreatitis
Pulmonary	Pleurisy, pleural effusion, chest pain, shortness of breath, pulmonary parenchyma, pulmonary hypertension
Cardiovascular	Pericarditis, noninfective endocarditis (Libman-Sacks), myocarditis, chest pain, arrhythmia, valve abnormalities
Reticuloendothelial	Lymphadenopathy, splenomegaly, hepatomegaly
Hematologic	Anemia, autoimmune thrombocytopenia purpura or thrombocytopenia as a consequence of antiphospholipid antibody syndrome, leukopenia with lymphopenia
Ocular	**Anterior uveitis, iridocyclitis,** retinal vasculitis, central retinal artery occlusion, central retinal vein occlusion, ischemic optic neuropathy, xerostomia with keratoconjunctivitis sicca
Neuropsychiatric	Cerebrovascular accidents, seizure, organic effective disorders, personality disorder, psychosis, coma, vascular or migraine headaches, organic brain syndrome, dementia, cranial neuropathies, peripheral neuropathies
Secondary Antiphospholipid Antibody Syndrome	Recurrent arterial and venous thrombosis, thrombocytopenia, fecal wastage, skin mottling (livedo reticularis), myocardial infarction, miscarriages particularly in the second trimester

Reprinted with permission from Gurenlian JR: Systemic lupus erythematosus, *Access* 15(8):50-53, 2001; Belmont HM: *Lupus: clinical overview.* Available at http://cerebel.com/lupus/overview.html, Accessed on August 13, 2005. Louis PJ, Fernandes R: Review of systemic lupus erythematosus, *Oral Surg Oral Med Oral Pathol Oral Radiol Endod* 91(5):512-516, 2001; American College of Rheumatology Ad Hoc Committee on Systemic Lupus Erythematosus Guidelines: Guidelines for referral and management of systemic lupus erythematosus in adults, *Arthritis Rheum* 42:1785-1796, 1999; Merrill JT: The antiphospholipid syndrome: what we know today and what the future holds, *Lupus News* 20(5):14-16, 2000; Cawson RA, Odell EW: *Essentials of oral pathology and oral medicine,* ed 6, Edinburgh, 1998, Churchill Livingstone; Neville BW et al: *Oral & maxillofacial pathology,* ed 2, Philadelphia, 2002, WB Saunders.

schedules with their appropriate specialists (i.e., rheumatologists, cardiologists, nephrologists). Regular testing, including blood assays and urinalysis, will need to be performed to monitor disease activity and effects of therapy.[41]

Many of the drugs used to manage RA are used to treat SLE. Aspirin and NSAIDs are used to manage mild forms of the disease. Antimalarials, such as hydroxychloroquine (Plaquenil), are used to treat the dermatologic conditions related to SLE; steroids are used for the treatment of severe symptoms. Cytotoxic agents are used when symptoms are unresponsive to other forms of treatment or as adjunctive therapies in severe forms of the disease.[67]

Discoid lupus is a condition confined to the skin, with skin lesions and oral lesions that are a mixture of inflammation, ulceration, keratosis, and atrophy. These lesions respond well to topical corticosteroid therapy. Patients with severe organ involvement are treated with systemic glucocorticoids (Predni-sone) or glucocorticoids in combination with immunosuppressive drugs, such as azathioprine (Imuran) or cyclophosphamide (Cytoxan).[38]

ORAL SIGNS AND SYMPTOMS

Oral lesions of SLE can occur in up to 40% of cases.[79] Areas of involvement include the lips, buccal mucosa, attached gingiva, tongue, and palate. The vermillion border of the lip, particularly the mandibular lip, is known as *lupus cheilitis,* and appears as scaly, reddish lesions. Asymptomatic ulcerations that resemble erosive lichen planus may be present. These lesions have been described as "alternating parallel red and white lines in a radial arrangement at the margins."[5] As these lesions heal, they may produce fibrosis and scarring.

Other oral manifestations include xerostomia, stomatodynia, dysgeusia, and periodontal disease. Secondary infection of ulcerative lesions with candidiasis may occur, and the presence of ecchymosis, petechiae, and bleeding may be noted. The bleeding manifestations are associated with autoimmune hemolytic anemia or thrombocytopenia. Involvement of both major and minor salivary glands may occur secondary to SS.[5,79]

DENTAL CONSIDERATIONS

Physician consultations are recommended for patients who have SLE. These individuals may have significant organ involvement and experience side effects from medications. Particular attention should be provided for patients who have renal complications or a history of pericarditis or noninfective endocarditis **(Libman-Sacks endocarditis).** Prophylactic antibiotics may be indicated, especially for patients with low WBC counts, for those taking immunosuppressive medications, and for those with valve abnormalities. Supplemental steroid therapy will be indicated for patients with SLE taking long-term glucocorticoids in high doses. A platelet count and coagulation studies should be conducted before performing any procedures that result in significant bleeding for patients with SLE with a history of thrombocytopenia or those taking immunosuppressive medication. For SLE patients who experience renal failure, medication dose adjustments must be addressed with their specialists. If these patients are being treated with dialysis, then the clinician should use guidelines for management of any patient with renal failure.[5,41,67,68]

Once medical clearances have been provided, patients with SLE should be treated with caution throughout each appointment. Vital signs should be monitored and thorough oral examinations performed at each appointment to assess for oral manifestations of SLE. Patients with SLE who are taking long-term steroid medication also may develop osteoporosis, cataracts, hypertension, acne, hyperglycemia, delayed wound healing, and infection in addition to adrenal suppression. These conditions warrant further evaluation through careful review of the medical history and the oral assessment process.[41]

If oral ulcers are noted during the examination, then the clinician should treat with topical steroids or palliatively depending on the symptoms. Patients should be taught to avoid hot and spicy foods to prevent recurrence. Secondary *Candida* infections should be treated with antifungal medications. Periodontal assessment should be performed routinely at each appointment, because symptoms of oral infection may be masked by medications used to treat SLE. If patients with SLE have xerostomia, then the clinician should stress plaque biofilm control and consider recom-

---

Distinct Care Modifications

Patients with SLE may develop cardiac valve abnormalities that increase susceptibility to infectious endocarditis (IE). A physician consultation is needed to determine whether the patient is a candidate for antibiotic premedication. If necessary, the American Heart Association (AHA) guidelines for the prevention of endocarditis should be followed.

✦ CASE APPLICATION 46-1.1

Systemic Lupus Erythematosus

Patients with SLE frequently have multisystem involvement, and a physician consultation is necessary to determine the extent of the systemic manifestations of the disease. Cardiac assessment, including echocardiogram, is required to determine the presence of valve dysfunction and the need for antibiotic premedication. Cytotoxic and immunosuppressive medications lower WBC counts, posing a risk for infection. Patients receiving these drug therapies should have a WBC count performed before dental hygiene treatment is initiated; antibiotic premedication may be required. DMARDs increase the risk of thrombocytopenia, whereas aspirin and NSAIDs alter platelet function. A platelet count and bleeding time test may be necessary to ensure that initiation of treatment is safe and to provide information that dictates what preventive measures are needed to reduce the risk of posttreatment bleeding complications.

---

mending daily home fluoride therapy and saliva substitutes, depending on the severity of the condition and dental caries susceptibility.

In general, shorter appointments and more frequent prophylaxis and reevaluation appointments are indicated for patients with SLE. These appointments allow for opportunities to assess for healing and other signs of infection or disease.

Scleroderma

Scleroderma is a chronic disease of connective tissue affecting all organ systems secondary to fibrosis and vascular injury. The term is derived from the Greek words *skleros,* meaning hard or indurated, and *derma,* meaning skin. Two major types of scleroderma exist: (1) localized scleroderma and (2) **systemic scleroderma.** Both types have subgroups.

Localized types of scleroderma are those that are confined to the skin and muscle; internal organs are not affected. The two types of localized scleroderma are (1) morphea scleroderma and (2) linear scleroderma. **Morphea scleroderma** is characterized by local patches of skin that thicken into firm, oval-shaped areas. The center of the patch becomes ivory in color with violet borders. These patches appear primarily on the chest, stomach, and back but may occur on the face, arms, and legs. This condition can be localized or generalized. **Linear scleroderma** refers to single lines or bands of thickened, abnormally colored skin. These linear bands tend to run down the arm or leg and in some cases occur on the forehead.

Systemic scleroderma, also known as *systemic sclerosis,* affects the skin, the blood vessels, and major organs. Types of systemic scleroderma include the following:

- Limited scleroderma
- Diffuse scleroderma
- Sine scleroderma

Limited scleroderma tends to affect the skin in certain areas, such as the fingers, hands, face, lower arms, and legs.

Raynaud's phenomenon is common. CREST syndrome tends to be common in this type of scleroderma and refers to the following:

- **C**alcinosis (formation of calcium deposits in connective tissue)
- **R**aynaud's phenomenon
- **E**sophageal dysfunction
- **S**clerodactyly (thick and tight skin on the fingers)
- **T**elangiectasias (small red spots on the hands and face caused by swelling of blood vessels)

Diffuse scleroderma is characterized by sudden skin thickening throughout the body in a symmetrical pattern accompanied by organ damage. The heart, kidneys, stomach, and lungs experience advanced deterioration. **Sine scleroderma** may resemble either limited or diffuse scleroderma. The major difference is that this form of scleroderma does not affect the skin.

The prevalence of scleroderma in the United States is approximately 300,000 individuals, with 80,000 to 100,000 with the systemic form and the remainder experiencing the localized form. The disease occurs three to four times more often in women than men, and the onset tends to occur most frequently between the ages of 25 and 55 years.[101] Black women tend to experience more frequent and severe forms of systemic scleroderma.[61] Oklahoma Choctaw Indians have an incidence of 472 cases per million, which may reflect environmental exposures or genetic predisposition.[52]

PATHOGENESIS

Proposed pathogenic mechanisms for scleroderma include endothelial cell injury, fibroblast activation, and immunologic derangement. Environmental triggers that may be associated with this disease include silica exposure, solvent exposure, and human cytomegalovirus and human herpesvirus (HHV) 5.[52]

Symptoms of tissue fibrosis and occlusion of the microvasculature occur from excessive production and deposition of types I and III collagens. Macromolecules of connective tissue, including fibronectin, tenascin, and glycosaminoglycans, are increased. Some patients have a serine proteinase known as *granzyme A,* which is secreted by activated T cells, degrades type IV collagen, and may be responsible for the breakdown of the basal lamina. Other patients have serum with mediators for antibody-dependent cellular toxicity against endothelial cells. Serum antinuclear antibodies are present in 90% of patients with systemic scleroderma.[50,52,61]

Table 46-3	Clinical Features of Scleroderma
SYSTEM	**CLINICAL FEATURES**
Constitutional	Fatigue, weight loss
Skin	Diffuse pruritus, skin pigment changes (hyperpigmentation or hypopigmentation), skin tightness and induration, telangiectasias, calcinosis, edema
Ear, Nose, Throat	Sicca syndrome, tooth mobility, widening of the periodontal ligament, microstomia, anterior open bite, resorption of the mandible, concomitant Sjögren's syndrome
Musculoskeletal	Arthralgia, myalgia, loss of joint range of motion, carpal tunnel syndrome symptoms, flexion contractures
Gastrointestinal	Gastroesophageal reflux disease, dysphagia, dyspepsia, gastroparesis, diarrhea alternating with constipation, abdominal cramping, nausea, vomiting, severe esophagitis, candidiasis, watermelon stomach, primary biliary cirrhosis, malabsorption, diverticula
Cardiovascular	Dyspnea with pericardial effusion, congestive heart failure, or myocardial fibrosis, palpitations, and arrhythmias
Respiratory	Dyspnea, chest pain from pulmonary artery hypertension, cough from restrictive lung disease
Renal	Renal crisis, renal failure
Endocrine and Exocrine	Hypothyroidism, erectile dysfunction, vaginal dryness, **dyspareunia,** menstrual irregularities, xerostomia, xerophthalmia
Neurologic	Facial pain and hand paresthesias from nerve entrapment neuropathies, headache, stroke
Vascular	Raynaud's phenomenon; ischemic ulcerations of the fingers; ischemic resorption of the phalanges; gangrene of digits, lips, nose, and ears

Modified from Humes HD: *Kelley's essentials of internal medicine,* ed 2, Philadelphia, 2001, Lippincott Williams & Wilkins; Jimenez S, Koenig AS: *Scleroderma.* Available at www.emedicine.com/med/topic2076.htm. Accessed on 8/8/2005; National Institute of Arthritis and Musculoskeletal and Skin Diseases: *Handout on health: scleroderma.* Available at www.niams.nih.gov/hi/topics/scleroderma/scleroderma.htm. Accessed on 8/8/2005.

CLINICAL SIGNS AND SYMPTOMS

Scleroderma is variable in presentation and can affect multiple organs. The disease often occurs in conjunction with other autoimmune disorders including RA, SLE, and SS. The clinical features of scleroderma are summarized in Table 46-3.

TREATMENT

Treatment of scleroderma involves medication management, surgery in severe cases, and supportive care. Patients take multiple medications for symptom control and disease management, and thorough medical and pharmacologic history reviews are warranted before initiating dental hygiene treatment. The medications used to treat scleroderma are summarized in Table 46-4.

When digits become severely erosive or gangrenous, amputation is indicated. For those patients with significant cardiovascular or respiratory involvement (or with both), heart-lung or single-lung transplant may be needed.

Supportive measures include educating the patient to avoid cold exposure, stress, and smoking. Encouraging the patient to exercise regularly will improve flexibility and increase circulation.

ORAL SIGNS AND SYMPTOMS

Scleroderma has both clinical and radiographic oral manifestations. Collagen deposition in the perioral tissues results in **microstomia.** This causes a limitation in mandibular opening in up to 70% of cases. The lips tend to be thin and drawn in appearance. Teeth may protrude because of the tightness of the circumoral soft tissue. Destruction of the TMJ appears as erosion of the superior slope of the condyle. Buccal fibrosis contributes to the limited opening and pathologic resorption of the angles of the mandible. Xerostomia frequently occurs in patients with scleroderma and may occur in conjunction with secondary SS. Periodontal destruction leading to tooth mobility occurs, as well as multiple areas of gingival recession. Patients may exhibit anterior open bite, drug-induced gingival enlargement, and dysphagia because of a hypomobile tongue and inelastic esophagus.

Radiographic manifestations of the disease include diffuse symmetric widening of the periodontal ligament spaces. Osseous resorption of the mandibular angle, coronoid process, or condyle may be noted in 10% to 20% of cases.[79] Pathologic jaw fractures may occur late in the disease process.

DENTAL CONSIDERATIONS

Depending on the extent of the disease and the treatment used, a physician consult may be indicated. For those patients who experience gastrointestinal symptoms, a semi-reclined position is recommended.

Given that patients with scleroderma may have microstomia, oral hygiene may be compromised. Thorough assessment of the patient's oral health status and manifestations of the disease is imperative. Nutrition counseling should be conducted, and patients should be encouraged to limit their intake of cariogenic foods. The patient's mobility should be assessed, and recommendations for use of a powered toothbrush or modifications to a manual toothbrush should be made to allow for accessibility, grip, and control. Use of an antimicrobial mouthrinse and daily home fluoride will assist the patient in managing dental caries and periodontal concerns. Salivary substitutes may be indicated if chronic xerostomia occurs. Gradual and incremental isometric exercises can be recommended to help stretch the muscles of the face and head and make opening the mouth easier for the patient.[78]

Diabetes

Diabetes mellitus (DM) is a chronic endocrine disease that is associated with a triad of symptoms including polydipsia, polyuria, and polyphagia caused by a malfunction of insulin-dependent glucose homeostasis. The disease occurs in more than 18.2 million Americans; researchers estimate that approximately one third of these individuals are undiagnosed. One in three children born in the United States in 2000 will get diabetes, and between 45 and 50 million people will have diabetes by 2050.[72,77]

DM is the fourth leading cause of death in the United States.[27] DM is a major cause of cardiovascular disease and is a leading cause of adult blindness, nontraumatic lower extremity amputations, and end-stage renal disease. Among middle-aged people with diabetes, life expectancy is reduced by 5 to 10 years. For the entire population with diabetes, an estimated 13 years is lost by both men and women.[77]

Types of diabetes include type 1, type 2, secondary diabetes, maturity-onset diabetes of the young (MODY), and gestational diabetes mellitus (GDM). Type 1 diabetes was formerly referred to as *insulin-dependent diabetes* or *juvenile diabetes*. It occurs in approximately 5% to 10% of the population. The average onset of type 1 DM is 8 to 12 years of age. This type of DM primarily affects white individuals, and the male-to-female ratio is 1:1.

Type 2 diabetes was formerly known as *non–insulin-dependent diabetes mellitus (NIDDM)*, or *adult-onset diabetes*. It typically occurs in adults older than the age of 40 years; however, more recently this type of diabetes has been occurring in adolescents, likely because of a sedentary lifestyle and dietary factors. This type of diabetes occurs more in female subjects than male subjects and is more prevalent among Hispanic, Native American, black, and Asian-Pacific Islander racial groups.

Secondary diabetes is associated with other illnesses such as pancreatitis, cystic fibrosis, pancreatic cancer, acromegaly, and Cushing's syndrome, as well as drug-induced diabetes from the long-term use of phenytoin, glucocorticoids, and estrogens. MODY is a form of type 2 DM that affects many generations in the same family, with the onset occurring before the age of 25 years. Gestational diabetes refers to any degree of glucose intolerance with onset or first recognition during pregnancy. This type of diabetes can lead to complications during

Table 46-4   Medications Used to Treat Scleroderma

CONDITION	DRUG CLASS	EFFECT
Raynaud's Phenomenon	• Calcium channel blockers • Angiotensin II receptor antagonists • Alpha-I adrenergic blockers	• Relax blood vessels • Block vasoconstriction • Relax blood vessels
Gastroesophageal Reflux Disease (GERD)	• Antacids • H$_2$ blockers • Proton pump inhibitors • Sucralfate	• Neutralize stomach pH • Inhibit stomach acid secretion • Inhibit stomach acid secretion • Coats esophagus and stomach
Swallowing Problems	• Gastrointestinal stimulants	• Stimulate peristalsis; heartburn relief
Constipation	• Bulking agents • Softening agents • Laxatives	• Soften stool • Soften stool • Make bowels move
Small Intestine Dysfunction; Bacterial Overgrowth and Diarrhea	• Broad-spectrum antibiotics	• Decrease bacterial overgrowth
Joint and Tendon Pain	• Nonsteroidal antiinflammatory drugs (NSAIDs) • Analgesics • Narcotics	• Suppress inflammation • Relieve pain • Relieve severe pain
Pulmonary Fibrosis and Alveolitis	• Immunosuppressants	• Suppress immune response, impair lymphocytes
Pulmonary Arterial Hypertension	• Endothelin receptor antagonists • Prostaglandin derivatives • Calcium channel blockers	• Act on blood vessels • Act on blood vessels • Relax blood vessels
Renal Crisis and New-Onset Hypertension	• Angiotensin-converting enzyme (ACE) inhibitors	• Block vasoconstriction
Skin Fibrosis	• Immunosuppressants	• Suppress immune response, impair lymphocytes
Sjögren's Syndrome (SS)	• Cholinergic agonists • Salivary substitutes • Artificial tears	• Stimulate salivary secretion • Relieve xerostomia • Relieve xerophthalmia
Reactive Depression	• Selective serotonin reuptake inhibitors • Tricyclic antidepressants	• Improve symptoms of depression • Improve symptoms of depression and sleep
Localized Scleroderma	• Hydroxychloroquine • Methotrexate • Prednisone • Phenytoin • Potassium p-aminobenzoate • D-Penicillamine • Psoralen and ultraviolet light A (PUVA)	• Suppresses immune response • Suppresses inflammation • Unclear • Unclear • Inhibits collagen cross-linking • Decreases skin thickening • Phototherapy
Pruritus and Dryness	• Over-the-counter (OTC) skin lotions • Antihistamines • Colchicines	• Moisturize skin • Decrease itching • Reduce inflammation associated with calcinosis

Modified from The Scleroderma Foundation. Available at www.scleroderma.org/medical/medication.htm. Accessed on August 12, 2005. *H$_2$*, Histamine-2.

pregnancy and places both the infant and the mother at risk for developing diabetes later in life.

Because type 1 DM is the form of diabetes that represents an autoimmune process, the remainder of discussion pertains to this particular type of DM only.

PATHOGENESIS

The primary cause of type 1 DM is the marked inability of the pancreas to secrete insulin because of autoimmune destruction of the beta cells (B cells). The existing pancreatic islet cells contain A cells, which produce glucagons; D cells, which produce somatostatin; and PP cells, which produce pancreatic polypeptide.[50] However, with progressive destruction of the B cells, the disease produces hyperglycemia that leads to ketosis (i.e., accumulation of large quantities of ketone bodies that are acids in the blood and tissues), and eventually ketoacidosis develops. Patients with type 1 DM are insulin dependent in that they produce no endogenous insulin.

The development of type 1 DM begins with a genetic susceptibility to the disease. More than 90% of patients with type 1 DM express genes DR3 or DR4 class II HLA molecules (or they express both).[50]

CLINICAL SIGNS AND SYMPTOMS

Type 2 DM can be present for more than 10 years before individuals are diagnosed with the disease. Symptoms may be overt or subtle. However, in patients with type 1 DM, the symptoms are more profound. Signs of DM include the following:

- **Polyuria** (excessive urination)
- **Nocturia** (urination at night)
- **Polyphagia** (increased appetite)
- **Polydipsia** (extreme thirst)
- **Glucosuria** (glucose in the urine)
- **Pruritus** (itchy, dry skin)
- Unexplained weight loss
- General fatigue
- Increased infections, including frequent bladder or vaginal infections
- Leg cramps or paresthesia of the fingers and toes
- Blurred vision
- Impotence

TREATMENT

Insulin is the drug of choice for the treatment of type 1 diabetes and is the primary hormone required for proper glucose use in normal metabolic processes. Drug preparations are derived from beef or pork pancreas or via a biosynthetic process that converts pork insulin to human insulin. Insulin is characterized by its duration and intensity of action. Patients use short-acting and intermediate or long-acting insulin preparations,

depending on the clinical circumstance. Duration also depends on the type of preparation used, the route of administration, and patient-dependent factors. In general, the larger the dose of insulin, the longer the duration of activity.[118] Insulin preparations are summarized in Table 46-5.

Several drug interactions occur with insulin that are significant to dentistry. Corticosteroids may enhance blood glucose levels, which may require an increase in insulin dosing. Large doses of salicylates and NSAIDs may enhance the hypoglycemic effects of insulin.

Table 46-5	Insulin Preparations		
INSULIN PREPARATION	**ONSET**	**PEAK EFFECT**	**DURATION**
Insulin Aspart (NovoLog)	0.17-0.33 hours	1-3 hours	3-5 hours
Insulin Lispro (Humalog), Insulin Glulisine (Apidra)	0.25 hours	0.5-1.5 hours	6-8 hours
Insulin, Regular (Novolin R)	0.5-1.0 hours	2-3 hours	8-12 hours
Isophane Insulin Suspension (NPH) (Novolin N)	1.0-1.5 hours	4-12 hours	24 hours
Insulin Zinc Suspension (Lente)	1.0-2.5 hours	8-12 hours	18-24 hours
Isophane Insulin Suspension and Regular Insulin Injection (Novolin 70/30)	0.5 hours	2-12 hours	24 hours
Extended Insulin Zinc Suspension (Ultralente)	4-8 hours	16-18 hours	>36 hours
Insulin Glargine (Lantus)			24 hours

From Wynn RD, Meiller TF, Crossley HL: *Drug information handbook for dentistry,* ed 10, Hudson, 2005, Lexi-Comp Inc.

ORAL SIGNS AND SYMPTOMS

Oral signs and symptoms of diabetes vary and include the following:

- Xerostomia
- Burning mouth syndrome
- Gingival proliferation
- Abnormal wound healing
- Multiple carious lesions

Prevention

Epinephrine is an insulin antagonist; thus caution must be used when administering local anesthetics containing vasoconstrictors. When hemostasis is necessary, the clinician should use a vasoconstrictor at the lowest dose and at the lowest concentration available to produce the desired effects. Patients should be monitored for signs of hyperglycemia.[118]

- Gingivitis
- Periodontitis
- Periodontal abscesses
- Candidal infection
- Acetone (fruity) breath
- Tooth loss
- Impaired ability to wear dental prostheses
- Taste impairment
- Increased salivary viscosity
- Asymptomatic parotid gland swelling[40,110]

These findings may be related to the excessive loss of fluids through frequent urination, the altered response to infection, microvascular changes, and increased glucose concentrations in saliva.[67,110]

Studies of patients with type 1 DM and chronic poor metabolic control reveal they have more extensive and severe periodontal disease than those patients who maintain rigorous control of their disease. Moreover, patients who have type 1 DM for longer durations with periodontitis are more likely to develop long-term complications of retinopathy, ketoacidosis, and neuropathy.[32,49,96,106,107]

The periodontal changes of diabetes reflect host-response abnormalities such as nonenzymatic glycation and oxidation, imbalance in lipid metabolism, altered collagen metabolism, and neutrophil dysfunction.[97] Bacterial invasion of the gingiva stimulates the formation of inflammatory mediators including IL-1, TNF-α, prostaglandins, and cytokines. These inflammatory mediators produce and activate enzymes that destroy gingival connective tissue and resorb bone. In diabetes it appears that the production of new bone is impaired after bone loss. The cytokines that stimulate loss of tissue, most notably TNF-α, may be responsible for killing cells that repair damaged connective tissue or bone. Furthermore, more TNF-α may be produced, which can lead to even less ability to repair periodontal tissues.[36,44]

DENTAL CONSIDERATIONS

When scheduling dental and dental hygiene appointments for individuals with DM, morning appointments should be offered. If the clinician anticipates that the appointment may be lengthy, then he or she should offer the patient a short break or a nutritious snack.

For type 1 DM patients, the clinician should document the type of insulin being used, how often the insulin is administered, when peak insulin activity occurs, and the type of carbohydrate consumed before the scheduled appointment. A blood glucose reading should be obtained at each appointment and noted in the dental chart.

Oral care for patients with DM includes frequent oral debridement to minimize infection. The dental hygienist will need to determine a continuing care schedule based on individual needs, signs of peri-

Note

The clinician should not provide oral health care if the patient reports that he or she has not eaten or taken his or her medications or if blood glucose readings are below 70 mg/dl or above 150 mg/dl.[27]

odontal disease, and response to treatment. Periodontal disease should be treated aggressively using host-modulation therapy, such as antibiotic therapy or a subantimicrobial agent. Wound healing and response to debridement therapy should be monitored 4 to 6 weeks posttreatment. For those patients whose glycemic levels are poorly controlled, prophylactic antibiotic therapies may be indicated before periodontal debridement. Clinicians should follow the AHA guidelines for endocarditis prophylaxis for these individuals.[39,67,110]

Oral health recommendations should include reinforcement of the need for proper nutrition, exercise, adherence to medication regimens, and regular monitoring of blood glucose levels. Patients should be advised to brush, floss, and use an antiseptic mouthrinse twice daily. Peridex and Listerine are the only two antiseptic mouthrinses that have been approved by the American Dental Association (ADA) Council on Scientific Affairs. Similarly, Colgate Total is the only ADA-approved toothpaste that contains triclosan, an antibacterial ingredient that adheres to the mucosa for 12 hours and directly inhibits potent mediators responsible for gingival inflammation.[23,123] Given its antiinflammatory effects, this toothpaste would be an excellent recommendation for individuals with diabetes. Recommendations for use of power toothbrushes, daily fluoride therapy, home irrigation, and host-modulation therapy should be based on clinical presentation, response to initial therapy, and scientific evidence that supports their use.[44]

Although most emphasis will be placed on the prevention of oral manifestations of diabetes, the clinician should educate patients with diabetes about strategies to achieve and maintain total health and adequate glycemic control. Box 46-2 includes key health messages for individuals with diabetes. These messages can be customized and offered throughout a series of periodontal therapy appointments.[44]

During each dental and dental hygiene appointment, the clinician should monitor the patient's vital signs and evaluate for signs of medical emergency. Patients who are taking insulin are at risk for hypoglycemia and insulin shock, especially if they report that they have not eaten at a regularly scheduled mealtime.[88] Signs of hypoglycemia and insulin shock include the following:

- Weakness
- Hunger
- Trembling
- Sweating
- Tachycardia
- Confusion
- Anxiety

These symptoms can progress to combativeness and incoherence, which can lead to unconsciousness, sweating, seizures, hypotension, and hypothermia. In these situations, patients need to be treated immediately with the administration of glucose. If the patient is conscious, then the clinician should administer 15 g of carbohydrate (e.g., 4 to 5 oz of juice or cola, 4

Prevention

The clinician should avoid providing treatment to patients with type 1 DM during peak insulin activity, because these patients are at risk for hypoglycemia.

BOX 46-2

KEY HEALTH MESSAGES FOR INDIVIDUALS WITH DIABETES[13]

Eye Care

- Monitor recent changes in eyesight: blurred vision, blindness, floaters, flashlights, signs of infections (red, painful eyes).
- Remind patient to seek dilated-eye examination yearly or immediately if above eye changes occur.
- Remind patient to keep eyeglasses and contact lens prescriptions current.

Foot Care

- Remind patient to inspect feet daily for signs of infection of neuropathy (foot ulcers, redness, burning, tingling, numb or cold feet).
- Remind patient to have periodic examinations (every 3 to 4 months) with foot care specialist and not to cut toenails or self-treat foot problems.
- Remind patient to remove shoes every time he or she sees a medical primary care provider.

Pharmacy

- Remind patient to take all medications as prescribed.
- Remind patient to ask pharmacist whether any prescribed medications, vitamins, or herbal products will affect diabetes.

Oral Care

- Encourage patient to maintain daily mouth care, brushing teeth after eating to remove plaque biofilm and flossing at least once each day.
- Remind patient to conduct a monthly self-examination and to contact the dental hygienist or dentist if he or she notices signs of infection, such as sore, swollen, or bleeding gums or mouth ulcers.
- Encourage patient to eat healthful snacks, choosing foods that are low in sugar and fat.
- Remind patient to have periodic dental and periodontal examinations, every 3 months or more, as recommended by his or her oral health professional.
- Encourage patient to achieve the best glycemic control possible. (Controlled diabetes improves oral health, and maintaining good oral health helps control diabetes.)

Other Health Messages

- Do not smoke or chew tobacco.
- Have blood pressure and cholesterol checks performed regularly.
- Exercise regularly.
- Reduce stress.
- Eat a healthy diet.
- Get vaccinated to protect against pneumonia and flu.

From Centers for Disease Control and Prevention: *Working together to manage diabetes: a guide for pharmacists, podiatrists, optometrists, and dental professionals,* Atlanta, 2004, US Department of Health and Human Resources, Public Health Service, Centers for Disease Control and Prevention, National Center for Chronic Disease Prevention and Health Promotion[13]; Gurenlian JR: *Diabetes mellitus: strategies for providing comprehensive care,* Continuing Education for the Healthcare Professional (CEHP), City, 2005, Sullivan-Schein (course reference # 05AS2904).

teaspoons of table sugar or cake icing). Patients who are combative and hostile may resist attempts to eat and drink. When patients become uncooperative, a relatively small window of time exists for the patient to ingest a carbohydrate before seizing and losing consciousness. The clinician must determine whether the patient is coherent enough to swallow before placing anything in the mouth to reduce the risk of choking. If the patient is sedated, then the clinician should administer 20 to 25 ml 50% dextrose intravenously (IV), 1 mg glucagon intramuscularly (IM) or subcutaneously (SQ), or 1 mg glucagon IV.

Patients who are using an insulin pump must be monitored for signs of hyperglycemia, which can lead to diabetic ketoacidosis and diabetic coma. Signs of diabetic ketoacidosis include nausea, abdominal cramping, disorientation, and fatigue. In this circumstance, the patient requires a small bolus of insulin to treat the hyperglycemia. If insulin is not available in the dental office, then the dental hygienist should call 911 for immediate medical assistance. If the hyperglycemia persists after insulin administration, then the patient's physician should be contacted and the patient should be referred for immediate medical evaluation. If the condition worsens, then the clinician should provide basic life support, call 911, and allow the emergency medical service (EMS) personnel to perform necessary care.[44]

Hyperthyroidism

The thyroid gland is one of the largest endocrine glands in the body and is located below the larynx on each side of and anterior to the trachea. The gland secretes two hormones, thyroxine (T_4) and triiodothyronine (T_3), both of which have a profound effect on regulating the body's metabolic rate. Secretion of thyroid hormone (TH) from the thyroid gland is controlled by thyroid-stimulating hormone (TSH), which is secreted by the anterior pituitary gland. Regulation of TH secretion is controlled by a neurochemical feedback signaling mechanism via the hypothalamic-pituitary axis in the brain.[45]

Iodine-deficiency goiter is the most common thyroid disorder and may develop into either hypothyroidism or hyperthyroidism. However, in the United States, where iodine is readily available in the diet, the prevalence of this disorder is very small—ranging from 0.5% to 7.0%.[67] In the United States, both hypothyroidism and hyperthyroidism are four to five times more common in women than in men.[37,109] Both hyperthyroidism and hypothyroidism have multiple causes; however, only those conditions caused by autoimmune dysfunction are discussed here.

Studies show that hyperthyroidism is 10 times more common in women than in men, with an incidence of three cases per 10,000 U.S. women per year.[109] Among patients with hyperthyroidism, 60% to 80% of them have **Graves' disease.**[114] In women, the age of onset of Graves' disease typically occurs between the ages of 40 and 60 years.[114] Prevalence of Graves' disease is similar among whites and Asians and is lower among blacks.[114]

PATHOGENESIS

Hyperthyroidism is also known as **thyrotoxicosis,** which is defined as an excess of T_4 and T_3 in the bloodstream.[67] The underlying etiology of Graves' disease is not fully understood; however, Graves' disease is considered to be an autoimmune disorder.[113] In most patients with hyperthyroidism, the thyroid gland itself is two to three times its normal size, with an increased number of cells composing its structure. Each cell significantly increases its rate of secretion, often at rates that are 5 to 15 times normal. These physiologic changes are similar to what is caused by excessive TSH, which overstimulates the thyroid gland. However, in almost all patients with hyperthyroidism, plasma TSH concentrations are lower than normal, and at times, the level is close to zero. Other substances are found in the blood that mimic the stimulatory effects of TSH. These substances are immunoglobulin antibodies that bind with the same membrane receptors that bind TSH; they are collectively known as *thyroid-stimulating immunoglobulin (TSI).* TSI continuously activates cyclic adenosine monophosphate (cAMP) in thyroid cells, with the resultant development of hyperthyroidism. TSI produces a prolonged stimulatory effect that persists for up to 12 hours, in contrast to the stimulatory effects of TSH that last for 1 hour. The high level of TH secretion produced by this TSI hyperstimulation in turn suppresses the anterior pituitary formation of TSH. This mechanism explains why plasma levels of TSH are very low.[45]

The antibodies that cause hyperthyroidism are formed as a result of autoimmunity that has developed against the thyroid tissue, presumably from the release of excess thyroid cell antigens from the thyroid cells themselves.[45] Several autoantibodies are most often involved with autoimmune thyroid disease: TSHRAb (TSH receptor antibodies), TPOAb (thyroid peroxidase antibodies), and TgAb (thyroglobulin antibodies).[91] The vast majority of patients with Graves' disease (80% to 95%) possess TSHRAb, and most are stimulatory, causing a release of TH. However, other antibodies have an inhibitory effect on TH. TSHR-blocking Ab blocks the release of TH and the binding of TSH to its receptors. The ratio of these stimulating antibodies to the blocking antibodies (TSHR-blocking Ab) determines the clinical status of the patient and overall thyroid function.[67,91,113,114] Patients with Graves' disease often have high serum titers of TSHRAb and low titers of TSHR-blocking Ab, although the level of TSHRAb does not correlate with the severity of disease symptoms.[67]

TgAb are found in 50% to 70% of patients with Graves' disease, and TPOAb are present in 50% to 80% of patients with Graves' disease.[91] Radioimmunoassay techniques are available for measuring TSHRAb, TSHR-blocking Ab, TPOAb, and TgAb.[45,91,102,113]

The primary risk factor for Graves' disease is female gender. A familial tendency also occurs, with an increased incidence in **monozygotic** twins. No single gene is causative for Graves' disease, although associations have been linked with HLA alleles and with polymorphisms of the cytotoxic T-lymphocyte antigen 4 (CTLA-4) gene in several racial groups. HLA-DR3 and HLA-DQA*0501 are associated with Graves' disease in whites.[114]

CLINICAL SIGNS AND SYMPTOMS

The primary role of TH is to activate nuclear transcription in large numbers of genes. In most cells of the body, TH produces increased synthesis of protein enzymes, structural proteins, and transport proteins. This result is a generalized increase in functional activity throughout the body.[45] TH has an effect on multiple body systems; therefore alteration in thyroid function causes many signs and symptoms. The most common signs and symptoms are summarized in Table 46-6.

TH stimulates virtually all aspects of carbohydrate and fat metabolism. Increased TH secretion lowers plasma levels of cholesterol, phospholipids, and triglycerides. Increased TH almost always decreases weight; however, it also stimulates appetite, gastrointestinal motility, and secretion of digestive juices. Increased metabolic rate increases oxygen demand and thus respiratory rate increases. Vasodilation occurs to improve oxygen delivery to the tissues and to facilitate heat elimination from the body.[45]

Table 46-6	Common Signs and Symptoms of Thyroid Disease	
HYPERTHYROIDISM		**HYPOTHYROIDISM**
Pernicious anemia		Anemia
Thin, fine hair and soft nails		Brittle hair and nails
Diarrhea		Constipation
Exophthalmos		
Lid lag and stare		Edema of eyelids
Goiter		Goiter
Osteoporosis		
Hyperactivity and excitability		Drowsiness
Nervousness and anxiety		Slowed mental acuity
Difficulty sleeping		Somnolence
Increased appetite		Decreased appetite
Weight loss		Weight gain
Muscle weakness		Muscle weakness
Fatigue		Fatigue
Palpitations and arrhythmias		
Tachycardia		Bradycardia, slowed pulse
Hyperventilation, dyspnea		Hypoventilation
Sweating		
Hand tremors		Arthritis
Warm, flushed skin		Dry, thick skin
Heat intolerance		Cold intolerance

From Guyton AC, Hall JE, eds: *Textbook of medical physiology,* ed 10, Philadelphia, 2000, WB Saunders; Little JW et al: *Dental management of the medically compromised patient,* ed 6, St Louis, 2002, Mosby.

Increased blood flow increases cardiac output, heart rate, and the force of myocardial contraction. In hyperthyroidism, heart muscle strength actually becomes depressed because of long-term, excessive protein catabolism. Patients with severe thyrotoxicosis may die of cardiac decompensation secondary to heart failure and the increased cardiac load from increased cardiac output.[45]

TH improves skeletal muscle contraction; however, excessive TH weakens muscles because of excess protein catabolism. A characteristic sign of hyperthyroidism is muscle tremor caused by increased reactivity of synapses in the spinal cord that control muscle tone. Neuronal excitability in the CNS produces nervousness, anxiety, and other psychologic disorders. Constant excitability of the neurons, coupled with excitatory effects on the musculature, make hyperthyroid patients feel tired but unable to sleep.[45]

TH increases the quantities of many enzymes and coenzymes that are composed, in part, by vitamins. Therefore vitamin deficiencies can occur with hyperthyroidism unless the intake of vitamins is adequate.[45] Vitamin B_{12} and folic acid requirements increase because of an increase in the total number of red blood cells (RBCs) needed to carry the additional oxygen required to meet the metabolic demands of hyperthyroidism.[67]

Most people with hyperthyroidism exhibit **exophthalmos,** or protrusion of the eyeballs. Immunoglobulins that destroy the eye muscles are found in higher concentrations in the blood in hyperthyroid patients who also have elevated levels of plasma TSIs. Exophthalmos is considered to be an autoimmune process unto itself. Treatment for hyperthyroidism greatly reduces exophthalmos, although vision damage and damage to the corneas persist, causing long-term vision disability in these patients.[45,67,114]

The other characteristic finding is goiter. Iodine is necessary for the formation of TH, via an oxidation reaction within thyroglobulin molecules that are stored in the follicles of the thyroid gland. Thus iodine deficiency leads to a decrease in TH production. Decreased TH levels are detected by the hypothalamus, which causes the anterior pituitary to secrete excessive quantities of TSH. TSH then stimulates the thyroid cells to secrete large amounts of thyroglobulin into the follicles, which enlarges the follicle size, and the gland begins to grow. The thyroid gland may enlarge to 10 to 20 times its normal size. Iodized salt has greatly reduced this type of goiter, known as an *endemic goiter.*[45]

TREATMENT

Treatment for hyperthyroidism is varied. Antithyroid medications are used to decrease the formation of TH and include propylthiouracil and methimazole (Tapazole). These medications are typically used for up to 18 months, although the length of time varies depending on the severity of the disease, tolerance of side effects, and response to treatment. Antithyroid medications cause multiple adverse side effects, some of which are serious, but rare. These side effects include leukopenia and agranulocytosis, although treatment is not stopped unless the WBC count becomes more severely depressed. If the patient also develops a fever, sore throat, or mouth ulcers, then treatment is stopped until the WBC count can be assessed.[67,91,113] Other adverse side effects include skin rash, poor wound healing, oral ulceration, oral infections, facial paresthesias, and taste loss.[118]

Nonselective beta-blockers, most notably propranolol (Inderal), are used to reduce the symptoms associated with adrenergic stimulation, including tachycardia, heart palpitations, sweating, and hand tremors.[67,118]

Potassium iodide (Iosat, Pima, SSKI) is administered to decrease thyroid activity, reduce the rate of TH formation, and reduce the size of the thyroid gland. Iodides also decrease the blood supply to the thyroid gland and are often administered for 2 to 3 weeks before thyroid surgery to decrease both the amount of bleeding and the amount of surgery necessary.[45]

The primary treatment for Graves' disease is with radioactive iodine (iodine is tagged with a radioactive nucleotide and swallowed for the partial destruction of the thyroid gland). Because iodine receptors are located on the thyroid gland, the drug binds to the thyroid gland and produces localized radiation that eventually destroys the glandular tissue, thus the entire body is not subjected to the radiation effects. This treatment is contraindicated in pregnant and lactating women. The outcome of this treatment is hypothyroidism: patients who undergo this procedure will be required to take TH replacement therapy for life.[45,67]

> **Prevention**
> Caution must be used when administering epinephrine to patients taking this medication, because propranolol may enhance the pressor response to epinephrine, resulting in an initial episode of hypertension followed by bradycardia.[118]

ORAL SIGNS AND SYMPTOMS

Patients with hyperthyroidism may have a mild tremor in the tongue. Hyperthyroidism is a known risk factor for osteoporosis; if the condition is left untreated, then changes in normal bone structure will be found within both the peripheral and axial skeleton, including the skull. Children may exhibit premature loss of deciduous teeth and accelerated tooth eruption, and the bones of the jaws develop more quickly. In adults, signs may include marked loss of the alveolar process and a diffuse demineralization of the mandible. Periodontal disease may progress rapidly. Patients may also experience lingual thyroid tissue on the posterior dorsal region of the tongue, just below the area of the foramen cecum.[67,91,113]

DENTAL CONSIDERATIONS

Patients with thyroid disease require a careful medical history review and a detailed physical assessment to determine the extent and severity of their illness and compliance with medication use. The thyroid gland should be inspected carefully, with notations made regarding enlargement, the presence of nodules, and pain and tenderness on palpation. Caution must be taken not to overpalpate the gland to reduce additional secretion of TH into the circulation and to reduce the risk of causing a thyroid storm.

Patients with hyperthyroidism are more difficult to manage in the dental environment than patients with hypothyroidism. These patients may be more sensitive to pain and also demonstrate an increased sensitivity to catecholamines, including epinephrine. Although it may be tempting to use more local anesthetic to achieve adequate pain control, extreme caution must be used when administering a vasoconstrictor.

> *Note*
>
> Uncontrolled or poorly controlled hyperthyroidism is one of the few occasions in dentistry in which epinephrine is absolutely contraindicated.

Well-controlled hyperthyroid patients may receive vasoconstrictors, but careful monitoring is warranted. Hyperthyroid patients are also more tolerant to drugs that are CNS depressants and therefore may require higher doses of sedatives and analgesic medications.

Perhaps the greatest risk with treating hyperthyroid patients is **thyrotoxic crisis,** also known as a *thyroid storm.* Untreated or poorly treated hyperthyroidism makes individuals more susceptible to this medical emergency. Stress, oral and systemic infections, and invasive procedures can trigger this adverse event. The patient will experience the following:

- Restlessness
- Fever
- Tachycardia
- Arrhythmias
- Pulmonary edema
- Tremor
- Sweating
- Nausea
- Vomiting
- Abdominal pain
- Stupor

If left untreated, then the patient develops congestive heart failure (CHF), eventual coma, and death. During the initial stage of a thyroid storm, the patient may appear to be having a heart attack, because many of the initial symptoms are the same. However, thyroid storm appears to be associated with adrenocortical insufficiency.[67,91,113]

Treatment for thyroid storm includes antithyroid medications, potassium iodide, propranolol, hydrocortisone, dexamethasone, intravenous glucose, vitamin B complex, wet packs, fans, and ice packs. Vital signs must be monitored, and cardiopulmonary resuscitation (CPR) may be required. Emergency medical assistance is required for any patient who develops this condition while in the dental office. Risk reduction strategies for this condition include proper disease management, compliance with antithyroid medications, good oral and total body hygiene, and stress reduction.[67,91,113]

Hypothyroidism

In the United States, hypothyroidism is five to six times more common than hyperthyroidism. More than 10% of women older than 40 years have a TH deficiency caused by autoimmune thyroid disease.[7] **Hashimoto's thyroiditis** is the most common autoimmune inflammatory thyroid disease. It primarily affects middle-aged women and has an increasing prevalence in the United States. Hashimoto's thyroiditis may coexist with other autoimmune disorders, including type 1 DM and SS.[67,91,113]

PATHOGENESIS

Autoimmunity against the thyroid gland initiates hypothyroidism; however, the effects are destructive versus stimulatory. Patients with hypothyroidism typically first demonstrate autoimmune thyroiditis, or an inflammation of the thyroid gland. The inflammatory changes cause progressive gland deterioration leading to fibrosis and diminished or absent secretion of TH.[45] Hormone synthesis is impaired because of cellular destruction and a defect in the binding of thyroid iodine.[67]

The autoantibodies that are most often involved with autoimmune thyroid disease are TSHRAb, TPOAb, and TgAb.[91] TSHRAb are found in 10% to 20% of patients, TgAb are found in 80% to 90% of patients, and TPOAb are present in 90% to 100% of patients with autoimmune thyroiditis.[91]

CLINICAL SIGNS AND SYMPTOMS

In patients with hypothyroidism, increased concentrations of cholesterol, phospholipids, and triglycerides are found in the plasma, which results in fat deposition in the liver and large circulating quantities of cholesterol in the blood. These changes are associated with arteriosclerosis, which makes hypothyroidism a known risk factor for heart disease.[45]

Decreased TH allows for weight gain because of a slower metabolic rate. The appetite is suppressed, with decreased gastrointestinal motility, decreased secretion of digestive juices, and constipation.[45] In hypothyroidism, cardiac output may drop by as much as 50%. Lack of TH causes muscles to contact and relax more slowly.

Hypothyroid patients often report a slowed reaction time, difficulty with cognitive tasks, or decreased mental acuity, and may sleep for periods of up to 12 hours or more each day.

Enlarged thyroid glands also occur in those without iodine deficiency, which are known as *idiopathic nontoxic colloid goiters.* Idiopathic goiters are associated with patients with mild thyroiditis. The thyroiditis causes slight hypothyroidism, which increases TSH secretion and causes progressive growth of the noninflamed portions of the gland. This can also contribute to nodular growth while the inflammation is destroying other portions of the gland.[45]

TREATMENT

Treatment for hypothyroidism is accomplished with TH replacement therapy. The most commonly prescribed medication for this disorder is levothyroxine sodium (Levothroid, Levoxyl, Novothyrox, Synthroid, and Unithroid). Other medications include liothyronine sodium (Cytomel, Triostat), liotrix (Thyrolar), and thyroid (Armour Thyroid, Nature-Throid NT, Westhroid). These medications are well tolerated and pose no significant dental treatment complications. The efficacy of these medications in controlling basal metabolic rate is dependent on compliance. Medications are taken daily, at the same time each day. Patients should have their thyroid function tested annually to ensure that the replacement therapy is adequate to meet their needs.

ORAL SIGNS AND SYMPTOMS

Children with hypothyroidism may exhibit an enlarged tongue, delayed eruption patterns, and malocclusion. Adult patients show few oral side effects but may have a hoarse voice, enlarged tongue, and swelling of the facial features.[67]

DENTAL CONSIDERATIONS

Patients with well-controlled hypothyroidism are easily managed in the dental office. These patients are more sensitive to CNS depressants, including narcotic analgesics and sedatives; therefore the dose may need to be lowered. Older patients with severe hypothyroidism need to be treated with caution, because a hypothyroid (myxedema) coma may be precipitated by surgery, stress, trauma, infections, and CNS depressants. This emergency is more common in the winter months and has a high mortality rate. Treatment includes parenteral levothyroxin, steroids, artificial respiration, intravenous glucose, and intravenous saline.[67,91,113]

Pernicious Anemia

Failure of the stomach to produce intrinsic factor and a lack of cobalamin, or vitamin B_{12}, results in **pernicious anemia.** This condition occurs most frequently in late adulthood, usually after the age of 50, and is not gender specific. However, it does tend to occur 20 times more frequently in family members who have this condition than in the general population.

Pernicious anemia is associated with autoimmune atrophic gastritis in some cases. Pernicious anemia is also associated with malabsorption syndromes, inadequate vitamin-B_{12} intake because of vegetarian diets, myxedema (hypothyroidism), and patients who have undergone gastrectomy. Cobalamin, or extrinsic factor, is an essential factor in the maturation of blood cells, is present in meat and animal protein, and is stored in the liver. Absorption of this vitamin occurs in the ileum and requires the presence of intrinsic factor, a specific glycoprotein secreted by parietal cells of the fundus of the stomach. When the stomach fails to produce intrinsic factor and the patient lacks cobalamin, pernicious anemia occurs.[61,79,92]

Signs and symptoms of pernicious anemia include the following:

- Painful, red, burning tongue with atrophy of the papillae
- Generalized weakness
- Tingling of extremities
- Anorexia
- Yellowish skin pigmentation
- Abdominal pain and weight loss
- Cerebral disturbances (headache, dizziness, and tinnitus)

- Gastrointestinal manifestations (nausea, diarrhea, and stomatitis)

The incidence of gastric cancer is increased in cases associated with atrophic gastritis.[61,92]

Treatment of pernicious anemia consists of vitamin B_{12} injections in amounts sufficient to provide daily requirements such that the hematologic abnormality is corrected. Monthly maintenance doses are then administered for life. Oral ulcerations may be treated with topical antiinflammatory medications including diphenhydramine (Benadryl) elixir, fluocinonide (Lidex) gel 0.01%, or clobetasol (Temovate) gel.

Myasthenia Gravis

MG is a chronic autoimmune disease that affects the neuromuscular system. Willis first described it in the 1600s.[116] The disease represents a decrease of AChRs in muscle fibers that results in progressive fatigability and abnormality of skeletal muscles. The disease occurs more frequently in women than men with a ratio of 3:2.[119] The prevalence of MG is between 50 and 125 per million in Western countries and 142 per million in the United States.[24,87]

The muscle weakness and fatigue of MG may be associated with autoantibodies against the AChR. These antibodies reduce the number of available AChRs at the neuromuscular junction by "accelerated endocytosis and degradation of the receptors, functional blockade of the acetylcholine-binding sites, and complement-mediated damage to the acetylcholine receptors."[119] Researchers estimate that approximately 75% of patients have thymic abnormalities including thymus hyperplasia or thymoma.[79,119] Almost half of the patients with MG have at least one other autoimmune disorder, usually of the thyroid gland.[79]

In the initial stages of MG, weakness of the extraocular muscles is noted, which causes drooping eyelids (ptosis) and double vision (diplopia). The disease may remain restricted to the extraocular muscles in approximately 15% of cases or become widespread, causing generalized weakness in 85% of cases. The weakness fluctuates with repeated muscle contractions, and patients are more affected as the day progresses. The muscles of mastication are affected, making chewing difficult. As the disease progresses, patients experience **dysphagia, dysarthria,** soft palate weakness, impaired lip movement, and an aberrant voice with a nasal tone. In some cases, patients experience such weakness of the muscles of mastication that they have to support the lower jaw during and between meals to prevent a spontaneous dropping of the lower jaw and opening of the mouth. Severe involvement affects the respiratory muscles and can lead to respiratory compromise or myasthenic crisis—a life-threatening respiratory collapse that requires mechanical ventilation.

Treatment of MG consists of anticholinesterase agents, thymectomy, and use of immunosuppressive therapy. Anticholinesterase agents are the preferred treatment. Pyridostigmine (Mestinon) is administered in varying doses and times based on individual need. Thymectomy is an option performed on adults with generalized MG. This treatment reduces the quantity of AChR antibodies.[60] For those patients who do not respond to anticholinesterase agents, steroids or other immunosuppressive medications such as azathioprine (Imuran), cyclosporine (Sandimmune), tacrolimus (Prograf), or mycophenolate mofetil (CellCept)—in conjunction with steroid therapy or as monotherapy—have been used.*

Dental Considerations

Medication and patient consultations are necessary to avoid medical and functional complications during oral health care. Scheduling short, early-morning appointments is important to take advantage of the greater strength that occurs during morning hours.[86] To maximize the dental or dental hygiene appointment, oral anticholinesterase agents should be administered 1½ hours before the treatment session.[115] To avoid aspiration of saliva or dental debris, use of a rubber dam, evacuation, and mouth props may be helpful.

Amide-type local anesthetics, such as lidocaine or mepivacaine, may be administered safely. Nitrous oxide and oxygen sedation may also be used and is helpful in reducing stress and anxiety during dental and dental hygiene treatment. The clinician should consult with the patient's neurologist before prescribing antibiotics or muscle relaxants to patients with MG. These patients have increased sensitivity to the effects of muscle relaxants, and some antibiotics have muscle-relaxing properties.[119] Edentulous patients with MG may have difficulty wearing dentures. Implant-supported complete dentures may represent a better option for these patients.

Psoriasis

Psoriasis is a common chronic dermatologic condition affecting 1% to 2% of the U.S. population. Approximately 4 million people have psoriasis, and 250,000 new cases are diagnosed each year.[79] The disease tends to occur during the second or third decade of life, affects both sexes equally, and is characterized by periods of exacerbations and remission. Lesions tend to improve during the summer and become worse during the winter, possibly because of the amount of exposure to UV light.

Psoriasis involves epidermal changes that are related to an increased proliferation of cutaneous keratinocytes. Activated T lymphocytes initiate the disease by interacting with APCs in the skin. Cytokines, chemotactic polypeptides, and growth factors are involved in the cascade that results in inflammation and angiogenesis. Triggering factors may include systemic infections, stress, and drugs. Genetic factors may also be responsible for a component of this disease, because a strong association

exists between psoriasis and HLA-C. Approximately two thirds of patients carry the HLA-Cw*0602 allele. However, only 10% of carriers develop psoriasis, indicating that other factors are influencing the pathogenesis of this disease.[61,79,92]

The classic presentation of psoriasis is a well-demarcated, erythematous plaque with a silver-white scale on the surface of the lesion. These lesions are typically asymptomatic, but occasional itching may be reported. When the scales are removed, small areas of bleeding occur, known as *Auspitz sign*. Psoriasis most often occurs on the skin of the elbows, knees, scalp, and back. Nail changes occur in 30% of cases of psoriasis. Characteristics include discoloration, thickening, pitting, and separation of the nail plate from the nail bed. Pustular psoriasis is a rare form of the disease that manifests as multiple small pustules on erythematous plaques.

Oral manifestations of psoriasis are rare. Lesions may appear as white plaques, red plaques, mixed red and white lesions, pustules, vesicles, or ulcerations.[121] In some cases geographic tongue may be a coincident finding.[92]

Treatment of psoriasis depends on the severity of the disease. A wide variety of agents and combinations may be used. Coal tar derivatives, calcipotriene (a vitamin D_3 analog), and tazarotone (a retinoid compound) have been used for mild to moderate cases. PUVA (psoralen and ultraviolet light A) therapy or UV B therapy, methotrexate, and cyclosporine have been used for severe disease.

Rheumatic Heart Disease

Rheumatic heart disease (RHD) results from a throat or ear infection caused by Group A beta-hemolytic streptococci, leading to acute rheumatic fever (ARF). Symptoms include fever, inflamed or painful joints (or both), and rash. Typically a latent period of several weeks is seen between the streptococcal infection and the development of ARF. Rheumatic fever is an autoimmune disease that is caused by a reaction between the patient's antibodies against the streptococcal antigens. All portions of the heart may be affected, with the mitral valve most frequently affected by the antigen-antibody complex, as well as the aortic semilunar value.[54,74]

Streptococcal pharyngitis primarily affects children and young adults. Approximately 3% of people who have not had their infection treated with antibiotics will go on to develop ARF several weeks later.[54,67] The incidence of ARF has decreased considerably, with approximately 1 in 100,000 persons affected in the United States.[63] Decreased incidence is attributed to widespread antibiotic use in treating streptococcal infections.[74]

Carditis, or inflammation of the heart, is the most serious manifestation of ARF.[67] As a result of the infection, the heart valves become inflamed and clotting elements are deposited on the valves. Vegetations form on the cusp tips, which then thicken and adhere to one another. Valve adhesions cause the opening to narrow, resulting in mitral valve stenosis. Stenosis slows blood flow from the left atrium to the left ventricle, which may cause thrombus formation. Occasionally the valve

---

*References 14, 15, 24, 26, 100, 108, 120.

cusps retract and no longer meet, and the value is unable to close. This condition is known as **valvular insufficiency,** allowing a backflow of blood, or regurgitation from the left ventricle to the left atrium.[74] Approximately 50% of patients with carditis develop RHD with heart murmur.[54]

In approximately 20% of cases, a single episode of ARF results in heart damage (i.e., RHD). If a patient has more than one episode of ARF, then the chance that RHD is present is nearly 100%.[67] Patients with a history of RHD are more susceptible to IE and require antibiotic premedication according to AHA guidelines.[18]

Antibiotic premedication is not required for patients with a history of ARF without RHD.[67]

The cardiac status of the patient reporting a history of ARF must be confirmed with the patient's physician before initiating treatment. Evaluation includes auscultation, electrocardiogram, echocardiogram, and a chest radiograph. Treatment for RHD includes NSAIDs and steroids to reduce pain and inflammation, diuretics as needed, and bed rest.[74]

Multiple Sclerosis

Multiple sclerosis (MS) is the most common autoimmune disease affecting the nervous system. The disease is characterized by demyelination of nerves in the CNS because of chronic inflammation; the peripheral nervous system is not affected.[67,74] Women are twice as likely to develop this disease as men, with the age of onset between 20 and 40 years. In the United States, approximately 300,000 persons have MS, with a prevalence of 58 per 100,000 persons.[62]

MS is a progressive disease with an unknown etiology. Suggested causes include viruses, immunologic reactions to viruses, bacteria, trauma, autoimmunity, and heredity.[74] HHV 6 has been found in active demyelinated regions of the CNS in patients with MS. Researchers believe that this form of herpesvirus in combination with host genetic factors causes immune-mediated demyelination; however, not all patients infected with HHV 6 develop MS. This suggests that other factors must play a role in the initiation of disease.[8,58] Risk for MS is higher among monozygotic twins.[25]

Demyelination of the neuronal sheath occurs in the white matter of the brain, resulting in patchy areas that become sclerotic. Affected brain regions reveal inflammatory demyelination with accumulation of macrophages, B and T lymphocytes, and plasma cells. Cytokines and immunoglobulins induce macrophages to destroy the myelin.[104] Immunoglobulin levels in the cerebrospinal fluid are increased in the majority of patients. Degeneration of the myelin sheath impairs nerve conduction, with the optic nerve, periventricular cerebral white matter, and cervical spinal cord most affected. Demyelination of the nerve fibers is apparent with magnetic resonance imaging (MRI) of the brain.[67,74]

Initially the disease manifests as muscle impairment and loss of coordination and balance. Paresthesia with tremors, muscle weakness, speech difficulties, and bladder dysfunction are all symptoms in the early stages of MS. Visual disturbances frequently accompany this disease. Fatigue is a major symptom that worsens as the day progresses. Oral manifestations occur in 2% to 3% of MS patients and include paresthesia, difficulty with speech, orofacial numbness, and trigeminal neuralgia.[67,74]

MS appears in cycles of activity and remission; relapses are unpredictable as is the extent of recovery. Heat and dehydration exacerbate symptoms. Recovery is usually temporary, because the myelin sheath does not regenerate. Repeated attacks cause permanent damage; however, intellectual function remains the same. Depression and anxiety challenge patients in coping with their disease.[67,74]

No effective treatment for MS exists. Nonpharmacologic measures include physical therapy, occupational therapy, and counseling.[74] Patients with MS take multiple medications and require comprehensive medical and pharmacologic history reviews to ensure safety before initiating treatment. Steroids are used to block the release of cytokines and to reduce inflammation. Interferons are used to reduce the proliferation of T cells and TNF, and they are administered during periods of remission to reduce the rate of relapse.[67,82] Muscle spasticity is treated with gamma-aminobutyric acid (GABA) agonists, benzodiazepines, and α_2-adrenergic agonists. Bladder dysfunction is treated with oxybutynin (Ditropan) or tolterodine tartrate (Detrol). Stimulants, such as methylphenidate (Ritalin), can be used to combat fatigue, and anticonvulsants are prescribed for extraneous movements and seizure activity. Antidepressants are also frequently prescribed.[67]

DENTAL CONSIDERATIONS

MS patients should be scheduled for short morning appointments and should be treated only during periods of remission. Patients in an active period of MS should not receive routine dental care. Patients who are stable can receive routine dental care with little modification needed. Long-term steroid use may dictate the need for steroid supplementation during stressful or surgical procedures.[67]

Patients may require assistance with walking to the operatory and transferring to the dental chair. Drug-induced xerostomia is a chronic oral complication that requires dental hygiene intervention. Use of powered oral hygiene devices, fluorides, and antimicrobials are all beneficial in helping MS patients maintain adequate oral hygiene.

Chronic Fatigue Syndrome

Chronic fatigue syndrome (CFS) is a debilitating and complex disorder characterized by profound fatigue that is not improved with bed rest and is worsened by physical or mental activity.[12] CFS is nicknamed the "yuppie flu," because it primarily affects young, professional people. The cause and cure remain unknown. Initially researchers believed that the cause was psychosomatic or occurred as a result of depression; however, alterations in the patient's immune system have been identified. Blood tests reveal an immune response consistent with viral infection. Some, but not all, patients with CFS have antibodies to Epstein-Barr virus or herpesvirus B.[74]

Patients with CFS function at a lower level of activity than that before the onset of illness. Other nonspecific symptoms include weakness, muscle pain, impaired memory or mental concentration, insomnia, and postexertional fatigue that persists for more than 24 hours.

Diagnosis of CFS is difficult, because no specific diagnostic tests are available and many other conditions include fatigue as a symptom. To receive a diagnosis of CFS, two criteria must be satisfied:

1. The patient must have severe chronic fatigue of 6 months or longer duration with other known medical conditions excluded by clinical diagnosis.
2. The patient must have four or more of the following symptoms concurrently: substantial impairment in short-term memory or concentration; sore throat; tender lymph nodes; muscle pain; multijoint pain without swelling or redness; headaches of a new type, pattern, or severity; unrefreshing sleep; and postexertional malaise lasting more than 24 hours.[74]

These are considered to be the eight defining symptoms of CFS. Other symptoms affect between 20% and 50% of patients and are summarized in Table 46-7.

Treatment of CFS is aimed at improving symptoms and restoring function and well-being to the patient. Many proposed treatments are unproven and may be harmful. Patients should be encouraged to discuss treatment options with a qualified health professional to design a treatment regimen that will provide the best relief. Nonpharmacologic therapies include carefully paced exercise, such as aquatic therapy, yoga, or Tai Chi. Massage therapy, acupuncture, chiropractic care, and therapeutic touch may also be helpful for some patients. Pharmacologic therapies include NSAIDs for pain relief, tricyclic antidepressants to improve sleep and to relieve mild pain, anxiolytic medications to manage anxiety, and stimulants to improve daytime sleepiness. Sedating antihistamines, such as diphenhydramine, can be helpful at bedtime.[12]

Patients who arrive at the dental office with undiagnosed CFS may inquire about their symptoms of headaches, jaw pain, and xerostomia. A thorough medical history evaluation, physical assessment, and patient interview should reveal other nondental defining characteristics of CFS. A suspicious history of CFS warrants referral to the patient's physician. Many patients experience frustration while in the process of obtaining a formal CFS diagnosis.

Note
The dental hygienist plays an important role as an advocate for the patient and can assist the patient in obtaining educational resources, referral networks, and support programs in the local area.

Table 46-7	Other Common Symptoms of Chronic Fatigue Syndrome
SYSTEM	**SYMPTOM**
HEENT	Xerostomia, xerophthalmia, earaches, jaw pain, chronic cough
Gastrointestinal	Abdominal pain, bloating, diarrhea, nausea
Respiratory	Shortness of breath
Cardiovascular	Chest pain, irregular heartbeat
Neurologic	Dizziness, skin sensations, tingling sensations, depression, irritability, anxiety, panic attacks, alcohol intolerance
Musculoskeletal	Morning stiffness
Endocrine	Night sweats, weight loss

HEENT, Head, eyes, ears, nose, and throat.
From Centers for Disease Control and Prevention: *Chronic fatigue syndrome.* Available at www.cdc.gov/cfs/cfssymptomsHCP.htm#other. Accessed on August 13, 2005.

Fibromyalgia

Fibromyalgia syndrome (FMS) is a widespread musculoskeletal disorder characterized by pain in the muscles, ligaments, and joints, as well as fatigue. The cause remains unknown but is a frequent comorbidity with other autoimmune conditions, including CFS, RA, SLE, and hypothyroidism. Proposed causative factors include abnormally elevated cytokines, alteration in pain-producing neurotransmitters, abnormal sleep patterns, and hormonal irregularities. Triggering events, such as infections or trauma, are not causative; instead they precipitate the onset of the underlying condition.[28]

Symptoms include deep muscle aching and pain, with periods of intense burning sensation, and morning pain and stiffness. Fatigue, sleep disorders, irritable bowel syndrome, premenstrual syndrome, cognitive and memory impairment, skin sensitivity, numbness, tingling sensations, edema of the extremities, and chest pain may also occur.

Changes in weather, infection, allergies, stress, depression, anxiety, and overexertion may increase symptoms. Orofacial symptoms frequently include TMJ dysfunction, face and head pain, and xerostomia.[28]

Treatment is aimed at improving sleep and reducing pain. Antidepressants that elevate serotonin are used to improve sleep quality, including citalopram (Celexa) and trazodone (Desyrel). Zolpidem (Ambien) or the benzodiazepine clonazepam (Klonopin) can also be used to improve sleep. Amitriptyline (Elavil) is a tricyclic antidepressant that improves sleep, elevates mood, and acts as an analgesic. Skeletal muscle relaxants, such as cyclobenzaprine (Flexeril), and analgesics are used for pain relief. Nonpharmacologic treatment methods include physical and occupational therapy, acupuncture, acupressure, relaxation techniques, chiropractic care, therapeutic massage, exercise, and trigger point injections with lidocaine.[28]

Acquired Immunodeficiency Syndrome

Acquired immunodeficiency syndrome (AIDS) is not caused by autoimmunity like the others previously described but rather is a disease caused by the **human immunodeficiency virus** (HIV), resulting in destruction of the person's immune system. The HIV retrovirus carries its genetic information as RNA versus DNA. The virus infects CD4+ T lymphocytes, macrophages, and dendritic cells. After infecting CD4+ T lymphocytes, the RNA is released, then it is copied into the host cell's DNA. The integrated viral DNA is a provirus that can remain latent within the infected cells or can become activated by a stimulus. Activation of the provirus increases the production of viral RNA and proteins, allowing the virus to shed its host cell as an infectious viral particle, which is then ready to infect another cell. Viral gene production and protein synthesis interfere with normal T-cell function, resulting in death of the T cells. Normally the T lymphocytes activate antibody-producing B-cell lymphocytes; however, because infectious viral production kills the CD4+ T cells, the body's immune response is adversely affected. Viral production also kills uninfected lymphocytes. During HIV infection, most viral particles are found in activated CD4+ T cells, whereas macrophages and dendritic cells serve as reservoirs for infection. Patients with the resultant immune deficiency become highly susceptible to infections and certain types of cancers. The reader is referred to Chapter 47 on HIV infection and AIDS for a more detailed discussion of this clinical syndrome.[1,74]

Adrenal Insufficiency

The adrenal glands are located on top of each kidney and are composed of two distinct parts: (1) the cortex that secretes steroid hormones and (2) the medulla that secretes epinephrine and norepinephrine. Steroid hormones are classified into three groups: (1) mineralocorticoids that regulate salt and water balance; (2) glucocorticoids that regulate carbohydrate, fat, and protein metabolism; and (3) the sex hormones, androgens, and estrogens. Epinephrine and norepinephrine are secreted in stressful situations when additional energy and strength are needed and promote vasoconstriction to shunt blood and oxygen to vital organs.[74]

The primary glucocorticoid hormone is cortisol, also known as *hydrocortisone*. Regulation of cortisol secretion is controlled by the hypothalamic-pituitary-adrenal axis. Virtually any type of stress, whether physical or psychologic, causes an immediate increase of pituitary secretion of adrenocorticotropic hormone (ACTH) that stimulates the adrenal cortex to produce and secrete cortisol. Surgery is one of the greatest stressors that produces this response.[83]

In autoimmune diseases the inflammation is often more damaging to the tissues than the disease itself. Cortisol administration can block inflammation and potentially reverse the effects once it has begun. When large amounts of cortisol are either secreted or injected into the body, it produces two primary antiinflammatory effects: (1) it blocks the early stages of the inflammatory process before inflammation actually begins; (2) if inflammation has already begun, then it promotes a rapid resolution of inflammation and speeds the rate of healing.[45]

Cortisol prevents the development of inflammation by reducing the quantity of lysosomal enzymes released by damaged cells that initiate inflammation; decreases the formation of prostaglandins and leukotrienes that decreases vascular permeability and migration of WBCs; and suppresses the reproduction of T lymphocytes, which lessens the antibodies in the inflamed area and the resultant tissue reactions associated with the inflammatory process. If inflammation is already established, then the administration of cortisol can reduce inflammation within 24 hours.[45]

Cortisol decreases the number of eosinophils and lymphocytes in the blood within minutes after injection. Large doses cause atrophy of the lymphoid tissues, which decreases T cells and antibodies, decreasing the level of immunity and increasing risk for infection. However, decreasing immunologic reactions is another benefit of cortisol therapy for autoimmune diseases.[45]

Primary adrenal insufficiency is known as *hypoadrenalism,* or **Addison's disease.** This disease is caused by destruction of the adrenal glands via infections, cancer, or the chronic use of steroid hormones. The adrenal glands fail to produce the corticosteroids aldosterone and cortisol, resulting in dehydration, decreased cardiac output, hypoglycemia, impaired protein and fat metabolism, and generalized weakness. Increased melanin pigmentation may be seen on the lips, mucous membranes, and skin. If left untreated, then the person dies within 2 weeks from circulatory shock or deterioration in response to a stressor, such as infection.[45]

Fortunately, these patients respond well to daily administration of mineralocorticoids and glucocorticoids. Because the patient with Addison's disease does not secrete increased glucocorticoids in times of severe stress, such as dental surgery, the patient is at risk for **addisonian crisis,** which may require the administration of 10 or more times the amount of glucocorticoids necessary to prevent death.[45] Dental professionals must be aware of this risk before performing surgery on patients with this disease.

Secondary adrenal insufficiency is most often caused by chronic use of glucocorticoid medications.[67] Systemic cortisone medication use suppresses the endogenous production of cortisone, because the hypothalamic-pituitary axis senses adequate levels of cortisol in the circulation. One method used to minimize this suppression is to administer cortisone on alternating days, with higher doses used to maintain adequate serum levels, while still allowing the body to secrete its own cortisone on opposing days. The amount of suppression found with alternate-day dosing is less than the typical twice-a-day therapy; however, this approach often does not provide adequate symptom control for patients.[67]

Topically applied and inhaled glucocorticoids rarely produce adrenal suppression, although caution must be used when topical products are applied over large inflamed surface areas or inhaled steroids are used in high, frequent doses[17,47,69,90] (Box 46-3). When drug therapy is discontinued, normal adrenal secretion is restored within 2 weeks.[33] Testing is available to determine the degree of adrenal suppression.

Dental professionals must determine whether patients receiving chronic glucocorticoid therapy require steroid supplementation before treatment. The literature suggests that other than major surgical procedures, most of these patients do not require supplementation for general or routine dental procedures. Even for minor surgeries, patients taking their medications at their usual dose within 2 hours of the procedure should have enough exogenous and endogenous steroids to handle the procedure. Furthermore, local anesthesia or conscious sedation (or both) lowers the stress response to pain, which helps to eliminate the need for supplementation.[67]

Adrenal crisis is a rare, life-threatening condition caused by acute adrenal suppression. Treatment includes immediate intravenous injection of a 100-mg hydrocortisone bolus, as well as intravenous fluid and electrolyte replacement. Over the next 24 hours, 100 mg hydrocortisone is administered IV every 6 to 8 hours with additional fluid replacement and treatment for hypoglycemia as needed.[67] Four factors contribute to the risk of adrenal crisis during oral surgery: (1) the severity of the surgery, (2) the drugs used, (3) the health status of the patient, and (4) the degree of pain control.[6,9,67,99]

DENTAL CONSIDERATIONS

Patients receiving dental surgery should be scheduled first thing in the morning when cortisol levels are highest. Proper stress-reduction protocols should be implemented, including measures to reduce anxiety and pain. Blood pressure should be taken before the procedure, during the perioperative period, and before dismissing the patient. Minor oral and periodontal surgeries require supplementation of glucocorticoids at a 25-mg hydrocortisone equivalent per day, which is equal to a 6-mg dose of prednisone. The drug should be taken within 2 hours of the procedure. Patients undergoing major oral surgical procedures using general anesthesia, those lasting for more than 1 hour, or those involving significant blood loss should be supplemented at 50 to 100 mg hydrocortisone equivalent for the day of surgery, given intraoperatively and for at least 1 postoperative day; hospitalization may be required for these patients. Patients are instructed to take their normal dose and are supplemented to reach the 100-mg equivalent. Hydrocortisone (25 mg) is then given every 8 hours after the surgery for 24 to 48 hours, depending on the extent of the procedure and the degree of postoperative pain.[67]

Finally, monitoring blood pressure is a critical method used to recognize the onset of adrenal crisis. A blood pressure reading below 100/60 mm Hg indicates hypotension, and immediate action must be taken to ensure patient safety. The patient should be positioned with the feet elevated above the height of the head, with fluid replacement, administration of vasopressor, and treatment of hypoglycemia given as needed. Hydrocortisone (100 mg) is administered IV, and the patient is then transported to the hospital.[67,83]

BOX 46-3

TOPICAL GLUCOCORTICOIDS

Topical glucocorticoids are:
- Synthetic derivatives of hydrocortisone
- Used to treat inflammatory diseases that affect the oral mucosa
- Classified according to their potency

    Long-term or repeated use of topical glucocorticoids can result in resistance to their antiinflammatory effects.

    The most frequent oral complication of long-term use of topical glucocorticoids is oral candidiasis.

Data from Greenberg MS: Drugs used for connective-tissue disorders and oral mucosal diseases. In Ciancio SG, ed: *ADA guide to dental therapeutics*, ed 2, Chicago, 2000, ADA Publishing.

Distinct Care Modifications

Dental hygienists should monitor blood pressure before and after treatment in patients at risk for adrenal crisis. Proper pain control, using local anesthetics and nitrous oxide sedation, is an essential component of a stress-reduction protocol in patients with adrenal suppression.

References

1. Abbas AK, Lichtman AH: *Basic immunology: functions and disorders of the immune system*, ed 2, Philadelphia, 2004, Elsevier.
2. Adler J, Terregino CA: Systemic lupus erythematosus, *Emedicine Journal* January 26, 2001 2(1). Available at www.emedicine.com/emerg/topic564.htm. Accessed on June 14, 2001.
3. American College of Rheumatology Ad Hoc Committee on Systemic Lupus Erythematosus Guidelines: Guidelines for referral

and management of systemic lupus erythematosus in adults, *Arthritis Rheum* 42:1785-1796, 1999.

4. Belmont HM: *Lupus: clinical overview.* Available at http://cerebel.com/lupus/overview.html. Accessed on June 14, 2001.

5. Bricker SL, Langlais RP, Miller CS: *Oral diagnosis, oral medicine, and treatment planning,* ed 2, Philadelphia, 1994, Lea & Febiger.

6. Broutsas MG, Seldin R: Adrenal crisis after tooth extractions in an adrenalectomized patient: report of a case, *J Oral Surg* 30:301-302, 1972.

7. Carnell NE, Wilber JF: Primary hypothyroidism. In Bardin CW, ed: *Current therapy in endocrinology and metabolism,* ed 5, St Louis, 1994, Mosby.

8. Carrigan D, Harrington D, Knox K: Subacute leukoencephalitis caused by CNS infection with human herpesvirus-6 manifesting as acute multiple sclerosis, *Neurology* 47:145-148, 1996.

9. Cawson RA, James J: Adrenal crisis in a dental patient having systemic corticosteroids, *Br J Oral Surg* 10:305-309, 1973.

10. Cawson RA, Odell EW: *Essentials of oral pathology and oral medicine,* ed 6, Edinburgh, 1998, Churchill Livingstone.

11. Celiker R, Gokce-Kutsal Y, Eryilmaz M: Temporomandibular joint involvement in rheumatoid arthritis: relationship with disease activity, *Scand J Rheumatol* 24:22-25, 1995.

12. Centers for Disease Control and Prevention: *Chronic fatigue syndrome.* Available at www.cdc.gov/cfs. Accessed on August 13, 2005.

13. Centers for Disease Control and Prevention: *Working together to manage diabetes: a guide for pharmacists, podiatrists, optometrists, and dental professionals,* Atlanta, 2004, US Department of Health and Human Resources, Public Health Service, Centers for Disease Control and Prevention, National Center for Chronic Disease Prevention and Health Promotion.

14. Chaudhry V et al: Mycohenolate mofetil: a safe and promising immunosuppressant in neuromuscular diseases, *Neurology* 56:94-96, 2001.

15. Ciafaloni E et al: Mycophenolate mofetil for myasthenia gravis: an open-label pilot study, *Neurology* 56:97-99, 2001.

16. Ciancio SG, ed: Dental caries and chewing gum; plaque pH, dental caries and chewing gum; increase in salivary flow and remineralization with sugarless gum, *Biol Ther Dent* 5:5-8, 1989.

17. Coskey RJ: Adverse effects of corticosteroids: I—topical and intralesional, *Clin Dermatol* 4:155-160, 1986.

18. Dajani AS et al: Prevention of bacterial endocarditis: recommendations by the American Heart Association, *JAMA* 277:1794-1801, 1997.

19. Damjanov I: *Pathology for the health related professions,* ed 2, Philadelphia, 2000, WB Saunders.

20. Daniels TE: Labial salivary gland biopsy in Sjögren's syndrome: assessment as a diagnostic criterion in 362 suspected cases, *Arthritis Rheum* 27:147-156, 1984.

21. Daniels TE, Fox PC: Salivary and oral components of Sjögren's syndrome, *Rheum Dis Clin North Am* 8:571-589, 1992.

22. Daniels TE et al: The oral component of Sjögren's syndrome, *Oral Surg Oral Med Oral Pathol* 39:975-985, 1975.

23. DeVizio W, Davies R: Rationale for the daily use of a dentifrice containing triclosan in the maintenance of oral health, *Compend Contin Educ Dent* 25(7 suppl 1):54-57, 2004.

24. Drachman DB: Myasthenia gravis, *N Engl J Med* 330:1791-1810, 1994.

25. Ebers GC, Sadovnick AD, Risch NJ: A genetic basis for familial aggregation in multiple sclerosis, *Nature* 377:150-151, 1995.

26. Evoli A et al: Successful treatment of myasthenia gravis with tacrolimus, *Muscle Nerve* 25:111-114, 2002.

27. Fehrenbach MJ: Dental care for the diabetic patient, *The Prevention Angle* IV(III):1-5, 2005.

28. Fibromyalgia Network: *Fibromyalgia basics: symptoms, treatments and research.* Available at www.fmnetnews.com/pages/basics.html. Accessed on August 13, 2005.

29. Firestein GS: Evolving concepts of rheumatoid arthritis, *Nature* 423:356, 2003.

30. Fox, PC, Speight PM: Current concepts of autoimmune exocrinopathy: immunologic mechanisms in the salivary pathology of Sjögren's syndrome, *Crit Rev Oral Biol Med* 7:144-158, 1996.

31. Fox RI, Stern M: Sjögren's syndrome: mechanisms of pathogenesis involve interaction of immune and neurosecretory systems, *Scand J Rheumatol Suppl* 116:3-13, 2002.

32. Glavind L, Lund B, Löe H: The relationship between periodontal state and diabetes duration, insulin dosage and retinal changes, *J Periodontol* 39:341-347, 1968.

33. Glick M: Glucocorticosteroid replacement therapy: a literature review and suggested replacement therapy, *Oral Surg* 67:614-620, 1989.

34. Gluch J: Sugarfree chewing gums and caries prevention, *Cont Oral Hyg* 3:14-15, 2003.

35. Gravallese EM, Goldring SR: Cellular mechanisms and the role of cytokines in bone erosions in rheumatoid arthritis, *Arthritis Rheum* 43:2143, 2000.

36. Graves DA, Al-Mashat H, Liu R: Evidence that diabetes mellitus aggravates periodontal diseases and modified the response to an oral pathogen in animal models, *Compend Contin Educ Dent* 25(7 suppl 1):38-46, 2004.

37. Green MF: The endocrine system. In Pathy MSJ, ed: *Principles and practice of geriatric medicine,* ed 2, New York, 1991, John Wiley & Sons.

38. Greenberg MS: Drugs used for connective-tissue disorders and oral mucosal diseases. In Ciancio SG, ed: *ADA guide to dental therapeutics,* ed 2, Chicago, 2000, ADA Publishing.

39. Grossi SG, Genco RJ: Periodontal disease and diabetes mellitus: a two-way relationship, *Ann Periodontol* 3(1):51-61, 1998.

40. Gurenlian JR: Diabetes mellitus: overview and guidelines for providing oral health care, *Cont Oral Hyg* 1(1):14-20, 2001.

41. Gurenlian JR: Systemic lupus erythematosus, *Access* 15(8):50-53, 2001.

42. Gurenlian JR: Rheumatoid arthritis, *Access* 16(10):30-34, 2002.

43. Gurenlian JR: Sjögren's syndrome, *Access* 16(2):30-34, 2002.

44. Gurenlian JR: *Diabetes mellitus: strategies for providing comprehensive care,* Continuing Education for the Healthcare Professional (CEHP), Farmington Hills, Mich., 2005, Sullivan-Schein (course reference # 05AS2904).

45. Guyton AC, Hall JE: *Textbook of medical physiology,* ed 10, Philadelphia, 2000, WB Saunders.

46. Gynther GW, Tronje G, Holmlund AB: Radiographic changes in the temporomandibular joint in patients with generalized osteoarthritis and rheumatoid arthritis, *Oral Surg Oral Med Oral Pathol Oral Radiol Endod* 81:613-618, 1996.

47. Hanania NA, Chapman KR, Kesten S: Adverse effect of inhaled corticosteroids, *Am J Med* 98:196-208, 1995.

48. Holmlund AB, Gynther GW, Reinhold FP: Rheumatoid arthritis and disk derangement of the temporomandibular joint: a comparative arthroscopic study, *Oral Surg Oral Med Oral Pathol Oral Radiol Endod* 73:273-277, 1992.

49. Hugoson A et al: Periodontal conditions in insulin-dependent diabetes, *J Clin Periodontol* 16:215-223, 1989.

50. Humes HD: *Kelley's essentials of internal medicine,* ed 2, Philadelphia, 2001, Lippincott Williams & Wilkins.

51. Jacob LS: *The national medical series for independent study: pharmacology,* ed 4, Philadelphia, 1996, Williams & Wilkins.

52. Jimenez S, Koenig AS: *Scleroderma.* Available at www.emedicine. com/med/topic2076.htm. Accessed on August 8, 2005.

53. Jordan RCK, Speight PM: Lymphoma in Sjögren's syndrome: from histopathology to molecular pathology, *Oral Surg Oral Med Oral Pathol Oral Radiol Endod* 81:308-320, 1996.

54. Kaplan EL: Acute rheumatic fever. In Alexander RW, ed: *Hurst's the heart, arteries and veins,* vol 2, New York, 1998, McGraw-Hill.

55. Kassan S, Thomas T, Moutsopoulos HM: The increased risk of lymphoma in sicca syndrome, *Ann Intern Med* 89:888-892, 1978.

56. Kent JN, Carlton DM, Zide MF: Rheumatoid disease and related arthropathies: II—surgical rehabilitation of the temporomandibular joint, *Oral Surg* 61:423-439, 1986.

57. Khurshudian AV: A pilot study to test the efficacy of oral administration of interferon-α lozenges to patients with Sjögren's syndrome, *Oral Surg Oral Med Oral Pathol Oral Radiol Endod* 95: 38-44, 2003.

58. Knox KK et al: Human herpesvirus 6 and multiple sclerosis: systemic active infections in patients with early disease, *Clin Infect Dis* 31:894-903, 2000.

59. Koopman WJ: *Arthritis and related conditions,* Baltimore, 1997, Williams & Wilkins.

60. Kuks JBM, Oosterhuis HJGH, Limburg PC: The TH:anti-acetylcholine receptor antibodies decrease after thymectomy in patients with myasthenia gravis: clinical correlations, *J Autoimmun* 4:197-211, 1991.

61. Kumar V, Abbas AK, Fausto N: *Robbins and Cotran pathologic basis of disease,* ed 7, Philadelphia, 2005, Elsevier Saunders.

62. Kurtzke J: Epidemiology of MS. In Hallpike JF, Adams CWM, Tourtellote WE, eds: *Multiple sclerosis,* Baltimore, 1983, Williams & Wilkins.

63. Land MA, Bisno AL: Acute rheumatic fever: a vanishing disease, *JAMA* 249:895-898, 1983.

64. Larheim TA, Johannessen S, Tveito L: Abnormalities of the temporomandibular joint in adults with rheumatic disease: a comparison of panoramix, transcranial, and transpharyngeal radiography with tomography, *Dentomaxillofac Radiol* 17:109-113, 1988.

65. Lee DM, Weinblatt ME: Rhematoid arthritis, *Lancet* 358:903, 2001.

66. Levine MJ: Development of artificial salivas, *Crit Rev Oral Biol Med* 4:279-286, 1993.

67. Little JW et al: *Dental management of the medically compromised patient,* ed 6, St Louis, 2002, Mosby.

68. Louis PJ, Fernandes R: Review of systemic lupus erythematosus, *Oral Surg Oral Med Oral Pathol Oral Radiol Endod* 91(5):512-516, 2001.

69. Maxwell DL: Adverse effects of inhaled corticosteroids, *Biomed Pharmacother* 44:421-427, 1990.

70. McMahon RFT, Sloan P: *Essentials of pathology for dentistry,* Edinburgh, 2000, Churchill Livingstone.

71. Merrill JT: The antiphospholipid syndrome: what we know today and what the future holds, *Lupus News* 20(5):14-16, 2000.

72. Moore, PA, Zgibor JC, Dasanayake AP: Diabetes: a growing epidemic of all ages, *J Am Dent Assoc* 134:11S-15S, 2003.

73. Moutsopoulos HM et al: Association of serum IgM kappa monoclonality in patients with Sjögren's syndrome with an increased proportion of kappa positive plasma cells infiltrating the labial salivary glands, *Ann Rheum Dis* 49:929-931, 1990.

74. Mulvihill ML et al: *Human diseases: a systemic approach,* ed 5, Upper Saddle River, NJ, 2001, Prentice Hall.

75. Najera M et al: Prevalence of periodontal disease in patients with Sjögren's syndrome, *Oral Surg Oral Med Oral Pathol Oral Radiol Endod* 83:453-457, 1997.

76. National Institute of Arthritis and Musculoskeletal and Skin Diseases: *Handout on health: scleroderma.* Available at www.niams.nih. gov/hi/topics/scleroderma/scleroderma.htm. Accessed on August 8, 2005.

77. National Institute of Diabetes and Digestive and Kidney Diseases: *National Diabetes Statistics fact sheet: general information and national estimates on diabetes in the United States, 2005,* Bethesda, Md, 2005, US Department of Health and Human Services, National Institutes of Health.

78. Nauert P: *Scleroderma and dental health.* Available at www. scleroderma.org/medical/dental_articles/Nauert_1999a.htm. Accessed on August 8, 2005.

79. Neville BW et al: *Oral & maxillofacial pathology,* ed 2, Philadelphia, 2002, WB Saunders.

80. Nieuw Amerongen AV, Veerman ECI: Current therapies for xerostomia and salivary gland hypofunction associated with cancer therapies, *Support Care Cancer* 11:226-231, 2003.

81. Nikolaos GN et al: Primary Sjögren syndrome in childhood: report of a case and review of the literature, *Oral Surg Oral Med Oral Pathol Oral Radiol Endod* 96:42-47, 2003.

82. Noseworthy JH et al: Multiple sclerosis, *N Engl J Med* 343: 938-952, 2000.

83. Orth DN, Kovacs WJ, Debold CR: The adrenal cortex. In Wilson JD, Foster DW, eds: *Williams textbook of endocrinology,* ed 8, Philadelphia, 1992, WB Saunders.

84. Ostuni PA et al: Juvenile onset of primary Sjögren's syndrome: report of ten cases, *Clin Exp Rheumatol* 14(6):689-693, 1996.

85. Papas A, Stack KM, Spodak D: Sonic toothbrushing increases saliva flow rate in Sjögren's syndrome patients, *J Dent Res* (spec iss):981, 1998 (abstract #2795).

86. Patton LL, Howard JF Jr: Myasthenia gravis: dental treatment considerations, *Spec Care Dentist* 17:25-32, 1997.

87. Phillips LH: The epidemiology of myasthenia gravis, *Neurol Clin* 12:263-271, 1994.

88. Pickett F, Gurenlian JR: *The medical history: clinical implications and emergency prevention in dental settings,* Baltimore, 2005, Lippincott Williams & Wilkins.

89. Pisetsky DS: Systemic lupus erythematosus: A—epidemiology, pathology, and pathogenesis. In Schumacher HR Jr, ed: *Primer on rheumatic diseases,* ed 10, Atlanta, 1993, Arthritis Foundation.

90. Plemons JM, Rees TD, Zachariah NY: Absorption of a topical steroid and evaluation of adrenal suppression in patients with erosive lichen planus, *Oral Surg* 69:688-693, 1990.

91. Reed Larson P, Davies TF, Hay ID: The thyroid gland. In Wilson JD et al, eds: *Williams textbook of endocrinology,* ed 9, Philadelphia, 1998, WB Saunders.

92. Regezi JA, Sciubba JJ, Jordan RCK: *Oral pathology: clinical pathologic correlations,* ed 4, St Louis, 2003, Saunders.

93. Rhodus NL: Sjogren's syndrome, *Quintessence Int* 30:689-699, 1999.

94. Rhodus NL et al: *Candida albicans* levels in patients with Sjögren's syndrome before and after long-term use of pilocarpine hydrochloride, *Quintessence Int* 29:705-710, 1998.

95. Rhodus NL, Schuh MJ: Effect of pilocarpine on salivary flow in patients with Sjögren's syndrome, *Oral Surg Oral Med Oral Pathol* 72:545-549, 1991.

96. Rosenthal I, Abrams H, Kopczyck A: The relationship of inflammatory periodontal disease to diabetic status in insulin-dependent

diabetes mellitus patients, *J Clin Periodontol* 15:425-429, 1988.

97. Ryan ME, Carnu O, Kamer A: The influence of diabetes on the periodontal tissues, *J Am Dent Assoc* 134:34S-40S, 2003.

98. Saito T et al: Sjögren's syndrome in the adolescent, *Oral Surg Oral Med Oral Pathol* 77:368-372, 1994.

99. Schietler LE, Tucker WM, Christian DG: Adrenal insufficiency: report of a case, *Spec Care Dentist* 4:22-24, 1984.

100. Schneider C et al: Mycophenolate mofetil in the therapy of severe myasthenia gravis, *Eur Neurol* 46:79-82, 2001.

101. Scleroderma Foundation: *Medication information.* Available at www.scleroderma.org/medical/medication.shtm. Accessed on August 12, 2005.

102. Smallridge RC: Evaluation of thyroid function: blood tests. In Becker K, ed: *Principles and practice of endocrinology and metabolism,* Philadelphia, 1990, JB Lippincott.

103. Spolarich AE: Medication use and xerostomia, *Dimensions Dent Hyg* 3:22-24, 2005.

104. Steinman L: Multiple sclerosis: a coordinated immunological attack against myelin in the central nervous system, *Cell* 85: 299-302, 1996.

105. Sugahara T et al: Obstructive sleep apnea associated with temporomandibular joint destruction by rheumatoid arthritis: report of case, *J Oral Maxillofac Surg* 52:876-880, 1994.

106. Tervonen T, Karjalainen KM: Periodontal disease related to diabetic status: a pilot study of the response to periodontal therapy in type 1 diabetes, *J Clin Periodontol* 24:505-510, 1997.

107. Tervonen T, Oliver RC: Long-term control of diabetes mellitus and periodontitis, *J Clin Periodontol* 20:431-435, 1993.

108. Tindall RSA et al: A clinical therapeutic trial of cyclosporine in myasthenia gravis, *Ann N Y Acad Sci* 681:539-551, 1993.

109. Tunbridge WMG, Caldwell G: The epidemiology of thyroid disease. In Braverman LE, Utiger RD, eds: *Werner and Ingbar's the thyroid,* ed 6, Philadelphia, 1991, JB Lippincott.

110. Vernillo AT: Diabetes mellitus: relevance to dental treatment, *Oral Surg Oral Med Oral Pathol Oral Radiol Endod* 91(3): 263-270, 2001.

111. Vitali C: Classification criteria for Sjögren's syndrome, *Ann Rheum Dis* 62:94-95, 2003.

112. Wall GC, Magarity ML, Jundt JW: Pharmacotherapy of xerostomia in primary Sjögren's syndrome, *Pharmacotherapy* 22: 621-629, 2002.

113. Wartofsky L: Diseases of the thyroid. In Fauci AS et al, eds: *Harrison's principles of internal medicine,* ed 14, New York, 1998, McGraw-Hill.

114. Weetman AP: Graves' disease, *N Engl J Med* 343(17):1236-1248, 2000.

115. Weijnen FG et al: Masticatory performance in patients with myasthenia gravis, *Arch Oral Biol* 47:393-398, 2002.

116. Willis T: *De anima brutorum,* Oxford, 1672, Theatro Sheldoniano.

117. Wray D et al: *Textbook of general and oral medicine,* Edinburgh, 1999, Churchill Livingstone.

118. Wynn RD, Meiller TF, Crossley HL: *Drug information handbook for dentistry,* ed 10, Hudson, Ohio, 2005, Lexi-Comp Inc.

119. Yarom N et al: Dental management of patients with myasthenia gravis: a literature review, *Oral Surg Oral Med Oral Pathol Oral Radiol Endod* 100:158-163, 2005.

120. Yoshikawa H et al: FK506 prevents induction of rat experimental autoimmune myasthenia gravis, *J Autoimmun* 10:11-16, 1997.

121. Younai FS, Phelan JA: Oral mucositis with features of psoriasis: report of a case and review of the literature, *Oral Surg Oral Med Oral Pathol Oral Radiol Endod* 84:61-67, 1997.

122. Young W et al: Syndromes with salivary dysfunction predispose to tooth wear: case reports of congenital dysfunction of major salivary glands, Prader-Will, congenital rubella, and Sjögren's syndromes, *Oral Surg Oral Med Oral Pathol Oral Radiol Endod* 92:38-48, 2000.

123. Xu T et al: Effectiveness of a triclosan/copolymer dentifrice on microbiological and inflammatory parameters, *Compend Contin Educ Dent* 25(7 suppl 1):46-53, 2004.

HIV and AIDS

Eve Cuny • David A. Reznik • Helene Bednarsh

INSIGHT

As a disease of significant concern and impact, everyone must understand human immunodeficiency virus and acquired immunodeficiency syndrome. More importantly, as healthcare providers, dental hygienists must understand and recognize the oral manifestations, infection-control implications, and postexposure management associated with HIV disease.

✦ CASE STUDY 47-1 | Clinical Presentations of HIV

Sheila Jones is a 29-year-old female patient. She returns for a 6-month recall. As you update her medical history, she complains of fatigue, muscle aches, night sweats, and a loss of appetite. She reports no other changes in her medical history or any medications. She does reveal a new relationship in her life since her last visit; she says, "This is the one for me!" On oral examination, you note white-red mixed patches in her mouth, most notably on her hard palate. You question her, and she says that she has noticed them as well, but she cannot recall how long they have been there. Her gingival tissue is inflamed and appears to have a red banding along the gingival margin. You refer her back to her primary care provider to determine the cause of the symptoms.

KEY TERMS

acquired immunodeficiency
 syndrome
Americans with Disabilities Act
angular cheilitis
cytomegalovirus
erythematous candidiasis
exposure-prone invasive
 procedures

highly active antiretroviral therapy
human immunodeficiency virus
human papillomavirus
Kaposi's sarcoma
Kaposi's sarcoma–associated
 herpesvirus

linear gingival erythema
necrotizing ulcerative gingivitis
necrotizing ulcerative
 periodontitis
oral hairy leukoplakia
Pneumocystis carinii pneumonia

postexposure prophylaxis
pseudomembranous candidiasis
retrovirus
window period
zidovudine (azidothymidine)

LEARNING OUTCOMES

After reading this chapter the student will be able to:
1. Discuss the etiologic factors of HIV and AIDS.
2. Demonstrate an appreciation and understanding for the epidemiologic mechanisms of HIV and AIDS.
3. Relate the forms of prevention for HIV.
4. Compare and contrast the clinical characteristics of HIV and AIDS.
5. Develop a care plan for patients with HIV and AIDS.

History of Human Immunodeficiency Virus and Acquired Immunodeficiency Syndrome

In June and July 1981, unusual patterns of disease were reported by the Centers for Disease Control and Prevention (CDC) through the *Morbidity and Mortality Weekly Report (MMWR)*. Five young men were treated for biopsy-confirmed *Pneumocystis carinii* **pneumonia** at three different hospitals in Los Angeles, California, between October 1980 and May 1981.[6] All five patients had laboratory-confirmed previous or current **cytomegalovirus** (CMV) infection and candidal mucosal infections. On July 4, 1981, the CDC reported that during the previous 30 months, 26 cases of Kaposi's sarcoma were reported among gay men and that eight had died within 24 months of diagnosis.[5] An underlying cause of these unusual presentations in otherwise healthy young men was not immediately evident. As reports of infections continued, investigations for common associations began. In 1982, reports of infection in persons with hemophilia and recipients of blood transfusions suggested transmission via a blood-borne route. Since the first reports in 1981, more than 1.5 million people in the United States have been infected with HIV and more than 500,000 of them have died. Currently, approximately 40,000 new infections are reported each year, down from a one-time high of more than 150,000 per year in the 1980s.

Not until 1984 was a retrovirus discovered and determined to be the association researchers were seeking. A **retrovirus** replicates using ribonucleic acid (RNA) rather than deoxyribonucleic acid (DNA) and was thought to be rare in humans. The first isolates of what later would be known as **human immunodeficiency virus** (HIV) were discovered in France (lymphadenopathy-associated virus [LAV]) in 1983 and in the United States (human T-lymphotropic virus [HTLV]-III) in 1984. The identification of this agent enabled tests to be developed by 1985 to detect the presence of antibodies, a sign of infection, in individuals with the signs and symptoms of what we now refer to as **acquired immunodeficiency syndrome** (AIDS). Testing allowed for prevalence and incidence studies and demonstrated that infection was more common than in later-stage HIV. Testing also made it possible to screen blood and plasma donations, study the progression of disease, and provide surveillance of healthcare workers who are potentially exposed to the blood of persons infected with HIV. Surveillance is also useful for determining prevention and targeting populations who are at risk of infection by identifying modes of transmission, trends in the epidemic, and where to allocate resources to control the spread of infection. Thus surveillance takes on an importance in policy decisions.

HIV is composed of three significant components:
1. Envelope
2. RNA genome
3. Structural proteins

These components are important to the understanding of transmission in terms of where the virus attaches to the cell and how it enters, reverses cellular DNA, replicates, and exits to infect other cells. This understanding is also crucial to the development of drugs intended to prevent or control infection because antiretroviral agents target specific sites associated with the process of transmission and infection. The first antiretroviral medication, **zidovudine (azidothymidine [AZT]),** a reverse transcriptase inhibitor, was approved by the U.S. Food and Drug Administration (FDA) in 1987. Reverse transcriptase is the enzyme on which HIV relies to transcribe HIV RNA to DNA. Patients were required to take this medication every 4 hours around the clock. Not until the Concorde study was published in 1993 did researchers realize that AZT monotherapy taken early in the disease offered no benefit. The next class of drugs were not approved until 1995; these drugs had the ability to interrupt HIV replication and provide evidence of immune response through an increase in CD4+ cells, the primary measure of the extent of disease progression at that time.

The availability of potent antiretrovirals, in combinations rather than the monotherapy offered by AZT, had a dramatic affect on prolonging life. The number of AIDS-related deaths before the advent of combination therapy steadily increased, peaking in 1995 with more than 48,000 known deaths caused by AIDS in the United States. **Highly active antiretroviral therapy** (HAART) slowed the progression of HIV disease, and the death rate began to fall in 1996 to the present rate of approximately 18,000 per year. An important point to note is that, with the advent of HAART, HIV disease became a chronic disease that the medical community might manage through continual lifelong treatment. HAART slowed the progression of disease, but behaviors leading to infection still exist. Therefore more people are living with HIV/AIDS rather than dying from it.

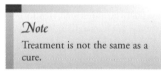

Note
Treatment is not the same as a cure.

HAART improves the immune system but does not eradicate the virus. Prevention remains the most critical element in reducing infection and death.

Prevention efforts are twofold.

An example of successful prevention is the progress the developed world has seen in the dramatic decrease of mother-to-child transmission. Through the use of antiretroviral therapy in pregnant women living with HIV, the risk of transmission has fallen from 25% to approximately 2%. Methods of prevention include the following:

Prevention
Primary prevention is designed to prevent HIV infection in the first place; secondary prevention efforts educate persons living with this disease in an attempt to limit the spread of the infection.

- Reducing behaviors associated with the risk of HIV infection
- Using barriers such as condoms for safer sex
- Having access to clean needles and syringes for injection drug users
- Treating sexually transmitted infections

Without a vaccine, reliance for prevention remains focused on methods that are proven to reduce the spread of infection.

AIDS is a reportable infection to the CDC, and some states report HIV infection as well. The latest surveillance reports from the CDC through the end of 2003 estimated that 1,039,000 to 1,185,000 persons in the United States are living with HIV/AIDS.[3]

The majority of new AIDS cases (71%) and new HIV cases (64%) in 2003 were among minorities. The highest incidence rates now occur among blacks, with AIDS being the third leading cause of death. In Hispanics, AIDS is the sixth leading cause of death. Heterosexual transmission increased from 3% in the mid-1980s to 31% in 2003, and women represent a growing proportion of new AIDS cases, increasing from 8% in the mid-1980s to 27% in 2003. In this same time period, cases among men who have sex with men decreased from 65% to 42%. Increases were also seen among injection drug users. Ten states accounted for 71% of all reported cases. However, many persons infected with HIV are not measured because many states do not have an HIV-reporting system accepted by the CDC and because many people have not sought testing.

Globally, the HIV/AIDS pandemic has killed at least 23 million of the more than 65 million people it has infected thus far, leaving 15 million orphans worldwide.

In 2003, almost 5 million people became infected, the greatest number ever in a single year, and 3.1 million died. Hardly any area in the world has not been touched by this pandemic. In sub-Saharan Africa, an estimated 3 million people were infected in 2003, and 25 million have HIV. Worldwide, women are at increased risk of infection, and young people account for nearly one half of all infections. Asia is an area of the largest growth in HIV infection with 8.5 million cases reported. Eastern Europe reports 1.3 million, Latin America 1.6 million, and the Caribbean approximately 430,000. Current projections predict that an additional 100 million will become infected and 45 million will die by the end of this decade unless the trends are reversed.[16] In developing countries, AIDS is reversing gains made in health, economic, political, and social progress.

Definition

HIV is characterized by deterioration of the immune system, as noted by decreases in CD4+ cells. CD4+ cells have an important role in immune response. HIV can replicate only within cells using the reverse transcriptase enzyme to convert their RNA into DNA, thus becoming part of the host cell. HIV is composed of a viral envelope, an RNA genome, and structural proteins. Proteins in the envelope facilitate HIV's entry and exit from CD4+ cells, and enzymes within the cell core control replication. Eight steps compose the replication cycle:

1. Attachment
2. Entry
3. Reverse transcriptase
4. Integration
5. Gene expression
6. Assembly
7. Budding
8. Maturation

HIV replicates by attaching to the cell surface of CD4+ cells and then entering the cell and beginning its life process. Once within the cell, RNA is converted into DNA through a process known as *reverse transcriptase.* The HIV DNA becomes integrated into the cell as a provirus. For the provirus to produce new viruses, RNA must be copied, and these copies are messenger RNA and are produced through the process known as *transcription.* Once the virus is translated in the cytoplasm, the new viral particles in long chains of viral proteins and enzymes can be assembled. Chains are cut into smaller pieces by the protease enzyme, and the virus buds and matures. Interference with any of these stages is the goal in treatment and prevention (Figure 47-1).

Once infection is established, HIV rapidly replicates. This early stage of HIV infection is referred to as *acute HIV syndrome,* producing symptoms such as fever, malaise, lymph node swelling, and other influenza-like symptoms. Early infection may not be recognized as HIV infection because the symptoms resemble other viral infections. During this time, antibodies to HIV are produced, although possibly not at detectable levels, and high levels of HIV RNA can be detected by viral load testing.

From this point, wide variation exists in the progression of disease. Individuals may remain asymptomatic, yet the virus continues to replicate and destroy or disable infected cells. As immune suppression progresses, symptoms may appear relative to infection. Opportunistic infections, those that take advantage of a suppressed immune system, appear.

The presence of certain conditions seen in association with disease progression distinguishes HIV infection from AIDS. These conditions are known as *AIDS-defining conditions,* and they established a case definition of AIDS (Box 47-1). The CDC's definition of AIDS includes fewer than 200 CD4+ cells and 26 other clinical conditions, including malignancies and fungal and viral infections. However, even in some individuals with fewer than 200 CD4+ cells, no identifiable symptoms may be present.[4]

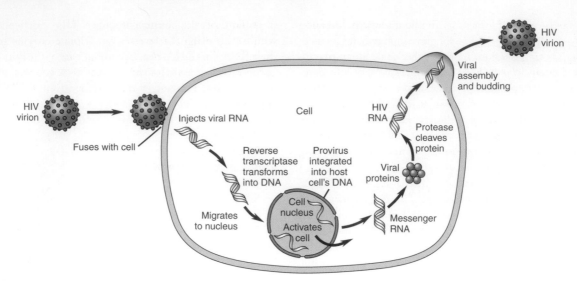

FIGURE 47-1
HIV life cycle. A schematic representation from the time of initial HIV fusion with a host cell, integration into the host cell's DNA, and ending with the replication of a new virion. (From Copstead LC, Banasik JL: *Pathophysiology*, ed 3, St Louis, 2005, WB Saunders.)

BOX 47-1

AIDS-Defining Conditions

AIDS-defining conditions include HIV infection plus any of the following:

- Candidiasis
- Invasive cervical cancer
- Cryptosporidiosis
- Cytomegalovirus
- HIV-related encephalopathy
- Herpes simplex
- Histoplasmosis
- Isosporiasis
- Kaposi's sarcoma
- Lymphoma
- *Mycobacterium avium* complex
- *Pneumocystis carinii* pneumonia
- Recurrent pneumonia
- Progressive multifocal leukoencephalopathy
- Recurrent salmonella
- Toxoplasmosis
- Tuberculosis
- Wasting syndrome

    Case definition* is not only important as a diagnostic tool, but also important in terms of eligibility for certain disability benefits.

---

*Refer to Reference #4 for specific case definitions on AIDS.

Testing

Testing for HIV infection searches for the presence of antibodies to HIV, not for the virus itself. A person with detectable antibodies is considered seropositive. Up to 3 months may be required for detectable antibodies to develop. This period between infection and antibody response is referred to as the window period. During this period, the individual is infected and may transmit infection but may not be clinically or symptomatically aware. HIV antibody testing is screening to detect infection through the use of an enzyme immune assay (EIA) or an enzyme-linked immunoabsorbent assay (ELISA). If the EIA is reactive, then the test is repeated on the same blood sample, and if still positive, then it is confirmed by the Western blot test. The Western blot is more specific than both EIA and ELISA and can differentiate between antibodies to HIV and other antibodies. Early in the epidemic, the Western blot test was the only test available to detect infection. Other tests are now available to detect infection with HIV, such as the viral load test. The viral load test identifies actual HIV viral particles in the blood, more specifically the p24 protein, and detects infection earlier than antibody testing. It has the advantage of not only earlier detection, but also measures expression of HIV and disease progression. This expression is a measure of the number of HIV copies in a milliliter of blood, and if the expression is high, then it indicates active reproduction and progression. A low viral load corresponds to less active reproduction and progression. An undetectable viral load means that the level of circulating virus is below the test's ability to detect but is not evidence of absence of HIV. HIV antibody testing is the preferred method of detecting HIV, whereas viral load testing is more important for disease progression, determining treatment regimens or modifying treatment, detecting failures in treatment, and making decisions about postexposure management in the event of an occupational exposure. Other types of testing include rapid testing for antibodies. Rapid testing produces results in 20 minutes compared with the 1 to 2 weeks for the EIA screening test and are considered as accurate. Rapid tests still require a confirmatory test before a specific

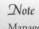

Note

Management of HIV infection relies on testing and early diagnosis.

diagnosis can be made. Home tests kits are under consideration as well.

Although testing is voluntary, it is recommended for persons known or thought to have been exposed to HIV and for pregnant women. Appropriate testing includes pretest and posttest counseling with informed consent. Counseling provides information on test interpretation and methods to avoid secondary transmission if the test is positive. Counseling can provide information on treatment and appropriate referral into medical care or other treatment programs.

Treatment to Suppress the Virus and Prevent Opportunistic Diseases

No known cure exists for HIV or AIDS; therefore the best attempts are to suppress the virus and prevent opportunistic disease occurrences. Antiretroviral agents suppress the virus. However, HIV-drug resistance is a major concern both in treating the infected individual and in determining the appropriate postexposure management. Resistance can be to individual drugs, to classes, or cross-resistance.

The FDA approves drugs for treating HIV infection. This rapidly evolving area has improved since the advent of combination therapy recommendations in the mid-1990s. The first classes of drugs approved act by interfering with the virus's ability to use specific enzymes, reverse transcriptase, and protease enzymes. Reverse transcriptase inhibitors interfere with the process by which HIV copies itself and are of two types: nucleoside and nucleotide, which interfere with the DNA chain, and nonnucleoside, which bind the virus to prevent it from copying. Protease inhibitors interfere with the protease enzyme to prevent viral particle production. The newest class of antiretrovirals are entry inhibitors, which block cell entry. Other drugs under development include categories designed to do the following:

- Interfere with cell integration
- Interfere with budding and assembly
- Interfere with replication
- Possibly modify genes to suppress replication

The goal in treatment is to reduce morbidity and mortality associated with HIV infection, to restore and preserve immune function, to suppress viral load, and to improve the quality of life.

DENTAL CONSIDERATIONS

Dental healthcare professionals have a key role in improving the quality of life by assisting patients in maintaining their oral health and in managing oral infection.

A patient with HIV may be taking several different drugs in the various classes or even in a clinical trial for a drug under development. Consultation with the healthcare provider for the person with HIV, with the appropriate informed consent, is necessary to determine any contraindications to care. In addition, patients may also be taking drugs to treat or prevent opportunistic infections.

Failure of drug treatment may be virologic, immunologic, or clinical. If failure is detected, then the provider may modify the treatment regimen.

What is the significance of this possibility to oral healthcare? As with any patient, dental healthcare professionals have a responsibility to manage oral care appropriately. This obligation includes a complete medical history, oral examination, review of systems, and attention paid to underlying medical conditions. HIV disease is but another underlying medical condition that may influence patient care. It is not a pretext to deny care or treat a patient in a manner of which all patients are deserving.

> **Distinct Care Modifications**
>
> An understanding of treatment that includes antiretroviral therapy, a thorough medical history and oral evaluation, and consultation with the patient's HIV provider is essential.

> **Prevention**
>
> The dental healthcare professional, through close clinical observation, may detect drug failure as the appearance of oral manifestations of HIV disease.

DENTAL CONSIDERATIONS

Dental healthcare professionals have a unique opportunity to detect and treat oral manifestations of HIV disease, to perhaps be the first to recognize symptoms associated with HIV infection, and to refer a patient to medical care if indicated.

Oral Manifestations of Human Immunodeficiency Virus Disease

47-1

Oral manifestations of HIV infection are a fundamental component of disease progression and occur in approximately 30% to 80% of the affected patient population.[2,7,14] Factors that predispose expression of oral lesions include CD4+ cell counts of less than 200/mcl, HIV RNA levels greater than 3000 copies/ml, xerostomia, poor oral hygiene, and smoking.[1,15] Oral lesions are differentiated as fungal, viral, and bacterial infections; as neoplasms such as Kaposi's sarcoma; and as nonspecific presentations such as aphthous ulcerations and salivary gland disease.

Overall prevalence of the oral manifestations of HIV disease has changed since the advent of HAART. One study noted a reduction of oral lesions from 47.6% pre-HAART to 37.5% during the HAART era.[14] The details of this study included a significant reduction in oral hairy leukoplakia and necrotizing ulcerative periodontitis, yet no significant change occurred in the incidence of oral candidiasis, oral ulcers, or Kaposi's sarcoma. This population did, however, have an increase in salivary gland disease. Other published reports show a markedly increased incidence of oral warts in the HAART era.[9,10]

Treatment of the oral diseases seen in association with HIV disease is reportedly low. A study of 1424 adults who participated in the AIDS Cost and Utilization Study revealed that only 9.1% reported treatment for oral manifestations. After adjusting for CD4+ cell count and other variables, blacks and Hispanics were significantly less likely than other groups to receive treatment. Factors that were significant with regard to receiving care for oral disease included more than a high school education, participation in clinical trials, and utilization of counseling services.[12] The ability to differentiate one manifestation from another and to manage some of the more common conditions are fundamental to the overall health care of this patient population. A description of the most common oral manifestations seen in association with HIV disease follows.

FUNGAL INFECTIONS

The most common fungal infection seen in association with HIV infection is oropharyngeal candidiasis. Three frequently observed forms of oral candidiasis have been found:

1. Erythematous candidiasis
2. Pseudomembranous candidiasis
3. Angular cheilitis

Erythematous candidiasis exhibits as a red, flat, subtle lesion on the dorsal surface of the tongue or the hard or soft palates (Figure 47-2). Erythematous candidiasis tends to be symptomatic, with patients complaining of oral burning most frequently while eating salty or spicy foods or drinking acidic beverages. Clinical diagnosis is based on appearance, taking into consideration the person's medical history and virologic status.

> ***Distinct Care Modifications***
> Because of the limited nature of erythematous candidiasis, treatment involves topical antifungal therapies.

Pseudomembranous candidiasis appears as creamy white curdlike plaques on the buccal mucosa, tongue, and other oral mucosal surfaces that will wipe away, leaving a red or bleeding underlying surface (Figure 47-3). The most common organism involved with the presentation of candidiasis is *Candida albicans.* However, reports of the increased incidence of nonalbicans species are increasing.[11] Although the prevalence of pseudomembranous candidiasis in the HAART era has declined, it is still one of the most common oral manifestations seen in HIV disease.

The clinical presentation of **angular cheilitis** is erythema or fissuring of the corners of the mouth (Figure 47-4). Angular cheilitis can occur with or without the presence of oral erythematous candidiasis or pseudomembranous candidiasis.

> ***Distinct Care Modifications***
> Treatment for pseudomembranous candidiasis should be based on the extent of the infection, with topical therapies (nystatin, clotrimazole) used for mild to moderate cases and systemic therapies (fluconazole) used for moderate to severe presentations. Antifungal therapy should last for 2 weeks to reduce the number of colony-forming units to the lowest level possible to prevent recurrence.

> ***Distinct Care Modifications***
> Treatment for angular cheilitis involves a topical antifungal cream directly applied to the affected areas four times a day for the 2-week treatment period.

★ CASE APPLICATION 47-1.1

Candidiasis Prescription

The dentist for whom you work wrote an appropriate prescription for candidiasis for Ms. Jones based on the white-red patches on the hard palate.

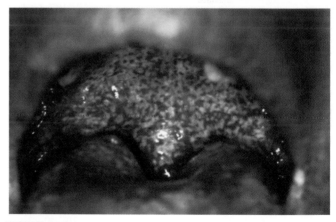

FIGURE 47-3
Pseudomembranous candidiasis.

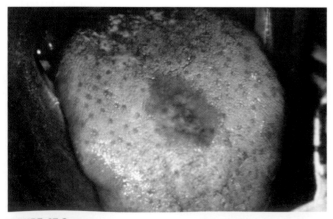

FIGURE 47-2
Erythematous candidiasis.

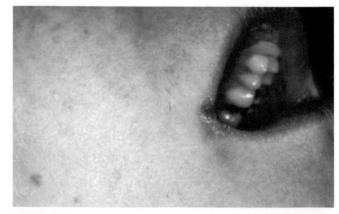

FIGURE 47-4
Angular cheilitis.

PERIODONTAL DISEASES

Whereas chronic adult periodontal disease occurs frequently in persons living with HIV disease, three unique presentations of periodontal disease have also been reported in this patient population:

1. Linear gingival erythema
2. Necrotizing ulcerative gingivitis
3. Necrotizing ulcerative periodontitis

Linear gingival erythema (LGE) exhibits as a red band along the gingival margin, which may or may not be accompanied by occasional bleeding and discomfort (Figure 47-5). Linear gingival erythema is seen most frequently in association with anterior teeth but commonly extends to the posterior teeth. LGE can also exist on attached and nonattached gingiva as petechia-like patches.

The demarcation between necrotizing gingivitis and necrotizing periodontitis was created to define the difference between the rapid destruction of soft (**necrotizing ulcerative gingivitis**) and hard (**necrotizing ulcerative periodontitis**) tissues. Whether necrotizing ulcerative gingivitis and necrotizing ulcerative periodontitis are the same or unique entities has yet to be determined, and both have been classified as *necrotizing*

periodontal diseases by the American Academy of Periodontology. Because of the lack of significant differences in the microbial profile of these two conditions and similarity in treatment, this discussion will focus on *necrotizing ulcerative periodontitis,* a marker of severe immune suppression[8] (Figure 47-6) and characterized by the following:

- Severe pain
- Loosening of teeth
- Bleeding
- Fetid odor
- Ulcerated gingival papillae
- Rapid loss of bone and soft tissue

Patients often refer to their pain as *deep jaw pain.*

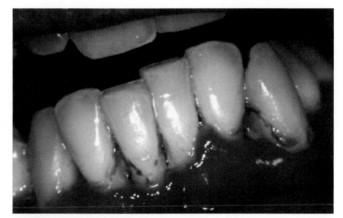

FIGURE 47-6
Necrotizing ulcerative periodontitis.

VIRAL DISEASES

Herpes simplex virus-1 infection is widespread, and oral manifestations of herpes lesions are common. In the United States, 17% of the population older than 12 years of age experienced an oral herpetic lesion over a 1-year period.[13] Recurrent intraoral herpes simplex starts as a small crop of vesicles that rupture to produce small, painful ulcerations that may coalesce (Figure 47-7). Although these herpetic ulcerations are often

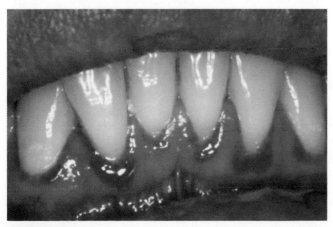

FIGURE 47-5
Linear gingival erythema.

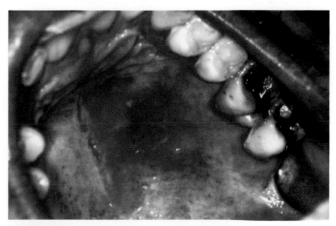

FIGURE 47-7
Herpetic ulceration.

self-limiting, the use of an antiviral medication such as acyclovir is sometimes necessary to control the outbreak.

Herpes zoster virus infection, a reactivation of the varicella zoster virus, can occur along any branch of the trigeminal nerve; therefore an intraoral or extraoral presentation along branches of this nerve is possible. The external lesions will start as vesicles, break open, and then crust over. The intraoral lesions will start as vesicles, burst, and then show as oral ulcerations. Because both of these presentations are along the trigeminal nerve, the patient's chief complaint may be toothache of unknown origin. Treatment options include higher doses of acyclovir (800 mg five times a day for 7 to 10 days) or famciclovir (500 mg three times a day for 7 days).

Oral hairy leukoplakia is caused by the Epstein-Barr virus and produces a white, corrugated, nonremovable lesion on the lateral borders of the tongue (Figure 47-8). Studies have shown a significant decrease in the incidence of oral hairy leukoplakia in the HAART era.[3,4] This condition is normally asymptomatic and does not require therapy unless cosmetic concerns exist.

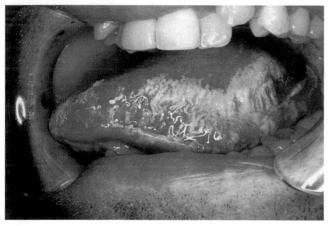

FIGURE 47-8
Oral hairy leukoplakia. (From Silverman S Jr: *Color atlas of oral manifestations of AIDS,* ed 2, St Louis, 1996, Mosby-Year Book.)

DENTAL CONSIDERATIONS

Patients who have oral hairy leukoplakia while receiving HAART may be experiencing a failure of their present antiretroviral regimen.

Oral warts from **human papillomavirus** (HPV) have dramatically increased in the HAART era.[9,10] One study noted that the risk of oral warts was associated with a 1-$\log_{10}$ or greater decrease in HIV RNA level in the 6 months before oral HPV diagnosis, which suggests that this condition may in part be related to immune reconstitution.[10] Oral warts may appear cauliflower-like, spiked, or raised with a flat surface (Figure 47-9). Treatment, which may involve surgery, laser surgery, or cryotherapy, is problematic because these lesions tend to recur.

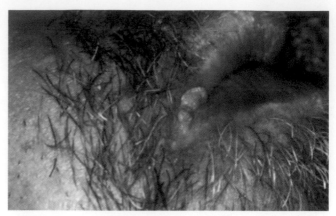

FIGURE 47-9
Oral warts from human papillomavirus.

NEOPLASTIC DISEASES
Kaposi's Sarcoma

Kaposi's sarcoma is the most frequent oral malignancy seen in association with HIV infection, although the incidence has dramatically decreased in the HAART era[15] (Figure 47-10). **Kaposi's sarcoma–associated herpesvirus** (KSHV) has been implicated as a cofactor in the presentation of Kaposi's sarcoma in persons living with HIV disease. The clinical appearance of Kaposi's sarcoma can be macular, nodular, or raised and ulcerated; the color can range from red to purple. Early lesions tend to be flat, red, and asymptomatic, with the color becoming darker as the lesion ages. As lesions

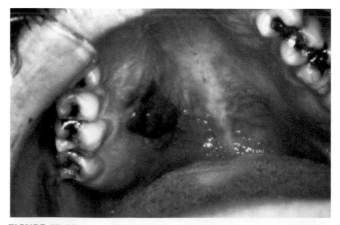

FIGURE 47-10
Kaposi's sarcoma.

progress, they can interfere with the normal functions of the oral cavity and become symptomatic secondary to trauma or infection. A biopsy is necessary for a definitive diagnosis.

Non-Hodgkin's Lymphoma

Non-Hodgkin's lymphoma is an AIDS-defining condition that, on occasion, exhibits in the oral cavity. This lesion tends to show as a large, painful, ulcerated mass on the palate or gingival tissues. A biopsy is necessary for a definitive diagnosis.

> *Distinct Care Modifications*
> The oral healthcare team should refer patients with a diagnosis of non-Hodgkin's lymphoma to an oncologist for treatment.

SALIVARY GLAND DISEASE AND XEROSTOMIA

Salivary gland disease is clinically apparent by an increase in the size of the major salivary glands, most notably the parotids. Biopsy of enlarged parotid salivary glands may reveal an increase in lymphocytic infiltrates, more specifically, CD8+ cells.

This condition usually exhibits as a bilateral enlargement of the parotid salivary glands and is often accompanied by symptoms of dry mouth. An increase in the presentation of salivary gland disease in the HAART era has been reported, which may be related to a reconstitution syndrome.[14]

Xerostomia, or dry mouth, is a common complaint among people living with HIV disease. Approximately 29% of those participating in the HIV Cost and Utilization Study cohort reported symptoms of xerostomia. Factors that proved to be significant in the presentation of xerostomia included the previously referenced salivary gland disease, use of medications to manage HIV and other conditions, smoking, and a viral load between 3,000 and 10,000 copies/ml.[1,15]

RECURRENT APHTHOUS ULCERATIONS

Recurrent aphthous ulcerations are a common occurrence, with approximately 17% of the U.S. population reporting an episode within a 12-month period.[13] Recurrent aphthous ulcerations are found on nonkeratinized or nonfixed tissues such as labial and buccal mucosa, floor of the mouth, ventral surface of the tongue, posterior oropharynx, and maxillary and mandibular vestibules. Recurrent aphthous ulcerations are characterized by a halo of inflammation and a yellow-gray pseudomembranous covering. Recurrent aphthous ulcerations, which last between 7 and 14 days in the general population, may last longer and be more painful in immunocompromised individuals.

The dental healthcare provider's main role, other than addressing the oral disease present, is to ensure that all potential causes of candidiasis, including HIV infection, have been ruled out.

> *Note*
> Many primary care providers still believe women are not at risk although more than 30% of AIDS cases are among women.

★ CASE APPLICATION 47-1.2

Recommending an HIV Test

You have scheduled Ms. Jones for a 3-month continuing supportive care appointment. The white patches are back, and the gingiva is fully inflamed with deep pockets. She reports feeling better than she did during the last visit when she had influenza-like symptoms, but she is just not quite herself. She went to her primary care provider who ran a battery of diagnostic tests. The results of the tests were insignificant, and she was told that she most likely had a viral infection. She is no longer seeing the love of her life because she found out he had many loves in his life. She seems concerned that he may also have occasionally used injection drugs, or so she has heard. You do the following:

1. Explain that her gingival condition has deteriorated, and you are concerned about the underlying cause.
2. Ask her whether she has taken or is considering taking an HIV test. Ask whether her primary care provider performed an HIV test at her previous visit.
3. Refer her to her primary care physician, and ask her to sign a written informed consent to discuss the oral findings with her medical provider.

All of the symptoms that Ms. Jones exhibited at the initial visit were consistent with HIV seroconversion illness. Even if her symptoms were seroconverting at the time of the primary care visit, chances are that an HIV diagnostic test would have been negative, given that up to 3 months are needed for antibodies to develop.

Infection Control

In the early years of the HIV pandemic, healthcare workers sometimes took extraordinary measures to prevent the transmission of the disease in their occupational settings. As a result mainly of a lack of understanding the mechanism of transmission and infectivity, practices such as double gloving, sterilizing instruments before cleaning and then sterilizing them again, screening patients and referring persons with HIV disease to other providers, and avoiding the use of certain devices such as ultrasonic scalers were commonplace. These practices may continue in some private settings in spite of the wealth of data indicating standard precautions are adequate to prevent the transmission of HIV. All of these practices, unless consistently applied regardless of the patient's HIV status, are potentially discriminatory and have not been proven necessary or more effective than standard precautions.

STANDARD PRECAUTIONS

The CDC first identified *universal precautions* to reduce the risk of transmission of blood-borne diseases in healthcare settings. These precautions were updated and expanded in 1996 and are referred to as *standard precautions*. Standard precautions apply to contact with all body fluids, secretions, and excretions whether or not they contain blood. The only body fluid to which this rule does not apply is sweat. Because universal precautions identified saliva in connection with dental procedures as a potentially infectious material, this change in terminology does not indicate a change of view regarding most body fluids encountered in dentistry. Therefore recommendations do not indicate any major changes in approaches to infection control in dental settings except for areas in which the science and knowledge developed over time warrant revision or additions to precautions.

A simplified means of understanding standard precautions is

> *Note*
>
> Selecting personal protective attire, sterilization, disinfection, and other infection-control practices does not consider the patient's infectious disease status, only the potential for workers or work surfaces to encounter body fluids.

that it requires healthcare providers to tailor their infection control precautions to the risk of encountering patient body fluids during a given procedure. It also means that providers do not base infection control precautions on the known or perceived infectious status of the patient.

Standard precautions, consistently applied, protect patients and healthcare providers during every procedure. Identifying the infectious status of every patient for any number of diseases, including HIV, hepatitis B virus (HBV), hepatitis C virus (HCV), and herpes simplex virus (HSV), is not possible. A health history is an important clinical tool, but because the patient self-reports the information, the dental health history is subject to censorship by the patient's fear of discrimination, denial of the disease itself, or lack of knowledge about his or her own infectious disease status.

Dental Considerations

Patients with HIV disease are often highly susceptible to infection because of their immune-compromised status. Therefore considering precautions directed toward protecting their health is indicated when in the dental care environment. Exposure to contaminants in the water, contaminants on environmental surfaces, and infections harbored by dental healthcare providers places these patients at heightened risk for potentially life-threatening illnesses.

Dental Waterlines

The scientific literature leaves no doubt to the fact that, if untreated, dental waterlines encourage the development and growth of biofilm. These biofilms typically contain a vast variety of microorganisms in a symbiotic environment that are resistant to chemical treatment and other means of control. These opportunistic organisms may include *Legionella* sp., *Pseudomonas aeruginosa*, *Moraxella* sp., and others. Ailments caused by these organisms may include respiratory infections, wound site infections, endocarditis, and a host of other illnesses. Reports of infections associated with dental waterlines are not widespread, but neither is conducting epidemiologic studies typical in dental healthcare settings. The extent to which biofilm-contaminated waterlines may pose a risk to patients, particularly those with immune system disorders, is largely unknown.

In recent years, numerous effective treatment methods have emerged on the dental market to control plaque biofilm and improve water quality exiting from dental waterlines attached to devices such as high-speed hand pieces, ultrasonic cleaners, and air/water syringes. The methods include filters, chemical treatment regimens, maintenance protocols, or some combination of these. Products are available for systems with independent water reservoirs (water bottles) and for those connected directly to the municipal water system. These devices and products are generally effective if used according to the manufacturer's instructions and if the proper equipment maintenance instructions are followed. The CDC identifies 500 colony-forming units of heterotrophic bacteria as an appropriate level of water purity. This identification is consistent with the standard that the U.S. Environmental Protection Agency sets for drinking water.

> *Note*
>
> Untreated dental waterlines typically produce water that cannot pass the water-purity standards for drinking water.

> *Distinct Care Modifications*
>
> The CDC recommends sterile irrigants in connection with periodontal and oral surgical procedures. Delivery of sterile irrigants through the dental waterline will compromise the sterility of the solutions. Therefore using sterile tubing or sterile irrigating syringes is necessary to deliver sterile irrigant during surgical procedures. Hand pieces, ultrasonic scaler tips, and other attachments used in surgery must also be sterile.

IMMUNIZATIONS AND WORK RESTRICTIONS

Vaccine-preventable diseases pose a significant risk to immunocompromised patients. Every healthcare worker should ensure that his or her immunizations are up to date before treating patients. Most adults receive the majority of the recommended vaccinations as children. Individuals who did not spend their childhood in the United States, who believe they may have missed some childhood immunizations, or who are uncertain regarding their status should seek the advice of a medical healthcare provider. The HBV vaccine did not become widely available until the early 1980s and became a routine childhood vaccination in the late 1980s.

Because of the potential for disease transmission, healthcare workers harboring certain infections should refrain from direct patient contact when incubating and when actively infected. The CDC has identified work restriction guidelines, which appear in Table 7-5.

> *Prevention*
>
> The HBV vaccine is particularly significant for dental healthcare providers because the scientific literature indicates that HBV is transmitted in dental healthcare settings from infected patients to nonimmunized workers. The other vaccine recommended for all healthcare workers is the annual influenza vaccine. Receiving this vaccine not only protects the dental provider from contracting influenza but also protects patients from potential exposure should the provider contract influenza and present to the workplace while contagious.

POSTEXPOSURE PROPHYLAXIS

Occupational exposure to a patient's body fluids via percutaneous injury, splash to the eye or other mucous membranes, or contact with nonintact skin carries some potential for HIV transmission. A significant number of factors, including the source patient status and the depth of the injury, as well as the amount of patient blood involved in the incident, affect the risk of disease transmission.

In spite of the fact that the risk of HIV transmission from patient to healthcare provider during dental procedures appears to be low, lowering the risk even further is possible with appropriate postexposure protocols. Immediately following the exposure, first aid, consisting of washing the area with soap and water and applying an antiseptic, is the first step. If the exposure is a splash to the eyes, then flushing with copious amounts of water suffices as first aid. A medical healthcare provider trained in postexposure management is an essential element of an effective protocol. The referral mechanism needs to be in place before an exposure occurs to ensure prompt follow-up. Testing of the source patient and the exposed dental healthcare provider should be part of the follow-up performed by the medical provider. If the patient's serostatus relative to bloodborne diseases (including HIV, HBV, and HCV) is known, then no testing is needed. **Postexposure prophylaxis** with antiretroviral drugs is believed to reduce the risk of HIV transmission by 74% or more. Inquiring as to which antiretrovirals the patient currently takes and to which he or she is resistant assists the medical provider in determining the appropriate medications for prophylaxis. The most common regimen for postexposure prophylaxis is 30 days taking whichever antiretroviral medications the medical professional determines are appropriate. In some instances, prophylaxis may not be indicated at all, such as with superficial injuries or exposures when no visible blood contamination postexposure exists.

Legal Issues

HIV, as well as other disabilities, is protected by state and federal legislation. This legislation protects both patients and oral healthcare professionals from discrimination as a result of actual or perceived HIV infection. The two major pieces of federal legislation are the **Americans with Disabilities Act** and the Rehabilitation Act of 1973. By federal definition, a disability is defined as having the following:

- A physical or mental impairment that substantially limits one or more major life activities of such individual
- A record of such impairment
- Being regarded as having such impairment

Passage of the Rehabilitation Act of 1973 was intended to provide national protection against discrimination on the basis of a *handicap*. In 1987 a clarifying position was added to Section 504, which implicitly acknowledges HIV infection as a handicapping condition covered under the Act (including asymptomatic infection). Section 504 prohibits discrimination against people with disabilities from places of public accommodation that receive federal funds, such as Medicare or Medicaid, among other funds. Places of public accommodation are those that are open to serve the public and entities that accept public patronage, including the private offices of dentists and physicians or hospitals that accept federal funds. A limitation to the extent of protection by places of public accommodation rested within their acceptance of federal funding.

Congress passed the Americans with Disabilities Act in 1990, and it was declared as "perhaps the most sweeping civil rights legislation passed since the Civil Rights Act of 1964 nearly 30 years before."[17] The Act is intended "to provide a clear and comprehensive national mandate for the elimination of discrimination against individuals with disabilities."[17] The Americans with Disabilities Act picks up where Section 504 left off in that coverage is extended to places not receiving federal funds.[17]

The Americans with Disabilities Act has three Titles.

- Title I prohibits employment discrimination.
- Title II prohibits discrimination by states and local government.
- Title III prohibits discrimination in places of public accommodation.

The Act makes clear that a place of public accommodation includes the "professional office of a healthcare provider."[17] Titles I and II carry the most significant meaning for dental offices.

Title III establishes the types of discrimination that are prohibited during the delivery of oral healthcare services, which are that it is illegal to do the following:

- Deny an HIV-positive patient the *full and equal enjoyment* of dental services or deny him or her the *opportunity to benefit* from the dental services in the same manner as other patients
- Establish *eligibility criteria* for receiving dental services if these criteria attempt to screen out individuals with HIV
- Provide *different or separate* services or fail to provide services in the most *integrated setting* to HIV-positive patients
- Deny equal services to a person who is known to have a *relationship* or *association* with person with HIV, such as a spouse, partner, child, or friend

Among the various types of discrimination cited are those such as the following:

- Illegal referrals (referrals based on a patient's HIV status for services otherwise performed)
- Refusing to treat someone perceived as having HIV infection
- Screening out patients with infectious disease that cannot be cured
- Referrals based in fear or out of concern that other patients will leave a practice that treats someone with HIV or because of simple refusals to treat

Courts have upheld individuals' rights to access dental care.

Many states have civil rights legislation that can be applied to persons with HIV or are specific to HIV. Some of the specific pieces of legislation include those that protect information relative to HIV infection from release without a written informed consent and testing without consent. Additional statutes may exist to protect the privacy of medical information, the confidentiality of medical information, or the improper release of medical information, including HIV-related information and not simply laboratory test results. Consulting individual laws in the state in which clinicians practice is important. In addition, the most stringent law prevails; therefore if the state legislation is stricter than the federal, then the clinician must comply with the state legislation.

Employment discrimination is covered under Title I. The Americans with Disabilities Act protects persons who are HIV positive or have AIDS from employment discrimination for employers with at least 15 employees (most states' protection is based on fewer employees). Employment decisions must be based on current fitness to perform job duties and not on the possibility that a person will become ill and unable to do the job in the future.

Under Titles I and III, an important exception exists: the direct threat defense. A direct threat is defined as a "significant risk to the health and safety of others that cannot be eliminated by a modification of policies, practices or procedures."[17] Assessment of a direct threat is made based on reasonable judgment that relies on current medical knowledge or on the best available objective evidence to ascertain the following:

- Nature, duration, and severity of risk
- Probability that potential injury will occur
- Whether reasonable modifications to policies, practices, and procedures will mitigate the risk

In cases under Title III, courts have almost uniformly ruled on behalf of the patient. Arguments using the direct threat have been countered with those emphasizing that, although the nature, duration, and severity of the risk are apparent, the probability of injury is low, and reasonable modifications are in place that mitigate the risk. Among the reasonable modifications cited are the following:

- Universal and standard precautions
- Engineering controls
- Work-practice controls
- Administrative controls
- Postexposure management
- Safety devices

Cases under Title I have not been so clear-cut, and decisions made on a case-by-case basis vary between judicial jurisdictions. Some courts have used the legal principle that healthcare workers have a special fiduciary duty to patients, which makes even a theoretical risk unacceptable, and cite the 1991 CDC *Recommendations for Preventing Transmission of Human Immunodeficiency Virus and Hepatitis B Virus to Patients During Exposure-Prone Invasive Procedures,*[4a] which leave room for facilities and institutions to restrict activities of healthcare workers who perform **exposure-prone invasive procedures.** Other courts have relied on the reasonable medical judgment of public health experts who have emphasized the risk to patients as being considered very low and rejected mandatory testing or restriction of work procedures

based on infection alone. These guidelines were based on the following considerations:

- Infected dental healthcare professionals who adhere to universal precautions and who do not perform invasive procedures pose no risk for transmitting HIV or HBV to patients.
- Infected dental healthcare professionals who adhere to universal precautions and who perform certain exposure-prone procedures pose a small risk for transmitting HBV to patients.
- HIV is transmitted much less readily than HBV.
- Mandatory testing for dental healthcare professionals for HIV, hepatitis B surface antigen (HBsAg), or hepatitis B e antigen (HBeAg) is not recommended.

These recommendations emphasized the importance of universal precautions in reducing any transmission risks, discussed training and education for all staff, and discussed the use of HBV vaccination and other appropriate methods to mitigate risk. Consensus remains that transmission can be prevented through HBV vaccination, strict adherence to standard precautions, the use of safer devices, and modification of work practices.

A thorough understanding of the disease of HIV and its accompanying manifestations, symptoms, and appropriate precautions, as well as the associated professional, ethical, and legal obligations are important to every healthcare provider.

References

1. Aguirre JM et al: Reduction of HIV-associated oral lesions after highly active antiretroviral therapy, *Oral Surg Oral Med Oral Pathol Oral Radiol Endod* 88:114-115, 1999.
2. Arendorf TM et al: Oral manifestations of HIV infection in 600 South African patients, *J Oral Pathol Med* 27:176-179, 1998.
3. Centers for Disease Control and Prevention: HIV/AIDS surveillance report—2003, *Morbid Mortal Wkly Rep* 15:1-46, 2004.
4. Centers for Disease Control and Prevention: *AIDS case definition change,* Atlanta, Ga, 1993, CDC.
4a. Centers for Disease Control and Prevention: Recommendations for Preventing Transmission of Human Immunodeficiency Virus and Hepatitis B Virus to Patients During Exposure-Prone Invasive Procedures, *Bull Am Coll Surg* 76(9):29-37, 1991.
5. Centers for Disease Control and Prevention: Kaposi's sarcoma and pneumocystis pneumonia among homosexual men: New York City and California, *Morbid Mortal Wkly* 30:305, July 1981.
6. Centers for Disease Control and Prevention: Pneumocystis pneumonia: Los Angeles, *Morbid Mortal Wkly* 30:250, July 1981.
7. Dios PD et al: Changing prevalence of human immunodeficiency virus-associated oral lesions, *Oral Surg Oral Med Oral Pathol Oral Radiol Endod* 90:403-404, 2000.
8. Glick M et al: Necrotizing ulcerative periodontitis: a marker for immune deterioration and a predictor for the diagnosis of AIDS, *J Periodontol* 65:393-397, 1994.
9. Greenspan D et al: Effect of highly active antiretroviral therapy on frequency of oral warts, *Lancet* 357:1411-1412, 2001.
10. King MD et al: Human papillomavirus-associated oral warts among human immunodeficiency virus-seropositive patients in the era of highly active antiretroviral therapy: an emerging infection, *Clin Infect Dis* 34:641-648, 2002.

11. Magaldi S et al: In vitro susceptibility of 137 *Candida* sp. isolates from HIV positive patients to several antifungal drugs, *Myco-pathologia* 149:63-68, 2001.

12. Mascarenhas AK, Smith SR: Factors associated with utilization of care for oral lesions in HIV disease, *Oral Surg Oral Med Oral Pathol Oral Radiol Endod* 87:708-713, 1999.

13. McDowell MA, Centers for Disease Control and Prevention, National Center for Health Statistics: 1996 Update: the Third National Health and Nutrition Examination Survey (NHANES III). Available at: http://www.nal.usda.gov/fnic/foodcomp/conf/NDBC21/p3-2.pdf. Accessed: May 26, 2005.

14. Patton LL et al: Changing prevalence of oral manifestations of human immuno-deficiency virus in the era of protease inhibitor therapy, *Oral Surg Oral Med Oral Pathol Oral Radiol Endod* 89:299-304, 2000.

15. Tappuni AR, Fleming GJ: The effect of antiretroviral therapy on the prevalence of oral manifestations in HIV-infected patients: a UK study, *Oral Surg Oral Med Oral Pathol Oral Radiol Endod* 92:623-628, 2001.

16. UNAIDS: *2004 Report on the global AIDS epidemic: executive summary*, Geneva, Switzerland, June 2004, UNAIDS.

17. US Department of Justice, Office of Justice Programs, National Institute of Justice: *The Americans with Disabilities Act and criminal justice: an overview*, Washington, DC, 1993, Institute of Justice.

Cancer and Treatment Effects on the Oral Cavity

Christina B. DeBiase

INSIGHT

Local and regional cancers involving the head and neck and systemic cancers such as leukemia are particularly relevant to the dental hygienist because both the disease and the treatment modalities (surgery, radiation, chemotherapy, and transplantation) adversely affect the oral soft and hard tissues. The dental hygienist must thoroughly evaluate the patient's medical history; determine the appropriate precautions that must be taken before dental treatment; recognize oral complications of the disease and its treatment; provide palliative measures to alleviate oral pain and discomfort; eliminate any potential sources of oral infection; and instruct the patient, caregiver, or both in appropriate home care to promote healing and prevent further complications.

✴ CASE STUDY 48-1 — Intraoral Considerations in the Dental Treatment of a Patient with Head and Neck Cancer

A hospital oncologist consulted Dr. Kay Matthews, a dentist, about a 22-year-old patient, E. Thomas Fitzgibbons, who was diagnosed 5 years earlier with nasopharyngeal carcinoma. The cancer was staged according to the tumor, node, metastasis (TNM) system as $T_2 N_0 M_0$. Mr. Fitzgibbons underwent a 6-week course of radiation therapy in another state. Although he had been scheduled numerous times for medical and dental follow-up, he left home after turning 18 years of age and had refused further treatment. The only remaining side effect of the treatment was severe xerostomia. Mr. Fitzgibbons had been cancer free and pain free until he appeared to begin developing trismus. His mouth opening was becoming progressively smaller, and he lost 15 pounds in 3 months. These symptoms prompted Mr. Fitzgibbons to seek care.

Extraoral palpation revealed what appeared to be a cervical node approximately the size of a dime. The oral opening was only 9 mm wide. A cursory assessment of the oral cavity revealed dry, inflamed mucosa and extensive carious lesions. Two premolars and one molar were present in the form of retained root tips.

Medical assessment revealed recurrence of the tumor, and Dr. Matthews advised Mr. Fitzgibbons to undergo another course of radiation therapy as soon as possible. Treating Mr. Fitzgibbons' dental needs was paramount, and radiation therapy could not begin until several extractions and extensive restorative procedures had been performed to eliminate oral infection. Because of Mr. Fitzgibbons' previous exposure to radiation, *hyperbaric oxygen* treatments were scheduled to flood the tissues with oxygen to increase the blood supply, particularly at the extraction sites to reduce the risk of osteoradionecrosis.

The oncologist, dentist, and dental hygienist spent considerable time explaining to Mr. Fitzgibbons the treatment regimen, and they required a commitment on his part to follow through with dental treatment before, during, and after *radiotherapy* to ensure that the risk of infection would be kept to a minimum.

✦ CASE STUDY 48-2   Intraoral Considerations in the Dental Treatment of a Patient with Leukemia

A hospital oncologist consulted Dr. Mark Edwards, a dentist, about Maggie Clarkson, a 4-year-old girl who had been complaining of leg pain for several weeks. She was experiencing malaise and persistent oral bleeding associated with the eruption of her first molars. After numerous blood draws and a bone marrow biopsy, Maggie was diagnosed with acute lymphoblastic leukemia.

Maggie was enrolled in an intensive chemotherapy protocol consisting of a series of stomatotoxic antineoplastic drugs, a steroid, and an antibiotic. She receives these drugs via an indwelling catheter. Early in her treatment, the dental team examined her. Her neutrophil count was 1500/mm^3, and her platelet count was 18,000/mm^3.

The oncologist, dentist, and dental hygienist spent considerable time explaining the treatment regimen to Maggie and her parents. The complications associated with chemotherapy were also described. The dentist and dental hygienist focused on the long-term developmental issues and the short-term oral side effects such as mucositis, bleeding, and infection. The healthcare providers required a commitment from Maggie and her family to follow through with dental treatment before, during, and after chemotherapy to ensure that the risk of complications, particularly infection, would be kept to a minimum.

KEY TERMS

benign	fractionation	mucositis	relapse
bone marrow transplantation	graft versus host disease	oncology	remission
brush biopsy	hyperalimentation	osteoradionecrosis	stages
cancer	hyperbaric oxygen	palliative	survival rate
carcinoma	*in situ*	photodynamic therapy	TNM classification system
centigray	interferon	prognosis	total body irradiation
chemotherapy	leukemia	radiation modifiers	trismus
dysgeusia	malignant	radioactive isotopes	tumor
dysplasia	metastasis	radiotherapy	xerostomia

LEARNING OUTCOMES

After reading this chapter the student will be able to:

1. Know the incidence and contributing factors of cancer.
2. Understand the terminology associated with head and neck cancer, radiation therapy, leukemia, chemotherapy, and bone marrow transplantation.
3. Understand the potential etiologies or risk factors of cancer, particularly those affecting the head and neck.
4. Identify head and neck cancer by its appearance, symptoms, and location, and be able to identify the stage of the disease.
5. Describe the early signs and symptoms of leukemia.
6. Identify the types of leukemia.
7. Discuss the various methods for evaluating head and neck lesions.
8. Explain the types of radiation therapy and the dosage regimens.
9. Identify the drug categories used in chemotherapy regimens.
10. Describe the process and types of bone marrow transplantation.
11. Describe the types of oral complications associated with radiation therapy and chemotherapy and their management.
12. Outline a typical oral care protocol for patients before, during, and after radiation therapy, chemotherapy, or both.

Incidence

Cancer is the second leading cause of death in the United States. **Cancer** or **carcinoma** refers to a complex group of more than 100 diseases that share the ability to spread **malignant** or abnormal cells uncontrollably throughout the body. Cells normally divide and grow in an orderly, controlled manner. Cancer cells grow haphazardly, forming a mass of tissue referred to as a **tumor.** Malignant tumors can spread to surrounding tissue, to other areas of the body, or into the bloodstream. The term for this spreading is **metastasis.** Not all tumors are cancerous.

When a tumor is not cancerous, it is called a **benign** tumor. Benign tumors can often be removed with surgery and usually do not reoccur.

The death rate for all cancers has declined. Lung cancer deaths among women have begun to level off after statistics showed increases over the last several decades. Deaths for all cancers among black men and women are

> *Note*
>
> The most common estimated new cancer cases by gender include: for women—breast, lung and bronchus, and colon; for men—prostate, lung and bronchus, colon, and urinary bladder.

higher than deaths among white men and women. In addition, minority populations are more likely than whites to be diagnosed when their disease in the advanced stages. Nonmelanoma skin cancers are on the rise nationally.

Oncology is the specialty that refers to the diagnosis and treatment of cancers. Cancers of the head and neck represented 2.14% of all estimated new cancer cases in the United States for 2005. Approximately one in four of these 30,000 individuals will die. Cancers of the oral cavity and pharynx compose approximately 2.7% of all new cancers in men and 1.55% in women. The mean age of onset for both sexes is 63 years of age.[21] In India, Southeast Asia, Africa, Brazil, and other developing countries, cancers of the head and neck are much more prevalent than other cancers. These cancers include malignant tumors of the upper aerodigestive tract; the paranasal sinuses; the major and minor salivary glands; the parathyroid and thyroid glands; and the skin, soft tissue, bone, and neurovascular structures in the head and neck region.

> *Note*
>
> More than 90% of all oral carcinomas are of squamous cell origin.[38]

Leukemia is an acute or chronic progressive, malignant neoplasm of the blood-forming organs that is characterized by a proliferation of abnormal white blood cells or leukocytes. In other words, the bone marrow of a person with leukemia produces abnormal white blood cells, known as *leukemic cells*. During 2005, leukemia accounted for approximately 2.5% of all estimated new cancer cases in the nation.[21] Although similar to cancers of the oral cavity and pharynx with regard to incidence, the estimated deaths annually for leukemia are much higher than those associated with cancers of the head and neck. Leukemias occur slightly more frequently in men than in women. The cure rates for leukemia in children have risen drastically over the last 25 years. Although the 5-year survival rate for acute myeloid leukemia continues to improve, it remains the lowest among childhood cancers.

Etiology and Contributing Factors

In many cases, the cause of a cancer is unknown. For some types of cancer, however, certain risk factors seem to make some people more susceptible to them. Several known risk factors include the following:

- Tobacco
- Alcohol
- Diets high in fat and processed foods
- Excessive exposure to sunlight and occupationally related agents such as dye, asbestos, and other substances

Many questions remain unanswered as to why other people can have the same risk factors and never develop cancer.

> *Note*
>
> The origin of leukemias, lymphomas, and sarcomas is uncertain.

Speculation suggests that exposure to high levels of radiation, benzene, and formaldehyde may be risk factors for leukemias, lymphomas, and sarcomas. Other risk factors include treatment with high-dose chemotherapy, Down syndrome, human T-cell leukemia virus, and myelodysplastic syndrome.

The etiology of oral cancer is also unknown, with an estimated 25% of cases in people who do not possess any of the risk factors for the disease. Several factors do, however, show a high correlation with the development of this disease. Smoking and other forms of tobacco use are usually associated with oral cancer or cancers of the head and neck.

DENTAL CONSIDERATIONS

The smoke and heat from cigarettes, cigars, and pipes irritate the oral mucosa, and smokeless tobacco products irritate these membranes through direct contact. Smokeless tobacco products should not be considered a safe alternative to smoking. A dose-response relationship exists between smokeless tobacco and health; the more tobacco that is used, the greater the risk is of cancer. Chewing tobacco may also be related to cancers of the upper digestive tract. Excessive alcohol intake, particularly in combination with smoking, has been associated with most cases of oral squamous cell carcinoma[36,39] (Figure 48-1).

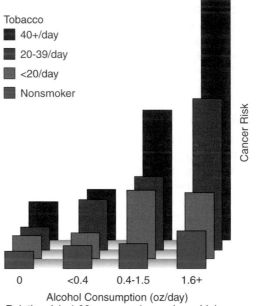

FIGURE 48-1
Relative risk of cancer related to alcohol consumption and tobacco use.

Individuals who are exposed to sunlight may be at risk for lip cancer. People at increased risk of head and neck carcinomas are those with congenital and acquired defects of the immune system and organ transplant patients. Controversy exists as to whether upper aerodigestive carcinomas become clinically evident only when the immune system is impaired.[26]

> *Note*
>
> New research suggests that viruses also are involved in the development of oral cancers.

The human papillomavirus and herpesviruses have been detected in oral cancer biopsies. Kaposi's sarcoma, which is related to acquired immuno-deficiency syndrome (AIDS), has a preference for the head and neck area, most commonly causing lesions on the hard palate and gingiva.[20,23]

Other risk factors that have been implicated previously in the development of some types of oral cancer are poor oral hygiene; nutritional deficiencies, particularly diets lacking in fruits and vegetables; heavy exposure to certain materials, such as wood and metal dust; and chronic thermal or physical trauma.[38,43] However, these risk factors are currently acknowledged to have little relevance to the development of oral or oropharyngeal squamous cell carcinoma.[26]

Some supplements and foods seem to reduce the risk of oral cancer.

Clinical Diagnosis

HEAD AND NECK CANCER

Carcinomas of the head and neck may appear clinically as red, speckled (mixed red and white), or white lesions that do not rub off. Histologically, these lesions may be described as hyperkeratosis, parakeratosis, atypia, **dysplasia,** carcinoma *in situ,* or varying grades of invasive cancer. The malignant potential of *white lesions* (traditionally referred to as *leukoplakias*) may range from 0.1% to 6%, depending on the source.[23,25,26] With *red lesions* (erythroplakias), the risk of the lesion developing into an oral carcinoma is three to five times greater than for leukoplakias.

Most early oral cancers are either small, asymptomatic, smooth red lesions or speckled, granular, red lesions with patchy areas of keratin or normal mucosa within or around the lesion. Approximately 60% of invasive oral carcinomas have a granular texture, whereas an equal percentage of carcinomas *in situ* are smooth.[25] The patient should be asked how long the lesion has been present to distinguish cancer from an inflammatory lesion, which normally lasts approximately 10 days to 2 weeks.

DENTAL CONSIDERATIONS

48-1

The most common sites for oral cancer are the floor of the mouth; the ventrolateral borders of the tongue; and the soft palate, including the uvula, lingual aspect of the retromolar trigone, and the anterior tonsillar pillars[8] (Figure 48-2). Individuals who use chewing tobacco are more prone to cancer of the buccal mucosa. Histologically, the tissues at high risk are not protected by keratin.

As a tumor enlarges, symptoms often appear. The tumor may ulcerate and bleed. Dysgeusia; ear pain; and difficulty opening the mouth, speaking, chewing, and swallowing may also develop.

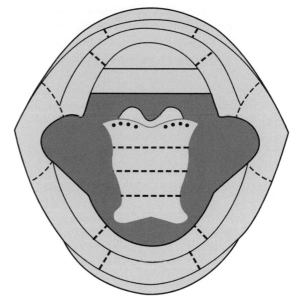

FIGURE 48-2
Shaded area shows the location of most oral cancers.

LEUKEMIA

The first signs and symptoms of leukemia are similar to those of influenza. The person may exhibit fatigue and fever. In acute leukemia, the blood cells are very abnormal and increase rapidly, causing the patient's condition to worsen quickly. A person with chronic leukemia may not experience any symptoms early in the disease process because the leukocytes appear well differentiated and able to mature, yet their immunologic capacity is compromised. Symptoms occur as the number of leukemic cells in the blood rises. The displacement of hematopoietic tissue in the bone marrow by abnormal leukocytes or blast cells results in a diminished production of platelets, erythrocytes, and normal leukocytes. Consequently, the patient may suffer spontaneous hemorrhage, anemia, malaise, and opportunistic infections.[8]

Staging

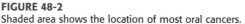
48-2

Head and neck carcinomas are staged to correlate treatment outcomes with the initial extent of the tumor.

Carcinoma *in situ,* as its name implies, is noninvasive but has the strong potential to become invasive if not treated.[27] The diagnosis of invasive squamous cell carcinoma is made when abnormal cells disrupt the basement membrane and extend into the underlying connective tissue. The deeper the primary tumor's invasion is, the greater the risk will be of lymph node involvement and the more adverse will be the effect on the **prognosis.**[26]

Note
The tumor is assessed by inspection, palpation, and histologic confirmation of the diagnosis.

The boundaries of an invasive carcinoma may be graded as G_1 (well differentiated), G_2 (moderately well differentiated), G_3 (poorly differentiated), and G_4 (undifferentiated).[2]

Well-differentiated tumors are usually considered less aggressive than poorly differentiated ones. However, the degree of differentiation and the biological behavior of a tumor are unpredictable, particularly in patients with an impaired immune response.[26,41]

The **stages** of a tumor are defined by the international tumor, node, metastasis **(TNM) classification system.** *T* refers to the *size* of the tumor; *N* refers to the *extent of lymph node involvement;* and *M* indicates whether *metastasis* has occurred[23] (Box 48-1).

✵ CASE APPLICATION 48-1.1

Applying the TNM Classification System

How would you describe Mr. Fitzgibbons' tumor according to the staging listed in Case Study 48-1?

Categories of Leukemia

Leukemia is grouped into types based on how quickly the disease develops and progresses. Leukemia is either chronic (slowly progressing) or acute (rapidly progressing). These types include the following:

- *Chronic lymphocytic leukemia* (chronic lymphoblastic leukemia, CLL) accounts for approximately 7000 new cases of leukemia each year. Most often, people diagnosed with the disease are older than age 55. It almost never affects children.
- *Chronic myeloid leukemia* (chronic myelogenous leukemia, CML) accounts for approximately 4400 new cases of leukemia each year. It affects mainly adults.
- *Acute lymphocytic leukemia* (acute lymphoblastic leukemia, ALL) accounts for approximately 3800 new cases of leukemia each year. It is the most common type of leukemia in young children. It also affects adults.

BOX 48-1

INTERNATIONAL TNM SYSTEM OF CLASSIFICATION AND STAGING OF ORAL CARCINOMAS

T: Size of tumor
T_{is}: Carcinoma *in situ*
T_1: Tumor <2 cm in size
T_2: Tumor <2 cm to >4 cm in size
T_3: Tumor >4 cm in size
T_4: Massive tumor with deep invasion into bone, muscle, or skin

N: Regional lymph node involvement
N_0: No palpable nodes
N_1: Single, homolateral palpable node <3 cm in diameter
N_2: Single, homolateral palpable node 3 to 6 cm
or
Multiple, homolateral nodes, none >6 cm
N_3: Single or multiple homolateral nodes, one >6 cm
or
Bilateral nodes (stage each side of neck)
or
Contralateral nodes

M: Metastases
M_0: No known distant metastasis
M_1: Distant metastasis
PUL (pulmonary)
OSS (osseous)
HEP (liver)
BRA (brain)

Stages*

Stage	Classification
I	T_1, N_0, M_0
II	T_2, N_0, M_0
III	T_3, N_0, M_0
	T_1, T_2, *or* T_3, N_1, M_0
IV	T_4, N_0, N_1, M_0
	Any T, N_2, N_3, M_0
	Any T, any N, M_1

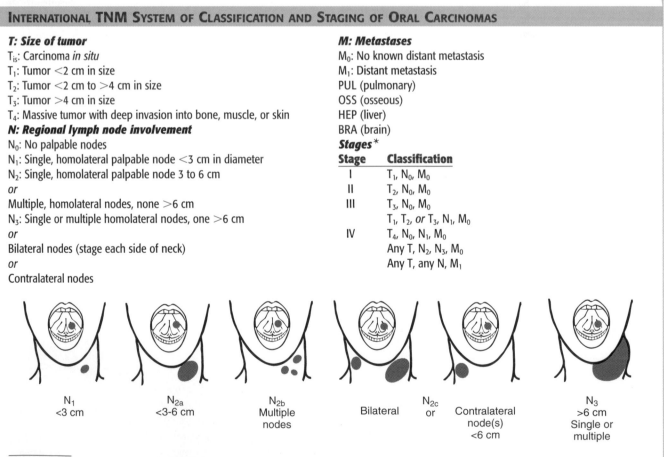

N_1 <3 cm
N_{2a} <3-6 cm
N_{2b} Multiple nodes
Bilateral
N_{2c} or Contralateral node(s) <6 cm
N_3 >6 cm Single or multiple

Data from Shah JP et al: Cervical lymph node metastasis, *Curr Probl Surg* 30(3):1-335, 1993.
Modified from Beahrs OH et al, eds: *American Joint Committee on Cancer: manual for staging cancer,* ed 4, Philadelphia, 1992, Lippincott.
*In text, these designations are written as T_1 N_0 M_0 or T_4 N_1 M_0, for example.

- *Acute myeloid leukemia* (acute myelogenous leukemia, AML) accounts for approximately 10,600 new cases of leukemia each year. It occurs in both adults and children.[29]

Early Detection

The role of the dental hygienist in early detection cannot be underestimated. Currently, the 5-year **survival rate** (time period without symptoms after treatment) is only 50% for persons diagnosed with oral cancer. In most patients, a primary tumor can be detected by a thorough intraoral and extraoral examination. This examination involves careful assessment of the skin of the face, scalp, and neck; the regional lymph nodes (Figure 48-3); the thyroid gland; the salivary glands; the oral cavity; and the oropharynx.

> *Patient Education Opportunity*
>
> Patients must be taught the importance of oral self-examination, how to perform it, when to perform it, and which findings may warrant a visit to a healthcare provider (Box 48-2).

BOX 48-2

SELF-EXAMINATION PROCEDURES FOR ORAL CANCER

Self-examination for oral cancer is an essential procedure for everyone. Oral cancers are painless in their initial stages and often go unnoticed. Take a few minutes and learn this easy three-step self-examination.

Before a well-lighted mirror observe each of the structures discussed below for any swelling, ulceration, or change in color or texture.

Lips

1 Look at your lips with your mouth closed and then opened; feel the lip for any hard swelling by pressing and rolling the lip between your index finger and thumb of the same hand.

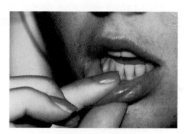

Retract your lips and slide your fingers all the way back, exposing the insides of your cheeks and gums. Observe for any differences in appearance.

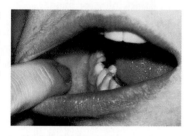

Tongue

2 Stick out your tongue and check for any swelling; ulcers; or changes in size, color, or texture.

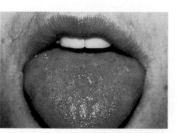

Pull the tip of your tongue to your right with a washcloth as you examine the left side of your tongue. Now examine the opposite side of the tongue by pulling the tip of the tongue to the left.

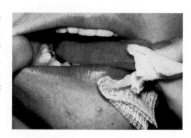

Floor of the Mouth

3 Touch the roof of your mouth with the tip of your tongue, open wide, and look at the bottom surface of the tongue and the floor of the mouth. Veins observed on the underside of the tongue are normal, so do not be alarmed. Notice the flow of saliva from the opening of the duct; it should be free flowing, watery, and clear.

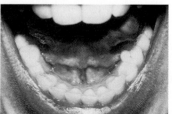

Modified from Bouquot J, DeBiase CB, Graves CE: *Self-exam procedures for oral cancer,* Morgantown, WV, 1987, Biomedical Communications, West Virginia University Press.

Continued

BOX 48-2

SELF-EXAMINATION PROCEDURES FOR ORAL CANCER—CONT'D

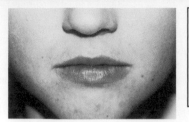

This simple three-step examination might save your life by helping you find oral cancer early, when it is most treatable.

Oral cancer affects almost 30,000 persons yearly. Approximately one third of these individuals will die. Tobacco usage, excessive consumption of alcohol, and overexposure to the sun increase your chances of developing a cancer of the mouth.

Q Why should you examine your mouth bimonthly?

Most people visit their dentist or physician once a year. Because oral cancers found early and treated promptly have a better prognosis, learning how to examine your mouth properly might help save your life. Follow the self-examination procedures shown here.

Q When is the best time to examine your mouth?

Every 2 months, right after brushing your teeth is the best guide. Following the self-examination procedures regularly will give you peace of mind, and seeing your dentist at least once a year will reassure you that there is nothing wrong.

Q What should you do if you find a sore, thickening, or lump?

If a sore, thickening, or lump is discovered during the self-examination procedures, you must consult with your dentist as soon as possible. Do not be frightened. Most changes are not cancer, but only your dentist or physician can make the diagnosis.

Know Oral Cancer's Warning Signals!

- Sore that bleeds easily or does not heal within a 2-week period
- Color change of the oral tissues
- Lump, thickening, rough spot, crust, or small eroded area
- Pain, tenderness, or numbness in the mouth or of the lips
- Difficulty chewing, swallowing, speaking, or moving the jaw or tongue
- Change in the way the teeth fit together
- Nagging cough or hoarseness

These signals may pertain to an oral cancer most often seen as one or more of the following:

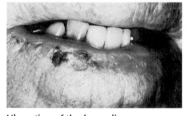

Ulceration of the lower lip

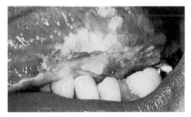

White area on the side of the tongue

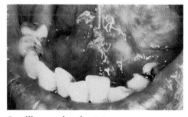

Swelling under the tongue

Modified from Bouquot J, DeBiase CB, Graves CE: *Self-exam procedures for oral cancer,* Morgantown, WV, 1987, Biomedical Communications, West Virginia University Press.

Good lighting and radiographs are essential for a complete examination (see Chapters 12 through 18). Delays in diagnosis may be attributed to the patient, the professional, or both.

Knowledge of the common locations and appearance of lesions that have the greatest carcinogenic potential is paramount in detecting cancers early. Unfortunately, many lesions are missed or considered innocuous.

Toluidine blue vital stain clinically stains malignant lesions; normal mucosa remains unchanged (Box 48-3). Although nonmalignant inflammatory areas may also stain, producing a false-positive result, restaining after 2 weeks may clarify the findings because inflammatory lesions should have resolved by then.

Patients with advanced lesions or those with typical malignant presentations should be referred for diagnosis.

Distinct Care Modifications
Toluidine blue stain can be used to rule out subjective clinical impressions of questionable lesions or as a screening rinse for patients who have high-risk behaviors, such as smoking and drinking.

Distinct Care Modifications
The **brush biopsy** has recently gained acceptance as a screening tool used to identify questionable oral lesions at an early stage (Box 48-4).

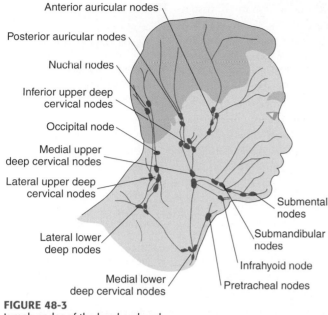

Anterior auricular nodes

Posterior auricular nodes

Nuchal nodes

Inferior upper deep cervical nodes

Occipital node

Medial upper deep cervical nodes

Lateral upper deep cervical nodes

Lateral lower deep nodes

Medial lower deep cervical nodes

Submental nodes

Submandibular nodes

Infrahyoid node

Pretracheal nodes

FIGURE 48-3
Lymph nodes of the head and neck.

Distinct Care Modifications
Biopsy diagnosis is required before the type and extent of therapy can be determined.[11,26]

The final diagnosis for oral lesions can be established only with a biopsy. *Incisional biopsy* is the method of choice for microscopic analysis of possible intraoral carcinoma. *Excisional biopsy* is recommended when the clinical examination indicates that a lesion most likely is *benign* but has the potential for functional impairment or when a malignant lesion is so small that it can be removed completely without compromising function.

BOX 48-3

TECHNIQUE FOR VISUAL STAINING

1. Rinse the mouth twice with water for 20 seconds.
2. Rinse the mouth vigorously with 1% acetic acid for 20 seconds.
3. Gently dry the areas with gauze.
4. Apply the 1% toluidine blue vital stain to the lesion.
5. Rinse with the acetic acid solution for 1 minute to remove the excess stain.
6. Rinse with water.

BOX 48-4

TECHNIQUE FOR ORAL BRUSH BIOPSY

1. Place the sterile brush against the surface of the lesion.
2. With firm pressure, rotate the brush 5 to 10 times. The tissue should appear pink or demonstrate pinpoint bleeding.
3. Transfer the sample of cells to the glass slide.
4. Flood the sample with the fixative agent.
5. Place the dried slide in the plastic container and mail to the appropriate laboratory for computerized image analysis.

The dental hygienist's role in early detection does not need to be limited to cancers of the head and neck.

Careful assessment includes the following:

Note
Leukemias and lymphomas may also be identified through a thorough examination of the head and neck both intraorally and extraorally.

1. Lymph nodes may reveal enlargement (see Figure 48-3).
2. Left and right sides of the face and neck may disclose an asymmetry.
3. Gingiva and intraoral soft tissues may expose pale, bulbous, and bleeding mucosa.

Treatment

An estimated one third or more of Americans diagnosed with cancer each year may develop painful and debilitating oral complications from their cancer treatment. Cancer therapies may be administered alone or in combination. The most common forms of therapy include:

- Surgery
- Radiation
- Chemotherapy
- Stem cell transplants

Therapies that most commonly elicit oral side effects include surgery, radiation, or both for a tumor involving the head and neck; chemotherapy; and bone marrow peripheral stem cell transplant.

SURGERY AND RADIOTHERAPY

Early cancers (stage I or stage II) are highly curable by surgery or **radiotherapy.** The mode of treatment is dictated by several factors, including the following:

- The tumor's stage, grade, and location
- The patient's age, overall health status, personal desires, and history of carcinoma and treatment
- The anticipated functional and cosmetic results of treatment
- Socioeconomic issues
- The availability of professional resources

The collaborative efforts of professionals specializing in rehabilitation; preventive, restorative, and prosthetic dentistry; and social services are an integral part of a patient's recovery plan.[18,26,28,45]

Surgery is usually the treatment of choice when neoplasms are not radiosensitive, such as those of the brain and spinal cord, or when the sequelae of radiation may be more debilitating than the healed surgical defects.

Combined therapy (surgery and radiation) is usually recommended for stage III and stage IV tumors and for early cancers that have poorly defined margins or a tumor depth greater than 5 mm. The risk of recurrence, particularly second primary tumors of the aerodigestive tract, increases for tumors that have advanced to these levels. **Radiation modifiers** or **chemotherapy** combined with surgery or radiation (or both) may be administered to limit local recurrence and distant metastases.[7,15,28]

An antineoplastic drug, 5-fluorouracil, applied topically in combination with laser surgery has been used to treat carcinoma *in situ*. **Photodynamic therapy** (PDT) is undergoing evaluation for the treatment of T_1 tumors, Kaposi's sarcoma, carcinoma in situ of the oral cavity, and laryngeal carcinoma.[43]

Generally, the higher the tumor's stage number is, the worse the prognosis will be. Because cancers of the lip are readily observable, most such lesions are detected and treated early with surgery or radiation. Cure rates are generally 90% to 100%. Other small lesions of the retromolar trigone, hard palate, and gingiva are equally curable by either treatment method. Small cancers of the anterior tongue, the floor of the mouth, and the buccal mucosa have cure rates of approximately 90% when treated with radiation therapy or surgery.[44]

Moderately advanced lesions without evidence of spread to the cervical lymph nodes are usually curable, with control rates of 90% for the retromolar trigone; 80% for lesions involving the hard palate, gingiva, and buccal mucosa; 70% for the floor of the mouth; and 65% for the anterior tongue.[42,44] Unfortunately, professional consultation is often delayed until the patient has some type of discomfort. By that time, in more than one half of these patients, the cancer has metastasized to the lymph nodes of the neck or axilla, reducing the 5-year survival rate to 30% to 40%.

The most important factor in determining the prognosis for a squamous cell carcinoma of the head and neck is whether metastasis to the lymph nodes has occurred.[37] The cure rate for patients with lymph involvement is one half that of an individual without nodal metastasis.

RADIATION THERAPY

48-3
48-4

Radiation can be delivered externally through ports (e.g., cobalt, linear accelerator) or internally by implantation of radioactive materials in tissues or body cavities. The body metabolizes these materials.

A simulator determines the field of radiation from an external source. The simulator is a diagnostic x-ray unit used to visualize the proposed treatment site. Masks or head holders are used to keep the head stabilized in the same position for all treatments. Field markings are placed on the masks, rather than on the skin, to alleviate the conspicuous facial tattoos that were once used in the past. Superficial lesions are usually treated through a single field; multiple fields are used for deep and large tumors. Multiple fields maximize the amount of radiation to the tumor and reduce the amount of scatter

radiation to normal tissues. Lead blocks, also used to protect vital body organs and tissues, are secured to a plastic tray and placed on the head of the treatment machine between the beam and the person receiving treatment.[5]

Radiation can directly damage deoxyribonucleic acid (DNA) or can interact with water and oxygen molecules, producing free radicals that indirectly cause cell death through DNA damage.[23,46] Unfortunately, normal tissues also are affected by the radiation, which creates side effects that serve as a dose-limiting gauge for determining tumor destruction and host survival. The frequency, severity, and duration of the damage in the irradiated tissues of the head and neck are a function of this radiobiological effect, the dosing schedule, the type and **fractionation** of the radiation administered, the host response, and the volume and radiosensitivity of the tissues involved. In general, rapidly dividing cells are more sensitive to radiation (Table 48-1).[37] Radiosensitizers are used to sensitize tumor cells to the effects of radiation so that the amount of radiation needed to kill tumor cells can be reduced, thereby limiting radiation injury to normal cells.[23]

Adjuvant radiation therapy can be administered preoperatively or postoperatively. Physicians rarely choose preoperative irradiation because of the dose limitations, impaired oxygenation and healing potential of the intended surgical site, and poor compliance by some patients on following through with surgery after radiation treatment. Postoperative irradiation, on the other hand, is highly recommended. The dose limitation is much higher, the complications associated with wound healing do not exist, and accurate pathologic staging of the tumor is possible.

Table 48-1	Degree of Organ Radiosensitivity
RADIOSENSITIVITY	**ORGAN**
Very High	Lymph, bone marrow, blood, testes, ovaries, intestines
High	Skin, oral cavity, esophagus, rectum, bladder, vagina, cervix, ureters, cornea
Moderate	Stomach, growing cartilage and bone, fine vasculature, optic lens
Moderately Low	Mature cartilage and bone, salivary glands, kidney, liver, pancreas, respiratory organs, thyroid, adrenals, pituitary gland
Low	Muscle, brain, spinal cord

Modified from Rubin P, Constantine L, Nelson D: Late effects of cancer treatment: radiation and drug toxicity. In Perez C, Brady LW, eds: *Principles and practice of radiation oncology*, ed 4, Philadelphia, 2003, Lippincott, pp 357-391.

Patients who smoke while undergoing radiation therapy have a diminished healing response and shorter survival duration than those who do not.[4]

Patients receiving radiation to the neck to kill oral cancer cells that have spread to the lymph nodes are five to six times more likely to have damaged carotid arteries, making them more vulnerable to strokes. These patients often drink or smoke heavily (or both), have hypertension, and have already developed *osteoradionecrosis* (bony destruction) of the mandible.[13]

Therapeutic doses of radiation normally range from 5000 to 7000 **centigray** (cGy) over a 6- to 7-week period. Doses are usually fractionated into 150 to 200 cGy on weekdays, leaving the weekends for normal cell repair.

Total body irradiation (TBI) is administered as part of a preparatory regimen for bone marrow transplantation. TBI (1000 cGy) and cyclophosphamide condition the graft recipient by inducing immunosuppression and killing all malignant cells. Bone marrow transplantation is not a suggested treatment for carcinomas of the head and neck.[23]

CHEMOTHERAPY

Chemotherapy differs from surgery and radiation in that it is almost always used as a systemic treatment, meaning that the drugs circulate throughout the body rather than being confined to one area to treat a localized cancer such as the oral cavity. This distinction is important because chemotherapy can reach cancer cells that may have spread to other parts of the body.

Note
Leukemia is a good example of a systemic form of cancer that responds best to chemotherapy.

More than 100 drugs are currently used for chemotherapy—either alone or in combination with other drugs or treatments. Many more drugs are expected to become available. These drugs vary widely in their chemical composition, mode of administration, usefulness in treating specific forms of cancer, and side effects.

Note
Factors that oncologists must consider when selecting which drugs to use for a chemotherapy regimen include the type of cancer, stage of the cancer, patient's age and general health status, other serious health problems (such as liver or kidney diseases), and other forms of cancer therapy administered in the past.

Usually, chemotherapy is given by mouth; by injection into a vein, skin, or muscle; or by mixing the drug into a solution and letting it flow into a vein for 30 minutes or longer. Chemotherapeutic drugs are usually placed into one of six categories[29]:

- Alkylating agents
- Antibiotics
- Antimetabolites
- Plant alkaloids
- Steroids and hormones
- Miscellaneous

IMMUNOTHERAPY

Immunotherapy stimulates or restores the ability of the immune system to fight cancer, infections, and other diseases. This form of therapy is also used to reduce certain side effects that may be caused by cancer treatment.

The therapy is given by injection into a vein. For some patients with CLL, the type of biological therapy used is a monoclonal antibody. This substance binds to the leukemia cells. This therapy enables the immune system to kill leukemia cells in the blood and bone marrow. For some patients with CML, the biological therapy is a natural substance called **interferon.** This substance can slow the growth of leukemia cells.[29]

Note
Immunotherapy is also referred to as biological therapy, biotherapy, or biological response modifier (BRM) therapy.

BLOOD AND MARROW TRANSPLANTATION

Hematopoietic or blood-forming stem cells are immature cells that can mature into blood cells. These stem cells are found in the bone marrow, bloodstream, or umbilical cord blood. **Bone marrow transplantation** (BMT) and *peripheral blood stem cell transplantation* (PBSCT) are procedures that restore stem cells that were destroyed by high doses of chemotherapy, radiation therapy, or both. Chemotherapy and radiation therapy generally target cells that divide rapidly. These therapies are used to treat cancer because cancer cells divide more often than most healthy cells. However, because bone marrow cells also divide frequently, high-dose treatments can severely damage or destroy the patient's bone marrow. Without healthy bone marrow, the patient is no longer able to make the blood cells needed to carry oxygen, fight infection, and prevent bleeding. BMT and PBSCT replace stem cells that were destroyed by treatment. The healthy, transplanted stem cells can restore the bone marrow's ability to produce the blood cells the patient needs.[34]

Three types of transplants include the following:

- *Autologous transplants*—patients receive their own stem cells.
- *Syngeneic transplants*—patients receive stem cells from their identical twin.
- *Allogeneic transplants*—patients receive stem cells from someone other than themselves or an identical twin. The patient's brother, sister, or parent may serve as the donor, or a person not related to the patient (an unrelated donor) may be used.

Oral Complications

RADIATION THERAPY

The vast majority of patients undergoing radiation therapy for malignancies of the head and neck experience oral complications associated with their treatment.[30] Radiation-induced oral complications can significantly affect morbidity, the patient's ability to tolerate treatment, and overall quality of life.[16,31]

DENTAL CONSIDERATIONS

The effects of radiation are cumulative; as the dose of radiation increases or the rate of delivery accelerates, the type and severity of oral complications increase.[10] Oral complications may become apparent as early as the first week of therapy and may continue for a few weeks or months after completion of therapy.

The early changes are caused by alterations in cellular division and maturation. They particularly affect epithelial and glandular tissue in the form of the following:

- Mucositis
- Ulcerations
- Salivary gland dysfunction
- Alterations in taste
- Dermatitis

Later complications are usually associated with tissues that have slower turnover rates, such as muscle or bone, and result in **trismus** or osteoradionecrosis (ORN).

> *Note*
>
> Salivary gland damage and vascular or osseous changes from irradiation usually are permanent.

The walls of blood vessels thicken, and the lumens narrow, reducing blood flow and oxygenation in the tissues. Consequently, the healing capacity of the tissues or bone is impaired, leading to necrosis in response to trauma or infection.[34]

If head and neck surgery is a treatment of choice, then the dental hygienist must recognize and manage the surgical site and tracheostomy (to reduce the risk of infections), **hyperalimentation** (tube feeding), pain, oral hygiene, limitations in movement, dysphasia, dermatitis, and speech alterations.

Mucositis

Chemotherapy given in conjunction with irradiation can accelerate the onset and increase the severity of **mucositis.*** Because oral mucosal cells have a life span of only 10 to 14 days, the basal cell layer is destroyed faster than it can reproduce. Consequently, mucositis clinically exhibits as edematous, erythematous tissue, after which, in more severe cases, the formation of ulcerations and pseudomembranes occurs. Mucositis usually is painful, and the involved mucosa is frequently sensitive to temperature extremes and pressure. A patient with dentures may not be able to tolerate wearing them. An unpleasant odor is common, caused by the sloughing necrotic tissue, bleeding, and plaque biofilm accumulation (Figure 48-4). Breaks in the mucosal integrity caused by mucositis become portals of entry for infection, compromising the patient's overall health. Mucositis may become so severe that radiation therapy is suspended temporarily and the patient is hospitalized for pain and infection control and intravenous fluid and nutritional support.[12] Mucositis usually heals approximately 6 weeks after therapy is complete. The epithelium never fully recovers

and tends to be thin and friable and minimal trauma may initiate ulceration.

DENTAL CONSIDERATIONS

Inflammation of the oral mucous membranes, with or without oral ulcerations, usually develops around the second week of radiation therapy, primarily on nonkeratinized tissues and the lateral borders of the tongue.

Management

Treatment of mucositis is primarily **palliative.** Brushing with an ultrasoft toothbrush is recommended. Although tooth swabs or sponges do not remove plaque biofilm, they may be used to apply rinsing agents to the teeth and sensitive oral tissues. Frequent rinsing with a baking soda solution, alone or with saline, throughout the day followed by a plain water rinse should make the patient more comfortable. Chlorhexidine rinsing reduces inflammation, particularly when the pain caused by mucositis hinders the removal of mechanical plaque biofilm. More recently, rinsing of the oral cavity with a povidone-iodine solution,[1] as well as the administration of narrow-spectrum antibacterial and antifungal agents, some in the form of lozenges, has shown some promise in the treatment of mucositis.*

> *Distinct Care Modifications*
>
> Mucositis may make mastication, swallowing, and speaking painful. Topical anesthetic or antiinflammatory rinses, gels, or ointments such as Orabase or 1-2-3 solution (mix of diphenhydramine elixir, milk of magnesia, and viscous lidocaine [Xylocaine]) may be applied before eating or speaking to increase comfort. Systemic analgesics may also become necessary. A soft, bland diet that is low in citric acid and served at room temperature is advised. Alcoholic beverages and smoking must be avoided.

Commercial mouthwashes with high alcohol content should not be used because of their drying, irritating effects. Hydrogen peroxide should be limited to short-term use and diluted with

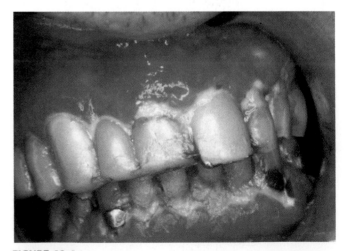

FIGURE 48-4
Oral mucositis in a patient receiving radiation therapy for cancer of the head and neck. (Courtesy JE Bouquot, DDS, Morgantown, WV.)

*References 3, 9, 23, 31, 33, 46.

*References 3, 9, 23, 29, 31, 32, 33, 46.

✦✦ **CASE APPLICATION 48-1.2**

Appropriate Management for Complications
Mr. Fitzgibbons has several complications associated with radiation treatments. What type of management would you recommend for each of these conditions?

water in a 1:4 concentration to prevent disruption of the normal flora.

Xerostomia

Radiation may cause permanent damage to the serous cells of the salivary glands if they are in the field of treatment.* Changes occur in the volume of saliva produced and its consistency according to the dose of radiation, the extent of gland involvement in the field, and the age of the patient.

---

*References 3, 9, 23, 31, 33, 46.

DENTAL CONSIDERATIONS

A 50% reduction in saliva may occur in the first week and may progress to a volume depletion of up to 90%. The saliva produced is also more acidic, which increases the risk of enamel demineralization and subsequent dental caries. *Radiation caries* is a term used to describe the rampant dental caries activity that may result from the reduction in salivary volume and pH and the increase in cariogenic bacteria. Clinically, this form of dental caries exhibits as a circumferential breakdown at the cervical margin of the teeth and may lead to tooth fracture at the gingival line in a matter of weeks or months (a finding consistent with the facts of Case Study 48-1) (Figures 48-5 and 48-6).

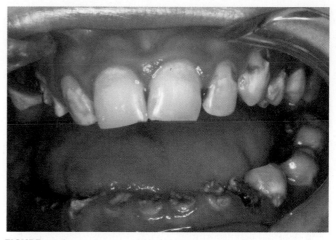

FIGURE 48-6
Advanced dental caries 2 years after radiation therapy in a noncompliant patient.

The increased viscosity of the saliva reduces its self-cleansing ability, making the patient more susceptible to periodontal and *Candida* infections. Dry, friable mucosa may be prone to cracking and bleeding (Figure 48-7), creating a portal of entry for infection, which increases the risk of ORN. Denture wearers may not be able to tolerate their prostheses because of reduced surface tension between the dry mucosa and the denture. Oral dryness can also compromise eating, taste, swallowing, and speech.

Management

Strategies for managing xerostomia include the following:
- Oral pilocarpine therapy[17,22]
- Artificial salivas
- Sugarless chewing gum
- Frequent sips of water
- Ice chips
- Humidifiers
- A diet of moist foods

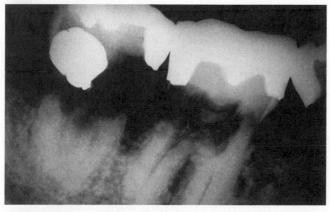

FIGURE 48-5
Radiograph showing *radiation caries,* the pattern of cervical decay that can develop in a patient with xerostomia that occurs secondary to irradiation of the salivary glands. (Courtesy JE Bouquot, DDS, Morgantown, WV.)

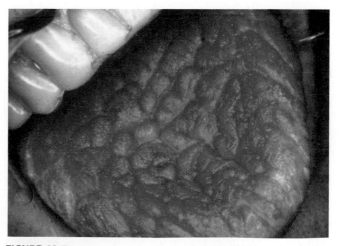

FIGURE 48-7
Effects of severe radiation-induced xerostomia on the tongue and other oral soft tissues. (Courtesy JE Bouquot, DDS, Morgantown, WV.)

Dentinal Hypersensitivity

Dentinal hypersensitivity is often a consequence of a lower salivary pH leading to enamel demineralization combined with open dentinal tubules from mechanical forces.

Management

Fluoride varnishes containing 5% sodium fluoride should be administered as an in-office treatment. The varnish is painted on demineralized, hypersensitive surfaces with a small brush. The yellowish film created by the varnish should be left undisturbed for at least 4 hours. The patient should be instructed not to eat or brush during this time period.

Infections

Candidiasis is the infection most often seen in patients with oral mucositis and hyposalivation.[3,23,46] These fungal lesions may be classified as pseudomembranous, erythematous, atrophic, or hyperplastic (Figure 48-8). The most frequently affected oral sites are the tongue, mucosa, and commissures of the lips. Bacterial, mycotic, and viral infections may also result, but these are more often associated with chemotherapy.

Management

Antifungal preparations containing sucrose should be avoided. In more extensive infections, ketoconazole, fluconazole, or amphotericin B may be indicated. The oral soft tissue should be examined frequently to assess for candidiasis.

Secondary infections caused by bacteria or viruses require proper diagnosis and subsequent treatment with organism-specific antibiotics and antivirals.

Dysgeusia

Dysgeusia, or loss of taste, is believed to occur as a result of damage to the microvilli and outer taste cells of the tongue or as a side effect of xerostomia and mucositis.[23,33,46]

Taste acuity for salt and sweet may be altered as therapy progresses. The symptoms usually appear within the first week of therapy, and the condition resolves 2 to 4 months after radiation is complete, if saliva is adequate. Permanent taste loss can occur when radiation doses exceed 6000 cGy. Dysgeusia often leads to a loss of appetite.

Management

Food aversions often develop with alterations in taste and smell. Patient education regarding dietary and preparation alternatives is important.

Dietary supplements of zinc have been prescribed to manage chronic taste loss.[40]

Dysphasia

Dysphasia, or difficulty swallowing, is not uncommon in patients who have received radiation to the head and neck. Videofluoroscopy has revealed prolonged pharyngeal transit times in postirradiation patients.[35]

DENTAL CONSIDERATIONS

Dysphasia is further complicated by xerostomia and results in eating and speaking difficulties.

Management

Taking small bites of food, eating a soft-to-semisoft diet, and taking frequent sips of liquids while eating can enhance swallowing.

Nutritional Deficiency

Xerostomia, mucositis, dysgeusia, and dysphasia trigger eating difficulties. Regardless of whether a loss of appetite is caused by

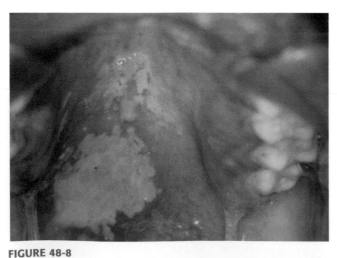

FIGURE 48-8
Oral candidiasis affecting the palatal mucosa in a patient undergoing radiation therapy for a tumor of the head and neck.

a sore mouth or a lack of desire, poor nutritional intake can lead to fatigue, dehydration, and compromised healing.

Management

> *Distinct Care Modifications*
> Unfortunately, nutritional liquid supplements contain sucrose, and dental caries assessments should be made frequently.

Nutritional liquid supplements are an ideal means of boosting calories in a patient who, for any reason, is not eating.

Foods that are easy to chew and swallow include cooked cereals, eggs, mashed potatoes, noodles, pureed meats, fruits and vegetables, milkshakes and puddings, gelatins, ice cream, sherbet, and sorbet.

Osteoradionecrosis

The bone, periosteum, connective tissue, and vascular epithelium in the field of radiation may become necrotic because irradiation has rendered the sites hypovascular, hypocellular, and hypoxic.* The result is a reduction in blood supply to the area, a change in the growth and repair potential of the bone, and a diminished resistance to infection.

DENTAL CONSIDERATIONS

Insults in the form of trauma (e.g., extraction, an ill-fitting appliance) or infection (e.g., periodontal disease, a dental abscess) may lead to the development of **osteoradionecrosis** (ORN). In response to trauma or infection, alveolar destruction may be progressive and extensive. Denture wearers are often advised to leave their prostheses out from the initiation of therapy to 6 months after completion of therapy to reduce the risk of ORN. Blood vessels in the periodontium and periosteum are similarly affected, resulting in a widening of the periodontal ligament space.

Symptoms may become apparent shortly after radiation therapy or may take years to develop. ORN has been reported to occur as late as 25 years after radiation therapy. The mandible is more susceptible to ORN because it is denser and less vascular than the maxilla and consequently absorbs more radiation. Patients undergoing radiation doses of more than 7000 cGy are also at greater risk. As in Case Study 48-1, the greatest risk is to the patient whose mandible has received extensive irradiation and who requires tooth extractions sometime after completion of radiation therapy.

Management

Before radiotherapy begins, a thorough assessment of the hard and soft oral tissues must be made to determine any possible risks of infection or trauma. All hopeless and questionable teeth (e.g., furcation involved; advanced periodontitis; impacted, nonrestorable im-

> *Prevention*
> The key to reducing the risk of ORN is prevention.

plants with an uncertain prognosis; root fragments; any potential soft tissue or bony pathologic condition) should be removed. If extractions are indicated, then a minimum of 14 days is required for primary closure of the socket before initiating radiotherapy. Periodontal care and restorations must be completed. A dentulous patient must practice meticulous oral hygiene before, during, and after radiotherapy. Daily fluoride gel applications using smooth, well-fitting custom fluoride trays are essential throughout the patient's life. Frequent supportive care to eliminate any sources of trauma or infection must be established. New prostheses may need to be fabricated after therapy to ensure smooth edges and a comfortable fit.[34]

Treatment of ORN requires conservative measures to promote healing. A series of **hyperbaric oxygen** (HBO) treatments to flood the tissue with oxygen is recommended before any invasive procedure on irradiated tissues is performed.

> *Distinct Care Modifications*
> Advanced cases may involve extended antibiotic therapy and surgery for the removal of bony sequestra or a portion of the mandible.

✦ CASE APPLICATION 48-1.3

Rationale for Hyperbaric Oxygen
What is the reason for using hyperbaric oxygen treatments on Mr. Fitzgibbons prior to radiation therapy?

Trismus

Trismus results from fibrosis of the muscles of mastication or the temporomandibular joint when these muscles are in the field of irradiation.[9,23,46] Patients with nasopharyngeal, maxillary sinus, and palatal tumors often develop trismus (as was suggested in Case Study 48-1). The usual onset of trismus is 3 to 6 months after completion of radiation therapy. Opening the mouth is difficult and often painful.

Management

A mouth block should be placed between the beam and the patient during irradiation to prevent scatter radiation to the muscles of the face.

Isometric exercises involve using opposing finger pressure on the incisal edges of the mandibular anterior teeth as the patient tries to open the mouth or opening against gentle pressure exerted by placing the fist against the midline of the mandible. Ten repetitions of finger pressure for 30 seconds five to six times daily is advised.

Mechanical stretching devices also are available.

> *Patient Education Opportunity*
> Instruct the patient to perform exercises designed to maintain or improve oral range of motion daily.

> *Distinct Care Modifications*
> The patient can also be given the maximal number of tongue blades that will comfortably stack between the maxillary and mandibular anterior teeth. One additional blade is then slid between the others to stretch the oral opening.

*References 3, 9, 10, 23, 31, 33, 46.

Developmental Anomalies

The extent of damage to the developing dentition depends on the total and fractional dose of radiation received and the stage of tooth development at the time of exposure. Irradiation of the developing dentition and facial bones with doses as low as 400 cGy may result in hypocalcification, enamel hypoplasia, delayed or arrested tooth development, premature closure of root apices, microdontia, complete or partial anodontia, micrognathia, retrognathia, and skeletal and dental malocclusion.[6,19,24]

Management

Parents must be alerted to the possible anomalies that may arise when their children receive radiation therapy to the head and neck. Long-term dental follow-up is necessary, and dental professionals should be diligent in observing and rehabilitating the dentition before, during, and after radiotherapy.

Several dental specialists are often required to restore the dentition.

Fluoride therapy must be monitored carefully to prevent fluorosis. Psychosocial issues related to facial deformity and delayed eruption or missing teeth should not be discounted.

> *Distinct Care Modifications*
> Before radiotherapy, mobile teeth should be extracted, and gingival opercula and orthodontic bands should be removed if they pose a risk of food entrapment, trauma, or infection.

> *Distinct Care Modifications*
> The importance of supervised, meticulous oral hygiene home care cannot be overemphasized.

Skin Erythema

The skin of the face and neck in the field of irradiation develop erythema as early as the second week of radiotherapy[8] (Figure 48-9). The skin becomes red, as if sunburned. Desquamation of the skin can occur, causing a breakdown of skin integrity and creating a portal of entry for infection. Radiation treatments may be postponed to allow for healing. In some cases, facial hair is lost.

Management

Patients should be instructed to shield the irradiated field from sunlight and ultraviolet rays and to avoid using soaps or lotions in the area because these products can contribute to necrosis of the skin. The treated area of the face and neck should not be exposed to temperature extremes of hot and cold; this includes heating pads and ice packs.

CHEMOTHERAPY

48-5

Although the risk for oral complications varies with the type of chemotherapy regimen, approximately one half of patients who are treated with chemotherapy will experience oral side effects of some form. The oral cavity can be affected because antineoplastic drugs function by suppressing the growth and spread of malignant cells. Unfortunately, normal cells are also adversely affected. Normal cells with the highest rate of mitotic activity are found in the following areas:

- Mouth
- Digestive tract
- Bone marrow
- Hair follicles
- Reproductive system

Cells in these areas are directly affected because chemotherapy interferes with cell production, maturation, and replacement. Indirect toxicity is caused by the *myelosuppressive* action of the drugs, resulting in a generalized *immunosuppression*. This action suggests *neutropenia, lymphocytopenia,* and *thrombocytopenia,* making the patient susceptible to oral infection and bleeding. Direct cytotoxic effects of the chemotherapy on the cells lining the oral cavity often result in mucositis and ulcerations.

DENTAL CONSIDERATIONS

Mouth pain, alterations in taste, transient **xerostomia,** *abnormal dental development, damaged tooth enamel,* and *neurotoxicity* are also common oral manifestations associated with chemotherapy.[30] (See the management suggestions on pages 906 to 910.)

Infection

Chemotherapeutic drugs target the cells of the bone marrow, increasing the patient's risk of infection resulting from a decline in the neutrophil count (neutropenia). Oral bacterial, fungal, and viral infections are considered opportunistic in the immunocompromised patient. Neutropenia also predisposes the patient to oral mucositis.

> *Note*
> Localized oral inflammation, ulceration, and infection can lead to pain, systemic infection, and nutritional compromise.

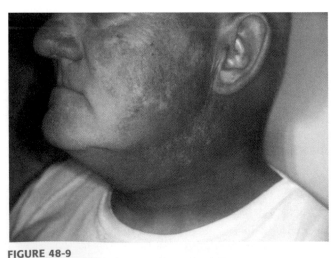

FIGURE 48-9
Skin erythema from exposure to therapeutic doses of radiation. (Courtesy JE Bouquot, DDS, Morgantown, WV.)

Management

Chemotherapy-induced mucositis and ulcerations (Figures 48-10 and 48-11) can be treated palliatively, as discussed in the management of radiation-induced mucositis.

Granulocyte colony–simulating factor (GCSF) initiates the production of neutrophils, eosinophils, and basophils.[32]

For dental procedures to be performed, the absolute neutrophil count must be at least 1000/mm^3. The patient's hematologic profile must be obtained within 24 hours of dental treatment. If surgical procedures are being scheduled, 7 to 10 days should be allowed for postoperative healing before the next cycle of chemotherapy.

Infections must be identified and treated early in the myelosuppressed patient, particularly when the patient is febrile. Gram-negative bacteria, *Candida* infections, and herpes simplex viruses (Figure 48-12) are common causes of morbidity and death in patients undergoing chemotherapy for acute leukemias.

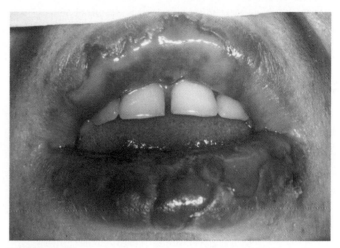

FIGURE 48-12
Severe case of oral herpes simplex virus in a patient undergoing chemotherapy.

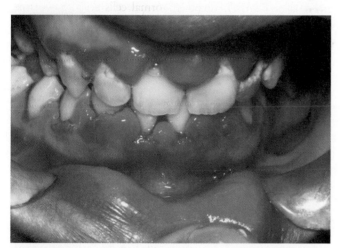

FIGURE 48-10
Chemotherapy-induced neutropenia and thrombocytopenia resulting in oral mucositis and bleeding.

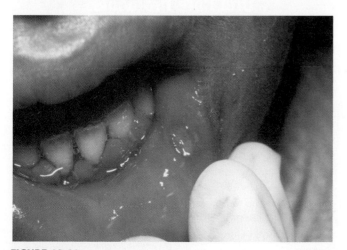

FIGURE 48-11
Oral ulcerations in the patient shown in Figure 48-10.

Bleeding

Oral manifestations of leukemia may exhibit as mucosal edema and pallor caused by infiltration of the gingiva by leukemic cells. In addition, a decrease in platelets (thrombocytopenia) may also be a sequela of chemotherapy.

DENTAL CONSIDERATIONS

Spontaneous mucosal bleeding can occur when the platelet count falls below 20,000/mm^3 or when the patient exhibits local factors such as poor oral hygiene, traumatic habits, preexisting periodontal conditions, mobile teeth, decayed or fractured teeth or restorations, or orthodontic bands or wires. A break in the mucosal integrity as a result of any of these local factors acts as a portal of entry for microbial infections, and a life-threatening septicemia might be a potential outcome.[34]

Management

If dental surgery is needed, then the patient should have a platelet count of at least 50,000/mm^3 to eliminate the risk of postoperative bleeding.

Platelet Count

Maggie had a platelet count of 18,000/mm³ and experienced persistent oral bleeding with the eruption of the first molars. What is the relationship between the two conditions? Should there be a concern about either symptom?

Distinct Care Modifications

When the patient's platelet count drops below 20,000/mm³, toothbrushing should involve using a supersoft nylon brush or gauze or cotton swabs dipped in warm water or 0.12% chlorhexidine gluconate.

Flossing should be avoided when the patient is neutropenic and thrombocytopenic to prevent unnecessary trauma.[34]

Neurotoxicity

The alkaloids have a toxic effect on the peripheral, autonomic, and cranial nerves and may be responsible for a persistent, deep aching, burning pain that mimics a toothache. The pain usually subsides when the course of chemotherapy is complete.[30]

Developmental Anomalies

Alterations in tooth development, craniofacial growth, and skeletal development are seen when children receive high-dose chemotherapy before the age of 9 years.[30]

Impaired Growth and Development

What factors in Maggie Clarkson's history cause her to be at significant risk for impaired growth and development?

Patient Education Opportunity

After a vomiting episode, the patient should be instructed to rinse the mouth with water, expectorate, and then follow with a few sips of cool water to rid the mouth of stomach acids that can irritate the oral mucosa and demineralize tooth enamel.

Note

An important point to remember is that vomitus and saliva of patients who are undergoing chemotherapy contain cytotoxic drugs. Family members and health care providers should handle these bodily fluids as hazardous waste material.[34]

Damaged Tooth Enamel

Repeated chemotherapy-induced nausea and vomiting may lead to enamel erosion.

Management

Some sources recommend a sodium bicarbonate rinse (baking soda and water) after vomiting to neutralize the acid.[30,34]

Eating small meals and avoiding drinking beverages with meals may help alleviate nausea and subsequent vomiting associated with chemotherapy. Sucking on sugar-free candies is recommended to reduce anticipatory vomiting and also has the potential to stimulate saliva.

BLOOD AND MARROW TRANSPLANTATION

Severe immunosuppression, resulting from high-dose TBI and intensive chemotherapy, is performed to prepare the recipient's body to accept the transplant from the donor. This pronounced immunosuppression can last up to 1 year, and therefore the risk of oral complications is relatively high, affecting approximately 75% of patients receiving blood or marrow transplants.[30] These complications include mucositis, ulceration, hemorrhage, infection, and xerostomia. Acute **graft versus host disease** (GVHD) may occur in the first 100 days after an allogeneic transplant because of the impaired immune system. The chronic form occurs after 100 days posttransplant. This condition, as its name implies, develops when the patient receiving the transplant *(host, recipient)* rejects the donor's cells *(graft)*. Engraftment is not successful and the rejection is characterized by fever, rash on the palms of the hands and the soles of the feet, anorexia or diarrhea (or both), and liver disease. Xerostomia and oral mucositis are commonly seen in the oral cavity of patients with GVHD. Cyclosporine and azathioprine (Imuran) are drugs given to transplant patients to reduce the risk of organ or marrow rejection. They function by suppressing the patient's immune system. Consequently, the patient is at risk of infection from these drugs.[29,34]

Management

Oral therapy involves (1) diagnostic testing to rule out any oral infections; (2) treating any oral infections of bacterial, viral; or fungal origin and pain management; and (3) managing xerostomia. The patient should also be monitored for cyclosporine-induced gingival overgrowth.[30,34]

Oral Care Protocols for Anticancer Therapies

BEFORE THERAPY

Persons who undergo cancer treatment are sometimes unaware that a dental examination is a critical initial step in maintaining their overall health. A treatment plan should be developed based on the patient's oral needs and the timetable for cancer therapy. At least 7 to 14 days should be allowed for healing from an oral surgical procedure before cancer therapy.[47]

Patient Education Opportunity

Patients should be instructed in proper oral hygiene techniques and the importance of oral hygiene as infection control. Custom fluoride trays should be fabricated for patients whose salivary gland or glands are in the field of radiation.

DURING THERAPY

Identification and management of oral complications associated with therapy are crucial at this time.

Precautions such as blood counts and prophylactic antibiotic coverage are particularly important for patients undergoing chemotherapy.

> *Prevention*
> Patients should be examined weekly during therapy.

> *Distinct Care Modifications*
> Invasive procedures are not recommended during this phase.

AFTER THERAPY

Patients who have previously received chemotherapy and are in **remission** (no longer experiencing symptoms of the disease) can resume regular dental treatment because their blood counts have returned to normal and their oral complications have subsided. Once an indwelling catheter has been removed, no modifications to dental treatment should be required. In the case of radiation therapy, some of the therapy-induced oral complications will persist temporarily after therapy, such as trismus, whereas some such as xerostomia may be permanent when the salivary glands are in the field of radiation.

> *Distinct Care Modifications*
> Lifelong daily fluoride therapy is indicated for the patient with severe permanent xerostomia.

> *Prevention*
> Frequent supportive care intervals are recommended to monitor oral hygiene; treat any restorative needs; and assess for infections, dental caries, or chronic GVHD.

> *Distinct Care Modifications*
> Precautions such as HBO therapy are often warranted before an extraction.

Patients should also be carefully monitored for secondary malignancies in the oral region. In some instances, signs of **relapse** (return of the disease) may be first evident in the oral cavity.

Precautions such as HBO therapy are often warranted before an extraction, for example, in a patient who has been previously irradiated to prevent ORN. Pediatric patients, in particular, should be followed long-term to assess growth and development.

References

1. Adamietz IA et al: Prophylaxis with povidone-iodine against inducing mucositis by radiochemotherapy, *Support Care Cancer* 6:373-377, 1998.
2. Bansberg SF, Olsen KD, Gaffey TA: High-grade carcinoma of the oral cavity, *Arch Otolaryngol Head Neck Surg* 100:41-48, 1989.
3. Barker GJ, Barker BF, Gier RE: *Oral management of the cancer patient: a guide for the health care professional,* Kansas City, Mo, 1996, Biomedical Communications.
4. Browman GP et al: Influence of cigarette smoking on the efficacy of radiation therapy in head and neck cancer, *N Engl J Med* 328:159-163, 1993.
5. Bushong SC: *Radiologic science for technologists,* ed 4, St Louis, 1988, Mosby.
6. Chin EA, Hopkins KP, Bowman LC: A brief overview of oral complications in pediatric oncology patients and suggested management strategies, *J Dent Child* 6:468-473, 1998.
7. Day GL, Blot WJ: Second primary tumors in patients with oral cancer, *Cancer* 70:14-19, 1992.
8. DeBiase CB: *Dental health education: theory and practice,* Philadelphia, 1991, Lea & Febiger.
9. DeBiase CB: The patient with cancer. In Wilkins EM, ed: *Clinical practice of the dental hygienist,* ed 8, Philadelphia, 1999, Lippincott Williams & Wilkins.
10. Epstein JB et al: Surgical periodontal treatment in the radiotherapy-treated head and neck cancer patient, *Spec Care Dent* 14:182-187, 1994.
11. Epstein JB, Scully C: Assessing the patient at risk for oral squamous cell carcinoma, *Spec Care Dent* 17:120-128, 1997.
12. Epstein JB, Van der Meij EH: Complicating mucosal reactions in patients receiving radiation therapy for head and neck cancer, *Spec Care Dent* 17:88-93, 1997.
13. Friedlander AH et al: Detection of radiation-induced accelerated atherosclerosis in patients with osteoradionecrosis by panoramic radiography, *J Maxillofac Surg* 56:455-459, 1998.
14. Garewall HS: Beta-carotene and vitamin E oral cancer prevention, *J Cell Biochem Suppl* 17(Suppl F):262-269, 1993.
15. Hong WK et al: Prevention of second primary tumors with isotretinoin in squamous cell carcinoma of the head and neck, *N Engl J Med* 323:795-801, 1990.
16. Jansma J, Vissink A, Spijkervet FKL: Protocol for the prevention and treatment of sequelae resulting from head and neck radiation therapy, *Cancer* 70:2171-2180, 1992.
17. Johnson JT et al: Oral pilocarpine for postirradiation xerostomia in patients with head and neck cancer, *N Engl J Med* 329:390-395, 1993.
18. Jones KR et al: Prognostic factors in the recurrence of stage I and II squamous cell cancer of the oral cavity, *Arch Otolaryngol Head Neck Surg* 118:483-485, 1992.
19. Kaste SC, Hopkins KP, Bowman LC: Dental abnormalities in long-term survivors of head and neck rhabdomyosarcoma, *Med Pediatr Oncol* 25:96-101, 1995.
20. Kelloff GJ et al: Progress in applied chemoprevention research, *Semin Oncol* 17:438-455, 1990.
21. Landis SH et al: Cancer statistics, *CA Cancer J Clin* 55(1):10-30, 2005.
22. LeVeque FG et al: A multicenter, randomized, double-blind, placebo-controlled, dose-titration study of pilocarpine for the treatment of radiation-induced xerostomia in head and neck cancer patients, *J Clin Oncol* 11:1124-1131, 1993.
23. Little JW et al: *Dental management of the medically compromised patient,* ed 6, St Louis, 2002, Mosby.
24. Maguire A et al: The long-term effect of treatment on the dental condition of children surviving malignant disease, *Cancer Nurs* 25:70-75, 1987.
25. Mashberg A, Feldman LJ: Clinical criteria for identifying early oral and oropharyngeal carcinoma: erythroplasia revisited, *Am J Surg* 156:273-275, 1988.
26. Mashberg A, Samit A: Early diagnosis of asymptomatic oral and oropharyngeal squamous cancers, *CA Cancer J Clin* 45:328-351, 1995.

27. Miller BF, Keane CB: *Encyclopedia and dictionary of medicine, nursing, and allied health,* ed 6, Philadelphia, 1997, WB Saunders.

28. Millon RR, Cassisi NJ, eds: *Management of head and neck cancer: a multidisciplinary approach,* St Louis, 1986, Mosby.

29. National Cancer Institute, National Institutes of Health: Cancer topics and statistics. Available at: www.cancer.gov. Accessed August 31, 2004.

30. National Institute of Dental and Craniofacial Research: *Oral complications of cancer treatment: what the oncology team can do,* NIH Publication No 02-4360, June 2002.

31. National Institutes of Health Consensus Development Conference Statements: oral complications of cancer therapies: diagnosis, prevention, and treatment, *NCI Monogr* 9:3-8, 1990.

32. Ord RA, Blanchaert RH: Current management of oral cancer, *J Am Dent Assoc* 132:19S-23S, 2001.

33. Peterson DE, D'Ambrosio JA: Nonsurgical management of head and neck cancer patients, *Dent Clin North Am* 38:425-445, 1994.

34. Rankin KV, Jones DL, eds: *Oral health in cancer therapy,* Austin, Tex, 1999, Texas Cancer Council.

35. Rhodus NL, Moller K: Dysphagia in postirradiation therapy head and neck cancer patients, *J Cancer Res Ther Control* 4:49-55, 1994.

36. Rothman K, Keller A: The effect of joint exposure to alcohol and tobacco on risk of cancer of the mouth and pharynx, *J Chron Dis* 25:711-716, 1972.

37. Rubin P, Constantine L, Nelson D: Late effects of cancer treatment: radiation and drug toxicity. In Perez C, Brady LW, eds: *Principles and practice of radiation oncology,* Philadelphia, 1992, JB Lippincott.

38. Shafer WG, Hine MK, Levy BM: *A textbook of oral pathology,* ed 4, Philadelphia, 1983, WB Saunders.

39. Shah JP, Lydiatt W: Treatment of cancer of the head and neck, *CA Cancer J Clin* 45:352-368, 1995.

40. Silverman S, ed: *Oral cancer,* ed 2, New York, 1985, American Cancer Society.

41. Spiro RH et al: Cervical node metastasis from epidermoid carcinoma of the oral cavity and oropharynx: a critical assessment of current staging, *Am J Surg* 128:562-567, 1974.

42. Takagi M et al: Causes of oral tongue cancer treatment failures: analysis of autopsy cases, *Cancer* 69:1081-1087, 1992.

43. US Department of Health, Education, and Welfare: *Management guidelines for head and neck cancer,* PHS Publication No 80-2037, Washington, DC, 1979, The Department.

44. Wallner PE et al: Patterns of care study: analysis of outcome survey data: anterior two-thirds of the tongue and floor of the mouth, *Am J Clin Oncol* 9:50-57, 1986.

45. Wang CC, ed: *Radiation therapy for head and neck neoplasms: indications, techniques and results,* ed 2, Littleton, Mass, 1990, John Wright-PSG.

46. Whitmeyer CC, Waskowski JC, Iffland HA: Radiotherapy and oral sequelae: prevention and management protocols, *J Dent Hyg* 71:23-29, 1997.

47. Wright WE: Pretreatment oral health care interventions for radiation patients, *NCI Monogr* 9:57-59, 1990.

Dental Hygiene Business Practice Management

Annette Ashley Linder

INSIGHT

Dental hygienists have a unique opportunity to positively affect the experience of each patient seeking dental hygiene services through professional practice management. Understanding the economic side of a dental practice is important as one prepares to exit the educational program and become a professional dental hygienist. Dentistry is a business; if employed in a traditional setting, then the dental hygienist will be expected to contribute to the productivity of the practice.

This chapter focuses on the following:
- Patient management including scheduling and appointments
- Marketing services offered by the dental practice
- Office operations that can increase productivity

Possessing an understanding of these concepts, in addition to clinical competence and appropriate communication skills, can improve one's value and marketability.

✦ CASE STUDY 49-1   Poor Self-Image Because of Appearance of Teeth

A school principal related the following story about his dental experience.

I had a poor self-image because of the problems with and appearance of my teeth. I considered leaving my position in education because it required public speaking and meeting with the public first-hand and close-up. I never had good teeth, had seen many dentists over the years, but had never had a positive dental experience. I was told that my ill-fitting partial was the "best

that could be done." I finally experienced a turnaround. I visited a new dental practice, established a positive professional relationship with the dental hygienist in the practice, and it ultimately helped me. The hygienist enabled me to have the confidence to go forward with the dental treatment. The dentist beautifully restored my mouth in the most clinically excellent and esthetic fashion. The dental experience in this office changed my life. I felt and looked like a new man because of my appearance.

✦ CASE STUDY 49-2   Concerns with Dental Hygiene Appointment Management

Annie, a recent graduate, has obtained employment in a general dental practice. She has been working for a month and notices an average of five broken or cancelled appointments a week. Annie inquires of the front desk staff whether they have any idea why so many cancellations occur. Joan replies, "The patient on Wednesday called and said he had something else he needed to do. I asked when he would like to reschedule, and he said he would call back." Annie asks, "What about Ms. Jones who was scheduled on Tuesday for the

second appointment in the series of four for completion of quadrant debridement? Did she provide a reason when she called to cancel?" Joan answers, "Ms. Jones did not call us, and she did not show. I forgot to confirm her appointment on Monday. I apologize." Jennifer, another front desk staff person, remarks, "You know calling and confirming patients is so time-consuming. Patients don't think having their teeth cleaned is important, so they don't remember."

KEY TERMS

CDT 4/5 codes	overhead	prescheduling	Supportive Care Appointment
chart audit	patient management	profitability	(SCA) reliability analysis
cotherapy	perceived value	risk management practice	time management
oral hygiene fitness report	practice economics		

LEARNING OUTCOMES

After reading this chapter the student will be able to:

1. Incorporate positive word choices into his or her vocabulary for communicating with patients, staff, peers, and employers with regard to dental hygiene services and appointments.
2. Identify ways of enhancing the patient's perceived value of the services provided.
3. Develop periodontal protocols for a dental hygiene department in a practice.
4. Determine the number of dental hygienists needed to provide dental hygiene services in a practice with 4500 patients of record.

5. Identify patient needs through the process of a chart review.
6. Discuss the relationship of the dental office and the service provider (dentist or dental hygienist) with a patient.
7. Explain the benefits of using the oral hygiene fitness report.
8. Discuss mechanisms for keeping patients informed of the services offered.

Being a caring provider is of utmost importance in the delivery of dental hygiene services. Exhibiting a caring attitude and genuine interest in the well-being of patients can result in an increase of patients in a dental practice. Patient care is a priority in the practice of dental hygiene. In addition, an understanding and application of practice management components is essential.

Increasing the Value of Dental Hygiene Services

How does one motivate patients to keep their scheduled appointments, maintain their daily oral hygiene, get excited about their dentistry, and be *willing and happy* to pay for it? The dental hygiene supportive care appointment (SCA) is a critical component to a dental practice. The SCA is often undervalued, underused, and misunderstood in dental practice. Often viewed by the patient as "just a cleaning and a checkup," this appointment is the easiest to cancel, break, or change. The reasons for these misperceptions, as well as strategies that will enable patients to understand, value, and actually get excited about coming to the dental office, are presented in the following paragraphs.

ENHANCING PERCEIVED VALUE

Building relationships with patients is one of the most rewarding aspects of professional dental hygiene practice. It also creates a patient-oriented practice that is necessary to be successful. For example, patients love to go to a practice where they feel special, valued, and as though they are the only priority.

In the past, every *individual* was viewed as a potential *patient*, but in today's competitive environment clinicians must think of each *patient* as an *individual*. The goal should be to make a patient feel as though he or she is the *only patient in the dental office;* this begins with what dental professionals say and do. By showing a personal interest, remembering important information reported by the patient (e.g., births, deaths, illness, family and work issues), clinicians and other staff members build trust and rapport with patients. Recording significant information reported by the patient (e.g., the daughter who started college, the husband's new job, particular dental care preferences) is a way to assist in developing a trusting, caring relationship.

Another way to enhance perception and one of the best ways to build value and patient commitment and to reduce the number of broken appointments and cancellations in the dental hygiene schedule is for the dental hygienist to schedule the next appointment at the completion of the current appointment. Before dismissal, the dental hygienist restates how much he or she enjoyed seeing the patient and the importance and the reason for the next appointment.

Successful dental practices have effective dental hygiene departments. These dental hygiene departments are responsible for 30% to 35% of practice productivity and are a primary source for patient education and case acceptance. Researchers estimate that between 50% and 85% of all restorative dentistry is generated at the hygiene appointment.[3]

SERVICES ROUTINELY PERFORMED AT THE SUPPORTIVE CARE APPOINTMENT

Regardless of the type of service, when a service is provided the recipient is charged a fee and money is exchanged. The provision of dental hygiene services is no exception to this concept.

While in the educational setting, some of these services may be packaged into a set

Note

The patient's **perceived value** of the appointment, dental hygiene services, and dental hygienist improves when the dental hygienist schedules the SCA. The patient's adherence to appointments increases.

Note

The clinician should never undervalue dental hygiene service and care provided to patients.

fee; however, this scenario will need to change in clinical practice. Many dental hygienists use professional knowledge and skills obtained through formal education and experience to provide patient services and then do not charge for some of these services. Although it may be customary to provide some services or procedures within the appointment, informing patients of each service and procedure is advisable. The clinic should provide the patient with a list of each service performed, even if the service is performed within the treatment code for an SCA. For example, the "Anatomy of the Supportive Care Appointment" provides a list of services and procedures performed at the SCA and is based on the standard of care and clinical responsibilities (Box 49-1). Taking a step-by-step look at the services and procedures performed during an SCA will provide a clear picture of the value the dental hygienist brings to oral health care.

BOX 49-1

ANATOMY OF THE SUPPORTIVE CARE APPOINTMENT

1. Audit chart
2. Greet and seat
3. Update health history
4. Update personal history
5. Vital signs and blood pressure screening
6. Oral cancer screening
7. Review and update radiographs if needed
8. Update dental concerns, using an intraoral camera if possible
9. Periodontal examination
10. Hard tissue examination
11. Discuss periodontal treatment
12. Periodontal therapy and debridement
13. Polish teeth
14. Patient education
15. Chart and document findings
16. Evaluate and discuss
17. Signal or wait for doctor
18. Review findings with doctor
19. Schedule next appointment(s)
20. Dispense oral healthcare aids
21. Record all clinical notes
22. Computer records (insurance)
23. Dismiss patient
24. Sterilize instruments
25. Infection control and prepare for next patient
26. Instrument sharpening

✵ CASE APPLICATION 49-1.1

Value of Services

While reading the next section, consider the value provided to each patient by these services and procedures.

At what point within the SCA would the discussion with the school principal in Case Study 49-1 have occurred?

What behaviors and procedures provided by the dental hygienist at the SCA would have led the school principal to consider esthetic dentistry?

AUDITING CHARTS AND RECORDS

One of the first steps in providing individualized patient care is to conduct a preappointment audit of the dental record. The dental hygienist can determine a great deal of information about a patient, such as the status of the following:

- Medical history and specific concerns
- Personal history notes
- Date of last radiographs
- Periodontal charting
- Incomplete restorative, esthetic, and comprehensive dental treatment recommendations
- Periodontal recommendations

A determination can be made regarding services that should be recommended to the patient. To help reinforce these areas to the patient, the dental hygienist might report findings from the audit at the daily planning meeting (some might refer to it as *the morning huddle*); then the entire dental team will be prepared to discuss the recommendations with the patient, if necessary. Patient needs can get overlooked if the chart or record is not audited. Not only will the patient's condition worsen but also thousands of dollars of productivity will be lost.

ESTABLISHING RAPPORT DURING THE GREETING

Building a positive environment of trust with patients is of great benefit to the dental hygienist and the entire dental practice (see Chapter 5). Focus group participants have reported that they return to a particular dental practice "because the dental hygienist is the best!" Patient comments include, "They know me and care about me," and "I am treated like family."[3] For some, good communication skills come naturally; however, most professionals need to work on the skills necessary to build positive relationships with patients. Verbal and nonverbal communication is essential in providing the best oral health care to patients (see Chapter 5).

> 𝒩ote
>
> Greeting the patient in a professional manner sets the stage for a positive experience for the patient and dental hygienist.

Recalling personal information, such as a hobby or child or grandchild's name, and asking about topics of interest can reduce patient anxiety and fear, make the patient feel important, and assist in building a relationship between the patient and dental hygienist.

UPDATING MEDICAL HISTORY

Ongoing research continues to demonstrate the significant relationship between the patient's systemic health and oral health. A comprehensive health history should be part of every dental record. (See Chapter 12 for a review of the Comprehensive Health History.) Patients of record need to complete a comprehensive health history at least every 3 years. For patients with complicated health problems, a comprehensive history may need to be completed more frequently. In addition to evaluating risk factors for disease and asking about existing medical and dental conditions, an updated health history should include—but not be limited to—the following questions (Figure 49-1):

- Have you seen your physician since we last saw you? If so, then for what reason?
- Do you have any allergies?
- What medications (including herbal and over-the counter [OTC] medications) are you currently taking?
- Have you been in the hospital or had any surgeries since your last visit? If yes, then for what purpose?
- Are you currently taking a hormone replacement or birth control pills? (When treating women)

A good **risk management practice** is to have patients sign the health history form to ensure the most current and accurate records have been obtained. (See Chapter 3 for more on legal issues.)

VITAL SIGNS AND BLOOD PRESSURE SCREENING

The opportunity to assess vital signs and health risks makes the SCA an important visit in oral health care. Patients who are on periodic supportive care visit the dental hygienist multiple times each year. At each of these visits the dental hygienist is given the opportunity to assess vital signs such as blood pressure, pulse, and respiration. Although recording height, weight, and temperature is not standard procedure in most dental practices, the visual physical assessment can provide information that can be used when assessing risk for diseases.

> *Patient Education Opportunity*
> With hypertension, obesity, and diabetes becoming more prevalent, the dental hygienist is in an important position to screen for potential health concerns, discuss health risks, and refer patients as needed.

All clinical members of the dental team can learn to assess and record blood pressure, pulse, and respiration. In addition to documenting this in the patient record, the clinician should place the results in the **oral hygiene fitness report** (OHFR) (Figure 49-2), on the business card, or on the next appointment card for the patient's benefit (see Chapter 12).

HEAD, NECK, AND ORAL CANCER SCREENING

In the United States, one person dies of oral cancer every hour. The Oral Cancer Foundation reported that 30,000 cases of oral cancer occur in the United States annually.[4] The dental hygienist plays a critical role in bringing awareness of this disease to patients and the public. An oral cancer screening is part of the supportive care and new patient appointment. The dental hygienist should teach patients to self-assess for changes from normal.

While the dental hygienist is performing the oral cancer screening (extraoral and intraoral soft tissue examination) the patient should be asked to watch in a mirror and observe the examination. The dental hygienist should describe for the patient structures being examined and what to look and feel for to determine possible abnormalities.

PROCESSING AND MOUNTING RADIOGRAPHS

Patients may express concern over exposure of dental radiographs. They have the misperception that radiographs are taken at every dental appointment. With the advent of digitized radiographic technology, the day is approaching when this will no longer be an issue. Until this technology becomes commonplace, the hygienist should respond to the issue by informing the patient of the date of the last radiographs and the reason for periodic images. A sample dialog might include the following:

"Mr. Smith, in reviewing your dental record, I noted that it has been 2 years since your last radiographs to detect dental caries and to evaluate the tooth-supporting periodontal tissues. To be able to do a thorough dental examination today, we need to update your radiographic images."

> *Note*
> All dental practices should follow the American Dental Association (ADA) guidelines for prescribing dental radiographs in dentistry.

UPDATING DENTAL CONCERNS AND EVALUATING AND DISCUSSING DENTISTRY

Auditing the patient record provides an opportunity to identify treatment needs that have been recommended but have not been completed. A good way to show these needs to the patient is to use the intraoral camera and "tour the mouth." This way the clinician can show and discuss any incomplete dental concerns (and options for addressing them), as well as pointing out any existing disease and the associated health risks. Dental hygienists who use the intraoral camera to allow the patient to see the infection, inflamed and bleeding gums, plaque biofilm, and calculus deposits will receive greater acceptance of planned treatment and adherence to the recommended self-care regimen. For example, the clinician should show the broken or fractured tooth and allow the patient to "see" exactly what is happening to the tooth (Figure 49-3). The esthetic options can be explained by comparing and contrasting what "could be."

EXAMINATION BY THE DENTIST-EMPLOYER

In most dental practices, patients will receive an oral examination by the dentist-employer some time during the SCA. Staying on schedule is a **time management** issue and one of the dental hygienist's greatest concerns. As a practice management issue, the interface between the dentist and dental hygiene patient examination takes time management skills and can be a cause of stress. An easy-to-implement practice protocol is to signal the dentist-employer once the data collection has been completed. This typically occurs in the first 10 to 15 minutes of the appointment. Rather than waiting until the end of the appointment, the dentist now has 15 or 20 minutes of flexibility to come to the dental hygiene treatment room and provide the examination.

The evaluation performed by the dentist at the SCA will depend on the supervision required by the particular state or country in which the clinic is located, as well as by the office policy.

PERIODONTAL EXAMINATION

Engaging the patient in the examination process is educational and encourages the patient to become responsible for his or her own health. The dental hygienist might use the following verbal skill:

"We perform the periodontal examination at each visit. Today, I invite you to do this examination with me and see how

Records Update #456 Office Use Only MEDICAL HISTORY UPDATE

SINCE YOUR LAST DENTAL APPOINTMENT: CONTACT PHONE NUMBERS:

CELL _____ WORK _____HOME _____
EMAIL _____ Tobacco Y_____N_____
Date of last visit to physician _____ For what purpose _____
Changes in your health history including weight gain/loss, allergies _____
Please list current medications including aspirin, vitamins, herbals_____
_____
Have you been hospitalized? No____ Yes, for what purpose_____
Please list any and all surgeries, specific replacement, hip, knee, cardiac
_____

Are you required /did you/ take medication (as prescribed by American Heart Association)
prior to treatment? Yes_____ No_____VS _____ BP_____
Date _____Signature _____

SINCE YOUR LAST DENTAL APPOINTMENT: CONTACT PHONE NUMBERS:

CELL _____ WORK _____HOME _____
EMAIL _____ Tobacco Y_____N_____
Date of last visit to physician _____ For what purpose _____
Changes in your health history including weight gain/loss, allergies _____
Please list current medications including aspirin, vitamins, herbals_____
_____
Have you been hospitalized? No____ Yes, for what purpose_____
Please list any and all surgeries, specific replacement, hip, knee, cardiac
_____

Are you required /did you/ take medication (as prescribed by American Heart Association)
prior to treatment? Yes_____ No_____VS _____ BP_____

Date _____Signature _____

SINCE YOUR LAST DENTAL APPOINTMENT: CONTACT PHONE NUMBERS:

CELL _____ WORK _____HOME _____
EMAIL _____ Tobacco Y_____N_____
Date of last visit to physician _____ For what purpose _____
Changes in your health history including weight gain/loss, allergies _____
Please list current medications including aspirin, vitamins, herbals_____
_____
Have you been hospitalized? No____ Yes, for what purpose_____
Please list any and all surgeries, specific replacement, hip, knee, cardiac
_____

Are you required /did you/ take medication (as prescribed by American Heart Association)
prior to treatment? Yes_____ No_____VS _____ BP_____
Date _____Signature _____

FIGURE 49-1
Medical history update.

Oral Hygiene Fitness Report (OHFR)

Dentist Name
Office Address
Office Phone Number

Prepared for _____ Date _____

We are happy to provide you with this information. At your dental appointment today the following was accomplished:

EXAMINATIONS, RISK ASSESSMENT, and CLINICAL PROCEDURES

☐ Medical History Update   ☐ Root Planing and Periodontal Scaling   ☐ Plaque Control Instructions

☐ Oral Cancer Screening   ☐ Quadrant, Sextant, Full Mouth   ☐ Polishing

☐ Blood Pressure Screening   ☐ Sealants, Custom Trays   ☐ Periodontal Debridement

☐ Plaque Index   ☐ Hard and Soft Tissue   ☐ Antimicrobial Therapy

☐ Radiographs   ☐ Cavity Detection   ☐ Fluoride Treatment

☐ Periodontal Therapy   ☐ Periodontal Screening   ☐ Diagnostic Study Models

☐ Vital Signs_____

☐ Other Evaluative Procedures_____

ORAL HYGIENE EVALUATION

☐ Good   Very little plaque, calculus, stain

☐ Satisfactory   Some plaque, food debris, light bleeding

☐ Needs Improvement   Plaque, calculus, stain present, inflammation

DISPENSED THE FOLLOWING

☐ Toothbrush   ☐ Mechanical Toothbrush   ☐ Power Irrigator

☐ Floss   ☐ Super Floss   ☐ Antimicrobials

☐ Proxabrush   ☐ Toothpaste   ☐ Fluorides

☐ Home Health Aids   ☐ Interdental Stimulator   ☐ Medicaments

☐ Patient Education Materials   ☐ Desensitizing Agent   ☐ Other_____

We have specifically purchased these oral health self-care products for you.
Please tell us of your experience with them.

TREATMENT RECOMMENDATIONS

☐ Maintenance therapy at 3 months, 4 months, 6 months _____

☐ Daily home care with attention to specific areas_____

☐ Please maintain dental hygiene appointments

☐ Periodontal therapy intervention _____

We thank you for choosing our dental office and look forward to serving your dental needs. We hope that you will continue to recommend our personalized dental care to your family and friends.

A

FIGURE 49-2
A, Oral hygiene fitness report (OHFR).

Dear _____   Date _____

The following time has been reserved exclusively for your supportive care appointment (SCA). The dental hygienist will review your health records, check blood pressure, perform preventive oral health examinations including oral cancer screening, and make recommendations regarding the appropriate treatment to maintain or return your oral tissues to health. We look forward to seeing you on_____.

Dental Hygienist Name

Dentist Name

Office Address

Office Phone Number

B

FIGURE 49-2—cont'd.
B, Recall reminder card.

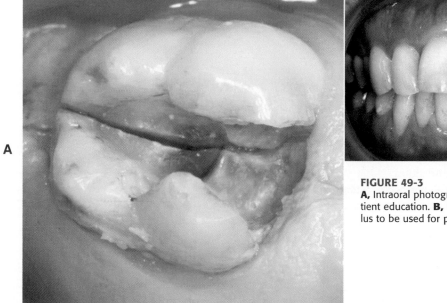

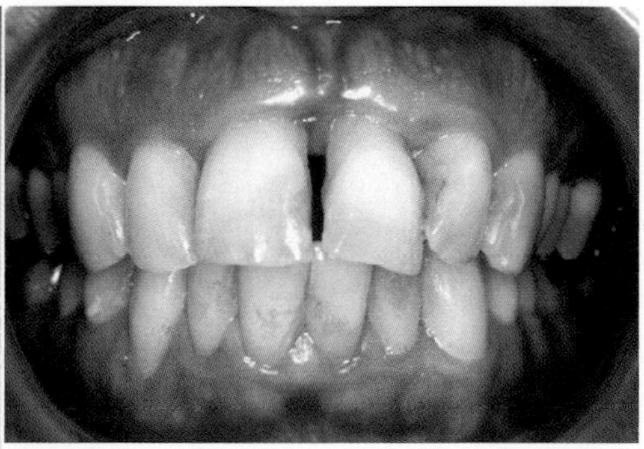

FIGURE 49-3
A, Intraoral photograph of a broken tooth for patient education. **B,** Intraoral photograph of calculus to be used for patient education.

healthy your gum or gingival tissues are. We have discovered that our patients like to know more about the examinations. I have found that my patients appreciate knowing more about their oral health status, and we can do this best when we are both involved in the examination process. If you have any questions during the examination, then please ask."

As oral healthcare providers and educators, dental hygienists are keenly aware of the importance of ongoing and continuous preventive care. Current research in periodontal diseases mandates the need for continuous periodontal evaluation and treatment.

> **Note**
>
> The most productive dental hygienists practice each day with clearly defined periodontal protocols agreed on by the dentist and understood by the entire dental team.

With the established link between periodontal inflammation and many systemic diseases such as coronary artery disease, cardiovascular disease, preterm low–birth-weight infants, and diabetes, the rationale for early intervention in treating periodontal disease is well founded.

This includes ongoing periodontal evaluation, documented examination, charting, and documentation of appropriate periodontal treatment.

Attempting to perform periodontal treatment without informing, advising, and involving the patient is both illegal and clinically ineffective. (See Informed Consent in Chapter 3.) A successful periodontal therapeutic outcome is dependent on patient participation. The clinician should inform the patient that, "the treatment plan involves **cotherapy,** and it will take both of us working together to achieve long-term health and stability." Meticulous daily self-care for disease control and commitment to dental appointments are two examples of working together.

ORAL HYGIENE FITNESS REPORT

The OHFR (see Figure 49-2) was developed using the anatomy of the SCA and can serve as an educational and motivational tool. This report helps redefine the SCA and demonstrates to the patient that services provided by the dental hygienist are more than just a cleaning and a checkup. This checklist is completed at the end of the appointment and given to the patient. It reviews services performed that day and provides an individualized evaluation of the patient's oral hygiene, products dispensed to patients for self-care, vital sign recordings, treatment provided, and self-care recommendations.

The area on the OHFR for identifying procedures and services completed allows for each service to be listed, including those provided as a line item on the bill. All items and products dispensed to the patient must be recorded, along with instructions for use of the products. Products dispensed are often a "hidden" value, but they are items that the office has to purchase. Some offices have chosen to select certain oral care products to sell directly to the patient. If the hygienist works in an office that decides to do this, then selection decisions and purchases should be based on clinical effectiveness evidence (see Chapter 4).

Clinical findings should be listed in the Treatment Recommendations section. The clinician can combine the personalized OHFR with a pamphlet on periodontal information. Giving both of these items to periodontal patients will help them gain a new perspective on the SCA.

One testimony for using the OHFR is as follows:

"I first implemented the OHFR in my own practice, where I had been treating patients for over 15 years. When I began giving each of these same patients their OHFR, the response was, 'Did you do all of this today? I didn't realize all this was part of the cleaning appointment.'"[3]

Dental hygienists know that much more occurs during the SCA than the removal of deposits from the teeth.

> *Patient Education Opportunity*
>
> Educating patients about the procedures performed can assist in improving their "dental knowledge" and help them understand why the term *SCA* is preferable to the term *cleaning appointment.*

CHANGING PERCEPTIONS OF SUPPORTIVE CARE APPOINTMENTS

As the dental team works to change patients' perceptions of the SCA, they should post the *anatomy of the SCA* at the front desk and in the dental hygiene treatment room as a reminder that the SCA is more than just a cleaning. In addition, this new approach should include the use of proper terms when discussing all functions of the SCA with team members and patients. Staff should replace the word *cleaning* with *supportive care,* or use *periodontal debridement* or *periodontal maintenance* when the patient is on periodic intervals for periodontal disease. (See Chapter 22 for more on this topic.) Table 49-1 is an example of preferred word choices when discussing supportive care.

> **Note**
>
> Clinicians cannot expect to change their patients' attitudes until they change their own perceptions.

> ⛤ **CASE APPLICATION 49-2.1**
>
> **Supportive Care Appointments**
>
> What advice would you have for Annie regarding the front desk staff's perception of the SCAs?

An example of a positive and well-defined SCA dialog includes the five concepts outlined in Box 49-2.

Integrating these management principles into daily practice will help maintain a full and productive dental hygiene schedule, as well as create a dental hygiene department that is clinically excellent, highly profitable, and professionally satisfying.

Clinicians should use the patients' periodontal and restorative charts as educational and motivational tools. Patients should be given a copy of their periodontal charting, and the

Table 49-1	Comparison of Effective (Positive) Communication Phrases with Ineffective (Negative) Phrases	
EFFECTIVE AND POSITIVE	**INEFFECTIVE AND NEGATIVE (INADEQUATE AND UNDERVALUES SERVICE)**
Periodontal instrumentation and comprehensive examination	Cleaning and checkup
Remove the bacterial infection	Just begin the cleaning
The areas in the mouth where infection is present	Just clean you up a bit . . . deeper cleaning
Today I will begin to remove the bacteria and deposits causing the inflammation, which will promote healing. This process will require more than this one appointment.	I cannot finish today; need you back again
Tooth lightening–whitening	Bleach your teeth
Continuing or supportive or preventive care, periodontal maintenance	Maintenance or recall
Professional removal of oral deposits	Cleaning
Dental hygiene appointment	Cleaning and checkup
This appointment time has been especially reserved for you.	Please call if this time is inconvenient.
Change in schedule	Cancellation
The doctor or dental hygienist can see you at 8 AM or 4 PM. Which do you prefer?	When do you want to come in?
Periodontal therapy	Scaling and root planing
Periodontal instrumentation	Deep scaling
Specific instrumentation	Deep scaling
Remove infection	Tartar and plaque biofilm buildup
Antimicrobial therapies, disinfect and sterilize	Subgingival irrigation
Monitor	Watch the area
Fee or investment in good health	Price or cost

BOX 49-2

CONCEPTS TO INCLUDE IN SUPPORTIVE CARE APPOINTMENT (SCA) DIALOG

The SCA is reserved for the following:
- Health assessment and risk for future disease
- Head and neck cancer and hypertension screening
- Examination for infectious diseases such as periodontitis and dental caries
- Continuous supportive care or periodontal maintenance therapy
- Determination of future oral needs based on assessment of risk

---

clinician should review the results of the periodontal examination with the patient at each appointment.

The chart provides a visual display of the patient's current periodontal status and gives both the clinician and the patient the opportunity to compare and contrast the probe depths, attachment levels, bleeding and plaque biofilm scores, and overall gingival health. Has there been an increase in pocket depth or gingival recession denoting bone loss? Is there active disease? Patients become more aware of what probe depths, gingival recession numbers, and bleeding scores mean when the dental hygienist explains these concepts to them. Of course, the dental hygienist should complete a thorough documentation of the conversation in the patient's progress notes to the dental team.

Communication: A Key Factor in Practice Building

COMMUNICATION AMONG THE DENTIST-EMPLOYER, DENTAL HYGIENIST, AND DENTAL TEAM

Many dental hygienists are unsure of the dentist-employer expectations with regard to discussing dentistry with patients, particularly those dental hygienists who are just beginning practice. This concern can and should be alleviated with a meeting between the dentist and the dental hygienist in a comfortable and supportive setting, answering questions and clarifying expectations. Staff meetings to review the latest in dental techniques and materials are needed. A regularly scheduled meeting provides the opportunity to explore new ideas, encourage initiative, and revisit goals.

> *Note*
>
> The most successful and productive practices are those in which the dental hygienist, dentist, and staff are a cohesive, communicative team.

Working in concert to share and promote the same vision results in maximum personal, professional, and productive rewards for everyone.

✦ CASE APPLICATION 49-2.2

Staff Meetings

The practice Annie is employed in does not have regularly scheduled meetings. How would regular meetings benefit Annie and the practice?

COMMUNICATION BETWEEN THE DENTAL HYGIENIST AND PATIENT

The dental hygienist is in a unique position to build trusting relationships with patients over time. Patients often look to the dental hygienist for help in decision making. Patients often ask for feedback after the dentist leaves the treatment room. "Do I really need that?" and "What would you do?" are frequently asked questions. Being knowledgeable and prepared to respond to these and other questions will enhance the value of the dental hygienist as a professional in the practice and with the patients.

> *Patient Education Opportunity*
> Positive statements about restorative and esthetic treatment provided can be an opening to a through discussion of the benefits of dental care.

Using positive language when speaking with patients is important to build trust and to get patients to understand and agree to dental treatments for improved health care (see Chapter 5).

Visual communication tools that are helpful when communicating with and educating the patient include the following:

- *Before* and *after* photographic images
- Radiographs of dental caries, bone loss, or impacted teeth
- Professional brochures and computer-based patient education programs

Box 49-3 provides examples of communications one might have with a patient regarding appointment management.

TECHNOLOGY TO STREAMLINE AND IMPROVE COMMUNICATION

Recording daily operations, patient records, and treatment documentation, as well as tracking supportive care intervals, pending information files, and notes are just some of the ways technology is being used in the delivery of dental hygiene and dental services. The use of this new and expanding technology contributes to overall practice efficiency.

Daily Operations

Electronic patient records stored in the computer include the following:

- Progress notes
- Medical and special needs
- Previous recommendations
- Periodontal and restorative chartings
- Comprehensive health history

These can be reviewed on the screen by scrolling through the file. Time and frustration are reduced when the dental hygienist and entire staff do not have to plow through several inches of a paper record filled with every piece of paper, radiograph, and insurance form since the patient first entered the practice.

Many offices use a customized appointment template to standardize the hygiene appointment and notes. In this way, all questions are answered and nothing is left out of the appointment. Computerized periodontal and dental chartings provide a spectacular visual display for the patient (Figure 49-4). At the same time, it allows the hygienist to easily store the data and view a comparative periodontal or hard tissue analysis.

Often the technology in many offices is not fully used. For example, the intraoral camera is typically used during the new patient appointment; then it gets placed in a storage closet or other inconvenient location where extra time is required to obtain and set it up. Two reasons given for lack of use include the following:

1. "I do not have the time."
2. "I'm not really sure how to use it. We learned when we first got the camera, but I don't use it regularly."

This problem can be remedied easily with a staff meeting in which all team members have an opportunity to be the patient. When was the last time you sat in the dental chair? How does it *feel* to be the patient? Staff should role-play with each other, have fun, and take turns being the patient in the chair. Office protocol for intraoral examination and *tour of the mouth* should be reviewed. Every member of the team is involved in this process and in the creation of a protocol for use. Once comfortable with how to use an intraoral camera, most dental hygienists will not part with it. This is because an intraoral camera is the best tool for the following:

- Education
- Motivation
- Case presentation
- Building patient adherence to appointments and self-care

Using technology to identify needed and desired treatment

The preappointment audit of the patient's record enables the dental hygienist (and the entire team) to identify planned treatment that has yet to be completed. The day should be planned and orchestrated so that all tools (e.g., camera, visual aids, staff) are in the treatment room and ready to provide treatment.

Audiovisual patient education programs with voice commentary and pictures are effective because the patient *listens* even when he or she is not *watching*. When the dentist arrives for the examination, the dental hygienist reports preliminary findings and patient concerns, and he or she provides the dentist with an overview of suggestions made to the patient. In this way the dentist-employer knows exactly what has occurred and can continue the timely reinforcement of the dialog.

Intraoffice Communications

When the dental hygienist posts services performed into the patient record during the appointment, the business coordinator at the front desk can view it. Insurance processing and payment calculations are completed by the time the patient reaches the front desk. Treatment plans and needed appointments can be communicated from the treatment room to the business desk. A patient consultation can be completed to ensure all questions are answered and treatment scheduled on the same day. Providers and business staff do not like having stacks of charts sitting around waiting for treatment plans to be typed and printed for the consultation and presentation visit. Using the computer for entry and retrieval improves time management, continuity of care, and productivity.

BOX 49-3

EXAMPLES OF COMMUNICATIONS ONE MIGHT HAVE DURING APPOINTMENT MANAGEMENT

Confirming Supportive Care Appointments (SCAs)

"Good morning, *Mr. or Ms. Patient.* This is_____ from Dr. ___'s office. How are you today?" *(Wait for response.)* "*Mr. or Ms. Patient,* I am calling to verify your appointment for _____ (preventive dental examination, supportive care, periodontal maintenance) with Dr. _____, as well as dental prophylaxis (i.e., professional dental cleaning), screening examinations for oral cancer, and periodontal health. We are looking forward to seeing you on ___ at ___."

If any doubts exist, the clinic employee should ask the following: "Do you have this on your calendar? I'll be happy to hold while you check."

Say "No" to Changes

"*Mr. or Ms. Patient,* Dr. _____ has given me the responsibility of scheduling all patients. We work very hard to accommodate the needs of all of our patients. We reserved this full hour on the doctor's (or hygienist's) schedule just for you. Although I have patients waiting for this time, at this point it will be extremely difficult for me to bring another patient into the office."

If any doubts exist, the clinic employee should ask the following: "What may I do to help you keep this appointment?"

Overdue Preventive Dental Care

"Good morning, *Mr. or Ms. Patient.* This is _____ from Dr. _____'s office. How are you today?" *(Wait for response.)* "*Mr. or Ms. Patient,* Dr. _____ was reviewing your record and found that it has been _____ since your last preventive oral health examination and professional dental cleaning (prophylaxis). Dr. _____ is very concerned and has asked me to call and schedule this important appointment for you. We have an available appointment on _____ at _____." *(Stop and listen for response.)*

Daily Reactivation and Chart Auditing

During patient checkout, review other family members and audit their files. Use computer routing information.

If overdue . . . "*Mr. or Ms. Patient,* in reviewing the records, I see that it has been _____(months) since your _____ (husband, wife, son, daughter, friend, other relative) last had an SCA and examination (or restorative appointment, if appropriate). Let's go ahead and schedule this appointment while you are here today. The doctor or hygienist will be able to see _____ on Monday at _____ or Wednesday at _____. Which time do you prefer?"

"*Mr. or Ms. Patient,* Dr. _____ was reviewing your record and has asked me to schedule your _____ (husband, wife, son, daughter, friend, other relative) for the _____ (crown, bridge, cosmetic procedure, restoration) that was discussed at the last visit. The doctor can see _____ on _____ at _____ or on _____ at _____. Which time do you prefer?"

Reactivating and Inviting

The patient responds that he or she does not wish to make an appointment *(find out why)*. Most patients respond this way for the following reasons: time, fear, lack of money, change of dentists. Review chart for clinical work.

"*Mr. or Ms. Patient,* the health of your mouth is very important to Dr. _____. Our work together (e.g., crown, root canal) on the lower right side of your mouth had such an excellent result. Through routine preventive examinations, professional supportive care, and periodontal maintenance, we help ensure good oral health." *(Pause)* "Is there anything that I may do to assist you in making this appointment?"

"I see that Dr. _____ has discussed with you _____ (necessary, recommended treatment)."

If the patient has a small cavity, the clinician should explain the need for restoring early: "Eliminating disease as soon as possible is always easier and is recommended to avoid further complications (e.g., fractured teeth, abscesses). How may I assist you in scheduling this appointment?"

Key Phrases
Appointments Policy

"At the request of our patients we have adopted an appointment policy that enables you to schedule and reserve appointments at the most convenient time for you. This time is reserved exclusively for you, and we find that our patients really appreciate this opportunity."

Chronic Canceller

"*Mr. or Ms. Patient,* it appears that you are having difficulty in keeping your regularly scheduled appointments. I would like to do this: I will place you on my priority scheduling list, call you when a change in the schedule occurs, and give you the first opportunity to take the appointment."

or

"Why don't you call me on Monday morning when you know that you will be in town for the week. I will do my very best to get you in as soon as possible. How does that sound?"

"Change in the Schedule" Replaces "Cancellation"

"The Doctor Can See You At" and "The Doctor Sees Emergencies At" Replaces *"When Do You Want to Come In?"*

Necessary Radiographs

"Dr. _____ was reviewing your record and found that it has been 10 years since we have taken a complete series of disease-detecting radiographs. The doctor has requested that we get these updated today."

Periodontal Case Presentation
Positive Communication

"Today I will begin to remove the bacteria and infection. The process will involve _____ (quadrant, half-mouth, full-mouth disinfection). The gum or gingival tissues will begin to heal as we proceed with the removal of deposits and bacteria. At your next appointment, we will continue these procedures. I will need to see you for approximately ___ appointments."

Negative Communication

"I will be unable to finish this today and will need to get you back. I will do what I can today in the remaining time, and we will get you back for another appointment." (This statement implies total responsibility for the success of treatment depends on the hygienist and how fast he or she can work.)

"Deep scaling or deeper cleaning takes more time; therefore I will need to see you for several more appointments." (Is "deep scaling or cleaning" the only reason the hygienist needs to see this patient for more therapy or treatment?)

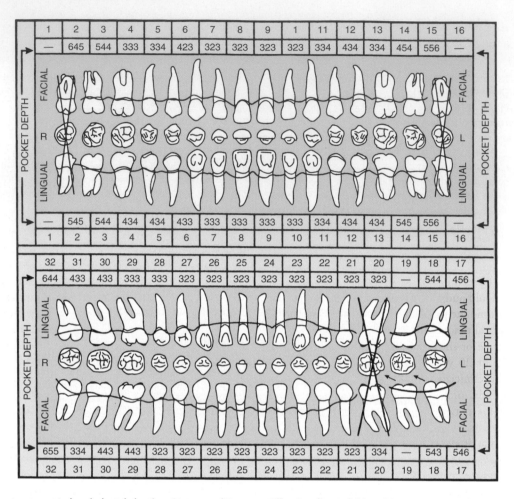

FIGURE 49-4
Example of a computer-generated periodontal charting. (Courtesy of Patterson Office Supplies, a division of Patterson Companies, Inc., 1-800-637-1140.)

Scheduling at the Chair

The success of the dental hygienist's schedule is directly related to the interaction that takes place between the dental hygienist and the patient when the patient is in the dental hygiene treatment room.

> **Note**
>
> Dental hygienists who preschedule and reserve future patient appointments have an opportunity to improve patient adherence to appointments.

Scheduling at the chair takes a few moments to complete and provides an opportunity for the dental hygienist to restate the importance of reserving the appointment now (at a time convenient to the patient for the amount of time needed) and to respond to any questions or concerns the patient may have. It also allows the hygienist to schedule appropriate time intervals for variations in patient need (i.e., longer appointments for a more complicated case and shorter appointments for an easy follow-up or healthy patient with few concerns). Business coordinators can then spend more time and energy on scheduling treatment needs and managing financial arrangements. Figure 49-2 contains an example of an SCA card.

★ CASE APPLICATION 49-2.3

Computerized Scheduling

Given Annie's recent knowledge of appointment scheduling and management, how could computerized scheduling benefit her and the patients?

Tracking SCAs, patient retention, and overdue SCA reports can be quickly computed and easily retrieved. Reports can be generated for an update on patient retention and those who need SCAs. A staff member can be delegated to spend a certain amount of time each day or each week working to ensure that needed SCAs have been scheduled. Appointment cards and letters can be printed directly from the computer scheduler, saving hours of time going through the schedule and writing cards. With the use of available technology, dental practices can function at a higher level of management efficiency. In treatment rooms, computers and other technology allow the dental hygienist to have more time to spend with patients on oral healthcare education, discussing the benefits of optimal oral health and setting the stage for case acceptance of the following:

- Periodontal procedures or the need for referral
- Restorative and esthetic dental procedures
- Orthodontic or other specialist treatment needs
- Other referrals

Appointment and Patient Management

Managing patients' needed care involves many activities by the

Note

Appointment and **patient man-agement** is directly linked to practice productivity.

dental hygienist and other office staff. For instance, one of these activities is to review charts of patients of record to determine the status of examinations. Criteria to use for this review can be seen in Box 49-4.

The clinician should audit the chart and patient record and determine the last time the patient received an updated examination. In most dental practices, the patient had a new patient examination when he or she first entered the practice (which may have been 15 or 20 years earlier). Because of time constraints at the SCA, clinicians tend to keep the patient in the system with a periodic oral examination only, not providing time to talk with the patient and update the comprehensive history and assessments.

The dentistry that is detected, presented, and accepted is amazing when ample time is allotted for a comprehensive examination to reassess treatment needs. Using any extra time in the schedule to do comprehensive and full-mouth examinations on dental hygiene patients can increase productivity and income. The dental hygienist can set the stage for a comprehensive status examination with the dentist-employer on the next visit. Time can be added to the SCA and scheduled to allow for the

examination. If time permits on that day, then the full examination can be included as part of the appointment services. If the dentist has a change in schedule and is left with open time, then that time should be allocated to the dental hygiene patient to perform a full examination. The same is true for any dental hygiene downtime. Extending time with the patient in the chair gives the dental hygienist the time to do the following:

- Update radiographs
- Complete the periodontal examination
- Evaluate the mouth with the intraoral camera
- Discuss various aspects of patient education for the patient or others
- Discuss and answer treatment options and questions

The 6-week periodontal posttreatment evaluation appointment, the appointment after periodontal instrumentation and before determining an appropriate interval of care for supportive periodontal maintenance, is a valuable appointment (see Chapter 22). At this time the dental hygienist can tour the mouth using the camera while describing the characteristics of the gingival tissues and additional needs the patient may have for professional care and self-care. This is an ideal time for a discussion regarding dental needs, appearance, and esthetic considerations. Ideally, the patient has been involved in the periodontal diagnosis and cotherapy, and the dental hygienist had the time to educate the patient during the course of treatment appointments. These patients are very receptive to learning about a variety of treatment options.

Some dental hygienists and dentists are not comfortable discussing treatment options with patients who simply want teeth that look better—whether whiter, straighter, or simply more functional. Following are reasons dental staff may not speak with patients about esthetic dentistry:

- "I don't want to overwhelm or scare patients off."
- "I don't like selling."
- "Insurance won't pay, so I won't recommend the procedure."
- "The patient cannot afford the needed treatment."
- "The patient just completed periodontal (or other dental treatment) and probably is tired of coming to the office."
- "The patient just retired, so why would he or she want to do it?"
- "The patient is not going to accept anyway, so why try?"

KEEPING PATIENTS INFORMED

Dental treatments available to patients should not be kept secret. When patients know the treatment options, they can make informed choices. At a recent focus group a patient stated the following[3]:

"One of my friends recently had a dental implant at another dental office in town. I am thinking of going to that dental office just for the implant."

Note

The clinician should never assume that patients "know" about dentistry and dental hygiene, as well as the services that can be provided. Box 49-5 provides some practical and easy ways to ensure that patients are kept informed of the procedures offered in the practice.

BOX 49-4

CRITERIA FOR PATIENT CHART REVIEW

- The patient has never had a full (comprehensive) patient examination (CDT 0150).
- It has been more than 3 years since full (comprehensive) patient examination.
- The patient has a treatment plan of incomplete and unscheduled needs (i.e., "incomplete dentistry").
- The patient has an interest in tooth whitening and esthetic dentistry.
- Time exists in the schedule to provide the full examination and needed services.
- A skilled clinician is available to see the patient.
  Note: If insufficient time is available that day, schedule patient to return for comprehensive examination at a more appropriate time. Schedule sufficient time for necessary components such as evaluation and recording of the patient's dental and medical history, a general health assessment, thorough charting, radiographs as indicated, and treatment planning and discussion.

BOX 49-5

METHODS FOR KEEPING PATIENTS INFORMED

- Practice brochure: Update practice brochure, welcome letter, or both to include all of the services offered to patients.
- Printouts and lists of evidence-based web sites for patients to seek additional information specific to their needs (e.g., National Institutes of Health [NIH], National Institute for Dental and Craniofacial Research [NIDCR], www.perio.org, www.adha.org).
- Books and individual professional procedures brochures: Many manufacturers provide professional and free informational patient brochures.
- Newsletters or office letters that include the following headline: *The Latest in Dentistry–Here's What We Can Do!*
- Display and distribution of this information at the desk, as well as in the reception and treatment rooms.
- Audiovisual displays in reception and clinical areas: A picture is worth a thousand words. Audiovisual patient education programs, including computer packages and video presentations, are available. Programs with voice commentary and pictures are most effective because patients may *listen* even when they are not *watching*.
- Intraoral camera and video-imaging systems.
- Before and after photos framed professionally and placed strategically on walls and tables, not buried in drawers or on shelves that patients never see. (Note: Patients must provide written permission before photos of them are displayed.)
- Before and after photo albums of real patients for use chairside. (Note: Patients must provide written permission before photos of them are displayed.)
- A smile evaluation form completed by all new and hygiene patients (see Figure 49-5).
- System in place to ensure that all questions have been answered regarding proposed treatment.
- System for tracking needed and incomplete dentistry in patient records.

When the patient was asked why she would go to another dental office, she said that she did not know that her dentist performed implants because no one had ever talked with her about it.

The clinician can educate the patient and set the stage with a Personalized Smile Evaluation Form (Figure 49-5). In the treatment room, the dental hygienist evaluates the information to be aware of patient concerns. Time is always a major factor, so discussions and ideas may be offered while performing clinical procedures. Asking open-ended, easy questions gives the patient the opportunity to reflect and think about esthetic dentistry and its effect on health, appearance, and personal or professional life.

Practice Economics

Clinically excellent and highly productive dental hygiene departments are desired by every dental practice. Those practices that can claim these characteristics adhere to the following attributes:

- The dental hygienist, as periodontal cotherapist, is current and up to date on the latest research regarding periodontal health and systemic health.
- The dental hygienist is skilled at providing exceptional and thorough clinical treatment.
- The dentist and dental hygienist are committed to educating patients in the concept of periodontal medicine.
- Treatment is offered based on patients' clinical requirements (including risk factors), rather than on what the dental hygienist thinks they want or what their insurance will cover.

PERIODONTAL PROTOCOLS AND IMPLEMENTATION

Current research regarding periodontal health and systemic health mandates the need for continuing periodontal evaluation, treatment, and maintenance. Researchers estimate that 75% of the adult population will, at some time, have some form of periodontal disease.[2] Given these data, the periodontal portion of the dental hygiene department should be seen as generating 30% to 40% of services. Clinics should track these data each month using the computer report category *Procedures Analysis (by Provider)* for the codes 4341, 4342, 4355, 4910, and 4381.

If the clinic's financial expectations and goals are not met for the time period being reviewed, then the team needs to gather and discuss periodontal protocols and implementation. The clinic should be up to date on the following[1]:

- Site specific treatment—Patients with isolated active periodontal disease (5 to 6 mm with bleeding) receive appropriate periodontal, mechanical, and chemotherapeutic treatment. The code 4342 is used when one to three teeth are involved as described in **CDT 4/5 codes.** The code 4341 is used for quadrants (four or more teeth). Some offices report success when filing insurance claims if they attach a periodontal chart, an intraoral photograph of bleeding and swollen gingiva with exudate around the gingival margin from the periodontal pockets, and supportive radiographic images. Periodontal scaling and root planing is not a once-in-a-lifetime procedure. Many insurance companies reimburse for 4341, if necessary, after a specific interval of time.
- Chemical antimicrobial agents—Localized delivery of antimicrobials and antibiotics such as minocycline microspheres and a chlorhexidine chip are placed when tissue healing does not occur. The code is 4381 for this adjunctive to scaling and root planing procedure (see Chapter 27). The progressive, state-of-the-art dental hygiene department uses evidence-based decision making to determine the best approach to care.[3]
- Treatment plan for the patient with generalized gingivitis—When a patient has inflamed tissue, generalized bleeding, plaque biofilm, and calculus but no pocket depth or bone loss, the patient requires more than an adult prophylaxis. The dentist and periodontal hygienist have clearly defined protocols for treating this patient. Rather

Personalized Smile Evaluation

First Name/Last Name_____

Date_____

Please take a moment to look at your teeth and gums carefully and then answer the following questions:

1. On a scale of 1 to 10, how do you feel about your teeth and smile?

2. Are your teeth crooked or crowded, and is that a concern? Please comment:

3. Do you have any spaces between your teeth that bother you? Please comment:

4. Do you like the color of your teeth? Please comment:

5. Do you like the shape of your teeth? Please comment:

6. What would you like to change about the appearance of your smile?

7. Have you ever considered how you might feel with a brighter smile? Please comment:

FIGURE 49-5
Personalized smile evaluation.

than running the risk (i.e., "waiting and watching"), wondering whether the patient will progress to periodontitis, an early intervention treatment protocol is presented. This includes a full-mouth ultrasonic debridement with medicaments, followed by a second appointment 4 to 6 weeks later to ensure healing and elimination of the inflammation. At this appointment, instrumentation of areas not responding to the first course of treatment and polishing

may occur. The patient is placed on a short interval of care. Typically the dental hygienist will see the patient every 3 months for periodontal maintenance to ensure health and stability. For all patients the interval of care is appropriately determined by clinical needs and risk factors of the patient, not just what his or her insurance will pay. The periodontal maintenance code 4910 is used after active therapy (4341). A full-mouth periodontal examination is performed, and retreatment of any active site is accomplished. Many offices struggle with patient compliance regarding periodontal maintenance appointments because of issues with the patient's insurance plan not paying for treatment. Having the periodontal patient accept treatment because he or she wants to be healthy (not because he or she wants the insurance company to pay first) is important. Success occurs when the dental hygienist educates the patient at each appointment during periodontal therapy so that by the end of the treatment regimen the patient knows as much about the disease process as possible.

Dental Insurance

Dental insurance has been and continues to be a great benefit for many patients. Clinicians should remember, however, that dental benefits are just that—a benefit to aid and *assist* the patient. In the United States, health insurance was never designed or created to cover 100% of the cost of treatment, and dental insurance is no different. Dental insurance provided by employers has assisted in making oral health care attainable for a portion of the population.

During the last 40 years, the maximum annual benefit paid by most dental insurance companies is approximately $1000 for the year. There have been no increases over time; however, procedures have been added that once were not covered by dental insurance such as dental sealants.

> ### Note
> The long-term success of the dental hygiene program and the health of the patient are directly related to patient attitude, perception, responsibility, and commitment to optimal oral health. The delivery of services is the responsibility of the dentist or dental hygienist and the patient.

Patients are motivated by the perceived need for treatment and good health.

Patients can develop a better understanding of dental benefits and become a proactive advocate for their health care. Examples of ways that dental teams communicate with patients can be seen in Box 49-6.

The dental hygienist has an important role in communicating effectively with the patient regarding dental benefits. Following are several positive and professional communications about dental insurance:

- "Our responsibility is to make recommendations based on what is in the best interest of your good health; it cannot be based on what your insurance company will pay."
- "We would be remiss in our responsibility to provide you with optimal dental care if we did not examine, assess, and advise you of the conditions in your mouth and recommend appropriate treatment to bring you into good health."

For the recall patient, the dental professional may say the following:

- "Our diagnosis and treatment recommendations are not—and never have been—based on the patient's insurance benefits."

BOX 49-6

THE RELATIONSHIP BETWEEN PARTIES INVOLVED IN INSURANCE BENEFITS

Dentist-Patient Relationship

The dentist has a direct and liable relationship with the patient.

- As a courtesy, the clinic prepares necessary claims paperwork, provides supportive documentation, and submits the file promptly.
- During a *free* consultation visit, business staff explains to the patient that any differences between the fee charged by the practice and the amount paid by the insurance is the result of the limitation in the contract (*not* because the clinic's fees are too high).
- Business staff explains to the patient the usual and customary reimbursement (UCR) is really a description of the dollar amount of benefits that his or her employer has purchased (otherwise, all insurance payments would be the same).

Patient-Employer Relationship

The patient has a direct relationship with his or her employer.

- The patient is advised that his or her employer has purchased the benefits plan.
- The patient may wish to inform his or her union official or employee benefits officer that the dental insurance purchased is not meeting the basic dental needs of employees (it does not enable them to maintain their oral health).

Employer-Insurance Carrier Relationship

The employer has a direct relationship with the insurance carrier.

- Insurance carriers have financial goals and objectives; they want to run efficient and successful businesses and make money. The carrier is not necessarily concerned with the health of each patient.
- Employers purchase services from insurance companies, cafeteria style, and may purchase any variety of benefits, depending on the amount they are willing to pay.

- "Your dental benefits coverage is between you, your employer, and your insurance company. We will, as always, do our very best to maximize your dental benefits."
- "We choose to make our treatment recommendations based on your specific needs and goals, rather than what the insurance company may or may not cover."
- Always use the term *estimated* when discussing dental benefits. In other words, "The estimated benefit for this procedure from your insurance policy is . . ."

Developing an Effective Dental Hygiene Schedule

The dental hygienist may have to determine the number of hours it would take to provide appropriate SCAs for all the patients in the practice. To determine how many hours and the number of dental hygienists needed to provide an effective schedule for these services, a formula must be used. The formula and discussion of each component are presented in the following sections.

KNOWING THE NUMBERS

The first step in creating a dental hygiene department that is economically viable is to understand the revenue potential in this sector of the business. The effectiveness of the SCA system determines the health of the practice. When patients do not maintain their SCA appointments, they will not have optimal oral care. On the business side, they do not see the dentist for restorative and esthetic dentistry. The **Supportive Care Appointment (SCA) reliability analysis** provides the data necessary to begin to create a business strategy that includes staffing and facility planning projections. Following are the steps for the analysis (an example of this can be seen in Box 49-7):

- Determine the core patient base (this is the heart of the practice, the business). An *active patient* is defined as a patient who has visited the practice within the last 18 to 24 months and has received at least two SCAs during this period. This number is multiplied by 2 (as in twice yearly prophylaxis and examination) and divided by 12 months. Multiply this number by 85% to allow for a *real world* 15% attrition rate (people who move or leave the practice).
- Determine the total monthly dental hygiene patients. Add the number of monthly new patients to the core patient base. Multiply that total by 25% to meet the periodontal requirement. This number allows for patients undergoing active periodontal therapy and those patients in periodontal maintenance (4910) (3-month supportive periodontal maintenance).
- Determine the annual dental hygiene patient requirement. Multiply the monthly dental hygiene patient requirement by 12 (months). Determine the current status by calculating the number of patients seen in the previous year in dental hygiene. This may be accomplished by running a computer procedure report for adult prophylaxis and periodontal procedure codes 1110, 4341, 4355, and 4910.
- Determine the supportive care requirement. Divide the annual requirements by daily patients that can be seen in hygiene.

An achievable productivity goal for the entry-level dental hygienist employed in an office with good scheduling protocols (i.e., confirming of patients, maintaining daily dental hygiene schedule) is 93% to 95%. This productivity is calculated weekly or monthly by taking the total units available for dental hygiene appointments and dividing by the actual number of patients treated.

This analysis should be run every quarter to determine whether the target goal for the practice is being met. Waiting until the end of the year to determine whether the goal for dental hygiene production has been met means that the dental hygienist may have lost 12 months of good production capabilities. In addition, this will negatively affect the dentist's production, resulting in fewer restorative patients seen and decline in total practice production. The clinician can analyze the data by asking the following questions:

- How many dental hygiene days or hours do I need to meet my patient base?
- If I do not have enough days, then what strategy should I explore?
  - Add another dental hygienist?
  - Add a dental hygiene assistant so that the dental hygienist can work with two treatment rooms?
  - Extend office hours to accommodate the patient volume?
  - Bring in another dentist?
- What percentage of dental hygiene production is generated by periodontal and other nonpreventive procedures?
- Is the practice growing? If so, then why?
- Is the practice shrinking? If so, then why and how can it be fixed?

BOX 49-7

SUPPORTIVE CARE RELIABILITY ANALYSIS

Steps to compute the number of patients and number of dental hygienists needed to meet the needs of patients in the practice:

Step 1

- Start with 1500 patients per year, times 2 visits per year = 3000 active patients.
- 3000 patients divided by 12 months = 250 patients per month.
- 250 patients per month multiplied by 85% (15% attrition rate is normal in the average practice) = 212 patients treated per month.

Step 2

- Add new patients per month (n = 20) to 212 active patients treated per month = 232 total.
- Of these 232 patients, 25% will be periodontal patients, not routine prophy patients. Multiply 232 times 25% = 58 patients per month needing some form of periodontal therapy.
- Add base patient volume (232) to those requiring periodontal therapy (58) = 290 total hygiene patients monthly.

Step 3

- Multiply the number of patients seen monthly (n = 290) by 12 months = 3480 patients treated annually.
- The number of patients required annually = 3480.
- Patients actually treated in this example practice = 1620.
- The shortfall (effectiveness of hygiene department) is 45%.

Step 4

- Divide 3480 patients annually by the average number of patient appointments per day (n = 8). It will take 435 days at 8 patients per day to provide treatment to the 3480 patients. This number will assist the practice in determining the number of dental hygiene days needed in the practice.

REDUCING CANCELLATIONS AND FAILURES

Step 2 in maximizing the dental hygiene schedule involves the following:

- Moving patients beyond "I only want what insurance pays" to gaining acceptance for the treatment that will provide optimal oral health.
- Creating a reason for returning to the practice and communicating that all patients are prescheduled builds value and importance into the appointment. The personal words coming from the dental hygienist when the patient is in the chair are critical to patient compliance, and review of the current supportive care program is essential.
- Reviewing the office written and verbal communications is important. Do the verbal and written communications that reflect the overall goal of the practice contain positive or negative messages? Negative messages such as, "This is to confirm your appointment for cleaning and checkup," and "Please call if this time is inconvenient" encourage and invite patients to cancel and break appointments (see Box 49-2).
- Focusing on dialog that emphasizes the positive reasons for returning is essential. Messages that define the functions of the hygiene appointment and replace negative statements (e.g., statements that send the message that missing or changing the appointment is acceptable) are helpful.
- Providing patients with written information and patient education regarding oral hygiene, periodontal diseases, and other systemic health issues reinforces the value and emphasis the practice places on each patient's health.

Examples of patient information material can include the following:

- Supportive care
- Hypertension screening
- Oral cancer screening
- Oral health examination
- Assessment of future health risk
- Examination for periodontal health
- Preventive dental health examination

MAXIMIZING THE DENTAL HYGIENE SCHEDULE

Not all patients require the same amount of time, yet many practices still appoint a standard 45- to 60-minute allotment, regardless of procedures to be performed. Just as the dentist schedules 6 units of time for the crown preparation, the productive dental hygienist schedules appointments based on the clinical requirements of each patient. Documentation of a realistic treatment plan and presentation to the patient is a necessary step in developing an appropriate appointment schedule. An appropriate fee is charged for services rendered, and time is reserved to properly assess, inform, discuss, educate, and instruct the patient. This is best accomplished at the completion of the appointment when the dental hygienist schedules her or his own appointments.

To create a need for the patient to return to see either the doctor or dental hygienist, the clinician might say, "I am concerned about the bleeding on the upper left," or "Dr. Jones is concerned about that lower right molar. We should schedule you for a return at 3 months to assess these areas."

Prescheduling allows the dental hygienist to see a full complement of patients—preventive and periodontal. Depending on the size of the practice, a minimum of one dental hygiene appointment each day should be reserved in the schedule. This production appointment can be used for the following situations:

- New patients (ideally, seeing the doctor first to have a full evaluation, charting, and treatment plan created)
- Patients needing active periodontal treatment
- Periodontal maintenance patients returning at 3 and 4 months

The appointment stays blocked until 2 days before it occurs. If it has not been filled, then it needs to be used to appoint any patient in need of treatment.

The practice should have written and understood protocols for broken and cancelled appointments. Dialog such as the following are helpful:

"We respect the importance of your time and work to schedule appointments that accommodate the busy scheduling needs of all of our patients. In return, we ask that patients make every effort not to change reserved dental appointments."

BRINGING PATIENTS OF RECORD BACK TO THE PRACTICE

The following example depicts today's typical dental hygiene department:

- One dental hygienist sees 8 to 9 patients per day (16 days per month or 190 days per year).
- The total dental hygiene patients treated for the year is 1600.
- In a practice with 2500 patients of record and dental hygiene hours to accommodate 1600 patients, requirements for 85% effectiveness would be 3400 annual patients.
- The result is a shortfall of dental hygiene hours. In this scenario, over time, patient retention and SCAs will not be able to support the patients and the entire practice suffers.

The typical dental practice in the United States has a patient interval return system that accommodates only 55% of the patients, with 40% to 50% of the patients overdue and unnoticed. This translates to 5.5 of every 10 patients in the practice not being seen, treated, or maintained with the level of care recommended by the healthcare team.[3]

Organized dentistry spends thousands of dollars each year recruiting new patients while ignoring the heart of the patient base. These are excellent, long-term patients of record who have had extensive dentistry in the past. The clinic staff should perform a **chart audit** and invite these patients back into the practice.

Increasing Profitability

The following two models should be considered, with and without an appropriate periodontal program.

EXAMPLE ONE

Dental hygiene department without a periodontal program:
- Ninety percent routine preventive appointments
- Ten percent supportive periodontal therapy appointments

Hygiene department without periodontal program (per 1000 patients):

90% Routine preventive = 900 patients × $65 = $58,500

10% Supportive therapy = 100 patients × $97 = $ 9,700

Total revenue= $68,200

Dental hygiene department with a periodontal program:
- Sixty-five percent routine preventive appointments
- Twenty-five percent supportive periodontal therapy (SPT) appointments
- Ten percent active periodontal therapy appointments

Hygiene department with periodontal program (per 1000 patients):

65% Routine preventive = 650 patients × $65 = $42,250

25% SPT = 250 patients × $97 = $24,250

10% Active periodontal therapy =

100 patients × $195 = $19,500

Total revenue = $86,000

(Plus site-specific therapies, antimicrobials, and localized delivery of antibiotics.)[5]

Through implementation of a clinically appropriate program for the detection, treatment, and ongoing management of periodontal disease, the practice achieved an increase in hygiene **profitability** of $17,800. The example illustrates how, with a conservative estimate of 35% of patients requiring either active periodontal treatment and/or supportive periodontal maintenance, the department increased hygiene production for periodontal services by 26%.

EXAMPLE TWO

One dental hygienist usually sees 8 patients per day and works 16 days per month. With a conservative estimate of 35% of the patients requiring active or supportive periodontal care, this practice increased hygiene production by 26%, or $27,000.

Note

Good communication skills; sound management principles; and organized periodontal, preventive, and supportive care protocols will enable the dental hygienist to build the hygiene department and the entire practice into a clinically excellent and profitable healthcare business, while helping patients achieve optimal oral health.

Determining Overhead for the Dental Hygiene Department

Knowing how to maximize efforts and increase profits does not give one the entire financial picture. Knowledge of the operating costs (**overhead**) of a dental hygiene department is required to have a clear picture of **practice economics.**

Dental hygienists use expendable and nonexpendable supplies. The capital investment in equipment and rent (or mortgage) for the owner of the practice must also be considered, as well as the cost of utilities, maintenance, and salaries of any support staff. This section focuses on the nonexpendable and expendable supplies used in dental hygiene services.

Expendable supplies are those that are replaced frequently because the items are used and disposed of with each patient visit. Nonexpendable items are those that can be used more than once and have a per item cost greater than that of expendable supplies; however, these items do not fall into the equipment category. Box 49-8 lists expendable and nonexpendable items.

Preparing the treatment room for patients requires many items. The clinician should consider the cost of the following:
- Chemicals used to disinfect and sanitize the area
- Wraps used on light handles, tubing, chair, hand pieces, and evacuation equipment
- Sterilization equipment and packaging supplies for instruments
- Radiographic film and holders
- Radiographic mounts

Hand pieces, powered instrument tips, and hand instruments used by the dental hygienist are all items that have to be replaced—but not after a single use on each patient.

One of the exercises located in the Critical Thinking Activities in the Clinical Companion Study Guide requires one to list

---

BOX 49-8

EXAMPLES OF EXPENDABLE AND NONEXPENDABLE SUPPLIES AND EQUIPMENT

Expendable*	Nonexpendable†
Gauze	Hand pieces
Patient napkins	Periodontal instruments
Saliva ejectors	Ultrasonic scalers
Plastic coverings	Ultrasonic cleaners
Air/water syringe tip	Autoclaves
Fluoride trays	Anesthetic syringes
Radiographic film	View boxes
Polishing agents	Curing light

*Single-use items (disposables).

†Multiple-use items.

the expendable supplies and nonexpendable supplies and identify the cost per patient for these items. This exercise provides an awareness of the costs per patient of operating the dental hygiene department. The clinician can multiply these costs by the number of patients per day per dental hygienist. Once these numbers have been identified and a proportion of the nonexpendable costs is added, the true picture emerges. This figure (the per patient cost) can be subtracted from the fee paid by the patient for a realistic estimation of income. This per patient overhead figure provides a starting point for determining what one would want the dental hygiene department to gross (i.e., total income).

Dental hygienists often fill the role of office manager in a dental practice. When this occurs, having knowledge of how to estimate costs per patient can be very beneficial to the owner of the practice. Being a good steward of resources by engaging in resource management is another way to enhance one's value within a practice.

This chapter focuses on the concept that dental hygiene is not entirely about providing excellent patient care. Having knowledge of the business aspects of a practice is an important asset and can enhance value and professional respect for the dental hygienist in the dental practice environment.

References

1. American Dental Association: *CDT codes,* Chicago, 2007, ADA.
2. Burt B, Research, Science and Therapy Committee of the American Academy of Periodontology: Position paper: epidemiology of periodontal diseases, *J Periodontol* 76:1406-1419, 2005.
3. Linder A: Personal communication and experiences as a practice management consultant, August 5, 2005.
4. Oral Cancer Foundation: *Oral cancer facts: rates of occurrence in the United States.* Available at www.oralcancerfoundation.org/facts/index.htm. Accessed on July 31, 2006.
5. Wilder R: Incorporating LAAs into perio therapy, *Dent Econ* 95(10):86-95, 2005.

Professional Development

Susan J. Daniel • Rebecca S. Wilder • Mary C. George

INSIGHT

Preparing for professional employment can be intimidating to recent graduates. Creating a resume and cover letter that a job seeker can submit for a position resulting in an invitation for an interview is what every prospective dental hygienist would like. This chapter will provide instructions on developing these tools and a portfolio for use during the interview. The dental hygienist is part of the healthcare professional team, and this topic, along with maintaining competence and methods for attaining continuing education, is covered in this chapter.

✦ CASE STUDY 50-1 Embracing the Dental Hygiene Profession

Jennifer Freeman, a 28-year-old dental hygienist, has been in practice for 4 years. She is the only dental hygienist in the mature (25-year) practice. Her primary responsibilities consist of performing clinical and radiographic assessments and providing preventive and therapeutic interventions. She is not a member of the American Dental Hygienists' Association and seldom attends professional meetings.

She obtains the necessary *continuing education* hours required to maintain an active license. However, Jennifer has become complacent with her position (provides the same treatment to all patients), is no longer satisfied with her job, and is questioning her career choice.

KEY TERMS

advanced degree	degree completion program	interview	portfolio
baccalaureate degree	distance education	maintaining competence	professional development
communication	empower	master of science degree	resume
continuing education	goal setting	philosophy	

LEARNING OUTCOMES

After reading this chapter the student will be able to:

1. Assess values, philosophy, and interpersonal needs.
2. Develop professional goals based on values, philosophy, and needs.
3. Determine attainment of goals.
4. Develop a resume and cover letter for professional employment.
5. Prepare for an employment interview.
6. Establish a respectful working relationship within the healthcare environment and on a dental team.
7. Identify ways to empower self and others.
8. Maintain competence.
9. Develop an educational career plan based on opportunities for advanced education.
10. Gain insight into the various options available to pursue an advanced degree.

Professional development is an integral part of being a healthcare professional and cannot exist without attention to the whole person. This chapter explores elements of professional development and the components that aid in personal development. Healthcare providers are held to a somewhat higher standard than individuals in other occupations. This public expectation requires this person to examine his or her values and **philosophy** as a healthcare provider and to assess and evaluate personal and professional goals, **communication** skills, and treatment and relationships with others.

Professional Self

50-A VALUES

Values are established early in life by a person's environment. Valuing quality of life is part of being human and is certainly essential to the competent dental hygienist, who plays an important role in health promotion and disease prevention as a member of the healthcare team. Value for life and health is a prerequisite for embarking on a healthcare career.

Providing health care also requires a desire to serve humankind, driven by the value for life and health. Not all people share the same values for health. Values determine a person's response in a given situation. Health care providers may experience internal conflict when providing health care to someone who does not value health in the same manner. Providing the service in a caring, professional manner is still essential. Learning to recognize this conflict and the cause may assist the healthcare provider in fostering self-improvement and professional growth.

50-B PHILOSOPHY OF PRACTICE

In addition to valuing quality of life and providing compassionate care, dental hygienists must examine their philosophy about the healthcare system. Various work environments and payment methods have led many healthcare providers to assess their philosophy about the delivery of health care. Many questions abound. Where should care be provided? Who should provide the services? Who should receive care? At what costs are questions being raised around healthcare issues? Each healthcare professional has to identify a personal philosophy to answer some of these issues. Typically, the philosophy will be based on personal values. When the chosen philosophy is based on something other than professional values, any performance or delivery of care will be compromised. An individual must either pursue this direction or begin to adjust what is valued. Adjusting a person's values will begin to erode self-image and self-worth. As a care provider, the dental hygienist must examine the philosophy of practice and weigh interpersonal needs into this examination.

50-C INTERPERSONAL NEEDS

Each person has certain needs that feed the mind, body, and soul. Maslow's hierarchy of needs is indeed true (Figure 50-1 and Box 50-1).[4]

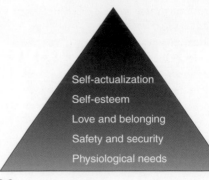

FIGURE 50-1
Maslow's hierarchy of needs.

BOX 50-1

DESCRIPTION OF MASLOW'S HIERARCHY OF NEEDS

Self-actualization: Need for fulfillment
Self-esteem: Need for recognition
Love and belonging: Needs for communication, affection, identity, modesty, companionship, and dependence
Safety and security: Needs for safety and accident prevention, religion and philosophy, and feelings of well-being
Physiological needs: Needs for personal hygiene, activity, sexuality, viral functions, eating and drinking, sleeping, and resting

---

Professional growth mandates an examination of interpersonal needs. A dental hygienist may consider the following questions:

- What are my needs?
- Are they being met?
- What adjustments are needed to have my needs met?
- Are my social outlets enough or the type I want?
- Can I adjust my professional setting or work responsibilities to meet my needs?

Exploring questions such as these may assist in achieving personal fulfillment. One of the primary steps in developing the professional self requires the meeting of interpersonal needs.

CAREER GOAL SETTING 50-D

Generating professional goals is impractical without also addressing components of personal life, such as family. **Goal setting** is the first step in measuring professional growth or accomplishments. Establishing both short- and long-term goals is appropriate and necessary. A professional who has identified deficits in interpersonal needs and has a vision for future attainment of these needs may begin setting goals. Immediate changes must sometimes be made in pursuit of goals. Small changes or steps toward a larger goal may need to

> *Note*
> In the pursuit of professional development, establishing goals is essential for success and personal satisfaction.

occur first. Outlining these steps is often necessary to achieving the anticipated change.

A professional may want to focus on more than one area of growth or change. Once these areas have been identified, writing a goal statement complete with action terms and measurable criteria is necessary. Developing a goal may involve creating an action plan, identifying strategies to reach the goal, or both. Implementing the strategies can be driven by a timeline.

50-E | MEASUREMENT OF GOALS

Articulating professional goals to others may often be helpful in the quest for professional growth. Some individuals perform best when they are accountable to others. Additionally, other persons may offer assistance, encouragement, and feedback during the process. An employer, co-worker, peer, spouse, parent, or anyone with whom the professional has a respectful, nurturing relationship can be a coach or mentor.

DEVELOPING A PROFESSIONAL CREDO

Developing nurturing relationships with professionals and others is an important part of developing the professional self. Establishing respectful, caring relationships with others is part of fully living a person's values and philosophy and meeting interpersonal needs. Some people have devised professional credos or codes for interacting with others. Box 50-2 provides an example of one of these credos. Each professional should establish a unique style of personal interaction based on personal values, philosophy, and needs.

Seeking Professional Employment

Completing a professional education and licensure marks the end of the first stage in the professional career. Now is the time to enter the profession and to identify values, needs, and goals. Once these components have been identified, the search for an employment situation consistent with the job seeker's values, needs, and goals can begin. Developing a resume, a cover letter, and a portfolio highlighting professional achievement and experiences is the next phase of professional development. In addition, now is the time to determine the salary and benefits required or expected. If the job seeker is unsure of how to calculate this value, resources are available to assist with this process.

DEVELOPING A RESUME

A **resume** is one of three marketing tools used when seeking employment that is discussed in this chapter. The resume is a short, one- or two-page document providing pertinent educational and employment information to prospective employers. The resume is the document that provides a prospective employer the impetus to invite the job seeker for an **interview.** A resume should include the following items:
- Name and contact information
- Educational experience
- Work experience

BOX 50-2

CREDO FOR RELATIONSHIPS WITH OTHERS

You and I are in a relationship, which I value and want to keep; yet each of us is a separate person with unique needs and the right to meet these needs.

When you are having problems meeting your needs, I will try to listen with genuine acceptance to facilitate your finding your own solutions instead of depending on mine. I also will try to respect your right to choose your own beliefs and develop your own values, different though they may be from mine.

However, when your behavior interferes with what I must do to get my own needs met, I will openly and honestly tell you how your behavior affects me, trusting that you respect my needs and feelings enough to try to change the behavior that is unacceptable to me. In addition, whenever some behavior of mine is unacceptable to you, I hope you will openly and honestly tell me your feelings. I will then listen and try to change my behavior.

At those times when we find that neither one of us can change a behavior to meet the other's needs, let us acknowledge that we have a conflict of needs that requires resolving. Let us then commit ourselves to resolve each such conflict without either one of us resorting to using power or authority to try to win at the expense of the other's losing. I respect your need, but I also must respect my own. Therefore let us always strive to search for a solution that will be acceptable to both of us. Your needs will be met, but so will mine—neither will lose, both will win.

In this way, you can continue to develop as a person through satisfying your needs, but so can I. Thus our relationship can be a healthy one in which each of us can strive to become what each is capable of being; and we can continue to relate to each other with mutual respect, love, and peace.

Modified from materials copyright 2000 by Thomas Gordon, PhD, Founder, Gordon Training International, Solana Beach, Calif. (Available at www.gordontraining.com.)

- Objective or goal indicating the type of position or practice the job seeker would like to obtain
- Professional or educational associations, honors, and awards

Many resources are available to assist in developing a resume. The job seeker should search the Internet for sites and sources that have examples. Information from the most reliable sources should be gathered, and a format that appears to be used consistently by healthcare professionals seeking employment should be followed. Resumes should be concise and usually do not exceed one or two pages. Good resources for resume writing and cover letters can be located on the Internet. One site with samples and resources is www.jobweb.com.

Note

Seek employment using the following tools:
- Resume
- Cover letter
- Portfolio

CREATING THE COVER LETTER

A cover letter (second tool) provides an introduction to a perspective employer. Content found in a cover letter includes the following:

- States the position for which the applicant is applying
- Emphasizes experiences the applicant has that meet the qualifications of the position, including what the applicant can bring to the practice
- Desire for the position
- The time the applicant would be available to begin the position
- Request for an interview

The cover letter should not exceed one page but should provide an introduction to the items listed previously. The applicant needs to remember that the purpose of the cover letter and resume is to obtain an interview.

INTERVIEW

The cover letter and resume served their purpose, the interview date is set, and now comes the preparation for the interview. The third tool is introduced during the interview—the professional education portfolio.

50-F PORTFOLIO

A portfolio is not an item the dental hygiene profession has used to assist in seeking employment, but it has been a valuable tool in other professions.

> *Note*
> The portfolio is a tool that can be used to gain a competitive edge over others seeking employment in the same market.

What can the portfolio provide that a cover letter and resume cannot?

The portfolio provides documentation of achievement and experiences that went into the applicant's professional development. However, items in the student portfolio may not be needed when using the tool for supportive documentation during an employment interview. The portfolio presented at an interview should include the following evidence:

- Copy of license to practice dental hygiene
- Copy of certifications (e.g., national board certificate or special certificates to administer local anesthesia, nitrous oxide–oxygen sedation, cardiopulmonary resuscitation, restorative or periodontal advanced functions).
- Documentation of experiences that would support skills and abilities to meet the requirements for the position, including the following:
  - Clinical experiences reflecting competence in the performance of patient care on the type of patients associated with the practice at which employment is sought
  - Health-promotion and disease-prevention activities within the community reflecting ability and interest in going outside the clinical practice environment to influence oral health care and health practices in general
  - Professional development activities that include

- membership and activities in professional associations
- Core values for others reflected by using evidence-based decision making in clinical services, awards or honors received, goals established, and comments from peers and recommendations from faculty and others

After the portfolio is readied for the interview, at what point during the interview is it introduced? The interviewer should notice that the applicant has a binder when he or she enters the interview; therefore, after the greetings have occurred, introducing the portfolio may occur next. The interviewer may ask about the item the applicant has, or he or she might begin by asking other questions or providing general information. Nonetheless, a point will come at which it will be appropriate to introduce the portfolio. How should this introduction occur? Simply stated, the applicant should say to the interviewer, "I have a portfolio documenting the educational experiences I have had that qualify me for this position. I would like to share this with you." Now is the time for the job applicant to market his or her skills and knowledge.

> *Note*
> An assertive, self-assured manner tells the interviewer that you are comfortable with new people in new settings and that you can talk with patients about oral care.

Most people will be impressed with the display of confidence.

The portfolio can also open the discussion of practice philosophy, management philosophy, office policies, and periodontal programs. This valuable tool can be used to sell the applicant's abilities and to generate discussion of healthcare issues, values, and topics that might not ordinarily occur in an interview. Each person in the interview (one or more interviewers and the applicant) will come away from the interview with more knowledge of each other than if the interview had been conducted using a list of questions generated and asked by the interviewer.

APPEARANCE, BEHAVIOR, AND DEMEANOR

Many people do not like discussing appearance in this *be yourself age,* but healthcare professionals are held to a higher standard, and guidelines in the clinical environment dictate to some extent a person's appearance. Therefore what does the applicant wear to an interview? The answer might be easy for some people, but the number of responses can be as many as the number of people who are seeking an interview. Certain points to consider follow.

- Health care requires meticulous personal hygiene from providers.
- How the applicant appears and the first impression someone has can greatly influence the outcome of an interview.
- Appearance needs to reflect the impression the applicant wants to make and the image the applicant leaves with others.
- The applicant should select business attire with traditional tailoring, appropriate fit (never too tight), and a color that flatters features.

- Hair should be clean and neat.
- Hands and fingernails should be clean and neat.

Note
Although first visual impressions can make a difference in acceptance, the applicant's behavior and demeanor will surely have an effect.

Good manners are always important, they speak volumes to an interviewer, and they can put others at ease. Manners, poise, and demeanor often reflect more about the applicant than appearance.

Before the interview, the job seeker should sit in front of a mirror and notice posture to determine whether changes are needed. The person should look into the mirror and talk as though talking to the interviewer and notice what would be eye contact if speaking to another person. Eye contact is important in an interview and conveys confidence or self-assuredness; it also allows the applicant to observe the interviewer's mannerisms.

Preparation for the interview also includes listing questions that should be asked or questions that the applicant would like to have answered during the interview. Interaction of staff and the relationship between staff and employer should be observed, if possible. The applicant should take mental notes of the office environment and if tension among staff is present in the office. The applicant should ask to see an office manual or position descriptions if available. This information will be good to know when making decisions concerning employment in this setting.

One question *not* to ask during the interview concerns salary. If the interviewer approaches the topic, okay, *but the applicant should not ask the question.* This question is reserved for the conversation that follows if the position is offered. A notepad should be taken along and notes should be made during the interview, or if the applicant has a good memory, then notes of observations and comments can be made after the interview.

POSTINTERVIEW

Immediately following the interview, notes should be made concerning impressions of the work environment, staff, and employer. Answers to the questions developed before the interview from information gained during the interview should be recorded. These notes, answers, thoughts, and feelings are then compared with the employment goals and values. This process will assist the job seeker in determining whether this employment opportunity appears to be the right one. Whether this employment setting is the right one or not, sending a *thank you* note would be appropriate. A hand-written note is personal; is appreciated; and, whether the position is offered, can influence the interviewer's opinion of the applicant.

ACCEPTING THE POSITION

The offer for employment has been extended. Now what? The job seeker should then ask, if not already, "Do I want this position?" If the answer is *yes,* then the discussion of salary and benefits can begin. This discussion may occur at the time of

notification of the position, and if so, then knowing in advance the needed salary and benefits will be most helpful in negotiations.

What forms of compensation are offered? Examples of compensation and benefits include the following:
- Salary or commission
- Base salary plus commission
- Benefits such as the following:
  - Health insurance—medical, dental, and ophthalmic
  - Profit sharing
  - Retirement
  - Paid vacation and sick leave days
  - Educational leave
  - Tuition for professional continuing education courses
  - Professional courtesies for care to self and family
  - Travel to and from work (fuel reimbursement for employees traveling long distances to work)

Not all practices offer all of these benefits. Some of the ones listed here might be more important than others and offer items for negotiation. Salary can be based on an hourly, daily, weekly, or some other rate. The compensation method used by the employer for dental hygienists should be identified, and if a different method is preferred, then the discussions can begin to work toward a solution. The various methods of compensation should be investigated by using Internet resources, seeking advice from dental practice consultants, and discussing the topic with other professionals. The prospective employee can now make an informed decision and negotiate, but he or she must be reasonable. Room for advancement, benefits, and salary increases should be discussed. A written work agreement or contact may be provided by the employer. Having expectations of job performance, periodic reviews, salary and benefits, and other matters clearly understood is important to the employer and employee. Negotiating from an understanding of the employee's skills and abilities and the benefit to the practice is best.

CASE APPLICATION 50-1.1

Ms. Freeman
Reflect on Ms. Freeman's situation. What elements is she missing in her professional life? What can she do to develop satisfaction in her career?

Interdisciplinary Approach to Health Care

As the complex healthcare delivery system in the United States has evolved, professional healthcare providers have realized that an interdisciplinary team approach is both efficient and effective in providing quality patient care. Unlike multidisciplinary healthcare, in which several professions work in parallel and often with separate goals, interdisciplinary health care coordinates health care and other fields in collaborations that include joint planning, decision making, and responsibility.[3]

The medical model for interdisciplinary teams capitalizes on disciplinary differences among team members, as well as overlapping roles. Team members in this role must consistently collaborate to solve patient problems that are too complex to solve independently. Building strong interdisciplinary teams requires careful planning; commitment; and an understanding of the education, core competencies, and scope of practice of different members of the healthcare team. Interdisciplinary team care for the patient improves care by increasing coordination of services and can **empower** patients as active partners in care.

Competencies that are necessary for a good interdisciplinary team include the following:

- Patient-centered focus that places the patient's needs as its first priority and that includes and respects the patient's values and preferences when making care decisions
- Ability to trust the work of others
- Flexibility in taking on assignments that are in the best interest of the patient
- Excellent communication both interpersonally and through effective record keeping
- Willingness to be held accountable for actions
- Constant evaluation of team effectiveness

An example of an interdisciplinary team of professionals dedicated to the care of the patient and family with cleft lip, cleft palate, and other craniofacial anomalies is the University of North Carolina Craniofacial Center interdisciplinary team. In addition to general dentistry team members, the team consists of specialists from the following fields:

- Audiology
- Genetics
- Neurosurgery
- Otolaryngology
- Oral and maxillofacial surgery
- Orthodontics
- Ophthalmology
- Pediatrics
- Pediatric dentistry
- Plastic surgery
- Prosthodontics
- Psychology
- Social work
- Speech-language pathology
- Speech pressure-flow assessments
- Other specialties as needed on a consultation basis[7]

Maintaining Competence

Health care requires of each professional person some form and amount of continued learning for updating and advancing in the field. These requirements are designed to keep providers competent in their respective field. Many options exist to maintain competence in professional skills and knowledge. These options range from professional **continuing education** courses awarding continuing education units to the pursuit of an advanced academic degree. Options for obtaining professional continuing education is provided in Box 50-3.

BOX 50-3

METHODS FOR OBTAINING CONTINUED PROFESSIONAL EDUCATION CREDITS

- Attending continuing education courses
- Self-instructional courses:
  - On line
  - Journals
  - DVDs and other videos
- Study clubs
- Presenting at professional meetings
- Publications
- Conventions
- Independent consulting
- Developing continuing education courses
- Cardiopulmonary resuscitation classes

Advanced Educational Opportunities Beyond Entry Level

The number of expanded roles for dental hygienists continues to increase. The American Dental Hygienists' Association (ADHA) web site lists the most updated version of the professional roles of the dental hygienist[1] (see Figure 1-7). The goal of this action is to create a clearly identified set of expectations for all licensed dental hygienists that will help facilitate further growth in the role of this vitally important frontline healthcare provider.

Although many dental hygienists are completely satisfied with clinical practice, many want to pursue other avenues of the profession during their lifetime. Fortunately, many opportunities exist for dental hygienists to stay in the profession and expand their career options and level of growth. For example, dental hygienists are actively employed in positions outside of clinical practice, including the following[2]:

- Faculty in dental hygiene programs
- Directors of dental hygiene programs
- Deans of health science colleges
- University presidents
- Corporate salespersons and managers
- Researchers
- Professional speakers, authors, and practice and industry consultants
- Community-based practitioners and managers
- Staff to professional organizations
- Business administrators for private dental offices

For most of these opportunities, an **advanced degree** will be required. Given that the majority of dental hygienist programs in the United States are 2-year entry programs, the first point of entry for an advanced degree is the **baccalaureate degree.** Currently, the ADHA lists approximately 60 degree completion programs that culminate in a bachelor's degree. The **degree completion program** is a means to acquire a baccalaureate degree after the 2-year or entry-level degree. This list may be accessed at www.adha.org/careerinfo/index.html.

Many of these programs are on-site programs, meaning that all coursework must be completed at the site of the school or via correspondence courses. An increasing number of programs offer on-line or distance-education options. **Distance education** is when the student receives the education from an off-site location via televideo or through the Internet.[6] Some programs offer a combination of on-site and distance-education options.

> *Note*
>
> Distance education is when the student receives the education from an off-site location via televideo or through the Internet.

In addition, most degree programs are part time, allowing the student to work while completing the degree.

Additional opportunities (above those that are available to graduates with a bachelor of science or art degree) exist when the dental hygienist has earned a **master of science degree.** Graduate education through a master of science program allows the dental hygienist to specialize in an area of interest and develop research skills.[2] It serves as a venue for new growth and development and expansion of the dental hygiene body of knowledge.

Employment opportunities expand with the master's degree. For example, academia is facing a critical shortage of dental hygiene faculty and administrators. Dental hygienists with graduate degrees are needed to fill these vacancies.[5,8]

> *Note*
>
> Academia is facing a critical shortage of dental hygiene faculty and administrators. Dental hygienists with graduate degrees are needed to fill these vacancies.

Currently, 11 masters programs are in dental hygiene or dental hygiene education. Additional programs with related disciplines and the on-line (distance) education programs may be accessed at www.adha.org/careerinfo/index.html. As with the degree-completion programs, graduate programs vary in the following options:

- Length
- Required number of credit hours
- Part-time or full-time options
- Affiliation with and without a dental school
- Requirements for research thesis
- Possibility of accelerated bachelor's to master's degree and higher

In the future, the profession will most likely have a doctoral degree in dental hygiene. Presently, though, dental hygienists who wish to pursue a doctorate do so in areas such as higher education and administration, public health, or allied health.

The interested dental hygiene student may wish to take the opportunity to investigate possible options while he or she is in school and make a career plan for the future. Resources are available for career development through the ADHA or through local colleges and universities.

Documentation and Evaluation of Professional Growth

Throughout this text and the CD-ROM, development of the educational **portfolio** has been encouraged. In Chapter 1, the concept of the portfolio was introduced as a mechanism for documenting the process of **maintaining competence.** The process and responsibility of maintaining competence to perform quality health care is continuous.

Documenting all aspects of continuing competence can be useful in evaluation, employment promotion, and renewal of the professional license. Goal setting is the first part of the process. Following a plan to attain the goals and documenting each step in the process are necessary to evaluate competence. Periodically, the dental hygienist should review the professional portfolio contents and assess whether the contents reflect the attainment of goals and maintaining competence. Once goals are met, new goals should be established.

Materials from the portfolio may be used to verify professional growth by documenting continuing education requirements for licensure. This portfolio might include the following information:

- Titles of continuing education course attended or taken (if through self-study)
- Name of presenter or presenters
- Location of presentation
- Continuing education certificate indicating hours awarded and entity awarding hours
- A brochure of the course, course description, or outline, if one is available

Some practice jurisdictions will periodically perform an audit of continuing education hours of licensees. The audit is often performed randomly and can require verification of continuing education hours received during a specific licensure period. Maintaining the information listed previously in an accessible file is important to eliminate frustration.

Although these contents are important, the professional portfolio should contain more of the rich evidence of professional growth such as the following:

- Participation in community service projects
- Publications
- Educational presentations
- The formation of study groups
- Oral care product inquiry
- Professional correspondence
- Mentoring
- Problem solving with staff
- Completed an academic course for enrichment
- Enrollment in an advanced degree program
- Participation as part of an interdisciplinary healthcare team
- Participation as a healthcare provider on a mission trip

- Developing patient communication materials or more efficient office patterns
- Documenting interesting patient cases that have provided new insights into health and disease
- Documenting ethical or legal dilemmas encountered, strategies implemented, and the respective outcomes

Professional development is the responsibility of each health-care professional. The desire to maintain competence, to pursue an advanced degree, and to maximize potential within a discipline is incumbent on all providers of patient care. As a direct care provider of oral health services, dental hygienists have the responsibility of being the most competent and professionally respected providers of oral health disease prevention and health promotion services.

References

1. American Dental Hygienists' Association: *Professional roles of the dental hygienist.* Available at: www.adha.org/careerinfo/roles.htm.
2. Darby M: Opening the door to opportunity, *Dimen Dent Hyg* 2(9):12-14, 16, 2004.
3. Drinka TJK, Clark PG: *Health care teamwork: interdisciplinary practice and teaching,* Westport, Conn, London, 2000, Auburn House.
4. Maslow AH: *Toward a psychology of being,* ed 2, New York, 1968, Van Nostrand Reinhol.
5. Nunn PJ et al: The current status of allied dental faculty: a survey report, *J Dent Educ* 68:329-344, 2004.
6 Stolberg R: Back to school, *Dimen Dent Hyg* 2(1):28-30, 2004.
7. University of North Carolina Craniofacial Center: Available at: www.dent.unc.edu/patient/clinics/craniofacial.
8. Wilder RS, Mann G, Tishk M: Dental hygiene program directors' perceptions of graduate dental hygiene education and future faculty needs, *J Dent Educ* 63:479-483, 1999.

Commitment and Vision

Susan J. Daniel • Sherry A. Harfst •

Rebecca S. Wilder • Mary C. George

INSIGHT

"By altering its present course, the dental hygiene profession can assume leadership in the risk-assessment movement by embracing novel, creative approaches to research and preventive dental medicine."[8] Knowing what the profession needs to advance in delivering health care is critical to the survival of dental hygiene. This chapter should be read while asking the question, *What can I do to direct the future course of dental hygiene?*

✦ CASE STUDY 51-1 | Vision of Oral Care in 2020

Use your imagination as you journey into the future. Make written notes after each question has been presented.

You have walked into a healthcare facility in the year 2020. Dental and medical care is being provided in the same facility. Imagine what the surroundings would look like.

- What type of healthcare equipment would be in this facility?
- What is the reception area like?
- What does the business area look like?
- What type of personnel would you see in this environment?

KEY TERMS

accreditation
advanced dental hygiene
    practitioner (ADHP)

commitment
distance learning
Human Genome Project

licensing examinations
licensure by credentials

National Dental Hygiene Research
    Agenda (NDHRA)
vision

LEARNING OUTCOMES

After reading this chapter the student will be able to:
1. Generate discussion of trends and future directions for the profession of dental hygiene in the following areas:
   - Clinical practice
   - Education, licensure, and portability
   - Research
   - Public health

2. Identify the relationship of technology to the profession of dental hygiene.
3. Identify methods for staying current with dental hygiene research.
4. Discuss the role of the dental hygiene profession in access to care.

Planning professional growth is an important step in ensuring a person's future as a dental professional. This type of planning helps dental hygienists reach higher levels of competence both as individuals and as a profession. Some happenings may appear to be serendipitous, but **vision** and **commitment** to a vision are essential to produce successful outcomes. Dental hygienists may take the first step in achieving their vision by visualizing themselves in a particular situation or at a particular place and time. Major developments in health care have occurred because some individuals had a strong vision, idea, or theory that was unwaveringly pursued. Some risk takers failed but learned from their mistakes and continued to pursue their goals. Successful individuals attribute their ability to persevere to those who encouraged or mentored them.

Gifted visionaries are not the only contributors to the field of dental hygiene. On the contrary, individuals who share the same vision and who commit themselves to seeing the vision materialize are necessary for implementing strategies to reach the vision. This chapter presents future trends in clinical practice, education and licensure, research, and public health.

Disease Prevention and Health Promotion

Healthcare delivery has been founded on the knowledge and understanding of basic sciences such as biology, anatomy and physiology, chemistry, physics, microbiology, and the psychosocial sciences. These sciences have provided information through scientific inquiry by people who are committed to improving human life. Without this information founded by scientists and practitioners, the field of dental hygiene would not be where it is today. The profession is still growing in all areas of identifying and preventing disease and promoting health. The role of the healthcare professional encompasses many facets of administration and practice:

- To further advancements in identifying diseases
- To develop new methods for preventing and curing disease
- To promote health

> *Note*
> Identifying possible disease before the manifestation of clinical signs and symptoms will be the next frontier.

Technological advances coupled with basic and clinical scientific inquiry is critical to future practice. A greater understanding now exists of the human body and the function of the immune system. The technology to locate specific enzymes and markers associated with specific diseases will move health care and dental hygiene forward to the next level.

Although some diseases can be identified through screening activities before the development of clinical signs and symptoms, the dental hygienist must always listen to what the patient says and how it is said. Listening to the patient and conducting a thorough assessment inquiry can provide invaluable information for the professional to:

- Be a more accurate diagnostician
- Provide appropriate healing arts
- Monitor progress toward health

The **Human Genome Project**[11] has provided science with the deoxyribonucleic acid (DNA) pattern for life, unlocking the doors of human discovery. Surrounding this incredible finding is controversy over the ethical application of the knowledge—another frontier to explore. Many unanswered questions exist about the affective human component such as the development of a person's soul, compassion, and heart or caring spirit—essential elements in the healthcare provider. The development or acquisition of affective behaviors is clearly not as certain as the physiologic development. Perhaps this component is what makes humans unique.

Future Direction

The literature is replete with publications on the following topics:

- Healthcare practices
- Association between systemic and oral disease
- Patient practices and trends in seeking health care
- Present and future healthcare needs

Trends and current practices can provide insight into the future directions and role of the dental hygiene profession. Opportunities abound for dental hygiene to provide the leadership in oral disease prevention and systemic disease recognition and detection. "By altering its present course, the dental hygiene profession can assume leadership in the risk-assessment movement by embracing novel, creative approaches to research and preventive dental medicine."[8] With insight, commitment, and leadership, a dental hygienist can assist the profession in establishing vision and seizing opportunities to improve human life.

To establish a framework of categories to address future direction, a traditional academic model will be used. The *three-legged stool* model to which academic institutions subscribe is that of teaching, service, and research. This model has been stabilized in some institutions with a fourth leg of patient care. The four-component academic model—teaching, service, research, and patient care—will morph into the framework for future directions in dental hygiene:

- Education
- Clinical practice
- Research
- Public health (Table 51-1)

This model reflects professional roles of the American Dental Hygienists' Association (ADHA) (see Figure 1-7). Dental hygienists with insight and leadership can be found in all four categories—education, clinical practice, research, and public health—and in taking on the roles of advocate in promoting the profession and in administration and management.

> *Note*
> Improving the public's health is the overarching goal for the profession no matter what the role, function, interest, or work environment.

Table 51-1	Using the Academic Model for Categories of Future Direction
ACADEMIC MODEL	**FRAMEWORK MODEL FOR DIRECTION**
Teaching	Education
Service	Public health
Research	Research
Patient care	Clinical practice

As technological advances are made, they will be incorporated into each of these four categories, and the dental hygienists will assume professional roles, resulting in major contributions in each category of the model.

EDUCATION

Educational oversight agencies will continue to demand accountability from educational institutions and programs for the product being produced (student and graduate). The American Dental Association's (ADA) Commission on Dental and Allied Dental **Accreditation** requires accountability from accredited educational programs. Additionally, to become licensed in 49 of the 50 states, students must successfully complete the National Board Dental Hygiene Examination administered by the ADA and pass the clinical and jurisprudence licensure examination for the state or region. Only students who have graduated from an ADA-accredited program can sit for the National Board Dental Hygiene Examination.[2]

Educational accountability occurs in primary, secondary, and higher education in the liberal arts and in the sciences. Holding educational institutions accountable for a competent end product (graduate) is one method of ensuring student outcomes and quality in health care and bettering the quality of life.

The ADA Commission on Dental and Allied Dental Accreditation requires each dental hygiene educational program to meet certain standards. The accreditation standards have undergone numerous revisions over the years. Currently, dental hygiene programs are required to establish competence for specific areas of education.[2] Students must be provided competency statements when entering the program, and these statements must be used as a measure for evaluating student performance. Documenting each competency by course and evaluation methods is required. For this reason, the educational portfolio was incorporated within this text and its accompanying CD-ROM to assist students in documenting educational development and for use after graduation to document professional development.

Another trend in higher education in general, including dental hygiene education, is **distance learning.** Continuing education may lead to career change and upward mobility. Individuals who want to pursue careers requiring additional education and skill development need flexibility in the procurement of this education. Technology has paved an avenue for persons who cannot put aside job and family responsibilities to pursue education from institutions at a distance or on a school-established schedule. (See Chapter 50 for additional information on advanced degrees.)

Distance learning is available in dental hygiene. Accessing video conferencing and using the Internet have increased opportunities for persons who wish to pursue a dental hygiene career. Using these technologies now and in the future will change the way traditional dental hygiene education is delivered. Accredited dental hygiene educational programs are currently offering distance-learning programs, and a listing of these can be obtained through the ADHA web site (www.adha.org).

LICENSURE AND PORTABILITY

Flexibility in the portability of dental and dental hygiene licenses to other jurisdictions is needed, and changes are occurring in state dental practice acts, affording professionals the option for **licensure by credentials** rather than requiring an additional examination of clinical skills. Licensure by credentials, when offered by a jurisdiction, may require the individual to provide some of the following:

- Certain documentation of licensure in another recognized jurisdiction
- Proof of the number of years of practice (designated by the regulatory board)
- Proof of graduation from an accredited dental hygiene program

A search of the National Practitioner Data Bank (NPDB) may be performed, and a fee must be paid for the application for licensure by credentials.

If all information satisfies the regulatory board, then the applicant usually has to complete an ethical and jurisprudence examination or any other written examination required for licensure successfully before the license can be issued.

The need for mobility of licensed dentists prompted the creation of regional licensing examination boards representing numerous states in each region. Some regional boards recognize and grant licensure to individuals who are licensed by other regional boards. At this time, only 10 states administer independent clinical licensure examinations, and only four regional testing agencies have been established.[1] (See Chapter 1 for a list of states using regional or independent testing agencies.)

The number of independent state **licensing examinations** will continue to decline with a movement toward national licensure, which may be in effect by the time of this writing. The reader is encouraged to consult the American Association of Dental Examiners web site for new information (see Suggested Agencies and Websites for this chapter on the Evolve website).

As dental professionals look toward the future, the concept of current clinical examinations for licensure will become passé.

With the accountability of competencies established for educational institutions, the need for a clinical examination for licensure will no longer be necessary. When this action is coupled with a simulated national board examination, only the need for jurisprudence and an ethical examination will be necessary for licensure. Ethics and law will continue to be the determining factors for licensure. Holding to a high ethical standard would make a dental hygienist less likely to perform functions that the professional is not competent to perform. Additionally, practicing outside the laws governing the dental hygiene profession would not be acceptable conduct of an ethical professional.

Clinical skills are taught, performed, and evaluated by each program, and students are deemed competent at graduation. The standards of competence and accountability are only as good as the people who teach and evaluate students, as well as those professionals who evaluate the accountability of educational programs and institutions. With the advent of this new pathway to licensure, dental hygiene faculty members would be given a greater responsibility for ensuring that those persons entering the profession are indeed competent healthcare professionals.

RESEARCH

Research will continue to be a vital part of the dental hygiene profession.

> **Note**
> Research facilitates the development of new clinical techniques, materials, and treatment modalities.

Research affects access to care, education, and public and private policies on oral health.[5]

Many different types of research are important to the dental hygiene profession. Some of the types of research about which dental hygienists might read in professional, peer-reviewed publications are based on basic or applied research. Hygienists may use qualitative or quantitative methods. Some of the typical types of oral health research are as follows:

- Laboratory research
- Clinical research
- Health services research
- Health-promotion and community-based research
- Epidemiologic research (e.g., National Health and Nutrition Examination Survey [NHANES])
- Dental practice–based research
- Educational research

> **Note**
> When tracking the progress of the profession of nursing or occupational therapy, clearly, each discipline established a specific body of knowledge that is unique to the profession.

The ADHA has created and implemented the **National Dental Hygiene Research Agenda (NDHRA),** which outlines the priority areas for research that will assist the growth of the dental hygiene profession. The NDHRA was first developed in the 1990s and was further revised and published in 2002.[9] The NDHRA will continually be updated and revised. The dental hygienist should stay abreast of the research priorities of the profession by reviewing the

NDHRA on the ADHA web site.[6]

Examples of evidence-based publications that contain original research articles are the *Journal of Dental Hygiene, International Journal of Dental Hygiene, Journal of Periodontology, Journal of Public Health Dentistry, Journal of the American Dental Association, Journal of Dental Education,* and *Journal of Evidence-Based Dental Practice,* among others. Even though dental hygienists receive many publications, some of which are based on research findings, frequently reading original works is prudent for professionals to base their decisions about treatments for their patients (see Chapter 4). As stated in the 2005 ADHA Dental Hygiene Focus on Advancing the Profession, "The decisions that they [dental hygienists] make every day must be firmly grounded in knowledge that is obtained from research and clinical experience, to improve their professional judgment and ultimately, to improve the quality of services provided."[3]

> **Note**
> Dental hygienists may also keep up with the latest original research by reading peer-reviewed publications that have been reviewed by blinded evaluators and accepted based on the quality of the research and the writing.

★ CASE APPLICATION 51-1.1

Applying Evidence-Based Decision Making (EBDM)

How will the dental hygienist of the future apply EBDM? Will it be an automatic response to use EBDM or will it be sporadically applied? Will you apply EBDM as standard practice?

Other professional associations and organizations have quality web sites and publications that assist dental hygienists in staying abreast of the latest research that will influence oral health. Examples are the National Institutes of Health, National Institute of Dental and Craniofacial Research, and the American Academy of Periodontology. In addition, dental hygienists may quickly access information via national databases such as PubMed, MEDLINE, CINAHL, and HealthSTAR.

Finally, the dental hygiene profession will need an increased number of researchers in the future. Although research typically requires an advanced degree (see the section, Advanced Educational Opportunities beyond Entry Level, in Chapter 50), the area is exciting, challenging, and a rewarding way to contribute to the growth of the dental hygiene profession.

CLINICAL PRACTICE

Technology has changed every area of health care. In dental hygiene practice, computers used for demonstrating patient oral self-care has provided greater reliability than traditional techniques and paper records.[7] Patient recall of historical data may often be flawed, and clinician notes may be sketchy or incomplete. A permanent record of health history findings and clinical data maintained in a database for future access assist the clinician in providing more efficient and effective patient care. Periodontal and dental chartings may be recorded at each visit and easily compared with previous findings for evaluating oral conditions and assessing components such as oral risks, preventive and intervention strategies, implementation, and evaluation.

Maintaining clinical and radiographic images electronically reduces the need for physical storage space and provides a ready comparison from previous images for assessing disease and patient oral care needs. These same images also provide an excellent means of educating and motivating the patient to perform better oral self-care and to accept the professional interventions needed to prevent further oral and systemic disease.

Many people within the United States do not have access to care, and many underserved do not have oral hygiene services. Nurses and other allied healthcare providers are beginning to step in to meet these needs, and dental hygienists who are the most knowledgeable and skilled to provide service are often not permitted to do so because of practice act restrictions. Changes are occurring in practice acts and in the future preparation of a new professional to meet the underserved needs. The ADHA has developed a proposal and curriculum for the **advanced dental hygiene practitioner (ADHP)** to meet the needs of the underserved within our population. Monies were appropriated from the federal government to be used by the Health Resources and Services Administration (HRSA) to:

explore alternative methods of delivering preventive and restorative oral health services in rural America. Specifically, the Committee encourages HRSA to explore development of an advanced dental hygiene practitioner who would be a graduate of an accredited dental hygiene program and complete an advanced educational curriculum, which prepares the dental hygienist to provide diagnostic, preventive, restorative and therapeutic services directly to the public in rural and underserved areas.[3]

This new healthcare professional has the potential for providing dental hygiene a larger presence in improving the overall health of the public and in interdisciplinary healthcare environments.

Screening for Disease Using Oral Fluids

If the mouth is the portal through which the body receives nourishment, then might it also hold the keys to help detect disease and monitor health? With this information in mind, who is more suited to screen, refer, and monitor patients than the oral care prevention specialist, the *dental hygienist?* Perhaps the name of this professional would change to encompass the expanded healthcare concept.

Patients would come in at regular intervals and, by way of either a saliva, plaque biofilm, or crevicular fluid sample, would leave the visit knowing whether they required further healthcare evaluations. The technology and science of dentistry are rapidly approaching the day when whole-health screening through an oral assessment will be a reality.

Might the specialized oral healthcare provider (the dental hygienist), who is equipped with a greater knowledge of oral medicine and screening for illness and disease from oral fluids, become the gatekeeper to entry into the healthcare

environment in the future? In other words, this professional known as the *dental hygienist, the preventive professional,* might become the individual who screens for diseases at supportive care intervals and makes referrals to appropriate healthcare providers based on the results of such screening tests. The reader is encouraged to think about the possible locations where dental hygienists would be able to screen for disease and then refer individuals to a dentist or internist for full assessments and diagnosis. Box 51-1 lists places where future screening activities might occur.

Dental hygienists currently screen for disease with vital signs; health histories; and clinical, periodontal, and radiographic examinations—the process known as *risk assessment.* This information is now being used to link oral health status with total health but not to the extent that will be possible in the future. The National Institute of Dental and Craniofacial Research has funded research for saliva biomarker discovery and salivary diagnostic technology development. Within the next 5 years, screening for diseases may be possible using saliva.

Risk-assessment screening by dental hygienists does not mean that providing professional oral care would be delegated to another dental healthcare professional. It means that the role of the dental hygienist will expand to more fully use the special knowledge, skills, abilities, and commitment that these professionals already possess.

Screening for total-body health can be performed in many settings in which dental hygienists are currently employed. This function would have an impact on public health, with an increase in the need for more advanced dental hygiene specialists.

> **Note**
>
> The opportunity to reach a larger portion of the population with healthcare screening would revolutionize the nation's health and healthcare system. The result would be a healthier society—one in which illness and disease are diagnosed early, resulting in decreased morbidity and mortality.

Box 51-1

FUTURE SETTINGS FOR SCREENING FOR DISEASE AND OTHER SERVICES

Private offices
Mobile clinics and vans
Public health clinics
Kiosks in public shopping areas
Spas
Homes
Institutions
Government buildings
Schools
Construction sites
Rural farm co-operatives

Health Promotion and Disease Prevention

What forms of health promotion and disease prevention would be performed in the healthcare environment of the future?

PUBLIC HEALTH

Public health dentistry offers an exciting and challenging future. Providing access to care, determining oral needs, and providing preventive and restorative services to the half of the population that does not receive consistent oral care are indeed part of the challenges. Although fluoride has significantly reduced dental caries, this disease is still the most prevalent disease in society. Periodontal diseases are also prevalent and exist in some form and extent in nearly all adults. Both diseases are considered infectious and have multifactorial etiologies. Emerging knowledge about the etiology of each disease results in new innovations, prevention methods, techniques, and treatments. The dental hygienists' education includes content on the etiology, prevention, and treatment for these widespread diseases.

Prevention

Imagine what the future holds for preventing systemic diseases and conditions such as heart disease, stroke, diabetes, and low–birth-weight babies. Might prevention of dental caries and periodontal diseases reduce and perhaps prevent life-threatening illnesses?

Historically, the public and the dental profession have viewed these oral diseases as less serious than heart disease and stroke. Current focus, however, is on the relationship between oral and systemic disease.

This question gives persons in public health dentistry and dental hygiene something exciting to explore. The public health dental hygienist might be the primary preventive healthcare professional. Programs once geared toward preventing oral disease might now focus on disease prevention and true whole-body health promotion.

School and community oral screening programs might expand to include other types of screening for persons with dental caries and evidence of gingival and periodontal concerns. Individuals might be referred for cholesterol and triglyceride screenings if the oral conditions related to systemic diseases were noted. In addition, vital signs might be assessed to determine the need for referral to a physician for followup. Integrating systemic and oral health into public health dentistry and dental hygiene creates an exciting future and integrates the dental hygienist into an interdisciplinary approach to health care.

DENTAL HYGIENIST'S ROLE IN ACCESS TO DENTAL CARE

Oral Health in America: A Report of the Surgeon General[12] released in May 2000 describes profound and far-reaching disparities in the oral health among the poor of all ages in the United States, with poor children and poor older persons, as well as members of racial and ethnic minority groups, being particularly vulnerable. Among the reasons for disparities cited in the report were socioeconomic factors, lack of community programs such as fluoridated water supplies, lack of transportation to a clinic and flexibility in getting time off from work to attend to health needs, and physical disability or other illness limiting access to services. Another major barrier to seeking and obtaining professional oral health care cited in the report relates to a lack of public understanding and awareness of the importance of oral health. The following are included among strategies to ensure adequate access to oral care:

- Adequate numbers of individuals to provide the care, as well as an equitable distribution of providers to ensure the availability for care
- Sufficient financial resources to support the delivery of and reimbursement for care
- Cultural competency of oral healthcare providers
- Sound public education programs that promote preventive oral health practices through self-care and professional oral care[12]

As specialists in preventing dental disease, dental hygienists play a critical role in eliminating oral health disparities, reducing barriers to care, and ensuring quality oral health care for all. Individuals in need of oral health care often lack knowledge regarding prevention of dental disease and awareness of their personal clinical needs. Dental hygienists can work with patients individually or in community health programs to develop oral healthcare treatment plans that manage oral infections.[4]

Note

A role for dental hygienists exists in working with public policy makers to assist them in better understanding the role of oral health as part of general health, thus potentially elevating oral health issues to a higher priority in public policy decisions.

Additional public policy inroads that can be made by dental hygienists include the following:

- Working with state legislative bodies to eliminate statutory and regulatory language in dental practice acts that restrict the public's access to oral health care provided by licensed dental hygienists
- Dental hygienists who can also seek out practice opportunities in areas where geographic disparity of oral health providers exists
- Being prepared to render culturally competent oral care to racially and ethnically diverse populations[10]

Best Possible Health Care

What would your role or roles be, and what types of personnel and who would you interact to provide patients with the best possible health care?

The Future

51-A

What tools and methods are needed for a future that holds great promise for delivering preventive care, monitoring disease, and providing appropriate interventions and referrals? Well-educated dental hygienists with knowledge of healthcare delivery, economics, and human needs are required. They must have well-developed communication skills, insight, and a commitment to capturing the opportunities that lie ahead. Dental hygienists are needed who believe that the oral environment is the portal to the body through which discoveries and advances in diagnosis and treatment of oral and systemic disease lie. Dental hygienists must present themselves as educated professionals to obtain respect within and outside the profession. Self-respect, values for health care, and continued competence are required to obtain respect from others. To embrace this future in health care, the successful dental hygienist will be one with the following attributes:

> **Note**
>
> Leaders in the future of dental hygiene must possess sound self-assessment skills and a keen awareness that vision cannot materialize unless others value the vision and are willing to work.

- Vision to generate ideas, concepts, and strategies
- Ability to organize and implement strategies to see visions come to fruition
- Interpersonal skills to encourage, support, evaluate, provide mentoring, and question the visionaries

Leaders are required in the following disciplines:

- Research and administration
- Education
- Public health
- Legislation
- Clinical practice

Leadership, personal insight, and commitment are necessary for dental hygiene and, more specifically, for the advancement of oral and systemic health care, resulting in a better quality of life for all.

Motivation and an element of risk taking are part of the development and implementation of a vision. With today's tremendous scientific advances, now is an opportune time to continue developing the path set by earlier dental hygiene professionals.

> **Note**
>
> Now is the time to embrace the vision of the future of health care by recognizing that the future lies in perhaps the yet-undiscovered components of the human body—the immune system in health and disease.

As dental hygiene professionals support the continued advancement of technology and research to unlock the mysteries of human health, the future will be limited only by the professionals' vision and wisdom. Insight and commitment to make changes and seize opportunities that present themselves will prove to be vital to the dental hygiene profession. Dental hygiene is now established as an integral component of health care, and the dental hygienist is clearly a valued professional integral to the identification and prevention of oral and systemic diseases.

✷ CASE APPLICATION 51-1.4

Vision of the Future

What can you and other dental hygienists do to shape this future vision?

References

1. American Association of Dental Examiners: *Listing of regional board examinations for licensure, reciprocity and licensure by credentials,* Chicago, 2001, The Association. Also available at: www.aadexam.org.
2. American Dental Association, Commission on Dental and Allied Dental Accreditation: *Accreditation standards for dental hygiene programs,* Chicago, 2000, American Dental Association.
3. American Dental Hygienists' Association: *ADHA focus on advancing the profession, 2005.* Available at: www.adha.org/downloads/adha_focus_report.pdf.
4. American Dental Hygienists' Association: *Access to care position paper 2001.* Available at: www.adha.org/profissues/access_to_care.htm.
5. American Dental Hygienists' Association: *Building the foundation—advancing the profession.* Available at: www.adha.org/research/index.html.
6. American Dental Hygienists' Association: *National Dental Hygiene Research Agenda.* Available at: www.adha.org/research/nra.htm.
7. Berthelsen CL, Stilley KR: Automated personal health inventory for dentistry: a pilot study, *J Am Dent Assoc* 131(1):59-66, 2000.
8. DePaola D: Thinking big, *Dimen Dent Hyg* 3:10, 12, 2005.
9. Gadbury-Amyot CC et al: Prioritization of the National Dental Hygiene Research Agenda 2000-2001 American Dental Hygienists' Association Council on Research, *J Dent Hyg* 76(2):157-166, 2002.
10. Haden NK et al: Improving the oral health status of all Americans: roles and responsibilities of academic dental institutions, *J Dent Educ* 67(5):563-583, 2003.
11. Scott B: Impact of the Human Genome Project on oral health care, *Access* 15:36-46, 2001.
12. US Department of Health and Human Services: *Oral health in America: a report of the Surgeon General. National Institute of Dental and Craniofacial Research,* Rockville, Md, 2000, National Institutes of Health.

Glossary

A

Abandonment: Once a healthcare professional establishes a relationship with a patient, services must continue to be provided for the patient. If the healthcare provider does not provide services and the patient's health is jeopardized, then a legal action of *abandonment* may be commenced against the healthcare provider.

Abfraction: Pathologic loss of hard tooth substance caused by biomechanical loading forces. Such loss is thought to be a result of flexure and chemical fatigue degradation of enamel or dentin at some location distant from the actual point of loading or both.

Abfraction lesions: Lesions thought to be caused by excessive facial or lingual occlusal load through either compression or tension in the cervical region of the tooth just above the bony support.

Abrasion: Wearing away of surface material as a result of friction.

Abrasive: Abrasives consist of particles of sufficient hardness and sharpness that cut or scratch a soft material when drawn across its surface. Abrasive materials are available in various particle sizes.

Abutment: Tooth, root, or implant used for the retention of a fixed or removable prosthesis.

Accreditation: Processes of approval, certification, or endorsement. For example, the American Dental Association can accredit a dental educational program.

Acellular cementum: First layers of cementum deposited without many embedded cementocytes.

Acid etchant: Concentration of 35% to 50% phosphoric acid applied to the occlusal pits and fissures to open the enamel tubules for receipt of a liquid sealant resin.

Acquired immunodeficiency syndrome (AIDS): Syndrome that (1) involves a defect in cell-mediated immunity that has a long incubation period, (2) follows a protracted and debilitating course, (3) is exhibited by various opportunistic infections, and (4) has a poor prognosis.

Acromegaly: Condition that is caused by hyperfunction of the pituitary gland in adults. An enlargement of the skeletal extremities, including the feet, hands, mandible, and nose, characterizes acromegaly.

Acrophobia: Fear of heights.

Acrylic test stick: Plastic rod-shaped device used to check instrument sharpness.

Activated partial thromboplastin time (aPTT) test: Laboratory test that evaluates the intrinsic clotting cascade. This test is primarily used to monitor anticoagulation with heparin therapy and to aid in the diagnosis of hemophilia; congenital deficiencies in intrinsic clotting factors II, V, VIII, IX, X, XI, and XII; vitamin K deficiency; and various congenital clotting abnormalities. The aPTT test uses a contact activator that is added to the patient's blood to measure the ability of the blood to clot.

Active caries: Condition in which a lesion leads to cavitation of the tooth structure. Active caries can be radiographically observed and feels *mushy* or *leathery* to the touch.

Active periodontal therapy: Therapy that brings periodontal disease into remission. Active periodontal therapy includes professional debridement and personal care instruction that may be used in conjunction with periodontal surgery.

Acute necrotizing ulcerative gingivitis (ANUG): Recurrent periodontal disease that primarily involves the interdental papillae, which undergoes necrosis and ulceration.

Acute-phase proteins: The body produces acute-phase proteins in response to inflammation. Common acute-phase proteins include C-reactive protein, fibrinogen, and serum-amyloid A protein. These substances bind to microbial cell walls and act as opsonins.

Adaptive immunity: Form of immunity that is mediated by lymphocytes and stimulated by exposure to infectious agents. Adaptive immunity is characterized by specificity for distinct macromolecules and for its memory, which is the ability to respond more vigorously to repeated exposure to the same microbe. Adaptive immunity is also known as *acquired immunity*.

Addiction: Compulsive behavior. See *Dependence*.

Addison's disease: Primary adrenal insufficiency, also known as *hypoadrenalism*, that is characterized by the destruction of the adrenal glands and a failure to produce and secrete the corticosteroids, aldosterone and cortisol. Symptoms include severe weakness, weight loss, low blood pressure, digestive disturbances, hypoglycemia, lowered resistance to infection, and abnormal pigmentation (e.g., bronze color of the skin with associated melanotic pigmentation of the oral mucous membranes, particularly of the gingival tissues).

Addisonian crisis: Emergency situation caused by extreme stress in a patient with Addison's disease who is unable to secrete the necessary corticosteroids for survival. Extreme stress causes hypoglycemia and circulatory shock, which are life-threatening conditions requiring the administration of glucocorticoids to prevent death.

Adenoid cystic carcinoma: Pseudoadenomatous basal cell carcinoma that originates from salivary glands, the cells of which resemble basal cells and form ductlike or cystlike structures. Adenoid cystic carcinoma grows slowly but is malignant.

Adenoma: Benign epithelial neoplasm or tumor with a basic glandular structure that suggests derivation from glandular tissue.

Adherence: Willingness and ability of a patient to perform those tasks specifically necessary to attain and maintain health.

Adrenal crisis: Rare, life-threatening condition caused by acute adrenal suppression. Risk is associated with adrenal suppression caused by the long-term use of glucocorticoid medications; consequently, on exposure to stress, the patient is unable to respond with enough endogenous cortical to manage the stress. Adrenal crisis may result in severe hypoglycemia and circulatory shock. Treatment includes intravenous (IV) hydrocortisone, fluid and electrolyte replacement, and glucose administration as needed.

Adrenocorticotropic hormone (ACTH): Hormone produced by basophilic cells of the anterior lobe of the pituitary gland, which exerts a reciprocal regulating influence on the production of corticosteroids by the adrenal cortex.

Advanced directive: Directive that indicates a person's wishes regarding his or her health care in advance of the need.

Agoraphobia: Anxiety about or avoidance of places or situations from which escape might be difficult or embarrassing or in which help may not be available in the event of experiencing paniclike symptoms.

Agranulocytosis: Symptom complex characterized by a significant decrease in the number of granulocytes and by lesions of the throat, mucous membranes, gastrointestinal (GI) tract, and skin.

Air-powder polisher: Air-powered device that uses air and water pressure to deliver a controlled stream of specially processed sodium bicarbonate slurry through the hand piece nozzle; also called *air abrasive, air polishing,* or *air-powered abrasive.*

Air turbine: Hand piece with a turbine powered by compressed air.

Ala: Wing or a winglike anatomical part or process.

ALARA principle: Concept of radiation protection that states that all exposure to radiation must be kept to a minimum or *as low as reasonably achievable.*

Alcohol-based hand rub: Alcohol-containing preparation designed to reduce the number of viable microorganisms on the hands.

Alginate: Flexible impression material in which the alginate in water (sol) reacts chemically with calcium ions to form insoluble calcium alginate (gel).

Algophobia: Fear of pain.

Allele: One of different forms of a gene present at a particular chromosomal locus.

Alopecia: Normal or abnormal deficiency of hair; baldness.

Alveolar bone proper: Bone lining the alveolus.

Alveolar crestal fibers: Alveolar crestal fibers run from the crest of the alveolar bone to the cementum in the region of the cementoenamel junction. Their primary function is to retain the tooth in the socket and to oppose lateral forces.

Alveolar mucosa: Portion of the oral mucosa immediately apical to the mucogingival junction.

Alveolar process: Extension of the maxilla and mandible that surrounds and supports the teeth to form the dental arches. The alveolar process is also known as the *alveolar ridge.*

Amalgam: Alloy in which mercury is one of the metals.

Analog format: Image produced by conventional x-ray film.

Anatomical charting forms: Charts used to indicate conditions of the mouth. In all charts, the teeth are presented as though looking into the patient's mouth.

Anatomical crown: Portion of crown covered by enamel.

Anemia: Reduction to less than normal of the number of red blood cells, quantity of hemoglobin, or volume of packed red blood cells in the blood.

Angina pectoris: Condition that is frequently a symptom of cardiovascular diseases and is characterized by a severe, viselike pain behind the sternum that sometimes radiates to the arms, neck, or mandible. Angina pectoris may also produce a sense of constriction or pressure of the chest. It is caused by exertion or excitement and is relieved by rest.

Angiogenesis: Process of forming new blood vessels.

Angioma: Benign tumor of vascular nature.

Angle's classification: System that is used to classify malocclusion initially and simply.

Angles: *90-degree (right) angle:* joining of a horizontal line to a vertical line from the same point; *110-degree angle:* line that is 20 degrees to the right or left of the right angle; *45-degree angle:* angle that is half of 90 degrees. These angles are used in periodontal instrumentation, instrument sharpening, radiologic studies, and other dental applications.

Angular cheilosis: Inflammation of the lip or lips with redness and the production of fissures that radiate from the angles of the mouth.

Angulation, horizontal: Position of the x-ray tubehead and central ray in a side-to-side (horizontal) plane.

Angulation, vertical: Position of the x-ray tubehead and central ray in an up-and-down (vertical) plane.

Anionic: Pertaining to a negatively charged ion.

Ankylosed: Joint or tooth that is immobile or abnormally fused as a result of injury, disease, or surgical procedure.

Anorexia: Partial or complete loss of appetite for food.

Anterior palate: Front or forward part of the palate that is hard and bony.

Anterior uveitis: Inflammation of the anterior portions of the iris, ciliary body, and choroid of the eye.

Antibodies: Protein molecules that are produced by plasma cells and react with a specific antigen.

Antibody: Glycoprotein molecule, also known as an *immunoglobulin,* that is produced by B lymphocytes that bind antigens with a high degree of specificity and affinity. Antibodies neutralize antigens, activate complement, and promote phagocytosis and the destruction of microbes.

Anticipatory guidance: Psychologic preparation of a person to help relieve fear and anxiety of an event expected to be stressful. An example of anticipatory guidance is the preparation of a child for surgery by explaining what will happen and what it will feel like and by showing equipment or the area of the hospital where the child will be. It is also used to prepare parents for the normal growth and development of their child.

Anticoagulant: Drug that delays or prevents coagulation of blood.

Antifungal agents: Agents that inhibit, control, or kill fungi. *Candida albicans* is the most common yeastlike fungus that occurs in or near the oral cavity.

Antigen: Molecule that binds to an antibody or a T-cell antigen receptor to induce an immune response.

Antimicrobial agent: Substance that kills or inhibits the growth or replication of microorganisms.

Antimicrobial soap: Detergent that contains an antiseptic agent.

Antiphospholipid antibody syndrome: Syndrome exhibited by high titers of circulating antibodies directed against anionic phospholipids. These antibodies interfere with the assembly of phospholipid complexes and inhibit coagulation in vitro. These antibodies induce a hypercoagulable state *in vivo.*

Antiseptic: Germicide used on skin or living tissue for the purpose of inhibiting or destroying microorganisms (e.g., alcohols, chlorhexidine, chlorine, hexachlorophene, iodine, chloroxylenol [PCMX], quaternary ammonium compounds, triclosan).

Anxiety: Diffuse emotional reaction disproportional to the issue at hand and typically directed at future problems and not toward present circumstances.

Apex: Anatomical end of a tooth root.

Apexification: Process in which an environment is created in the root canal and periapical tissues after the death of the pulp, which allows a calcified barrier to form across the open apex.

Apexogenesis: Normal development of the apex of a root of a tooth.

Aphthous ulcers: Recurring condition that is characterized by the eruption of painful sores (commonly called *canker sores*) on the mucous membranes of the mouth. The cause is unknown, but evidence suggests that aphthous ulcers are an immune reaction. Heredity, some foods, overenthusiastic toothbrushing, and emotional stress are also possible causes.

Apical fibers: Fibers that pertain to the periodontal ligament. These fibers radiate around the apex of the tooth at approximately right angles to their cementum attachment, extending into the bone at the bottom of the alveolus. These fibers resist forces that may lift the tooth from the socket and also help stabilize the tooth against tilting movements.

Area specific: Specific area on the tooth or a specific group of teeth. For example, an area-specific dental instrument indicates the instrument can be used only on a specific tooth surface).

Arkansas stone: Type of sharpening stone made of natural stone used to sharpen periodontal instruments.

Arrested caries: Dental decay in which the area of decay has stopped progressing and infection is not present but in which the demineralized area in the tooth remains.

Arthrograms: Radiograph of a joint usually with the introduction of a contrast compound into the joint capsule. In dentistry, an arthrogram usually involves the temporomandibular joint.

Asbestosis: Inflammation or fibrosis (or both) of the lungs caused by inhalation of asbestos fibers, sometimes complicated by pleural mesothelioma or bronchogenic carcinoma.

Aspiration: Ingestion of a foreign body into the airway tree; aspiration is also negative pressure in a hypodermic syringe.

Assessment: Evaluation of a potential or actual problem.

Astraphobia: Fear of thunder, lightning, winds, and heavy rain.

Atherosclerotic plaque: Yellowish deposits containing cholesterol, lipids, and lipophages that form in the intima and inner media of large- and medium-sized arteries.

Atrial arrhythmia: Abnormal cardiac rhythm or disturbance of rhythm that occurs in an atrium or heart chamber.

Atrophic: Characterized by a wasting of tissues, usually associated with general malnutrition or a specific disease state.

Attached gingiva: Gingiva that tightly adheres to the alveolar bone around the roots of the teeth.

Attachment apparatus: General term used to designate the cementum, periodontal ligament, and alveolar bone.

Attending: Paying attention to a patient. It involves observation, warmth, empathy, and interest.

Attrition: Wearing away of a tooth surface as a result of tooth-to-tooth contact.

Auscultation: Process of determining the condition of various parts of the body by listening to the sounds they emit.

Autoantibody: Antibody specific for a self-antigen.

Autoimmune: Pertaining to the development of an immune response to a person's own tissues.

Autoimmune deficiency syndromes: One of a large group of diseases that is characterized by the subversion or alteration of the function of the immune system of the body.

Autoimmune disease: Disease caused by a breakdown of self-tolerance, during which the immune system responds to self-antigens and mediates cell and tissue damage. Autoimmune diseases can be systemic or are organ specific.

Avoidant personality disorder: Long-standing pattern that is characterized by significant social discomfort, fear of negative social evaluation, and timidness. People with this disorder tend to be socially isolated although they desire to be liked by others and are often hurt by even the slightest sign of disapproval.

Avulsed: Torn away; extracted by force.

B

B Lymphocyte: The only cell that is capable of producing antibody molecules and participates in the humoral immune response. B lymphocytes are formed in the bone marrow; on maturation, B lymphocytes are found in lymphoid tissues, in bone marrow, and in the circulation.

BANA: Acronym for *benzoyl-arginine napthylamide,* which is an enzyme-based assay.

Basal lamina: Superficial portion of the basement membrane.

Bass method: Refers to a toothbrushing method named for Dr. C.C. Bass, an early pioneer in preventive dentistry. The Bass technique is the most generally recommended method for patients with and without routine periodontal involvement.

Battered child syndrome: Specific injury patterns that involve the skin and skeletal system and internal organ damage of a child.

Battery: Committing bodily harm to another individual. Battery can be a civil or criminal offense.

Beliefs: Concepts believed or accepted as true.

Beneficence: Promotion of well-being of both individuals and the public by engaging in health promotion and disease prevention activities.

Benign: Not malignant or recurrent; remains localized; favorable for recovery.

Beveled edge: Design feature of specific periodontal instruments in which the toe is flat and angled.

Bidi: Crude, unprocessed form of cigarette commonly manufactured in India. Cut tobacco is rolled in a temburni leaf and secured with a thread. Pronounced *bee-dee.*

Bidigital palpation: Palpation of the tissue with two fingers.

Bifurcation: Site where a single structure divides into two parts, as in two roots of a tooth.

Bilateral: Having or pertaining to two sides.

Bimanual palpation: Examination of soft tissue between the hands.

Bioburden: Microbiological load (i.e., number of viable organisms in or on an object or surface) or organic material on a surface or object before decontamination, or sterilization. Also known as *bioload* or *microbial load.*

Biocentric technique: Technique used by a dental professional to position the body while seated in the dental chair.

Biocompatibility: Degree to which the body's defense system tolerates the presence of foreign material. If something is biocompatible, then no toxic or injurious effects occur on biological function.

Biofeedback: Instrumental process or technique of learning voluntary control over automatically regulated body functions.

Biologic width: Combined width of connective tissue and epithelial attachment superior to the crestal bone.

Biomedical database: Database containing citations, abstracts, and/or full text of research articles that is relevant to the biomedical professions.

Biopsy: Removal and examination, usually microscopic, of tissue from the living body. A biopsy is usually performed to determine whether a tumor is malignant or benign.

Biopsychosocial: Pertaining to the complex of biological, psychologic, and sociologic aspects of life.

Bipolar mood disorder: Mood disorder characterized by episodes of mania and depression.

Bis-GMA: Acronym for *bisphenol A-glycidyl methacrylate.*

Bite-wing image: Intraoral image that is used to examine the interproximal areas of the maxillary and mandibular teeth.

Blepharitis: Inflammatory condition of the lash follicles and meibomian glands of the eyelids, characterized by swelling, redness, and crusts of dried mucus on the lids.

Bond: Linkage or adhesive force among atoms, as in a compound.

Bone: Rigid calcified connective tissue.

Borderline personality disorder: Enduring pattern of instability of mood, self-image, and interpersonal relationships. Frantic efforts often characterize this disorder to avoid real or perceived abandonment. Individuals with this disorder often hold views of significant others that vacillate between unrealistically positive and negative extremes.

Branchial cleft cyst: Typically occurs as the persistence of the second branchial groove, which forms a space lined by squamous epithelium. A branchial cleft cyst is most commonly observed in children younger than 10 years of age.

Breach of duty: Failure to observe the legal and ethical duties as described by law.

Brown spot lesion: Decalcification of enamel discolored by environmental pigmentation.

Bruit: Abnormal blowing sound or murmur heard during auscultation of a carotid artery, organ, or gland, such as the liver or thyroid.

Bruxism: Involuntary grinding or clenching of the teeth that damages both tooth surface and periodontal tissues.

Buccal: Pertaining to or adjacent to the cheek.

Buccal frenula: Area that passes from the oral mucosa of the outer surface of the maxillary arch to the inner surface of the cheek.

Buccal mucosa: Mucosa that lines the inner cheek.

Buccinator: Main muscle of the cheek. It is 1 of the 12 muscles of the mouth. The buccinator, innervated by buccal branches of the facial nerve, compresses the cheek, acting as an important accessory muscle of mastication by holding food on the chewing surfaces of the teeth.

Bulimia nervosa: Type of eating disorder characterized by episodes of binge eating, followed by purging.

Bulimic: Pertaining to bulimia.

Bupropion: Nonnicotine aid to smoking cessation originally developed and marketed as an antidepressant agent. Bupropion is chemically unrelated to other known antidepressant agents.

Burning mouth syndrome: Burning sensation in one or several parts of the mouth that often occurs with no obvious cause.

Burnished calculus: Extrinsic tooth deposit that has been smoothed by improper instrument adaptation, dullness, or inadequate pressure on the working stroke.

Burnishing: Smoothing the surface of a dental amalgam after initial carving or adapting margins of gold restorations by rubbing with a broad-surfaced metal instrument. Burnishing also refers to the rubbing of a medication into the dentinal tubules.

C

Calculus: Mineralized, hard deposits developed from plaque biofilm and salivary salts found on tooth surfaces above and below the gingiva and on dental appliances.

Calibration: Process of measuring or calibrating against an established standard, such as a deciliter or kilogram. Calibration is also applied to the process by which consistency is established among examiners.

Cancer: Neoplasm characterized by the uncontrolled growth of anaplastic cells that tend to invade surrounding tissue and to metastasize to distant body sites; any of a large group of neoplastic diseases characterized by the presence of malignant cells.

Candidiasis: Fungal infection caused by *Candida albicans* that appears as thrush or denture stomatitis in the mouth.

Cannula: Narrow-bore (metal) cylinder similar in appearance and size to a needle that permits entry of a fluid into a body opening.

Capillary action: Surface force that draws aqueous liquids into and along the lumen of a capillary tube.

Carcinoma: Malignant tumor of epithelial origin.

Cariogenic: Tending to produce dental caries.

Carious lesion: Tooth tissue that has sustained a loss of function or a discontinuity caused by dental caries or decay.

Carotid artery: Either of the two main right and left arteries of the neck.

Case-controlled studies: Retrospective studies in which participants who already have a certain condition or disease are compared with a representative group of disease-free individuals (control participants) who do not have the condition or disease. Case-controlled studies are less reliable than either randomized controlled trials or cohort studies. Simply because a statistical relationship exists between two conditions does not mean that one condition actually caused the other.

Case series and case report: Collection of reports on the treatment of several patients or a report on a single patient. Case series and case reports have no statistical validity because they do not use a specific research design to report observations and do not use a control group with which to compare outcomes. However, case series and reports can be extremely important in identifying new health concerns and generating hypotheses.

Casts: Gelled protein in the renal tubules that become molded to the tubular lumen.

Catabolism: Breakdown of complex compounds into simpler ones in the body.

Catatonia: Motor symptoms that include either immobility and extreme muscular rigidity or overactivity.

Catatonic type: Type of schizophrenia that is characterized by symptoms of motor immobility or excessive and purposeless motor activity.

Cationic: Pertaining to a positively charge ion.

Causal factors: Factors or variables that directly cause an event to occur.

Cavitation: Formation of cavities in the body or any cavity in the body, such as the pleural cavities.

Cavity sealers, liners, bases: Materials placed over the pulpal area of the preparation to soothe irritated or sensitive pulp.

Cavosurface: Surface of a cavity, such as in a tooth.

Cellular cementum: Outer layers of cementum that contain embedded cementocytes.

Cementum: Thin calcified tissue of ectomesenchyme origin that covers the root of a tooth. Colony-forming units (CFUs) can consist of pairs, chains, clusters, or single cells and are often expressed as CFUs per milliliter (CFUs/mL).

cGy (centigray): Unit of absorbed radiation dose; 1 cGy = 1 rad.

Chancre: Primary lesion of syphilis that is located at the site of entrance of the spirochete into the body and occurs approximately

3 weeks after contact. Chancre begins as a papule and develops into a clean-based shallow ulcer.

Charge-coupled device (CCD): Solid-state image detector that is found in the intraoral sensor in digital radiography.

Charters' method: Method of toothbrushing in which the toothbrush is held horizontally, with the bristles lying against the teeth and gingivae and pointed in a coronal direction at 45 degrees to ensure that the bristles lie half on the teeth and half on the gingivae. A vibratory cycle of a constricted diameter is negotiated, enabling the brush head to move circularly; however, the brush bristles remain fairly stationary while being agitated. The circular vibration loosens debris and pumps the bristles into interproximal areas to massage the tissues.

Charting: Use of a system that allows uniform interpretation of a patient's dental chart information. Symbols are used to indicate certain oral conditions.

Chemokines: Small proteins that act as chemoattractants for leukocytes. Chemokines help control the normal migration of cells through the tissues.

Chemotaxis: Unidirectional movement of white blood cells through the tissue to a site of inflammation. Chemical substances in the tissue attract the cells to migrate in this direction.

Chemotherapeutic: Refers to agents that affect microbial activity. *Chemotherapeutic* is used interchangeably with *pharmacotherapeutics,* which also includes agents that affect host response.

Chemotherapy: Treatment of an illness by chemical means (i.e., by drugs or medications).

Child abuse: Physical, sexual, or emotional maltreatment of a person younger than 18 years of age. Child abuse occurs predominantly with children younger than the age of 3 years. Symptoms include bruises, contusions, medical records of repeated trauma, radiographic evidence of fractures, emotional distress, and failure to thrive.

Chlorhexidine: Disinfectant with broad antibacterial action.

Chronic fatigue syndrome: Debilitating and complex autoimmune disorder characterized by profound fatigue that is not improved with bedrest and is worsened by physical or mental activity.

Chronic obstructive pulmonary disease (COPD): Progressive and irreversible condition characterized by diminished inspiratory and expiratory capacity of the lungs. An individual with COPD complains of dyspnea with physical exertion, difficulty in inhaling or exhaling deeply, and sometimes expresses a chronic cough.

CINAHL: Acronym for *Cumulative Index to Nursing & Allied Health,* which is a database that provides authoritative coverage of the literature related to nursing and allied health.

Circular fibers: Any one of many fibers in the free gingiva that encircle the teeth.

Circumferential: To carry around the perimeter of the tooth; with respect to scaling, circumferential is also the use of a horizontal stroke that moves around the tooth.

Circumvallate: Surrounded by a trench or ridge.

Claustrophobia: Fear of confinement or closed areas.

Cleft lip: Developmental disturbance of the upper lip caused by the failure of fusion of the maxillary processes with the medial nasal process.

Cleft palate: Developmental disturbance caused by failure of fusion of the palatal shelves with the primary palate or with each other.

Clinical crown: Portion of the anatomical crown that is visible in the oral cavity and not covered by the gingiva.

Clinical trial: Organized study that provides large bodies of clinical data for statistically valid evaluation of treatment.

Clinician: Professional who directly provides healthcare assistance.

Cochrane Collaboration: International endeavor in which clinicians and researchers collaborate to systematically find, appraise, and review available evidence from randomized controlled trials (RCTs) to answer specific clinical questions. The reports are then published and indexed in the Cochrane Database of Systematic Reviews to make this information readily available to clinicians and other decision makers at all levels of healthcare systems (www.cochrange.org/).

Cochrane Database of Systematic Reviews: Database of the full text of the regularly updated systematic reviews prepared by the Cochrane Collaboration.

Cohort studies: Cohort studies make observations about the association between a particular exposure or risk factor (e.g., tobacco) and the subsequent development of a disease or condition (e.g., lung cancer). In these studies, participants do not presently have the condition of interest (e.g., lung cancer) and are followed over time to determine at what frequency the participants develop the disease or condition as compared with a group of control participants who are not exposed to the risk factor (e.g., tobacco) under investigation. If the end point frequency significantly differs between the two groups, then an *association* between exposure and end point is present. A disadvantage of cohort studies is that the conditions of interest can take a long time to develop.

Collagenase: Enzyme that degrades body protein collagen in connective tissue.

Colony-forming unit (CFU): Minimum number (i.e., tens of millions) of separable cells on the surface of or in semisolid agar medium that give rise to a visible colony of progeny.

Commissure: Point of union or junction, especially between two anatomical parts.

Commitment: Civil commitment; the legal proceeding by which an individual is involuntarily confined to a mental hospital or made to undergo outpatient treatment.

Communication: Act of giving or exchanging information through speech, gestures, or written text.

Competence: Measure of the degree of a person's ability to cope with all aspects of the environment.

Complaint: In law, complaint denotes the legal document that is filed with a court of law that initiates a lawsuit against an individual. Complaint also can denote the instance in which an individual contacts a dental board with a concern about treatment of a licensee.

Complete dentures: Removable dental prosthesis that replaces the entire dentition and associated structures of the maxilla or mandible.

Compliance: See *Adherence.*

Composite: Resinous filling material formed by a reaction of an ether bisphenol A with acrylic resin monomers. Composite is initiated by a benzoyl peroxide amine system to which inorganic fillers—glass beads and rods of aluminum, silicate, quartz, or tricalcium phosphate—are added.

Comprehensive dental history: Provides information about previous treatment and dental experiences and is often a component of the health questionnaire.

Comprehensive health history: Collection of data provided by the patient about his or her general health and an important means of preventing medical emergencies.

Computed tomographic (CT) scans: Radiographic body scanning technique in which thin or narrow layer sections of the body can be imaged for diagnostic purposes. The technique uses a computer-linked x-ray machine to focus the radiographs on a particular section of the body to be viewed.

Computer-assisted charting: Digital charting of hard tissue and periodontal findings are printed as computer images.

Condyle: Articular prominence of a bone (e.g., in the mandible, an ellipsoidal projection of bone) usually for articulation with another bone.

Cone-beam imaging: Three-dimensional imaging technique that uses a cone-shaped radiation beam to acquire a digital image.

Confidentiality: A principle that demands that a healthcare professional hold in strict confidence all information gained regarding a patient in the course of treatment.

Congestive heart failure: Abnormal condition characterized by circulatory congestion (i.e., retention of fluids) caused by cardiac or kidney disorders. Congestive heart failure usually develops chronically in association with the retention of sodium and water by the kidneys. Acute congestive heart failure may result from myocardial infarction of the left ventricle.

Congruity: Agreement of verbal and nonverbal cues.

Conjunctiva: Mucous membrane that lines the inner surfaces of the eyelids and anterior part of the sclera.

Connective tissue: Tissue of mesodermal origin that is rich in interlacing processes, which supports or binds together other tissues.

Consistency: Coherence among parts; reliability of successive events or results.

Context: Whole situation or background that is relevant to a particular event.

Contraangle: Angle that deviates from a vertical line.

Controlled delivery device: Refers to delivery systems and agents that are pharmaceutically active for more than 1 day.

Convenience form: Methods and space needed to gain access to the cavity preparation to insert and finish the restorative material.

Coping skills: Mechanisms that assist individuals in adjusting to changes in their lives and environments. Coping skills include helping patients identify sociologic, psychologic, and environmental conditions that stimulate a desire to use tobacco and developing a way to manage each. Examples include helping the patient resolve living with someone who smokes, managing stress, managing weight, and avoiding places and events where tobacco use is common.

Coronal polishing: Polishing of the tooth surface coronal to the gingival margin to remove bacterial plaque biofilm and extrinsic stains. Coronal polishing does not involve calculus removal.

Corrosion: Action, process, or effect of corroding; a product of corroding; the loss of elemental constituents to the adjacent environment.

Cortisol: Endogenous steroid secreted by the adrenal cortex that produces multiple antiinflammatory effects.

Cracked tooth syndrome: Transient acute pain that is difficult to locate and to reproduce and is occasionally experienced while chewing. The syndrome usually exhibits a vertical crack or split that extends across the marginal ridge of a tooth through the crown and into the root involving the pulp. Cracked teeth are visible by transilluminated light or with the use of disclosing dyes.

Cracking: Incomplete splitting or breaking.

Crepitus: Cracking or popping sound, such as that produced by rubbing together fragments of a fractured bone or by moving air in a tissue space.

Crevicular fluid: Fluid that seeps through the crevicular epithelium. Crevicular fluid usually increases in the presence of inflammation.

Cricoid cartilage: Lowest cartilage of the larynx.

Crohn's disease: Chronic inflammatory bowel disease of unknown origin that usually affects the ileum, colon, or another part of the GI tract.

Crossover studies: Multipart research projects, tests, or experiments in which each participant is tested with each or most of the treatments being compared in turn and in random order.

Cross-section: View of an object cut through at a right angle to visualize the object internally.

Crown elongation: Surgical process by which gingival tissue is removed to increase the crown length. Crown elongation is usually performed before a crown preparation to obtain enough tooth structure to allow the crown to seat properly.

Crown fracture: Microscopic or macroscopic cleavage in the coronal portion of a tooth.

Cultural sensitivity: Recognition, understanding, and consideration of customs, norms, and behaviors different from an individual's own.

Culture: Ideas, customs, and skills of a given group of people.

Curet: Periodontal scaling instrument designed to remove calculus from above and below the gingival margin and to remove endotoxins from the root surface.

Curing: To process a material from a plastic or raw state to a hard state or finish, usually by means of heat or chemical treatment such as polymerization.

Cushing's disease (primary aldosteronism): Complex syndrome associated with an excess of adrenal steroids of all types that results from hyperplasia of the adrenal cortex, malignant neoplasms, pituitary basophilia, or prolonged administration of adrenal cortical thyroid hormone. Manifestations include hypertension, buffalo obesity, diabetes mellitus, osteoporosis, purple striae of the skin in areas of tension, and disorders of glucose tolerance.

Cusp fracture: Crack or break in a notably pointed or rounded eminence on or near the masticating surface of a tooth.

Custodial care: Services and care of a nonmedical nature given to an individual to care for another on a long-term basis.

Custom fabricated: Prosthesis made specifically for an individual, based on an individual's specific anatomy.

Cutting edge: Found on the working end of periodontal scaling instruments. The joining of the face of the blade with the lateral side of the working end forms the cutting edge.

Cyanosis: Characteristic bluish tinge or color of the skin and mucous membranes associated with the reduction in hemoglobin as a result of inadequate respiratory change.

Cycles per second (cps): Unit of measurement of wave frequency equal to 1 cycle per second; also called *hertz*.

Cynophobia: Fear of dogs.

Cysts: Abnormal pathologic sacs or cavities that are lined with epithelium and are enclosed in a connective tissue capsule.

Cytokines: One of a large group of low–molecular-weight proteins secreted by various cell types. Cytokines are involved in cell-to-cell communication, coordination of antibody and T-cell immune interactions, and amplification of immune reactivity. Cytokines include colony-stimulating factors; interferons; interleukins; and lymphokines, which are secreted by lymphocytes.

Cytotoxic T cell: Specialized type of T lymphocyte that kills invading organisms by secreting toxic substances directly into the microorganism or by secreting perforans, which are proteins that create holes in the cell membrane of the organism, allowing for fluid influx that eventually kills the organism. These cells are also known as *killer cells* and are effective at destroying viruses, cancerous and foreign cells, and bacteria.

D

Darkfield microscopy: Examination with a darkfield microscope, in which the specimen is illuminated by a peripheral light source.

Organisms in specimens that have been prepared for use with a darkfield microscope appear to glow against a dark background.

Debonding: Removal of the attachment and all adhesive resin from the tooth and restoration of the surface as closely as possible to its pretreatment condition without inducing iatrogenic damage.

Decontamination: Use of physical or chemical means to remove, inactivate, or destroy pathogens on a surface or item so that they are no longer capable of transmitting infectious particles; the surface or item is rendered safe for handling, use, or disposal.

Defendant: Individual or party against whom a lawsuit for recovery is brought in a civil case, or the accused in a criminal case.

Delivery system: Means by which an agent is made available to the body, which includes the drug carrier, route, and target.

Demineralization: Removal of minerals from tooth structures.

Demophobia: Fear of crowds.

Dental caries: Infectious disease that results in the demineralization of teeth by microbial acids.

Dental history: Record of all aspects of a person's oral health, previous evaluations, and treatments, as well as the state of general physical and mental health.

Dental neglect: Lack of attendance to oral care needs.

Dental sealant: Plastic film coating that is applied to pits and fissures of teeth to prevent plaque biofilm, food, and bacteria from entering.

Dental trauma: Result of injury by force to the oral cavity.

Dental treatment water: Nonsterile water used during dental treatment, including irrigation of nonsurgical operative sites and cooling of high-speed rotary and ultrasonic instruments.

Dentifrice: Pharmaceutical abrasive preparation provided as a paste, gel, or powder and used in conjunction with a toothbrush to clean and polish the teeth.

Dentin: Portion of the tooth that lies subjacent to the enamel and cementum. Dentin consists of an organic matrix on which mineral (calcific) salts are deposited. It can be pierced by tubules that contain filamentous protoplasmic processes of the odontoblasts that line the pulpal chamber and canal. Dentin has a mesodermal origin.

Dentinal hypersensitivity: Common intermittent pain sensation that affects many people when they eat or drink or touch the teeth. The pain can be caused by mechanical, chemical, thermal, or bacterial stimuli.

Dentinal tubule: Microscopic channel that extends from the pulp through the dentin.

Dentoalveolar (dentoperiosteal) fibers: Fibers that extend facially and lingually from the cementum. These fibers pass over the crest of the alveolar bone and then insert into the periosteum of the alveolar process. Their primary function is to support the tooth and gingiva.

Denture adhesive: Material that is used to adhere a denture to the oral mucosa.

Denture stomatitis: Irritation and inflammation of the palate covered by the denture.

Dependence: Compulsive reliance on a drug after a period of use, with consequences of use being, in part, adverse.

Dependent personality disorder: Pattern of submissive and dependent behavior. Those who exhibit this disorder depend on others for advice and reassurance and often have difficulty making everyday decisions on their own.

Depression: Mood disorder characterized by feelings of profound sadness, despair, loss of energy, sleeping difficulties, and change in eating habits that are persistent and significantly interfere with social, work, and personal activities.

Dermoid cyst: Tumor derived from embryonic tissues that consist of a fibrous wall lined with epithelium and a cavity containing fatty material, hair, teeth, bits of bone, and cartilage.

Desensitizing: Deprivation of sensation; paralyzing a sensory nerve by section or blocking.

Diabetes mellitus (DM): Chronic syndrome of impaired carbohydrate, protein, and fat metabolism owing to insufficient secretion of insulin or to target tissue insulin resistance. DM occurs in two major forms: type 1 or type 2, which differ in cause, pathologic characteristics, genetics, age of onset, and treatment.

Diapedesis: Process by which white blood cells leave a blood vessel by squeezing through pores in the walls of the vessel.

Diastema: Space between teeth that is *not* the result of a missing tooth.

DICOM: Acronym for *digital imaging* and *communications* in *medicine.*

Differential diagnosis: Distinguishing between two diseases or among several diseases with similar symptoms by systemically comparing signs and symptoms.

Diffuse scleroderma: Form of systemic scleroderma characterized by sudden skin thickening throughout the body in a symmetrical pattern accompanied by organ damage.

Digastrics: Having two bellies. In dentistry, digastrics refers to the anterior belly and posterior belly of the facial nerve (cranial nerve VII). The anterior belly originates from the lower border of the mandible, and the posterior belly originates from the mastoid process of the temporal bone.

Digital format: Image composed of pixels.

Digital radiography: Filmless imaging system that uses a sensor and presents the image through a computer.

Diopter magnification: Magnification device that helps the eyes focus at a close range. Diopter magnification is available in three basic types: (1) hand held, (2) headband, and (3) clip on. Diopter magnification is also called *first generation.*

Discipline: Corrective action taken by a state dental board against a licensee.

Disclosing tablet: Coloring agent that, when chewed, adheres to the teeth to reveal dental plaque biofilm.

Disclosure: Act of revealing facts that are unknown or not understood.

Discoid lupus: Condition confined to the skin, with skin lesions and oral lesions that are a mixture of inflammation, ulceration, keratosis, and atrophy.

Discretionary calorie allowance: Number of calories beyond the amount needed for growth, maintenance, and repair. All calories in candy, soft drinks, alcohol, and solid fats are discretionary calories.

Disease: Abnormal body condition that impairs functioning. Disease exhibits a group of clinical signs, symptoms, and laboratory findings distinctive to a sickness.

Disease prevention: Activities designed to protect patients or other members of the public from actual or potential health threats and their harmful consequences.

Disinfectant: Chemical agent used on inanimate objects (e.g., floors, walls, sinks) to destroy virtually all recognized pathogenic microorganisms but not necessarily all microbial forms (e.g., bacterial endospores). The U.S. Environmental Protection Agency (EPA) groups disinfectants on the basis of whether the product label claims limited, general, or hospital disinfectant capabilities.

Disinfection: Destruction of pathogenic and other kinds of microorganisms by physical or chemical means. Disinfection is less lethal than sterilization because it destroys the majority of microorganisms.

Disorder: Abnormal state of mind or body.

Distance: Comfortable distance or space between communicants.

Distance learning: Learning derived from a source that is not originating in the learner's physical presence.

Distraction: In dentistry, an unusual width of the dental arch; the placement of the teeth or other maxillary or mandibular structures farther than normal from the median plane.

Documentation: Act or instance of furnishing or authenticating with documents. Process by which events and words or images or both are recorded to reflect the aspects of preventive or therapeutic care.

Dorsal surface: Pertaining to the back or to the posterior part of a surface.

Double-blind design: Experimental design for drug testing in which neither the patients receiving the drugs nor the individuals conducting the test know which participants are receiving a new drug and which are receiving a placebo or sugar pill.

Drifted teeth: Teeth that have migrated from their normal positions in the dental arches as a result of factors such as loss of proximal support, loss of functional antagonists, occlusal traumatic tooth relationships, inflammatory and retrograde changes in the attachment apparatus, and oral habits.

Droplet nuclei: Particles less than 5 mcm in diameter formed by dehydration of airborne droplets containing microorganisms that can remain suspended in the air for long periods.

Droplets: Small particles of moisture (e.g., spatter) generated when a person coughs or sneezes or when water is converted to a fine mist by an aerator or showerhead. These particles, intermediate in size between drops and droplet nuclei, can contain infectious microorganisms and tend to settle quickly from the air in such a way that risk of disease transmission is usually limited to those in close proximity to the droplet source.

Duty: Obligation of care that one party owes to another.

Dysarthria: Imperfect articulation of speech caused by disturbances of muscular control that are the result of central or peripheral nervous system damage.

Dysgeusia: Distortion of the sense of taste.

Dyspareunia: Difficult or painful coitus in women.

Dysphagia: Difficulty in swallowing.

Dysplasia: Abnormality of development; in pathologic characteristics, an alteration in size, shape, and organization of the adult cells.

Dyspnea: Difficulty breathing.

Dysuria: Painful urination that is usually caused by a bacterial infection or obstructive condition in the urinary tract.

E

Early childhood caries: Rampant tooth decay associated with inappropriate feeding practices in infants and toddlers.

Ecchymosis: Small, flat, hemorrhagic patch that is larger than a petechia and found on the skin or mucous membranes.

Edema: Swelling that is usually caused by the accumulation of fluid in the tissues.

Edentulism: Condition of being without teeth; usually means having lost all natural teeth.

Efficacy studies: Clinical studies designed to determine the outcome of a specific procedure, drug, intervention, or other similar event to establish whether the entity being observed does what it was intended to do.

Electric pulp tester: Diagnostic device used to determine tooth vitality.

Embolus: Free-floating clot that is caused by high-velocity blood flow dislodging the attached thrombus from the vessel wall. Emboli that travel in the circulation pose a risk for causing adverse ischemic events such as stroke.

Embrasure: Opening, as in a wall. Space between the curved proximal surfaces of the teeth.

Empathy: Ability to share in another's feelings or emotions.

Empowerment: Giving the authority to perform to others; the provision to an individual of what that individual needs to perform a certain act or job.

Enamel: Hard outer layer of the crown of a tooth.

Enamel flaking: Process by which layers of enamel separate and fall off.

Endocrine: Pertaining to a process in which a group of cells secrete into the blood or lymph circulation a substance (e.g., insulin) that has a specific effect on tissues in another part of the body.

Endodontics lesion: Pathologic or traumatic injury or loss of function to the dental pulp, tooth root, or periapical tissue.

Endogenous: Produced within or caused by factors within.

Endosteum: Lining of the medullary cavity of bone.

Enzyme-linked immunosorbent assay (ELISA): Laboratory technique for detecting specific antigens or antibodies that uses enzyme-labeled immunoreactants and a solid-phase binding support, such as a test tube. ELISA is nearly as sensitive as radioimmunoassay and more sensitive than complement fixation, agglutination, and other techniques. ELISA is commonly used in the diagnosis of human immunodeficiency virus (HIV) infections.

Epidermal cyst: Abnormal closed cavity in the epidermis, which is lined by epithelium that contains a liquid or semisolid material.

Epistaxis: Bleeding from the nose.

Epithelium: Basic tissue type that covers and lines the external and internal body surfaces.

Ergonomics: Scientific discipline devoted to the study and analysis of human work, especially as it is affected by individual anatomical, psychologic, and other human characteristics.

Erosion: Chemical or mechanical destruction of tooth tissue. Erosion can create concavities of various shapes at the cementoenamel junction of teeth.

Erythema: Redness of the skin or mucosa.

Erythroplakia: Clinical red mucosal lesions that are not inflammatory and that cannot be otherwise clinically diagnosed by location, specific morphologic structure, or history.

Essential oil: Volatile oil that emits a distinctive odor or flavor.

Esthetics: Branch of philosophy that deals with beauty, especially with the components of color and form.

Estrogen: Natural or artificial substance that induces the development of female sex characteristics.

Estrogenicity: Affects the production, metabolism, and activity of estrogens.

Ethics: Code of morals or standards of conduct. Each health profession defines professional ethics in written standards of professional behavior (see Box 3-3).

Ethyl chloride: Colorless liquid local anesthetic of short duration. Its action is accomplished by rapid vaporization from the skin, producing superficial freezing. Ethyl chloride is occasionally used in inhalation therapy as a rapid, fleeting general anesthetic, comparable with nitrous oxide but somewhat more dangerous.

Evidence-based decision making (EBDM): Formalized process and structure for solving clinical problems to allow the best scientific evidence to be considered along with clinical expertise and patient values when making patient care decisions.

Evidence-based decision-making (EBDM) skills: Abilities to define patient-centered questions, to locate valid evidence to answer the questions, to appraise critically the evidence for its validity and applicability, to apply the evidence correctly to decisions made about patient care, and to evaluate performance of the process.

Evidence-based journals: Journals that publish concise summaries of original research articles and of systematic reviews selected from the biomedical literature with the goal of providing practitioners with clinically relevant evidence in a user-friendly format. Typically, a one- to two-page structured abstract along with an expert commentary is provided, highlighting the most relevant and practical information.

Evidence-based practice: Provision of clinical care based on documented efficacious treatment, procedures, and techniques.

Evidence-based teaching: Teaching using documented effective methodologies to deliver content based on efficacious clinical outcomes.

Exfoliating: Peeling and shedding of tissue cells. In dentistry, exfoliating refers to the loss of the primary dentition.

Exocrine gland: Gland having a duct associated with it.

Exofoliative cytology: Nonsurgical technique that is helpful in the diagnosis of oral lesions. The surface of the lesion is scraped or wiped to gather a sample of the cells. The cells are then spread on a glass slide for microscopic examination.

Exogenous: Originating outside or caused by factors outside.

Exophthalmos: Protrusion of the eyeballs caused by the swelling of the tissues surrounding the orbits and degeneration of the ocular muscles; an autoimmune disease process associated with Graves' disease.

Explorer: Diagnostic instrument used to examine and evaluate tooth structure irregularities and defective margins of restorations.

Exposure: Concept that an individual may be vulnerable to legal action.

Extension for prevention: Principle of cavity preparation as stated by G.V. Black in 1891. To prevent the recurrence of decay, Black advocated the extension of the preparation subgingivally, axially, and occlusally into an area that is readily polished and cleaned.

External auditory meatus: Canal of the external ear that consists of bone and cartilage and extends from the auricle to the tympanic membrane.

Extrinsic: Derived from or situated on the outside; external.

Eye loupes: Convex lenses used for low magnification of minute objects at close range; they may be monocular, binocular, or mounted on spectacles.

F

Face: In dentistry, portion of the working end of a periodontal scaling instrument that joins with the lateral side to create the cutting edge.

Facet joint: Synovial joint between articular processes (zygapophytes) of the vertebrae. Also called *zygapophyseal joint.*

Facial prosthesis: Removable prosthesis that artificially replaces a portion of the face lost as a result of surgery, trauma, or congenital absence.

Fainting (syncope): Loss of consciousness because of transient cerebral hypoxia. A sensation of lightheadedness usually precedes fainting, and lying down or sitting with the head between the knees may often prevent fainting. Fainting may be caused by many different factors, including emotional stress, vascular pooling in the legs, or sudden change in environmental temperature or body position.

Fallible: Liable to be mistaken; capable of error.

Family history: An essential part of a patient's medical history in which he or she is asked about the health of members of the immediate family in a series of specific questions to discover any disorders to which the patient may be susceptible. Hereditary and familial diseases are especially noted. The age and health of each person, age at death, and causes of death are charted. The family health history is obtained from the patient or family in the initial interview and becomes a part of the permanent record.

Fauces: Opening posteriorly from the oral cavity proper into the pharynx.

Fear: Emotion, generally considered negative and unpleasant, that is a reaction to a real or threatened danger; fright. Fear is distinguished from anxiety, which is a reaction to an unreal or imagined danger.

Feedback: Loop of command action. An idea is demonstrated, questions are posed, or input is solicited; then action is accomplished.

Fermentable carbohydrate: Element that can be metabolized by bacteria in plaque biofilm to decrease the pH to a level at which demineralization occurs.

Fiberoptic examination: Technical process by which an internal organ or cavity can be viewed through the use of glass or plastic fibers to transmit light through a specially designed tube and to reflect a magnified image.

Fibrinolysis: Continual process of fibrin decomposition by fibrinolysin, which is the normal mechanism for the removal of small fibrin clots. Fibrinolysis is stimulated by anoxia, inflammatory reactions, and other kinds of stress.

Fibromyalgia: Form of nonarticular rheumatism characterized by musculoskeletal pain, spasm and stiffness, fatigue, and severe sleep disturbance. Common sites of pain or stiffness can be palpated in the lower back, neck, shoulder region, arms, hands, knees, hips, thighs, legs, and feet. These sites are known as *trigger points.*

File: Periodontal scaling instrument designed to crush and remove heavy calculus deposits.

Filiform: Thread shaped; in dentistry, filiform refers to threadlike elevations that cover most of the tongue's surface.

Filled resin: Contains fillers such as glass, quartz, and silica. Filled resin is used in composite restorations to make sealants more resistant to wear.

Fixed bridge: Partial denture that is luted or otherwise securely retained to natural teeth, tooth roots, and/or dental implant abutments that furnish the primary support for the prosthesis.

Flap (periodontal or surgical): Oral tissue that has, by incision, been partially detached from its surrounding vasculature and nutrient supply.

Floss: Waxed or unwaxed dental tape that is used to clean the interproximal tooth surfaces, subgingivally and supragingivally.

Fluconazole: Oral antifungal tablet used in the treatment of oral candidiasis.

Fluctuant: Pertaining to a wavelike motion that is detected when a structure that contains a liquid is palpated.

Focal trough: Image layer that is used in extraoral radiography in which structures are reasonably well defined.

Folate: Salt of folic acid; any of a group of substances found in some foods and in mammalian cells that act as co-enzymes and promote the chemical transfer of single carbon units from one molecule to another. Folates are often used as a dietary supplement during pregnancy to prevent birth defects such as spina bifida.

Follow-up: Scheduled contacts made by the clinician with patients.

Fones' method: Toothbrushing technique named after Dr. Alfred Fones.

Foramen cecum: Small pitlike depression located where the sulcus terminalis points backward toward the pharynx.

Fordyce granules: Normal variations sometimes appearing on the buccal mucosa and lips that are caused by the entrapment of fat cells clinically observed as small yellowish elevations.

Fractionation: Division of the total dose of radiation into small doses given at intervals.

Free gingival groove: Shallow line or depression on the gum surface at the junction of the free and attached gingiva.

Free gingival margin: Unattached gingiva surrounding the teeth in a collarlike fashion and demarcated from the attached gingiva by a shallow curvilinear depression that mirrors the gingival margin.

Free soft tissue graft: Living tissue detached from its vascular and nutrient supply, removed from its origin, and transplanted to a recipient site within the oral cavity.

Frena: Restraining portion or structure. See also *Frenum.*

Frenectomy: Excision or removal of a frenum.

Frenum: Fold of mucous membrane attaching the cheeks and lips to the upper and lower arches, in some instances limiting the motions of the lips and cheeks.

Fulcrum: Stabilization of an instrument; the pad of the ring finger serves as a finger rest.

Full denture: Removable dental prosthesis that replaces the entire dentition and associated structures of the maxillae or mandible.

Full gold crown (FGC): Gold crown that completely covers the anatomical crown of an individual tooth to restore the tooth to its original contour and function.

Full-mouth disinfection: Process within a 24-hour period during which the oral cavity is debrided and the oral tissues, including the pharyngeal area, are scrubbed, rinsed, and/or irrigated with an antimicrobial solution. Full-mouth disinfection results in a total bacterial count drop throughout the oral cavity.

Full-thickness periodontal (mucoperiosteal) flap: Surgical flap that includes epithelium, connective tissue, periosteum, and their components. A full-thickness flap reflection exposes the underlying osseous structure.

Fungiform: Papilla on the dorsum of the tongue that is shaped like a mushroom.

Furcation: Area between two or more root branches before they divide from the root trunk.

G

GV Black caries classification: Dental caries and cavity classification system developed by GV Black that remains in use today. Carious lesions are categorized as Class I, II, III, IV, V, or VI.

Galvanic reaction: Shock that occurs when an electrical current is present in the oral cavity as a result of the coming together of several conditions: (1) saliva that contains salt, which makes it a good conductor of electricity; (2) two metallic components of different composition that act as the battery (two restorations or a metal object such as a fork placed in the mouth); (3) electrical current, which occurs through the saliva.

Generalized anxiety disorder: Persistent and excessive anxiety or worry that lasts for at least 6 months.

Genome: Complete set of genes in the chromosomes of each cell of a specific organism.

Genuine: Sincere, frank, and honest.

Geometric angle: Figure formed by two lines that extend from the same point.

Geometric charting forms: Charting forms that use a geometric design to represent a tooth with each surface represented.

Gingiva: Mucous membrane tissue that immediately surrounds a tooth.

Gingiva or implant interface: Space where the implant and gingival tissue intersect.

Gingival recession: Apical migration of the gingiva from the cementoenamel junction, resulting in root surface exposure.

Gingival sulcus: Shallow furrow formed from the gingival margin to the junctional epithelium between the tooth and sulcular epithelium.

Gingivitis: Inflammation of the gingiva.

Glass ionomer: Cement, luting, or restorative agent consisting of an acid-soluble glass, polyacrylic acid, and water that sets via an acid-base reaction.

Glomerulonephritis: Form of kidney disease characterized by inflammation of the capillary loops in the renal glomeruli.

Glossitis: Inflammation of the tongue.

Glossodynia: Painful sensations in the tongue; a sensation of burning in the tongue; a sore tongue.

Glucosuria: Glucose in the urine.

Glycosaminoglycans: Any of several high–molecular-weight linear heteropolysaccharides that have disaccharide-repeating units that contain an *N*-acetylhexosamine and a hexose or hexuronic acid. Either or both residues may be sulfated.

Glycosylated hemoglobin: Hemoglobin A molecule with a glucose group on the *N*-terminal valine amino acid unit of the beta chain. The glycosylated hemoglobin concentration represents the average blood glucose level during the previous several weeks. In controlled DM the concentration of glycosylated hemoglobin is within the normal range, but in uncontrolled cases, the level may be three to four times the normal concentration.

Goal setting: Determination of what a clinician wishes to accomplish, both personally and professionally, based on talents, values, and personal philosophy.

Goiter: Enlarged thyroid gland.

Gold foil (GF): Pure gold that has been thinned to a small thickness and is used in direct gold cavity restorations.

Gold inlay (GI): Intracoronal cast restoration of gold alloy that restores one or more tooth surfaces.

Gold onlay (GO): Extracoronal cast restoration of gold alloy that restores the occlusal surface extending over the cusp and marginal ridges.

Grade: Attempt to describe the extent to which tumor cells resemble their normal counterparts in histologic appearance and biological behavior.

Gram-negative infections: Infections caused by gram-negative bacteria. Some of the most common gram-negative pathogenic bacteria include *Bacteroides fragilis, Brucella abortus, Escherichia coli, Haemophilus influenzae, Klebsiella pneumoniae, Neisseria gonorrhoeae, Proteus vulgaris, Pseudomonas aeruginosa, Salmonella typhi, Shigella dysenteriae,* and *Yersinia pestis.*

Graves' disease: Form of hyperthyroidism caused by autoimmune disease.

Grit: With reference to abrasive agents, grit is the particle size.

Ground substance: Basic substance from which a specific organ or kind of tissue develops.

Growth factors: Molecules that initiate cellular signaling mechanisms and regulate growth, proliferation, and maturation of cells.

Guardian ad litem: Individual appointed by a court of law to act on behalf of another (e.g., a minor) who is not legally capable of making decisions.

Gutta-percha: Plastic type of filling material used in endodontic treatment.

Gynecomastia: Abnormal enlargement of one or both breasts in a man.

H

Halitosis: Offensive odor of the breath resulting from local and metabolic conditions (e.g., poor oral hygiene, periodontal disease, sinusitis, tonsillitis, suppurative bronchopulmonary disease, acidosis, uremia).

Hand hygiene: Applies to handwashing, antiseptic handwash, antiseptic hand rub, or surgical hand antisepsis.

Handle: Portion of a dental hygiene instrument that is held by the clinician.

Haptephobia: Fear of being touched.

Hard palate: Anterior portion of the palate.

Hashimoto's thyroiditis: Most common autoimmune inflammatory thyroid disease that frequently exists with other autoimmune diseases; inflammation of the thyroid gland associated with hypothyroidism.

Health: Complete state of physical, mental, emotional, spiritual, and social well-being and not simply the absence of infirmity. Health includes actions taken to protect or enhance health and legal, fiscal, educational, and social measures.

Health education: Any combination of learning experiences designed to facilitate voluntary actions conducive to health.

Health promotion: Any planned combination of educational, political, regulatory, and organizational support for actions and conditions of living conducive to the health of individuals, groups, or communities. One component of health promotion also includes actions to protect or enhance health and legal, fiscal, educational, and social measures.

Helper T cell: Specialized type of T lymphocyte whose main effector functions are to activate macrophages in cell-mediated immune responses and to promote B-cell antibody production in humoral immune responses.

Hematuria: Blood in the urine.

Hemidesmosomal attachment: Mechanism that attaches epithelial cells to the tooth surface.

Hemodialysis: Procedure in which impurities or wastes are removed from the blood. Hemodialysis is used to treat renal failure and various toxic conditions.

Hemolysis: Breakdown of red blood cells and the release of hemoglobin that normally occur at the end of the life span of a red cell.

Hemostasis: Stoppage or cessation of bleeding.

Hepatitis: Inflammation of the liver.

Hepatitis B e antigen (HBeAg): Secreted product of the nucleocapsid gene of hepatitis B virus (HBV) found in serum during acute and chronic HBV infection. Its presence indicates that the virus is replicating.

Hepatitis B immune globulin (HBIG): Product used for prophylaxis against HBV infection. HBIG is prepared from plasma containing high titers of hepatitis B surface antibody (anti-HBs) and provides protection for 3 to 6 months.

Hepatitis B surface antibody (anti-HBs): Protective antibody against hepatitis B surface antigen (HBsAg). Presence in the blood can indicate past infection with and immunity to HBV.

Hepatitis B surface antigen (HBsAg): Serologic marker on the surface of HBV detected in high levels during acute or chronic hepatitis. The body normally produces antibodies to surface hepatitis B vaccine.

Herniated or slipped disc: Rupture of the fibrocartilage surrounding an intervertebral disc, releasing the nucleus pulposus that cushions the vertebrae above and below. The resultant pressure on spinal nerve roots may cause considerable pain and damage to the nerves. A herniated or slipped disc most frequently occurs in the lumbar region.

Hertz (Hz): Unit of frequency equal to 1 cycle per second.

High-level disinfection: Disinfection process that inactivates vegetative bacteria, mycobacteria, fungi, and viruses but not necessarily high numbers of bacterial spores. The U.S. Food and Drug Administration (FDA) further defines a high-level disinfectant as a sterilant used for a shorter contact time.

Hirsutism: Increased body or facial hair, which is especially noted in women.

Histoplasmosis: Disease caused by the fungus *Histoplasma capsulatum* that affects the reticuloendothelial system. Ulceration of the oral mucosa may occur.

History of illnesses: Account obtained during the interview with the patient of the onset, duration, and character of the present illness, as well as any acts or factors that aggravate or ameliorate the symptoms. The patient is asked what he or she considers to be the cause of the symptoms and whether a similar condition has occurred in the past.

History of present oral condition: History of the chief concern or complaint.

HIV infection: Infection of the host with the HIV-1.

Honing machine: Bench-type device in which sharpening stones are mechanically rotated across an instrument blade.

Horizontal fibers: Fibers that run at right angles to the long axis of the tooth, from the cementum to the bone. Their primary function is to restrain lateral tooth movement.

Hormonal gingivitis: Inflammation of the gingiva (gums) relating to hormones.

Hormones: Biologically active substances that are released into the circulation and produce an effect in cells that are distant from the site of secretion.

Hospital disinfectant: Germicide registered by the U.S. Environmental Protection Agency (EPA) for use on inanimate objects in hospitals, clinics, dental offices, and other medical-related facilities. Efficacy is demonstrated against *Salmonella choleraesuis, Staphylococcus aureus,* and *Pseudomonas aeruginosa.*

Host response: Immune response of a host when cells receive an invader or insult.

Human immunodeficiency virus (HIV): Retrovirus that causes acquired immunodeficiency syndrome (AIDS).

Human leukocyte antigens (HLAs): Major histocompatibility complex molecules expressed on the surface of human cells.

Hydrodynamic theory: Theory most accepted for the transmission of a pain stimulus with dentinal tubules.

Hydrolysis: Reaction between the ions of salt and those of water to form an acid and a base, one or both of which is only slightly dissociated. Hydrolysis is a process during which a large molecule is split by the addition of water.

Hyoid: Pertaining to the hyoid bone.

Hyperbaric oxygen: Placing a patient in a sealed chamber and administering pure oxygen through a facemask. At the same time, compressed air is introduced into the chamber to raise the atmospheric pressure to several times the normal level, which equalizes the pressure inside and outside the body and thereby floods the tissues with oxygen. An increase in oxygen to the irradiated tissues can temporarily compensate for the reduction in circulation.

Hyperkeratinization: Abnormal thickening of the epithelium from excessive friction, trauma, or use.

Hypertelorism: Abnormally increased distance between two organs or parts. *Orbital* or *ocular hypertelorism* is an abnormally increased distance between the orbits.

Hypertension: Abnormal elevation of systolic or diastolic (or both) arterial pressures.

Hyperthyroidism: Metabolic abnormality that results from an elevation of the thyroid hormone.

Hyperventilation: Abnormally prolonged, rapid, and deep breathing; hyperventilation is also the condition produced by overbreathing of oxygen at high pressures.

Hypnosis: Condition of artificially induced sleep or of a trance resembling sleep induced by drugs, psychologic means, or both. Hypnosis generally creates a condition of heightened suggestibility in the participant.

Hypochromic microcytic anemia: Group of anemias characterized by a decreased concentration of hemoglobin in the red blood cells.

Hypofunction: Diminished or inadequate level of activity of an organ system or its parts.

Hypomineralized: Pertaining to a deficiency of mineral elements in the body.

Hypoplasia: Incomplete development or underdevelopment of an organ or tissue.

Hypothyroidism: Diminished activity of the thyroid gland with decreased secretion of thyroxin that results in a lowered basal metabolic rate, lethargy, sleepiness, dysmenorrhea in women, and tendency toward obesity.

Hypoxia: Low oxygen content or tension.

I

Iatrogenic: An iatrogenic disorder is a condition induced inadvertently by healthcare personnel (HCP), medical (including dental) treatment, or diagnostic procedures, including fears instilled in patients by remarks or questions of examining physicians. Used particularly in reference to an infectious disease or other complication.

Icteric: Jaundiced.

Imaging: Production of diagnostic images, including radiography, ultrasonography, photography, or scintigraphy.

Immune system: Biochemical complex that protects the body against pathogenic organisms and other foreign bodies. The immune system incorporates the humoral immune response, which produces antibodies to react with specific antigens, and the cell-mediated response, which uses T cells to mobilize tissue macrophages in the presence of a foreign body.

Immunity: Resistance to infectious disease. The cells, tissues, and molecules that make up the immune system act together to mediate resistance to disease in a process known as the *immune response*. The function of the immune system is to prevent and eliminate infections.

Immunization: Process by which a person becomes immune or protected against a disease. Vaccination is defined as the process of administering a killed or weakened infectious organism or toxoid; however, vaccination does not always result in immunity.

Immunoassays: Competitive-binding assays in which the binding protein is an antibody.

Immunocompromised: Weakened immune response caused by a disease or an immunosuppressive agent.

Immunoglobulin: Synonymous with antibody.

Immunologic and inflammatory responses: Tissue reactions to an injury or antigen. These responses may include pain, swelling, itching, redness, heat, loss of function, or a combination of these symptoms.

Immunologic tolerance: Lack of response to antigens that is induced by the exposure of lymphocytes to these antigens.

Immunosuppression: Act or action of lowering or reducing the immune response.

Implant abutments: Portions of dental implants that serve to support and retain any prosthesis.

Implant-borne prosthesis: Prosthesis that fits on a dental implant, such as an overdenture.

Implementation: Deliberate action performed to achieve a goal, such as carrying out a plan in the care of a patient.

Implied consent: After agreeing to treatment, the patient is presumed to have consented to all procedures required for such treatment.

In situ: In its normal place; confined to the site of origin.

In vitro: Occurring in a laboratory apparatus.

Inactive caries: Condition in which lesions do not progress; inactive caries may remineralize and appear small on radiographs.

Incidence: Number of times an event occurs.

Incision: Cut or wound created by the separation of adjacent tissue with a sharp instrument.

Incisive canal: Opening in the anterior palate through which the nasopalatine nerve and blood vessels exit.

Incompetent: Individual who does not possess the knowledge or skills necessary to perform a professional function to the expected standard.

India stone: Type of a sharpening stone that is made of man-made materials and is used to sharpen periodontal instruments.

Indices: Methods by which clinical disease parameters are quantitatively recorded.

Inferior: Situated below or lower than a point of reference.

Inflammation: Complex reaction of the innate immune system in vascularized tissues that involves accumulation and activation of leukocytes and plasma proteins at a site of infection, toxin exposure, or cell injury. Inflammation is initiated by changes in blood vessels that promote leukocyte recruitment. Local adaptive immune responses can promote inflammation. Although inflammation serves a protective function in controlling infections and promoting tissue repair, it can also cause tissue damage and disease.

Informed consent: Patient's consent to medical or dental treatment given after the patient understands the nature of his or her condition, treatment options, risks involved in treatment, and risks if no treatment is sought.

Informed refusal: Individual's election not to accept treatment after being fully educated about the risks and benefits associated with the treatment.

Innate immunity: Natural immunity that provides the initial protection against infection that relies on mechanisms that exist before infection. Innate immune responses are capable of rapid response to microbial invasion and react the same way to repeat exposures.

Insulin: Peptide hormone produced in the pancreas by the beta cells in the islets of Langerhans. Insulin regulates glucose metabolism and is the major fuel-regulating hormone.

Insulin-dependent diabetes mellitus (IDDM): Inability to metabolize carbohydrate caused by an absolute insulin deficiency. IDDM occurs in children and adults and is characterized by excessive thirst, increased urination, increased desire to eat, loss of weight, diminished strength, and marked irritability.

Interdental: Between the proximal surfaces of the teeth within the same arch.

Interdental papilla: Projection of the gingiva filling the space between the proximal surfaces of two adjacent teeth.

Interexaminer reliability: Consistency of measurement between two or more examiners who are evaluating the same event.

Interleukins: Large groups of cytokines produced mainly by T cells or in some cases by mononuclear phagocytes or other cells. Most interleukins direct other cells to divide and differentiate. Each acts on a particular group of cells that express receptors specific for that interleukin.

Intermediate-level disinfectant: Liquid chemical germicide registered with the EPA as a hospital disinfectant and with a label claim of potency as tuberculocidal.

Intermediate-level disinfection: Process that inactivates vegetative bacteria, majority of fungi, mycobacteria, and majority of viruses (particularly enveloped viruses) but not bacterial spores.

Internal jugular: One of a pair of veins in the neck. Each internal jugular vein is continuous with the transverse sinus in the posterior part of the jugular foramen at the base of the skull.

International normalized ratio (INR): Laboratory test used to monitor the effects of anticoagulation therapy. The INR test uses the World Health Organization international reference preparation of thromboplastin as the laboratory standard. The INR is the patient's prothrombin time (PT) divided by the mean normal PT for the laboratory (prothrombin time ratio [PTR]) with additional adjustment for the reactivity of the reagents (International Sensitivity Index [ISI]). The INR makes it possible to target the same therapeutic ranges while using different laboratory reagents.

International system: System used in more than one country; in dentistry, the international system is a specific charting system.

Interproximal: Between the proximal surfaces of adjoining teeth.

Interradicular fibers: Fibers that are found only in multirooted teeth. Interradicular fibers run from the cementum of the root and insert into the interradicular septum. Their primary function is to aid in the resistance of tipping and twisting.

Interstitial nephritis: Primary or secondary disease of the renal interstitial tissue.

Interval: Specified length of time between healthcare visits when patients manage their chronic conditions. In periodontal maintenance, the most common interval is 3 months between visits, although any interval should be tailored to the patient's current health status.

Intervention: Step or measure designed to halt or significantly alter the current course of an event.

Intimate: Close physical proximity (0 to 18 inches).

Intraexaminer reliability: Internal consistency of one individual during the rating or evaluation of a specific event more than once.

Intrinsic: Situated entirely within.

Iridocyclitis: Inflammation of the iris and ciliary body of the eye.

Irreversible hydrocolloid impression material: Material that cannot return to the sol state after it becomes a gel. The change in the physical state results from a chemical change in the material.

Irrigation: Flushing of an area. Irrigation can be a steady stream of liquid or it can be pulsed. A daily pulsed or fractionated, intermittent stream of water has been shown to be of therapeutic benefit in the treatment of gingivitis.

ISO: Designation system of the International Standards Organization.

J

Jargon: Vocabulary specific to a profession.

Jugulodigastric: Name for a lymph node, based on its location in the neck.

Junctional epithelium: Single or multiple layer of nonkeratinizing cells that adhere to the tooth surface at the base of the gingival crevice by hemidesmosomes.

Juvenile periodontitis: Distinct form of periodontal disease that may exhibit either localized or generalized inflammatory changes in the periodontium at prepubescence and adolescence.

K

Keratinized: Formation of a protein layer (keratin) on the surface of some epithelia.

Keratoconjunctivitis sicca: Dryness of the cornea caused by a deficiency of tear secretion in which the corneal surface appears dull and rough and the eye feels gritty and irritated.

Ketoacidosis: Accumulation of acid in the body resulting from the accumulation of ketone bodies.

Ketoconazole: Broad-spectrum synthetic antifungal agent applied to the skin to inhibit the growth of dermatophytes and yeasts. It is effective in *Candida* infections and in the treatment of seborrheic dermatitis.

Keyes' technique: Use of salt, baking soda, and hydrogen peroxide to prevent or control periodontal disease.

Knurl: One in a series of small ridges or beads on a metal surface that aids in gripping.

Koch's postulates: Prerequisites for experimentally establishing that a specific microorganism causes a particular disease.

Kretek: Clove- and tobacco-mixed product.

Kyphosis: Abnormal curvature of the spine with the convexity backward.

L

Labial mucosa: Mucosal lining of the inner portions of the lips.

Lactobacillus: Any one of a group of nonpathogenic, gram-positive, rod-shaped bacteria that produce lactic acid from carbohydrates.

Lamina densa: Layer of epithelial basal lamina that appears dark in electron micrographs.

Lamina lucida: Layer of epithelial basal lamina that appears light or clear in electron micrographs.

Lamina propria: Layer of connective tissue that lies just under the epithelium of the mucous membrane.

Lateral: Toward the side.

Lateral jaw: Radiographic image of one side of the jaw obtained via external film placement.

Lateral pressure: Force activated by wrist motion that is applied to secure the instrument's working end against the tooth surface.

Lateral sides: Portion of the working end of a periodontal scaling instrument located on either side of the face. The lateral sides join the face at either side to form the cutting edges.

Legal accountability: Legal responsibility for one's actions.

Leukemia: Condition caused by the uncontrolled production of white blood cells. Leukemia is caused by cancerous mutation of either myelogenous or lymphogenous cells.

Leukocyte: White blood cell.

Leukocytosis: Elevated white cell count that is a characteristic sign of infection. During infection, the bone marrow and lymph tissues increase the production and release the leukocytes, which may elevate the white blood cell count to 30,000 or higher per microliter of blood.

Leukodema: Innocuous oral condition characterized by a filmy, opalescent, white covering of the buccal mucosa that consists of a thickened layer of parakeratotic cells. It is most commonly associated with mechanical and chemical irritation.

Leukopenia: Condition characterized by the reduced production of white blood cells by the bone marrow.

Levels of evidence: Levels, or hierarchy, of evidence that are based on the research design's ability to control for bias and demonstrate cause and effect in humans. Although each level may contribute to the total body of knowledge, not all levels are equally useful in making patient care decisions. Evidence is judged on its methodologic rigor, and the level of evidence is directly related to the type of questions asked, such as those derived from issues of therapy and prevention, diagnosis, etiologic factors, and prognosis. For example, the highest level of evidence associated with questions about therapy or prevention will be from systematic reviews of RCT studies, whereas the highest level of evidence associated with questions about prognosis will be from systematic reviews of inception cohort studies

Liability: Responsibility for a breach of duty.

Libman-Sacks disease: Formation of sterile vegetations on heart valve leaflets made up of fibrin and platelets known as *Libman-Sacks verrucae*. Verrucae cause the valves to thicken and become functionally impaired, often causing regurgitation and increasing the risk for endocarditis.

Licensing examinations: Practical examinations that are administered to graduates of professional schools to determine whether each individual is qualified to practice the profession.

Licensure: Process whereby a competent authority issues permission to perform a certain act or engage in a specific business that would otherwise be unlawful.

Ligaments: Tough, fibrous connective tissue bands that connect bones or support viscera.

Limited scleroderma: Form of systemic scleroderma that affects the skin of the fingers, face, lower arms, and legs; Raynaud's phenomenon commonly occurs.

Line angle: Point at which two lines join; in dentistry, the point at which the facial surface joins to form the mesial surface of a tooth.

Linea alba: White ridge of raised keratinized epithelial tissue on the facial mucosa that extends horizontally at the level where the teeth occlude.

Linear scleroderma: Localized form of scleroderma characterized by single lines or bands of thickened, abnormally colored skin, typically found on the arms, legs, and forehead.

Lingual tonsils: Irregular mass of tonsillar tissue posteriorly located on the lateral surfaces of the tongue.

Lipoma: Benign tumor characterized by fat cells.

Lipopolysaccharides: Part of the outer layer of the cell wall in gram-negative bacteria.

Listening: Element of communication that involves hearing, speaking, and paying attention to the spoken word.

Litigation: Court proceedings to determine legal issues regarding the rights and responsibilities among the parties.

Long axis: Imaginary straight line with respect to which a body is symmetric; the axis of a tooth divides the tooth in half from crown to apex.

Lordosis: Anteroposterior curvature of the spine with the convexity facing forward.

Loss of attachment: Placement of the junctional epithelium that is apical to the cementoenamel junction.

Low-level disinfectant: Liquid chemical germicide registered with the EPA as a hospital disinfectant. The Occupational Safety and Health Administration (OSHA) requires low-level hospital disinfectants to also have a label claim for potency against HIV and HBV if used for disinfecting clinical contact surfaces.

Low-level disinfection: Process that inactivates the majority of vegetative bacteria, certain fungi, and certain viruses but cannot be relied on to inactivate resistant microorganisms.

Lumen: Opening. Oral irrigators have a lumen at the end of the tip or on the side of the tip.

Lupus: Autoimmune disease of the skin and mucous membrane.

Luxation: Dislocation or displacement of the condyle in the temporomandibular fossa or tooth from the alveolus.

Lymph nodes: Bean-shaped bodies grouped in clusters along the connecting lymphatic vessels that are positioned to filter toxic products from the lymph.

Lymphadenectomy: Excision of one or more lymph nodes.

Lymphatic system: Vast, complex network of capillaries, vessels, valves, ducts, nodes, and organs that helps protect and maintain the internal fluid environment of the entire body by producing, filtering, and conveying lymph and by producing various blood cells. The lymphatic network also transports fats, proteins, and other substances to the blood system and restores 60% of the fluid that filters from the blood capillaries into interstitial spaces during normal metabolism.

Lymphocytes: Leukocytes (white blood cells) found in large numbers in lymphoid tissues that contribute to immunity.

Lymphoma: Any neoplasm consisting of lymphoid tissue.

Lysosomes: Intracellular sacs found in the cytoplasm of macrophages that contain toxins used during phagocytosis.

M

Macrophages: Phagocytic leukocytes found in tissues.

Magnetostrictive: Mechanism used to convert electrical energy into ultrasonic movement.

Maintaining competence: Act of keeping one's skills and knowledge current to ensure quality performance.

Major depression: Severe form of depression that interferes with concentration, decision making, and social functioning.

Major histocompatibility complex (MHC) genes: Molecules that encode cytokines and are recognized by T lymphocytes for antigen processing.

Malignant: Cancerous tumor.

Malpractice: Negligent conduct of a professional individual or a breach of a standard of care.

Mandibular: Pertaining to the lower jaw.

Mandibular tori: Bony, hard, painless lesions that attach to the jaws and are frequently lobulated. Mandibular tori are usually bilateral and attach to the mandible, lingual to the bicuspid roots.

Mandrel-mounted stones: Small cylindrical or conical stones mounted to a slow-speed handpiece that is used to sharpen periodontal instruments.

Mania: Mood disturbance characterized by symptoms such as elation, inflated self-esteem, hyperactivity, and accelerated speaking and thinking. Mania is often associated with bipolar disorder.

Marginal breakdown: Breakdown of the integrity of the margin of a restoration, creating a trap for bacterial and potential dental caries activity.

Marginal irrigation: Flushing the pocket area by inserting a soft, flexible rubber tip approximately 3 mm below the gingival margin. Marginal irrigation is used daily at home.

Margination: Phenomenon that occurs when white blood cells, especially neutrophils that have traveled in the blood to the inflamed site, begin to accumulate along the inner walls of the blood vessels.

Masseter: One of the four muscles of mastication. The masseter is a thick rectangular muscle in the cheek that functions to close the jaw.

Masticatory mucosa: Mucosa associated with keratinized stratified squamous epithelium.

Materia alba: Soft white deposit around the necks of the teeth, which is usually associated with poor oral hygiene. Materia alba is composed of food debris, dead tissue elements, and purulent matter and serves as a medium for bacterial growth.

Maxillary tuberosity: Bony extension posterior to the maxillary teeth.

Mechanical: Pertaining to or accomplished by mechanical or physical forces; performed by means of some artificial mechanism.

Medial: In a direction toward or forward of the midline or middle of an object or the body.

Median lingual sulcus: Midline depression on the dorsal surface of the tongue.

Median palatine raphe: Ridge of tissue covering the palatine suture.

Mediators: Plasma proteins released from mast cells that regulate chemical events.

Medical history: Record of the state of health and medical history of a patient.

Megaloblastic anemia: Anemia characterized by hyperplastic bone marrow changes and maturation arrest that is the result of a dietary deficiency, impaired absorption, impaired storage and modification, or impaired use of one or more hematopoietic factors.

Melanocytes: Dendritic cells of the gingival epithelium that, when functional, cause pigmentation regardless of race.

Menopause: Period that marks the permanent cessation of menstrual activity, usually occurring between ages 35 and 58 years.

Mesothelioma: Rare, malignant neoplasm derived from the lining cells of the pleura and peritoneum, which grows as a thick sheet covering the viscera.

Meta-analysis: Statistical process commonly used with systematic reviews, involving a combination of the statistical analyses and a summary of the results of several individual studies into one analysis. When data from multiple studies are pooled, the sample size and power usually increase.

Metastasis: Transfer of disease from one organ or part to another not directly connected with it (e.g., regional or distant spread of cancer cells from the site primarily involved).

Microcrystals: Extremely minute crystals.

Microleakage: Seepage of fluids, debris, and microorganisms along the interface between a restoration and the walls of a cavity preparation.

Micron: One-thousandth part of a millimeter or the one-millionth part of an 0 symbol: mcm.

Microradiography: Process by which a radiograph of a small object is produced on fine-grained photographic film under conditions that permit subsequent microscopic examination.

Microstreaming: Phenomenon associated with ultrasonic scaling instruments whereby the water hitting the lip causes a hydrodynamic shear stress close to the oscillating tip.

Microvasculature: Portion of the circulatory system that is composed of the capillary network.

Minor: Individual who has not reached the age of legal competence—usually 21 years of age.

Mobility: Distance that a tooth moves in its socket beyond normal physiologic movement.

Modified Stillman's method: Toothbrushing technique developed to massage the gingiva only; the modified Stillman's method now includes cleaning the entire tooth.

Monoclonality: Pertaining to cells or cell products derived from a single clone.

Monofilament: Made of a single strand of material.

Monomer: Simplest molecular form of a substance.

Mononucleosis: Acute infectious viral disease that most commonly affects young adults and older children.

Monophobia: Fear of being alone.

Monostotic: Affecting a single bone.

Monozygotic: Derived from a single zygote (fertilized ovum); denotes identical twins.

Mood disorder: Disturbances in emotions severe enough to interfere with normal living.

Morphea scleroderma: Localized form of scleroderma characterized by local patches of skin that thicken into firm, oval-shaped areas.

Motivation: Provision of encouragement, support, and direction.

Mount and Hume classification system: Proposed classification for cavity designs that allows the introduction of smaller, more conservative dental caries than are possible with G.V. Black classification while allowing for the more extensive cavities that are the inevitable end result of continuing replacement restorative dentistry.

Mouthguard: Resilient intraoral device worn during participation in contact sports to reduce the potential for injury to teeth and associated tissue.

MRI: Acronym for *magnetic resonance imaging*.

Mucocutaneous: Of or pertaining to the mucous membrane and skin.

Mucoepidermoid carcinoma: Malignant neoplasm of glandular tissues, especially the ducts of the salivary glands. Mucoepidermoid carcinoma contains mucinous and epidermoid squamous cells.

Mucogingival junction: Line that separates the attached gingiva from the alveolar mucosa. The mucogingival junction is relatively loose, thin, and movable.

Mucoperiosteal full-thickness flap: All soft tissue in an area that is incised and elevated.

Mucoperiosteal split-thickness flap: Epithelium and part of the underlying connective tissue that are incised and separated from the remaining connective tissue and periosteum.

Mucositis: Oral inflammation.

Mucous membrane: Membrane composed of epithelium and lamina propria that lines the oral cavity and other canals. The mucous membrane also includes cavities of the body that communicate with external air.

Multiaxial: Classification system developed by the American Psychiatric Association in which an individual is evaluated with regard to multiple variables rather than from a single aspect of assessment.

Multifilament: Consisting of several filaments or strands that are braided or twisted together.

Multilevel brush design: Toothbrush in which the head contains bristles of varying lengths.

Multiple sclerosis: Most common autoimmune disease affecting the nervous system. Multiple sclerosis is characterized by the demyelination of nerves in the central nervous system as a result of chronic inflammation.

Muscles of mastication: Powerful muscles that elevate and rotate the mandible to enable the opposing teeth to occlude for mastication.

Musculoskeletal disorders (MSD):   Disorders affecting muscle and skeletal tissues resulting from inappropriate positioning, usually during repetitive use.

Mutans streptococci: Group of *Streptococcus*, specifically with properties similar to *Streptococcus mutans* (e.g., *Streptococcus sobrinus*, *Streptococcus cricetus*, *Streptococcus rattus*, *Streptococcus ferus*, *Streptococcus macacae*).

Myasthenia gravis: Abnormal condition characterized by chronic fatigability and muscle weakness, especially in the face and throat, as a result of a defect in the conduction of nerve impulses at the myoneural junction (e.g., mycobacteria, bacterial spores).

Mylohyoid muscle: One of a pair of flat triangular muscles that form the floor of the cavity of the mouth. The mylohyoid muscle is innervated by the mylohyoid nerve and acts to raise both the hyoid bone and the tongue.

Myocardial infarction: Occlusion or blockage of one or more arteries supplying the muscle of the heart that results in injury or necrosis of the heart muscle.

Mysophobia: Fear of germs.

N

Nadir: Lowest point, such as the blood count after it has been depressed by chemotherapy, of the item being measured.

Narcissistic personality disorder: Pattern of thinking and behavior characterized by a person's sense of grandiosity and preoccupation with his or her own achievements and abilities.

Nasal septum: Thin, vertical, bony septum separating the right and left nasal cavities.

Nasogastric tube: Tube placed through the nose into the stomach to introduce nutrients in a liquid form or to relieve gastric distension by removing gas, gastric secretions, or food or to obtain a specimen for laboratory analysis.

Nasolabial sulcus: Groove formed by the labial surface of the upper lip at the midline and the inferior border of the nose. The nasolabial sulcus is a measure of the relative protrusion of the upper lip.

Necrotizing ulcerative periodontitis: Massive tissue destruction of the bone and connective tissue attachment in which the gingiva appears red and ulcerative with punched-out papillae.

Neglect: Failure to do something that an individual is bound to do; lack of due care.

Negligence: Failure to use such care as a reasonable and careful person would use under similar circumstances.

Neonatal: Period covering the first 28 days after birth.

Neoplasia: Process of the formation of tumors by the uncontrolled proliferation of cells.

Neoplasm: Any new and abnormal growth, specifically one in which cell multiplication is controlled and progressive; may be benign or malignant.

Neuroleptic: Type of antipsychotic medication with associated side effects that resemble Parkinson's disease.

Neurotoxicity: Ability of a drug or other agent to destroy or damage nervous tissue.

Neurotransmitters: Chemicals that are activated to transmit signals from one neuron to another (neural pathways) and to other tissues. The neurotransmitters primarily activated by nicotine are acetylcholine, norepinephrine, dopamine, serotonin, vasopressin, beta-endorphin, growth hormones, and adrenal cortical thyroid hormone.

Neutral position: Position of a dental clinician in which an appendage is not moved from or directed toward the body's midline, including during monitoring or twisting.

Nicotine: Tertiary amine composed of a pyridine and a pyrrolidine ring. Nicotine is the chief alkaloid in tobacco products and is rapidly absorbed through the skin and respiratory tract.

Nicotine replacement agents, products, and drugs: Nicotine in a form that is free of tobacco; can be taken as a gum, transdermal patch through the skin, nasal spray, or oral inhaler to supply nicotine to the central nervous system to reduce the intensity and duration of some withdrawal symptoms.

Nicotinic stomatitis: Whitish lesion on the hard palate caused by the heat from smoking or consuming hot liquid.

Night guard: Any removable artificial occlusal surface used for diagnosis or therapy that affects the relationship of the mandible to the maxillae. A night guard may be used for occlusal stabilization, treatment of temporomandibular disorders, or prevention of dentition wear.

Nocturia: Urination at night.

Non–insulin-dependent diabetes mellitus (NIDDM): Type of diabetes mellitus in which patients are not insulin dependent or prone to ketosis, although they may use insulin to correct symptomatic or persistent hyperglycemia. These patients can develop ketosis under special circumstances, such as infection or stress. Onset is usually after 40 years of age but can occur at any age. Two subclasses are the presence or absence of obesity.

Nonkeratinized: Movable and compressible; soft and smooth to the touch.

Nonmaleficence: Obligation to provide services in a manner that protects the patient and results in the prevention of harm.

Nonspecific plaque hypothesis: Hypothesis associated with the cause of periodontal disease based on the quality of plaque biofilm present, *not* on specific organisms.

Nonverbal cues: Gestures, facial expressions, or body posture used to convey a message.

Normochromic normocytic anemia: Anemia associated with disturbances of red cell formation and related to endocrine deficiencies, chronic inflammation, and carcinomatosis.

Nosocomial: Infection acquired in a hospital as a result of medical care.

Nuchal: Referring to the neck.

Nucleic acid probes: Microbiological assay that uses deoxyribonucleic acid (DNA) and ribonucleic acid (RNA) to identify oral microorganisms.

Nucleus pulposus: Central part of each intervertebral disc consisting of a pulpy elastic substance that loses some of its resiliency with age. The nucleus pulposus may be suddenly compressed and squeezed out through the annular fibrocartilage, which causes a herniated disc and extreme pain.

Nyctophobia: Fear of darkness or night.

Nystagmus: State of oscillatory movements of an organ or part, especially the eyeballs; irregular jerking movement of the eyes. Each movement of the cycle consists of a slow component in one direction and a rapid component in the opposite direction.

O

Oblique: Either perpendicular or parallel; inclined.

Oblique fibers: Any of the collagenous filaments that are bundled obliquely together in the periodontal ligament, inserted into the cementum, and extended more occlusally in the alveolus. These fibers compose approximately two thirds of the periodontal fibers.

Observing: To notice or pay attention to; watching in a nonverbal manner.

Obsessions: Ideas or thoughts that involuntarily and constantly intrude into awareness and are generally pointless.

Obsessive-compulsive disorder: Characterized by obsessions that provoke clinically significant anxiety and by compulsions that act to neutralize the anxiety.

Obturation: Act of closing or occluding.

Obturator: Device used to restore the continuity of the hard or soft palate or both.

Occipital: Back part of the head.

Occlude: To close or bring the teeth together.

Occlusal plane: Average plane established by the incisal and occlusal surfaces of the teeth. Generally, the occlusal plane represents the planar mean of the curvature of these surfaces.

Occlusal radiograph: Intraoral radiograph made with occlusal film placed on the occlusal surfaces of one of the arches. Occlusal radiograph shows the relationship of teeth to the underlying structures, such as cysts and abscesses, in the alveolar process.

Occupational exposure: Reasonably anticipated skin, eye, mucous membrane, or parenteral contact with blood or other potentially infectious materials (OPIM) that can result from the performance of an employee's duties.

Odontoblast: Cell that forms the surface layer of the dental papilla that forms dentin of the tooth. Odontoblasts continue production for years after eruption of recognized pathogenic microorganisms but not necessarily all microbial forms (e.g., bacterial spores). Disinfection does not ensure the degree of safety associated with sterilization processes of treatment.

Oligoclonality: Referring to cells cloned or derived from one or a few cells or molecules.

Omohyoid: Pertaining to the shoulder and hyoid bone.

Oncology: Sum of knowledge regarding tumors; the study of tumors.

Operator positioning: Operator's chair position changes in relation to the area of the mouth that is being treated. A change in the position of the operator within the zone of activity can improve visibility and reduce back and neck strain caused by bending and leaning.

OPIM: OSHA term that refers to *other potentially infectious materials.* OPIM refers to the following: (1) body fluids including semen, vaginal secretions, cerebrospinal fluid, synovial fluid, pleural fluid, pericardial fluid, peritoneal fluid, amniotic fluid, saliva in dental procedures; any body fluid visibly contaminated with blood; and all body fluids in situations where differentiation among body fluids is difficult or impossible; (2) any unfixed tissue or organ (other than intact skin) from a human (living or dead); and (3) HIV-containing cell, tissue cultures, or organ.

Opsonin: Macromolecule that becomes attached to the surface of a microbe that can be recognized by surface receptors of neutrophils and macrophages and that increases the efficiency of phagocytosis of the microbe. Opsonins include immunoglobulin G (IgG) antibodies and fragments of complement proteins.

Opsonization: Process of attaching opsonins, such as IgG or complement fragments, to microbial surfaces to target microbes for phagocytosis.

Oral candidiasis: Infection caused by a species of *Candida,* usually *Candida albicans.* Pruritus (e.g., white exudate), peeling, and easy bleeding characterize this infection. Oral candidiasis without a history of recent antibiotic therapy, chemotherapy, corticosteroid therapy, or radiation therapy to the head and neck or other immunosuppressive disorders may indicate the possibility of HIV infection.

Oral human papillomavirus infection: Warts caused by the human papillomavirus (HPV) that may be scattered throughout the mouth or localized in one area; they frequently recur. Oral warts are associated with AIDS infection.

Oral irrigator: Powered device for personal use that delivers an intermittent stream of water or an antimicrobial agent at the tooth or below the gingival margin.

Oral nystatin: Antifungal antibiotic taken by mouth.

Oral physiotherapy aids: Any oral cleaning device, such as a toothbrush or floss.

Organ system: Part of the body having a special or specific function.

Orofacial: Pertaining to the mouth and face.

Oropharyngeal isthmus: Narrow opening between the mouth and pharynx.

Oropharynx: Oral division of the pharynx that is located between the soft palate and the opening of the larynx.

Orthopnea: Inability to breathe except in an upright position.

OSHA: Acronym for *Occupational Safety and Health Administration.*

Osmolarity: Osmotic pressure of a solution expressed in osmols or milliosmols per liter of the solution.

Osmotic: Pertaining to osmosis.

Osseous: Bony.

Osseous defect: Imperfection, failure, or absence of bone.

Osseous surgery: Portion of periodontal surgery that modifies bone in an attempt to correct osseous defects and deformities.

Osteoblast: Cuboidal cells associated with the growth and development of bone. In active growth, osteoblasts form a continuous layer on old bone similar to a sheet of epithelial cells. When the bone growth is arrested, osteoblast cells assume an elongated appearance similar to fibroblasts.

Osteoporosis: Disease process that results in reduction in the mass of bone.

Outline form: Shape of the area of the tooth surface included within the cavosurface margins of a prepared cavity.

Overbite: Vertical overlapping of maxillary over mandibular teeth that is usually measured perpendicular to the occlusal plane.

Overdenture: Complete or partial removable denture supported by retained roots to provide improved support, stability, and tactile sensation and to reduce ridge resorption.

Overjet: Horizontal projection of maxillary teeth beyond the mandibular teeth, usually measured parallel to the occlusal plane.

P

Pain: Subjective unpleasant sensory and emotional experience associated with actual or potential tissue damage or described in terms of such damage.

Pain stimulus: Event that precipitates the conduction of the pain response.

Palatal lift: Vault-shaped muscular structure forming the soft palate between the mouth and the nasopharynx.

Palatine fovea: Small pits in the mucosa on each side of the midline where the soft and hard palates meet.

Palatine rugae: Irregular ridges or folds of masticatory mucosa extending laterally from the incisive papilla and the anterior part of the palatine raphe.

Palatine tonsil: One of a pair of almond-shaped masses of lymphoid tissue between the palatoglossal and the palatopharyngeal arches on each side of the fauces. Palatine tonsils are covered with mucous membrane and contain numerous lymph follicles and various crypts.

Palatopharyngeal fold: Sphincteric action that seals the oral cavity from the nasal cavity by the synchronous movement of the soft palate superiorly, the lateral pharyngeal wall medially, and the posterior wall of the pharynx anteriorly.

Palliative: Affording relief but not curing.

Palmer's tooth notation: Tooth-numbering system that codes the teeth with numbers and letters using brackets to indicate the arch.

Palpation: Act of feeling with the hand.

Panic attack: Sudden, overwhelming sense of terror. Unlike anxiety, which involves a more generalized stimulus for onset, a panic attack has a more focused precipitant.

Panoramic: Radiographic method in which a continuous image of both the maxillary and the mandibular dental arches, as well as associated structures, are obtained.

Panoramic image: Extraoral image used to examine the maxilla, mandible, and surrounding structures on one film.

Papilla: Gingiva filling the interproximal spaces between adjacent teeth; projections located on the dorsum of the tongue that contain receptors for the sense of taste.

Parallel: Two straight lines of equal distance apart that will never meet.

Paranoid personality disorder: Pattern of thinking and behavior characterized by inappropriate suspiciousness of the motives and behaviors of others.

Paranoid type: Type of schizophrenia characterized by persecutory delusions.

Paraphrase: Rewording of the meaning expressed in something spoken.

Parathormone: Tradename for parathyroid hormone (PTH).

Parenteral: Means of piercing mucous membranes or skin barrier through such events as needlesticks, human bites, cuts, or abrasions.

Paresis: Progressive psychosis associated with neurosyphilis.

Paresthesia: Extended period of numbness.

Parotid: Pertaining to the parotid gland, which is one type of salivary gland.

Partial denture: Prosthetic device containing artificial teeth supported on a framework and attached to natural teeth by means of clasps.

Partial gold crown (¾ GC): Gold crown that does not cover the entire anatomical crown. The tooth is prepared to ensure that the facial surface of the tooth is unchanged. When the partial gold crown is placed, the natural enamel on the facial surface is visible and the crown covers the prepared portion.

Partial split-thickness periodontal flap: See *Mucoperiosteal full-thickness flap* and *Mucoperiosteal split-thickness flap.*

Partially erupted tooth: Tooth that has only a portion of the anatomical crown exposed in the oral cavity.

Pastille: Gelatin-based sweetened and molded medication impregnated with a therapeutic substance intended to be sucked. Chemically treated paper disk that undergoes color changes when exposed to radiation.

Pathogenesis: Source or cause of an illness or abnormal condition.

Pathophobia: Fear of disease.

Patient positioning: Arrangement of the patient in the dental chair and the relationship of the chair to the workspace and clinician.

Pavementing: After margination, white blood cells stick to the surface of the capillary endothelium in preparation for diapedesis.

Pellagra: Nutritional deficiency that is the result of faulty intake or metabolism of nicotinic acid, a vitamin B–complex factor. Pellagra is characterized by glossitis and dermatitis of sun-exposed surfaces, stomatitis, diarrhea, and dementia.

Pellicle: Thin, saliva-based, protein layer that coats the teeth and forms the base over which dental plaque biofilm develops.

Percussion: Examination by striking an area and evaluating the sounds and sensations.

Performance logic positioning: Clinician positioning during patient care, based on the elimination of musculoskeletal strain.

Periapical image: Intraoral image used to examine the entire tooth and surrounding bone.

Periapical radiolucency (PAR): Translucent area observed at the apex of a tooth, depicting reduced calcification, usually the result of infection.

Pericoronitis: Inflammation of the tissue flap over a partially erupted tooth, commonly a third molar.

Perimenopause: Phase before the onset of menopause.

Periodontal debridement: Removal of plaque biofilm, calculus, and endotoxins from the root surface of the tooth.

Periodontal disease: Infectious disease that results in the destruction of the soft tissue or bone or both that support the teeth (e.g., gingivitis, periodontitis).

Periodontal dressing (pack): Protective material applied postoperatively to the surface of a wound created by a periodontal surgical procedure.

Periodontal ligament: Connective tissue fibers that surround the root of the tooth and attach it to the alveolar process.

Periodontal maintenance (PM): Term accepted by the *American Academy of Periodontology* in 2000 to replace the term *supportive periodontal therapy.*

Periodontal surgery: Surgical procedure used to modify the periodontium in an attempt to treat or prevent periodontal disease.

Periodontitis: Inflammation of the supporting tissues of the teeth, resulting in attachment loss.

Periodontium: Tissues that invest or help invest and support the teeth (i.e., gingiva, cementum of the tooth, periodontal ligament, alveolar and supporting bone).

Pernicious anemia: Macrocytic-normochromic, megaloblastic anemia associated with achlorhydria and a lack of a gastric intrinsic factor necessary for the binding and absorption of vitamin B_{12}, which is an erythrocyte-maturing factor.

Perpendicular: Two straight lines that meet at a right angle.

Personal space: Distance between two people that is neither threatening nor too distant so as not to be heard.

Personality disorder: Maladaptive patterns of personality that result in either social or occupational problems and in significant distress to the person.

Petechiae: Minute red spots on the skin or mucous membranes, resulting from escape of a small amount of blood.

Phagocytosis: Process by which certain cells of the innate immune system, including macrophages and neutrophils, engulf large particles such as intact microbes. The cell surrounds the particle with extensions of its plasma membrane, leading to the formation of an intracellular vesicle called a *phagosome,* which contains the ingested particle.

Phagosome: Membrane-bound intracellular vesicle that contains microbes or particulate material from the extracellular environment. Phagosomes are formed during the process of phagocytosis and fuse with other vesicular structures such as lysosomes, leading to the enzymatic degradation of the ingested material.

Pharyngeal: Pertaining to the pharynx.

Phase-contrast microscopy: Microscope with a special condenser and objective that contains a phase-shifting ring through which small differences in the index of refraction become visible. The use of phase-contrast capabilities allows for direct viewing of transparent live cells and tissues.

Philtrum: Vertical groove on the midline of the upper lip that extends downward from the nasal septum to the tubercle of the upper lip.

Phobia: Persistent and irrational fear associated with a specific object or situation.

Photodynamic therapy (PDT): Cancer treatment modality that uses a photosensitizing drug and laser.

PICO: Components—**p**roblem, **i**ntervention, **c**omparison, **o**utcome—of a well-built clinical question used in the evidence-based decision-making process.

Piezoelectric: Type of ultrasonic powered scaler used in dentistry. The conversion of electrical power to tip motion is by way of ceramic crystal vibrations.

Pilocarpine (Salagen): Alkaloid that causes parasympathetic effects (e.g., secretion of the salivary, bronchial, and gastrointestinal glands). Pilocarpine stimulates the sweat glands and also causes vasodilation and cardiac inhibition.

Pits and fissures: Result of noncoalescence of enamel during tooth formation.

Pixel: Discrete unit of information used in digital electronic images.

Placebo: Substance that resembles medicine superficially and is believed by the patient to be medicine; however, a placebo has no intrinsic drug activity.

Plaintiff: Party who sues in a civil action and is named on the record of the lawsuit. In a criminal action the plaintiff would be the person or persons of the state in a state action or the people of the United States in a federal action.

Plaque-associated gingivitis: Inflammation of the gingivae directly related to the presence of bacterial plaque biofilm on the tooth surface and the amount of time during which the plaque biofilm is allowed to remain undisturbed.

Plaque biofilm: Microcosm of bacteria, various food particles, salivary proteins, and polysaccharides that accumulate on the teeth.

Plaque index: Standardized mechanism used to categorize or quantify the amount and location of plaque biofilm in the oral cavity.

Platelet count: Laboratory test that measures the number of platelets in the systemic circulation.

Platelets: Fragments of megakaryocytes that are synthesized in the bone marrow and play an essential role in blood clotting.

Plica fimbriata: Fringelike projections on the ventral surface of the tongue in the location of the lingual veins.

Plica lingualis: Fingerlike tissue projections along the top of the sublingual fold.

Point angle: Angle formed by the junction of three walls at a common point; designated by combining the names of the walls that form the angle.

Polarized light microscopy: Microscopy in which polarized light is used for special diagnostic purposes, such as examining crystals of chemicals found in patients with gout and related disorders. Polarized light is light in which the radiation waves occur in only one direction in the vibration plane and not at random.

Polishing: Production, especially by friction, of a smooth, glossy, mirrorlike surface that reflects light; a fine agent is used for polishing after a coarser agent is used for cleaning.

Polishing agent: Any material used to impart luster to a surface.

Polycythemia: Increase in the total red blood cell mass in the blood.

Polydipsia: Abnormally increased thirst.

Polymer: Product formed by joining together many small molecules (monomers).

Polymerization: Reaction in which a complex molecule of relatively high molecular weight is formed by the union of a number of simpler molecules, which may be alike.

Polymerization shrinkage: Pulling away or contraction of polymerized composite resins.

Polymyositis: Inflammation of many muscles, usually accompanied by deformity, edema, insomnia, pain, sweating, and tension. Some forms of polymyositis are associated with malignancy.

Polyostotic: Affecting more than one bone.

Polyphagia: Excessive uncontrolled eating.

Polyuria: Passage of an abnormally increased volume of urine. Polyuria may be the result of increased intake of fluids, inadequate renal function, uncontrolled diabetes mellitus or diabetes insipidus, diuresis of edema fluid, or ascites.

Pontic: Artificial tooth on a fixed partial denture that replaces a missing natural tooth, restores its function, and usually fills the space previously occupied by the clinical crown.

Porcelain fused to metal (PFM): Fixed restoration that uses a metal substructure on which a ceramic veneer is fused.

Porcelain jacket crown (PJC): Ceramic crown made on a platinum matrix.

Porte polisher: Hand instrument constructed to hold a wooden point. A Porte polisher is used in a dental engine to burnish and apply polishing paste to teeth.

Postauricular: Portion posterior to the ear.

Postmenopause: Phase after the completion of menopause.

Postprandial: After a meal.

Posttraumatic stress disorder: Reexperience of an extremely traumatic event accompanied by increased arousal and by the avoidance of stimuli associated with the trauma.

Postural syndrome: Condition that occurs from the repetitive maintenance of muscles in a position other than the neutral position for long periods, ultimately resulting in pain.

Potassium nitrate: Compound occurring as a white granular or crystalline powder or as colorless transparent prisms; used as a food preservative and formerly used as an oral diuretic. Also called *niter* and *saltpeter.*

Power driven: Energy of movement from an external source (e.g., electricity).

Powered toothbrush: Toothbrush powered by batteries or electricity that uses one or several motions such as back and forth, up and down, or circular.

Practice act: Combined state statutory regulations and agency laws.

Practice philosophy: Way of thinking that underpins an individual's clinical practice or patient care.

Preauricular: Located anterior to the auricle of the ear.

Preceptorship: Commonly called *on-the-job training,* preceptorship is the learning of a new career on the job. The employer assumes the role of teacher. In dentistry, preceptorship relates to the training of the dental hygienist by the dentist.

Precipitate: Insoluble solid substance that forms from chemical reactions between solutions.

Premature ventricular contractions (PVCs): Cardiac sinus conducted arrhythmia characterized by ventricular depolarization that occurs earlier than expected. PVCs are shown on the electrocardiogram as an early, wide QRS complex without a preceding related P wave.

Prepubertal periodontitis: Disease of the periodontium that occurs early in life, affecting both deciduous and permanent teeth and usually resulting in early edentulism. Patients with prepubertal periodontitis often have white blood cell defects.

Presentation: (1) Something presented as a symbol or image that represents something; (2) something offered or given (e.g., gift); (3) something set forth for the attention of the mind; (4) a descriptive or persuasive account. Case presentation is a symbol that represents a case and a persuasive account of the strategies within the case for the intent of learning more about the actual care of a patient.

Prevalence: Number of people infected with a particular disease at any one time.

Prevention: Method that prevents an expected or anticipated event from occurring.

Prevention strategy: Action plan directed to prevent illness and promote health so as to eliminate the need for secondary or tertiary health care.

Primary care provider: Practitioner in one of the health professions (e.g., medicine; nursing; psychology; dentistry or oral health; physical, occupational, respiratory therapy) who provides health-care services.

Primary intention: Process of wound healing that occurs when a narrow incisional space fills with clotted blood, resulting in clot formation and a scab that covers the wound. The edges of the wound are brought together in close approximation, typically with sutures. Healing by primary intention is also known as *primary union.*

Primary source: Original research publications that have not been filtered or synthesized and include randomized controlled trials, cohort studies, and case studies.

Principal fibers: Collagen fibers organized into groups based on their orientation to the tooth and related function.

Professional portfolio: Method by which an individual's achievements, work, or performance is documented.

Progesterone: Steroid hormone responsible for changes in the endometrium in the second half of the menstrual cycle.

Prognosis: Forecast of the probable course and outcome of an attack of disease and the prospects of recovery as indicated by the nature of the disease and reported symptoms of the patient.

Prophylaxis: Pertaining to the cleaning and polishing of teeth.

Proprioceptive: Describes the feeling of muscle movement associated with operator positioning and movement during patient care.

Prostaglandins: Group of potent hormonelike substances that produce a wide range of body responses such as changing capillary permeability, smoothing muscle tone, clumping of platelets, and endocrine and exocrine functions. Prostaglandins may be used in some instances to terminate a pregnancy.

Proteinase: Proteolytic enzyme that splits protein molecules at central linkages.

Proteoglycans: Any of a group of polysaccharide-protein conjugates primarily occurring in the matrix of connective tissue and cartilage. Proteoglycans are composed mainly of polysaccharide chains—particularly glycosaminoglycans—and minor protein components.

Prothrombin time (PT) test: Laboratory test that measures the extrinsic pathway of coagulation. The PT test assesses reduced levels or activity of the clotting factors II, V, VII, and X and fibrinogen.

Pruritus: Itching.

psi: Abbreviation for *pounds per square inch.*

Psoriasis: Chronic, hereditary, recurrent skin condition marked by discrete, vivid red macules, papules, or plaques covered with silvery lamellated scales.

Psychoactive chemicals or drugs: Substances that produce signals in the brain's limbic and cortical systems and produce strong sensations of liking, well-being, or pleasure. Such signals, needed for thriving and survival, are reinforcing; consequently, when artificially stimulated, psychoactive chemicals or drugs tend to upset and distort natural balances of consciousness, reason, and behavior.

Pterygoid: Pertaining to a winglike structure. Pterygoid plates are part of the sphenoid bone of the skull.

Pterygomandibular raphe: Tendinous line between the buccinator and constrictor pharynges superior muscles, from which the middle portions of both muscles originate.

Ptosis: Abnormal condition of one or both upper eyelids in which the eyelid droops because of a congenital or acquired weakness of the levator muscle or paralysis of cranial nerve III.

Puberty: Stage in life when members of both sexes become functionally capable of reproduction.

Public: Term used to express a formal status.

PubMed: Developed by the National Center for Biotechnology Information (NCBI) at the National Library of Medicine (NLM), PubMed is an on-line database that provides access to MEDLINE and other biomedical literature citations, as well as links to full-text journals at web sites of participating publishers (www.pubmed.gov/).

Pulpitis: Inflammation of the pulp of a tooth.

Pulsating: Intermittent or fractionated stream of water or irrigant.

Pulse rhythm: Rhythmic expansion of an artery as the heart beats; pulse rhythm can be felt with slight finger pressure on the surface of the skin in several areas of the body.

Pumice: Type of volcanic glass used as an abrasive. Pumice is prepared in various grits and used for finishing and polishing.

Purpura: Group of disorders characterized by purplish or brownish-red discolorations caused by bleeding into the skin or tissues.

Purulent: Containing or forming pus.

Purview: Body and scope of an act or bill.

Pyogenic granuloma: Small nonmalignant mass of excessive granulation tissue that is usually found at the site of an injury. Most often a dull red color, pyogenic granuloma contains numerous capillaries, bleeds readily, and is tender. It may be attached by a narrow stalk.

Pyrophobia: Fear of fire.

Q

Quiescence: State of inactivity, quiet, or rest; latency or dormancy.

Quit day: Day of a given cessation attempt during which a patient tries to abstain totally from tobacco use.

R

Radiation caries: Decay, mostly at the cervical margins, that is caused by the loss of minerals that results from radiation therapy.

Radiation modifiers: Agents such as beta-carotene and 13 cis-retinoic acid believed to have value as chemopreventive agents in the reduction of tumors.

Radiation osteomyelitis or osteonecrosis: Damage or destruction of the blood supply to the bone as a result of radiation therapy.

Radiolucency: Characteristic of materials of relatively low atomic number that have low attenuation characteristics, which allows most x-rays to pass through them and thus produces relatively dark images.

Radiolucent: Substance that allows radiant energy to pass through it, producing black areas on radiographs.

Radiopacity: Quality of being radiopaque or having the ability to stop or reduce the passage of radiation.

Radiopaque: Substance that does not allow radiant energy to pass through it, producing light areas on radiographs.

Radiotherapy: Treatment of disease by ionizing radiation; may be external megavoltage or internal by use of interstitial implantation of an isotope (radium).

Radium: Highly radioactive chemical element found in uranium minerals. Radium is used in the treatment of malignant tumors in the form of needles or pellets for interstitial implantation.

Radon: Colorless gas produced by the disintegration of radium.

Randomized controlled trials (RCTs): Trial in which participants are randomly assigned to two groups: (1) an experimental group, which receives the intervention that is being tested, and (2) the comparison or control group, which receives an alternative treatment, a placebo, or no treatment. The two groups are then followed to see whether any different results occur between them.

Rapidly progressive periodontitis: Condition that occurs in young adults ages 20 to 30 years that is characterized by gingival inflammation and rapid loss of bone and supporting tissues.

Rapport: Creation and enhancement of a positive relationship.

Raynaud's phenomenon: Intermittent attacks of ischemia of the extremities of the body, especially the fingers, toes, ears, and nose, caused by exposure to cold or by emotional stimuli. The attacks are characterized by severe blanching of the extremities, followed by cyanosis, then redness; numbness, tingling, and burning; pain usually accompanies the attacks. Normal color and sensation are restored by heat.

Recession: Loss of part or all of the gingiva over the root of a tooth.

Reciprocity: Professional licensure valid in one state based on the fact that the individual requesting the license is validly licensed in another state.

Recurrent or secondary caries: Dental caries occurring at the restoration-tooth interface or under an existing restoration.

Refractory periodontitis: Progressive inflammatory destruction of the periodontal attachment that resists conventional mechanical treatment.

Regulation: Criterion described in laws that outlines what a practitioner can do under an act or statute.

Relapse: Return to tobacco use after a period of hours, days, weeks, months, or years by an individual who had at one time been a tobacco user (100 or more cigarettes in an individual's life or a regular user of any tobacco product or combination of tobacco products). Same process occurs in other chemical addictions.

Relaxation: Reduction of tension, such as when a muscle relaxes between contractions.

Remineralization: Process of restoring minerals to a mineralized tissue that has been demineralized.

Removable partial denture: Prosthesis that replaces one or more teeth in a partially dentate arch and is removable from the mouth.

Reparative dentin: Dentin of an irregular nature formed below a carious lesion as a means of preserving pulpal integrity.

Repetitive strain injuries (RSIs): Tissue damage to the neck and arms associated with tasks that require repeated manipulations of the hands, such as meat cutting, computer keyboarding, playing musical instruments, or practicing dentistry or dental hygiene.

Resistance form: Shape that is given to a cavity to provide a filling that has the ability to withstand the stress brought on with mastication.

Respect: To look with or to show consideration, regard, or esteem.

Retainer: Device used to hold something in place; the attachment or abutments of a fixed or removable prosthesis; an appliance for maintaining the positions of the teeth and jaws immediately after the completion of orthodontic treatment.

Retention: Act of retaining or holding back; the fixation or stabilization.

Retention form: Shaping the remaining enamel and dentin to strengthen the tooth and restoration.

Retinopathy: Noninflammatory eye disorder resulting from changes in the retinal blood vessels.

Retroauricular: Pertaining to a location behind the ear.

Retromolar pad: Dense pad of tissue just distal to the last tooth of the mandibular arch.

Revocation: Act of terminating an individual's license to practice a profession such as dental hygiene. This action is delegated to the regulatory agency that governs a profession.

Rheumatic heart disease (RHD): Damage to the heart muscle and valves caused by episodes of rheumatic fever. When a susceptible person acquires a group A beta-hemolytic streptococcal infection, an autoimmune reaction may occur in the heart tissue, which results in permanent deformities of heart valves or chordae tendineae.

Rheumatoid arthritis: Chronic inflammatory disease characterized by pain, swelling, stiffness, and loss of function that affects the joints of the body.

Rhomboidal: Resembling the shape of an oblique equilateral parallelogram, such as in a rhomboid muscle.

Rinsing: Act of vigorously forcing liquid from side to side in the oral cavity by closing the lips and flexing the cheeks and tongue.

Risk: Probability of an event occurring, such as a loss or injury.

Risk assessment: Survey designed to determine the degree to which an individual is placed at risk for developing a condition or a disease.

Risk factors: Conditions or behaviors associated with risk occurrence.

Risk in a health event: Probability of experiencing a change in health status over time.

Rolling stroke: Toothbrushing method characterized by the rolling of the brush head to clean the facial and lingual tooth surfaces.

Root canal (RC): Space occupied by the nerves, blood vessels, and lymph in the radicular part of the tooth; procedures associated with the removal of the components within the canal and filling with a material.

Rotated teeth: Movement of teeth to the left or right from normal alignment.

Rounded edge: Instrument edge that may or may not be sharp and contains no angles.

rpm: Abbreviation for *revolutions per minute.*

Rubber dam: Material used in the patient's mouth for protection, to ensure access and visibility in the operating field, and for the efficient use of operating time.

Rubber dam clamp: Device made of spring metal that is used to retain a rubber dam in place or to improve the operating field by isolating it from the oral environment.

S

Salivary gland acini: Any small saclike structure that is found in the salivary glands.

Salivary glands: Glands that produce saliva.

Sanguinarine: Benzophenanthridine alkaloid thought to be useful in reducing plaque biofilm and gingivitis.

Schizoid personality disorder: Pattern of thinking and behavior characterized by indifference to other people, coupled with a diminished range of emotional experience and expression.

Scleroderma: Collagen disease of unknown cause. Skin lesions are characterized by thickening, rigidity, and pigmentation in patches or diffuse areas.

Sclerosis: Hardening. As applied to the jaws, sclerosis usually indicates an increased calcification centrally with radiopacity. Tracts of increased density in the dentin are called *areas of dentinal sclerosis.* Sclerosis occurs beneath dental caries and with abrasion, attrition, or erosion.

Sclerotic dentin: Hardening or induration of the chief material of teeth, which surrounds the pulp and is situated inside the enamel and cementum.

Sealant: Resin that bonds to enamel surface by mechanical retention via tiny openings created by acid etching the enamel surface.

Sebaceous cyst: Misnomer for epidermoid cyst or pilar cyst.

Secondary adrenal insufficiency: Condition commonly caused by chronic use of glucocorticoid medications that suppress the hypothalamic-pituitary axis and the normal secretion of endogenous cortisol; also known as *adrenal suppression*.

Secondary intention: Process of wound healing associated with wounds that have separated edges, causing extensive granulation tissue formation from the margins and the base of the wound. Healing by secondary intention is also known as *secondary union*.

Secondary source: Synthesized publications of the primary literature (already published original research). Secondary sources include systematic reviews and meta-analyses, evidence-based article reviews, and clinical practice guidelines and protocols.

Self-help: Treatment methods that are not aided by a clinician.

Self-regulation: A profession's assumption of the responsibility for controlling its members through licensure and enforcement of the rules and regulations governing it.

Self-tolerance: Unresponsiveness of the immune system to self-antigens; function of the normal immune system. Failure of self-tolerance results in autoimmune diseases.

Semisupine position: Pertaining to a posture that is between a mid-position and the supine position.

Sensitivity: State of responsiveness to external influences or sensations such as heat or trauma; susceptibility to a substance, such as a drug or antigen.

Sensor: Small detector that is intraorally placed in digital radiography to capture a radiographic image.

Sequelae: Any abnormal condition that follows and is the result of a disease, treatment, or injury, such as paralysis after poliomyelitis, deafness after treatment with an ototoxic drug, or scar formation after a laceration.

Shank: Portion of a dental hygiene instrument that joins the handle with the working end. The shank can be straight or contraangled.

Sharpey's fibers: Collagen fibers from the periodontal ligament that are partially inserted into the cementum and bone.

Sialadenitis: Any inflammation of one or more of the salivary glands.

Sialadenopathy: Disease of a salivary gland.

Sialograms: Radiographic films taken after injection of a radiopaque medium that determine the presence or absence of calcareous deposits in a salivary gland or its ducts.

Sialolith: Calcification in the salivary gland.

Sicca syndrome: Abnormal dryness of the mouth, eyes, or other mucous membranes. Sicca syndrome is observed in patients with Sjögren's syndrome, sarcoidosis, amyloidosis, and deficiencies of vitamins A and C.

Sickle: Periodontal scaling instrument designed to remove calculus deposits from the coronal tooth surface.

Side port: The lumens on the irrigator tip are located on the side of the tip or side port.

Sine scleroderma: Form of systemic scleroderma that does not affect the skin; sine scleroderma resembles limited and diffuse scleroderma.

Single-blind study: Experiment in which the person collecting data knows whether the participant is in the control group or in the experimental group; the participants do not know the group in which they are participating.

Sinus bradycardia: Slow beating of the sinus node at rates of fewer than 60 beats per minute.

Sinus rhythm: Cardiac rhythm stimulated by the sinus (sinoatrial) node. A rate of 60 to 100 beats per minute is normal.

Sinus tachycardia: Rapid heart rate generated by the discharge of the sinoatrial pacemaker. The rate is generally 100 to 180 beats per minute in the adult, 140 to 200 beats per minute in a child, and greater than 200 beats per minute in an infant.

Site specific: Localized to a particular area.

Sjögren's syndrome: Condition related to deficient secretion of salivary, sweat, lacrimal, and mucous glands (e.g., xerostomia, keratoconjunctivitis, rhinitis, dysphagia), increased size of salivary glands, and polyarthritis.

Slow-speed hand piece: Dental hand piece used to hold rotary instruments that operates at 6000 to 10,000 rpm.

Sludge: Collection of metal fragments and oil from grinding a stone against an instrument.

Smear layer: Thin (5 to 10 microns) organic film of organic debris that adheres to dentin as a result of cavity preparation or burnishing action on exposed dentin.

Snyder colorimetric test: Method of determining the concentration of acid-producing bacteria in the saliva by the use of bromcresol green in a culture medium.

Social history: Patient's activities that could have an effect on disease risk.

Social phobia: Clinically significant anxiety provoked by exposure to certain types of social or performance situations, which often leads to avoidance behavior.

Sodium benzoate: Sodium salt of benzoic acid that is used as an antifungal preservative in pharmaceutical preparations and foods. Sodium benzoate may also be used as a test for liver function, administered orally or intravenously.

Sodium bicarbonate: Antacid, electrolyte, and urinary alkalinizing agent. Sodium bicarbonate is prescribed in the treatment of acidosis, gastric acidity, peptic ulcer, and indigestion.

Sodium citrate: Trisodium salt of citric acid used as an anticoagulant for blood or plasma that is to be fractionated or for blood that is to be stored.

Sodium fluoride: Dental caries–preventive agent, occurring as a white powder. Sodium flouride is used in the fluoridation of water and applied topically to the teeth.

Sodium laurel sulfate: Anionic surfactant that is used as a wetting agent, emulsifying aid, and detergent in various cosmetic and dermatologic preparations and as an ingredient in toothpastes.

Soft palate: Posterior portion of the palate.

Solubility: Extent to which a substance (solute) dissolves in a liquid (solvent) to produce a homogeneous system (solution).

Sonic scaler: Type of instrument for scaling that is driven by air, which produces vibrations in the sonic range of 3000 to 8000 cps.

Specific phobia: Avoidance behavior and clinically significant anxiety provoked by exposure to a specific feared object or situation.

Specific plaque biofilm hypothesis: Hypothesis associated with the cause of specific forms of periodontal disease that is based on specified form or forms of bacteria.

Specificity: Quality of being distinctive. Kinds of specificity may include group, species, and type.

Specificity rate: Statistical rates in which the events in both the numerator and the denominator are restricted to a specific subgroup of a population.

Sphygmomanometer: Blood pressure cuff used to measure the systolic and diastolic blood pressures indirectly.

Spinal accessory nerve: Either of a pair of cranial nerves essential for speech, swallowing, and certain movements of the head and shoulders. Each nerve has cranial and spinal portions, communicates with certain cervical nerves, and connects to the nucleus ambiguous of the brain.

Spit tobacco: Referred to as *smokeless tobacco* by the tobacco industry and in most scientific forums. Spit tobacco is tobacco that is not burned but used primarily in the oral cavity, where nicotine and other chemicals are absorbed through the oral mucosa.

Staging: Classification of neoplasms according to the extent of the tumor.

Standard precautions: The relevance of universal precautions to other aspects of disease transmission has been recognized for many years. In 1996 the Centers for Disease Control and Prevention (CDC) expanded the concept and changed the term to *standard precautions*. Standard precautions integrate and expand the elements of universal precautions into standards of care designed to protect HCPs and patients from pathogens that can be spread by blood or any other body fluid, excretion, or secretion. Standard precautions apply to contact with the following: (1) blood; (2) all body fluids, secretions, and excretions (except sweat), regardless of whether they contain blood; (3) nonintact skin; and (4) mucous membranes. Saliva has always been considered a potentially infectious material in dental infection control; thus no operational difference exists in clinical dental practice between universal precautions and standard precautions.

Stannous fluoride: Fluoride salt of tin used in toothpaste and mouthrinses to reduce dental caries and as an anti–plaque biofilm agent.

Staphylococcus: Species of spherical, gram-positive bacteria that grows in grapelike clusters. *Staphylococcus* is of low pathogenicity, although occasional strains may be coagulase-positive and produce hemolysis. *Staphylococcus* is normally present as part of the oral flora and mucosa-lined cavities, such as the mouth and nasal cavity. It can be isolated, along with *S. aureus,* streptococci, pneumococci, fusiform bacilli, *Borrelia vincentii,* molds, and yeasts, from the gingival crevice by cultural examination.

Statutes: Laws that are enacted and written by federal and state legislatures.

Stensen's duct: Excretory duct of the parotid gland. The Stensen's duct passes lateral to the masseter muscle and enters the oral cavity through the buccal tissues adjacent to the maxillary first and second molars.

Sternocleidomastoid: Muscle of the neck that is attached to the mastoid process of the temporal bone and superior nuchal line and by separate heads to the sternum and clavicle. The muscles function together to flex the head.

Stimuli: Chemical, thermal, electrical, or mechanical influences that change the normal environment of irritable tissue and create an impulse.

Stimulus generalization: Tendency to give conditioned or learned responses to stimuli (e.g., situations, objects) that are similar to the original stimulus.

Stippling: Pinpoint depressions present on the surface of the attached gingiva.

Stock: Security certificate that represents an equity ownership in a corporation.

Storage phosphor imaging: Method of obtaining a digital image in which the image is recorded on phosphor-coated plates; the plates are placed into a laser-scanning device, and the image is produced on the computer monitor.

Stratified: Arranged in layers.

Stratified squamous: Epithelial cells that include the superficial layers of the skin and oral mucosa.

Stratum basale: Deepest of the five layers of the epidermis, which is composed of tall cylindrical cells. The stratum basale provides new cells by mitotic cell division.

Stratum corneum: Horny, outermost layer of the skin composed of dead flat cells converted to keratin, which continually flakes away. The thickness of the layer is correlated with the normal wear of the area it covers. The stratum corneum is thick on the palms of the hands and soles of the feet but relatively thin over most other areas.

Stratum granulosum: One of the layers of the epidermis situated immediately below the stratum corneum.

Stratum spinosum: One of the layers of the epidermis situated immediately beneath the stratum granulosum.

Streptococcus mutans: Cariogenic bacteria found in dental plaque biofilm and one of two of the index organisms (e.g., *Lactobacillus*) used to assess dental caries susceptibility.

Strontium chloride: Chloride salt of strontium 89, a calcium analog that concentrates in areas of increased osteogenesis; used as a local radiation source for palliative treatment of bone pain in patients with metastatic bone lesions; administered intravenously.

Subgingival: Below the gingival margin.

Subgingival irrigation: Delivery of water or an antimicrobial agent to a deep periodontal pocket, usually by insertion of a cannula.

Sublingual: Pertaining to the region or structures located beneath the tongue.

Sublingual caruncle: Small papilla at the anterior end of each sublingual fold that contains openings of the submandibular glands.

Subluxation: Partial dislocation of both temporomandibular joints.

Submandibular: Below the mandible.

Submargination: When a deficiency of contour at the margin of a restoration or pattern is present.

Submental: Situated below the chin.

Substantivity: Ability of an agent to adhere to oral soft tissues, thereby permitting continued antimicrobial action; resists dilution by salivary action or gingival crevicular fluid.

Sulci: Grooves or depressions on the surface of a tooth or in a portion of the oral cavity.

Sulcular epithelium: Epithelium that stands away from the tooth, creating a gingival sulcus.

Supererupted teeth: Teeth where the projection lies beyond the normal occlusal plane.

Superior: In a direction above or higher than a specified point.

Supervision: Denotes that the dentist must accept responsibility for the services provided by the dental hygienist. Supervision implies that the dentist will review or evaluate the procedures performed, depending on the level of supervision required.

Supine position: Lying on the back.

Supporting alveolar bone: Part of the bone that is considered best suited to bear the forces of mastication with functioning dentures.

Supportive care: Practice of frequent professional supervision and monitoring of a person with a chronic disease.

Supportive periodontal care (SPC): Describes three levels of periodontal care: (1) preventive, (2) posttreatment, and (3) palliative. *Preventive care* preserves the healthy periodontium; *posttreatment care* is specific and regular professional care after periodontal treatment; and *palliative care* is the optimal possible treatment for patients who are not adherent. Supportive periodontal care was defined at the first European Workshop on Periodontology in 1989.

Supportive periodontal therapy (SPT):   Described at the 1989 World Workshop in Clinical Periodontics; SPT was replaced by the term *periodontal maintenance* in 2000. SPT means the same as SPC, which is used in Europe.

Suppressor T cell: Specialized form of T lymphocyte that blocks the activation and functions of other T lymphocytes. Some suppressor cells produce cytokines that inhibit the immune response.

Suppurating: Producing or discharging pus.

Suppuration: Formation and discharge of pus.

Supraclavicular: Pertaining to the area above the clavicle or collarbone.

Supragingival: Pertaining to the area above the gingival margin.

Supragingival irrigation: Flushing of the gingival sulcus by directing a stream of water or irrigant at right angles to the long axis of the tooth. Flushing is accomplished with the use of an irrigating tip with a lumen at the end.

Surgeon's knot: Mechanical technique that unites opposite ends of suture material.

Surgical stent: Device used to hold a skin graft in place to maintain a body orifice, cavity, or space. A surgical stent is also an acrylic resin appliance used as a positioning guide or support.

Survival rate: Time describing years alive after diagnosis. The survival rate is normally defined as 5 years.

Sustained-release device: Refers to delivery systems and agents that are pharmaceutically active for less than 24 hours.

Suture: Material (e.g., silk, gut) used to approximate or unite surfaces.

Synaptic junction: Space between two nerve cells where the release of neurotransmitters from a transmitting (presynaptic) neuron briefly allow an ion flow that activates a signal in the receiving (postsynaptic) neuron.

Synovial joints: Freely movable joints in which contiguous bony surfaces are covered by articular cartilage and connected by a fibrous connective tissue capsule lined with synovial membrane.

Systematic review: Summary of individual research studies that have investigated the same phenomenon or question using explicit criteria for retrieval, assessment, and synthesis of evidence from individual RCTs and other well-controlled methods.

Systemic: Pertains to the entire body.

Systemic desensitization: Technique used in behavior therapy to eliminate maladaptive anxiety associated with phobias. Systemic desensitization involves the construction by the person of a hierarchy of anxiety-producing stimuli and the general presentation of these stimuli until they no longer elicit the initial response of fear.

Systemic lupus erythematosus: Chronic inflammatory disease of unknown origin affecting the skin, joints, kidneys, nervous system, serous membranes, and often other organs of the body.

Systemic scleroderma: Condition that affects the skin, blood vessels, and major organs; also known as *systemic sclerosis.*

T

T Lymphocytes: Cell type involved in cell-mediated immune responses in the adaptive immune system. T cells mature in the thymus gland, circulate in the blood, and are found in lymphoid tissues. T cells are recruited to peripheral sites of antigen exposure.

Tachypnea: Excessively rapid respiration; a respiratory neurosis marked by quick, shallow breathing.

Tactile sensitivity: Sensitivity relating to the sense of touch.

Taste buds: Barrel-shaped organs of taste associated with certain lingual papilla of the tongue.

Telangiectasia: Dilation of the capillaries and small arteries of a region. A hereditary form (e.g., hereditary hemorrhagic telangiectasia) may appear intraorally. In addition, telangiectasia is a disorder characterized by cutaneous and mucosal vascular macules, nodules, and arterial spiders that tend to bleed sporadically.

Telescopic loupes: Surgical telescopes that can improve visual activity.

Temporalis: Broad radiating muscle that acts to close the jaws and retract the mandible.

Temporomandibular disorders: Abnormal, incomplete, or impaired function of the temporomandibular joints. The symptoms can include headache around the vertex and occiput, tinnitus, pain around the ear, impaired hearing, and pain around the tongue.

Temporomandibular joint: Joint formed by the two condyles of the mandible. The structures that make up the temporomandibular joint include the mandibular fossae of the temporal bones, articular discs, mandibular condyles, and articular tubercles of the zygomatic process of the temporal bone.

Teratogens: Drugs or substances that cause congenital deformities.

Terminal shank: Portion of a periodontal scaling instrument just above the working end.

Therapeutic alliance: Cooperation and contribution between the patient and the oral care professional in achieving health stability for the patient.

Therapeutic intervention strategy: Specific procedure or set of procedures designed to intervene in the disease process to produce a therapeutic benefit.

Therapeutic polishing: Polishing of the tooth surface to remove or disrupt bacterial agents responsible for disease.

Therapeutic privilege: Exception to informed consent; based on disclosure harming the emotional well-being of the patient and contraindicated from a medical point of view.

Thermal stimulus: Stimulus that causes a pain sensation with either heat or cold.

Thoracic outlet syndrome (TOS):   Abnormal condition and type of mononeuropathy characterized by paresthesia. TOS may be caused by a nerve root compression by a cervical disc.

Thrombocytopenia: Reduction in the number of platelets. A decreased production of platelets, decreased survival of platelets, and increased consumption of platelets or splenomegaly may occur. Thrombocytopenia is the most common cause of bleeding disorders.

Thromboxane: Compound synthesized by platelets and other cells that cause platelet aggregation and vasoconstriction.

Thrombus: Abnormal clot that forms in a blood vessel.

Thyroglossal duct cyst: Tube that connects the thyroid gland with the base of the tongue during prenatal development. The thyroglossal duct cyst later becomes obliterated.

Thyroid cartilage: Includes the midline prominence of the larynx.

Thyroid gland: Endocrine gland in the neck.

Thyrotoxic crisis: Emergency situation with rapid onset caused by increased thyroid hormone in the circulation. Condition is precipitated by infections, trauma, stress, or surgery. Symptoms include GI symptoms, sweating, tachycardia, and arrhythmias. Without intervention, the patient develops congestive heart failure, coma, and dies. Treatment includes antithyroid drugs, systemic steroids, glucose administered intravenously, and interventions to keep the patient cool; also known as *thyroid storm.*

Thyrotoxicosis: Excess thyroxine (T_4) and triiodothyronine (T_3) in the bloodstream; also known as *hyperthyroidism.*

Tinnitus: Noise in the ears, often described as ringing or roaring.

Tip: Portion of the working end of a periodontal instrument that should be placed against the tooth at all times to ensure proper instrument adaptation.

Tobacco abstinence: State of being tobacco free either as an individual who never used tobacco or an individual who no longer uses tobacco.

Tobacco user: Individual who regularly uses tobacco, usually measured as daily use among adults (age 18 and older) and as any use in the past month among children and youths (younger than age 18).

Toe: End portion of the working end of a curet. The toe is usually round.

Tofflemire universal matrix system: Mechanism composed of two components: (1) retainer and (2) band. The Tofflemire universal matrix system is used to hold and form the restorative material (amalgam) during the packing and carving of the amalgam restoration.

Tomogram: Radiograph made with a tomograph.

Tongue: Muscular organ that is the main articulatory element in the production of speech and accounts for the clarity and fluidity of speech.

Tonsillectomy: Surgical removal of the tonsils, which are a rounded mass of tissue, usually of a lymphoid nature (especially the palatine tonsil).

Tooth-colored (TC) restoration: Restorative material that matches the color of a tooth. TC restorative material is usually a resin or ceramic.

Topical: On the surface.

Tort: Civil wrong or injury, other than a breach of contract, for which the plaintiff is monetarily compensated for the unreasonable harm he or she has sustained.

Trabecular: Irregular meshwork of joined matrix pieces forming a lattice in cancellous bone or when bands of connective tissue in a lymph node separate the node into lymphatic nodules.

Traditional literature review: Report on a broad range of issues on a given topic rather than answering a specific question in depth as found in a *systematic review*. Literature reviews can be a subjective assessment in that literature can be selected to support a desired conclusion.

Tragus of the ears: Prominence in front of the opening of the external ear.

Transdermal nicotine: Nicotine diffusion through the skin, usually by the use of a nicotine patch.

Transient ischemic attacks (TIAs): Episodes of cerebrovascular insufficiencies, usually associated with partial occlusion of an artery by an atherosclerotic plaque or embolism. The symptoms vary with the site and degree of the occlusion. Disturbance of normal vision in one or both eyes, dizziness, weakness, dysphasia, numbness, or unconsciousness may occur. TIAs are usually brief, lasting only a few minutes; symptoms rarely continue for several hours.

Transmucosal nicotine: Nicotine diffusion through the oral mucosa, usually by the use of a nicotine gum (e.g., nicotine polacrilex) or oral inhaler.

Transseptal fibers: Part of the gingival fiber system that extends horizontally from the supraalveolar cementum of one tooth through the interdental attached gingiva above the septum of the alveolar bone to the cementum of the adjacent tooth.

Trapezius: Large, flat triangular muscle of the shoulder and upper back. The trapezius arises from the occipital bone, ligamentum nuchae, and spinous processes of the seventh cervical and all the thoracic vertebrae. It acts to rotate the scapula, raise the shoulder, and abduct and flex the arm.

Triage: Process during which patients are sorted according to their need for care. The kind of illness or injury, the severity of the problem, and the facilities available govern the process, as in a hospital emergency room.

Triclosan: Antibacterial effective against gram-positive and most gram-negative organisms. Triclosan exhibits slight activity against yeasts and fungi; it is used as a detergent in surgical scrubs, soaps, and deodorants.

Trifurcation: Areas in a three-rooted tooth where the roots divide.

Trigeminal neuralgia (cranial nerve V): Fifth cranial nerve, which provides motor innervation to the muscles of mastication and sensory innervation to the face, jaws, and teeth.

Trismus: Limitations of opening because of spasm or fibrosis of the muscles of mastication or temporomandibular joint.

Tuberculosis: Infectious disease caused by *Mycobacterium tuberculosis* and characterized by the formation of tubercles in the tissues.

Tubule: Nodule or a small eminence, such as that on a bone. In addition, a tubule is a nodule that is especially elevated from the skin and larger than a papule.

Tumor necrosis factor alpha: Natural body protein with anticancer effects; is also produced synthetically. The body produces tumor necrosis factor alpha in response to the presence of toxic substances such as bacterial toxins. Adverse effects are toxic shock and cachexia.

Type 1 diabetes: See *Insulin-dependent diabetes mellitus.*

Type 2 diabetes: See *Non–insulin-dependent diabetes mellitus.*

Type II herpes: Infection caused by a herpes simplex virus (HSV), which has an affinity for the skin and nervous system and usually produces small, transient, irritating, and sometimes painful fluid-filled blisters on the skin and mucous membranes. Type II herpes *(herpes genitalis)* infections are usually limited to the genital region.

U

Ulcerative stomatitis: Periodic episodes of aphthous lesions (canker sores) ranging from 1 week to several months. Trauma, menses, immunologic factors, upper respiratory tract infections, herpes simplex, and other causes have been suggested. The single or multiple discrete or confluent ulcers have a well-defined marginal erythema and central area of necrosis with sloughing. The herpetic appearance suggests a common mechanism with herpes simplex, but no known infectious agents have been demonstrated.

Ultrasonic instruments: Instruments that use high-frequency sound waves, instrument vibrations, and water lavage to remove plaque biofilm, calculus, and endotoxins from the root surface.

Unerupted teeth: Teeth not having perforated the oral mucosa. In dentistry, used with reference to a normal developing tooth, an embedded tooth, or an impacted tooth.

Unilateral: One-sided.

Universal: Ability to be used on all tooth surfaces.

Upper respiratory infections (URIs): Any infectious disease of the upper respiratory tract. URIs include the common cold, laryngitis, pharyngitis, rhinitis, sinusitis, and tonsillitis.

Urticaria: Pruritic skin eruption that is characterized by transient wheals of varying shapes and sizes with well-defined erythematous margins and pale centers. Urticaria is caused by capillary dilation in the dermis that results from the release of vasoactive mediators, including histamine, kinin, and the slow reactive substance of anaphylaxis associated with antigen-antibody reaction. Drugs, food, insect bites, inhalants, emotional stress, exposure to heat or cold, and exercise may cause urticaria. Urticaria is also called *hives.*

Uvula: Midline muscular structure that hangs down from the posterior margin of the soft palate.

V

Values: Social principles, goals, or standards accepted by a society.

Valvular insufficiency: Condition of the heart when the valve cusps retract and no longer meet, allowing for backflow of blood or regurgitation.

Varnish: Resin-surface coating formed by evaporation of a solvent.

Vasculitis: Inflammation of a blood vessel.

Vasovagal syncope: Sudden loss of consciousness, resulting from cerebral ischemia; secondary to decreased cardiac output, peripheral vasodilation, and bradycardia; and associated with vagal activity. Vasovagal syncope may be triggered by pain, fright, or trauma and is accompanied by symptoms of nausea, pallor, and perspiration.

Ventral surface: Position more toward the belly surface than some other object of reference; the anterior surface.

Ventricular fibrillation: Cardiac arrhythmia marked by rapid disorganized depolarizations of the ventricular myocardium. Ventricular fibrillation is characterized by a complete lack of organized electric activity and ventricular contraction. Blood pressure falls to zero, resulting in unconsciousness. Death may occur within 4 minutes. Cardiopulmonary resuscitation must be immediately initiated with defibrillation and resuscitative medications given per advance cardiac life support protocol.

Vermillion border (zone): Transition zone where the lips are outlined from the surrounding skin.

Vertical: Upright; perpendicular to the horizon.

Vertical bite-wing image: Intraoral image used to examine the interproximal areas of the maxillary and mandibular teeth and the level of the alveolar bone.

Vesiculobullous disease (desquamative gingivitis): Gingival inflammation characterized by peeling of the surface epithelium. In its chronic state, vesiculobullous disease is most frequently caused by the hormonal changes associated with menopause. It may also be associated with any biological stress, such as trauma to the epithelium.

Vestibule: Space or cavity that serves as the entrance to a passageway, such as the vestibule of the vagina or the vestibule of the ear.

Vibrating line: Imaginary line across the posterior part of the palate, marking the division between the movable and immovable tissues of the soft palate. This line can be identified when the movable tissues are functioning.

Videofluoroscopy: Dynamic radiographs recorded on videotape.

Viscosity: Resistance that a liquid exhibits to the flow of one layer over another.

Vision: Sight; the faculty of seeing.

Vital signs: Measurement of pulse rate, respiration rate, body temperature, and tobacco use.

Vital staining: Dyeing process used to impart color to tissues or cells of living organisms.

W

Wall: Outside layer of material surrounding an object or space; a paries.

Wharton's duct: Excretory duct of the submandibular glands; opens into the oral cavity at the sublingual caruncle of the mucous membrane of the floor of the mouth behind the lower incisor teeth.

White spot lesion: Lesions found on the mucosa that have a white coating. White spot lesions require differential diagnosis because they may indicate trauma, infection, or a cancerous process.

Wicking: Absorption of a liquid by capillary action along a thread or through the material (e.g., penetration of liquids through undetected holes in a glove).

Wire edge: Unsupported metal fragments extending beyond the cutting edge.

Within normal limits (WNL): Clinical measurements and radiographs that are within the health parameters; findings are noncontributory to disease.

Working end: Portion of the instrument that comes into contact with the tooth and performs the intended task.

Work-related musculoskeletal disorders (WMSD): Musculoskeletal disorders of the neck, back, and shoulder, as well as carpal tunnel syndrome and thoracic outlet syndrome, resulting from repetitive appropriate body mechanics during the performance of work activities.

X

Xerostomia: Dry mouth caused by a decreased production of saliva.

Z

Zoophobia: Fear of animals.

Zygomatic: Pertaining to the cheekbone or malar bone of the face.

American Academy of Periodontology Report: Guidelines for the Management of Patients with Periodontal Diseases

In 2005, the American Academy of Periodontology undertook the development of guidelines for the management of patients with periodontitis. The development process took into consideration the latest research in the field of periodontics, comments from Academy members, and input from other dental organizations. The final product—*Guidelines for the Management of Patients With Periodontal Diseases*—is published in this issue of the *Journal,* September 2006.

Today, there is greater public awareness about periodontal diseases and more treatment options for patients than ever before. However, as advancements in periodontal therapy continue to develop at a record-breaking pace, periodontal diseases remain the most common cause of adult tooth loss. In addition, accumulating research is further defining the links between periodontal diseases and other systemic conditions such as diabetes, adverse pregnancy outcomes, and cardiovascular diseases. Patients are beginning to understand that good periodontal health is more important than ever before.

It is the Academy's hope that these *Guidelines* will help to improve the periodontal health of all patients with periodontitis. Evidence suggests that an increasing number of patients would benefit from periodontal specialty care. Clearly, there has been some confusion regarding periodontal treatment and continued reevaluation of its effectiveness and when a periodontist should be consulted as a member of the patient's treatment team. These *Guidelines* can help the entire dental team in the timely identification of patients with periodontal diseases and those most appropriate for specialty care.

Patients at risk for periodontal diseases can often be overlooked during a routine dental examination because they appear to be in a state of periodontal health, yet there can be underlying risk factors that could increase the probability of periodontitis in the future. Many practitioners are aware that the concept of risk in the treatment of chronic diseases is rapidly becoming an important component of patient care and will ultimately drive treatment decisions and appropriate referrals in the healthcare community. For example, we know that a patient in excellent cardiovascular health today may be at high risk for developing the disease at some point in the future based on certain genetic or behavioral factors. The same is true for periodontal diseases. These *Guidelines* are meant to help identify patients who are at greatest risk early and, therefore, would benefit from specialty care. The *Guidelines* are in no way meant to replace a practitioner's knowledge, skills, or abilities; a "one-size-fits-all" treatment plan for periodontal diseases does not exist. The diagnosis and treatment of periodontal diseases continue to present significant challenges to all practitioners regardless of experience level.

We encourage periodontists to take these *Guidelines* and incorporate them into their daily routine and share them with their referring colleagues. These *Guidelines* provide a basis for strengthening existing relationships and building new ones. Periodontists have a unique relationship with general dentists because they are the only specialists who work with the restorative community throughout a patient's life. There are many times that we hear from our referring colleagues that they have referred patients for specialty care, but, for one reason or another, the patient never follows through. We urge you to take the time to develop protocols with your referring colleagues for periodontal specialty care and to help optimize the health of your patients.

This is an exciting time in periodontics. We encourage you to share these *Guidelines* with all members of your dental team and work to incorporate them into the management of your periodontal patients. The Academy hopes that the adoption of the *Guidelines* into everyday practice will help to provide guidance and perspective to the dental community. Together, we can work to enhance and ensure the periodontal health of all.

Kenneth A. Krebs, DMD, President, American Academy of Periodontology, 2005-2006

Donald S. Clem III, DDS, Chair, Task Force to Develop the *Guidelines*

doi: 10.1902/jop.2006.069001

Guidelines for the Management of Patients with Periodontal Disease

Periodontal diseases present significant challenges for the public and dental profession. They are the major cause of tooth loss in adults, and they can have a devastating impact on oral function and appearance. Emerging research suggests possible links between inflammation caused by periodontal diseases and other adverse health conditions, such as heart attacks, strokes, diabetes, and preterm and low-weight births.

Some patients can be well managed within the general dental practice, whereas others would benefit from comanagement with a periodontist. Determining if and when a patient should be referred to a periodontist are sometimes difficult issues.

Communication between the referring dentist and periodontist is especially important in establishing responsibilities for periodontal treatment and maintenance. The education, experience, and interest of individual practitioners vary, and, therefore, specialty referral may occur at different stages of a patient's disease state and risk level. The chronic nature of inflammatory periodontal diseases requires that the clinician regularly reassess patients for appropriate lifelong disease management. Because periodontal diseases can affect soft and hard tissues, practitioners are cautioned to address both soft tissue lesions and bone involvement. This is particularly true for practices that administer "soft tissue management" programs, as the limited approach of these programs may lead to inappropriate treatment of the patient's periodontal diseases.

Risk assessment is increasingly important in periodontal treatment planning and should be part of every comprehensive dental and periodontal evaluation. This evolving paradigm in the treatment of chronic diseases, such as periodontal diseases, not only identifies the existence of disease and its severity, but also considers factors that may influence future progression of disease.

The American Academy of Periodontology recognizes that the periodontist–dental team partnership is unique in that it enables long-term comanagement of periodontal patients. This concept of comanagement may occur at different intervals of a patient's treatment depending on risk factors that may contribute to the progression of periodontal diseases and its consequences. The following *Guidelines* are provided to assist in the timely identification of patients who would benefit from co-

management and the unique partnership between a periodontist and referring dentist. From time to time, the Academy will update these *Guidelines*.

An explanation of terms is included as part of the *Guidelines*, and research supporting the content of the *Guidelines* is available on the American Academy of Periodontology's Web site at http://www.perio.org.

LEVEL 3: PATIENTS WHO SHOULD BE TREATED BY A PERIODONTIST

Any patient with:
  Severe chronic periodontitis
  Furcation involvement
  Vertical/angular bony defect(s)
  Aggressive periodontitis (formerly known as juvenile, early-onset, or rapidly progressive periodontitis)
  Periodontal abscess and other acute periodontal conditions
  Significant root surface exposure and/or progressive gingival recession
  Peri-implant disease

Any patient with periodontal diseases, regardless of severity, whom the referring dentist prefers not to treat.

LEVEL 2: PATIENTS WHO WOULD LIKELY BENEFIT FROM COMANAGEMENT BY THE REFERRING DENTIST AND THE PERIODONTIST

Any patient with periodontitis who demonstrates at reevaluation or any dental examination one or more of the following risk factors/indicators* known to contribute to the progression of periodontal diseases:

Periodontal Risk Factors/Indicators
  Early onset of periodontal diseases (prior to the age of 35 years)
  Unresolved inflammation at any site (e.g., bleeding upon probing, pus, and/or redness)
  Pocket depths ≥5 mm
  Vertical bone defects
  Radiographic evidence of progressive bone loss
  Progressive tooth mobility
  Progressive attachment loss
  Anatomic gingival deformities
  Exposed root surfaces
  A deteriorating risk profile

Medical or Behavioral Risk Factors/Indicators
  Smoking/tobacco use
  Diabetes
  Osteoporosis/osteopenia

---

* It should be noted that a combination of two or more of these risk factors/indicators may make even slight to moderate periodontitis particularly difficult to manage (e.g., a patient under 35 years of age who smokes).

Drug-induced gingival conditions (e.g., phenytoins, calcium channel blockers, immunosuppressants, and long-term systemic steroids)

Compromised immune system, either acquired or drug induced

A deteriorating risk profile

LEVEL 1: PATIENTS WHO MAY BENEFIT FROM COMANAGEMENT BY THE REFERRING DENTIST AND THE PERIODONTIST

Any patient with periodontal inflammation/infection and the following systemic conditions:

Diabetes
Pregnancy
Cardiovascular disease
Chronic respiratory disease

Any patient who is a candidate for the following therapies who might be exposed to risk from periodontal infection, including but not limited to the following treatments:

Cancer therapy
Cardiovascular surgery
Joint-replacement surgery
Organ transplantation

FREQUENTLY ASKED QUESTIONS (FAQS)

The American Academy of Periodontology's Guidelines for the Management of Patients with Periodontal Diseases

What are the *Guidelines?*

- The *Guidelines* provide information to assist in the timely identification of patients who would benefit from comanagement by the referring dentist and the periodontist.

Why did the Academy develop the *Guidelines?*

- The Academy's objective is to encourage referring dentists and periodontists to work together to optimize the health of patients. Determining if and when a patient should be referred to a periodontist are sometimes difficult issues. These *Guidelines* are intended to help the general practitioner in the rapid identification of those patients at greater risk for the consequences of periodontal inflammation and infection and, therefore, those patients most appropriate for specialty referral.

- Despite recent advancements in periodontal therapy, periodontal diseases continue to present significant challenges for the public and dental profession. Periodontal diseases remain a major cause of tooth loss in adults. In addition, periodontal diseases are associated with systemic conditions, such as cardiovascular disease, diabetes, adverse pregnancy outcomes, and respiratory disease. Periodontists are experts in assessing and treating periodontal diseases.

- Accumulating evidence, including recent literature, suggests that an increasing number of patients would benefit from periodontal specialty care. This evidence also suggests that these patients are being referred later in the disease process than in the past.

Who needs/benefits from the *Guidelines?*

- All dental teams and their patients need and will benefit from the *Guidelines.*

How were the *Guidelines* developed, and who developed them? Did the Academy collaborate with organized dentistry or any other groups or individuals on these *Guidelines?*

- A Board of Trustees—appointed task force consisting of periodontal practitioners, academicians, and researchers developed the *Guidelines.*

- The Academy distributed a draft version of the *Guidelines* to all members, the American Dental Association, Academy of General Dentistry, and American Dental Hygienists' Association for commentary.

- All organizations and more than 375 members provided commentary.

- The task force revised the *Guidelines* based on the comments received.

What are the benefits of using the *Guidelines?*

The *Guidelines* will:

- Help the practitioner in triaging patients who currently have or who are at risk for the development of periodontal diseases.

- Help the general practitioner more effectively address the association of periodontal diseases and systemic diseases/conditions.

- Assist the general dentist and hygienist in the management of periodontal diseases.

- Result in appropriate and timely treatment of periodontal diseases.

In addition, the *Guidelines:*

- Should enhance the restorative outcome of dental treatment by establishing and maintaining a healthy periodontal foundation.

- Are clear, concise, and should be easy to incorporate into daily practice and will enhance the partnership between periodontists and referring dentists.

Where do the *Guidelines* fit in the process of care?

- The *Guidelines* will become an integral part of patient management.

- The *Guidelines* do not replace the knowledge, skills, and abilities of the dental team.

The *Guidelines* mention the concept of risk assessment. What is risk assessment, and why is it so important?

- Risk assessment is the process of determining the qualitative or quantitative estimation of the likelihood of adverse events that may result from exposure to specified health hazards or from the absence of beneficial influences. Upon dental examination, many practitioners incorrectly assume that a patient in a state of periodontal health is not at risk for developingperiodontitis. Indeed, the patient may have risk factors/indicators (e.g., a smoking habit, diabetes, and young age) that could increase the probability of the occurrence of periodontitis in the future. Therefore, risk assessment helps predict a patient's disease state at some future point in time or the rate of progression of current disease.

Why are patients with furcation involvement considered among those patients who "should be treated by a periodontist"?

- Periodontists are specialists trained to assess and treat the more advanced forms of periodontal diseases and associated lesions. Furcation involvements are among the most problematic periodontal lesions. Therefore, it is often appropriate that earlier manifestations of these lesions be evaluated and managed by a periodontist.

The *Guidelines* suggest that certain patients can only be treated by a periodontist. Is this true?

- No. Some patients can be well managed within the general dental practice, whereas others would benefit from comanagement with a periodontist. The Academy understands that the education, experience, and interests of individual general-practitioner dentists vary, and, therefore, specialty referral may occur at different stages of a patient's disease state and risk level.
- Referral is not only associated with treatment but also includes consultation.

Do all patients who are referred to periodontists require surgery?

- No. Comprehensive care by a periodontist includes nonsurgical and/or surgical therapies depending on the needs of the individual patient.

Dental implants, oral reconstructive and corrective procedures, and tissue engineering are not included in the *Guidelines*. Why aren't these procedures included?

- These *Guidelines* are focused on the management of patients with periodontitis. They do not include all areas of periodontal specialty care or specific treatment modalities.
- Dental implants, periodontal plastic surgery, oral reconstructive surgery, and tissue-engineering procedures are currently performed by periodontists.
- The development of clinical guidelines for these other areas of periodontics is being considered by the Board of Trustees.

Where is the research to support statements made in the *Guidelines*?

- The Academy's web site includes many resources that support the *Guidelines for the Management of Patients With Periodontal Diseases*. These resources are located at http://www.perio.org/resources-products/posppr2.html.

Is the Academy implying a medicolegal standard with the dissemination of these *Guidelines*?

- This document is intended to serve as a guide for the dental team in managing patients with periodontal diseases.
- The Academy believes that all dentists have the right to practice according to their education, training, and experience.

Clearly, each dentist has an obligation to render treatment in the best interests of the patient.

- It is hoped that this document will help dentists identify patients at greatest risk for periodontal diseases so that these patients receive appropriate and timely periodontal care.

EXPLANATION OF TERMS

- **May:** A choice to act or not; indicates freedom or liberty to follow a suggested alternative.
- **Should:** A highly desirable direction but does not mean mandatory.
- **Must:** Used to express a command; indicates an imperative or duty. This term does not appear in the document and is provided as a comparison to the terms "may" and "should."
- **Comanagement:** A shared responsibility for patient care between a periodontist and referring dentist. This patient management may consist of consultation and/or treatment.
- **Reevaluation:** Assessment of a patient's periodontal status and risk profile after therapy to be used as a basis for subsequent patient management.
- **Deteriorating Risk Profile:** Adverse changes in risk factors/indicators suggestive of disease onset or progression.
- **Disease Definitions:** For disease definitions such as Severe Chronic Periodontitis, Aggressive Periodontitis, and Acute Periodontal Conditions, please refer to volume 4 of the *Annals of Periodontology* at http://www.perio.org/resources-products/classification.htm.
- **Peri-Implant Disease:** Chronic inflammation and/or bone loss around dental implants that may influence implant status.
- **Periodontal Inflammation:** Most periodontal diseases including chronic and aggressive periodontitis are inflammatory diseases. Chronic periodontitis has an infectious etiology from the endogenous plaque biofilm. This type of opportunistic infection results in a chronic release of inflammatory cytokines, prostaglandins, and destructive enzymes from neutrophils and mononuclear cells in the periodontium. The ensuing chronic inflammation in the tissue is what leads to the pathologic anatomic changes clinically detectable as periodontal pockets and alveolar bone loss. Furthermore, some microorganisms of the biofilm and inflammatory mediators from the affected tissue may adversely affect systemic chronic inflammatory diseases and pregnancy outcomes.
- **Significant Root Surface Exposure:** Gingival recession of sufficient magnitude that results in the loss of tooth structure, sensitivity, esthetic concerns, or attachment loss.

Glossary of Selected Centers for Disease Control and Prevention Terms

To help integrate the Centers for Disease Control and Prevention's (CDC's) *Guidelines for Infection Control in Dental Health-Care Settings—2003,* the following CDC definitions are applied:

Alcohol-based hand rub: Alcohol-containing preparation designed to reduce the number of viable microorganisms on the hands.

Antimicrobial soap: Detergent that contains an antiseptic agent.

Antiseptic: Germicide used on skin or living tissue for the purpose of inhibiting or destroying microorganisms (e.g., alcohols, chlorhexidine, chlorine, hexachlorophene, iodine, chloroxylenol, quaternary ammonium compounds, triclosan).

Bioburden: Microbiological load (i.e., number of viable organisms in or on an object or surface) or organic material on a surface or object before decontamination or sterilization. Is also known as *bioload* or *microbial load.*

Colony-forming unit (CFU): Minimum number (i.e., tens of millions) of separable cells on the surface of or in a semisolid agar medium that give rise to a visible colony of progeny. CFUs can consist of pairs, chains, clusters, or single cells and are often expressed as colony-forming units per milliliter (CFUs/ml).

Decontamination: Use of physical or chemical means to remove, inactivate, or destroy pathogens on a surface or item to ensure that they are no longer capable of transmitting infectious particles and that the surface or item is rendered safe for handling, use, or disposal.

Dental treatment water: Nonsterile water used during dental treatment, including irrigation of nonsurgical operative sites and cooling of high-speed rotary and ultrasonic instruments.

Disinfectant: Chemical agent used on inanimate objects (e.g., floors, walls, sinks) that destroys virtually all recognized pathogenic microorganisms but not necessarily all microbial forms (e.g., bacterial endospores). The Environmental Protection Agency (EPA) groups disinfectants on the basis of whether the product label claims limited, general, or hospital disinfectant capabilities.

Disinfection: Destruction of pathogenic and other kinds of microorganisms by physical or chemical means. Disinfection is less lethal than sterilization because it destroys the majority of recognized pathogenic microorganisms but not necessarily all microbial forms (e.g., bacterial spores). Disinfection does not ensure the degree of safety associated with sterilization processes.

Droplet nuclei: Particles less than 5 mcm in diameter formed by dehydration of airborne droplets containing microorganisms that can remain suspended in the air for long periods.

Droplets: Small particles of moisture (e.g., spatter) generated when a person coughs or sneezes or when water is converted to a fine mist by an aerator or showerhead. These particles, intermediate in size between drops and droplet nuclei, can contain infectious microorganisms and tend to settle from the air quickly, resulting in risk of disease transmission to be usually limited to persons in close proximity to the droplet source.

Hand hygiene: General term that applies to handwashing, antiseptic handwash, antiseptic hand rub, or surgical hand antisepsis.

Hepatitis B e antigen (HBeAg): Secreted product of the nucleocapsid gene of hepatitis B virus (HBV) found in serum during acute and chronic HBV infection. Its presence indicates that the virus is replicating and serves as a marker of increased infectivity.

Hepatitis B immune globulin (HBIG): Product used for prophylaxis against HBV infection. HBIG is prepared from plasma containing high titers of hepatitis B surface antibody and provides protection for 3 to 6 months.

Hepatitis B surface antibody (anti-HB): Protective antibody against hepatitis B surface antigen. Presence in the blood can indicate past infection with and immunity to HBV or an immune response from hepatitis B vaccine.

Hepatitis B surface antigen (HBsAg): Serologic marker on the surface of HBV detected in high levels during acute or chronic hepatitis. The body normally produces antibodies to surface antigen as a normal immune response to infection.

High-level disinfection: Process that inactivates vegetative bacteria, mycobacteria, fungi, and viruses but not necessarily high numbers of bacterial spores. The U.S. Food and Drug Administration (FDA) further defines a high-level disinfectant as a sterilant used for a shorter contact time.

Hospital disinfectant: Germicide registered by the EPA for use on inanimate objects in hospitals, clinics, dental offices, and other medical-related facilities. Efficacy is demonstrated against *Salmonella choleraesuis, Staphylococcus aureus,* and *Pseudomonas aeruginosa.*

Iatrogenic: Induced inadvertently by health-care personnel (HCP), medical (including dental) treatment, or diagnostic procedures. Used particularly in reference to an infectious disease or other complications of treatment.

Immunization: Process by which a person becomes immune or protected against a disease. Vaccination is defined as the process of administering a killed or weakened infectious organism or a toxoid; however, vaccination does not always result in immunity.

Intermediate-level disinfection: Process that inactivates vegetative bacteria, the majority of fungi, mycobacteria, and the majority of viruses (particularly enveloped viruses) but not bacterial spores.

Intermediate-level disinfectant: Liquid chemical germicide registered with the EPA as a hospital disinfectant with a label claim of potency as a tuberculocidal disinfectant.

Low-level disinfectant: Liquid chemical germicide registered with the EPA as a hospital disinfectant. Occupational Safety and Health Administration (OSHA) requires low-level hospital disinfectants to also have a label claim for potency against HIV and HBV if the product is to be used for disinfecting clinical contact surfaces.

Low-level disinfection: Process that inactivates the majority of vegetative bacteria, certain fungi, and certain viruses but cannot be relied on to inactivate resistant microorganisms (e.g., mycobacteria, bacterial spores).

Nosocomial: Infection acquired in a hospital as an unintended result of medical care.

Occupational exposure: Reasonably anticipated skin, eye, mucous membrane, or parenteral contact with blood or other potentially infectious materials (OPIM) that can result from the performance of an employee's duties.

OPIM: An OSHA acronym that includes the following:
1. Body fluids, including semen, vaginal secretions, cerebrospinal fluid, synovial fluid, pleural fluid, pericardial fluid, peritoneal fluid, amniotic fluid, saliva in dental procedures; any body fluid visibly contaminated with blood; and all body fluids in situations where differentiation among body fluids is difficult or impossible

2. Any unfixed tissue or organ (other than intact skin) from a human (living or dead)
3. HIV-containing cell or tissue cultures, organ cultures, and HIV- or HBV-containing culture medium or other solutions, as well as blood, organs, or other tissues from experimental animals infected with HIV or HBV

Parenteral: Means of piercing mucous membranes or skin barrier through such events as needlesticks, human bites, cuts, and abrasions.

Standard precautions: When the relevance of universal precautions to all aspects of disease transmission was recognized (1996), the CDC expanded the concept and changed the term to *standard precautions*. No operational difference exists in clinical dental practice between universal precautions and standard precautions. Standard precautions integrate and expand the elements of universal precautions into a standard of care designed to protect HCP and patients from pathogens that can be spread by blood or any other body fluid, excretion, or secretion. Standard precautions apply to contact with the following:
1. Blood
2. All body fluids, secretions, and excretions (except sweat), regardless of whether they contain blood
3. Nonintact skin
4. Mucous membranes (Saliva has always been considered a potentially infectious material in dental infection control.)

Wicking: Absorption of a liquid by capillary action along a thread or through material (e.g., penetration of liquids through undetected holes in a glove).

Page numbers followed by *f* indicate figures; *t,* tables; *b,* boxes.

982

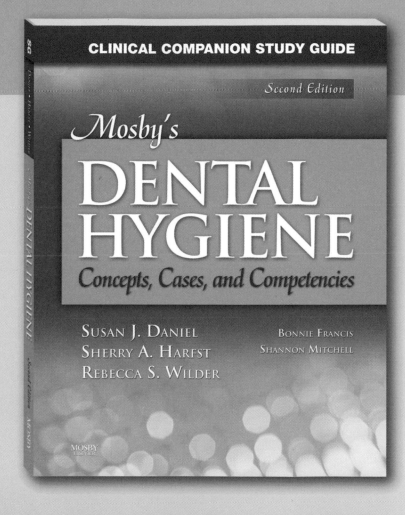
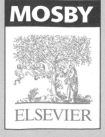